Contents

GET CONNECTED

To Content Updates, Study Tools, and More!

Meet **MERLIN** 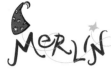 Your online companion

sign on at:

http://www.mosby.com/MERLIN/Stuart

what you will receive:

Use this passcode to access the many features of this website. Whether you're a student, an instructor, or a clinician, you'll find information just for you. Things like:

- Worksheets
- "Drug of the Month" Updates
- "Citing the Evidence" Updates
- Critical Thinking Activities and Exercises
- Annotated Suggested Readings
- More!

plus:

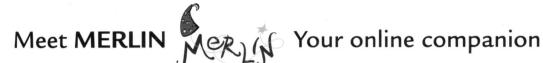

Lift here.
PASSCODE INSIDE
MOSBY

Web Links

Use this passcode to access hundreds of active websites keyed specifically to the contents of this book. **The web links are updated continually, with new ones added as they develop.**

If passcode sticker is removed, this textbook cannot be returned to Mosby, Inc.

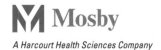
A Harcourt Health Sciences Company

Principles and Practice of
PSYCHIATRIC
NURSING

SEVENTH EDITION

Principles and Practice of
PSYCHIATRIC NURSING

Gail W. Stuart, PhD, RN, CS, FAAN

Professor, College of Nursing,
Director of Doctoral Studies,
Coordinator of the Psychiatric-Mental Health
 Nursing Graduate Program;
Professor, College of Medicine,
Department of Psychiatry and Behavioral Sciences,
Medical University of South Carolina,
Charleston, South Carolina

Michele T. Laraia, PhD, RN, CS

Associate Professor,
Department of Primary Care,
Division of Mental Health Nursing,
School of Nursing,
Oregon Health Sciences University,
Portland, Oregon

with 193 illustrations

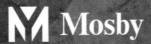

Mosby

A Harcourt Health Sciences Company

St. Louis   London   Philadelphia   Sydney   Toronto

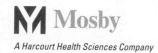

A Harcourt Health Sciences Company

Vice President, Nursing Editorial Director   *Sally Schrefer*
Senior Editor   *Terri Wood*
Developmental Editor   *Tom Stringer*
Project Manager   *Deborah L. Vogel*
Senior Production Editor   *Sarah E. Fike*
Design Manager   *Amy Buxton*

Mosby, Inc.
A Harcourt Health Sciences Company
11830 Westline Industrial Drive
St. Louis, Missouri 63146

Printed in the United States of America

International Standard Book Number 0-323-01254-X

01   02   03   04   GW / KPT   9   8   7   6   5   4   3   2

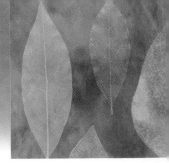

About the authors

Dr. Gail Stuart is a tenured professor in the College of Nursing and a professor in the College of Medicine in the Department of Psychiatry and Behavioral Sciences at the Medical University of South Carolina. She received her bachelor of science in nursing degree from Georgetown University, her master of science degree in psychiatric nursing from the University of Maryland, and her doctorate in behavioral sciences from Johns Hopkins University, School of Hygiene and Public Health. She is an American Nurses' Association Certified Specialist in psychiatric and mental health nursing, a fellow in the American Academy of Nursing, a member of Sigma Theta Tau and the American College of Mental Health Administration, a Distinguished Practitioner in the National Academies of Practice, and past-president of the American Psychiatric Nurses Association. She has also been a van Ameringen fellow at the Beck Institute of Cognitive Therapy and Research and is a visiting professor at King's College, Institute of Psychiatry at the Maudsley in London.

Dr. Stuart's current position at the Medical University of South Carolina is in the College of Nursing, where she is the Director of Doctoral Studies and Coordinator of the Psychiatric-Mental Health Nursing Graduate Program. She was previously the associate director of the Center for Health Care Research, where she worked as a member of an interdisciplinary research team focusing on issues of access, resource utilization, outcomes, and health-care delivery systems. She was also the administrator and chief executive officer of the Institute of Psychiatry at the Medical University, where she was responsible for all clinical, fiscal, and human operations across the continuum of psychiatric care. Dr. Stuart has taught in undergraduate, graduate, and doctoral programs in nursing. She serves on numerous academic, pharmaceutical, and governmental boards and represents nursing on a number of National Institutes of Health policy and research panels. She is a strong advocate for the specialty and is in great demand to speak and consult both nationally and internationally. She is a prolific writer and has published numerous articles, textbooks, and media productions. She has received many awards, including the American Nurses' Association Distinguished Contribution to Psychiatric Nursing Award and the Psychiatric Nurse of the Year Award from the American Psychiatric Nurses Association. Dr. Stuart's clinical and research interests involve the study of depression, anxiety disorders, clinical outcomes, and mental health delivery systems.

Dr. Michele Laraia is an associate professor in the Department of Primary Care, Division of Mental Health Nursing, in the School of Nursing at Oregon Health Sciences University, Portland, Oregon. She received her bachelor of science degree in nursing from D'Youville College, Buffalo, New York; her master of science degree in psychiatric mental health nursing from the University of Virginia, Charlottesville, Virginia; and her doctorate in public health at the University of South Carolina, Columbia, South Carolina. Dr. Laraia has more than 25 years' experience in psychiatric mental health nursing, including teaching, conducting research, and treating persons with psychiatric disorders. She has taught at the undergraduate, master's, and doctoral levels of nursing education. Her particular areas of expertise include psychobiology and psychopharmacology, for which she has a national reputation in the field. Her research has a focus in the areas of panic and other anxiety disorders, depression, and health services. She specializes in the treatment of persons with mood and anxiety disorders. She is certified as a cognitive therapist from the Beck Institute for Cognitive Therapy and Research, Bala Cynwyd, Pennsylvania. She is also certified as an advanced practice registered nurse by the American Nursing Credentialing Center. Dr. Laraia presents at a variety of psychiatric nursing conferences throughout the United States and has published and produced teaching materials for the psychiatric mental health nursing specialty. She received the American Psychiatric Nurses Association Award for Excellence in Research and has held several national and local consultant and advisory positions. Most notably, Dr. Laraia chaired the American Nurses' Association Psychopharmacology Task Force for Psychiatric Mental Health Nurses.

Contributors

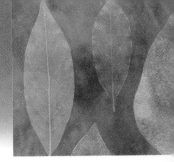

Carole F. Bennett, PhD, RN, CS
Private Practice and Consultation,
Charleston, South Carolina

Sandra E. Benter, DNSC, ARNP, CS
Psychiatric Nurse Practitioner,
Private Practice and Consultation,
Boca Raton, Florida

Carol M. Burns, MSN, RN, CS
Electroconvulsive Therapy (ECT) Program
  Coordinator,
Department of Psychiatry and Behavioral Sciences,
Medical University of South Carolina,
Charleston, South Carolina

Jacquelyn C. Campbell, PhD, RN, FAAN
Anna D. Wolf Endowed Professor,
Associate Dean for the PhD Program and
  Research,
Johns Hopkins University School of Nursing,
Baltimore, Maryland

Carolyn E. Cochrane, PhD, RN, CS
Assistant Professor,
Center for Drug & Alcohol Programs and Eating
  Disorder Program,
Department of Psychiatry and Behavioral Sciences,
Medical University of South Carolina,
Charleston, South Carolina

Victoria Conn, MN, MA, RPRP
Curriculum Consultant,
NAMI PA Training Institute,
Philadelphia, Pennsylvania

Nancy Fishwick, PhD, RN, CS
Associate Professor,
School of Nursing,
University of Maine,
Orono, Maine

Suzanne D. Friedman, MS, RN, CSP
Psychiatric Clinical Nurse Specialist,
Ellicot City, Maryland

Beth Gage Greco, MSN, RN, CS
Geropsychiatric Clinical Nurse Specialist,
Life Program, University of Pennsylvania;
Psychiatric Consult Liaison Advance Practice
  Nurse,
Visiting Nurse Association of Greater Philadelphia,
Philadelphia, Pennsylvania

Christine Diane Hamolia, MS, RN, CS
Manager, Eating Disorders Program,
Institute of Psychiatry,
Medical University of South Carolina,
Charleston, South Carolina

Patricia E. Helm, MSN, CS
West Haven, Connecticut

Linda V. Jefferson, PhD, RN, CS-P, CNAA
Director of Nursing,
Spring Grove Hospital Center,
Catonsville, Maryland

Therese K. Killeen, PhD, RN, CS
Project Coordinator,
Center for Alcohol and Drug Programs,
Institute of Psychiatry,
Medical University of South Carolina,
Charleston, South Carolina

Arthur J. LaSalle, EDD
Partner, LaSalle Counseling Associates,
Psychotherapist, Consultant, Trainer,
Ellicott City, Maryland

Paula C. LaSalle, MS, RN-P, CS, LCPC
Partner, LaSalle Counseling Associates,
Psychotherapist, Consultant, Trainer,
Ellicott City, Maryland

Elizabeth G. Maree, MSN, RN, CS
Director, Westcott Center,
Behavioral Health Services,
Hamilton Medical Center,
Dalton, Georgia

Mary D. Moller, MSN, APRN, CS, RPRP
Administrator, Sunerest Wellness Center;
CEO, Psychiatric Rehabilitation Nurses, Inc.,
Nine Mile Falls, Washington;
Adjunct Faculty,
Washington State University,
College of Nursing,
Spokane, Washington

Millene F. Murphy, PhD, APRN, LMFT, CS, RPRP
Professor Emeritus,
Brigham Young University,
Provo, Utah;
President,
Psychiatric Rehabilitation Nursing, Inc.,
Nine Mile Falls, Washington;
CEO,
Wellness Consultation and Education,
Richfield, Utah

Linda D. Oakley, PhD, RN
Associate Professor,
School of Nursing,
University of Wisconsin,
Madison, Wisconsin

Barbara Parker, RN, PhD, FAAN
Professor and Director,
Center for Nursing Research and Doctoral Program,
University of Virginia,
Charlottesville, Virginia

Carol K. Perlin, MS, RN, CS
Psychotherapist,
Baltimore, Maryland

Susan G. Poorman, PhD, RN, CS
Associate Professor,
Department of Nursing and Allied Health Professions,
Indiana University of Pennsylvania,
Indiana, Pennsylvania

Audrey Redston-Iselin, MA, RN, CS
Clinical Specialist,
Children's Services of Soundview Throgs Neck;
Community Mental Health Center of Albert Einstein
  College of Medicine;
Psychotherapist and Consultant–Private Practice,
White Plains, New York

Georgia L. Stevens, PhD, RN, CS
Psychotherapist and Consultant,
PAL (Partners in Aging and Long-term Caregiving)
  Associates;
Adjunct Assistant Professor,
School of Nursing,
The Catholic University of America,
Washington, DC

Sandra J. Sundeen, MS, RN, CNAA
Chief, Division of Staff Development & Training,
Maryland Mental Hygiene Administration;
Adjunct Assistant Professor,
University of Maryland School of Nursing,
Baltimore, Maryland

Nancy K. Worley, PhD, RN
Charleston, South Carolina

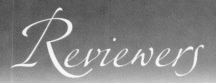
Reviewers

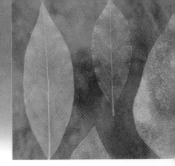

Cynthia Hoppe Allen, RN, MPH, MN
Associate Professor in Nursing,
Charity School of Nursing,
Delgado Community College,
New Orleans, Louisiana

Kathleen Barrett, RN, MSN, ARNP-CS
Cancer Case Manager,
Via Christi Regional Medical Center,
Wichita, Kansas

Barbara Mathews Blanton, MSN, RN
Clinical Instructor,
Texas Women's University College of Nursing,
Denton, Texas

Jeri L. Brandt, PhD, RN
Associate Professor of Nursing,
Nebraska Wesleyan University,
Lincoln, Nebraska

Yvonne E. Darr, RN, C, BA, MS, MN
Associate Professor of Nursing,
Kansas City Community College,
Kansas City, Kansas

Mavonne A. Gansen, MA, RNC
Nursing Instructor, Mental Health Nursing,
Northeast Iowa Community College,
Peosta, Iowa

Netha O'Meara, RN, CNS, MSN
Consultant and Adjunct Faculty,
Greater Houston Area Schools,
Houston, Texas

Linda S. Smith, DSN, RN
Assistant Professor,
Oregon Health Sciences University,
Klamath Falls, Oregon

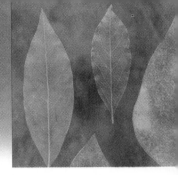

Preface

Welcome to the seventh edition of *Principles and Practice of Psychiatric Nursing*—the "living text." We hope that beginning with the verdant cover design and continuing with the rich visual images on each page, you will sense the transformation and emergence of the new ideas captured in this edition. The elements of growth and evolution permeate both its content and design and underscore the fact that with its interactive website, the seventh edition of *Principles and Practice of Psychiatric Nursing* has taken on a living form that reaches out to the reader in a contemporary and ongoing way.

There are many reasons this text is the well-established leader in its field. It has an outstanding reputation of being comprehensive, engaging, and futuristic. This new edition builds on this legacy of excellence while launching forward to further define evidence based psychiatric nursing practice in a rapidly changing health-care environment. Thus the seventh edition continues to use the Stuart Stress Adaptation Model to organize content, which is based on a holistic biopsychosocial approach to psychiatric nursing care. It also continues to emphasize the full continuum of care; the broad range of preventive, crisis, and rehabilitative nursing activities; and the strong partnerships that psychiatric nurses form with patients and their families. These elements are the foundation of both contemporary and future psychiatric nursing practice. To these elements we have added the latest scientific knowledge on neurobiology and psychopharmacology and new information on alternative and complementary therapies, treatment algorithms, and the new American Nurses' Association (ANA) standards for the specialty. We have also developed a MERLIN website for the text that contains valuable web links, annotated readings, drug updates, worksheets, research questions, and many other features. Our goal with this edition, therefore, is to help psychiatric nurses and nursing students stay abreast with state-of-the-art knowledge to foster competent caring in their work with patients and families.

CONTENT ORGANIZATION

This book is divided into six units. Unit 1 presents psychiatric nursing principles that are fundamental to practice. First, the contemporary psychiatric nurse's roles and functions are addressed, followed by a chapter on therapeutic relationship skills. Conceptual models of psychiatric treatment, including the Stuart Stress Adaptation Model of psychiatric nursing care, are then presented. A new chapter to this edition describes evidence based psychiatric nursing practice and is followed by separate chapters devoted to the biological, psychological, sociocultural, environmental, and legal-ethical contexts of practice. Finally, the two ending chapters in this unit focus on the ANA professional practice and performance standards for 2000.

Unit 2 addresses the continuum of care, including mental health promotion and illness prevention, crisis intervention, and psychiatric rehabilitation. These topics, unique to this textbook, are more important than ever because health-care reform focuses on nontraditional settings and a wide range of treatment strategies. This unit concludes with an important chapter on the family's perspective of the continuum of mental health care, further reinforcing the importance of families that is reflected throughout the text.

Unit 3 applies psychiatric nursing principles to specific clinical disorders, based on a continuum of adaptive-maladaptive coping responses, the six-step nursing process, and the diagnoses of the *Diagnostic and Statistical Manual of Mental Disorders (DSM–IV–TR)* and North American Nursing Diagnosis Association (NANDA). There are separate chapters on anxiety, somatoform and sleep, dissociative, mood, psychotic, personality, substance abuse, eating, sexual, and organic mood disorders as well as suicidal behavior. The information in this unit has been completely updated and includes all *DSM–IV–TR* diagnostic categories.

Unit 4 describes various modalities of psychiatric treatment, including chapters on psychopharmacology, somatic therapies, cognitive behavioral therapy, and managing aggressive behavior. A new chapter describes alternative and complementary therapies in psychiatric care from an evidence based approach. Each of these areas is of importance in the field, and together they join with chapters on therapeutic groups and family interventions to round out the repertoire of psychiatric nursing practice.

Unit 5 begins with chapters on hospital-based and community-based psychiatric nursing care that reflect the most recent developments and current practice in these settings. Also included is a chapter on home care because health-care reform emphasizes the psychiatric nurse's abilities to collaborate, advise, and manage patients in the home.

Unit 6 concludes the text with a discussion of the unique issues and concerns in the psychiatric treatment of special populations and includes revised chapters on children, adolescents, the elderly, survivors of abuse and violence, and patients with HIV/AIDS.

SPECIAL FEATURES

We hope by now your appetite has been stimulated and you are ready to embark with us on this fascinating journey through the art and science of psychiatric nursing. On the way, look for other signposts and special features that we have included to illuminate your journey. Many of the special features have been highlighted with a special design or logo to enhance the teaching-learning process. These features are described in the "To the Student" preface located just before the detailed table of contents. In addition:

- The six steps of the nursing process are highlighted with the following special headings as they are discussed in the disorders chapters:
  Assessment
  Nursing Diagnosis
  Outcome Identification
  Planning
  Implementation
  Evaluation
- Tables and boxes that address specific pharmacology information emphasize its importance in the treatment of psychiatric illnesses.
- Learning objectives and a topical outline at the beginning of each chapter inform the students of the basic concepts and organization of the chapter, and a chapter summary includes key points at the end of each chapter to help students grasp important concepts.
- Key terms are highlighted in color and are included in the glossary at the back of the book.

We wish to communicate our respect for individuals and the roles they enact, regardless of their gender. To that end, we have attempted to avoid pronouns that express bias and to give recognition and support for the commitment of both men and women to the nursing profession. However, this sometimes creates difficult and tedious language for the reader. Therefore, for clarity and simplicity, the nurse is referred to in the third person, female gender, and the patient in the third person, masculine gender, when necessary. It should also be noted that Ms. is used instead of Miss or Mrs. in examples used in the text.

TEACHING AND LEARNING PACKAGE
Computerized Test Bank/Image Collection CD-ROM

The Computerized Test Bank/Image Collection CD-ROM for *Principles and Practice of Psychiatric Nursing*, seventh edition, is designed to help you, the instructor, develop lectures and evaluate student comprehension. The Computerized Test Bank, featuring more than 950 test items in NCLEX format, can generate tests for you or allow you to customize your own tests and perform online testing. An answer key is included, along with the rationales for correct answers, the cognitive level of each question, and the corresponding stages of the nursing process. The electronic Image Collection provides PowerPoint presentations with more than 180 slides, including four-color images from the text.

MERLIN (Mosby's Electronic Resource Links and Information Network)

We wish to remind you of the wealth of information that is available to students, instructors, and clinicians on the book's companion MERLIN website. Students will find a valuable resource in worksheets, critical thinking activities and exercises, annotated suggested readings, and "Citing the Evidence" and "Drug of the Month" updates. In addition to the same information available to students, instructors are able to access suggested course outlines and a syllabus conversion guide.

This completes your introduction to the journey that lies ahead. We invite you now to open the pages beneath your fingers and join us in a world of new ideas, challenging beliefs, and expanding competencies. We wish you well as you actualize the ideas of this living text in your own psychiatric nursing practice.

Gail Wiscarz Stuart
Michele T. Laraia

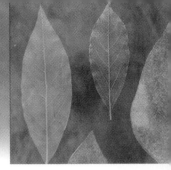

Special features

To the Student *This book offers special features that will aid your learning of the material and provide you with quick reference guides.*

Clinical Examples are taken from actual clinical situations. Many provide samples of nursing diagnoses related to the particular clinical situation (see page 301).

Case Studies are in-depth examples of clinical scenarios that discuss each step of the nursing process, providing you with realistic application of the nursing process (see page 133).

 Critical Thinking questions throughout each chapter promote independent clinical reasoning and encourage you to integrate the text material with your own understanding of the world and nursing (see page 21).

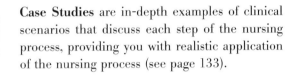 boxes help you to understand the latest clinical research and apply it in practice (see page 737).

 Critical Thinking about Contemporary Issues boxes present discussions about current controversial issues (see page 288).

Medical and Nursing Diagnoses and **Detailed Diagnoses** boxes present examples of NANDA diagnoses applicable for a specific disorder and describe the essential features of related *DSM–IV–TR* diagnoses (see pages 332 and 333).

Therapeutic Dialogues provide samples of appropriate verbal therapeutic interactions with patients (see page 33).

 A Patient Speaks and **A Family Speaks** boxes offer you a better understanding of the patient's and family's perspectives on treatment (see pages 452 and 325).

Patient Education Plans and **Family Education Plans** guide you in educating the patient and family about important treatment issues (see pages 306 and 430).

Nursing Treatment Plan Summaries guide you in the nursing care related to the treatment of major disorders (see page 433).

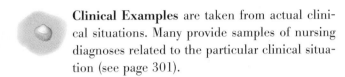 **A Clinical Exemplar of a Psychiatric Nurse** are featured boxes written by practicing psychiatric nurses who share their clinical experiences and personal insights (see page 776).

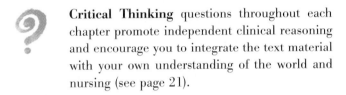 help you to review important points and master the chapter's content (see page 742).

 Be sure to visit the **MERLIN** online ancillary to find a wealth of information that reinforces and expands on the discussions in each chapter. The website is updated regularly to provide the most up-to-date information on evidence based practice and psychotropic drugs. Interactive exercises help you to master the chapter contents.

Contents

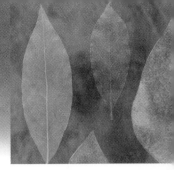

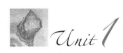

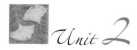

Continuum of Care

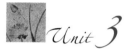

Applying Principles in Nursing Practice

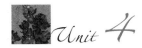

Unit 4

Treatment Modalities

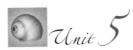

Unit 5

Treatment Settings

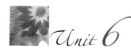

Unit 6

Special Populations in Psychiatry

41 Care of Survivors of Abuse and Violence, *824*

Nancy Fishwick
Barbara Parker
Jacqueline C. Campbell

42 Psychological Care of the Patient with HIV/AIDS, *842*

Paula C. LaSalle
Arthur J. LaSalle

Glossary, *857*

Appendices

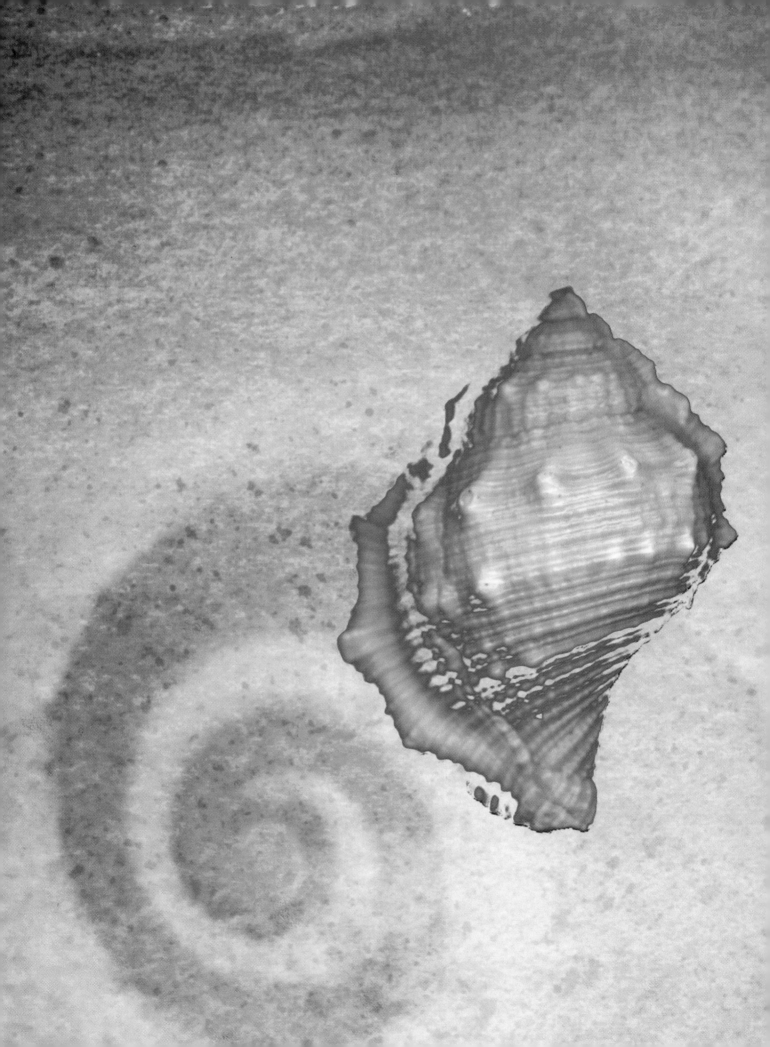

Unit 1

Principles of Psychiatric Nursing Care

You are about to begin a voyage to places you have never been before: the world of psychiatric and mental health nursing. In the old days of nursing, students learned about pieces of people—an infected toe, a congested lung, a troubling twitch, or maybe even a broken heart—but pieces nonetheless. Today, students learn about the wholeness of people: a physically ill child struggling for safety in an abusive family, an adolescent coping with eating problems and self-esteem, a young adult grieving over the diagnosis of HIV/AIDS, or an elder confused and disoriented at times but frightened at the thought of going to a nursing home. This is the exciting world of today's psychiatric nurse. It integrates the biological, psychological, sociocultural, environmental, legal, and ethical realities of life and weaves them together in a rich tapestry called psychiatric nursing practice.

This unit introduces you to parts of this world that may be new to you. It will help you explore how patients think, feel, and behave. It will help you learn how to talk with patients and families as partners in the caregiving process. It will suggest that you think about people in terms of their overall functioning and adaptation rather than of the symptoms of their specific illness. Most importantly, it will define for you the responsibilities you have as a professional health care provider. We hope you are ready to begin your journey, and we wish you curiosity about human nature, openness to new ways of thinking, and delight in the process of learning.

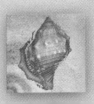

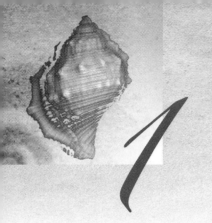

Roles and Functions of Psychiatric Nurses: Competent Caring

Gail W. Stuart

And what they dare to dream of, dare to do.

JAMES RUSSELL LOWELL

Nursing, or caring for the sick, has existed since the beginning of civilization. Before 1860 the emphasis in psychiatric institutions was on custodial care, and attendants were hired to maintain control of the patients. Often these attendants were little more than jailers or cellkeepers with little training, and psychiatric care was poor. Nursing as a profession began to emerge in the late nineteenth century, and by the twentieth century it had evolved into a specialty with unique roles and functions.

HISTORICAL PERSPECTIVES

In 1873 Linda Richards graduated from the New England Hospital for Women and Children in Boston. She developed better nursing care in psychiatric hospitals and organized nursing services and educational programs in state mental hospitals in Illinois. For these activities she is called the first American psychiatric nurse. Basic to Richards' theory of care was her statement, "It stands to reason that the mentally sick should be at least as well cared for as the physically sick" (Doona, 1984).

The first school to prepare nurses to care for the mentally ill opened at McLean Hospital in Waverly, Massachusetts, in 1882. It was a 2-year program, but few psychological skills were addressed; the care was mainly custodial. Nurses took care of the patients' physical needs, such as medications, nutrition, hygiene, and ward activities. Until the end of the

nineteenth century little changed in the role of psychiatric nurses. They had limited training in psychiatry, and they primarily adapted the principles of medical-surgical nursing to the psychiatric setting. At that time psychological care consisted of kindness and tolerance toward the patients.

One of Linda Richards' more important contributions was her emphasis on assessing both the physical and emotional needs of the patients. In this early period of nursing history, nursing education separated these two needs; nurses were taught either in the general hospital or in the psychiatric hospital. In 1913 Johns Hopkins became the first school of nursing to include a fully developed course for psychiatric nursing in the curriculum. Other schools soon followed. It was not until the late 1930s that nursing education recognized the importance of psychiatric knowledge in general nursing care for all illnesses (Box 1-1).

An important factor in the development of psychiatric nursing was the emergence of various somatic therapies, including insulin shock therapy (1935), psychosurgery (1936), and electroconvulsive therapy (1937). These techniques all required the medical-surgical skills of nurses. Although these therapies did not help the patient understand his or her problems, they did control behavior and make the pa-

Evolutionary Timeline in Psychiatric Nursing

SOCIAL ENVIRONMENT		PSYCHIATRIC NURSING
	1873	Linda Richards graduated from New England Hospital for Women and Children
	1882	First school to prepare nurses to care for the mentally ill opened at McLean Hospital in Massachusetts
American Journal of Nursing first published	1900	
Florence Nightingale died	1910	
	1913	Johns Hopkins was first school of nursing to include a course on psychiatric nursing in its curriculum
Electroconvulsive therapy developed	1937	
National Mental Health Act passed by Congress, creating National Institute of Mental Health (NIMH) and providing training funds for psychiatric nursing education	1946	
	1950	National League for Nursing (NLN) required that to be accredited schools of nursing must provide an experience in psychiatric nursing
	1952	Hildegard Peplau published *Interpersonal Relations in Nursing*
Maxwell Jones published *The Therapeutic Community*	1953	
Development of major tranquilizers	1954	
Community Mental Health Centers Act passed	1963	*Perspectives in Psychiatric Care* published; *Journal of Psychiatric Nursing and Mental Health Services* published
	1973	*Standards of Psychiatric-Mental Health Nursing Practice* published; certification of psychiatric mental health nurse generalists established by American Nurses' Association (ANA)
Report of the President's Commission on Mental Health	1978	
	1979	*Issues in Mental Health Nursing* published; certification of psychiatric-mental health nurse specialists established by ANA
Nursing: A Social Policy Statement published by ANA	1980	
Mental Health Systems Act passed		
Mental Health Systems Act repealed	1981	
National Center for Nursing Research created in National Institutes of Health (NIH)	1985	*Standards of Child and Adolescent Psychiatric and Mental Health Nursing Practice* published by ANA
	1986	American Psychiatric Nurses Association (APNA) established
	1987	*Archives of Psychiatric Nursing* published; *Journal of Child and Adolescent Psychiatric and Mental Health Nursing* published
	1988	*Standards of Addictions Nursing Practice* published by ANA
	1990	*Standards of Psychiatric Consultation Liaison Nursing Practice* published by ANA
Center for Mental Health Services created	1992	
	1994	Revised *Standards of Psychiatric-Mental Health Clinical Nursing Practice* published by ANA
	1994	*Psychopharmacology Guidelines for Psychiatric-Mental Health Nurses* published by ANA
Revised *Nursing's Social Policy Statement* published by ANA	1995	*Journal of the American Psychiatric Nurses Association (JAPNA)* published
Report of the Surgeon General on Mental Health	1999	Hildegard Peplau died
	2000	Revised *Scope and Standards of Psychiatric-Mental Health Clinical Nursing Practice* published by ANA

Box **1-1**

A Nurse Speaks

We do not hesitate to emphasize the need of some psychiatric training in the life of every nurse who would represent her profession on the basis of modern standards. The psychiatrically trained nurse must remember, on the other hand, that all symptoms are not of mental origin. This fact has been long recognized, so nurses trained in mental hospitals have wisely requested affiliation in general hospitals, thus avoiding the danger of overspecialization. Does it not seem rational, therefore, that the general hospital shall guarantee its nurse an equivalent knowledge of the workings of the patient's mind as the psychiatric nurse has of the workings of his body? Modern psychology reveals the close interrelation of the two; it recognizes the ceaseless interaction of one on the other. Should we not then more consistently work toward the ideal that every hospital shall graduate nurses trained in preventive and curative methods of caring for the inevitably associated physically and mentally ill?

Annie L. Crawford, RN, BS
South Carolina Nurses' Association
Annual Convention Presentation
October 6, 1934

Box **1-2**

A Physician Speaks

I have spent all of my professional career in close association with, and close dependency on, nurses, and like many of my faculty colleagues, I've done a lot of worrying about the relationship between medicine and nursing.

The doctors worry that nurses are trying to move away from their historical responsibilities to medicine (meaning, really, to the doctors' orders). The nurses assert that they are their own profession, responsible for their own standards, coequal colleagues with physicians, and they do not wish to become mere ward administrators or technicians.

My discovery as a patient is that the institution is held together, *glued* together, enabled to function as an organism, by the nurses and by nobody else.

The nurses make it their business to know everything that is going on. They spot errors before errors can be launched. They know everything written on the chart. Most important of all, they know their patients as unique human beings, and they soon get to know the close relatives and friends. Because of this knowledge, they are quick to sense apprehensions and act on them. The average sick person in a large hospital feels at risk of getting lost, with no identity left beyond a name and a string of numbers on a plastic wristband, in danger always of being whisked off on a litter to the wrong place to have the wrong procedure done, or worse still, *not* being whisked off at the right time. The attending physician or the house officer, on rounds and usually in a hurry, can murmur a few reassuring words on his way out the door, but it takes a confident, competent, and cheerful nurse, there all day long and in and out of the room on one chore or another through the night, to bolster one's confidence that the situation is indeed manageable and not about to get out of hand.

Knowing what I know, I am all for the nurses. If they are to continue their professional feud with the doctors, if they want their professional status enhanced and their pay increased, if they infuriate the doctors by their claims to be equal professionals, if they ask for the moon, I am on their side.

Lewis Thomas, MD
The Youngest Science
New York, 1983, Viking Press

tient more amenable to psychotherapy. Somatic therapies also increased the demand for improved psychological treatment for patients who did not respond.

As nurses became more involved with somatic therapies, they began the struggle to define their role as psychiatric nurses. An editorial in the *American Journal of Nursing* in 1940 described the conflict between nurses and physicians as nurses tried to implement what they saw as appropriate care for psychiatric patients. This conflict continues to demand attention in current nursing practice (Box 1-2).

The period after World War II was one of major growth and change in psychiatric nursing. Because of the large number of service-related psychiatric problems and the increase in treatment programs offered by the Veterans Administration, psychiatric nurses with advanced preparation were in demand. The content of psychiatric nursing had now become an integral part of the generic nursing curriculum; its principles were applied to other areas of nursing practice, including general medical, pediatric, and public health nursing. By 1947 eight graduate programs in psychiatric nursing had been started.

Role Emergence

The role of psychiatric nursing began to emerge in the early 1950s. In 1947 Weiss published an article in the *American Journal of Nursing* that reemphasized the shortage of psychiatric nurses and outlined the differences between psychiatric and general duty nurses. She described "attitude therapy" as the nurse's directed use of attitudes that contribute to the patient's recovery. In implementing this therapy the nurse observes the patient for small and fleeting changes, demonstrates acceptance, respect, and understanding of the patient,

and promotes the patient's interest and participation in reality.

An article by Bennett and Eaton in the *American Journal of Psychiatry* in 1951 identified the following three problems affecting psychiatric nurses:

- The scarcity of qualified psychiatric nurses
- The underuse of their abilities
- The fact that "very little real psychiatric nursing is carried out in otherwise good psychiatric hospitals and units"

These psychiatrists believed that the psychiatric nurse should join mental health societies, consult with welfare agencies, work in outpatient clinics, practice preventive psychiatry, engage in research, and help educate the public. They supported the nurse's participation in individual and group psychotherapy and stated, "Despite the fact that most psychiatrists seem to ignore the role of the psychiatric nurse in psychotherapy, all nurses in psychiatric wards do psychotherapy of one kind or another by their contacts with patients "(Bennett & Eaton, 1951). Many of the issues raised in the article were debated years later.

> *Do you think that the problems affecting psychiatric nurses described by Bennett and Eaton in 1951 continue to exist in the specialty today?*

Also in 1951 Mellow wrote of the work she did with schizophrenic patients. She called these activities "nursing therapy." A year later, Tudor (Tudor, 1952) published a study in which she described the nurse-patient relationships she established, which were characterized by unconditional care, few demands, and the anticipation of her patients' needs. These articles were some of the earliest descriptions by psychiatric nurses of the nurse-patient relationship and the nature of its therapeutic process.

As nurses engaged in these kinds of activities, many questions arose. Are these activities therapeutic or are they therapy? What is a therapeutic relationship or a one-to-one nurse-patient relationship? How does it differ from psychotherapy? These questions were addressed by Dr. Hildegard Peplau, a dynamic nursing leader whose ideas and beliefs shaped psychiatric nursing.

In 1952 Peplau published a book, *Interpersonal Relations in Nursing,* in which she described the skills, activities, and role of psychiatric nurses. It was the first systematic, theoretical framework developed for psychiatric nursing. Peplau defined nursing as a "significant, therapeutic process." While she studied the nursing process, she saw nurses emerge in various roles: as a resource person; a teacher; a leader in local, national, and international situations; a surrogate parent; and a counselor. She wrote, "Counseling in nursing has to do with helping the patient remember and to understand fully what is happening to him in the present situation, so that the experience can be integrated with rather than dissociated from other experiences in life" (Peplau, 1952).

> *Compare the roles of psychiatric nurses identified by Hildegard Peplau in 1952 with your observations of contemporary psychiatric nursing practice.*

Finally, two significant developments in psychiatry in the 1950s also affected nursing's role for years to come. The first was Jones' publication of *The Therapeutic Community: A New Treatment Method in Psychiatry* in 1953. It encouraged using the patient's social environment to provide a therapeutic experience. The patient was to be an active participant in care and become involved in the daily problems of the community. All patients were to help solve problems, plan activities, and develop the necessary rules and regulations. Therapeutic communities became the preferred environment for psychiatric patients.

The second significant development in psychiatry in the early 1950s was the use of psychotropic drugs. With these drugs more patients became treatable, and fewer environmental constraints such as locked doors and straitjackets were required. Also, more personnel were needed to provide therapy, and the roles of various psychiatric practitioners were expanded, including the nurse's role.

Evolving Functions

In 1958 the following functions of psychiatric nurses were described (Hays, 1975):

- Dealing with patients' problems of attitude, mood, and interpretation of reality
- Exploring disturbing and conflicting thoughts and feelings
- Using the patient's positive feelings toward the therapist to bring about psychophysiological homeostasis
- Counseling patients in emergencies, including panic and fear
- Strengthening the well part of patients

The nurse-patient relationship was referred to by a variety of terms, including "therapeutic nurse-patient relationship," "psychiatric nursing therapy," "supportive psychotherapy," "rehabilitation therapies," and "nondirective counseling." The distinction between these terms and the exact nature of the nurse's role remained hazy.

Once again Peplau clarified psychiatric nursing's position and directed its future growth. In *"Interpersonal Techniques: The Crux of Psychiatric Nursing,"* published in 1962, she identified the heart of psychiatric nursing as the role of counselor or psychotherapist. In her article Peplau differentiated between general practitioners who were staff nurses working on psychiatric units and psychiatric nurses who were specialists and expert clinical practitioners with graduate degrees in psychiatric nursing. Thus from an undefined role involving primarily physical care, psychiatric nursing was evolving into a role of clinical competence based on interpersonal techniques and use of the nursing process.

In the 1960s the focus of psychiatric nursing began to shift to primary prevention and implementation of care and consultation in the community. Representative of these changes was the shift in the name of the field from **psychiatric nursing** to **psychiatric and mental health nursing.** This focus was stimulated by the Community Mental Health Centers Act of 1963, which made federal money available to states to plan, construct, and staff community mental health centers. This legislation was prompted by growing awareness of the value of treating people in the community and preventing hospitalization whenever possible. It also encouraged the formation of multidisciplinary treatment teams by combining the skills of many professions to alleviate illness and promote mental health. This team approach continues to be negotiated. The issues of territoriality, professionalism, authority structure, consumer rights, and the use of paraprofessionals are still being debated.

The 1970s gave rise to the further development of the specialty. Psychiatric nurses became the pacesetters in specialty nursing practice. They were the first to:

- Develop standards and statements on scope of practice
- Establish generalist and specialist certification

At this same time, the nursing profession was defining caring as a core element of all nursing practice, and the contributions of psychiatric nurses were embraced by nurses of all specialty groups. Partly as a result of this broader definition of psychiatric nursing and the perceived skills of psychiatric nurses, nursing education reorganized its curriculum and began to integrate psychiatric nursing content into nonpsychiatric courses. This blending of content was evident in the second change in the name of the field in the 1970s from **psychiatric and mental health nursing** to **psychosocial nursing.** Clinical rotations focusing on the psychiatric illnesses of patients in psychiatric settings were often replaced by clinical rotations integrating psychosocial aspects of the care of physically ill patients in general medical-surgical units. Unfortunately, this trend often did not provide students with an opportunity to care for patients with psychiatric illnesses and learn about new information that was emerging in the field of psychiatry and the broader behavioral sciences.

It has been proposed that psychiatric nursing content can be learned by taking care of patients in medical-surgical settings, because patients in these settings have depression, anxiety, and other psychiatric problems. How do the problems of these patients differ from those experienced by psychiatric patients? If there are no differences, why could not medical-surgical nursing content be learned by taking care of psychiatric patients because patients in these settings have diabetes, cancer, heart disease and other medical problems?

The 1980s were years of exciting scientific growth in the area of psychobiology.

Advancements occurred in five basic areas:

- Brain imaging techniques
- Neurotransmitters and neuronal receptors
- Psychobiology of emotions
- Understanding the brain
- Molecular genetics related to psychobiology

Although this information explosion advanced knowledge in the field, it lacked integration and was often of limited clinical usefulness. It has also been observed that psychiatric nurses in the 1980s were slow to make the shift away from primarily psychodynamic models of the mind to more balanced psychobiological models of psychiatric care (Abraham et al, 1992; McEnany, 1991).

Psychiatric nurses thus entered the 1990s faced with the challenge of integrating the expanding bases of neuroscience into the holistic biopsychosocial practice of psychiatric nursing. Advances in understanding the relationships of the brain, behavior, emotion, and cognition offered new opportunities for psychiatric nursing (Hays, 1995). Psychiatric nurses saw the need to become realigned with care and caring, which represent the art of psychiatric nursing and complement the high technology of current health care practices (McBride, 1996).

The new millennium brings with it issues of balance, differentiation, and integration. The knowledge base of the specialty is rooted in the integration of the biological, psychological, spiritual, social, and environmental realms of the human experience. As Flaskerud and Wuerker (1999) note: "The philosophical and ethical challenge to nursing is to integrate the biological and behavioral concepts into the nursing care of mentally ill people while remaining centered in the nursing domain and maintaining our focus on caring and our sensitivity to the human condition."

Compare the length of your clinical rotation in psychiatric nursing with your clinicals in medicine, surgery, and pediatrics. Given the high prevalence of mental health problems such as depression and substance abuse, do you feel you have sufficient learning time in psychiatric nursing?

CONTEMPORARY PRACTICE

Psychiatric nursing is an interpersonal process that promotes and maintains patient behavior that contributes to integrated functioning. The patient may be an individual, family, group, organization, or community. The American Nurses' Association *Scope and Standards of Psychiatric-Mental Health Clinical Nursing Practice* defines psychiatric nursing as "a specialized area of nursing practice, employing the wide range of explanatory theories of human behavior as its science and purposeful use of self as its art" (American Nurses' Association, 2000). The Center for Mental Health Services officially recognizes psychiatric nursing as one of the five core mental health disciplines. The other four disciplines are marriage and family therapy, psychiatry, psychology, and social work.

The current practice of psychiatric nursing is based on a number of underlying premises or beliefs. The philosophical beliefs of psychiatric nursing practice on which this text is based are described in Box 1-3. The psychiatric nurse uses knowledge from the psychosocial and biophysical sciences and theories of personality and human behavior. From these sources the nurse derives a theoretical framework on which to base nursing practice. Various models of psychiatric treatment are described in Chapter 3. Chapter 4 presents the Stuart Stress Adaptation Model of psychiatric nursing care that is used as the organizing framework for this text.

The contemporary practice of psychiatric nursing occurs within a social and environmental context (see Critical Thinking about Contemporary Issues). Thus the nurse-patient **relationship** has evolved into a nurse-patient **partnership** that expands the dimensions of the professional psychiatric nursing role. These elements include **clinical competence, patient-family advocacy, fiscal responsibility, interdisciplinary collaboration, social accountability,** and

Box **1-3**

Philosophical Beliefs of Psychiatric Nursing Practice

- The individual has intrinsic worth and dignity and each person is worthy of respect.
- The goal of the individual is one of growth, health, autonomy, and self-actualization.
- Every individual has the potential to change.
- Each person functions as a holistic being who acts on, interacts with, and reacts to the environment as a whole person.
- All people have common, basic human needs. These needs include physical requirements, safety, love, belonging, esteem, and self-actualization.
- All behavior of the individual is meaningful. It arises from personal needs and goals and can be understood only from the person's internal frame of reference and within the context in which it occurs.
- Behavior consists of perceptions, thoughts, feelings, and actions. From one's perceptions thoughts arise, emotions are felt, and actions are conceived. Disruptions may occur in any of these areas.
- Individuals vary in their coping capacities, which depend on genetic endowment, environmental influences, nature and degree of stress, and available resources. All individuals have the potential for both health and illness.

- Illness can be a growth-producing experience for the individual.
- All people have a right to an equal opportunity for adequate health care regardless of gender, race, religion, ethics, sexual orientation, or cultural background.
- Mental health is a critical component of comprehensive health care services.
- The individual has the right to participate in decision making regarding physical and mental health.
- The person has the right to self-determination, including the decision to pursue health or illness.
- The goal of nursing care is to promote wellness, maximize integrated functioning, and enhance self-actualization. Nursing care is based on health care needs and expected treatment outcomes mutually determined with individuals, families, groups, and communities.
- An interpersonal relationship can produce change and growth within the individual. It is the vehicle for the application of the nursing process and the attainment of the goal of nursing care.

 CRITICAL THINKING about **CONTEMPORARY ISSUES**

Are Psychiatric Nurses Vulnerable or Valuable as Mental Health Care Providers?

One question that is often raised when nurses talk about the health care environment is whether psychiatric nurses will be vulnerable to being replaced as expensive and outdated providers or be valued as competent clinicians who can function in a world of changing needs, processes, and structures. Potential areas of vulnerability have been identified and include the following (Stuart, 2001):

- Fewer nurses are attracted to psychiatric nursing as compared with other specialty areas.
- Content devoted to understanding psychiatric illnesses and working with psychiatric patients in nursing education programs has decreased steadily during the past decade.
- Graduate programs are moving toward the preparation of nurse practitioners who have significantly less course work related to the diagnosis and treatment of psychiatric illnesses.
- Biopsychosocial skills and expertise of psychiatric nurses are often underused in mental health care systems.
- Psychiatric nurses often are viewed as expensive health care providers who can be replaced by two or more less costly personnel.
- There are increasing threats to nursing autonomy as state boards of nursing and other regulatory bodies attempt to establish separate advanced practice licensure and examinations, and require advanced practice nurses to be under the full supervision of physicians.
- There are few outcome studies that document the nature, extent, and effectiveness of care delivered by psychiatric nurses.

- Psychiatric nurses have difficulty receiving direct reimbursement for services, despite the 1997 achievement of Medicare reimbursement.
- The specialty is struggling with the education and certification of advanced practice psychiatric-mental health nurses in clinical nurse specialist, nurse practitioner, and combined roles.
- Role differentiation for psychiatric nurses based on education and experience is often lacking in the position descriptions, job responsibilities, and reward programs of the health care systems in which nurses practice.
- APRNs-PMH are underused in managed care and primary care delivery systems.

Each of these issues must be addressed if psychiatric nursing is to continue to develop as a specialty area. Nurses need to move into the continuum of care and clearly articulate their skills, functions, and abilities. They must also demonstrate their cost effectiveness and establish differentiated levels of practice based on education, experience, and credentials. Other survival skills needed by psychiatric nurses in the future include management of negative emotionality, achievement of collegial unity, understanding the nature of transitions, revising career trajectories, and marketing skills and functions (Thomas, 1999). Such strategies will position psychiatric nurses as visible, interdependent, central, and collaborating professionals who have much to offer a reformed health care system.

legal-ethical parameters (Fig. 1-1). No longer can psychiatric nurses focus exclusively on bedside care and the immediacy of patient needs. Rather, they must broaden the context of their care and the responsibility and understanding they bring to the caregiving situation. The current practice of psychiatric nursing requires greater sensitivity to the social environment and the advocacy needs of patients and their families. It also mandates thoughtful consideration of complex legal and ethical dilemmas that arise from a delivery system that is focused on the efficiencies of managed care, which can disadvantage and discriminate against those with mental illness. New models of mental health care also require greater skill in interdisciplinary collaboration that is built on the psychiatric nurse's clinical competence and professional self-assertion and balanced by a clear understanding of the costs of psychiatric care in general and psychiatric nursing care in particular. Each of these elements must influence the education, research, and clinical components of contemporary psychiatric nursing practice.

Continuum of Care

Traditional settings for psychiatric nurses include psychiatric facilities, community mental health centers, psychiatric units in the general hospital, residential facilities, and private practice. More recently, alternative treatment settings have emerged throughout the continuum of mental health care. Hospitals are being transformed into integrated clinical systems that provide inpatient care, partial hospitalization or day treatment, residential care, home care, and outpatient or ambulatory care (Fig. 1-2). Psychiatric nurses who continue to work within inpatient units have seen the goals, processes and structures of care change drastically. Nurses who staff inpatient units no longer have their responsibilities limited to activities delivered exclusively in the hospital setting. Rather, they are likely to be flexibly assigned on a daily basis to other settings in the continuum of mental health care based on fluctuating patient census and organizational need.

In addition, community-based treatment settings have expanded to include foster care or group homes, hospices, visiting nurse associations, home health agencies, emergency departments, nursing homes, shelters, primary care clinics, schools, prisons, industrial settings, managed care facilities, and health maintenance organizations.

The new opportunities for psychiatric nursing practice that are emerging throughout the continuum of mental health care are very exciting (Shea et al, 1999). They allow psychiatric nurses to be proactive in demonstrating their expertise in designing interventions, planning programs, implementing treatment strategies, and managing staff in a variety of traditional and nontraditional settings. Psychiatric nurses must also continue to demonstrate flexibility, accountability, and self-direction as they move into these expanding areas of practice.

Primary Mental Health Care

Primary mental health care is the "care that is provided to those at risk for or already in need of mental health services. It begins before or at the first point of contact with the mental health care delivery system. Such care involves all of the continuous and comprehensive services necessary for the promotion of optimal health, prevention of mental illness, and health maintenance, and includes the management of and/or referral for mental health and general health problems" (Haber & Billings, 1995). Primary mental health care is important because many people are not receiving the mental health care they need. Some are undiagnosed in general medical settings. Others are correctly diagnosed but lack a consistent care provider. Still others have problems with their prescribed treatments and have relapses that could have been prevented.

Psychiatric nurses are moving into the domain of primary care and working with other nurses and physicians to diagnose and treat psychiatric illness in patients with somatic complaints (Haber & Mitchell, 1997). Cardiovascular, gynecological, respiratory, gastrointestinal, and family practice settings are appropriate for assessing patients for anxiety, depression, and substance abuse disorders. As health-care initiatives continue to move into schools and other community settings, psychiatric nurses are assuming leadership roles in providing expertise through consultation and evaluation.

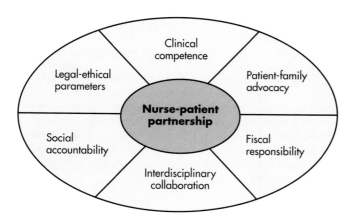

Fig. 1-1 Elements of the psychiatric nursing role.

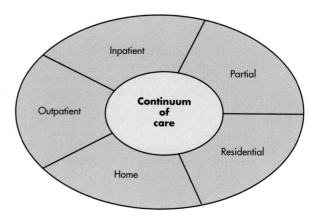

Fig. 1-2 Continuum of mental health-care settings.

Psychiatric nurses are very well suited to provide comprehensive health care to patients in both psychiatric settings and primary care environments. In particular, advanced practice psychiatric nurses acting as consultants to nonpsychiatric providers in hospital-based or outpatient clinics are in a unique position to assess and triage these patients on the basis of the immediacy of their needs. Early assessment and triage can minimize the length of time between psychiatric referral and intervention. By identifying patients in crisis and intervening in a timely fashion, psychiatric nurses may reduce failed appointments and enhance the efficacy of treatment (Wilkinson et al, 1995).

Psychiatric nurses are also providing medical and medication management for selected groups of patients in collaborative practices. For example, patients who are having difficulty being stabilized on their medications or who have comorbid medical illnesses are seen in a psychiatric nursing clinic in which nurses and physicians collaborate to provide high-quality patient care. Psychiatric nurses who obtain prescriptive authority can further expand the services they provide and deliver cost-effective psychiatric care to communities that do not have access to a psychiatrist.

Competent Caring

There are three domains of contemporary psychiatric nursing practice: direct care, communication, and management. Within these overlapping domains of practice, the **teaching, coordinating, delegating,** and **collaborating** functions of the nursing role are expressed (Fig. 1-3). Often the communication and management domains of practice are overlooked when discussing the psychiatric nursing role. However, these integrating activities are critically important and very time-consuming aspects of a nurse's role. They have become even more important in a reformed health care system that places emphasis on efficient patient triage and management.

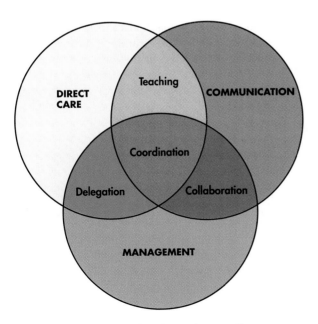

Fig. 1-3 Psychiatric nursing practice.

Box 1-4 lists specific psychiatric nursing activities that reflect the current nature and scope of competent caring functions performed by psychiatric nurses. Not all nurses perform all of these activities. Psychiatric nurses participate in these activities based on their education and experience. In addition, psychiatric nurses are able to:

- Make culturally sensitive biopsychosocial health assessments
- Design and implement treatment plans for patients and families with complex health problems and comorbid conditions
- Engage in case management activities such as organizing, accessing, negotiating, coordinating, and integrating services and benefits for individuals and families
- Provide a "health care map" for individuals, families, and groups to guide them to community resources for mental health, including the most appropriate providers, agencies, technologies, and social systems
- Promote and maintain mental health and manage the effects of mental illness through teaching and counseling
- Provide care for the physically ill with psychological problems and the psychiatrically ill with physical problems
- Manage and coordinate systems of care integrating the needs of patients, families, staff, and regulators.

Psychiatric nurses need to be able to articulate both the general and the specific aspects of their practice to patients, families, other professionals, administrators, and legislators. Only when such skills are identified will psychiatric nurses be able to ensure their appropriate roles, adequate compensation for the nursing care provided, and the most efficient use of scarce human resources in the delivery of mental health care.

LEVEL OF PERFORMANCE

A description of psychiatric nursing roles and activities includes a wide variation in levels of performance. Not all psychiatric nurses perform each of these functions. Individual nurses have primary responsibility and accountability for their own practice; one aspect of this accountability is that nurses define and adhere to the legitimate scope of their practice. Four major factors—laws, qualifications, setting, and personal initiative—play a part in determining the roles engaged in by each nurse.

Laws

Laws are the primary factor affecting the level of nursing practice. Each state has its own nursing practice act, which regulates entry into the profession and defines the legal limits of nursing practice that must be adhered to by all nurses. Nurse practice acts also address aspects of advanced practice, including prescriptive authority (Pearson, 2000). Nurses must be familiar with the nursing practice act of their state and define and limit their practice accordingly.

Qualifications

A nurse's qualifications include education, work experience, and certification. Two levels of psychiatric-mental health

Box **1-4**

Domains of Psychiatric Nursing Practice

DIRECT CARE ACTIVITIES

Activity therapy
Advocacy
Aftercare follow-up
Behavioral treatments
Case consultation
Case management
Cognitive treatments
Community assessment
Community-based care
Community education
Complementary interventions
Compliance counseling
Counseling
Crisis intervention
Discharge planning
Environmental change
Environmental safety
Family interventions
Group work
Health maintenance
Health promotion
Health teaching
High-risk assessment
Holistic interventions
Home health care
Individual counseling
Informed consent acquisition
Intake screening and evaluation
Interpreting diagnostic and laboratory tests
Medication administration
Medication management
Mental health promotion
Mental illness prevention
Milieu therapy
Nutritional counseling
Ordering diagnostic and laboratory tests
Parent education
Patient triage
Physical assessment
Physiological treatments
Play therapy
Prescription of medications
Promotion of self-care activities
Provision of environmental safety
Psychiatric rehabilitation
Psychobiological interventions
Psychoeducation
Psychosocial assessment
Psychotherapy
Rehabilitation counseling
Relapse prevention
Research implementation
Social action

Social skills training
Somatic treatments
Stress management
Support of social systems
Telehealth

COMMUNICATION ACTIVITIES

Clinical case conferences
Development of treatment plans
Documentation of care
Forensic testimony
Interagency liaison
Peer review
Professional nurse networking
Report preparation
Staff meetings
Transcription of orders
Treatment team meetings
Verbal reports of care

MANAGEMENT ACTIVITIES

Budgeting and resource allocation
Clinical supervision
Collaboration
Committee participation
Community action
Consultation/liaison
Contract negotiation
Coordination of services
Delegation of assignments
Grant writing
Marketing and public relations
Mediation and conflict resolution
Mentorship
Needs assessment and forecasting
Organizational governance
Outcomes management
Performance evaluations
Policy and procedure development
Practice guidelines formulation
Professional presentations
Program evaluation
Program planning
Publications
Quality improvement activities
Recruitment and retention activities
Regulatory agency activities
Risk management
Software development
Staff scheduling
Staff and student education
Strategic planning
Unit governance
Utilization review

clinical nursing practice, basic and advanced, have been identified (American Nurses' Association, 2000).

1. Basic Level

   Psychiatric-Mental Health Registered Nurse. Registered nurses at the basic level have completed a nursing program and passed the state licensure examination. Registered nurses, who practice in psychiatric-mental health nursing, care for mental health patients in various settings. Basic level nurses work as staff nurses, case managers, nurse managers and other nursing roles in the psychiatric-mental health field.

   Psychiatric-Mental Health Registered Nurse, Certified (RN,C). After acquiring experience and ongoing continuing education in the specialty, the basic level nurse may become certified as a psychiatric mental health nurse. Certification is a formal process that validates the clinical competence of the basic level nurse. This certification demonstrates that the basic level nurse has met the profession's standards of knowledge and experience in the specialty, exceeding those of a beginning RN or a novice in the specialty. The letter "C," placed after the RN (i.e., RN,C) is the initial that designates basic-level certification status.

2. Advanced Level

   Advanced Practice Registered Nurse—Psychiatric-Mental Health (APRN-PMH). The Advanced Practice Registered Nurse in Psychiatric-Mental Health (APRN-PMH) is a licensed Registered Nurse (RN) who is educationally prepared at least at the master's degree level in the specialty. The nurse's graduate level preparation is distinguished by a depth of knowledge of theory and practice, validated experience in clinical practice, and competence in advanced clinical nursing skills. The APRN-PMH focuses clinical practice on persons with diagnosed psychiatric disorders or those at risk of mental health disorders, and applies knowledge, skills, and experience autonomously to complex mental health problems. The term APRN-PMH applies to either the clinical nurse specialist or the nurse practitioner whose education and experience in psychiatric nursing practice meets criteria established by the profession.

   Advanced Practice Registered Nurse–Psychiatric-Mental Health, Certified Specialist (RN,CS). The designated certification for advanced clinical practice by either the clinical nurse specialist or the nurse practitioner in any area of nursing is that of Registered Nurse, Certified Specialist (RN,CS). In psychiatric-mental health nursing, the Certified Specialist designation indicates certified advanced practice in the specialty by a PMH clinical nurse specialist or a PMH nurse practitioner.

Another qualification is the nurse's work experience. Although work experience does not replace education, it does provide an added and necessary dimension to the nurse's level of competence and ability to function therapeutically.

Practice Setting

Psychiatric nurses may practice in settings that vary widely in purpose, type, location, and administration. They may be employed by an organization or self-employed in private practice (Lambert & Lambert, 1996). Nurses employed by an organization are paid for their services on a salaried or fee-for-service basis. Most nurses work in such organized settings. The administrative policies of these organizations can either foster or limit full use of the psychiatric nurse's potential. Nurses who are self-employed are paid for their services through third-party payment and direct patient fees. Some self-employed advanced practice psychiatric nurses maintain staff privileges with institutional facilities.

The role of a nurse in any psychiatric–mental health setting depends on the following:

- Philosophy, mission, values, and goals of the treatment setting
- Definitions of mental health and mental illness that prevail in the setting
- Needs of the consumers of the mental health services
- Number of clinical staff available and the services they are able to provide
- Organizational structure and reporting relationships in the setting
- Consensus reached by the mental health care providers regarding their respective roles and responsibilities
- Resources and revenues available to offset the cost of care needed and provided
- Presence of strong nursing leadership and mentorship

A supportive environment for psychiatric nurses is one in which there is open and honest communication among staff, interdisciplinary respect, recognition of nurses' contributions, nursing involvement in decision making about both clinical care and the work environment, delegation of nonessential nursing tasks, opportunity to expand into new roles and responsibilities, and the encouragement of involvement in professional psychiatric nursing activities and organizations.

What specific characteristics would you look for in an organization to see whether it promoted professional psychiatric nursing practice?

Personal Initiative

The personal competence and initiative of the individual nurse determine one's interpretation of the nursing role and the success of its implementation. The importance of this final factor should not be ignored; without a realization of clinical competence and the assumption of professional initiative, the psychiatric nurse's performance is significantly limited.

One strategy for enhancing the personal growth and competence of the psychiatric nurse is the use of support groups. Examples of the purposes and possible activities of a professional support group are described in Table 1-1.

Psychiatric nurses also benefit from networking. Networks are groups of people drawn together by common concerns to support and help one another. Networks range from informal friendships and small groups providing contacts to larger open groups providing emotional support and local and na-

Table **1-1**

Psychiatric Nursing Support Groups	
Purpose	**Related Activities**
PROVIDE PRACTICAL HELP AND PROFESSIONAL FEEDBACK	Review clinical cases Evaluate documentation methods Analyze staff interactions and performance Develop nursing practice guidelines Discuss changes in one's role and work setting Describe successful interventions Share difficult work experiences
EXCHANGE INFORMATION AND STIMULATE IDEAS	Report on conferences attended Distribute articles for reading and discussion Update on new developments in psychiatric nursing Review nursing practice legislative issues Share organizational policies and procedures Suggest resources for new information and problem solving

Citing the Evidence on

Outcome Evaluation

BACKGROUND: Contemporary mental health care requires Advanced Practice Registered Nurses in Psychiatric-Mental Health (APRN-PMH) to identify and evaluate the outcomes of their practices. This survey of 364 certified clinical nurse specialists documents the outcomes used by these nurses.

RESULTS: Approximately one third of respondents stated or inferred that they did not use any outcome measures. The most frequently mentioned outcome related to relieving a variety of symptoms. The use of patient and treatment goals and the use of patient self-report as criteria of outcome evaluation was common. Specific changes in behavior, functional status, length of stay, quality of life, satisfaction with care, compliance with treatment and family burden were also important. The use of service outcomes was mentioned inconsistently.

IMPLICATIONS: Despite the recent emphasis on outcome evaluation, it appears that many clinical specialists have not yet incorporated formal outcome evaluations into their practice. Still, nurses in the study were interested in being informed of available tools to use in the measurement of their practices. Nurse educators and administrators, together with professional organizations, need to provide greater assistance to practicing clinicians in the evaluation of their practices.

Barrell L, Merwin E, Poster E: Patient outcomes used by advanced practice psychiatric nurses to evaluate effectiveness of practice, *Arch Psychiatr Nurs* 11:184, 1997.

tional organizations representing one's specialty. Forming networks can help nurses to unite and to value their profession. Networking at the staff nurse level is crucial to the unity and survival of the profession. It helps nurses to care for one another and to influence their work environment.

What networks do you have in your life at this time and how do they help you? How might professional networks help you when you graduate?

PSYCHIATRIC NURSING AGENDA

Psychiatric nursing will continue to grow and evolve in the years ahead. There are more than 82,000 registered nurses working in mental health organizations in the United States, and over 17,000 of them have graduate degrees (Manderscheid & Henderson, 1999). Health care reform, patient and family needs, scientific developments, economic realities, and societal expectations will shape the future roles and functions of psychiatric nurses. To best meet the challenges of the next decade, psychiatric nurses need to focus their energies on three areas: outcome evaluation, leadership skills, and political action.

Outcome Evaluation

Psychiatric nurses need to be able to identify, describe, and measure the effect of the care they provide patients, families, and communities. Outcome studies documenting the quality, cost, and effectiveness of psychiatric nursing practice are an important part of the psychiatric nursing agenda (see Citing the Evidence). These studies should be able to stand up to the scientific review of the broader community of mental health professionals by being methodologically sound, empirically grounded, and replicated across the continuum of psychiatric care settings (Merwin & Mauck, 1995).

Focusing on ways to critically evaluate the outcomes of psychiatric nursing activities is a task for every psychiatric nurse regardless of role, qualifications, or practice setting. Psychiatric nurse clinicians, educators, administrators, and researchers all must assume responsibility for answering the question, "What difference does psychiatric nurse caring make?"

Leadership Skills

Psychiatric nurses need knowledge and strategies that enable them to exercise leadership and management in their work (Krejci & Malin, 1997). Such leadership has an effect on the care patients receive; it also strengthens and expands the contribution of psychiatric nursing to the larger health care system (Lanza, 1997a; Lanza, 1997b). Psychiatric nurses should use their leadership skills and work as change agents. Mental health consumers need adequate, humane, and socially acceptable care. To this end nurses can initiate change; assist by supporting, participating, or implementing change; engage in joint ventures for planned change; and evaluate completed change.

Another form of leadership is demonstrated by nurses who join their specialty organization (Carter et al, 1997). The American Psychiatric Nurses Association (APNA), located in Washington, D.C., is the largest organization of psychiatric nurses in the United States, representing more than 4000 registered nurses in both basic and advanced psychiatric nursing practice. Mental health nurses in Canada belong to the Canadian Federation of Mental Health Nurses (CFMHN). Nurses in Australia and New Zealand belong to the Australian & New Zealand College of Mental Health Nurses (ANZ-PSYCH). Organizations such as APNA, CFMHN, and ANZ-PSYCH can also provide informational networks to psychiatric nurses that are essential for consumer advocacy, continuing education, and effective political action.

> *Talk with some of the staff nurses who work in psychiatry and ask whether they know about APNA. Are they members? If not, what would it take for them to join?*

Political Action

Psychiatric nurses can be significant forces in the process of shaping the future of society. To do so, they must learn to use their power and resources in the political arena—one of the most important targets for nursing action. Increasing psychiatric nurses' political awareness and skills is necessary to bring about needed changes in the mental health care delivery system. The political empowerment of nursing involves the development of many dimensions:

- Raising consciousness of sociocultural realities
- Building coalitions
- Developing positive self-esteem
- Adopting feminist theory as empowering rather than threatening
- Acquiring proactive political skills

These dimensions are overlapping and interactive and form the basis of political action by psychiatric nurses that is respectful of others, confirming of self, and directed toward the common good.

It is essential that psychiatric nurses recognize the value and legitimacy of their own voices. Nurses must become educated in legislative and regulatory processes, involved in political campaigns, and testify in legislative hearings. Psychiatric nurses can then assert their right to an equitable share of the resources, given the value of the services they provide. Passive acceptance of decisions made by legislators, insurers, managed care companies, and other professionals should be replaced with proactive strategies. In this way the psychiatric nursing agenda of the next decade will advance nursing's commitment to caring in a mental health delivery system that is fair, sensitive, and responsible in meeting the biopsychosocial needs of patients, families, and communities.

Summary

1. Psychiatric nursing began to emerge as a profession in the late nineteenth century, and by the twentieth century it had evolved into a specialty with unique roles and functions.

2. Psychiatric nursing is an interpersonal process that promotes and maintains behaviors that contribute to integrated functioning. The patient may be an individual, family, group, organization, or community. The three domains of psychiatric nursing practice are direct care, communication, and management.

3. Four factors that help to determine the level of a psychiatric nurse's performance are the law, the nurse's qualifications, the practice setting, and the nurse's personal initiative.

4. To best meet the challenges of the next decade, psychiatric nurses need to focus their energies on three areas: outcome evaluation, leadership skills, and political action.

 Visit MERLIN: www.mosby.com/MERLIN/Stuart to find these additional materials and student activities.

- **Worksheets**
- **"Drug of the Month" Updates**
- **"Citing the Evidence" Updates**
- **Critical Thinking Activities and Exercises**
- **Annotated Suggested Readings**
- **Web Links**
- **More!**

Chapter Review Questions

1. **Fill in the blanks.**

A. _____ is known as the first American psychiatric nurse.

B. The book *Interpersonal Relations in Nursing* was written by _____.

C. The three domains of contemporary psychiatric nursing practice are _____, _____, and _____.

D. The two levels of psychiatric–mental health clinical practice are _____ and _____.

E. The largest organization of psychiatric nurses in the United States is the _____.

2. **Identify whether the following statements are true (T) or false (F).**

____ A. The psychiatric nursing role evolved from primarily physical care to clinical competence based on interpersonal techniques and use of the nursing process.

____ B. Psychiatric nursing was the first specialty to establish generalist (C) and specialty (CS) certification.

____ C. Psychiatric hospitals are being transformed into integrated clinical systems that provide the full continuum of psychiatric care.

____ D. Each state has its own nursing practice act that regulates entry into the profession and defines the legal limits of nursing practice.

____ E. Fewer than 50,000 registered nurses work in mental health organizations in the United States.

____ F. There are numerous published studies of the nature and outcome of psychiatric nursing care.

3. **Provide short answers for the following questions.**

A. Why was the development of psychotropic drugs so important in the treatment of people with mental illness?

B. List the five core mental health disciplines.

C. Identify the six dimensions of the nurse-patient partnership that characterize today's psychiatric nursing role.

D. Access APNA on the World Wide Web at **http://www.apna.org**. Do you think that having information about this nursing organization on the Internet is a service to psychiatric nurses?

REFERENCES

Abraham I et al: Integrating the bio into the biopsychosocial understanding and treating biological phenomena in psychiatric-mental health nursing, *Arch Psychiatr Nurs* 6:296, 1992.

American Nurses' Association: *Scope and standards of psychiatric-mental health clinical nursing practice,* Washington, DC, 2000, The Association.

Bennett A, Eaton J: The role of the psychiatric nurse in the newer therapies, *Am J Psychiatry* 108:167, 1951.

Carter E et al: The ins and outs of psychiatric-mental health nursing and the American Nurses Association, *J Am Psych Nurses Assoc* 3: 10, 1997.

Doona M: At least as well cared for . . . Linda Richards and the mentally ill, *Image* 16:51, 1984.

Editorial, *Am J Nurs* 40:23, 1940.

Flaskerud J, Wuerker A: Mental health nursing in the 21st century, *Issues Ment Health Nurs* 20: 5, 1999.

Haber J, Billings C: Primary mental health care: a model for psychiatric-mental health nursing, *J Am Psych Nurses Assoc* 1:154, 1995.

Haber J, Mitchell G: *Primary care meets mental health: tools for the 21st century,* Tiburon, California, 1997, CentraLink.

Hayes A: Psychiatric nursing: what does biology have to do with it? *Arch Psychiatr Nurs* 9:216, 1995.

Hays D: Suggested clinical practice of psychiatric nurses recorded in the literature between 1946 and 1958. In *Psychiatric nursing 1946 to 1974: a report on the state of the art,* New York, 1975, American Journal of Nursing.

Jones M: *The therapeutic community: a new treatment method in psychiatry,* New York, 1953, Basic Books.

Krejci J, Malin S: Impact of leadership development on competencies, *Nurs Econ* 15:235, 1997.

Lambert V, Lambert C: Advanced practice nurses: starting an independent practice, *Nurs Forum* 31:11, 1996.

Lanza M: Power and leadership in psychiatric nursing: directions for the next century, part I, *Perspect Psychiatr Care* 33(1):5, 1997a.

Lanza M: Power and leadership in psychiatric nursing: directions for the next century, part II, *Perspect Psychiatr Care* 33(2):5, 1997b.

Manderscheid R, Henderson M, editors: *Mental health United States, 1998,* Washington, DC, 1999, Department of Health and Human Services, Center for Mental Health Services.

McBride A: Psychiatric-mental health nursing in the twenty-first century. In McBride A, Austin J, editors: *Psychiatric-mental health nursing: integrating the behavioral and biological sciences,* Philadelphia, 1996, WB Saunders.

McEnany G: Psychobiology and psychiatric nursing: a philosophical matrix, *Arch Psychiatr Nurs* 5:255, 1991.

Mellow J: Nursing therapy, *Am J Nurs* 68:2365, 1968.

Merwin E, Mauck A: Psychiatric nursing outcome research: the state of the science, *Arch Psychiatr Nurs* 9:311, 1995.

Pearson L: Annual update of how each state stands on legislative issues affecting advanced nursing practice, *Nurse Pract* 25:16, 2000.

Peplau H: *Interpersonal relations in nursing,* New York, 1952, GP Putnam's Sons.

Peplau H: Interpersonal techniques: the crux of psychiatric nursing, *Am J Nurs* 62:53, 1962.

Shea C et al: *Advanced practice nursing in psychiatric and mental health care,* St Louis, 1999, Mosby.

Stuart G: Recent changes and current issues in psychiatric nursing. In McCloskey J, editor: *Current issues in nursing,* St Louis, 2001, Mosby.

Thomas S: Surrounded by banana peels: is psychiatric nursing slipping? *J Am Psych Nurses Assoc* 5:88, 1999.

Tudor G: Sociopsychiatric nursing approach to intervention in a problem of mutual withdrawal on a mental hospital ward, *Psychiatry* 15:193, 1952.

Weiss MO: The skills of psychiatric nursing, *Am J Nurs* 47:174, 1947.

Wilkinson L et al: Mental health problems in hospital-based clinics: patient profile and referral patterns, *J Am Psych Nurses Assoc* 1:140, 1995.

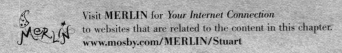
Visit **MERLIN** for *Your Internet Connection*
to websites that are related to the content in this chapter.
www.mosby.com/MERLIN/Stuart

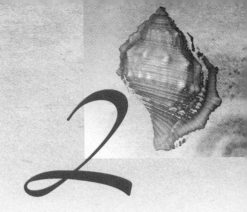

Therapeutic Nurse-Patient Relationship

Gail W. Stuart

When we treat man as he is, we make him worse than he is. When we treat him as if he already were what he potentially could be, we make him what he should be.

JOHANN WOLFGANG VON GOETHE

The therapeutic nurse-patient relationship is a mutual learning experience and a corrective emotional experience for the patient. It is based on the underlying humanity of nurse and patient, with mutual respect and acceptance of ethnocultural differences. In this relationship the nurse uses personal attributes and clinical techniques in working with the patient to bring about insight and behavioral change.

CHARACTERISTICS OF THE RELATIONSHIP

The goals of a therapeutic relationship are directed toward the patient's growth and include the following:

- Self-realization, self-acceptance, and an increased genuine self-respect
- A clear sense of personal identity and an improved level of personal integration
- An ability to form an intimate, interdependent, interpersonal relationship with a capacity to give and receive love
- Improved functioning and increased ability to satisfy needs and achieve realistic personal goals

To achieve these goals, various aspects of the patient's life experiences are explored. The nurse allows the patient to express thoughts and feelings and relates these to observed and reported actions, clarifying areas of conflict and anxiety. The nurse identifies and maximizes the patient's ego strengths and encourages socialization and family relatedness. Together the patient and nurse correct communication problems and modify maladaptive behavior patterns by testing new patterns of behavior and more adaptive coping mechanisms.

In the nurse-patient relationship, differing values are respected. The two communicate through a dialogue, or discussion, not a monologue, affirming the patient's reality and worth and allowing the patient to more fully define ego identity. In Box 2-1, Rogers (1961) summarizes the charac-

---

Box 2-1

Characteristics that Facilitate Growth in Helping Relationships

- Can I be in some way that will be perceived by the other person as trustworthy, as dependable, or consistent in some deep sense?
- Can I be expressive enough as a person that what I am will be communicated unambiguously?
- Can I let myself experience positive attitudes toward this other person—attitudes of warmth, caring, liking, interest, and respect?
- Can I be strong enough as a person to be separate from the other?
- Am I secure enough within myself to permit him his separateness?
- Can I let myself enter fully into the world of his feelings and personal meaning and see these as he does?
- Can I be acceptant of each facet of the other person that he presents to me? Can I receive him as he is?
- Can I communicate this attitude? Or can I only receive him conditionally, acceptant of some aspects of his feelings and silently or openly disapproving of others?
- Can I act with sufficient sensitivity in the relationship that my behavior will not be perceived as a threat?
- Can I free him from the threat of external evaluation?
- Can I meet this other individual as a person who is in the process of *becoming*, or will I be bound by his past and my past?

From Rogers C: *On becoming a person*, Boston, 1961, Houghton Mifflin.

---

teristics of a helping relationship that facilitate growth. All nurses working with patients may ask themselves these questions; their answers largely determine the progress of the relationship.

The therapeutic nurse-patient relationship is complex (Sundeen et al, 1998). Evidence exists that the therapeutic alliance in the context of psychotherapy has a positive effect on patient outcomes (Connors et al, 1997; Krupnick et al, 1996; Saunders, 1999). Similar research is needed to document the impact of the therapeutic nurse-patient relationship on clinical outcomes. This chapter examines the personal qualities of the nurse as helper, the phases of the relationship, facilitative communication, responsive and action dimensions, therapeutic impasses, and the therapeutic outcome (Fig. 2-1). Each of these factors influences the nurse's effectiveness.

PERSONAL QUALITIES OF THE NURSE

The key therapeutic tool the psychiatric nurse uses is oneself. Thus self-analysis is the first building block in providing quality nursing care.

Now, if a nurse is afraid or even ignorant of her own self, she is highly likely to be threatened by a patient's real-self expressions. . . . A nurse who is more aware of the breadth and depth of her own real self is in a much better position to empathize with her patients and to encourage (or at least not block) their self-disclosures (Jourard, 1971).

Research suggests some essential qualities needed to help others. These qualities are necessary characteristics for all nurses who wish to be therapeutic. They also help the nurse set goals for future growth.

Awareness of Self

Effective helpers must be able to answer the question, Who am I? Nurses who care for the biological, psychological, and sociocultural needs of patients see a broad range of human experiences. They must learn to deal with anxiety, anger, sadness, and joy in helping patients throughout the health-illness continuum.

Self-awareness is a key part of the psychiatric nursing experience. The nurse's goal is to achieve authentic, open, and personal communication. The nurse must be able to examine personal feelings, actions, and reactions. This also has been described as **emotional competence** (MacCulloch,

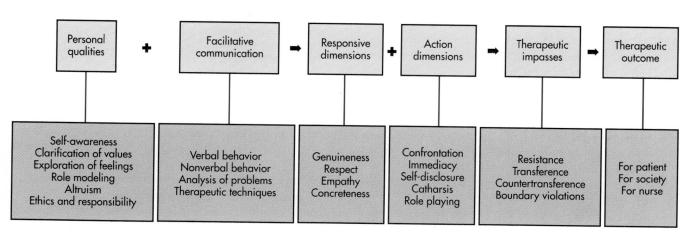

Fig. 2-1 Elements affecting the nurse's ability to be therapeutic.

1998). A good understanding and acceptance of self allow the nurse to acknowledge a patient's differences and uniqueness.

Campbell (1980) has identified a holistic nursing model of self-awareness that consists of four interconnected components: psychological, physical, environmental, and philosophical.

- The **psychological** component includes knowledge of emotions, motivations, self-concept, and personality. Being psychologically self-aware means being sensitive to feelings and outside events that affect those feelings.
- The **physical** component is the knowledge of personal and general physiology, as well as of bodily sensations, body image, and physical potential.
- The **environmental** component consists of the sociocultural environment, relationships with others, and knowledge of the relationship between humans and nature.
- The **philosophical** component is the sense of life having meaning. A personal philosophy of life and death may or may not include a superior being, but it does take into account responsibility to the world and the ethics of behavior.

Together these components provide a model that can be used to promote the self-awareness and self-growth of nurses and the patients for whom they care.

Increasing Self-Awareness. No one ever completely knows the inner self, as shown in the Johari window (Fig. 2-2). Quadrant 1 is the open quadrant; it includes the behaviors, feelings, and thoughts known to the individual and others. Quadrant 2 is called the blind quadrant because it includes all the things that others know but the individual does not know. Quadrant 3 is the hidden quadrant; it includes the things about the self that only the individual knows. Quadrant 4 is the unknown quadrant, containing aspects of the self that are unknown to the individual and to others. Taken together, these quadrants represent the total self. The following three principles help explain how the self functions:

- A change in any one quadrant affects all other quadrants.
- The smaller quadrant 1, the poorer the communication.
- Interpersonal learning means that a change has taken place, so quadrant 1 is larger and one or more of the other quadrants is smaller.

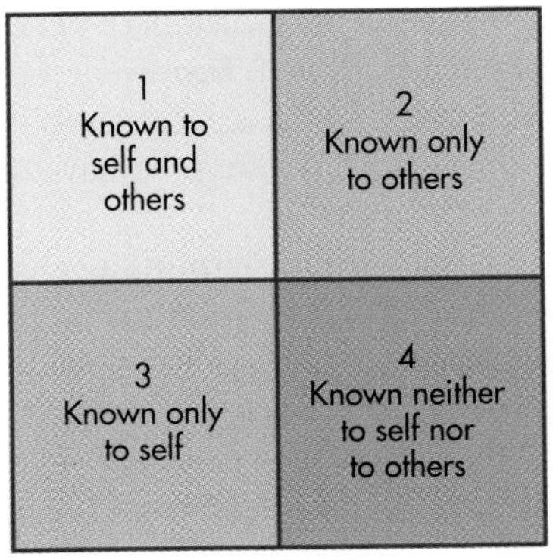

The goal of increasing self-awareness is to enlarge the area of quadrant 1 while reducing the size of the other three quadrants. To increase self-knowledge, it is necessary to **listen to the self.** This means the individual allows genuine emotions to be experienced; identifies and accepts personal needs; and moves the body in free, joyful, and spontaneous ways. It includes exploring personal thoughts, feelings, memories, and impulses.

The next step in the process is to reduce the size of quadrant 2 by **listening to and learning from others.** Knowledge of self is not possible alone. As we relate to others, we broaden our perceptions of self, but such learning requires active listening and openness to the feedback others provide.

The final step involves reducing the size of quadrant 3 by **self-disclosing,** or revealing to others important aspects of the self. Self-disclosure is both a sign of personality health and a means of achieving healthy personality.

Compare *A* and *B* of Fig. 2-3. *A* represents a person with little self-awareness whose behaviors and feelings are limited. *B*, however, shows an individual with great openness to the world. Much of this person's potential is being developed and realized. *B* represents an individual who has an increased capacity for experiences of all kinds: joy, hate, work, and love. This person also has few defenses and can interact more spontaneously and honestly with others. This configuration is a worthy goal for the nurse to pursue.

Draw your own Johari window. What changes would you like to make to any of the quadrants?

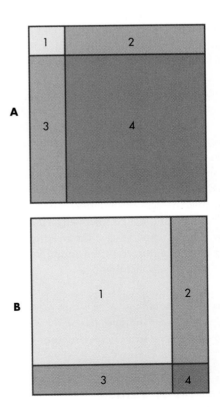

Fig. 2-3 Johari windows showing varying degrees of self-awareness.

Fig. 2-2 Johari window. Each quadrant, or windowpane, describes one aspect of the self.

The Nurse and Self-Growth. Nurses need time to explore and define the many parts of their personalities. If nursing does involve perceiving, feeling, and thinking, nursing students should have the time and opportunity to study their own experiences. Authenticity in relationships must be learned, and nurses must first experience openness and authenticity in relationships with instructors and supervisors. The student and instructor can participate in a relationship that accepts and respects their individual differences. Instructors can help students by facilitating students' self-awareness, increasing their level of functioning, stimulating more self-direction, and enabling students to cope more effectively with stressors.

Authenticity also involves being open to self-exploration of thoughts, needs, emotions, values, defenses, actions, communications, problems, and goals. Nursing students have many new experiences that provide opportunities for self-learning. Feelings related to these experiences should be focused on and discussed. Students might enter clinical settings with high ideals and unrealistic images. Perhaps they view nurses as all-knowing, all-caring "miracle workers." During initial encounters students may feel fearful, anxious, and inadequate, wondering how a nurse gains the necessary knowledge. Nursing students might devalue their abilities and feel like an imposition on patients. At another time, nurses may identify closely with patients and feel anger at the impersonal system and unresponsive personnel. The feelings involved in all of these situations should be identified, verbalized, and analyzed. Only then can nurses resolve them in a constructive manner.

A career in nursing is not easy if the nurse is still in adolescence. As a nurse, the student will be faced with many adult situations, such as disease, bizarre behavior, complex problems, and even death, when most of the student's friends are focusing on youth, enjoyment, and the future. This might alienate the nurse from some friends. Feelings of loneliness and sadness should be shared so that the nurse can work through personal needs.

Throughout the growing process the student needs the support and guidance of a noncritical but challenging instructor. Together they can analyze the student's behavior, and the student can assess personal strengths and limitations. Also, it is often helpful to share these experiences with a peer group. Students can empathize, critique, and support each other as they learn more about themselves.

Finally, objective self-examination is not easy or pleasant, particularly when findings conflict with self-ideals. However, like many painful experiences, discovering self-awareness presents a challenge: to accept self-limitations or to change the behaviors that support them.

> **?** *Think back over the courses you have taken in your nursing program. How much time and emphasis were placed on developing your self-awareness as a person and a nurse?*

Clarification of Values

Nurses should be able to answer the question, What is important to me? Awareness helps the nurse to be honest and to avoid the unethical use of patients to meet personal needs. Nurses should avoid the temptation to use patients for the pursuit of personal satisfaction or security. If nurses do not have sufficient personal fulfillment, they should realize it; their sources of dissatisfaction should then be clarified so that they do not interfere with the success of the nurse-patient relationship.

Value Systems. Values are concepts that are formed as a result of life experiences with family, friends, culture, education, work, and relaxation. The word value has positive connotations, because it denotes worth or significance. Yet values also imply negatives. If we value honesty, then it follows that we do not value dishonesty. People are likely to hold strong values related to religious beliefs, family ties, sexual preferences, other ethnic groups, and gender role beliefs.

One of the many challenges facing psychiatric nurses today is the need to provide care for patients from many different ethnocultural backgrounds. Because the goals of treatment are determined greatly by beliefs and values, establishing a therapeutic relationship with patients from different ethnocultural backgrounds requires particular skill and sensitivity (see Chapter 8).

Value systems provide the framework for many daily decisions and actions. By being aware of their value systems, nurses can identify situations in which value systems are in conflict. Clarification of values also provides some insurance against the tendency to project values onto other people. Many therapeutic relationships test the nurse's values. For example, a patient may describe a sexual behavior that the nurse finds unacceptable; a patient may talk about divorce, whereas the nurse may strongly believe that marriage contracts should not be broken; or a patient may be a "born-again" Christian, but the nurse may not believe in God or religion.

> **?** *Can a nurse empathize with and help a patient solve a problem while maintaining personal values that are different from the values of the patient?*

Value Clarification Process. Understanding personal values may be promoted by value clarification, which allows individuals to discover their values by assessing, exploring, and determining what those values are and what priority they hold in decision-making processes. Value clarification does not determine what the individual's values should be or what values should be followed. To prevent the imposition of values, value clarification focuses exclusively on the **process** of valuing, or on how people come to have the values they have.

Seven criteria are used to determine a value. These criteria should be considered in relation to a person's strongest value and tested against the person's own definition of a value. The seven criteria are broadly grouped into the three steps listed in Box 2-2.

The three criteria of **choosing** rely on the person's cognitive abilities, the two criteria of **prizing** emphasize the emotional or affective level, and the two criteria of **acting** have a behavioral focus.

Box **2-2**

Steps in the Value Clarification Process

CHOOSING	Freely From alternatives After thoughtful consideration of the consequences of each alternative
PRIZING	Cherishing, being happy with the choice Willing to affirm the choice publicly
ACTING	Doing something with the choice Repeatedly, in some pattern of life

A change takes place when certain contradictions are perceived in the person's value system. To eliminate the distress that follows such a realization, the person realigns values to coincide with the new view of self.

The Mature Valuing Process. The valuing process in the mature person is complex, and the choices are often perplexing and difficult. There is no guarantee that the choice made will prove to be self-actualizing. The valuing process in the mature person has the following characteristics (Kirschenbaum & Simon, 1973):

- It is fluid and flexible, based on the particular moment and the degree to which the moment is enhancing, enriching, and actualizing. Values are continually changing.
- The valuing experience is tied to a particular time and experience.
- Personal experience provides the value information. Although the person is open to all evidence obtained from other sources, outside evidence is not considered as important as subjective responses. The psychologically mature adult trusts and uses personal wisdom.
- In the valuing process the person is open to the immediacy of experience, trying to sense and clarify all its complex meanings. However, the immediate impact of the moment is colored by experiences from the past and conjecture about the future.

Exploration of Feelings

It is often assumed that helping others requires complete objectivity and detachment. This is definitely not true. Complete objectivity and detachment describe someone who is unresponsive, false, unapproachable, impersonal, and self-alienated—qualities that block the establishment of a therapeutic relationship. Rather, nurses should be open to, aware of, and in control of their feelings so that they can be used to help patients.

The feelings that nurses have serve an important purpose. They are barometers for feedback about themselves and their relationships with others. In helping others, nurses have many feelings: elation at seeing a patient improve, disappointment when a patient regresses, distress when a patient refuses help, anger when a patient is demanding or manipulative, and power when a patient expresses strong dependence on the nurse.

Nurses who are open to their feelings understand how they are responding to patients and how they appear to patients. The nurse's feelings are valuable clues to the patient's problems. For example, despite the patient's statement that "things are going real well," the nurse might perceive a strong sense of despair or anger. So too, nurses should be aware of the feelings they convey to the patient. Is the nurse's mood one of hopelessness or frustration? If nurses view feelings as barometers and feedback instruments, their effectiveness as helpers will improve.

Serving as Role Model

Formal helpers have a strong influence on those they help, and nurses function as role models for their patients. Research has shown the power of role models in molding socially adaptive, as well as maladaptive, behavior. Thus a nurse has an obligation to model adaptive and growth-producing behavior. If a nurse has a chaotic personal life, it will show in the nurse's work with patients, decreasing the effectiveness of care. The nurse's credibility as a helper also will be questioned. The nurse may object, saying that it is possible to separate one's personal life from one's professional life, but in caring for patients this is not possible because psychiatric nursing *is* the therapeutic use of self.

This is not to suggest that the nurse must conform totally to local community norms or must live a happy, fully contented life. What is suggested is that the effective nurse has a fulfilling and satisfying personal life that is not dominated by conflict, distress, or denial and that the nurse's approach to life conveys a sense of growing, hopefulness, and adapting.

 Who have been role models in your life, and what qualities did you most admire about them?

Altruism

It is important for nurses to have an answer to the question, Why do I want to help others? Obviously, an effective helper is interested in people and tends to help out of a deep love for humanity. It also is true that everyone seeks a certain amount of personal satisfaction and fulfillment from work. The goal is to maintain a balance between these two needs. Helping motives can become destructive tools in the hands of naive or zealous users.

Another danger lies in adopting an extreme view of altruism. Altruism is concern for the welfare of others. It does not mean that an altruistic person should not expect adequate compensation and recognition or must practice denial or self-sacrifice. Only if personal needs have been appropriately met can the nurse expect to be maximally therapeutic.

Finally, a sense of altruism also can apply to changing social conditions to meet human welfare needs. One goal of all helping professionals should be to create a people-serving and growth-facilitating society. Thus a legitimate and necessary role for the nurse is to work to change the larger structure and process of society in ways that will promote the individual's health and well-being.

Ethics and Responsibility

Personal beliefs about people and society can serve as conscious guidelines for action. The Code for Nurses reflects common values regarding nurse-patient relationships and responsibilities and serves as a frame of reference for all nurses in their judgments about patient welfare and social responsibility. For psychiatric nurses, decisions are a part of daily functioning. Responsible ethical choice involves accountability, risk, commitment, and justice.

Related to the nurse's sense of ethics is the need to assume responsibility for behavior. This involves knowing limitations and strengths and being accountable for them. As a member of a health care team, the nurse has ready access to the knowledge and expertise of other people; these resources should be used appropriately.

PHASES OF THE RELATIONSHIP

A vital characteristic of the nurse-patient relationship is the sharing of behaviors, thoughts, and feelings. As such, it is important to distinguish between social support and professional support (Hupcey & Morse, 1997). In social support, two people are part of a natural social network and the rela-

tionship is based on reciprocal trust and congruent expectations. In contrast, the relationship between a professional and a patient is based on clear role expectations. The support requested and ultimately provided should be within the domain of the nurse's role as a professional caregiver. It also is important to remember that the elements of a therapeutic nurse-patient relationship apply to all clinical settings. Thus nurses working in medical, surgical, obstetrical, oncological, and other specialty areas also need to understand and be able to use therapeutic nurse-patient relationship skills.

Four phases of the nurse-patient relationship have been identified: preinteraction phase; introductory, or orientation, phase; working phase; and termination phase. Each phase builds on the preceding one and is characterized by specific tasks.

Preinteraction Phase

Concerns of New Nurses. The preinteraction phase begins before the nurse's first contact with the patient. The nurse's initial task is one of self-exploration. This is no small task as the psychiatric nursing clinical experience can bring both stress and challenge to the student (see Citing the Evidence). In the first experience working with psychiatric patients, the nurse brings the misconceptions and prejudices of the general public, in addition to feelings and fears common to all novices (Box 2-3). An overriding one usually is anxiety or nervousness, which is common to new experiences of any kind. A related feeling is ambivalence or uncertainty; nurses may see the need for working with these patients but feel unclear about their ability.

The informal nature of psychiatric settings also may threaten the nurse's role identity. A common first reaction among students is a feeling of panic when they realize that they "can't tell the patients from the staff." It also is unsettling for many students to give up their uniforms, stethoscopes, and scissors. Doing so dramatically emphasizes that, in this nursing setting, the most important tools are the abil-

---

Citing the Evidence on

Psychiatric Nursing Clinical Experiences

BACKGROUND: Few studies have focused on the stress of clinical practice at the completion of a course. This research examined the stress and challenge of psychiatric nursing clinical experiences in 12 randomly selected associate and baccalaureate nursing programs at the end of the course.

RESULTS: Students in psychiatric courses experienced moderate stress. Students in all other clinical specialties reported more stress in their clinical practice than they did in psychiatric nursing courses. They rarely reported negative emotions in caring for psychiatric patients and described the psychiatric clinical experiences as stimulating and promoting the development of confidence in clinical practice. However the psychiatric clinical courses were identified as among the least challenging.

IMPLICATIONS: Clinical learning activities need to promote the development of knowledge, skills, and values essential for the care of psychiatric patients and at the same time be stimulating and challenging for students. Findings suggest the need for innovative clinical teaching strategies that challenge students and extend their thinking about psychiatric patients. This will be significant as students consider their choice of a clinical practice specialty upon graduation.

Oermann M, Sperling S: Stress and challenge of psychiatric nursing clinical experiences, *Arch Psych Nurs* 13:74, 1999.

Box 2-3

Common Concerns of Psychiatric Nursing Students

- Acutely self-conscious
- Afraid of being rejected by the patients
- Anxious because of the newness of the experience
- Concerned about personally overidentifying with psychiatric patients
- Doubtful of the effectiveness of skills or coping ability
- Fearful of physical danger or violence
- Insecure in therapeutic use of self
- Suspicious of psychiatric patients stereotyped as "different"
- Threatened in nursing role identity
- Uncertain about ability to make a unique contribution
- Uncomfortable about the lack of physical tasks and treatments
- Vulnerable to emotionally painful experiences
- Worried about hurting the patient psychologically

ity to communicate, empathize, and solve problems. Without a tangible physical illness to care for, new students are likely to feel acutely self-conscious and hesitant about introducing themselves to a patient and initiating a conversation.

Many nurses express feelings of inadequacy and fears of hurting or exploiting the patient. They worry about saying the wrong thing, which might drive the patient "over the brink." With their limited knowledge and experience, they doubt that they will be of any value. They wonder how they can help or whether they can really make a difference. Some nurses perceive the plight of psychiatric patients as hopeful; others perceive it as hopeless.

A common fear of nurses is related to the stereotype of psychiatric patients as violent. Because this is the picture portrayed by the media, many nurses are afraid of being physically hurt by a patient's outburst of aggressive behavior. Some nurses fear being psychologically hurt by a patient through rejection or silence. A final fear is related to nurses' questioning their own mental health status. Nurses may fear mental illness and worry that exposure to psychiatric patients might cause them to lose their own grasp on reality. Nurses who are working on their own crises of identity and intimacy may fear overidentifying with patients and using patients to meet their own needs.

The following clinical example contains many of the feelings and fears expressed by one nursing student in the preinteraction phase of self-analysis, as reported in the notes from her diary of her psychiatric rotation.

 CLINICAL EXAMPLE

When first told that I would have a clinical psychiatric nursing experience, I received this information with a blank mind. Mental overload, denial, repression, or whatever it was made me hear the words but put off dealing with it. Then, when given a chance to sort through my thoughts and feelings, I thought more about what this experience would entail. Having never been personally involved with any people who were psychiatrically ill before, I was unable to rely on past personal experiences. I did, however, have quite a "pseudo-knowledge base" from my novels, television, and movie encounters. Do places like the hospitals in *One Flew Over the Cuckoo's Nest* or *Frances* really exist? Was the portrayal of *Sybil* accurate? How could I possibly help someone who has so many problems, like the boy in *Ordinary People* or the young women in *Girl, Interrupted*? After all, I have problems myself. I'm afraid these thoughts have raised more questions in me than they have answered.

Three things scare me the most about this experience. First, I feel that the behavior of a psychiatric patient is quite unpredictable. Would they get violent or aggressive without any warning? Would this aggression be directed toward me? If so, would I be hurt? Did I provoke them, and was I wrong in my actions that caused this sudden shift?

The second, related to the first, is my feeling of inadequacy. I've been exposed to physically ill people and have learned how to respond to them. But, the psychiatrically ill are almost totally alien to me. How can I help? What if I do, or say, or infer something they could take offense to? Will I have the patience to persevere? I just don't know, and my not knowing makes me even more nervous.

My third fear is how seeing and being in contact with the psychiatrically ill will affect me. Although I know it's not contagious, the more exposure and knowledge I acquire in this area, the more I may begin to doubt my own stability and sanity. I mean, adolescence hasn't been easy for me, and I feel like I'm just now beginning to see things more clearly and feel better about myself. Will this experience stir up any past fears and doubts and, if so, how will I handle it? I am beginning to realize that there is a fine line between health and illness and that the psychiatric patients we'll meet have been unable to gather enough resources from within to cope with their problems. Help, reassurance, and understanding are their needs. I'm hoping I can help them . . . but I'm just not sure.

 What feelings, fears, and fantasies do you have about working with psychiatric patients?

Self-Assessment. Experienced nurses benefit by asking themselves the following questions:

- Do I label patients with the stereotype of a group?
- Is my need to be liked so great that I become angry or hurt when a patient is rude, hostile, or uncooperative?
- Am I afraid of the responsibility I must assume for the relationship, and do I therefore limit my independent functions?
- Do I cover feelings of inferiority with a front of superiority?
- Do I require sympathy, warmth, and protection so much that I become too sympathetic or too protective toward patients?
- Do I fear closeness so much that I am indifferent, rejecting, or cold?
- Do I need to feel important and keep patients dependent on me?

The self-analysis of the preinteraction phase is a necessary task. To be effective, nurses should have a reasonably stable self-concept and an adequate amount of self-esteem. They should engage in constructive relationships with others and face reality to help patients do likewise. If they are aware of and in control of what they convey to their patients verbally and nonverbally, nurses can function as role models. To do this, however, some nurses abandon their personal strengths and assume a facade of "professionalism" that alienates their authentic self. This facade immobilizes them and acts as a barrier to establishing mutuality with patients.

Other tasks of this phase include gathering data about the patient if information is available and planning for the first interaction with the patient. The nursing assessment is begun, but most of the work related to it is done with the patient in the second phase of the relationship. Finally, nurses review general goals of a therapeutic relationship and consider what they have to offer patients.

Introductory, or Orientation, Phase

It is during the introductory phase that the nurse and patient first meet. One of the nurse's primary concerns is to find out

Table **2-1**

Analysis of Why Patients Seek Psychiatric Help		
Reasons for Patients' Seeking Psychiatric Care	Appropriate Nursing Approach	Sample Response
ENVIRONMENTAL CHANGE FROM HOME TO TREATMENT SETTING		
They desire protection, comfort, rest, and freedom from demands of their home and work environments.	Emphasize the ability of the environment to provide protection and comfort while the healing process of the mind occurs.	"Tell me what it was at home/on the job that made you feel so overwhelmed."
NURTURANCE		
They wish for someone to care for them, cure their illnesses, and make them feel better.	Acknowledge their nurturance needs and assure them that help and caring are available.	"I'm here to help you feel better."
CONTROL		
They are aware of their destructive impulses to themselves or others but lack internal control.	Offer sources of internal control such as medication, if prescribed; reinforce external controls available through the staff.	"We're not going to let you hurt yourself. Tell us when these thoughts come to mind, and someone will stay with you."
PSYCHIATRIC SYMPTOMS		
They describe symptoms of depression, nervousness, or crying spells and actively want to help themselves.	Ask for clarification of symptom and strive to understand life experiences of patient.	"I can see that you're nervous and upset. Can you tell me about how things are at home/on the job so I can better understand?"
PROBLEM SOLVING		
They identify a specific problem or area of conflict and express desire to reason it out and change.	Help patient look at problem objectively; use problem-solving process.	"How has drinking affected your life?"
ADVISED TO SEEK HELP		
Family member, friend, or health professional has convinced them to get treatment. They may feel angry, ambivalent, or indifferent.	Confirm facts surrounding seeking of help and set appropriate limits.	"I see that you're angry about being here. I hope that after we talk you might feel differently."

Modified from Burgess A, Burns J: Why patients seek care, *Am J Nurs* 73:314, 1973.

Box **2-4**

Elements of a Nurse-Patient Contract

- Names of individuals
- Roles of nurse and patient
- Responsibilities of nurse and patient
- Expectations of nurse and patient
- Purpose of the relationship
- Meeting location and time
- Conditions for termination
- Confidentiality

why the patient sought help and whether it was voluntary (Table 2-1). The reason for seeking help forms the basis of the nursing assessment and helps the nurse to focus on the patient's problem and to determine patient motivation.

Formulating a Contract. The tasks in this phase of the relationship are to establish a climate of trust, understanding, acceptance, and open communication and formulate a contract with the patient. Box 2-4 lists the elements of a nurse-patient contract. The contract begins with the introduction of the nurse and patient, exchange of names, and explanation of roles. An explanation of roles includes the responsibilities and expectations of the patient and nurse, with a description of what the nurse can and cannot do. This is followed by a discussion of the purpose of the relationship, in which the nurse emphasizes that the focus of it will be the patient and the patient's life experiences and areas of conflict. Because establishing the contract is a mutual process, it is a good opportunity to clarify misperceptions held by either the nurse or patient.

With the "who" and the "why" determined, the "where, when, and how long" are discussed. Where will they meet? How often and how long will the meetings be? The conditions for termination should be reviewed and may include a specified length of time, attainment of mutual goals, or the discharge of the patient from the treatment setting. The issue of confidentiality is an important one to discuss with the patient at this time. Confidentiality involves the disclosure of

Box 2-5

Reasons Patients Have Difficulty Seeking Help

- It may be difficult to see or admit one's difficulties, first to oneself and then to another.
- It is not easy to trust or be open with strangers.
- Sometimes problems seem too large, too overwhelming, or too unique to share them easily.
- Sharing personal problems with another person can threaten one's sense of independence, autonomy, and self-esteem.
- Solving a problem involves thinking about some things that may be unpleasant, viewing life realistically, deciding on a plan of action, and then, most important, carrying out whatever it takes to bring about a change. These activities place great demands on the patient's energy and commitment.

certain information only to another specifically authorized person (see Chapter 10). This means that information about the patient will be shared only with people who are directly involved in the patient's care in the form of verbal reports and written notes. This is important in providing for the continuity and comprehensiveness of patient care and should be clearly explained to the patient.

Establishing a contract is a mutual process in which the patient participates as fully as possible. In some cases, such as with the psychotic or severely withdrawn patient, the patient may be unable to fully participate, and the nurse must take the initiative in establishing the contract. As the patient's contact with reality increases, the nurse should review the elements of the contract when appropriate and strive to attain mutuality.

Exploring Feelings. Both the nurse and patient may experience some degree of discomfort and nervousness in the introductory phase. Reasons why patients may have difficulty receiving help are listed in Box 2-5. The nurse may be well aware of personal anxieties and fears, but the patient's difficulty in receiving help may be overlooked.

Other tasks of the nurse in the orientation phase of the relationship include the following:

- To explore the patient's perceptions, thoughts, feelings, and actions
- To identify pertinent patient problems
- To define mutual, specific goals with the patient

Patients also may display manipulative or testing behavior during this phase as they explore the nurse's consistency and intent. They may show temporary regressions as reactions to a large amount of self-disclosure in a previous meeting or to the anxiety created by a particular topic.

Finally, nurses need to be flexible in anticipating the length of time required for the orientation phase, particularly for patients who have a serious and persistent mental illness. Nurses might expect that more time will be required for patients who have had many or lengthy hospitalizations in the past (Forchuk, 1995). Also, staff changes affect the patient's ability to progress in the therapeutic relationship and should be taken into account when planning nursing care.

Talk with a friend or family member who has sought counseling. Why did they do so? Did anything make them uncomfortable about asking for help? What did the clinician do to put them at ease?

Working Phase

Most of the therapeutic work is carried out during the working phase. The nurse and the patient explore stressors and promote the **development of insight** in the patient by linking perceptions, thoughts, feelings, and actions. These insights should be translated into action and a change in behavior. They can then be integrated into the individual's life experiences. The nurse helps the patient to master anxieties, increase independence and self-responsibility, and develop constructive coping mechanisms. Actual **behavioral change** is the focus of this phase.

Patients often display resistance behaviors during this phase because it involves the greater part of the problem-solving process. As the relationship develops, the patient begins to feel close to the nurse and responds by clinging to defensive structures and resisting the nurse's attempts to move forward. An impasse or plateau in the relationship results. Because overcoming resistance behaviors is crucial to the progress of the therapeutic relationship, these behaviors are discussed in greater detail later in this chapter.

Termination Phase

Termination is one of the most difficult but most important phases of the therapeutic nurse-patient relationship. During the termination phase, learning is maximized for both the patient and the nurse. It is a time to exchange feelings and memories and to evaluate mutually the patient's progress and goal attainment. Levels of trust and intimacy are heightened, reflecting the quality of the relationship and the sense of loss experienced by both nurse and patient. Box 2-6 lists criteria that can be used to determine whether the patient is ready to terminate.

Although agreement between the patient and the nurse is desirable in deciding when to terminate, this is not always possible. Nonetheless, the nurse's tasks during this phase revolve around establishing the reality of the separation. Together the nurse and the patient review the progress made in treatment and the attainment of specified goals. Feelings of rejection, loss, sadness, and anger are expressed and explored. It may be helpful to prepare the patient for termination by decreasing the number of visits, incorporating others into the meetings, or changing the location of the meetings. The reasons behind a change should be clarified so that the patient does not interpret it as rejection by the nurse. It also may be appropriate to make referrals at this time for continued care or treatment.

Successful termination requires that the patient work through feelings related to separation from emotionally significant people. The nurse can help by allowing the patient to experience and feel the effects of the anticipated loss, to express the feelings generated by the impending

Box **2-6**

Criteria for Determining Patient Readiness for Termination

- The patient experiences relief from the presenting problem.
- The patient's functioning has improved.
- The patient has increased self-esteem and a stronger sense of identity.
- The patient uses more adaptive coping responses.
- The patient has achieved the planned treatment outcomes.
- An impasse has been reached in the nurse-patient relationship that cannot be resolved.

Table **2-2**

Nurse's Tasks in Each Phase of the Relationship Process

Phase	Task
Preinteraction	Explore own feelings, fantasies, and fears
	Analyze own professional strengths and limitations
	Gather data about patient when possible
	Plan for first meeting with patient
Introductory, or orientation	Determine why patient sought help
	Establish trust, acceptance, and open communication
	Mutually formulate a contract
	Explore patient's thoughts, feelings, and actions
	Identify patient's problems
	Define goals with patient
Working	Explore relevant stressors
	Promote patient's development of insight and use of constructive coping mechanisms
	Overcome resistance behaviors
Termination	Establish reality of separation
	Review progress of therapy and attainment of goals
	Mutually explore feelings of rejection, loss, sadness, and anger and related behaviors

separation, and to relate those feelings to former symbolic or real losses.

Reactions to Termination. Patients react to termination in different ways. They may deny the separation or deny the significance of the relationship, perhaps causing the inexperienced nurse to feel rejected by the patient. Patients may express anger and hostility, either overtly and verbally or covertly through lateness, missed meetings, or superficial talk. These patients may view the termination as personal rejection, which reinforces their negative self-concept. Patients who feel rejected by the nurse may terminate prematurely by rejecting the nurse before the nurse rejects them. It also is common to see the patient regress to an earlier behavior pattern, hoping to convince the nurse not to terminate because of the need for further help.

The nurse should be aware of these possible reactions and discuss them with the patient if they occur. For some patients, termination is a critical therapeutic experience because many of their past relationships were terminated in a negative way that left them with unresolved feelings of abandonment, rejection, hurt, and anger.

All these patient reactions have a similar goal: to cope with the anxiety about the separation and to delay the termination process. The patient's response will be significantly affected by the nurse's ability to remain open, sensitive, empathic, and responsive to the patient's changing needs. Helping the patient to work and grow through the termination process is an essential goal of each relationship. It is important that the nurse does not deny the reality of it or allow the patient to repeatedly delay the process. Particularly in this phase of the relationship, as in the orientation phase, the patient will be testing the nurse's judgment, and the issues of trust and acceptance will again predominate.

During the course of the relationship and with the attainment of nursing goals, the nurse and the patient come to realize a growing sense of equality. The impending termination therefore can be as difficult for the nurse as for the patient. Nurses who can begin reviewing their thoughts, feelings, and experiences will be more aware of personal motivation and more responsive to patients' needs.

Learning to bear the sorrow of the loss while working positive aspects of the relationship into one's life is the goal of termination for both the nurse and the patient. At the conclusion of the relationship students can be assisted in guided reflection to gain insight into their psychiatric nursing clinical experience and to better appreciate the roles of psychiatric nurses (McAllister, 1995). The major tasks of the nurse during each phase of the nurse-patient relationship are summarized in Table 2-2.

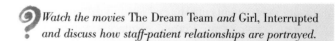 *Watch the movies* The Dream Team *and* Girl, Interrupted *and discuss how staff-patient relationships are portrayed.*

FACILITATIVE COMMUNICATION

Communication can either facilitate the development of a therapeutic relationship or serve as a barrier to it. Everyone communicates constantly from birth until death. All behavior is communication, and all communication affects behavior. This reciprocity is central to the communication process. Communication is critical to nursing practice because of the following:

- Communication is the vehicle for establishing a therapeutic relationship.
- Communication is the means by which people influence the behavior of another, leading to the successful outcome of nursing intervention.
- Communication is the relationship itself because without it, a therapeutic nurse-patient relationship is impossible.

Verbal Communication

Communication takes place on two levels: verbal and nonverbal. Verbal communication occurs through words, spoken or written. Taken alone, verbal communication can convey factual information accurately and efficiently. It is a less-effective means of communicating feelings or nuances of meaning, and it represents only a small part of total human communication.

Another limitation of verbal communication is that words can change meaning with different cultural groups or subgroups because words have both denotative and connotative meanings. The **denotative** meaning of a word is its actual or concrete meaning. For example, the denotative meaning of the word "bread" is "a food made of a flour or grain dough that is kneaded, shaped, allowed to rise, and baked." The **connotative** meaning of a word, in contrast, is its implied or suggested meaning. Thus the word *bread* can conjure up many different connotative or personalized meanings. Depending on a person's experiences, preferences, and present frame of reference, he or she may think of French bread, rye bread, a sesame seed roll, or perhaps pita bread. When used as slang, "give me some bread" may be understood to mean "give me some money." Thus the characteristics of the speaker and the context in which the phrase is used influence the specific meaning of verbal language.

When communicating verbally, many people assume that they are "on the same wavelength" as the listener. But because words are only symbols, they seldom mean precisely the same thing to two people. And if the word represents an abstract idea such as "depressed" or "hurt," the chance of misunderstanding or misinterpretation may be great. In addition, many feeling states or personal thoughts cannot be put into words easily. Nurses should try to overcome these problems by checking their interpretation and incorporating information from the nonverbal level as well.

Finally, today more than ever before, nurses need to be prepared to communicate effectively with people from a variety of ethnocultural backgrounds (Oquendo, 1996). For example, psychiatric patients may be evaluated in their second language, yet competence in a second language varies depending on the individual and the stage of illness. In addition, there are cultural nuances in language that are not often conveyed in translation, even when the patient uses similar words in the second language. Patients also may use a second language as a form of resistance to avoid intense feelings or conflicting thoughts, and events that may have occurred before a person learned English may not be easily communicated.

The effective psychiatric nurse uses verbal communication sensitively to promote mutual respect based on understanding and acceptance of cultural differences. The nurse also may communicate respect for the patient's dialect by adapting to the patient's linguistic style by using fewer words, more gestures, or more expressive facial behaviors.

> *Think of someone you know whose cultural background is different from your own. How does this difference influence your verbal and nonverbal communication?*

Nonverbal Communication

Nonverbal communication includes everything that does not involve the spoken or written word, including all of the five senses. It has been estimated that about 7% of meaning is transmitted by words, 38% is transmitted by paralinguistic cues such as voice, and 55% is transmitted by body cues. Nonverbal communication is often unconsciously motivated and may more accurately indicate a person's meaning than the words being spoken. People tend to say what they think the receiver wants to hear, whereas less acceptable or more honest messages may be communicated by the nonverbal route.

Types of Nonverbal Behaviors. There are various types of nonverbal behaviors. Each of these is greatly influenced by sociocultural background. Following are brief descriptions of five categories of nonverbal communication.

Vocal cues, or paralinguistic cues, include all the nonverbal qualities of speech. Some examples include pitch; tone of voice; quality of voice; loudness or intensity; rate and rhythm of talking; and unrelated nonverbal sounds such as laughing, groaning, nervous coughing, and sounds of hesitation ("um," "uh"). These are particularly vital cues of emotion and can be powerful conveyors of information.

Action cues are body movements, sometimes referred to as **kinetics**. They include automatic reflexes, posture, facial expression, gestures, mannerisms, and actions of any kind. Facial movements and posture can be particularly significant in interpreting the speaker's mood.

Object cues are the speaker's intentional and nonintentional use of all objects. Dress, furnishings, and possessions all communicate something to the observer about the speaker's sense of self. These cues often are consciously selected by the individual, however, and therefore may be chosen to convey a certain look or message. Thus they can be less accurate than other types of nonverbal communication.

Space provides another clue to the nature of the relationship between two people. It must be examined based on sociocultural norms and customs. The following four zones of space are evident interpersonally in North America:

- Intimate space: up to 18 inches. This allows for maximum interpersonal sensory stimulation.
- Personal space: 18 inches to 4 feet. This is used for close relationships and touching distance. Visual sensation is improved over the intimate range.
- Social-consultative space: 9 to 12 feet. This is less personal and less dependent. Speech must be louder.
- Public space: 12 feet and more. This is used in speech giving and other public occasions.

Observation of seating arrangements and use of space by patients can yield valuable information to the nurse, with implications for both the nurse's assessment of the patient and the way the nursing intervention should be implemented.

Touch involves both personal space and action. It is possibly the most personal of the nonverbal messages (Smith et al, 1997). A person's response to it is influenced by setting, cultural background, type of relationship, gender of communicators, ages, and expectations. Touch can express a desire to connect with another person as a way of meeting them or relating to them. It can be a way of expressing or conveying something to another, such as concern, empathy, or caring. Touch also can be used as a way of sensing, perceiving, or allowing someone else to leave an imprint on another person. Finally, there is the concept of therapeutic touch, or the nurse's laying hands on or close to the body of an ill person for the purpose of helping or healing. Touch continues to be the imprimatur of nursing, and the therapeutic, comforting effects of touch are often overlooked. Thus touch is a universal and basic aspect of all nurse-patient relationships. It is often described as the first and most fundamental means of communication.

Interpreting Nonverbal Behavior. All types of nonverbal messages are important, but interpreting them correctly can present problems for the nurse. It is impossible to examine nonverbal messages out of context, and sometimes the individual's body reveals a number of different and perhaps conflicting feelings at the same time.

Sociocultural background also is a major influence on the meaning of nonverbal behavior. In the United States, with its diverse ethnic communities, messages between people of different upbringing can easily be misinterpreted. For instance, Arab-Americans tend to stand closer together when speaking, and Asian-Americans tend to touch more; touching in the United States is often minimized because of perceived sexual overtones or because of Puritan heritage. Because the meaning attached to nonverbal behavior is so subjective, it is essential that the nurse check its meaning.

Nurses should respond to the variety of nonverbal behaviors displayed by the patient, particularly voice inflections, body movements, gestures, facial expression, posture, and physical energy levels. Incongruent behavior and contradictory messages are especially significant. The nurse should refer to the specific behavior observed and attempt to confirm its meaning and significance with the patient. The nurse may use the following three kinds of responses to the patient:

1. Questions or statements intended to increase the patient's awareness
2. Content reflections
3. Statements reflecting the nurse's responsiveness

These possible responses are illustrated in the following interaction.

 THERAPEUTIC DIALOGUE

PATIENT *(Shifting nervously in his chair, eyes scanning the room and avoiding the nurse)* What . . . what do you want to talk about today?

NURSE RESPONSE #1 *I sense that you are uncomfortable talking to me. Could you describe to me how you are feeling?*

NURSE RESPONSE #2 *You're not sure what we should be talking about, and you want me to start us off?*

NURSE RESPONSE #3 *You look very nervous, and I can feel those same feelings in me as I sit here with you.*

The nurse's first possible response is a reflection and attempt to validate the patient's feelings. The purpose is to communicate to the patient the nurse's awareness of his feelings, to show acceptance of those feelings, and to request that he focus on them and elaborate on them. The nurse's second possible response deals with the content of the patient's message. The nurse is clarifying what the patient is trying to say. The third possible response shares both the nurse's perception of her patient's feelings and the personal disclosure that she has some of those same feelings. This type of response may help the patient feel that the nurse accepts and understands him.

Implications for Nursing Care. Besides responding to patients' nonverbal behavior, nurses should incorporate aspects of it into patient care. For example, patients who resist closeness will be disturbed by entry into their intimate space. The nurse can assess the patient's level of spatial tolerance by observing the distance the patient maintains with other people. The nurse also can be alert to the patient's response during their interaction. If the nurse sits next to the patient on the sofa, does the patient get up and move to a chair? If the nurse moves closer to the patient does the patient move away to re-establish the original space? Sometimes increasing the space between the nurse and an anxious patient can reduce the anxiety enough to allow the interaction to continue. A decrease in the distance the patient chooses to maintain from others may indicate a decrease in interpersonal anxiety.

Height may communicate dominance and submission. Communication is made easier when both participants are at similar levels. Orientation of the participants' body positions also is significant. Face-to-face confrontation is more threatening than oblique (sideways) body positions. The physical setting also has spatial meaning. Control issues are minimized when communication takes place in a neutral area that belongs to neither participant. However, people quickly identify their own turf, even in unfamiliar settings, and then begin to exert ownership rights over this area. A common example of this can be observed in most classroom settings. At the beginning of the semester, people sit randomly, but the arrangement usually solidifies after a couple of classes. Students then feel vaguely annoyed if they arrive in class to find another person in "their seat." They are experiencing an invasion of personal space.

Touch also should be used carefully. Patients who are sensitive to issues of closeness may experience a casual touch as an invasion or an invitation to intimacy, which may be even more frightening. Physical contact with a person of the same gender may be experienced by the patient as a homosexual advance and may precipitate a panic reaction. If procedures requiring physical contact must be carried out, careful explanations should be given both before and during the procedure. In addition, the nurse should always be aware of the potential for touch to be interpreted in a sexual way, thus creating problems related to the sexual conduct of the nurse within the nurse-patient relationship.

Despite these issues, touch is a significant part of psychiatric nursing practice. Reasons why nurses use touch include the following:

- Establishing contact with the patient
- Enhancing communication
- Communicating caring, interest, and recognition
- Providing reassurance and comfort

Nurses also must be aware of not only patients' nonverbal cues but also of their own. The nurse's nonverbal cues can communicate interest, respect, and genuineness or disinterest, lack of respect, and an impersonal facade. Affiliative nonverbal behaviors include smiles, positive head nods, gestures, eye contact, and a forward body lean.

> *Follow the treatment team making patient rounds and observe body positions. Are staff and patients at eye level? What personal space is maintained? Is touch used at all?*

The Communication Process

There are three elements of the communication process: perception, evaluation, and transmission. Perception occurs by activating the sensory end organs of the receiver. The impulse is then transmitted to the brain. Human beings mostly rely on visual and auditory stimuli for communications.

When the sensory impulse reaches the brain, evaluation takes place. Personal experience allows for the evaluation of the new experience. If the person encounters a new experience for which there is no frame of reference, confusion results. Evaluation results in two responses: a cognitive response related to the informational aspect of the message and an affective response related to the relationship aspect of the message. Most messages stimulate both types of responses.

When the evaluation of the message is complete, transmission takes place. This is perceived by the sender as feedback, thereby influencing the continued course of the communication cycle. It is impossible not to transmit some kind of feedback. Even lack of any visible response is feedback to the sender that the message did not get through, was considered unimportant, or was an undesirable interruption. Feedback stimulates perception, evaluation, and transmission by the original sender. The cycle continues until the participants agree to end it or one participant physically leaves the setting.

Theoretical models of the communication process show visual relationships more clearly and can aid in finding and correcting communication breakdowns or problems. Two models, the structural and transactional analysis models, are presented because each gives a valuable but different perspective on the communication process.

Structural Model. The structural model has five functional components in communication: the sender, the message, the receiver, the feedback, and the context (Fig. 2-4). The sender is the originator of the message. The message is the information that is transmitted from the sender to the receiver. The receiver is the perceiver of the message. The verbal or behavioral response of the receiver is feedback to the sender. The fifth structural element of communication is the context. This is the setting in which the communication takes place. Knowledge of context is necessary to understand the meaning of the communication. For example, the phrase "I don't understand what you mean" may have different meanings in the context of a classroom or a courtroom. Context involves more than the physical setting for communication, however. It also includes the psychosocial setting, which includes the relationship between the sender and the receiver, their past experiences with each other, their past experiences with similar situations, and cultural values and norms. Consider again the meaning of "I don't understand what you mean" in the following contexts: two college students discussing a philosophy assignment, a wife responding to her husband's accusation of infidelity, and a Japanese tourist asking directions in San Francisco. Although the content of the message is the same, its meaning is different, depending on the context in which the communication takes place.

In evaluating communication from the perspective of the structural model, specific problems can be identified (Table 2-3). If the sender is communicating the same message on both the verbal and nonverbal levels, then the communication is congruent. However, if the levels are not in agreement, the communication is incongruent, which can be problematic.

THERAPEUTIC DIALOGUE

Congruent Communication

VERBAL LEVEL *I'm pleased to see you.*
NONVERBAL LEVEL *Warm tone of voice, continuous eye contact, smile.*

Incongruent Communication

VERBAL LEVEL *I'm pleased to see you.*
NONVERBAL LEVEL *Cold and distant tone of voice, little eye contact, neutral facial expression.*

Incongruent, or double-level, messages produce a dilemma for the listener, who does not know to which level to respond, the verbal or nonverbal. Because both levels cannot be responded to, the listener is likely to feel frustrated, angry, or confused. Obviously, both patients and nurses can display

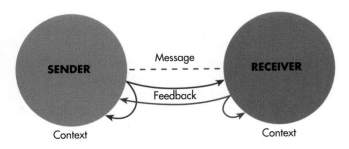

Fig. 2-4 Components of communication.

Table **2-3**

Problems with the Structural Elements of the Communication Process		
Structural Element	Communication Problem	Definition
Sender	Incongruent communication	Lack of agreement between the verbal and nonverbal levels of communication
	Inflexible communication	Exaggerated control or permissiveness by the sender
Message	Ineffective messages	Messages that are not goal directed or purposeful
	Inappropriate messages	Messages not relevant to the progress of the relationship
	Inadequate messages	Messages that lack a sufficient amount of information
	Inefficient messages	Messages that lack clarity, simplicity, and directness
Receiver	Errors of perception	Various forms of listening problems
	Errors of evaluation	Misinterpretation due to personal beliefs and values
Feedback	Misinformation	Communication of incorrect information
	Lack of validation	Failure to clarify and ratify understanding of the message
Context	Constraints of physical setting	Noise, temperature, or various distractions
	Constraints of psychosocial setting	Impaired previous relationship between the communicators

incongruent communication if they are not aware of their internal feeling states and the nature of their communication.

Another problem initiated by the sender is inflexible communication that is either too rigid or too permissive. A rigid approach by the nurse does not allow for spontaneous expression by the patient, nor does it allow the patient to contribute to the flow or direction of the interaction. Exaggerated permissiveness, on the other hand, refers to the lack of a direction and mutuality in the interaction established by the nurse. The patient may interpret the nurse's behavior as incompetence or lack of interest.

The message of the communication process also can pose problems. Messages can be ineffective, inappropriate, inadequate, or inefficient. Ineffective messages serve at least to distract and at most to prevent the objectives of the nurse-patient relationship from being met. Inappropriate messages are not relevant to the progress of the relationship. They may include failures in timing, stereotyping the receiver, or overlooking important information. Inadequate messages lack sufficient information. In this case, senders assume that receivers know more than they actually do. Inefficient messages lack clarity, simplicity, and directness. Using more energy than is necessary, these messages confuse or complicate the information.

The third element, the receiver, may experience errors of perception. The receiver may miss nonverbal cues, respond only to content and ignore messages of affect, be selectively inattentive to the speaker's message because of physical or psychological discomfort, be preoccupied with other thoughts, or have a physiological hearing impairment. These errors are problems of listening. The receiver also may have problems in evaluating the message. The meaning of the message may be misinterpreted because the receiver views it in terms of the receiver's value system rather than that of the speaker.

Errors in the feedback element include all of those that apply to the message. Feedback also can convey to the sender incorrect information about the message. Another serious error exists when the receiver fails to use feedback to validate understanding of the message. Although feedback is the last step, it has the potential for correcting previous errors and clarifying the nature of the communication.

The fifth element, context, also can contribute to communication problems. The setting may be physically noisy, cold, or distracting to one or both parties. The psychosocial context, or past relationship between the communicators, may be one of mistrust or harbored resentment. This analysis shows the complexity of the communication process. It may seem surprising that successful communication can occur, given all of these vulnerable areas. However, it does occur among people who understand the process and use appropriate techniques.

Transactional Analysis Model. Transactional analysis (TA) is the study of the communication or transactions that take place between people; it uncovers the sometimes unconscious and destructive ways ("games") in which people relate to each other. This approach to personality was developed by Berne (1964), a psychiatrist who made transactional analysis a popular theory through his classic book, *Games People Play: The Psychology of Human Relationships*. It is a method of therapy as well as a model of communication.

The cornerstone of this theory is that each person's personality is made up of three distinct components called ego states. An ego state is a consistent pattern of feeling, experiencing, and behaving. The three ego states that make up personality are the parent ego state, adult ego state, and child ego state. It is as though three people reside in each person; the "parent" incorporates all the attitudes and behaviors the individual was taught (directly or indirectly) by parents; the "child" contains all the feelings the individual had as a child; and the "adult" deals with reality in a logical, rational, computerlike manner.

The parent and child ego states are made up of the feelings, attitudes, and behaviors that are remnants of the past but can be re-experienced under certain conditions. The parent ego state consists of all the nurturing, critical, and prejudicial attitudes, behaviors, and experiences learned from other people, especially parents and teachers. The adult ego state is the reality-oriented part of the personality. It gathers and processes information about the world and is objective, emotionless, and intelligent in its approach to problem solving. The child ego state is the feeling part of the

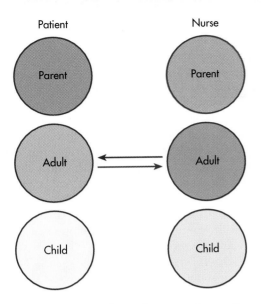

Fig. 2-5   Diagram of complementary transaction.

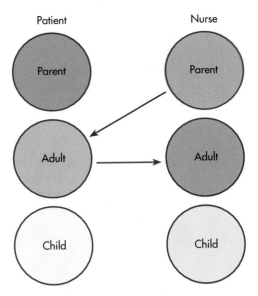

Fig. 2-6   Diagram of a crossed transaction.

personality. In it resides feelings of happiness, joy, sadness, depression, and anxiety.

Berne's model of communication makes it possible to diagram transactions using these ego states. A transaction or communication between two people can be complementary, crossed, or ulterior. In a complementary transaction (Fig. 2-5), the arrows in the ego state diagram are parallel, and the communication flows smoothly.

 THERAPEUTIC DIALOGUE

Complementary Transaction

PATIENT   *I know that when I get mad at my boss, I take it out on my wife and kids.*

NURSE   *Are you ready to think about some other ways you can handle your anger?*

If the arrows in the ego state diagram cross, however, communication breaks down (Fig. 2-6).

 THERAPEUTIC DIALOGUE

Crossed Transaction

PATIENT   *I know that when I get mad at my boss, I take it out on my wife and kids.*

NURSE   *Men always think that's OK, but the women have to suffer for it.*

The third type of transaction is ulterior transaction (Fig. 2-7). It takes place on two levels: the social, or overt, level and the psychological, or covert, level. These transactions tend to be destructive because the communicators conceal their true motivations. One of the best known examples of this is the "Why Don't You . . . Yes But" game. This game involves one person asking for a solution to a problem; how-

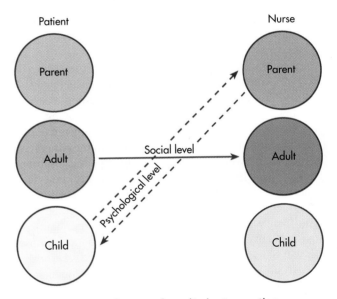

Fig. 2-7   Diagram of an ulterior transaction.

ever, every suggested solution is negated, until the helper is silenced. On the surface, the interaction is two adults problem solving; in reality, one person is using the child ego state to show what a bad parent the other person is.

 THERAPEUTIC DIALOGUE

Ulterior Transaction

PATIENT   *I know that when I get mad at my boss, I take it out on my wife and kids, but I don't know what else to do.*

NURSE   *Do you think you could let your boss know how you're feeling?*

PATIENT   *He'll fire me for sure.*

NURSE   *Perhaps you could talk it over with a co-worker.*

PATIENT   *I don't have time to chat on the job like that. Besides, no one cares about someone else's beefs.*

NURSE   *Sometimes physical exercise helps people get rid of their anger. Have you ever tried it?*

PATIENT   *Sure. I work out a lot, but it doesn't help.*

NURSE   *Perhaps you can explain all this to your family.*

PATIENT   *My wife's tired of "all my talk" as she puts it. She says she wants some action.*

The transactional analysis model of communication provides a framework for the nurse to use in exploring the patient's recurrent behaviors, identifying patterns, thinking about causes, and planning alternative ways to respond. Thus nonproductive communication patterns can be stopped and new, healthier ones learned.

> *Using the transactional analysis model, diagram a recent conversation you have had with a friend, your instructor, and a patient.*

Therapeutic Communication Techniques

The following are the two requirements for effective communication:

1. All communication must be aimed at preserving the self-respect of both the helper and the helpee
2. The communication of understanding should precede any suggestions of information or advice giving

The collection of data and the planning, implementation, and evaluation activities are carried out **with** the patient, not **for** the patient, when the nurse uses therapeutic communication skills. Although simple on the surface, these techniques are difficult and require practice. Because they are techniques, they are only as effective as the person using them. If they are used appropriately, they can enhance the nurse's effectiveness. If they are used as automatic responses, they will block the formation of a therapeutic relationship, negate both the nurse's and the patient's individuality, and divest them of their dignity.

To ensure that the nurse is using these skills effectively, the nurse needs to record interactions with the patient in some way and then analyze them. The nurse also should seek feedback from others. The nurse can benefit from maintaining a diary of thoughts, feelings, and impressions in relation to clinical work. This can prove valuable in working through difficult aspects of termination or counter-transference reactions.

The advantages and disadvantages of the various methods of recording nurse-patient interactions must be considered, along with the nurse's and patient's preferences, before a particular method is chosen. Some form of recording that is as objective and comprehensive as possible is necessary. Only by analyzing the interaction can the nurse evaluate the degree of success in using therapeutic communication techniques (Sundeen et al, 1998). Some of the more helpful techniques are now described.

Listening.   Listening is essential if the nurse is to reach any understanding of the patient. The only person who can tell the nurse about the patient's feelings, thoughts, and perception of the self is the patient. Therefore the first rule of a therapeutic relationship is to listen to the patient. It is the foundation on which all other therapeutic skills are built (Nichols, 1995).

Inexperienced nurses often find it difficult not to talk. This may be caused by their anxiety, the need to prove themselves, or their usual way of social interaction. It is helpful to remember that the patient should be talking more than the nurse during the interaction; the task of the nurse is to listen.

Real listening is difficult. It is an active, not a passive, process. The nurse should give complete attention to the patient and should not be preoccupied. The nurse should suspend thinking of personal experiences and problems and personal judgments of the patient. Listening is a sign of respect for the patient and is a powerful reinforcer. It reinforces verbalization by the patient, without which the relationship could not progress.

Broad Openings.   Broad openings such as "What are you thinking about?," "Can you tell me more about that?," and "What shall we discuss today?" confirm the presence of the patient and encourage the patient to select topics to discuss. They also can indicate that the nurse is there, listening to and following the patient. Also serving in this way are acceptance responses, such as "I understand," "And then what happened?," "Uh huh," or "I follow you."

Restating.   Restating is the nurse's repeating of the main thought the patient has expressed. It also indicates that the nurse is listening. Sometimes only a part of the patient's statement is repeated. This technique can serve as a reinforcer or bring attention to something important that might otherwise have been passed over.

Clarification.   Clarification occurs when the nurse attempts to put into words vague ideas or thoughts that are implicit or explicit in the patient's talking. It is necessary because statements about emotions and behaviors are rarely straightforward. The patient's verbalizations, especially if the patient is upset or overwhelmed with feelings, are not always clear and obvious. Nothing should be allowed to pass that the nurse does not hear or understand. Because of this uncertainty, clarification responses often are tentative or phrased as questions, such as "I'm not sure what you mean. Are you saying that...?" or "Could you go over that again?" This technique is important because two functions of the nurse-patient relationship are to help clarify feelings, ideas, and perceptions and to provide an explicit link between them and the patient's actions.

Reflection.   Reflection of content is also called **validation**; it lets the patient know that the nurse has heard what was said and understands the content. It consists of repeating in fewer and fresher words the essential ideas of the patient and is like paraphrasing. Sometimes it helps to repeat a patient's statement, emphasizing a key word.

THERAPEUTIC DIALOGUE

PATIENT   *When I walked into the room, I felt like I was going to faint. I knew I had tried to do too much too quickly, and I just wasn't ready for it.*

NURSE   *You thought you were ready to put yourself to the test, but when you got there, you realized it was too much too soon.*

Reflection of feelings consists of responses to the patient's feelings about the content. These responses let the patient know that the nurse is aware of what the patient is feeling. Broad openings, restatements, clarifications, and reflections of content need not represent empathic understanding. But reflection of feeling signifies understanding, empathy, interest, and respect for the patient. It increases the level of involvement between the nurse and patient.

The purpose of reflecting feelings is to focus on feeling rather than content to bring the patient's vaguely expressed feelings into clear awareness; it helps the patient accept or own those feelings. The steps in reflection of feelings are to determine what feelings the patient is expressing, describe these feelings clearly, observe the effect, and judge by the patient's reaction whether the reflection was correct. Sometimes even inaccurate reflections can be useful because the patient may correct the nurse and state feelings more clearly.

 THERAPEUTIC DIALOGUE

PATIENT *It's not so much that I mind changing jobs. It's just that I let down all the people working for me . . . relying on me.*
NURSE *You feel responsible for your employees and so you're both sad and guilty about what has happened at work.*
PATIENT *Yes—sad, guilty . . . and pretty angry now that we're talking about it.*

Although reflecting techniques are some of the most useful, the nurse also can use them incorrectly. One common error is stereotyping of responses; that is, the nurse begins reflections in the same monotonous way, such as "You think" or "You feel." A second error is in timing. Reflecting back almost everything the patient says provokes feelings of irritation, anger, and frustration in the patient because the nurse appears to be insincere and fails to be therapeutic. Other nurses may have trouble interrupting patients who continue talking in long monologues. Not only is it difficult to capture a feeling after it has passed, but also the nurse is failing to be a responsible, active partner in the relationship. Interruptions may at times be productive and necessary. Another error is inappropriate depth of feeling. The nurse fails by being either too superficial or too deep in assessing the patient's feelings. The final error is use of language that is inappropriate to the patient's sociocultural experience and educational level. Effective language is language that is natural to the nurse and readily understood by the patient.

Focusing. Focusing helps the patient expand on a topic of importance. Effectively used, it can help the patient become more specific, move from vagueness to clarity, and focus on reality.

By avoiding abstractions and generalizations, focusing helps the patient face problems and analyze them in detail. It helps a patient talk about life experiences or problem areas and accept the responsibility for improving them. If the goal is to change thoughts, feelings, or beliefs, the patient must first identify and own them.

 THERAPEUTIC DIALOGUE

PATIENT *Women always get put down. It's as if we don't count at all.*
NURSE *Tell me how you feel as a woman.*

Encouraging a description of the patient's perceptions, encouraging comparisons, and placing events in time sequence are focusing techniques that promote specificity and problem analysis.

Sharing Perceptions. Sharing perceptions involves asking the patient to verify the nurse's understanding of what the patient is thinking or feeling. The nurse can ask for feedback from the patient while possibly providing new information. Perception checking can consist of paraphrasing what the patient is saying or doing, asking the patient to confirm the nurse's understanding, and allowing the patient to correct that perception if necessary. Perception checking also can note the implied feelings of nonverbal language. It is best to describe the observed behavior first and then reflect on its meaning.

 THERAPEUTIC DIALOGUE

PATIENT *She was such a good girl . . . and really seemed to care about other people. I don't know what's happened to her . . . what I could have done differently.*
NURSE *You seem to be very disappointed with your daughter, and maybe with yourself. Am I right about that?*

Perception checking is also a way to explore incongruent or double-blind communication. "You're smiling, but I sense that you're really angry with me." Perception checking conveys understanding to the patient and clears up confusing communication.

Theme Identification. Themes are underlying issues or problems experienced by the patient that emerge repeatedly during the course of the nurse-patient relationship. Once the nurse has identified the patient's basic themes, he or she can better decide which of the patient's many feelings, thoughts, and beliefs to respond to and pursue. Important themes tend to be repeated throughout the relationship. They can relate to feelings (depression or anxiety), behavior (rebelling against authority or withdrawal), experiences (being loved, hurt, or raped), or combinations of all three.

Silence. Silence on the part of the nurse has varying effects, depending on how the patient perceives it. To a vocal patient, silence on the part of the nurse may be welcome, as long as the patient knows the nurse is listening. When patients pause, they often expect and want the nurse to respond. If the nurse does not, patients may perceive this as rejection, hostility, or disinterest. With a depressed or withdrawn patient, the nurse's silence may convey support, understanding, and acceptance. In this case, verbalization by the nurse may be perceived as pressure or frustration.

Silence can prompt the patient to talk. Some introverted people find out that they can be quiet but still be liked. Silence allows the patient time to think and to gain insights. Finally, silence can slow the pace of the interaction. In general, the nurse should allow the patient to break a silence, particularly when the patient has introduced it. Obviously, sensitivity is called for in this regard, and silence should not develop into a contest. However, if the nurse is unsure how to respond to a patient's comments, a safe approach is to maintain silence. If the nurse's nonverbal behavior communicates interest and involvement, the patient often will elaborate or discuss a related issue.

As a general technique, direct questioning has limited usefulness in the therapeutic relationship. Repetitive questioning takes on the tone of an interrogation and negates the element of mutuality. "Why" questions are particularly ineffective and are to be avoided, as are questions that can be answered yes or no. One consequence of these type of questions is that patients do not take the initiative and are discouraged or prevented from engaging in the process of exploration.

Humor. Humor is a basic part of the personality and has a place within the therapeutic relationship. As a part of interpersonal relationships, it is a constructive coping behavior. By learning to express humor, a patient may be able to learn to express other feelings. As a planned approach to nursing intervention, humor can promote insight by making conscious repressed material. A change in the expression of humor and the quality of interpersonal relationships may be indicators of significant change in the patient.

Humor can serve many functions within the nurse-patient relationship (Box 2-7). These can be either positive or negative. There are no rules for determining how, when, or where humor should be used in the therapeutic relationship. It depends on the nature and quality of the relationship, the patient's receptivity to such themes, and the relevance of the tale or witticism. Humor may be of therapeutic value in the following situations:

- When the patient is experiencing mild to moderate levels of anxiety, humor serves as a tension reducer. It is inappropriate if a patient has severe or panic anxiety levels.

- When it helps a patient cope more effectively, facilitates learning, puts life situations in perspective, decreases social distance, and is understood by the patient for its therapeutic value. It is inappropriate when it promotes maladaptive coping responses, masks feelings, increases social distance, and helps the individual avoid dealing with difficult situations.

- When it is consistent with the social and cultural values of the patient and when it allows the patient to laugh at life, the human situation, or a particular set of stressors. It is inappropriate when it violates a patient's values, ridicules people, or belittles others.

The nurse also must be aware of the dangerous ways it can be used to hide conflicts, ward off anxiety, manipulate the patient, and serve the nurse's own need to be liked and admired. If it is used indiscriminately, humor meets only the nurse's needs and may be destructive to the relationship and frightening to the patient.

Informing. Informing, or information giving, is an essential nursing technique in which the nurse shares simple facts with the patient. It is a skill used by nurses in health teaching or patient education, such as in informing a patient when to take medication and about necessary precautions and side effects. Giving information must be distinguished from giving suggestions or advice.

Suggesting. Suggesting is the presentation of alternative ideas. As a therapeutic technique, it is a useful intervention in the working phase of the relationship when the patient has analyzed the problem area and is exploring alternative coping mechanisms. At that time, suggestions by the nurse will increase the patient's perceived options.

Suggesting, or giving advice, also can be nontherapeutic. Some patients who seek help expect some pronouncement from the health care professional on what to do. Likewise, nursing students often perceive their function as giving "common sense" advice. In these instances giving advice shifts responsibility to the nurse and reinforces the patient's dependence.

Another limitation is that the patient may take the nurse's advice and still have an unsuccessful outcome. The patient then returns to blame the nurse for failure. Most commonly, though, patients do not follow the advice offered by others, as in the transactional analysis model. The request for advice is often a child's expression of dependency, and the patient really knows what to do. The nurse who falls into the trap and responds with advice receives the patient's anger and contempt. A more productive strategy is for the nurse to deal with the patient's feelings first—feelings of indecision, dependence, and perhaps fear. Then the request for advice can be looked at and responded to in its proper perspective.

Suggesting also is nontherapeutic if it occurs early in the relationship before the patient has analyzed personal conflicts or if it is a technique the nurse uses frequently. Then it negates the possibility of mutuality and implies that the patient is incapable of assuming responsibility for thoughts and actions. Suggestion by the nurse also is nontherapeutic when it is really covert coercion, as the nurse tells patients how they **ought** to live their lives.

Box **2-7**

Functions of Humor

- Establishes relationships
- Reduces stress and tension
- Promotes social closeness
- Provides social control
- Permits cognitive reframing
- Reflects social change
- Provides perspective
- Expresses emotion
- Facilitates learning
- Reinforces self-concept
- Voices social conflict
- Avoids conflict
- Facilitates enculturation
- Instills hope

The nurse's intent in using the suggesting technique should be to provide feasible alternatives and allow the patient to explore his or her potential value. The nurse can then focus on helping the patient explore the advantages and disadvantages and the meaning and implications of the alternatives. In this way suggestions can be offered in a nonauthoritarian manner with such phrases as "Some people have tried. . . . Do you think that would work for you?" When using the technique of suggesting, nurses must be careful about both the timing of their intervention and their underlying motivation.

The therapeutic communication techniques presented in this chapter are summarized in Box 2-8.

Which therapeutic communication techniques listed in Box 2-8 are you skilled in using? Which techniques are more difficult for you?

RESPONSIVE DIMENSIONS

The nurse must possess certain skills or qualities to establish and maintain a therapeutic relationship. Specific core conditions for facilitative interpersonal relationships can be divided into responsive dimensions and action dimensions (Carkhoff, 1969; Carkhoff & Berenson,1967; Carkhoff & Truax, 1967).

The responsive dimensions include genuineness, respect, empathic understanding, and concreteness. One study suggests reports that patients had much anxiety when interacting with psychiatric nurses, although they found them to be friendly and caring. However, they also experienced psychiatric nurses as lacking in empathy and intimacy and thought that they related to patients in stereotypical ways, acting as custodians and enforcers of rules (Muller & Poggenpoel, 1996). The helping process can therefore impede the patient's growth rather than enhance it, depending on the level of the nurse's responsive and facilitative skills.

The responsive dimensions are crucial in a therapeutic relationship to establish trust and open communication. The nurse's goal is to understand the patient and to help the patient gain self-understanding and insight. These responsive conditions then continue to be useful throughout the working and termination phases.

Genuineness

Genuineness means that the nurse is an open, honest, sincere person who is actively involved in the relationship. Genuineness is the opposite of self-alienation, which occurs when many of an individual's real, spontaneous reactions to life are suppressed. Genuineness means that the nurse's response is sincere, that the nurse is not thinking and feeling one thing and saying something different. It is an essential quality because nurses cannot expect openness, self-acceptance, and personal freedom in patients if they lack these qualities themselves. Whatever the nurse shows must be real and not merely a "professional" response that has been learned and repeated. In focusing on the patient, much of the nurse's personal need system is put aside, as well as some of the usual ways of relating to others.

Following is an example of genuineness.

 ## THERAPEUTIC DIALOGUE

PATIENT   *I'd like my parents to give me my freedom and let me do my own thing. If I need them or want their advice, I'll ask them. Why don't they trust what they taught me? Why do parents have to make it so hard—like it's all or nothing?*

NURSE   *I know what you mean. My parents acted the same way. They offered advice, but what they expected was obedience. When they saw I could handle things on my own and used good judgment, they began to accept me as an individual. There are still times when they slip back into their old ways, but we understand each other better now. Do you think you and your parents need to share more openly and honestly your feelings and ideas?*

Respect

Respect, also called **nonpossessive warmth** or **unconditional positive regard**, does not depend on the patient's behavior. **Caring, liking,** and **valuing** are other terms for respect. The patient is regarded as a person of worth and is respected. The nurse's attitude is nonjudgmental; it is without criticism, ridicule, or reservation. This does not mean that the nurse condones or accepts all aspects of the patient's behavior as desirable or likable. Patients are accepted for who they are, as they are. The nurse does not demand that the patient change or be perfect to be accepted. Imperfections are accepted along with mistakes and weaknesses as part of the human condition. The inexperienced nurse may have difficulty accepting the patient without transferring feelings about the patient's thoughts or actions. However, acceptance means viewing the patient's actions as coping behaviors that will change as the patient becomes less threatened and learns more adaptive ways. It involves viewing the patient's behavior as natural, normal, and expected, given the circumstances.

Although there should be a basic respect for the patient simply as a person, respect is increased with understanding of the patient's uniqueness. Respect can be communicated in many different ways: by sitting silently with a patient who is crying, by genuine laughter with the patient over a particular event, by accepting the patient's request not to share a certain experience, by apologizing for the hurt unintentionally caused by a particular phrase, or by being open enough to communicate anger or hurt caused by the patient. Being genuine with and listening to the patient also are signs of respect.

When nurses communicate conditional warmth, they foster feelings of dependency in patients because nurses become the evaluator and superior in the relationship, making mutuality impossible. If dependency feelings arise in patients, nurses can effectively deal with them by acknowledging and exploring these feelings with patients.

Box **2-8**

Therapeutic Communication Techniques

TECHNIQUE: LISTENING

Definition: An active process of receiving information and examining reaction to the messages received
Example: Maintaining eye contact and receptive nonverbal communication
Therapeutic value: Nonverbally communicates to the patient the nurse's interest and acceptance
Nontherapeutic threat: Failure to listen

TECHNIQUE: BROAD OPENINGS

Definition: Encouraging the patient to select topics for discussion
Example: "What are you thinking about?"
Therapeutic value: Indicates acceptance by the nurse and the value of the patient's initiative
Nontherapeutic threat: Domination of the interaction by the nurse; rejecting responses

TECHNIQUE: RESTATING

Definition: Repeating the main thought the patient expressed
Example: "You say that your mother left you when you were 5 years old."
Therapeutic value: Indicates that the nurse is listening and validates, reinforces, or calls attention to something important that has been said
Nontherapeutic threat: Lack of validation of the nurse's interpretation of the message; being judgmental; reassuring; defending

TECHNIQUE: CLARIFICATION

Definition: Attempting to put into words vague ideas or unclear thoughts of the patient to enhance the nurse's understanding or asking the patient to explain what he or she means
Example: "I'm not sure what you mean. Could you tell me about that again?"
Therapeutic value: Helps to clarify feelings, ideas, and perceptions of the patient and provide an explicit correlation between them and the patient's actions
Nontherapeutic threat: Failure to probe; assumed understanding

TECHNIQUE: REFLECTION

Definition: Directing back the patient's ideas, feelings, questions, or content
Example: "You're feeling tense and anxious and it's related to a conversation you had with your husband last night?"
Therapeutic value: Validates the nurse's understanding of what the patient is saying and signifies empathy, interest, and respect for the patient
Nontherapeutic threat: Stereotyping the patient's responses; inappropriate timing of reflections; inappropriate depth of feeling of the reflections; inappropriate to the cultural experience and educational level of the patient

TECHNIQUE: HUMOR

Definition: The discharge of energy through the comic enjoyment of the imperfect

Example: "That gives a whole new meaning to the word *nervous*," said with shared kidding between the nurse and patient
Therapeutic value: Can promote insight by making conscious repressed material, resolving paradoxes, tempering aggression, and revealing new options; a socially acceptable form of sublimation
Nontherapeutic threat: Indiscriminate use; belittling patient; screen to avoid therapeutic intimacy

TECHNIQUE: INFORMING

Definition: The skill of information giving
Example: "I think you need to know more about how your medication works."
Therapeutic value: Helpful in health teaching or patient education about relevant aspects of patient's well-being and self-care
Nontherapeutic threat: Giving advice

TECHNIQUE: FOCUSING

Definition: Questions or statements that help the patient expand on a topic of importance
Example: "I think that we should talk more about your relationship with your father."
Therapeutic value: Allows the patient to discuss central issues and keeps the communication process goal-directed
Nontherapeutic threat: Allowing abstractions and generalizations; changing topics

TECHNIQUE: SHARING PERCEPTIONS

Definition: Asking the patient to verify the nurse's understanding of what the patient is thinking or feeling
Example: "You're smiling, but I sense that you are really very angry with me."
Therapeutic value: Conveys the nurse's understanding to the patient and has the potential for clearing up confusing communication
Nontherapeutic threat: Challenging the patient; accepting literal responses; reassuring; testing; defending

TECHNIQUE: THEME IDENTIFICATION

Definition: Underlying issues or problems experienced by the patient that emerge repeatedly during the course of the nurse-patient relationship
Example: "I've noticed that in all of the relationships that you have described, you've been hurt or rejected by the man. Do you think this is an underlying issue?"
Therapeutic value: Allows the nurse to best promote the patient's exploration and understanding of important problems
Nontherapeutic threat: Giving advice; reassuring; disapproving

TECHNIQUE: SILENCE

Definition: Lack of verbal communication for a therapeutic reason
Example: Sitting with a patient and nonverbally communicating interest and involvement
Therapeutic value: Allows the patient time to think and gain insights, slows the pace of the interaction, and en-

Box 2-8

Therapeutic Communication Techniques—cont'd

TECHNIQUE: SILENCE—CONT'D

courages the patient to initiate conversation, while conveying the nurse's support, understanding, and acceptance
Nontherapeutic threat: Questioning the patient; asking for "why" responses; failure to break a nontherapeutic silence

TECHNIQUE: SUGGESTING

Definition: Presentation of alternative ideas for the patient's consideration relative to problem solving

Example: "Have you thought about responding to your boss in a different way when he raises that issue with you? For example, you could ask him whether a specific problem has occurred."
Therapeutic value: Increases the patient's perceived options or choices
Nontherapeutic threat: Giving advice; inappropriate timing; being judgmental

---

There is a common expression that "respect needs to be learned." How does this idea affect the lives of psychiatric patients?

Empathic Understanding

Empathy is the ability to enter into the life of another person and to accurately perceive his or her current feelings and their meanings. It is an essential part of the therapeutic process (Bohart & Greenberg, 1997). When communicated, it forms the basis for a helping relationship between nurse and patient. Rogers (1975) described it as "to sense the client's private world as if it were your own, but without losing the 'as if' quality. A high degree of empathy is one of the most potent factors in bringing about change and learning—one of the most delicate and powerful ways we have of using ourselves."

Accurate empathy involves more than knowing what the patient means. It also involves sensitivity to the patient's current feelings and the verbal ability to communicate this understanding in a language attuned to the patient. It means frequently confirming with the patient the accuracy of personal perceptions and being guided by the patient's responses. It requires that the nurse lay aside personal views and values to enter another's world without prejudice.

There are two types of empathy (Alligood, 1992) The first type is basic empathy. It involves the natural, universal human capacity to feel for others. The second type is trained empathy, which is taught and learned in relation to helping others. Trained empathy also is called clinical empathy or professional empathy. Unfortunately, these two types of empathy are often confused when empathy is discussed in terms of the nurse-patient relationship. It is important to first assess a baseline of empathic ability in nursing students. New approaches can then be used to facilitate students' discovery of their basic empathy and the impact it may have on the outcome of psychiatric nursing care (see Citing the Evidence).

Development of Empathy

Empathic understanding consists of a number of stages. If patients allow nurses to enter their private world and attempt to communicate their perceptions and feelings, nurses must be receptive to this communication. Next, nurses must

---

Citing the Evidence on

Empathy

BACKGROUND: The purpose of this study was to examine the differences between basic and trained empathy and to measure the endurance of empathy scores. Data were collected from 106 nursing students before, during, and after completion of a baccalaureate degree in nursing.

RESULTS: Analysis confirmed the existence of these two kinds of empathy and the fact that students enter nursing education with significantly different levels of basic and trained empathy. Results suggest that basic empathy cannot be taught but can be identified, reinforced, and refined to develop expertise. Trained empathy lacked endurance in caregiving situations.

IMPLICATIONS: The findings from this study call into question the long-standing practice of teaching empathy techniques. There may be a potential for harm if nurses rely on the rote behaviors learned superficially as trained empathy. Understanding in complex situations requires the multidimensional depth of empathy that uses moral, affective, developmental, and cognitive aspects of the caregiver. Findings suggest that educational approaches may need to be altered so that students who have low levels of basic empathy can develop other interpersonal strengths.

Evans G, Wilt D, Alligood M, O'Neil M: Empathy: a study of two types, *Issues Mental Health Nurs* 19:453, 1998.

---

understand the patient's communication by putting themselves in the patient's place. Nurses must then step back into their own role and communicate understanding to the patient. It is not necessary or desirable for nurses to feel the same emotion as the patient. Empathy should not be confused with sympathy. Instead, it is an appreciation and awareness of the patient's feelings. A good deal of research has been conducted on empathy. The findings presented in Box 2-9 underscore its importance in counseling.

Box **2-9**

Research Findings about Empathy

- Empathy is related to positive clinical outcome.
- The ideal therapist is first of all empathic.
- Empathy is correlated with self-exploration and self-acceptance.
- Empathy early in the relationship predicts later success.
- Understanding is provided by, not drawn from, the therapist.
- More experienced therapists are more likely to be empathic.
- Empathy is a special quality in a relationship, and therapists offer more of it than even helpful friends.
- The better self-integrated the therapist, the higher the degree of empathy.
- Experienced therapists often fall far short of being empathic. Brilliance and diagnostic perceptiveness are unrelated to empathy.
- An empathic way of being can be learned from empathic people.

Rogers (1975) expands on the profound consequences empathy can have in promoting constructive learning and change. In the first place, it dissolves the patient's sense of alienation by connecting the patient on some level to a part of the human race. The patient can perceive that "I make sense to another human being . . . so I must not be so strange or alien. . . . And if I am in touch with someone else, I am not so alone." On the other hand, if not responded to empathically, the patient may believe, "If no one understands me, if no one can see what I'm experiencing, then I must be very bad off. . . . I'm sicker than even I thought." Another benefit of empathy is that the patient can feel valued, cared for, and accepted as a person. Then perhaps he or she will come to think, "If this other person thinks I'm worthwhile, maybe I could value and care for myself. . . . Maybe I am worthwhile after all."

Empathic Responses. First, the nurse needs to provide genuineness and unconditional positive regard for the patient. Then the understanding conveyed to the patient through empathy gives him or her personhood or identity. The patient incorporates these aspects into a new, changing self-concept. Once self-concept changes, behavior also changes, thus producing the positive clinical outcome of therapy.

Nursing research has demonstrated a connection between nurse-expressed empathy and positive patient outcomes (Olson, 1995). One nursing study identified the following specific verbal and nonverbal behaviors that conveyed high levels of empathy to the patient (Mansfield, 1973):

- Having nurses introduce themselves to patients
- Head and body positions turned toward the patient and occasionally leaning forward
- Verbal responses to the patient's comments and responses that focus on strengths and resources
- Consistent eye contact and response to the patient's nonverbal cues such as sighs, tone of voice, restlessness, and facial expressions

- Conveyance of interest, concern, and warmth by the nurse's own facial expressions
- A tone of voice consistent with facial expression and verbal response
- Mirror imaging of body position and gestures between the nurse and patient

Additional studies are needed in nursing to identify the behavioral indicators and outcomes of this important aspect of nursing care.

Empathic Functioning Scale. Kalisch (1973) devised the Nurse-Patient Empathic Functioning Scale, which describes five categories of empathy. High levels of empathy (categories 3 and 4) communicate "I am with you"; the nurse's responses fit perfectly with the patient's conspicuous current feelings and content. The nurse's responses also serve to expand the patient's awareness of hidden feelings through the use of clarification and reflection. Such empathy is communicated by the language used, voice qualities, and nonverbal behavior, all of which reflect the nurse's seriousness and depth of feeling.

At low levels of empathy (categories 0 and 1), the nurse ignores the patient's feelings, goes off on a tangent, or misinterprets what the patient is feeling. The nurse at this level may be uninterested in the patient or concentrating on the "facts" of what the patient says rather than on current feelings and experiences. The nurse is doing something other than listening, such as evaluating the patient, giving advice, sermonizing, or thinking about personal problems or needs. A middle level of empathy (category 2) shows that the nurse is making an effort to understand the patient's feelings.

Empathic responses must be properly timed within the nurse-patient relationship. Category 4 responses in the orientation phase may be viewed as too intense and intrusive. Usually a number of category 2 responses are required initially to build an atmosphere of trust and openness. In the later stages of the orientation phase and most particularly in the working phase, categories 3 and 4 responses are appropriate and most effective. Responses from categories 0 and 1 are nontherapeutic at all times and block the development of the relationship.

The various levels of empathy are evident in the following example:

 THERAPEUTIC DIALOGUE

PATIENT *I'm really jittery today, and I hope I can get things out right. It started when I saw Bob on Friday, and it's been building up since then.*

NURSE *You're feeling tense and anxious, and it's related to a talk you had with Bob on Friday. (Category 2.)*

PATIENT *Yes. He began putting pressure on me to have sex with him again.*

NURSE *It sounds like you resent it when he pressures you for sex. (Category 3.)*

PATIENT *I do. Why does he think things always have to be his way? I guess he knows I'm a pushover.*

NURSE   *It makes you angry when he wants his way even though he knows you feel differently. But you usually give in and then you wind up disappointed in yourself and feeling like a failure. (Category 4.)*
PATIENT   *It happens just like that over and over. It's as if I never learn.*
NURSE   *So when the incident's all over, you're left blaming yourself and wallowing in self-pity. (Category 4.)*
PATIENT   *I guess that's right.*

Finally, sociocultural differences between nurses and patients can be barriers to empathy if nurses are not sensitive to them. Differences in gender, age, income, belief systems, education, and ethnicity can block the development of empathic understanding. However, the greater the nurse's cultural sensitivity and the greater the openness to the world view of others, the greater will be the potential for understanding people.

Identical or similar experiences are not essential for empathy. No man can really experience what it is like to be a woman; no white person can experience what it is like to be a black person. It is not necessary to be exactly like another, but it is desirable for nurses to prepare themselves in any way they can to understand potential patients. It also is important for nurses to realize that empathy can be learned and enhanced in a variety of ways, including staff development programs.

> *Evaluate a recent interaction you had with a patient based on the empathy scale described. Use it again at the end of your psychiatric nursing experience and note any differences.*

Concreteness

Concreteness involves using specific terminology rather than abstractions when discussing the patient's feelings, experiences, and behavior. It avoids vagueness and ambiguity and is the opposite of generalizing, categorizing, classifying, and labeling the patient's experiences. It has three functions: to keep the nurse's responses close to the patient's feelings and experiences, to foster accuracy of understanding by the nurse, and to encourage the patient to attend to specific problem areas.

The level of concreteness should vary during the various phases of the nurse-patient relationship (Fig. 2-8). In the orientation phase, concreteness should be high; at this time it can contribute to empathic understanding. It is essential for the formulation of specific goals and plans. As patients explore various feelings and perceptions related to their problems in the working phase of the relationship, concreteness should be at a low level to facilitate a thorough self-exploration. High levels of concreteness are again desirable at the end of the working phase, when patients are engaging in action, and during the termination phase.

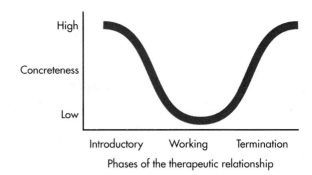

Fig. 2-8   Levels of concreteness in the therapeutic relationship.

Concreteness is evident in the following examples:

THERAPEUTIC DIALOGUE

Example 1
PATIENT   *I wouldn't have any problems if people would quit bothering me. They like to upset me because they know I'm high strung.*
NURSE   *What people try to upset you?*
PATIENT   *My family. People think being from a large family is a blessing. I think it's a curse.*
NURSE   *Could you give me an example of something someone in your family did that upset you?*

Example 2
PATIENT   *I don't know what the problem is between us. My wife and I just don't get along anymore. We seem to disagree about everything. I think I love her, but she isn't affectionate or caring—hasn't been for a long time.*
NURSE   *You say you're not sure what the problem is, and you think you love your wife. But the two of you argue often and she hasn't given you any sign of love or affection. Have you felt affectionate toward her, and when was the last time you let her know how you felt?*

These four responsive dimensions or conditions—genuineness, respect, empathic understanding, and concreteness—facilitate the formation of a therapeutic relationship. The therapeutic level at which nurses function is unknown at present (Holyoake, 1998). Additional research is needed on nurse-patient interactions because there is little evidence on which to base scientific practice in this area.

ACTION DIMENSIONS
The action-oriented conditions for facilitative interpersonal relationships are confrontation, immediacy, therapist self-disclosure, catharsis, and role playing. The separation of these therapeutic conditions into two groups—the understanding, or responsive conditions and the initiating, or action conditions—is not a distinct separation. To some extent all the dimensions are present throughout the therapeutic relationship. The action dimensions must have a context of warmth and understanding. This is important for inexperienced nurses to remember because they may be tempted to

move into high levels of action dimensions without having established adequate understanding, empathy, warmth, or respect. The responsive dimensions allow the patient to achieve insight, but this is not enough. With the action dimensions, the nurse moves the therapeutic relationship upward and outward by identifying obstacles to the patient's progress and the need for both internal understanding and external action.

Confrontation

Confrontation usually implies venting anger and aggressive behavior. However, confrontation as a therapeutic action dimension is an assertive rather than aggressive action. Confrontation is an expression by the nurse of perceived discrepancies in the patient's behavior. The three categories of confrontation are listed in the following (Carkhoff, 1969):

- Discrepancies between the patient's expression of what he or she is (self-concept) and what he or she wants to be (self-ideal)
- Discrepancies between the patient's verbal self-expression and nonverbal behavior
- Discrepancies between the patient's expressed experience of himself or herself and the nurse's experience of him or her

Confrontation is an attempt by the nurse to make the patient aware of incongruence in his or her feelings, attitudes, beliefs, and behaviors. It also may lead to the discovery of ambivalent feelings in the patient. Confrontation is not limited to negative aspects of the patient. It includes pointing out discrepancies involving resources and strengths that are unrecognized and unused. It requires that the nurse collect sufficient data about the patient's history and accumulate sufficient perceptions and observations of verbal and nonverbal communication so that validation of reality is possible.

The nurse must have developed an understanding of the patient to perceive discrepancies, inconsistencies in word and deed, distortions, defenses, and evasions. The nurse must be willing and able to work through the crisis after confronting the patient. Without this commitment the confrontation lacks therapeutic potential and can be damaging to both nurse and patient. Without question, the effects of confrontation are challenge, exposure, risk, and the possibility for growth. The nurse who uses confrontation is modeling an active role to the patient; the nurse is using insight and understanding to remove ambiguity and inconsistency and thus seek deeper understanding.

Timing in Relationships. Before confrontation, nurses should assess the following factors:

- The trust level in the relationship
- The timing
- The patient's stress level
- The strength of the patient's defense mechanisms
- The patient's perceived need for personal space or closeness
- The patient's level of rage and tolerance for hearing another perception

Patients have the capacity to deny or accept nurses' observations, and their response to the confrontation can serve as a measure of its success or failure. Acceptance indicates appropriate timing and patient readiness. Denial serves to allay any threat that the confrontation posed to the patient. It provides nurses with additional information; it tells them that patients are resisting change and are unwilling to enlarge their view of reality at this time.

Confrontation also must be appropriately timed to be effective (Fig. 2-9). In the orientation phase of the relationship, the nurse should use confrontation infrequently and pose it as an observation of incongruent behavior. A simple mirroring of the discrepancy between a patient's actions and words is the most nonthreatening type of confrontation. The nurse might say, "You seem to be saying two different things." This type of confrontation closely resembles clarification at this time. Nurses also might identify discrepancies between how they and patients are experiencing their relationship, point out unnoticed patient strengths or untapped resources, or provide patients with objective but perhaps different information about their world. Finally, to be effective, confrontation requires high levels of empathy and respect.

In the working phase of the relationship, more direct confrontations may focus on specific patient discrepancies. The nurse may confront the patient with areas of weakness or shortcomings or may focus on the discrepancy between the nurse's perception of the patient and the patient's self-perception. This expands the patient's awareness and helps the patient move to higher levels of functioning. Confrontation is especially important in pointing out when the patient has developed insight but has not changed behavior. This encourages the patient to act in a reasonable and constructive manner, rather than assuming a dependent and passive stance toward life.

Research indicates that effective counselors use confrontation frequently, confronting patients with their assets more often in earlier interviews and with their limitations in later interviews. In the initial interview, these confrontations were based on attempts to clarify the relationship, eliminate misconceptions, give patients more objective information about themselves and their world, and emphasize patient strengths and resources.

Inexperienced nurses often avoid confrontation. It can be nontherapeutic when it is not associated with empathy or warmth or when it is used to vent the nurse's feelings of anger, frustration, and aggressiveness. However, carefully

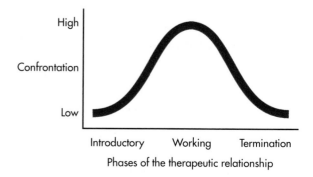

Fig. 2-9 Levels of confrontation in the therapeutic relationship.

monitored confrontation can be viewed as an extension of genuineness and concreteness. It is a useful therapeutic intervention that can further the patient's growth and progress.

Following are examples of confrontation:

 THERAPEUTIC DIALOGUE

Example 1

NURSE *I see you as someone who has a lot of strength. You've been able to give a tremendous amount of emotional support to your children at a time when they needed it very much.*

Example 2

NURSE *You say you want to feel better and go back to work, but you're not taking your medicine, which will help you to do that.*

Example 3

NURSE *The fact that Sue didn't accept your date for Friday night doesn't necessarily mean she never wants to go out with you. She could have had another date or other plans with her family or girlfriends. But if you don't ask her, you'll never find out why she refused you or if she'll accept in the future.*

Example 4

NURSE *You tell me that your parents don't trust you and never give you any responsibility, but each week you also tell me how you stayed out beyond your curfew or had friends over when your parents weren't home. Do you see a connection between the two?*

Example 5

NURSE *We've been talking for 3 weeks now about your need to get out and try to meet some people. We even talked of different ways to do that. But so far you haven't made any effort to join aerobics, take a class, or do any of the other ideas we had.*

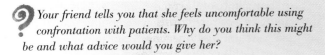 *Your friend tells you that she feels uncomfortable using confrontation with patients. Why do you think this might be and what advice would you give her?*

Immediacy

Immediacy involves focusing on the current interaction of the nurse and the patient in the relationship. It is a significant dimension because the patient's behavior and functioning in the relationship are indicative of functioning in other interpersonal relationships. Most patients experience difficulty in interpersonal relationships; thus the patient's functioning in the nurse-patient relationship must be evaluated. The nurse has the opportunity to intervene directly with the patient's problem behavior, and the patient has the opportunity to learn and change behavior.

Immediacy involves sensitivity to the patient's feelings and a willingness to deal with these feelings rather than ignore them. This is particularly difficult when the nurse must recognize and respond to negative feelings the patient ex-

presses toward the nurse. The difficulty is compounded by the fact that patients often express these messages indirectly and conceal them in references to other people.

It is not possible or appropriate for the nurse to focus continually on the immediacy of the relationship. It is most appropriate to do so when the relationship seems to be stalled or is not progressing. It also is helpful to look at immediacy when the relationship is progressing particularly well. In both instances the patient is actively involved in describing what is helping or hindering the relationship.

As with the other dimensions, high-level immediacy responses should not be suddenly presented to the patient. The nurse must first know and understand the patient and have developed a good, open relationship. The nurse's initial expressions of immediacy should be tentatively phrased, such as "Are you trying to tell me how you feel about our relationship?" As the relationship progresses, observations related to immediacy can be made more directly, and as communication improves, the need for immediacy responses may decrease.

Following are two examples of immediacy:

 THERAPEUTIC DIALOGUE

Example 1

PATIENT *I've been thinking about our meetings, and I'm really too busy now to keep coming. Besides, I don't see the point in them, and we don't seem to be getting anywhere.*

NURSE *Are you trying to say you're feeling discouraged and you feel our meetings aren't helping you?*

Example 2

PATIENT *The staff here couldn't care less about us patients. They treat us like children instead of adults.*

NURSE *I'm wondering if you feel that I don't care about you or perhaps I don't value your opinion?*

Nurse Self-Disclosure

Self-disclosures are subjectively true, personal statements about the self, intentionally revealed to another person. The nurse may share experiences or feelings that are similar to those of the patient and may emphasize both the similarities and differences. This kind of self-disclosure is an index of the closeness of the relationship and involves a particular kind of respect for the patient. It is an expression of genuineness and honesty by the nurse and is an aspect of empathy.

The research literature provides significant evidence that therapist self-disclosure increases the likelihood of patient self-disclosure. Patient self-disclosure is necessary for a successful therapeutic outcome. However, the nurse must use self-disclosure judiciously, and this is determined by the quality, quantity, and appropriateness of the disclosures (Deering,1999). Criteria for self-disclosure include the following:

- To model and educate
- To foster the therapeutic alliance
- To validate reality
- To encourage the patient's autonomy

The number of self-disclosures appears to be crucial to the success of the therapy. Too few nurse self-disclosures may fail to produce patient self-disclosures, whereas too many may decrease the time available for patient disclosure or may alienate the patient. The problem for the nurse is knowing where the middle ground is. Clinical experience is necessary to determine the optimum therapeutic level.

The appropriateness or relevance of the nurse's self-disclosure also is important. The nurse should self-disclose in response to statements made by the patient. If the nurse's disclosure is far from what the patient is experiencing, it can distract the patient from the problem or cause feelings of alienation. A patient who is experiencing severe anxiety may feel threatened or frightened by the nurse's self-disclosure. In these cases the nurse must be careful not to burden a patient with self-disclosures. Above all, disclosure by the nurse is always for the patient's benefit. The nurse does not disclose to meet personal needs or to feel better. When self-disclosing, the nurse should have a particular therapeutic goal in mind.

Guidelines that nurses can use to evaluate the potential usefulness of their self-disclosure are listed in Box 2-10. These guidelines govern the "dosage" and timing of self-disclosures and help the nurse assess the appropriateness, effectiveness, and anticipated response of the patient to the disclosure.

Self-disclosure by the nurse is evident in the following example:

 THERAPEUTIC DIALOGUE

PATIENT *When he told me he didn't want to see me again, I felt like slapping him and hugging him at the same time. But then I knew the problem was really me and no one could ever love me.*

NURSE *When I broke off with a man I had been seeing, I felt the anger, hurt, and bitterness you just described. I remember thinking I would never date another man.*

In this example the nurse self-disclosed to emphasize that the patient's feelings were natural. She also reinforced the external cause for the separation (boyfriend's decision to leave

versus the patient's inadequacy) and implied that, with time, the patient will be able to resolve the loss.

Emotional Catharsis

Emotional catharsis occurs when the patient is encouraged to talk about things that are most bothersome. Catharsis brings fears, feelings, and experiences out into the open so that they can be examined and discussed with the nurse. The expression of feelings can be very therapeutic in itself, even if behavioral change does not result. The previously described responsive dimensions create an atmosphere within the nurse-patient relationship in which emotional catharsis is possible. The patient's responsiveness depends on the confidence and trust the patient has in the nurse.

The nurse must be able to recognize cues from the patient concerning readiness for discussion of problems. It is important that the nurse proceed at the rate chosen by the patient and provide support during discussion of difficult areas. Forcing emotional catharsis on the patient could precipitate a panic episode because the patient's defenses are attacked without sufficient alternative coping mechanisms available.

Patients are often uncomfortable about expressing feelings. Nurses may be equally uncomfortable with expressing feelings, particularly sadness or anger. Nurses often assume that they know the patient's feelings and do not attempt to specifically validate them. The dimensions of empathy and immediacy require the nurse to notice and express emotions. Unresolved feelings and feelings that are avoided can cause stalls or barriers in the nurse-patient relationship. Specific examples are transference and countertransference phenomena, which are discussed later in the chapter.

If patients have difficulty in expressing feelings, nurses may help by suggesting how they or others might feel in the patient's specific situation. Some patients respond directly to the question, "How did that make you feel?" Others intellectualize and avoid the emotional element in their answer. When patients realize they can express their feelings within an accepting relationship, they expand their awareness and potential acceptance of themselves.

The following example illustrates emotional catharsis:

 THERAPEUTIC DIALOGUE

NURSE *How did you feel when your boss corrected you in front of all those customers?*

PATIENT *Well, I understood that he needed to set me straight, and he's the type that flies off the handle pretty easily anyhow.*

NURSE *It sounds like you're defending his behavior. I was wondering how you felt at that moment.*

PATIENT *Awkward . . . uh . . . upset, I guess (pause).*

NURSE *That would have made me pretty angry if it had happened to me.*

PATIENT *Well, I was. But you can't let it show, you know. You have to keep it all in because of the customers. But he can let it out. Oh sure (**emphatically**)! He can tell **me** anything he wants. Just once I'd like him to know how **I** feel.*

Role Playing

Role playing involves acting out a particular situation. It increases the patient's insight into human relations and can deepen the ability to see the situation from another person's point of view. The purpose of role playing is to closely represent real-life behavior that involves individuals holistically, to focus attention on a problem, and to permit individuals to see themselves in action in a neutral situation. It provides a bridge between thought and action in a safe environment in which the patient can feel free to experiment with new behavior. It is a method of learning that makes actual behavior the focus of study. It is action oriented and provides immediately available information. Role playing consists of the following steps:

1. Defining the problem
2. Creating a readiness for role playing
3. Establishing the situation
4. Casting the characters
5. Briefing and warming up
6. Acting
7. Stopping
8. Analyzing and discussing
9. Evaluating

When role playing is used for attitude change, it relies heavily on role reversal. The patient may be asked to assume the role of a certain person in a specific situation or to play the role of someone with opposing beliefs. Role reversal can help a person re-evaluate the other person's intentions and become more understanding of the other person's position. After role reversal, patients may be more receptive to modifying their own attitudes.

As a method of promoting self-awareness and conflict resolution, role playing may help the patient experience a situation rather than just talk about it. Role playing can elicit feelings in the patient that are similar to those experienced in the actual situation. It provides an opportunity for insight and for the expression of affect. For these reasons it is a useful method for heightening a patient's awareness of feelings about a situation.

One of the specific ways in which role playing can be used to resolve conflicts and increase self-awareness is through a dialogue that requires the patient to take the part of each person or each side of a problem. If the conflict is internal, the dialogue occurs in the present tense between the patient's conflicting selves until one part of the conflict outweighs the other. If the conflict involves a second person, the patient is instructed to "imagine that the other person is sitting in the chair across from you." The patient is told to begin the dialogue by expressing wants and resentments about the other person. Then the patient changes chairs, assumes the role of the other person, and responds to what was just said. The patient assumes the first role again and responds to the other person. Using dialogue in this way not only serves as practice for the patient in expressing feelings and opinions but also gives a reality base for the probable response from the other party involved in the conflict. This can often remove the barrier that is keeping the patient from making a decision and acting on it.

Role playing is included as an action dimension because it can help the patient develop insight. Nurses need a variety of intervention skills. Role playing can be effective when an impasse has been reached in the patient's progress or when it is difficult for the patient to translate insight into action. In these instances it can reduce tension and give the patient the opportunity to practice or test new behaviors for future use.

Table 2-4 summarizes the responsive and action dimensions for therapeutic nurse-patient relationships. It is important to remember that the nurse's effectiveness is based on openness to learning what works best with particular kinds of patients in particular situations. Both the use of communication techniques and the therapeutic conditions must be individualized to the nurse's personality and the patient's needs. The nurse needs to be willing to try other approaches that can be helpful if the current approach is ineffective.

THERAPEUTIC IMPASSES

Therapeutic impasses are blocks in the progress of the nurse-patient relationship. They arise for a variety of reasons, but they all create stalls in the therapeutic relationship. Impasses provoke intense feelings in both the nurse and the patient that may range from anxiety and apprehension to frustration, love, or intense anger. Four specific therapeutic impasses and ways to overcome them are discussed here: resistance, transference, countertransference, and boundary violations.

Resistance

Resistance is the patient's reluctance or avoidance of verbalizing or experiencing troubling aspects of oneself. The term resistance was initially introduced by Freud to mean the patient's unconscious opposition to exploring or recognizing unconscious or even preconscious material. Resistance is often caused by the patient's unwillingness to change when the need for change is recognized. Patients usually display resistance behaviors during the working phase of the relationship, because the greater part of the problem-solving process occurs during this phase.

Resistance also may be a reaction by the patient to the nurse who has moved too rapidly or too deeply into the patient's feelings or who has intentionally or unintentionally communicated a lack of respect. It also may simply be the result of a patient who is working with a nurse who is an inappropriate role model for therapeutic behavior.

Secondary gain is another cause of resistance. Favorable environmental, interpersonal, and situational changes occur, and material advantages may be obtained as a result of the illness. Types of secondary gain include financial compensation, avoiding unpleasant situations, increased sympathy or attention, escape from work or other responsibilities, attempted control of people, and lessening of social pressures. Secondary gain can become a powerful force in perpetuating an illness because it makes the environment more comfortable.

Table **2-4**

Responsive and Action Dimensions for Therapeutic Nurse-Patient Relationships	
Dimension	Characteristics
RESPONSIVE	
Genuineness	Implies that the nurse is an open person who is self-congruent, authentic, and transparent
Respect	Suggests that the patient is regarded as a person of worth who is valued and accepted without qualification
Empathic understanding	Viewing the patient's world from the patient's internal frame of reference, with sensitivity to the patient's current feelings and the verbal ability to communicate this understanding in a language attuned to the patient
Concreteness	Involves the use of specific terminology rather than abstractions in the discussion of the patient's feelings, experiences, and behavior
ACTION	
Confrontation	The expression by the nurse of perceived discrepancies in the patient's behavior to expand self-awareness
Immediacy	Occurs when the current interaction of the nurse and patient is focused on and is used to learn about the patient's functioning in other interpersonal relationships
Nurse self-disclosure	Evident when the nurse reveals personal information, ideas, values, feelings, and attitudes to facilitate the patient's cooperation, learning, catharsis, or support
Emotional catharsis	Takes place when the patient is encouraged to talk about things that are most bothersome
Role playing	The acting out of a particular situation to increase the patient's insight into human relations and deepen the ability to see a situation from another point of view. It also allows the patient to experiment with new behavior in a safe environment

Box **2-11**

Forms of Resistance Displayed by Patients

- Suppression and repression of pertinent information
- Intensification of symptoms
- Self-devaluation and a hopeless outlook on the future
- Forced flight into health where there is a sudden, but short-lived recovery by the patient
- Intellectual inhibitions, which may be evident when the patient says she has "nothing on her mind" or that she is "unable to think about her problems" or when she breaks appointments, is late for sessions, or is forgetful, silent, or sleepy
- Acting out or irrational behavior
- Superficial talk
- Intellectual insight in which the patient verbalizes self-understanding with correct use of terminology yet continues destructive behavior or uses the defense of intellectualization where there is no insight
- Contempt for normality, which is evident when the patient has developed insight but refuses to assume the responsibility for change on the grounds that normality "isn't so great"
- Transference reactions

Resistance may take many forms. Box 2-11 lists some of the forms of resistance that patients display (Wolberg, 1988).

Transference

Transference is an unconscious response in which the patient experiences feelings and attitudes toward the nurse that were originally associated with other significant figures in his or her life. They may be triggered by a superficial similarity, such as a facial feature or manner of speech, or by a personality style or trait. These reactions are the patient's attempt to reduce anxiety. The important trait defining transference is the inappropriate intensity of the patient's response.

Transference reduces self-awareness by allowing the patient to maintain an inaccurate view of the world in which all people are seen in similar terms. Thus the nurse may be viewed as an authority figure from the past, such as a parent figure, or as a lost loved object, such as a former spouse. Transference reactions are harmful to the therapeutic process only if they remain ignored and unexamined.

Two types of transference are particularly problematic in the nurse-patient relationship. The first is the hostile transference. If the patient internalizes anger and hostility, this resistance may be expressed as depression and discouragement. The patient may ask to terminate the relationship on the grounds that there is no chance of getting well. If the hostility is externalized, the patient may become critical, defiant, and irritable and may express doubts about the nurse's training, experience, or competence. The patient may attempt to compete with the nurse by reading books on psychology and debating intellectual issues rather than working on real life problems.

Hostility also may be expressed by the patient in detachment, forgetfulness, irrelevant chatter, or preoccupation with childhood experiences. An extreme form of uncooperativeness and negativism is evident in prolonged silences. Some of the most frustrating moments for the nurse are those spent in total silence with a patient. This is not the therapeutic silence that communicates mutuality and understanding. Rather, it is the silence that seems to be hostile, oppressive, and eternal. It is particularly disturbing for the nurse in the orientation phase, before a relationship has been established. The nurse's task is to understand the meaning of the patient's silence and decide how to deal with it despite feeling somewhat awkward and uncertain.

A second difficult type of transference is the dependent reaction transference. This resistance is characterized by patients who are submissive, subordinate, and ingratiating and who regard the nurse as a godlike figure. The patient overvalues the nurse's characteristics and qualities, and their relationship is in jeopardy because the patient views it as magical. In this reaction the nurse must live up to the patient's overwhelming expectations, which is impossible because these expectations are completely unrealistic. The patient continues to demand more of the nurse, and when these needs are not met, the patient is filled with hostility and contempt.

Overcoming Resistance and Transference

Resistances and transferences can be difficult problems for the nurse. The psychiatric nurse must be prepared to be exposed to powerful negative and positive emotional feelings coming from the patient, often on an irrational basis. The relationship can become stalled and nonbeneficial if the nurse is not prepared to deal with the patient's feelings.

Sometimes resistances occur because the nurse and patient have not arrived at mutually acceptable goals or plans of action. This may occur if the contract was not clearly defined in the orientation stage of the relationship. The appropriate action here is to return to the goals, purposes, and roles of the nurse and patient in the relationship.

Whatever the patient's motivations, the analysis of the resistance or transference is geared toward the patient gaining awareness of these motivations and learning about being completely responsible for all actions and behavior. The first thing the nurse must do is listen. When the nurse recognizes the resistance, clarification and reflection of feeling can be used. Clarification gives the nurse a more focused idea of what is happening. Reflection of content may help patients become aware of what has been going on in their own minds. Reflection of feeling acknowledges the resistance and mirrors it to the patient. The nurse may say, "I sense that you're struggling with yourself. Part of you wants to explore the issue of your marriage and another part says 'No—I'm not ready yet.'"

However, it is not sufficient to merely identify that resistance is occurring. The behavior must be explored and possible reasons for its occurrence analyzed. The depth of exploration and analysis engaged in by nurse and patient are related to the nurse's experience and knowledge base.

Countertransference

Countertransference is a therapeutic impasse created by the nurse's specific emotional response to the qualities of the patient. This response is inappropriate to the content and context of the therapeutic relationship and inappropriate in the degree of intensity of emotion. It is transference applied to the nurse. Inappropriateness is the important element, as it is with transference, because it is natural that the nurse will have a warmth toward or liking for some patients more than others.

Box 2-12

Forms of Countertransference Displayed by Nurses

- Difficulty empathizing with the patient in certain problem areas
- Feelings of depression during or after the session
- Carelessness about implementing the contract by being late, running overtime, etc.
- Drowsiness during the sessions
- Feelings of anger or impatience because of the patient's unwillingness to change
- Encouragement of the patient's dependency, praise, or affection
- Arguments with the patient or a tendency to push before the patient is ready
- Attempts to help the patient in matters not related to the identified nursing goals
- Personal or social involvement with the patient
- Dreams about or preoccupation with the patient
- Sexual or aggressive fantasies toward the patient
- Recurrent anxiety, unease, or guilt related to the patient
- Tendency to focus on only one aspect or way of looking at information presented by the patient
- Need to defend nursing interventions with the patient to others

---

The nurse also will be genuinely angry about the actions of certain patients. But in countertransference, the nurse's responses are not justified by reality. In this case, nurses identify the patient with individuals from their past, and personal needs interfere with their therapeutic effectiveness.

Countertransference reactions are usually of the following three types:

- Reactions of intense love or caring
- Reactions of intense disgust or hostility
- Reactions of intense anxiety often in response to resistance by the patient

Through the use of immediacy the nurse can identify countertransference in one of its various forms (Box 2-12).

Countertransference occurs because the nurse is involved with the patient as a participant observer and not as a detached bystander. These reactions can be powerful tools for exploring and uncovering inner states. They are destructive only if they are ignored or not taken seriously (Ens, 1998, 1999).

If studied objectively, these reactions can lead to further information about the patient. The ability to remain objective does not mean that the nurse may not at times become irritated or dislike what the patient says. The patient's resistance to acquiring insight and transforming it into action and the refusal to change maladaptive and destructive coping mechanisms can be frustrating. However, the nurse's ability to understand these feelings helps to maintain a working relationship with the patient.

Countertransference also can be a group phenomenon. Psychiatric staff members can become involved in countertransference reactions when they over-react to a patient's aggressive behavior, ignore available patient data that would promote understanding, or become locked in a power struggle with a patient. Other types of countertransference might include ignoring patient behavior that does not fit the staff's diagnosis, minimizing a patient's behavior, joking about or criticizing a patient, or becoming caught up in intimidation.

The experienced nurse is constantly on the lookout for countertransference, becomes aware of it when it occurs, and works with it to promote the therapeutic goals. In identifying a countertransference, the nurse applies the same standards of honest self-appraisal personally that are expected of the patient. The nurse should use self-examination throughout the course of the relationship, particularly when the patient attacks or criticizes. The following questions may be helpful:

- How do I feel about the patient?
- Do I look forward to seeing the patient?
- Do I feel sorry for or sympathetic toward the patient?
- Am I bored with the patient and believe that we are not progressing?
- Am I afraid of the patient?
- Do I get extreme pleasure out of seeing the patient?
- Do I want to protect, reject, or punish the patient?
- Do I dread meeting the patient and feel nervous during the sessions?
- Am I impressed by or try to impress the patient?
- Does the patient make me very angry or frustrated?

If any of these questions suggests a problem, the nurse should pursue it. What is the patient doing to provoke these feelings? Who does the patient remind me of? The nurse must discover the source of the problem. Because countertransference can be harmful to the relationship, it should be dealt with as soon as possible. When it is recognized, the nurse can exercise control over it. If the nurse needs help in dealing with countertransference, individual or group supervision can be most helpful.

Problem Patients. Countertransference problems are most evident when a patient is labeled a "problem or difficult patient." Usually such a patient elicits strong negative feelings such as anger, fear, and helplessness and is often described by nurses as manipulative, dependent, inappropriate, and demanding. The label **problem patient** implies that the patient's behavior should change for the sake of the helper rather than for the patient's own benefit. This labeling often causes the patient and nurse to become adversaries, and the nurse avoids contact.

It is more productive for a nurse to view a "problem patient" as one who poses problems for the nurse. This turns the responsibility for action back onto the nurse (see Citing the Evidence). It forces the nurse to explore responses to the patient that reinforce the patient's unproductive behavior. In this way the nurse also makes patients responsible for their behavior. By stepping back and reviewing again the patient's needs and problems, the nurse can become aware of failing to use the responsive dimensions of genuineness, respect, empathic understanding, and concreteness. Without this groundwork, a therapeutic outcome is impossible.

Boundary Violations

A final but very important therapeutic impasse is that of boundary violations. These occur when a nurse goes outside the boundaries of the therapeutic relationship and establishes a social, economic, or personal relationship with a patient. As a general rule, whenever the nurse is doing or thinking of doing something special, different, or unusual for a patient, often a boundary violation is involved. A nurse should consider the possibility of a boundary violation if he or she encounters the following:

- Receives feedback that his or her behavior is intrusive with patients or their families
- Has difficulty setting limits with a patient
- Relates to a patient like a friend or family member
- Has sexual feelings toward a patient
- Feels that he or she is the only one who understands the patient
- Receives feedback that he or she is too involved with a patient or family
- Feels that other staff are too critical of a particular patient

---

Citing the Evidence on

Problem Patients

BACKGROUND: Although there is increasing recognition of the existence of "difficult" patients who present particular challenges to mental health nurses, no research has been conducted into their perceptions of services and their experience of care. This study had three aims: first to identify people currently using services who mental health nurses defined as "difficult," second to explore the experiences of these patients, and third to develop an understanding of the "difficult" nurse-patient relationship, which might suggest a therapeutic approach acceptable to both parties.

RESULTS: "Difficult" patients were found to be those who challenged nurses' competence and control. Despite their different roles, both nurses and "difficult" patients were aware of the struggle to gain or retain a notion of control. Feelings of anger were reduced where nurses were perceived to demonstrate respect, time, skilled care, and a willingness to give patients some control and choice in their own care.

IMPLICATIONS: The external validity of the study is limited by the small sample size. Nonetheless, study findings suggest that "difficult" patients engender feelings of powerlessness in the nurse. In return, the nurse increases control over the patient and engages in a struggle with him or her. Skills that need to be present in order for nurses to empower patients are trust, knowledge, concern, communication, caring, respect, and courtesy. It is suggested that control is linked to the concept of "power over," whereas competence can be seen as "power to." Psychiatric nurses need to minimize the former and maximize the latter.

Breeze J, Repper J: Struggling for control: the care experiences of "difficult" patients in mental health services, *J Adv Nurs* 28:1301, 1998.

Box **2-13**

Possible Boundary Violations Related to Psychiatric Nurses

- The patient takes the nurse out to lunch or dinner
- The professional relationship turns into a social relationship
- The nurse attends a party at a patient's invitation
- The nurse regularly reveals personal information to the patient
- The patient introduces the nurse to family members, such as a son or daughter, for the purpose of a social relationship
- The nurse accepts free gifts from the patient's business
- The nurse agrees to meet the patient for treatment outside of the usual setting without therapeutic justification
- The nurse attends social functions of the patient
- The patient gives the nurse an expensive gift
- The nurse routinely hugs or has physical contact with the patient
- The nurse does business with or purchases services from the patient

- Believes that other staff members are jealous of his or her relationship with a patient

Specific examples of possible boundary violations are listed in Box 2-13.

Boundary violations can occur in the following categories (Gallop, 1998; Gutheil & Gabbard, 1993; Reid, 1999; Simon, 1999; Simon & Williams, 1999):

- **Role boundaries:** These are related to the psychiatric nurse's role. They are reflected in the question, Is this what a professional psychiatric nurse does? Problems with role boundaries require the insight of the nurse and the setting of firm therapeutic limits with the patient.
- **Time boundaries:** These relate to the time of day that the nurse implements treatment. Odd and unusual treatment hours that have no therapeutic necessity must be evaluated as potential boundary violations.
- **Place and space boundaries:** These are related to where treatment takes place. An office or hospital unit is the usual locale for most treatment. Treatment out of the office usually merits special scrutiny. Most often treatment over lunch, in the car, or in the patient's home must have a good therapeutic rationale and explicit treatment goals. In an inpatient setting, any time spent by a nurse in a patient's room should be done so only if indicated and with appropriate action taken to respect boundary concerns, such as with the door open and in the presence of other staff.
- **Money boundaries:** These relate to evaluating the compensation for treatment between the nurse and patient. Bartering or seeing an indigent patient for free should be carefully reviewed for potential boundary violations.
- **Gifts and services boundaries:** Gift giving is a controversial issue in nursing (see Critical Thinking about Contemporary Issues). Gifts that are obvious boundary violations place undue obligations on the patient for the

benefit of the nurse. Gifts can be divided into the following five types (Morse, 1991):
  - Gifts to reciprocate for care given
  - Gifts intended to manipulate or change the quality of care given or the nature of the nurse-patient relationship
  - Gifts given as perceived obligation by the patient
  - Serendipitous gifts or gifts received by chance
  - Gifts given to the organization to recognize excellence of care received
- **Clothing boundaries:** These pertain to the nurse's need to dress in an appropriate therapeutic manner. Suggestive or seductive clothing of the nurse is unacceptable, and limits should be set on inappropriate dress by patients as well.
- **Language boundaries:** This boundary raises questions of when patients should be addressed by their first or last names, the tone that the nurse uses when talking with the patient, and the nurse's choice of words in implementing care. Too familiar, sexual, off-color, or leading language constitutes a boundary violation.
- **Self-disclosure boundaries:** Inappropriately timed self-disclosure by the nurse and nurse self-disclosure that lacks therapeutic value are suspect for boundary violations, as discussed previously in this chapter.
- **Postdischarge social boundaries:** Postdischarge social contact with a patient by the nurse always raises questions of boundary violation. Such contacts confuse social support from professional support, can place the patient at risk, and disregards the basic tenets of the professional role.
- **Physical contact boundaries:** All physical contact with a patient must be evaluated for possible boundary violations. Sexual contact of any kind is **never therapeutic** and **never acceptable** within the nurse-patient relationship.

The nurse must carefully consider how to respond to each of these categories based on the possibility of boundary violations. Clinical supervision can be helpful in anticipating and heading off possible boundary violations (Walker & Clark, 1999).

What unique situations and customs may complicate the task of maintaining treatment boundaries in small communities and rural areas? How should they be handled?

THERAPEUTIC OUTCOME

The nurse's effectiveness in working with psychiatric patients is related to knowledge base, clinical skills, and capacity for introspection and self-evaluation. The nurse and patient, as participants in an interpersonal relationship, are entwined in a pattern of reciprocal emotions that directly affect the therapeutic outcome. The nurse conveys feelings to the patient. Some of these are in response to the patient; others arise from the nurse's personal life and are not necessarily associated with the patient.

Many painful feelings arise within the nurse because of the nature of the therapeutic process, which can be stressful. These

CRITICAL THINKING about **CONTEMPORARY ISSUES**

Is Gift Giving Acceptable Behavior in the Therapeutic Nurse-Patient Relationship?

Gift giving is a controversial issue in nursing. There has been a long-accepted taboo in nursing on accepting gifts from patients. On the other hand, some have questioned the theoretical rationale for this position and suggest that gift giving can sometimes serve discrete therapeutic purposes (Morse, 1991).

Gifts can take many forms. They can be tangible or intangible, lasting or temporary. Tangible gifts may include such items as a box of candy, a bouquet of flowers, a hand-knit scarf, or a hand-painted picture. Intangible gifts can be the expression of thanks to a nurse by a patient who is about to be discharged or a family member's sense of relief and gratitude at being able to share an emotional burden with another caring person. The underlying element of all of these gifts is that something of value is voluntarily offered to another person, usually to convey gratitude.

Because gifts can be so varied, it is inappropriate to lump them all together in deciding upon a nursing action. Rather, the nurse's response to gift giving and the role it plays in the therapeutic relationship depends on the timing of the particular situation, the intent of the giver, and the meaning of the giving of the gift. Occasionally it may be most appropriate and therapeutic for the nurse to accept a patient's gift; on other occasions it may be quite inappropriate and detrimental to the relationship.

The timing of the gift giving is an important consideration. In the introductory, or orientation, phase of the relationship, nurses may be asked, "Do you have a cigarette I can borrow?" or "Will you buy me a cup of coffee?" These seemingly minor requests may make the nurse feel uncomfortable refusing them. The nurse may rationalize compliance by thinking that it indicates interest in the patient and may help win his or her trust. However, these responses indicate the nurse's failure to examine the patient's underlying need and the nurse's own needs in complying with it.

Also, in this early phase of the relationship, the nurse may be the one to initiate gift giving by giving the patient a book, plant, or some other item that expresses interest in the patient.

In the orientation phase of the relationship, gift giving can be harmful if it meets personal needs rather than therapeutic goals. By giving a gift, the patient may be trying to manipulate the nurse and control the relationship. In contrast, by giving gifts to the patient, the nurse may be attempting to relate through objects instead of the therapeutic use of self and to avoid exploring possible feelings of inadequacy or frustration.

As the relationship progresses, gift giving may take on a different significance. In the working phase, for example, the patient may one day offer to buy the nurse a cup of coffee. This can be a sign of the patient's respect for the nurse and of belief in their work together. As an isolated incident, the nurse's acceptance of it can enhance the patient's confidence, self-esteem, and sense of responsibility.

Gift giving most often arises in the termination phase of the relationship, and it is in this phase that the meaning behind it can be the most complex and difficult to determine. At this time, gift giving can be tangible or intangible and can reflect a patient's need to make the nurse feel guilty, delay the termination process, compensate for feelings of inadequacy, or attempt to transform the therapeutic nurse-patient relationship into a social one that can possibly go on indefinitely. The nurse can initiate gift giving for similar reasons. The feelings evoked during the termination process can be very powerful, and they must be acknowledged and explored if termination is to be a learning experience for both participants. If feelings are identified and clarified, then a small gift that reflects gratitude and remembrance can be exchanged, accepted, and valued.

"normal" stresses are caused by a variety of factors. Although it is necessary to be a skilled listener, it is inappropriate for the nurse to discuss personal conflicts or responses, except when they may help the patient. This bottling up of emotions can be painful. The nurse is expected to empathize with the patient's emotions and feelings. At the same time, however, the nurse is expected to retain objectivity and not be caught up in a sympathetic response. This can create a kind of double bind.

Termination poses another stress when the nurse must separate from a patient she or he has come to know well and care for deeply. It is common to experience a grief reaction in response to the loss. Many nurses find it emotionally draining when a patient communicates a prolonged and intense expression of emotion, such as sadness, despair, or anger. Discomfort also arises when the nurse feels unable to help a patient who is in great distress. Suicide dramatizes this situation. Treating suicidal individuals can arouse intense and prolonged anxiety in the nurse.

The painful nature of these emotional responses makes the practice of psychiatric nursing challenging and stressful. The therapeutic use of self involves the nurse's total person-ality, and total involvement is not an easy task. It is essential that the nurse be aware of personal feelings and responses and receive guidance and support.

Summary

1. The therapeutic nurse-patient relationship is a mutual learning experience and a corrective emotional experience for the patient. The nurse uses personal attributes and specified clinical techniques in working with the patient to bring about behavioral change.

2. The qualities needed by nurses to be effective helpers include awareness of self, clarification of values, exploration of feelings, ability to serve as a role model, altruism, and a sense of ethics and responsibility.

3. The structural and transactional analysis models were used to examine components of the communication process and to identify common problems. Helpful therapeutic communication techniques also were discussed.

4. The responsive dimensions of genuineness, respect, empathic understanding, and concreteness were presented.

5. The action dimensions of confrontation, immediacy, nurse self-disclosure, catharsis, and role playing stimulate and contribute to patient insight.
6. Therapeutic impasses such as resistance, transference, countertransference, and boundary violations are roadblocks in the progress of the nurse-patient relationship.
7. The therapeutic outcome in working with psychiatric patients is related to the nurse's knowledge base, clinical skills, and capacity for introspection and self-evaluation.

MeRLiN Visit **MERLIN: www.mosby.com/MERLIN/Stuart** to find these additional materials and student activities.

- **Worksheets**
- **"Drug of the Month" Updates**
- **"Citing the Evidence" Updates**
- **Critical Thinking Activities and Exercises**
- **Annotated Suggested Readings**
- **Web Links**
- **More!**

Chapter Review Questions

1. **For each of the activities described below, select the correct phase of the therapeutic relationship.**

Orientation   Termination
Preinteraction   Working

A. _____ Analyze own feelings and fears
B. _____ Define goals with the patient
C. _____ Determine why the patient sought help
D. _____ Explore feelings of loss and separation
E. _____ Evaluate patient stressors
F. _____ Formulate a contract
G. _____ Gather data about the patient
H. _____ Overcome resistance
I. _____ Promote insight and behavioral change
J. _____ Review goal attainment

2. **Fill in the blanks.**

A. When a person sends double messages or verbal and nonverbal messages that do not agree, it is called _____ communication.
B. Reflection of the content of a patient's communication back to him is called _____.
C. The responsive dimension of _____ is the ability to see the patient's world from her point of view and to communicate this to the patient.
D. A _____ occurs when a nurse goes outside the limits of the therapeutic relationship and establishes a social, economic, or personal relationship with a patient.

3. **Provide short answers for the following questions.**

A. Identify four guidelines that should be used to evaluate the potential usefulness of nurse self-disclosure.
B. List elements that should be included in a nurse-patient contract.
C. Describe how the items listed below apply to a social and a therapeutic relationship.
   Use of feelings
       Social _____
       Therapeutic _____
   Content of interaction
       Social _____
       Therapeutic _____
   Confidentiality
       Social _____
       Therapeutic _____
   Termination
       Social _____
       Therapeutic _____
D. Think of a patient you recently cared for as a nurse. Evaluate how well you demonstrated each of the responsive dimensions of the therapeutic nurse-patient relationship described in this chapter.
E. Have you observed any boundary violations among your nursing colleagues? If so, have you talked with them about it? If not, why not?

4. Match the terms in Column A with the correct example in Column B.

Column A	Column B
____Altruism	**A.** Dependency by a patient on the nurse for getting better and coping with life.
____Catharsis	**B.** Encouraging a patient to talk about her feelings related to her brother's death.
____Confrontation	**C.** Having the patient assume the part of her husband when talking with the nurse about her marital problems.
____Countertransference	**D.** Irritation and disgust evidenced by a nurse toward a patient who is not responding to the treatment plan.
____Resistance	**E.** Refusal by a patient to discuss early events as they relate to her current depression.
____Role playing	**F.** Sharing the observation with a patient that he asks to be treated as a responsible adult but he has not been able to keep his last three jobs longer than a month.
____Transference	**G.** Volunteering to prepare and serve meals at a local homeless shelter.

REFERENCES

Alligood M: Empathy: the importance of recognizing two types, *J Psychosoc Nurs* 30:14, 1992.

Berne E: *Games people play: the psychology of human relationships,* New York, 1964, Grove Press.

Bohart A, Greenberg L: *Empathy reconsidered,* Washington DC, 1997, American Psychological Association.

Campbell J: The relationship of nursing and self-awareness, *Adv Nurs Sci* 2:15, 1980.

Carkhoff R: *Helping and human relations,* vols 1 and 2, New York, 1969, Holt, Rinehart & Winston.

Carkhoff R, Berenson B: *Beyond counseling and therapy,* New York, 1967, Holt, Rinehart & Winston.

Carkhoff R, Truax C: *Toward effective counseling and psychotherapy,* Chicago, 1967, Aldine Publishing.

Connors G et al: The therapeutic alliance and its relationship to alcoholism treatment participation and outcome, *J Consul Clinic Psychol,* 65:588, 1997.

Deering C: To speak or not to speak: self-disclosure with patients, *Am J Nurs* 99:34, 1999.

Ens I: An analysis of the concept of countertransference, *Archives Psych Nurs* 12:273, 1998.

Ens I: The lived experience of countertransference in psychiatric/mental health nurses, *Arch Psych Nurs* 13:321, 1999.

Forchuk C: Development of nurse-client relationships: what helps?, *J Am Psych Nurs Assoc* 1:146, 1995.

Gallop R: Postdischarge social contact: a potential area for boundary violation, *J Am Psychiatr Nurses Assoc* 4:105, 1998.

Guthiel T, Gabbard G: The concept of boundaries in clinical practice: theoretical and risk-management dimensions, *Am J Psychiatry* 150:188, 1993.

Holyoake D: Observing nurse-patient interaction, *Nurs Standard* 12:35, 1998.

Hupcey J, Morse J: Can a professional relationship be considered social support? *Nurs Outlook* 45:270, 1997.

Jourard S: *The transparent self,* New York, 1971, Litton Educational Publishing.

Kalisch B: What is empathy? *Am J Nurs* 73:1548, 1973.

Kirschenbaum H, Simon S, editors: *Readings in values clarification,* Minneapolis, 1973, Winston Press.

Krupnick J et al: The role of the therapeutic alliance in psychotherapy and pharmacotherapy outcome, *J Consult Clin Psychol* 64:532, 1996.

MacCulloch T: Emotional competence in professional communication, *Austral N Zealand J Mental Health Nurs* 7:60, 1998.

Mansfield E: Empathy: concept and identified psychiatric nursing behavior, *Nurs Res* 22:525, 1973.

McAllister M: The nurse as a tour guide: a metaphor for debriefing students in mental health nursing, *Issues Ment Health Nurs* 16:395, 1995.

Morse J: The structure and function of gift giving in the patient-nurse relationship, *West J Nurs Res* 13:597, 1991.

Muller A, Poggenpoel M: Patients' internal world experiences of interacting with psychiatric nurses, *Arch Psychiatr Nurs* 10:143, 1996.

Nichols M: *The lost art of listening,* New York, 1995, The Guilford Press.

Olson J: Relationships between nurse-expressed empathy, patient-perceived empathy and patient distress, *Image* 27:317, 1995.

Oquendo M: Psychiatric evaluation and psychotherapy in the patient's second language, *Psychiatr Serv* 47:614, 1996.

Reid W: Boundary issues and violations, *J Prac Psych Behav Health* 4:173, 1999.

Rogers C: *On becoming a person,* Boston, 1961, Houghton Mifflin.

Rogers C: Empathic: an unappreciated way of being, *J Counsel Psychol* 5:2, 1975.

Saunders S: Clients' assessment of the affective environment of the psychotherapy session: relationship to session quality and treatment effectiveness, *J Clin Psychol* 55:597, 1999.

Simon R: Therapist-patient sex, *Psych Clinics North America* 22:31, 1999.

Simon R, Williams I: Maintaining treatment boundaries in small communities and rural areas, *Psychiatric Services* 50:1440, 1999.

Smith E et al: *Touch in psychotherapy: theory, research and practice,* New York, 1997, Guilford Press.

Sundeen S et al: *Nurse-client interaction: implementing the nursing process,* ed 6, St Louis, 1998, Mosby.

Walker R, Clark J: Heading off boundary problems: clinical supervision as risk management, *Psychiatric Services* 50:1435, 1999.

Wolberg L: *The technique of psychotherapy,* ed 4, Orlando, Fla, 1988, Grune & Stratton.

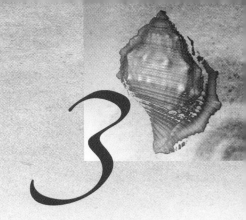

Visit **MERLIN** for *Your Internet Connection*
to websites that are related to the content in this chapter.
www.mosby.com/MERLIN/Stuart

Conceptual Models of Psychiatric Treatment

Gail W. Stuart

Though this be madness, yet there is method in't.

WILLIAM SHAKESPEARE *HAMLET,* ACT II

Mental health professionals should base their practice on a conceptual model of psychiatric treatment. A model is a way of organizing a complex body of knowledge, such as concepts related to human behavior. Models help clinicians by suggesting:

- Reasons for observed behavior
- Therapeutic treatment strategies
- Appropriate roles for patient and therapist

Models also provide for the organization of data. Organization allows the clinician to measure the effectiveness of the treatment process and facilitates research into human behavior.

This chapter presents an overview of some of the conceptual models used by mental health professionals, including the psychoanalytical, interpersonal, social, existential, supportive, and medical models. Other models often used by nurses are discussed in other chapters of this text including cognitive behavioral (Chapter 32, group (Chapter 33), and family (Chapter 34). Finally, the Stuart Stress Adaptation Model of psychiatric nursing, which is the organizing conceptual framework for this text, is presented in detail in Chapter 4.

PSYCHOANALYTICAL MODEL

Psychoanalytical theory was developed by Sigmund Freud (Fig. 3-1) in the late nineteenth and early twentieth centuries (1974). It focused on the nature of deviant behavior and proposed a new perspective on human development. Many of Freud's ideas were controversial, particularly in the Victorian society of that time. Objective observation of human behavior was a great contribution of the psychoanalysts, as was the identification of a mental structure. Such concepts as id, ego, superego, and ego defense mechanisms are still widely used. Most people also accept the existence of an unconscious level of mental functioning, first introduced by Freud.

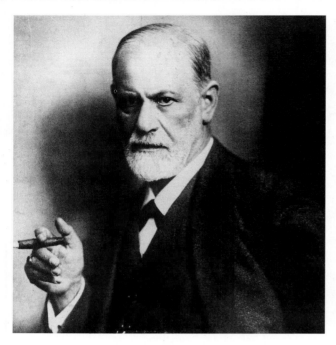

Fig. 3-1 Sigmund Freud. (From the Bettman Archive.)

View of Behavioral Deviations

Psychoanalysts trace disrupted behavior in the adult to earlier developmental stages. Each stage of development has a task that must be accomplished. If too much emphasis is placed on any stage or if unusual difficulty arises in dealing with the associated conflicts, psychological energy (libido) becomes fixated in an attempt to deal with anxiety.

Psychoanalysts believe that neurotic symptoms arise when so much energy goes into controlling anxiety that it interferes with the individual's ability to function. They believe that everyone is neurotic to some extent. Everyone carries the burden of childhood conflicts and is influenced in adulthood by childhood experiences. Psychoanalysts in training must undergo personal analysis so that their own neurotic behavior does not hinder their objectivity as therapists.

According to psychoanalytic theory, symptoms are symbols of the original conflict. For instance, compulsive hand washing may represent the person's attempt to cleanse the self of impulses that a parent labeled unclean during the anal stage of development. However, the meaning of the behavior is hidden from the conscious awareness of the person, who usually is upset about these uncontrollable feelings.

Freud developed most of his theories around neurotic symptoms. His theory is less well developed in the area of psychosis. However, other psychoanalytical theorists such as Frieda Fromm-Reichmann (1950) have successfully worked with patients with psychosis. They believe that the psychotic symptom arises when the ego must invest most or all of the libido to defend against primitive id impulses. This leaves little energy to deal with external reality and leads to the lack of reality testing seen in psychosis.

Psychoanalytical Therapeutic Process

Psychoanalysis uses free association and dream analysis to reconstruct the personality. Free association is the verbaliza-

tion of thoughts while they occur, without any conscious screening or censorship. Of course, there is always unconscious censorship of thoughts and impulses that threaten the ego. The psychoanalyst searches for patterns in the areas that are unconsciously avoided. Conflicting areas that the patient does not discuss or recognize are identified as resistances. Analysis of the patient's dreams can provide additional insight into the nature of the resistances because dreams symbolically communicate areas of intrapsychic conflict.

The therapist helps the patient recognize intrapsychic conflicts by using interpretation. Interpretation involves explaining to the patient the meaning of dream symbolism and the significance of the issues that are discussed or avoided. However, the process is complicated by transference, which occurs when the patient develops strong positive or negative feelings toward the analyst. These feelings are unrelated to the analyst's current behavior or characteristics; they represent the patient's past response to a significant other, usually a parent. Strong positive transference causes the patient to want to please the therapist and to accept the therapist's interpretations of the patient's behavior. Strong negative transference may impede the progress of therapy as the patient actively resists the therapist's interventions. Countertransference, or the therapist's response to the patient, can also interfere with therapy if the analyst is unaware of it or unable to deal with it.

Because the therapist can temporarily replace the significant other of the patient's early life, previously unresolved conflicts can be brought into the therapeutic situation. These conflicts can be worked through to a healthier resolution and more mature adult functioning. Psychoanalytical therapy is usually long term. The patient is often seen five times a week for several years. This approach is therefore time consuming and expensive.

Roles of Patient and Psychoanalyst

The roles of the patient and the psychoanalyst were defined by Freud. The patient was to be an active participant, freely revealing all thoughts exactly as they occurred and describing all dreams. The patient often lies down during therapy to induce relaxation, which facilitates free association.

The psychoanalyst is a shadow person. The patient is expected to reveal all private thoughts and feelings, and the analyst reveals nothing personal. The analyst usually is out of the patient's sight, to ensure that nonverbal responses do not influence the patient. The analyst keeps his or her verbal responses brief and noncommittal in order to prevent interference with the associative flow. For instance, the analyst might respond with "Uh huh," "Go on," or "Tell me more."

The therapist changes this communication style when interpreting behavior. Interpretations are presented for the patient to accept or reject, but rejections suggest resistance. Likewise, frustration that the patient expresses toward the analyst is interpreted as transference. By the end of therapy, the patient should be able to view the analyst realistically, having worked through conflicts and dependency needs.

❓ Do you think that the roles of the patient and psychoanalyst support patient empowerment or patient dependency?

Box **3-1**

Contemporary Psychoanalytical Theorists

ERIK ERIKSON (1963): Expanded Freud's theory of psychosocial development to encompass the entire life cycle

ANNA FREUD (1966): Expanded psychoanalytical theory in the area of child psychology

MELANIE KLEIN (1949): Extended the use of psychoanalytical techniques to work with young children through development of play therapy

KAREN HORNEY (1950): Focused on psychoanalytical theory in terms of cultural and interpersonal factors; rejected Freud's view of feminine sexuality

FRIEDA FROMM-REICHMANN (1950): Used psychoanalytical techniques with psychotic patients

KARL MENNINGER (1963): Applied the concepts of dynamic equilibrium and coping to mental functioning

Other Psychoanalytical Theorists

Much of Freud's theory is still used by psychotherapists. The theorists who followed him have modified and built on the original psychoanalytical theories.

Box 3-1 lists several contemporary psychoanalytical theorists and a brief statement identifying their major contributions.

INTERPERSONAL MODEL

Interpersonal therapy has been found to be an effective form of treatment for patients with a wide variety of psychiatric disorders (see Citing the Evidence). The theorist who originated the interpersonal model is Harry Stack Sullivan, a twentieth-century American therapist (1953, 1954). Since then it has been further developed and refined by Gerald Klerman (1993). Attention is also given to the interpersonal nursing theory of Hildegard Peplau (1952) (Fig. 3-2). Her work on the psychotherapeutic role of the nurse in the interpersonal relationship is a milestone in the field.

The goal of interpersonal therapy is to reduce symptoms, improve social functioning, and assist the person in developing more adaptive ways of relating to others. It is particularly effective in issues related to grief, role disputes, role transitions, and interpersonal deficits.

View of Behavioral Deviations

Interpersonal theorists believe that behavior evolves around interpersonal relationships. Whereas Freudian theory emphasizes a person's intrapsychic experience, interpersonal theory emphasizes social or interpersonal experience (Evans, 1996). Sullivan, like Freud, traces a progression of psychological development. Sullivan's theory states that the person bases behavior on two drives: the drive for satisfaction and the drive for security. Satisfaction includes the basic human drives of hunger, sleep, lust, and loneliness. Security relates

Citing the Evidence on

Interpersonal Therapy

BACKGROUND: It is known that a small number of patients with mental health problems have chronic disorders and account for a disproportionate amount of mental health costs. This randomized controlled trial evaluated the cost-effectiveness of interpersonal therapy versus usual care by psychiatrists in patients with mental health problems who were unresponsive to usual treatment.

RESULTS: Subjects randomized to interpersonal therapy had a significantly greater improvement than controls in psychological distress and social functioning 6 months after the trial. Baseline costs were similar for both groups. Interpersonal therapy subjects showed significant reductions in the cost of health care use in the 6 months after treatment compared with controls.

IMPLICATIONS: Clinicians need to carefully evaluate the type of treatment they provide as "usual care." They should use validated treatment approaches whenever possible to provide the highest quality of care and to maximize the health outcomes of their patients.

Guthrie E et al: Cost-effectiveness of brief psychodynamic-interpersonal therapy in high utilizers of psychiatric services, *Arch Gen Psychiatry* 56:519, 1999.

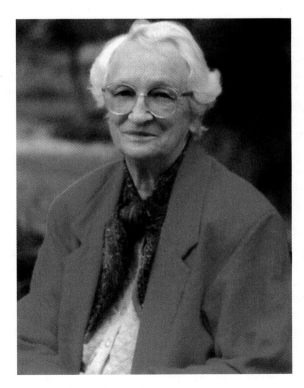

Fig. 3-2 Hildegard E. Peplau. (Courtesy Hildegard E. Peplau.)

to culturally defined needs such as conformity to the social norms and value system of the individual's reference group. Sullivan states that when a person's self-system interferes with the ability to meet the need for satisfaction or security, the person becomes mentally ill.

When Peplau defined nursing as an interpersonal process, she also discussed the importance of basic human needs. Needs must be met if a healthy state is to be achieved and maintained. For Peplau, the two interacting components of health are physiological demands and interpersonal conditions. These components may be seen as parallel to the drives of satisfaction and security identified by Sullivan, as is evident in the following clinical example.

 ## CLINICAL EXAMPLE

Ms. Y, an attractive 26-year-old woman, appeared at a psychiatric outpatient clinic requesting therapy. She said, "I can't get close to people." She said that her childhood was happy and that she had loving parents and liked her sister. Her family was devout members of a fundamentalist Protestant church, so most of her activities were church related. She had many friends during childhood and then one close girlfriend in early adolescence. She thought that her fear of closeness began when she slept over at her friend's house. During the night her friend began to fondle her in a way that she interpreted as sexual. She became very frightened and felt guilty. She did not tell her parents because of her feelings of guilt and, in fact, had told no one before entering therapy. Although she attended college, she never dated and participated only in superficial social contacts. She realized that this was not healthy young adult behavior and, because the behavior continued into her twenties, Ms. Y decided to seek help.

From an interpersonal perspective, Ms. Y was unable to fulfill her needs for friendship and sexual love. Interpersonal theorists would view the unfulfilled sexual love dynamism as a lack of satisfaction, and her fear that she had deviated from the norm as a lack of security. Her anxiety stemmed from her conviction that her parents would disown her if they heard what had happened. This belief was based on their earlier responses to childhood sexual play. The therapist decided that Ms. Y first needed to experience intimacy on a nonsexual level. This need was approached in therapy. After Ms. Y began to feel comfortable sharing closeness with the therapist, she gradually explored friendships and later began dating.

Interpersonal Therapeutic Process

The interpersonal therapist focuses on the "here and now," uses exploratory and behavioral change techniques, and encourages the expression of affect. The crux of the therapeutic process is the corrective interpersonal experience. The idea is that by experiencing a healthy relationship with the therapist, the patient can learn to have more satisfying interpersonal relationships. The therapist actively encourages the development of trust by relating authentically to the patient and sharing feelings and reactions with the patient. The process of therapy is a process of reeducation.

The therapist helps the patient identify interpersonal problems and then encourages attempts at more successful styles of relating. For example, patients often have a fear of intimacy. The therapist allows the patient to become close while showing him or her that there is no threat of sexual involvement. It is believed that closeness within the therapeutic relationship builds trust, facilitates empathy, enhances self-esteem, and fosters growth toward healthy behavior. Peplau describes this process as "psychological mothering," which includes the following steps:

1. The patient is accepted unconditionally as a participant in a relationship that satisfies needs.
2. There is recognition of and response to the patient's readiness for growth, as initiated by the patient.
3. Power in the relationship shifts to the patient, as the patient is able to delay gratification and to invest energy in goal achievement.

Therapy is complete when the patient can establish satisfying human relationships, thereby meeting basic needs. Termination is a significant part of the relationship that must be shared by the therapist and the patient. The patient learns that leaving a significant other involves pain but can also be an opportunity for growth.

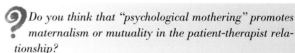
Do you think that "psychological mothering" promotes maternalism or mutuality in the patient-therapist relationship?

Roles of Patient and Interpersonal Therapist

The patient-therapist dyad is viewed as a partnership in interpersonal therapy. Sullivan describes the therapist as a "participant observer" whose role is to engage the patient, establish trust, and empathize. There is an active effort to help the patient realize that other people have similar perceptions and concerns. An atmosphere of uncritical acceptance encourages the patient to speak openly. The therapist interacts as a real person who also has beliefs, values, thoughts, and feelings. The patient's role is to share concerns with the therapist and to participate as fully as possible in the relationship. The relationship itself serves as a model of adaptive interpersonal relationships. While the patient matures in the ability to relate, life experiences with people outside the therapeutic situation are enhanced.

Interpersonal nursing roles have been identified by Peplau and are listed in Box 3-2. These roles may be assumed by the nurse or assigned to others. The therapist helps the patient meet the goals of therapy: need satisfaction and personal growth. In addition, through role performance the nurse also experiences growth and self-discovery. Self-awareness is essential to success as an interpersonal therapist.

SOCIAL MODEL

The two preceding models focused on the individual and intrapsychic processes and interpersonal experiences. The

Box 3-2

Interpersonal Nursing Roles Identified by Peplau

Stranger: the role assumed by both nurse and patient when they first meet

Resource person: provides health information to a patient who has assumed the consumer role

Teacher: helps the patient to grow and learn from experience with the health care system

Leader: helps the patient to participate in a democratically implemented nursing process

Surrogate: assumes roles that have been assigned by the patient, based on significant past relationships, as in the psychoanalytical phenomenon of transference

Counselor: helps the patient integrate the facts and feelings associated with an episode of illness into the patient's total life experience

social model moves beyond the individual to consider the social environment as it affects the person and the person's life experience (see Chapter 8). Psychoanalytical theory has been criticized for not extending to other cultures and times. For example, Freud's view of women has been repeatedly challenged, particularly by feminists. Some theorists such as Thomas Szasz (1961, 1987, 1993) and Gerald Caplan (1964) believe that the culture itself is useful in defining mental illness, prescribing therapy, and determining the patient's future. Others contend that the social realm is intrinsic to concepts of mind and mental illness and can complement or correct the prevailing assumptions of purely biological models (Cohen, 2000). In addition, the community mental health movement is an example of a government effort to respond to the philosophy of the social theorists (see Chapter 36).

View of Behavioral Deviations

According to the social theorists, social conditions are largely responsible for deviant behavior. Deviance is culturally defined. Behavior considered normal in one cultural setting may be eccentric in another and psychotic in a third. An example is the African exchange student described in the following clinical example.

 CLINICAL EXAMPLE

Early in the fall semester a black male exchange student from Africa was brought to the psychiatric emergency room. He had been walking around the campus carrying a spear and had been apprehended by the university security patrol. His speech was heavily accented and they could not understand his explanation of his behavior. Later evaluation revealed that in his culture one never went walking at night without a spear to defend against attack by wild beasts or hostile neighboring tribes. He was sent back to his dormitory after being convinced that his spear was not appropriate to the culture of the American college campus.

From this point of view Szasz (1961) writes of the "myth of mental illness." He believes that society must find a way to manage "undesirables," so it labels them as mentally ill. People who are so labeled usually are unable or refuse to conform to social norms, and their behavior usually leads to confinement. If these people then conform to social expectations, they are considered to have recovered and are allowed to return to the community. Confinement performs the dual function of removing deviant members from the community and exerting social control over their behavior.

Szasz believes that people are responsible for their behavior. The person has control over whether to conform to social expectations. Those labeled as mentally ill may be scapegoats, but they participate in the scapegoating process by inviting it or by allowing it to occur. Szasz objects to describing deviant behavior as illness. He believes that illness can occur and that diseases of the body (such as brain tumors) can influence behavior, but that no physiological disruption can be demonstrated to cause most deviancy. He distinguishes between the biological condition that is central to illness and the social role that is the focus of deviance.

Caplan also has studied deviant behavior from a social perspective. He has extended the public health model of primary, secondary, and tertiary prevention to the mental health field. He has focused particularly on primary prevention because much attention has been given to the secondary and tertiary levels. Lack of understanding of the cause of deviant behavior has hindered the development of primary prevention techniques.

Caplan believes that social situations can predispose a person to mental illness. Such situations include poverty, family instability, and inadequate education. Deprivation throughout the life cycle results in limited ability to cope with stress. The person has few environmental supports. The result is a predisposition to maladaptive coping responses.

> *How do you distinguish between social deviance and psychiatric illness? How do your friends and family define them?*

Social Therapeutic Process

Szasz advocates freedom of choice for psychiatric patients. People should be allowed to select their own therapeutic modalities and therapists. This freedom requires a well-informed consumer who can base this decision on knowledge of available modes of therapy (see Critical Thinking about Contemporary Issues). Szasz does not believe in involuntary hospitalization of people with mental illness. He questions whether any psychiatric hospitalization is truly voluntary. Szasz disapproves of the community mental health movement to place mental health care within the reach of every American. He questions government involvement in what he views as a private concern.

Caplan, on the other hand, supports community psychiatry. He sees the mental health professional using consultation to combat societal problems. He believes that future

What Kind of Psychotherapy Works Best, for Whom, under What Circumstances, and at What Cost?

Competition among the various models of psychiatric treatment has tended to distract attention from questions about what model of psychotherapy works best, for what type of patient, under what life conditions, and at what cost. Answering these questions has been difficult, but preliminary work suggests that psychotherapy does help (Consumer Reports, 1995); that it may be possible to predict patients' responses to psychotherapy (Leon et al, 1999) and that psychotherapy can reduce the total costs of care (Gabbard et al, 1997). Evaluating the outcomes of treatment is also a topic of research interest, but studies in this area have proven to be less exact and more subjective because of one or more of the following factors:

- The therapist's evaluation of changes that have occurred
- The patient's report of changes
- Reports from the patient's family and friends
- Comparison of pretreatment and posttreatment behavioral rating scale scores
- Measures of changes in selected symptoms or behaviors

Unfortunately, each of these sources has serious limitations. In addition, these studies often fail to measure other important aspects of treatment, such as the nature of the therapeutic alliance, health belief systems of the patient and therapist, cost of treatment, and impact of treatment on the patient's overall biopsychosocial functioning and quality of life. What is needed is greater specificity about the people and problems for which psychotherapy can provide the greatest benefit, the methodology that would be most useful in providing these data, and comprehensive quantification of the indications for, cost of, and outcomes produced by psychotherapy.

psychiatric patients would benefit indirectly from positive social change.

Roles of Patient and Social Therapist

Szasz believes that a therapist can help the patient only if the patient requests help. The patient initiates therapy and defines the problem to be solved. The patient also has the right to approve or reject the recommended therapeutic intervention. Therapy is successfully completed when the patient is satisfied with the changes in his or her life. The therapist collaborates with the patient to promote change. This change includes making recommendations about possible means of effecting behavioral adjustment, but it does not include any element of coercion, particularly the threat of hospitalization if the patient does not agree with the therapist's recommendations. The therapist's role also may involve protecting the patient from social demands for coercive treatment.

Caplan believes that society has a moral obligation to provide a wide range of therapeutic services covering all three levels of prevention. The patient has a consumer role and selects the appropriate level of help from a wide array of services. Ideally, effective primary preventive services decrease the need for secondary or tertiary care.

According to this model, therapists may be professionals or nonprofessionals with professional consultation. People such as clergy, police, bartenders, and beauticians can be trained to listen and to refer people who need professional help to appropriate resources. The therapist in the social context is not tied to the office but is involved in the community. Activities may include home visits, lectures to community groups, or consultation with other agencies. The rationale for this approach is that the more involved therapists are in the community, the greater the impact on the community's mental health. Community involvement also enhances the therapist's understanding of patients who live in that environment.

 Do you think bartenders and beauticians can be effective therapists? Why or why not?

EXISTENTIAL MODEL

The existential model focuses on the person's experience in the here and now, with much less attention to the person's past than in other theoretical models.

View of Behavioral Deviations

Existentialist theorists believe that behavioral deviations result when one is out of touch with oneself or the environment. This alienation is caused by self-imposed restrictions. The individual is not free to choose from among all alternative behaviors. Deviant behavior often is a way of avoiding more socially acceptable or more responsible behavior.

The person who is self-alienated feels helpless, sad, and lonely. Self-criticism and lack of self-awareness prevent participation in authentic, rewarding relationships with others. Theoretically, the person has many choices in terms of behavior. However, existentialists believe that people tend to avoid being real and instead surrender to the demands of others.

Existential Therapeutic Process

There are several existential therapies, all of which assume that the patient must be able to choose freely from what life has to offer. Although the approaches are somewhat different, the goal is to return the patient to an authentic awareness of being.

The existential therapeutic process focuses on the encounter. The encounter is not merely the meeting of two or more people; it also involves their appreciation of the total existence of each other. Through the encounter the patient is helped to accept and understand personal history, to live fully in the present, and to look forward to the future. Table 3-1 presents an overview of several existential therapies.

Table **3-1**

Overview of Existential Therapies		
Therapy	Therapist	Process
Rational-emotive therapy (RET)	Albert Ellis (1989)	An active-directive, cognitively oriented therapy. Confrontation is used to force patient to assume responsibility for behavior. Patients are encouraged to accept themselves as they are and are taught to try out new behavior.
Logotherapy	Viktor E. Frankl (1959)	A future-oriented therapy. The search for meaning (logos) is viewed as a primary life force. Without a sense of meaning, life becomes an "existential vacuum." The aim of therapy is to help patients assume personal responsibility.
Reality therapy	William Glasser (1965)	Central theme is the need for identity, which is reached by loving, feeling worthwhile, and behaving responsibly. Patients are helped to recognize life goals and ways in which they keep themselves from accomplishing goals.
Gestalt therapy	Frederick S. Perls (1969)	Emphasizes the here and now. The patient is encouraged to identify feelings and become more sensitive to other aspects of existence. Self-awareness is expected to lead to self-acceptance.
Encounter group therapy	Carl Rogers (1951, 1970)	Focuses on establishing intimate interactions in a group setting. Therapy is oriented to the here and now. The patient is expected to assume responsibility for behavior. Feeling is stressed; intellectualization is discouraged.

Roles of Patient and Existential Therapist

Existential theorists emphasize that the therapist and the patient are equal in their common humanity. The therapist acts as a guide to the patient, who has gone astray in the search for authenticity. The therapist is direct in specifying areas where the patient should consider changing, but caring and warmth are also emphasized. The therapist and the patient are to be open and honest. The therapeutic experience is a model for the patient; new behaviors can be tested before risks are taken in daily life.

The patient is expected to assume and accept responsibility for behavior. Dependence on the therapist generally is not encouraged. The patient is treated as an adult. Often, illness is deemphasized. The patient is viewed as a person who is alienated from the self and others but for whom there is hope if he or she trusts the therapist and follows directions. The patient is always active in therapy, working to meet the challenge presented by the therapist.

SUPPORTIVE THERAPY MODEL

Supportive therapy is a newer mode of psychotherapy that is widely used in hospital and community-based psychiatric treatment settings. It differs from other models in that it does not depend on any overriding concept or theory. Instead, it uses many psychodynamic theories to understand how people change. The aims of supportive psychotherapy include the following:

- Promote a supportive patient-therapist relationship
- Enhance patient's strengths, coping skills, and ability to use coping resources
- Reduce the patient's subjective distress and maladaptive coping responses
- Help the patient achieve the greatest independence possible based on the specific psychiatric or physical illness

- Foster the greatest amount of autonomy in treatment decisions with the patient

Controlled studies have shown supportive therapy to be effective in treating schizophrenia, borderline conditions, and affective, anxiety, posttraumatic stress, eating, and substance abuse disorders, as well as the psychological component of many physical illnesses (Rockland, 1993).

View of Behavioral Deviations

Supportive therapists are psychodynamically based, and they describe behavioral deviations as neurotic, borderline, or psychotic. They believe in the concepts of id, ego, and superego and emphasize the important role of psychological defenses in adaptive functioning (Rockland, 1989). Compared with those of other therapists, however, their focus is more behavior oriented. They emphasize current biopsychosocial coping responses and the person's ability to use available coping resources.

Supportive Therapeutic Process

Supportive therapy is an eclectic form of psychotherapy; that is, it is not based on a particular theory of psychopathology. Rather, it can draw as needed from other models and may address different symptoms with different therapeutic methods. Supportive therapy is equally applicable to high-functioning patients in crisis and low-functioning patients with psychosis or persistent mental illness. Its emphasis is on improving behavior and subjective feelings of distress rather than on achieving insight or self-understanding.

Principles of supportive therapy include the following:

- Immediate help to the patient, which may include a variety of treatment modalities
- Family and social support system involvement

- Focus on the present
- Anxiety reduction through supportive measures and medication if necessary
- Clarification and problem solving using a variety of approaches including advice, supportive confrontation, limit setting, education, and environmental change
- Helping the patient to avoid future crises and seek help early when under stress

Roles of Patient and Supportive Therapist

In supportive therapy the therapist plays an active and directive role in helping the patient improve social functioning and coping skills. The setting for supportive therapy should allow for a moderate to high level of activity by both the patient and the therapist. Communication is seen as an active two-way process, and the use of medications or other therapies is encouraged.

The therapist builds a therapeutic alliance with the patient. Expressing empathy, concern, and nonjudgmental acceptance of the patient are important therapist qualities. The therapist supports the patient's healthy adaptive efforts, conveys a willingness to understand, respects the patient as a unique human being, and takes a genuine interest in the patient's life activities and well-being. The therapist regards the patient as a partner in treatment and encourages the patient's autonomy to make treatment and life decisions. In turn, the patient is expected to show a willingness to talk about life events, accept the therapist's supportive role, participate in the therapeutic program, and adhere to the therapeutic structure.

 What aspects of supportive therapy are similar to those of the therapeutic nurse-patient relationship? In what ways are they different?

MEDICAL MODEL

The medical model refers to psychiatric care that is based on the traditional physician-patient relationship. It focuses on the diagnosis of a mental illness, and subsequent treatment is based on this diagnosis. Somatic treatments, including pharmacotherapy and electroconvulsive therapy, are important components of the treatment process. The interpersonal aspect of the medical model varies widely, from intensive insight-oriented intervention to brief sessions involving management of medications.

The medical model dominates much of modern psychiatric care. Other health professionals may be involved in interagency referrals, family assessment, and health teaching, but physicians are seen as the leaders of the team under this model. Elements of other models of care may be used in conjunction with the medical model. For instance, a patient with schizophrenia may be treated with phenothiazine medication. This patient may also be in supportive therapy to develop adaptive social skills.

A positive contribution of the medical model has been the continuous exploration for causes of mental illness using the scientific process. Recently great strides have been made in learning about the functioning of the brain and nervous system (see Chapter 6). This progress has led to greater understanding of the probable physiological components of many behavioral disorders and more effective psychiatric treatment.

What problems might the medical model pose for interdisciplinary collaboration in psychiatric treatment?

View of Behavioral Deviations

The medical model proposes that all mental processes, even the most complex psychological processes, derive from operations of the brain, and deviant behavior is a symptom of a brain disorder (Kandel, 1998). There are several types of brain disorders that could lead to mental illness: loss of nerve cells, excesses or deficits in chemical transmission, abnormal patterns of brain circuitry, problems in the command centers, and disruptions in the movement of messages along nerves. In addition, the medical model proposes that genes, and combinations of genes, exert significant control over behavior.

Currently it is thought that disorders such as bipolar disorder, major depression, and schizophrenia involve an abnormality in the transmission of neural impulses. It is believed that this problem occurs at the synaptic level and involves neurochemicals such as dopamine, serotonin, and norepinephrine (see Chapter 6). Much research into the brain's involvement in emotional response is under way.

Medical Therapeutic Process

The medical process of therapy is well defined and familiar to most patients. The examination of the patient includes the history of the present illness, social history, medical history, review of body systems, physical examination, and mental status examination. Additional data may be collected from significant others, and medical records are reviewed if available. A preliminary diagnosis is then formulated, pending further diagnostic studies and observation of the patient's behavior. This process may take place on an ambulatory or an inpatient basis, depending on the patient's condition.

The diagnosis is classified according to the *Diagnostic and Statistical Manual of Mental Disorders,* fourth edition, text revision (*DSM–IV–TR*) of the American Psychiatric Association (2000). The names of the illnesses are accompanied by a description of diagnostic criteria, associated general medical and psychiatric features, diagrams showing the longitudinal course of the disorder, and specific gender, age, and cultural aspects of each illness. Changes in the manual reflect changes in the medical model of psychiatric care. *DSM-I* was first published in 1952 (Grob, 1991), and *DSM-IV–TR,* published in 2000, is the most up-to-date edition.

After the diagnosis is made, treatment begins. The physician-patient relationship is developed to foster trust in the physician and compliance with the treatment plan. Other health team members may contribute their expertise. Response to treatment is evaluated on the basis of the patient's subjective assessment and the physician's objective observa-

tions of symptomatic behavior. Therapy is terminated when the patient's symptoms have remitted. For instance, most people who experience depression are able to return to their usual lifestyles after a course of medication and supportive therapy. Other patients may require long-term therapy, often including pharmacotherapy and periodic laboratory studies.

Roles of Patient and Medical Therapist

The roles of physician and patient have been well defined by tradition. The physician, as the healer, identifies the patient's illness and formulates a treatment plan. The patient may have some say about the plan, but the physician prescribes the therapy.

The role of the patient involves admitting being ill, which can be a problem in psychiatry. Patients sometimes are not aware of their disturbed behavior and may actively resist treatment. This is not congruent with the medical model. The patient is expected to comply with the treatment program and try to get well. If observable improvement does not occur, caregivers and significant others often suspect that the patient is not trying hard enough. This can be frustrating to a patient who is trying to get well and is disappointed with the lack of progress. The patient may also have difficulty letting people extend care while being self-sufficient.

> *How would each conceptual model described in this chapter view the issue of patient nonadherence to the psychiatric treatment plan?*

Summary

MODEL (MAJOR THEORISTS)	VIEW OF BEHAVIORAL DEVIATION	THERAPEUTIC PROCESS	ROLES OF PATIENT AND THERAPIST
Psychoanalytical (S. Freud, Erikson, A. Freud, Klein, Horney, Fromm-Reichmann, Menninger)	Based on inadequate resolution of developmental conflicts. Ego defenses unable to control anxiety. Symptoms result in effort to deal with anxiety and are related to unresolved conflicts.	Uses techniques of free association and dream analysis. Identifies problem areas through interpretation of patient's resistances and transferences.	Patient verbalizes all thoughts and dreams; considers therapist's interpretations. Therapist remains remote to encourage development of transference and interprets patient's thoughts and dreams.
Interpersonal (Sullivan, Klerman, Peplau)	Anxiety arises and is experienced interpersonally. Basic fear is fear of rejection. Person needs security and satisfaction that result from positive interpersonal relationships.	Relationship between therapist and patient builds feeling of security. Therapist helps patient experience trusting relationship and gain interpersonal satisfaction.	Patient shares anxieties and feelings with therapist. Therapist uses empathy to perceive patient's feelings, and uses relationship as a corrective interpersonal experience.
Social (Szasz, Caplan)	Social and environmental factors create stress, which causes anxiety and symptoms. Unacceptable (deviant) behavior is socially defined.	Patient helped to deal with social system. May use crisis intervention, environmental manipulation, and social supports.	Patient presents problem to therapist, works with therapist, and uses community resources. Therapist explores patient's social system and resources available.
Existential (Perls, Glasser, Ellis, Rogers, Frankl)	Life is meaningful when the person can fully experience and accept the self. The self can be experienced through authentic relationships with other people.	Person aided to experience authenticity in relationships. Therapy often conducted in groups. Patient encouraged to accept self and to assume control of behavior.	Patient participates in meaningful experiences to learn about real self. Therapist helps patient recognize value of self, clarify realities of situation, and explore feelings.
Supportive therapy (Wermon, Rockland)	Problems are a result of biopsychosocial factors. Emphasis on current maladaptive coping responses.	Reality testing and self-esteem-enhancing measures. Social supports are enlisted and adaptive coping responses are reinforced.	Patient actively involved in treatment. Therapist is warm, empathic, and allied with patient.
Medical (Meyer, Kraeplin, Spitzer, Frances)	Behavioral disruptions result from a biological disease process. Symptoms result from a combination of physiological, genetic, environmental, and social factors.	Treatment is related to diagnosis and includes somatic therapies and various interpersonal techniques. Treatment approach adjusted depending on symptomatic response.	Patient complies with prescribed therapy and reports effects of therapy to therapist. Therapist diagnoses illness and prescribes therapeutic approach.

MERLIN Visit MERLIN: **www.mosby.com/MERLIN/Stuart** to find these additional materials and student activities.

- **Worksheets**
- **"Drug of the Month" Updates**
- **"Citing the Evidence" Updates**
- **Critical Thinking Activities and Exercises**
- **Annotated Suggested Readings**
- **Web Links**
- **More!**

Chapter Review Questions

1. Match the theorists in Column A with the model of psychiatric treatment in Column B.

Column A	Column B
____Freud	A. Existential
____Rockland	B. Interpersonal
____Rogers	C. Medical
____Spitzer	D. Psychoanalytical
____Sullivan	E. Social
____Szasz	F. Supportive

2. Fill in the blanks.

A. Psychoanalysts believe that behavior problems in adulthood are caused by _____.

B. _____ is the verbalization of thoughts as they occur without any conscious screening or censorship.

C. Interpersonal theorists believe that behavior problems arise from _____.

D. The drives for _____ and _____ are critical to a person's psychological health according to the interpersonal model.

E. Social theorists believe that deviant behavior is caused by _____.

F. The community mental health movement is an example of the _____ model of psychiatric treatment.

G. Existential theorists believe that behavior problems arise when _____.

H. Encounter groups are an example of therapy from the _____ model of psychiatric treatment.

I. Supportive therapy theorists believe that behavior problems arise from _____.

J. In supportive therapy a therapist plays an _____ role and regards the patient as a _____ in the treatment process.

K. Medical model theorists believe that behavior problems arise from _____.

L. A significant contribution of the medical model has been _____.

M. The classification system used in the medical model to diagnose psychiatric illness is the _____.

3. Provide short answers for the following questions.

A. What purposes do dreams serve in psychoanalysis and how are dreams seen by people today?

B. Describe the six nursing roles identified by Peplau.

C. What model of psychiatric treatment do you think is most culture-bound? Which is the most culture-free? Defend your answer.

D. On a scale of 1 to 5, rank order your preference for the five models of psychiatric treatment described in this chapter. Explain your ranking.

REFERENCES

American Psychiatric Association: *Diagnostic and statistical manual of mental disorders,* Fourth Edition, Text Revision. Washington, DC, American Psychiatric Association, 2000.

Caplan G: *Principles of preventive psychiatry,* New York, 1964, Basic Books.

Cohen C: Overcoming social amnesia: the role of a social perspective in psychiatric research and practice, *Psychiatr Serv* 51(1):72, 2000.

Consumer Reports, p 734, November 1995.

Ellis A: *Inside rational emotive therapy,* San Diego, 1989, Academic Press.

Erikson E: *Childhood and society,* ed 2, New York, 1963, WW Norton.

Evans F: *Harry Stack Sullivan: interpersonal theory and psychotherapy,* New York, 1996, Routledge.

Frankl V: *Man's search for meaning,* New York, 1959, Beacon Press.

Freud A: *The ego and the mechanisms of defense,* New York, 1966, International Universities Press.

Freud S: In Strachey J, editor: *The standard edition of the complete psychological works of Sigmund Freud,* London, 1953-1974, Hogarth Press.

Fromm-Reichmann F: *Principles of intensive psychotherapy,* Chicago, 1950, University of Chicago Press.

Gabbard G et al: The economic impact of psychotherapy: a review, *Am J Psychiatry* 154:147, 1997.

Glasser W: *Reality therapy: a new approach to psychiatry,* New York, 1965, Harper & Row.

Grob G: Origins of DSM-I: a study in appearance and reality, *Am J Psychiatry* 148:421, 1991.

Horney K: *The collected works of Karen Horney,* vols 1 and 2, New York, 1950, WW Norton.

Kandel E: A new intellectual framework for psychiatry, *Am J Psychiatry*, 155(4):457, 1998.

Klein M: *The psychoanalysis of children*, London, 1949, Hogarth Press.

Klerman G, Weissman M: *New applications of interpersonal psychotherapy*, Washington, DC, 1993, American Psychiatric Press.

Leon S et al: Predicting patients' responses to psychotherapy: are some more predictable than others? *J Consult Clin Psychol* 67(5):698, 1999.

Menninger KA: *The vital balance*, New York, 1963, Viking Press.

Peplau HE: *Interpersonal relations in nursing*, New York, 1952, GP Putnam.

Perls FS: *In and out of the garbage pail*, Lafayette, Calif, 1969, Real People Press.

Rockland L: *Supportive therapy: a psychodynamic approach*, New York, 1989, Basic Books.

Rockland L: A review of supportive psychotherapy, 1986-1992, *Hosp Community Psychiatry* 44:1053, 1993.

Rogers CR: *Client-centered therapy*, Boston, 1951, Houghton Mifflin.

Rogers CR: *Carl Rogers on encounter groups*, New York, 1970, Harper & Row.

Sullivan HS: *The interpersonal theory of psychiatry*, New York, 1953, WW Norton.

Sullivan HS: *The psychiatric interview*, New York, 1954, WW Norton.

Szasz T: *The myth of mental illness*, New York, 1961, Hoeber-Harper.

Szasz T: *Insanity: the idea and its consequences*, New York, 1987, Wiley.

Szasz T: *A lexicon of lunacy*, New Brunswick, NJ, 1993, Transactional Publishers.

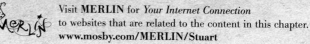

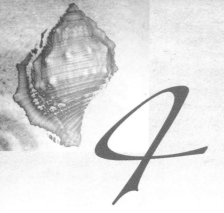

The Stuart Stress Adaptation Model of Psychiatric Nursing Care

Gail W. Stuart

Much madness is Divinest Sense—To a discerning eye.
EMILY DICKINSON

Models serve many purposes. They can help clarify relationships, generate hypotheses, and give perspective to an abstract idea. They also can provide a structure for thinking, observing, and interpreting what is seen. Conceptual nursing models are frames of reference within which patients, their environments and health states, and nursing activities are described. They explain in general terms why individuals respond to stress as they do and help to provide an understanding of the process and desired outcomes of nursing interventions. Psychiatric nurses can enhance their practice if their actions are based on a model of psychiatric nursing care that is inclusive, holistic, and relevant to the needs of patients, families, groups, and communities.

This text is based on the Stuart Stress Adaptation Model of psychiatric nursing care, which integrates biological, psychological, sociocultural, environmental, and legal-ethical aspects of patient care into a unified framework for practice. It was originally developed by Gail Stuart in the 1980s as a synthesis of diverse bodies of knowledge from the perspective of psychiatric nursing and, equally important, as an application of this knowledge to clinical practice. Since then the model has been revised and expanded to include rapidly emerging theoretical and scientific discoveries, as well as a clearer and more complete reflection of the process, content, and context of contemporary psychiatric nursing care.

THEORETICAL ASSUMPTIONS

The **first assumption** of the Stuart Stress Adaptation Model is that nature is ordered as a social hierarchy from the simplest unit to the most complex (Fig. 4-1). Each level of this hierarchy represents an organized whole with distinct properties. Each level also is a part of the next higher level, so nothing exists in isolation. Thus the individual is a component of family, group, community, society, and the larger biosphere. Material and information flow across levels, and each level is influenced by all the others. For this reason, one level of organization, such as the individual, cannot be seen as a dynamic system without incorporating the other levels of the social hierarchy. The most basic level of nursing intervention is the individual level. However, in working with the individual level, the nurse must include its relationship to the whole because wholeness is the essence of psychiatric nursing practice.

The **second assumption** of the model is that nursing care is provided within a biological, psychological, sociocultural,

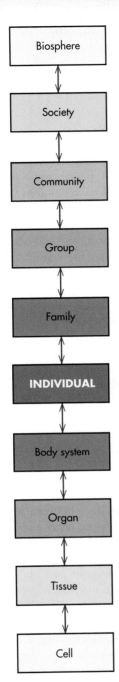

Fig. 4-1 Levels of organization that make up the social hierarchy.

environmental, and legal-ethical context. Each of these aspects of care is described in detail in Chapters 6 to 10. The nurse must understand and integrate them in order to provide competent, holistic psychiatric nursing care. The theoretical basis for psychiatric nursing practice is derived from nursing science as well as from the behavioral, social, and biological sciences. The range of theories used by psychiatric nurses includes nursing, developmental psychology, neurobiology, pharmacology, psychopathology, learning, sociocultural, cognitive, behavioral, economic, organizational, political, legal-ethical, interpersonal, group, family, and milieu. Psychiatric nursing practice requires the use of many theories because of the variation in patients' responses, the philosophical backgrounds of psychiatric nurses, and the settings in which nurses work. No one theory is universally applicable to all patients. Rather, the appropriate theory should be selected for its relevance to a particular patient, the presenting problem, and the environment of caregiving.

The **third assumption** of the model is that health/illness and adaptation/maladaptation are two distinct continuums. The health/illness continuum derives from a medical world view. The adaptation/maladaptation continuum derives from a nursing world view. This means that a person with a medically diagnosed illness may be adapting well to it. An example of this is the adaptive coping responses used by some people who have chronic physical or psychiatric illnesses. In contrast, a person without a medically diagnosed illness may have many maladaptive coping responses. This can been seen in the adolescent whose problematic behaviors reflect poor coping responses to the many issues that must be resolved during adolescence. These two continuums thus reflect the complementary nature of the nursing and medical models of practice.

The **fourth assumption** is that the model includes the primary, secondary, and tertiary levels of prevention by describing four discrete stages of psychiatric treatment: crisis, acute, maintenance, and health promotion. For each stage of treatment the model suggests a treatment goal, a focus of the nursing assessment, the nature of nursing interventions, and the expected outcome of nursing care. This aspect of the model is particularly useful in organizing one's practice, as well as in creating a structure for documenting both the process and outcome of psychiatric nursing care. It also embraces the full continuum of psychiatric care and can direct nursing practice in hospital, community, and home settings.

The **fifth assumption** of the Stuart Stress Adaptation Model is that it is based on the use of the nursing process described in Chapter 11 and professional role behavior discussed in Chapter 12. Psychiatric nursing care is provided through assessment, diagnosis, outcome identification, planning, implementation, and evaluation. Each step of the process is critically important, and the nurse assumes full responsibility for all nursing actions implemented and the enactment of a professional nursing role.

In summary, the Stuart Stress Adaptation Model is unique in that it does the following:

- Views nature as ordered on a social hierarchy
- Assumes a holistic biopsychosocial approach to psychiatric nursing practice
- Regards adaptation/maladaptation as distinct from health/illness
- Incorporates elements of primary, secondary, and tertiary levels of prevention
- Identifies four stages of psychiatric treatment and related nursing activities
- Can be used across psychiatric settings throughout the continuum of care
- Is based on standards of psychiatric nursing care and professional performance

DESCRIBING MENTAL HEALTH AND ILLNESS

The mental health–mental illness continuum is asymmetrical. The standards of mental health are less clear than those of mental illness. Problems arise with viewing mental health as the average or mean of a group because what is average is not necessarily healthy. It is similarly dangerous to equate social alternatives with illness, such as when an unusual lifestyle is regarded as sick or when aberrant behavior is taken to be a sign of personal abnormality. These problems can be avoided if it is recognized that health/illness and conformity/deviance are independent variables. Combining them generates four patterns: the healthy conformist, the healthy deviant, the unhealthy conformist, and the unhealthy deviant (Fig. 4-2). Psychiatric nurses must carefully consider the meaning of an individual's behavior and its context because it may reflect an adaptation to realistic forces in the individual's life or conformity to group norms.

Defining Mental Health

Mental health is often spoken of as a state of well-being associated with happiness, contentment, satisfaction, achievement, optimism, or hope (Bruckbauer & Ward, 1993; Lykken & Tellegen, 1996). These are difficult terms to define, and their meanings change by person and life situation. Some have suggested that the idea of any single criterion of mental health should be abandoned because mental health cannot be confined to a simple concept or a single aspect of behavior. Instead, mental health consists of a number of criteria that exist on a continuum with gradients or degrees. These criteria form the basis of the optimum of mental health. They are not absolute, however, and each person has limits. Although no one reaches the ideal in all the criteria, most people can approach the optimum.

> *Do you think that a person with diabetes that is controlled with medication can still be regarded as healthy? How does this compare with a person who has schizophrenia that is controlled with medication?*

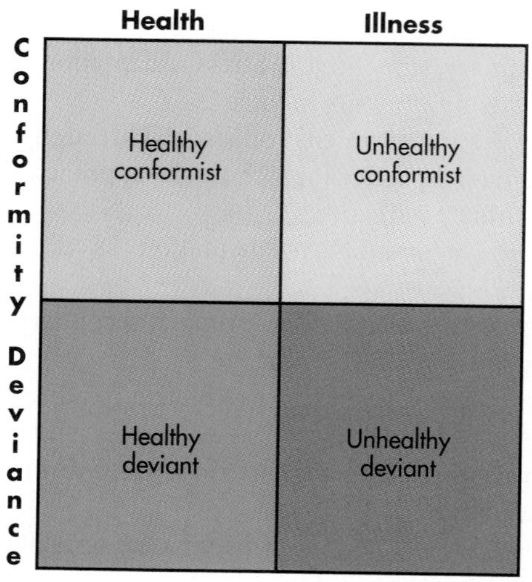

Fig. 4-2 Patterns of behavior.

Criteria of Mental Health. The following six criteria are indicators of mental health:

- Positive attitudes toward self
- Growth, development, and self-actualization
- Integration
- Autonomy
- Reality perception
- Environmental mastery

Positive attitudes toward self include an acceptance of self and self-awareness. A person must have some objectivity about the self and realistic aspirations that necessarily change with age. A healthy person also must have a sense of identity, wholeness, belongingness, security, and meaningfulness.

Growth, development, and **self-actualization** have been the objects of considerable research. Maslow (1958) and Rogers (1961), for example, developed theories on the realization of the human potential. Maslow describes the concept of self-actualization, and Rogers emphasizes the fully functioning person. Both theories focus on the entire range of human adjustment. They describe a self as being engaged in a constant quest, always seeking new growth, development, and challenges. These theories focus on the total person and whether the person has the following characteristics:

- Is adequately in touch with one's self to use the resources one has
- Has free access to personal feelings and can integrate them with thoughts and behaviors
- Can interact freely and openly with the environment
- Can share with other people and grow from such experiences

Integration is a balance between what is expressed and what is repressed, between outer and inner conflicts. It includes the regulation of moods, emotional responsiveness and control, and a unified philosophy of life. This criterion can be measured at least in part by the person's ability to withstand stress and cope with anxiety. A strong but not rigid ego enables the person to handle change and grow from it.

Autonomy involves self-determination, a balance between dependence and independence, and acceptance of the consequences of one's actions. It implies that the person is self-responsible for decisions, actions, thoughts, and feelings. As a result, the person can respect autonomy and freedom in others.

Reality perception is the individual's ability to test assumptions about the world by empirical thought. The mentally healthy person can change perceptions in light of new information. This criterion includes empathy or social sensitivity, a respect for the feelings and attitudes of others.

Environmental mastery enables a mentally healthy person to feel success in an approved role in society. The person can deal effectively with the world, work out personal problems, and obtain satisfaction from life. The person should be able to cope with loneliness, aggression, and frustration without being overwhelmed. The mentally healthy person can respond to others, love and be loved, and cope with reciprocal relationships. This individual can build new friendships and have satisfactory social group involvement.

Finally, a person should not be assessed against some vague or ideal notion of health. Rather, each person should be seen in a group context and an individual context. The issue is not how well someone fits an arbitrary sociocultural standard, but rather what is reasonable for a particular person. Is there continuity or discontinuity with the past? Does the person adapt to changing needs throughout the life cycle? Such a view incorporates the concept of **psychobiological resilience**, which proposes that humans must weather periods of stress and change throughout life (Dyer & McGuinness, 1996). Successfully weathering each period of disruption and reintegration leaves the person better able to deal with the next change.

Dimensions of Mental Illness

Mental disorders are a major contributor to the burden of illness in the United States. Nearly 50% of all people ages 15 to 54 have had a psychiatric or substance abuse disorder in their lifetimes, and close to 30% had one of these disorders in the past year (Fig. 4-3). Most importantly, more than half of all lifetime disorders occur in the 14% of the population who have a history of three or more co-existing disorders (Kessler et al, 1994). This group includes most of the people with severe psychiatric illness and represents a very vulnerable portion of the population. The seriousness and persistence of some disorders cause great strain on affected individuals, their families and communities, and the larger health care system. In addition, the increased risk of premature death from natural and unnatural causes for the common mental disorders has been documented (Dembling et al, 1999; Harris & Barraclough, 1998). Key facts about mental illness prepared by the National Institute of Mental Health (1993) are presented in Box 4-1.

Identify two key facts about mental illness from Box 4-1 that you did not know. How will these facts change your views about needed health care reform in this country?

In 1996, the Global Burden of Disease Study examined the disabling outcomes of 107 diseases around the world. Of the 15 specific leading causes of disability in developed countries, five are mental health problems: (1) unipolar major depressive disorder, (2) alcohol use, (3) schizophrenia, (4) self-inflicted injuries, and (5) bipolar disorder (Murray & Lopez, 1996). With regard to years lived with disability, depressive disorders as a single diagnostic category were the leading cause of disability worldwide. The Global Burden of Disease Study thus revealed the true magnitude of the long underestimated impact of mental health problems. Furthermore, by the year 2020, mental disorders are projected to increase, and unipolar major depression is predicted to become the second leading factor in disease burden. The Global Burden of Disease Study has thus been eye-opening for public health in terms of mainstreaming mental health, and it has highlighted the public significance of mental disorders (Neugebauer, 1999; Ustun, 1999).

BIOPSYCHOSOCIAL COMPONENTS

The Stuart Stress Adaptation Model of psychiatric nursing care views human behavior from a holistic perspective that integrates biological, psychological, and sociocultural aspects of care. For instance, a man who has had a myocardial infarction also may be severely depressed because he fears he

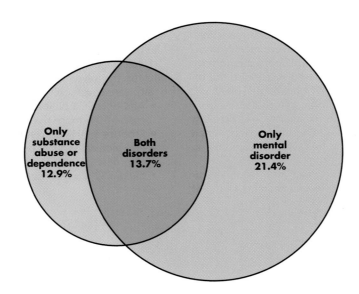

	Lifetime	Past Year
Any Substance Abuse or Mental Disorder	**48.0%**	**29.5%**
Only substance abuse or dependence	12.9	6.6
Only mental disorder	21.4	18.2
Both substance abuse and mental disorder	13.7	4.7

Fig. 4-3 Percentage of population with substance abuse, mental disorder, or both disorders, ages 15 to 54. (Redrawn from Kessler et al: Lifetime and 12-month prevalence of DSM-III-R psychiatric disorders in the US, *Arch Gen Psychiatry* 51:8, 1994.)

Box **4-1**

Key Facts about Mental Illness

EXTENT AND SEVERITY OF THE PROBLEM

The full spectrum of mental disorders affects 25% of the adult population in a given year. This figure refers to **all** mental disorders and is comparable to rates for "physical disorders" when similarly broadly defined (for example, respiratory disorders affect 50% of adults, and cardiovascular diseases affect 20%).

Severe mental disorders, such as schizophrenia, manic depressive illness and severe forms of depression, panic disorder, and obsessive compulsive disorder affect 2.8% of the adult population (approximately 5 million people) and account for 25% of all federal disability payments.

About 1 in 5 children in the United States younger than 18 years have a mental health problem severe enough to require treatment.

Approximately 18 million people in the United States 18 years of age and older have problems as a result of alcohol use; 10.6 million of these suffer from alcoholism.

An estimated 23 million people in the United States currently use illicit drugs.

At least two thirds of elderly nursing home residents have a diagnosis of a mental disorder, such as major depression.

Nearly one third of the nation's estimated 600,000 homeless people are believed to be adults with severe mental illness.

More than one in four jail inmates has a mental disorder. 29% of the nation's jails routinely hold people with a mental illness without any criminal charges.

COST OF MENTAL DISORDERS

In 1990 the nation's health care bill was $670 billion; the direct cost of treating all mental disorders was 10%, or $67 billion. Treatment plus indirect costs for all mental disorders was $148 billion in 1990 compared with $159 billion for the total cost of cardiovascular system diseases in 1990.

The total direct treatment costs for severe mental disorders are $20 billion per year plus $7 billion for long-term nursing home care. Indirect and related costs bring the total for severe mental disorders to $74 billion per year.

It has been estimated that drug and alcohol abuse contribute to more than $163.6 billion in health care costs, lost productivity, and crime. Estimates of hospital beds occupied by patients whose physical condition is complicated by alcohol and drug problems range from 25% to 50%.

Alcohol or mental illness is involved in 94% of all suicides, and suicide ranks as the second leading cause of death among people ages 15-24.

Alcoholism is the third leading cause of illness and disability in the United States and accounts for 10% of all deaths.

TREATMENT EFFICACY

How effective are treatments for severe mental disorders as compared with treatments for physical illness?

DISORDER	TREATMENT SUCCESS RATE (%)
Panic	80
Bipolar	80
Major depression	65
Schizophrenia	60
Obsessive compulsive	60
Cardiovascular treatments	
Atherectomy	52
Angioplasty	41

The majority of alcoholics improve through treatment, and evidence suggests that alcoholism treatment is effective in containing costs throughout the health care system and increasing worker productivity.

REIMBURSEMENT

People who need help often cannot receive it. Approximately 30% of the 2.8 million people with severe mental illness receive active treatment in a given year; 70% to 80% of children needing mental health treatment do not receive appropriate services.

85% of all drug and alcohol abusers are not in treatment. Only 150,000 of an estimated 1.4 million intravenous drug abusers are currently in treatment.

Under insurance plans offering full, comprehensive, and equitable coverage for mental disorders, the percentage of cost represented by these disorders plateaus at about 10% to 11%. Inpatient care for treatment of severe psychiatric disorders has grown less rapidly than inpatient care for all health conditions.

Under health care reform, making mental health coverage for the severely mentally ill commensurate to other health care coverage would do the following:

- Add only $6.5 billion in new mental health care costs—10% more than is currently spent
- Produce a 10% decrease in the cost and use of general medical services by people with severe mental disorders
- Yield a $2.2 billion net saving for the United States

From National Advisory Mental Health Council: *Am J Psychiatry* 150:1447, 1993.

will lose his ability to work and to satisfy his wife sexually. He also may have a family history of depression. Likewise, a patient who seeks treatment for a major depression also may have gastric ulcers that are exacerbated by her depression. The holistic nature of psychiatric nursing practice examines all aspects of the individual and his or her environment. The specific biopsychosocial components of the Stuart Stress Adaptation Model are shown in Fig. 4-4.

Predisposing Factors

Predisposing factors are biological, psychological, and sociocultural in nature. They may be seen as conditioning or risk factors that influence both the type and amount of resources the person can use to handle stress.

Biological factors include genetic background, nutritional status, biological sensitivities, general health, and exposure to toxins. Psychological factors include intelligence;

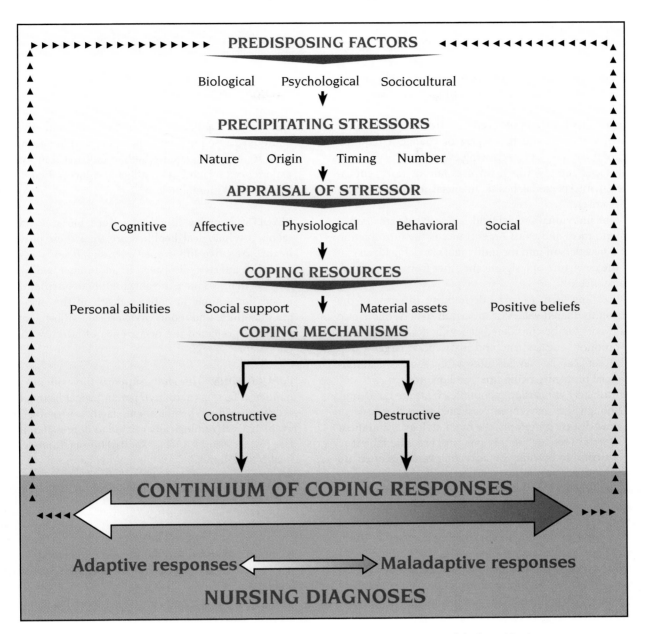

Fig. 4-4 Biopsychosocial components of the Stuart Stress Adaptation Model of psychiatric nursing care.

verbal skills; morale; personality; past experiences; self-concept, motivation; psychological defenses; and locus of control, or a sense of control over one's own fate. **Sociocultural characteristics** include age, gender, education, income, occupation, social position, cultural background, religious upbringing and beliefs, political affiliation, socialization experiences, and level of social integration or relatedness. Together these factors provide a link with higher and lower levels of the social hierarchy and a backdrop against which all current experiences are given meaning and value.

Explain why predisposing factors are also sometimes called risk factors.

Precipitating Stressors

Precipitating stressors are stimuli that the individual perceives as challenging, threatening, or demanding. They require excess energy and produce a state of tension and stress. They may be biological, psychological, or sociocultural in **nature,** and they may **originate** in the person's internal or external environment. Besides describing the nature and origin of a stressor, it is important to assess the **timing** of the stressor. Timing has many dimensions, such as when the stressor occurred, the duration of exposure to the stressor, and the frequency with which it occurs. A final factor to be considered is the **number** of stressors an individual experiences within a certain time period because events may be more difficult to deal with when they occur close together.

Stressful Life Events. One group of stressors that has received much attention in the health care literature is stressful life events. The relationship of stressful life events to the cause, onset, course, and outcomes of various psychiatric illnesses, such as schizophrenia, depression, and anxiety, has been the focus of much research.

Recent issues related to life events as stressors focus on the nature of the event and the degree of change it requires. There are three ways of categorizing events:

- By social activity, which involves family, work, educational, interpersonal, health, financial, legal, or community crises.
- By the individual's social field. These events are defined as entrances and exits. An entrance is the introduction of a new person into the individual's social field; an exit is the departure of a significant other from the person's social field.
- By relating them to social desirability. In terms of the currently shared values of American society, one group of events can be considered generally desirable, such as promotion, engagement, and marriage. A larger group of events can be viewed unfavorably, such as death, financial problems, being fired, and divorce.

Unfortunately, conclusions about life events are not definitive. Although they have been correlated with the onset of anxiety and disease symptoms, the methodological and theoretical aspects of research in this area have been the subject of much criticism. Intervening or mediating variables often are not taken into account in the research studies. Also, the particular events in the scales may not be the most relevant to certain groups, such as students, working mothers, the elderly, the poor, or the persistently mentally ill. Finally, the life-events approach provides no clues to the specific processes by which the events affect physical or mental health.

It may be more helpful, therefore, to suggest that stressful life events act along a continuum to influence the development of psychiatric illness. On one end of the continuum, they may act as triggers to precipitate an illness in people who would have developed the illness eventually for one reason or another. At the other end of the continuum, stressful life events may have a vulnerability effect in reducing an individual's resistance and coping resources and thus greatly advancing or bringing about psychiatric illness (see Citing the Evidence).

 What sociocultural norms and values must be considered in evaluating the impact of potentially stressful life events?

Life Strains and Hassles. Life-events theory is built on the idea of change. However, much stress arises from chronic conditions such as boredom, continuing family tension, job dissatisfaction, and loneliness. This aspect is reflected in the early work of Pearlin and Schooler (1978), who explored what people considered potential life strains. They identified four areas:

- Marital strains
- Parental strains associated with teenage and young adult children

Citing the Evidence on

Negative Life Events

BACKGROUND: One of the most controversial questions is, Do the stressful events of ordinary life, such as the death of a parent, unemployment, and divorce definitely cause physical or psychological impairment? This study investigated whether negative life events experienced by adult men affected subjects' long-term physical and mental health.

RESULTS: Negative life events were found to affect men's psychological health more than their physical health. Negative life events were significantly associated with affective disorders. In addition, a family history of depression, a bleak childhood environment, mood fluctuations in college, death of the maternal grandmother, and poor psychosocial adjustment in youth all predicted the occurrence of affective disorders before age 52.

IMPLICATIONS: This study supports the evidence that biological factors (heredity), psychological factors (unstable personality), and social factors (negative life events) are all etiologically related to depression. It offers clear support for a biopsychosocial model of health and illness.

Cui X & Vaillant G: Antecedents and consequences of negative life events in adulthood: a longitudinal study, *Am J Psych* 153:21.

- Strains associated with household economics
- Overloads and dissatisfactions associated with the work role

These findings suggest more long-term life dissatisfactions than major episodic events.

Research indicates that small daily hassles or stresses may be more closely linked to and have a greater effect on a person's moods and health than do major misfortunes (Monat & Lazarus, 1991). Hassles are irritating, frustrating, or distressing incidents that occur in everyday life. Such incidents may include disagreements, disappointments, and unpleasant surprises such as losing a wallet; getting stuck in a traffic jam; or arguing with a teenage son or daughter. Research suggests that daily hassles may be better predictors of psychological and physical health than major life events. The more frequent and intense the hassles people reported, the poorer their overall mental and physical health. Major events did have some long-term effects, but these effects may be accounted for by the daily hassles they precipitate. A study of the specific hassles and their frequency among people with severe mental illness found that loneliness and boredom were serious concerns. Finances, crime, self-expression, and upward mobility also were important (Segal & VanderVoort, 1993).

A certain amount of stress is necessary for survival, and degrees of it can challenge the individual to grow in new ways. However, too much stress at inappropriate times can place excessive demands on the individual and interfere with integrated functioning. Stress does not reside within the particular life event itself or within the individual. Rather, it is in the interaction between the individual and situation. The questions that emerge are: How much stress is too much and what is a stressful life event? These questions lead the nurse to explore the significance of the event for the individual's value system.

Appraisal of Stressor

Appraisal of a stressor is the processing and comprehension of the stressful situation that takes place on many levels. Specifically, it involves cognitive, affective, physiological, behavioral, and social responses. Appraisal is an evaluation of the significance of an event for a person's well-being. The stressor assumes its meaning, intensity, and importance from the unique interpretation and significance given to it by the person at risk.

Cognitive appraisal is a critical part of this model (Monat & Lazarus, 1991). Cognitive factors play a central role in adaptation. They affect the impact of stressful events; the choice of coping patterns used; and the emotional, physiological, and behavioral reactions. Cognitive appraisal mediates psychologically between the person and the environment in any stressful encounter. That is, damage or potential damage is evaluated according to the person's understanding of the situation's power to produce harm and the resources the person has available to neutralize or tolerate the harm.

There are three types of primary cognitive appraisals to stress:

- **Harm/loss** that has already occurred
- **Threat,** or anticipated or future harm
- **Challenge,** in which the focus is placed on potential gain, growth, or mastery rather than on the possible risks

The perception of challenge may play an important role in psychological hardiness or resistance to stress. This theory proposes that psychologically hardy people are less likely than nonhardy people to fall ill as a result of stressful life events. Three parts of a hardy personality have been described and researched (Maddi & Kobasa, 1991; Tartasky, 1993). Hardy people are high in the following:

Commitment—the ability to involve oneself in whatever one is doing

Challenge—the belief that change rather than stability is to be expected in life, so events are seen as stimulating rather than threatening

Control—the tendency to feel and believe that they influence events, rather than feeling helpless in the face of life's problems

From this list one might conclude that stress-resistant people have a specific set of attitudes toward life, an openness to change, a feeling of involvement in whatever they are doing, and a sense of control over events (Friedman & VandenBos, 1992). Such differences in cognitive appraisal affect the person's response to events. Those who view stress as a challenge are more likely to transform events to their advantage and thus reduce their level of stress. With more pas-

sive, hostile, avoidant, or self-defeating tactics, the source of stress does not go away.

> *What is your level of hardiness as measured by the elements of commitment, challenge, and control? How will it influence your effectiveness as a nurse?*

An **affective** response is the arousal of a feeling. In the appraisal of a stressor, the predominant affective response is a nonspecific or generalized anxiety reaction.

This generalized anxiety response becomes expressed as emotions. These may include joy, sadness, fear, anger, acceptance, distrust, anticipation, or surprise. Emotions also may be classified according to type, duration, and intensity—characteristics that change over time and events. For example, when an emotion is prolonged over time, it can be classified as a mood; when prolonged over a longer time, it can be considered an attitude.

Physiological responses reflect the interaction of several neuroendocrine axes involving growth hormone, prolactin, adrenocorticotropic hormone (ACTH), luteinizing and follicle-stimulating hormones, thyroid-stimulating hormones, vasopressin, oxytocin, insulin, epinephrine, norepinephrine, and a variety of other neurotransmitters in the brain. The fight-or-flight physiological response stimulates the sympathetic division of the autonomic nervous system and increases activity of the pituitary-adrenal axis. Additionally, stress has been shown to affect the body's immune system, affecting one's ability to fight disease.

Behavioral responses reflect emotions and physiological changes as well as cognitive analysis of the stressful situation. Caplan (1981) described the following four phases of an individual's responses to a stressful event:

- Phase 1 is behavior that changes the stressful environment or allows the individual to escape from it.
- Phase 2 is behavior that allows the individual to change the external circumstances and their aftermath.
- Phase 3 is intrapsychic behavior to defend against unpleasant emotional arousal.
- Phase 4 is intrapsychic behavior to come to terms with the event and its sequelae by internal readjustment.

Finally, there are three aspects of a person's **social** response to stress and illness (Mechanic, 1977). The first aspect is the **search for meaning,** in which people seek information about their problem. This is necessary for devising a coping strategy because only through some idea of what is occurring can one come up with a reasonable response.

The second aspect of social response is **social attribution,** in which the person tries to identify the factors that contributed to the situation. Patients who see their problem as resulting from their own negligence may be blocked from an active coping response. They may see their problems as a sign of their personal failure and engage in self-blame and passive, withdrawn behavior. Thus the way patients and health professionals view cause can greatly affect successful coping.

The third aspect of social response is **social comparison,** in which people compare skills and capacities with those of others with similar problems. A person's self-assessment depends very much on those with whom comparisons are made. The outcome is an evaluation of the need for support from the person's social network or support system. Predisposing factors such as age, developmental level, and cultural background, as well as the characteristics of the precipitating stressor, determine the perceived need for social support.

In summary, the way a person appraises an event is the psychological key to understanding coping efforts and the nature and intensity of the stress response. Unfortunately, many nurses and other health professionals ignore this fact when they presume to know how certain stressors will affect a patient and thus provide "routine" care. Not only does this practice depersonalize the patient, but it also undermines the basis of nursing care. The patient's appraisal of life stressors, with its cognitive, affective, physiological, behavioral, and social components, must be an essential part of the psychiatric nurse's assessment.

How might social attribution influence a nurse's response to a rape victim, a person with a substance abuse disorder, or a patient with HIV?

Coping Resources

Coping resources, options, or strategies help to determine what can be done, as well as what is at stake. This component takes into account which coping options are available, the likelihood that a given option will accomplish what it is supposed to, and the likelihood that the person can apply a particular strategy effectively.

Coping resources include economic assets, abilities and skills, defensive techniques, social supports, and motivation. They incorporate all levels of the social hierarchy represented in Fig. 4-1 on p. 61. Relationships between the individual, family, group, and society assume critical importance at this point of the model. Other coping resources include health and energy, positive beliefs, problem-solving and social skills, social and material resources, and physical well-being.

Viewing oneself positively can serve as a basis of hope and can sustain a person's coping efforts under the most adverse circumstances. Problem-solving skills include the ability to search for information, identify the problem, weigh alternatives, and implement a plan of action. Social skills facilitate the solving of problems involving other people, increase the likelihood of getting cooperation and support from others, and give the individual greater social control. Finally, material assets refer to money and the goods and services that money can buy. Obviously, monetary resources greatly increase a person's coping options in almost any stressful situation.

Knowledge and intelligence are other coping resources that allow people to see different ways of dealing with stress. Finally, coping resources also include a strong ego identity, commitment to a social network, cultural stability, a stable system of values and beliefs, a preventive health orientation, and genetic or constitutional strength (Kendler, 1997).

Coping Mechanisms

It is at this point in the model that coping mechanisms emerge. This is an important time for nursing activities directed toward primary prevention. Coping mechanisms can be defined as any efforts directed at stress management. There are three main types of coping mechanisms:

- **Problem-focused** coping mechanisms, which involve tasks and direct efforts to cope with the threat itself. Examples include negotiation, confrontation, and seeking advice.
- **Cognitively focused** coping mechanisms, by which the person attempts to control the meaning of the problem and thus neutralize it. Examples include positive comparison, selective ignorance, substitution of rewards, and the devaluation of desired objects.
- **Emotion-focused** coping mechanisms, by which the patient is oriented to moderating emotional distress. Examples include the use of ego defense mechanisms such as denial, suppression, or projection. A detailed discussion of coping and defense mechanisms appears in Chapter 17.

Coping mechanisms can be constructive or destructive. They are **constructive** when anxiety is treated as a warning signal and the individual accepts it as a challenge to resolve the problem. In this respect anxiety can be compared to a fever: Both serve as warnings that the system is under attack. Once used successfully, constructive coping mechanisms modify the way past experiences are used to meet future threats. **Destructive** coping mechanisms ward off anxiety without resolving the conflict, using evasion instead of resolution.

PATTERNS OF RESPONSE

According to the Stuart Stress Adaptation Model, an individual's response to stress is based on specific predisposing factors, the nature of the stressor, the perception of the situation, and an analysis of coping resources and mechanisms. Coping responses of the patient are then evaluated on a continuum of adaptation/maladaptation (see Fig. 4-4). Responses that support integrated functioning are seen as adaptive. They lead to growth, learning, and goal achievement. Responses that block integrated functioning are seen as maladaptive. They prevent growth, decrease autonomy, and interfere with mastery of the environment.

Nursing Diagnoses

Responses to stress, whether actual or potential, are the subject of nursing diagnoses. A nursing diagnosis is a clinical judgment about individual, family, or community responses to stress (see Critical Thinking about Contemporary Issues). It is a statement of the patient's nursing problem that includes both the adaptive and maladaptive responses and contributing stressors. These responses may be overt, covert, existing, or potential and may lie anywhere on the continuum from adaptive to maladaptive. Formulating the diagnosis and implementing treatment are nursing functions for which the nurse is accountable. Box 4-2 lists the NANDA-approved nursing diagnoses.

Box 4-2

NANDA-Approved Nursing Diagnoses

Activity intolerance
Adaptive capacity, intracranial, decreased
Adjustment, impaired
Airway clearance, ineffective
Anxiety
Aspiration, risk for
Body image disturbance
Body temperature, altered, risk for
Bowel incontinence
Breastfeeding
Breathing pattern, ineffective
Cardiac output, decreased
Caregiver role strain
Communication, impaired verbal
Confusion
Constipation
Coping, defensive
Coping, community
Coping, family, ineffective
Coping, individual, ineffective
Death anxiety
Decisional conflict
Decreased cardiac output
Denial, ineffective
Dentition, altered
Development, risk for altered
Diarrhea
Disuse syndrome, risk for
Diversional activity deficit
Dysreflexia
Elimination, urinary, altered
Energy field disturbance
Environmental interpretation syndrome, impaired
Failure to thrive, adult
Family processes, altered
Fatigue
Fear
Feeding pattern, ineffective infant
Fluid volume
Gas exchange, impaired
Grieving
Growth, risk for altered
Growth and development, altered
Health maintenance, altered
Health-seeking behaviors
Home maintenance management, impaired
Hopelessness
Hyperthermia
Hypothermia
Incontinence, bowel
Incontinence, urinary
Infant behavior, disorganized
Infant feeding pattern, ineffective
Infection, risk for
Injury, risk for
Knowledge deficit
Latex allergy response

Loneliness, risk for
Management of the therapeutic regimen
Memory, impaired
Mobility, impaired
Nausea
Noncompliance
Nutrition, altered
Oral mucous membrane, altered
Pain
Parent/infant/child attachment, altered, risk for
Parental role conflict
Parenting, altered
Peripheral neurovascular dysfunction, risk for
Personal identity disturbance
Poisoning, risk for
Post-trauma syndrome
Powerlessness
Protection, altered
Rape-trauma syndrome
Relocation stress syndrome
Retention, urinary
Role conflict, parental
Role performance, altered
Self-care deficit
Self-esteem
Self-mutilation, risk for
Sensory/perceptual alterations
Sexual dysfunction
Sexuality patterns, altered
Skin integrity, impaired
Sleep deprivation
Sleep pattern disturbance
Social interaction, impaired
Social isolation
Sorrow, chronic
Spiritual distress
Spiritual well-being, potential for enhanced
Stress incontinence
Suffocation, risk for
Surgical recovery, delayed
Swallowing, impaired
Thermoregulation, ineffective
Thought processes, altered
Tissue integrity, impaired
Tissue perfusion, altered
Total incontinence
Transfer ability, impaired
Trauma, risk for
Unilateral neglect
Urge incontinence
Urinary elimination, altered
Urinary incontinence, reflex
Urinary retention
Ventilation, inability to sustain spontaneous
Ventilatory weaning response, dysfunctional
Violence, risk for
Walking, impaired

From NANDA: *Nursing diagnoses: definitions and classifications,* 1999-2000, Philadelphia, 1999, The Association.

? CRITICAL THINKING about CONTEMPORARY ISSUES

How Does Mind-Body Dualism Influence the Way Nurses Think about Patients and Their Illnesses?

In formulating diagnoses, psychiatric nurses must be careful to avoid the mind-body dualism that dominates the expression, diagnosis, and use of health care services in the United States (Consumer Reports, 1993). In most other cultures this division between mind and body does not exist. There is a wide range of behavior for expressing emotion and psychological disorders, and in America many people express their distress somatically and attribute their problems to physical illness rather than to psychological, social, or spiritual dilemmas. This can create a variety of problems.

One problem is that nurses can respond to patients' somatic complaints and treat them as problems of physical illness without questioning them about possible psychosocial causes. Many patients often want a somatic explanation and treatment, and react with fear or anger to the suggestion that there may be a psychological component to their problem. These patients may receive treatment that results in harm or not receive treatment that is needed for their underlying psychological problem. Conversely, a physical illness with affective or cognitive symptoms might be misdiagnosed and inappropriately treated as a psychological problem. Another mistake is for nurses to believe that if a patient's problem is psychiatric, then physical symptoms can be discounted or ignored.

As a consequence of mind-body dualism, patients are separated according to whether their illnesses are deemed to be psychological or physical. They are then sent to different hospitals and are seen by different kinds of health care providers. The practical consequence of this dualistic thinking is that it can interfere with a nurse's ability to holistically understand people's reactions to events in their lives and the ways in which they cope and adapt.

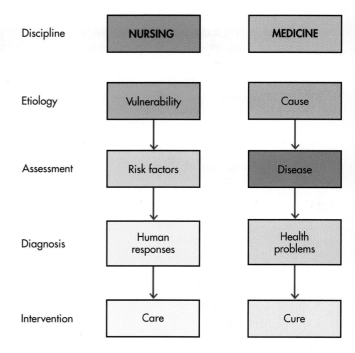

Fig. 4-5   Comparison of nursing and medical models of care.

whether or not a physician has diagnosed the presence of a psychiatric illness. Also, patients with a persistent psychiatric illness may be adapting well to it. People can successfully adapt to an illness without recovering from it. This is an important aspect of the Stuart Stress Adaptation Model because it suggests that psychiatric nurses can promote their patients' adaptive responses regardless of their health or illness state (Stuhlmiller, 1995).

Classifying Mental Disorders

Mental illnesses can be broadly differentiated as neurotic or psychotic. **Neuroses** have the following characteristics:

- A symptom or group of symptoms is distressing and is recognized as unacceptable and alien to the individual.
- Reality testing is grossly intact.
- Behavior does not violate major social norms (although functioning may be significantly impaired).
- The disturbance is enduring or recurrent without treatment and is not merely a transitory reaction to stressors.
- No demonstrable organic cause or factor is present.

In situations of severest conflict, however, the person may be powerless to cope with the threat by such patterns and may distort reality, as in **psychosis**. Psychosis consists of the following characteristics:

- Regressive behavior
- Personality disintegration
- A significant reduction in level of awareness
- Great difficulty in functioning adequately
- Gross impairment in reality testing

This last characteristic is critical. When people demonstrate gross impairment in reality testing, they incorrectly evaluate the accuracy of their perceptions and draw incorrect inferences about external reality, even in the face of con-

Relationship to Medical Diagnoses

Medical diagnosis is the health problem or disease state of the patient. In the medical model of psychiatry, these health problems are mental disorders or mental illnesses. It is important for psychiatric nurses to distinguish between nursing and medical models of care, as shown in Fig. 4-5. In particular, the following differences should be noted:

- Nurses assess **risk factors** and look for **vulnerabilities.**
- **Physicians assess disease states** and look for **causes.**
- Nursing diagnoses focus on the **adaptive/maladaptive coping continuum of human responses.**
- Medical diagnoses focus on the **health/illness continuum of health problems.**
- Nursing intervention consists of **caregiving activities.**
- Medical intervention consists of **curative treatments.**

A nurse may implement the nursing process for maladaptive responses based on the Stuart Stress Adaptation Model

trary evidence. Direct evidence of psychosis is the presence of delusions or hallucinations without insight into their pathological nature. Psychotic health problems reflect the most severe level of illness.

Medical diagnoses are classified according to the Diagnostic and Statistical Manual of Mental Disorders, fourth edition, text revision (DSM–IV–TR) of the American Psychiatric Association (2000). The various illnesses are accompanied by a description of diagnostic criteria, tested for reliability by psychiatric practitioners. It has been noted, however, that the DSM diagnoses are not as precise as the diagnostic processes in the rest of medicine (Tucker, 1998).

DSM–IV–TR uses a multiaxial system that gives attention to various mental disorders, general medical conditions, aspects of the environment, and areas of functioning that might be overlooked if the focus were exclusively on assessing a single presenting problem. The individual thus is evaluated on the following axes:

- Axis I: Clinical syndromes
- Axis II: Personality disorders
- Axis III: General medical conditions
- Axis IV: Psychosocial and environmental problems
- Axis V: Global assessment of functioning

Axes I-V are presented in Appendix A.

Axes I and II constitute the entire classification of mental disorders plus conditions that are not attributable to a mental disorder that are a focus of attention or treatment.

Axis III allows the clinician to identify any physical disorder potentially relevant to the understanding or treatment of the individual.

Axis IV is for reporting psychosocial and environmental problems that may affect the diagnosis, treatment, and prognosis of mental disorders.

Axis V is for reporting the clinician's judgment of the individual's overall level of functioning. This information is useful in planning treatment, measuring its impact, and predicting outcomes.

Psychiatric nurses use all five axes of the DSM–IV–TR and integrate the axes with related nursing diagnoses.

In addition to Axes I-V, the DSM–IV–TR has an outline for cultural formulation designed to help the clinician in systematically evaluating the person's cultural and social reference group and ways in which the cultural context is relevant to clinical care (see Chapter 8). It is suggested that the clinician provide a narrative summary of the evaluation of the categories listed in Box 4-3. The DSM–IV–TR also includes a list of culture-bound syndromes that are recurrent, locality-specific patterns of aberrant behavior and troubling experiences that may or may not be linked to a particular DSM–IV–TR diagnostic category. Although behaviors related to most DSM–IV–TR categories can be found throughout the world, the particular symptoms, course of illness, and social response are often influenced by cultural factors. In contrast, culture-bound syndromes are generally limited to specific societies or culture areas and are localized, folk, diagnostic categories that give coherent meanings for certain common, patterned, and troubling sets of experiences and observations.

Box 4-3

Outline for Cultural Formulation in Psychiatric Diagnosis

- Cultural identity of the individual
- Cultural explanations of the individual's illness
- Cultural factors related to one's psychosocial environment and levels of functioning
- Cultural elements of the relationship between the individual and clinician
- Overall cultural assessment for diagnosis and care

TREATMENT STAGES AND ACTIVITIES

The final aspect of the Stuart Stress Adaptation Model is the integration of the theoretical basis, biopsychosocial components, patterns of response, and nursing activities based on the patient's treatment stage. Once patterns of coping responses have been identified, the nurse determines which treatment stage the patient is in and implements the most appropriate nursing activities.

The model identifies four possible treatment stages: (1) health promotion, (2) maintenance, (3) acute, and (4) crisis. These stages reflect the range of the adaptive/maladaptive continuum and suggest a variety of nursing activities. For each stage the nurse identifies the treatment goal, focus of the nursing assessment, nature of the nursing intervention, and expected outcome of nursing care (Fig. 4-6).

Crisis Stage

- The nursing goal is the stabilization of the patient.
- The nursing assessment focuses on risk factors that threaten the patient's health and well-being.
- The nursing intervention is directed toward managing the environment to provide safety.
- The expected outcome of nursing care is that no harm will come to the patient or others.

Acute Stage

- The nursing goal is for the patient's illness to be placed in remission.
- The nursing assessment is focused on the patient's symptoms and maladaptive coping responses.
- The nursing intervention is directed toward treatment planning with the patient and the modeling and teaching of adaptive responses.
- The expected outcome of nursing care is symptom relief.

Maintenance Stage

- The nursing goal is the complete recovery of the patient.
- The nursing assessment is focused on the patient's functional status.
- The nursing intervention is directed toward reinforcement of the patient's adaptive coping responses and patient advocacy.
- The expected outcome of nursing care is improved patient functioning.

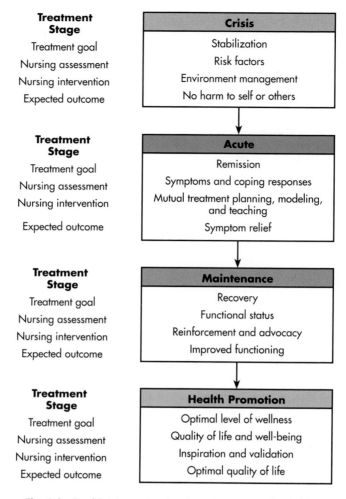

Fig. 4-6 Psychiatric nursing treatment stages and activities.

Table **4-1**

Stages of Treatment Related to Levels of Prevention and Clinical Chapters of the Text		
Stage of Treatment	**Level of Prevention**	**Clinical Chapter(s)**
Health promotion stage	Primary prevention	13: Mental Health Promotion
Crisis stage	Secondary prevention	14: Crisis Intervention
Acute stage	Secondary prevention	17-27: Coping responses chapters
Maintenance stage	Tertiary prevention	15: Psychiatric Rehabilitation

Health Promotion Stage

- The nursing goal is for the patient to achieve the optimal level of wellness.
- The nursing assessment is focused on the patient's quality of life and well-being.
- The nursing intervention is directed toward inspiring and validating the patient.
- The expected outcome of nursing care is that the patient will attain the optimal quality of life.

This aspect of the model moves the field of psychiatric nursing beyond the usual activities associated with the stabilization of patients in crisis and remission of the acutely ill patient's symptoms. It identifies nursing responsibilities in the maintenance and health promotion treatment stages as improving patients' functional status and enhancing their quality of life. These treatment stages are often overlooked in

traditional psychiatric nursing practice, yet they are essential aspects of the contemporary psychiatric nursing role. These stages also relate to the levels of prevention in psychiatric care and the clinical chapters of this text, as shown in Table 4-1.

The synthesis of all of the elements of the Stuart Stress Adaption Model of psychiatric nursing care can be seen in Fig. 4-7. They also are summarized in Table 4-2. Chapters 17 through 27 explore various maladaptive coping responses and related medical diagnoses. The phases of the nursing process are described for patients with maladaptive responses. Each chapter begins with a continuum of coping responses, followed by a discussion of behaviors, predisposing factors, precipitating stressors, appraisal of stressor, coping resources, coping mechanisms, nursing diagnoses, and related interventions. Through consistent application of the Stuart Stress Adaptation Model, the art and science of psychiatric nursing practice emerges.

The Stuart Stress Adaptation Model of Psychiatric Nursing Care

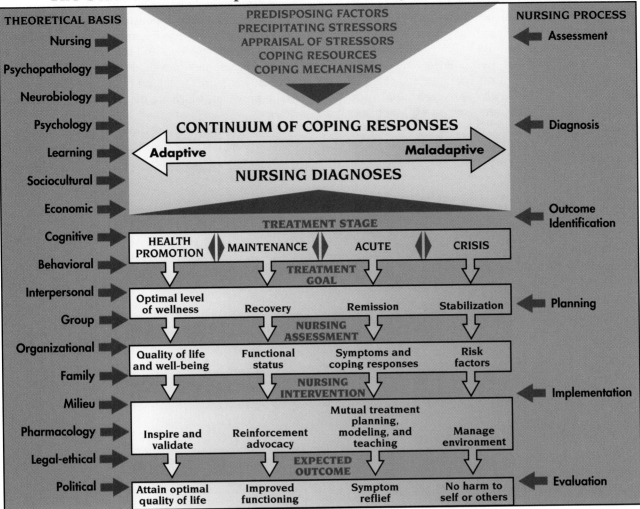

Fig. 4-7   The Stuart Stress Adaptation Model of psychiatric nursing care.

Table **4-2**

Summary of the Elements of the Stuart Stress Adaptation Model		
Element	**Definition**	**Examples**
Predisposing factors	Risk factors that influence both the type and amount of resources the person can elicit to cope with stress	Genetic background, intelligence, self-concept, age, ethnicity, education, gender, belief systems
Precipitating stressors	Stimuli that the person perceives as challenging, threatening, or demanding and that require excess energy for coping	Life events, injury, hassles, strains
Appraisal of stressor	An evaluation of the significance of a stressor for a person's well-being, considering the stressor's meaning, intensity, and importance	Hardiness, perceived seriousness, anxiety, attribution
Coping resources	An evaluation of a person's coping options and strategies	Finances, social support, ego integrity
Coping mechanisms	Any effort directed at stress management	Problem solving, compliance, defense mechanisms
Continuum of coping responses	A range of adaptive or maladaptive human responses	Social changes, physical symptoms, emotional well-being
Treatment stage activities	Range of nursing functions related to treatment goal, nursing assessment, nursing intervention, and expected outcome	Environment management, patient teaching, role modeling, advocacy

Summary

1. The Stuart Stress Adaptation Model assumes that nature is ordered as a social hierarchy; that psychiatric nursing care is provided through the nursing process within a biological, psychological, sociocultural, environmental, and legal-ethical context; that health/illness and adaptation/maladaptation are distinct concepts; and that primary, secondary, and tertiary levels of prevention are included in the four discrete stages of psychiatric treatment.

2. Standards of mental health are less clear than those for mental illness. Nearly one of every two people in the United States has had a psychiatric illness or substance abuse disorder in his or her lifetime.

3. The biopsychosocial components of the model include predisposing factors, precipitating stressors, appraisal of stressor, coping resources, and coping mechanisms.

4. Patterns of response include the individual's coping responses, which are the subject of nursing diagnoses, and health problems, which are the subject of medical diagnoses.

5. Psychiatric nursing activities were described for each of the four stages of treatment: crisis, acute, maintenance, and health promotion.

MERLIN Visit MERLIN: www.mosby.com/MERLIN/Stuart to find these additional materials and student activities.

- **Worksheets**
- **"Drug of the Month" Updates**
- **"Citing the Evidence" Updates**
- **Critical Thinking Activities and Exercises**
- **Annotated Suggested Readings**
- **Web Links**
- **More!**

Chapter Review Questions

1. Indicate whether the following statements are true (T) or false (F).

_____ A. The standards of mental health are less clear than those of mental illness.

_____ B. Approximately one out of every three people will experience a psychiatric or substance abuse problem in his or her lifetime.

_____ C. The treatment for depression is more effective than that for cardiovascular illness.

_____ D. The parasympathetic division of the autonomic nervous system is stimulated by the fight-or-flight response.

_____ E. A coping mechanism is considered to be constructive when it treats anxiety as a warning signal and the person accepts it as a challenge to solve the problem.

_____ F. Psychotic health problems reflect the most severe level of illness.

2. Fill in the blanks.

A. A person's ability to test assumptions about the world by empirical thought is called _____.

B. The concept of _____ proposes that humans must weather periods of stress and change throughout life.

C. Intelligence, morale, and self-concept are examples of _____ predisposing factors.

D. _____ is when a person tries to identify the unique factors that contributed to one's particular situation.

E. The three types of primary cognitive appraisals to stress are _____, _____, and _____.

F. Personality disorders are identified on Axis _____ of the *DSM-IV-TR*.

G. Recurrent, locality-specific patterns of aberrant behavior and troubling experience that may or may not be linked to a particular *DSM–IV–TR* diagnostic category are called _____.

3. Provide short answers for the following questions.

A. Describe the three parts of a hardy personality and the way in which they help a person cope with stress.

B. List the three types of coping mechanisms, and give an example of each.

C. Compare the nursing and medical models of care. Which model do you think currently receives more health care resources, research funding, and professional status? Defend your answer.

D. Identify the four stages of psychiatric treatment and the level of prevention related to each one.

REFERENCES

American Psychiatric Association: *Diagnostic and statistical manual of mental disorders,* Fourth Edition, Text Revision. Washington, DC, American Psychiatric Association, 2000.

Bruckbauer E, Ward S: Positive mental attitude and health: what the public believes, *Image J Nurs Sch* 25:311, 1993.

Caplan G: Mastery of stress: psychosocial aspects, *Am J Psychiatry* 13 8:41, 1981.

Consumer Reports: Can your mind heal your body? 58:107, 1993.

Dembling B et al: Life expectancy and causes of death in a population treated for serious mental illness, *Psych Services* 50:1036, 1999.

Dyer J, McGuinness T: Resilience: analysis of concept, *Arch Psychiatr Nurs* 10:276, 1996.

Friedman H, VandenBos G: Disease-prone and self-healing personalities, *Hosp Community Psychiatry* 43:1177, 1992.

Harris E, Barraclough: Excess mortality of mental disorder, *British J Psych* 173:11, 1998.

Kendler K: Social support: a genetic-epidemiologic analysis, *Am J Psych* 154:1398, 1997.

Kessler R et al: Lifetime and 12-month prevalence of DSM-R psychiatric disorders in the United States, *Arch Gen Psychiatry* 51:8, 1994.

Lykken D, Tellegen A: Happiness is a stochastic phenomenon, *Psychol Sci* 7:186, 1996.

Maddi S, Kobasa S: *Stress and coping: an anthology,* New York, 1991, Columbia University Press.

Maslow A: *Motivation and personality,* New York, 1958, Harper & Row.

Mechanic D: Illness behavior, social adaptation, and the management of illness, *J Nerv Ment Dis* 165:79, 1977.

Monat A, Lazarus R: *Stress and coping,* New York, 1991, Columbia University Press.

Murray C, Lopez A: *The global burden of disease: a comprehensive assessment of mortality and disability from disease, injuries, and risk factors in 1990 and projected to 2020,* Cambridge, Mass, Harvard University Press, 1996.

National Advisory Mental Health Council: health care reform for Americans with severe mental illnesses, *Am J Psychiatry* 150:1447, 1993.

Neugebauer R: Mind matters: the importance of mental disorders in public health's 21st century mission, *Am J Public Health* 89:1309, 1999.

Pearlin LI, Schooler C: The structure of coping, *J Health Soc Behav* 19:2, 1978.

Rogers C: *On becoming a person,* Boston, 1961, Houghton Mifflin.

Segal S, VanderVoort D: Daily hassles of persons with severe mental illness, *Hosp Community Psychiatry* 44:276, 1993.

Stuhlmiller C: The construction of disorders, *J Psychosoc Nurs* 33:20, 1995.

Tartasky D: Hardiness: conceptual and methodological issues, *Image J Nurs Sch* 25:225, 1993.

Tucker G: Putting DSM-IV in perspective, *Am J Psych* 155:159, 1998.

Ustun T: The global burden of mental disorders, *Am J Public Health* 89:1315, 1999.

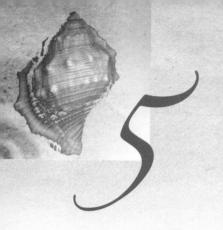

Visit **MERLIN** for *Your Internet Connection* to websites that are related to the content in this chapter. www.mosby.com/MERLIN/Stuart

Evidence Based Psychiatric Nursing Practice

Gail W. Stuart

Everything has changed but our ways of thinking, and if these do not change we drift toward unparalleled catastrophe.

ALBERT EINSTEIN

The *Report of the Surgeon General on Mental Health* is the first Surgeon General's report ever issued on the topic of mental health and mental illness. It is based on an extensive review of the scientific literature and on consultations with mental health providers and consumers. This landmark document concluded that (USDHHS, 1999):

- The efficacy of mental health treatments is well documented.
- A range of treatments exists for most mental disorders.

The challenges for psychiatric nurses stimulated by this report are three:

1. Do psychiatric nurses know the efficacy of the treatments and interventions they provide?
2. Are they practicing evidence based psychiatric nursing?
3. Is there documentation of the nature and outcomes of the care they provide?

The answers to these questions will be important in determining the contributions that nurses can make to mental health care. They will shape the present and future role nurses have in a specialty area that is growing in understandings of molecular and cell biology and genetics, as well as in the cognitive and behavioral sciences.

This text uses an evidence based approach to psychiatric nursing practice. It examines the research that supports psychiatric nursing care and highlights findings in the field using **Citing the Evidence** and **Summarizing the Evidence** boxes, as well as by providing **primary sources of evidence in the references** of each chapter. Another aspect of evidence based practice requires that the nurse continue to access current findings in the field. The web site of this text will be a useful resource to nurses who wish to stay abreast with new research findings and major developments in psychiatric and mental health care.

EVIDENCE BASED PRACTICE

Accountability for patient care outcomes is a basic responsibility of professional nurses. Central to this accountability is the ability to examine nursing practice patterns, evaluate the nature of the data supporting them and demonstrate sound clinical decision making in a way that can be empirically supported. This approach is the essence of evidence based practice. In the current health care environment, psychiatric nurses can no longer rely on opinion-based processes or unproven theories (see Critical Thinking about Contemporary Issues). They need to question their current practices and find better alternatives to improve patient care. To do so, nurses must learn to search the research literature, critically synthesize research findings, and apply relevant evidence to practice.

Evidence based practice is the conscientious, explicit and judicious use of the best evidence from systematic research to make decisions about the care of individual patients (Sackett et al, 1996). It blends a nurse's clinical expertise with the best available research evidence. Evidence based practice

How Effective are Mental Health Services and Providers?

In the last decade, behavioral health expenditures as a percentage of the total health care benefit dropped by 50%, and some argue that society has lost confidence in the mental health industry to deliver cost-effective services. This loss of confidence may result from a number of "myths" in the field including (Bickman, 2000):

- Clinicians improve with experience.
- Advanced-degree programs produce more effective clinicians.
- Continuing education improves the effectiveness of clinicians.
- Licensing helps ensure effective clinicians.
- Accreditation of health delivery organizations improves outcomes for consumers.
- Clinical supervision results in more effective clinicians.

Existing research does not support any of these commonly held beliefs. In fact, there is a growing consensus that training and education are failing the field at all levels. Specifically, it is noted that most clinicians are not taught evidence based assessment and treatment as a standard, and that proficiency and competency standards do not reflect current thinking in the field, particularly its increasing scientific basis.

Thus there has been a "call to action" issued to examine and reform the current accrediting and credentialing organizations and the academic training community to develop strategies around training and education, evidence based practice, and responsive competency standards (ACHMA, 2000). Other recommendations call for additional research and training on manualized treatments and practice guidelines, and the implementation of comprehensive outcome measurement and quality improvement systems. Failure to implement these recommendations may jeopardize the credibility and availability of mental health services for those who need them.

is also a method of self-directed, career-long learning while the nurse continuously seeks the best possible outcomes for patients through implementing effective interventions based on the most current research evidence. The evidence based paradigm is based on the following assumptions:

- It is risky to generalize from a small sample of patients or a single case to the universe of patients.
- It is not possible to rule out other aspects of the situation that may have caused the observed patient behavior but that are not known to the nurse.
- Information gathered from clinical practice tends to involve unsystematic observations.
- All clinicians have biases that influence clinical care.
- Even theories from respected colleagues must give rise to testable hypotheses and evidence of efficacy in order to be useful to clinical practice.
- Knowing that conclusions were reached through scientific methodology permits a higher level of confidence.

- Replication of findings increases confidence in their validity.
- Randomized controlled clinical trials are the "gold standard" of research methodologies.
- Nurses who are able to critically review the research literature related to a specific clinical question will be able to provide better nursing care.

Bases for Nursing Practice

There are four bases for nursing practice (Stetler, 1998):

1. The lowest level is the **traditional basis** for practice which includes rituals, unverified rules, anecdotes, customs, opinions, and unit culture.
2. The second level is the **regulatory basis** for practice which includes state practice acts, and reimbursement and other regulatory requirements.
3. The third level is the **philosophical or conceptual basis** for practice which includes the mission, values and vision of the organization, professional practice models, untested conceptual frameworks, and ethical frameworks and professional codes.
4. The fourth and highest level is **evidence based practice** which includes research findings, performance data, and consensus recommendations of recognized experts.

Apart from situations requiring a philosophical or regulatory basis, the best basis to substantiate clinical practice is the evidence of well-established research findings. Such evidence reflects verifiable, replicable facts and relationships that have been exposed to stringent scientific criteria. This research has less potential for bias than the other bases for practice, most particularly the traditional "that's how we've always done it" basis for practice.

It is also important to remember, however, that not all clinical practice is based on science. Many aspects will not or cannot be adequately tested empirically. Clinical experience is invaluable in these situations. Furthermore, clinical acumen or intuition is also important, particularly with certain patient problems (Benner, 1999). For example, if a patient situation is very complex, scientific inquiry will be unable to give clear guidance on many of the variables related to clinical decisions, so that the judgment developed from experience is essential to psychiatric nursing practice. Finally, there may be biases present in the analysis and interpretation of research data. Thus the nurse needs to critically evaluate studies from both a methodological and clinical perspective.

❓ *Think of one or two examples of psychiatric nursing interventions that have been "handed down" from colleague to colleague without empirical validation. Compare these to one or two nursing interventions that have a research basis.*

Developing Evidence Based Care

Evidence based psychiatric nursing practice involves the following series of activities (Fig. 5-1).

Defining the clinical question is the first step in the process. Clear answers require clear questions. The formula-

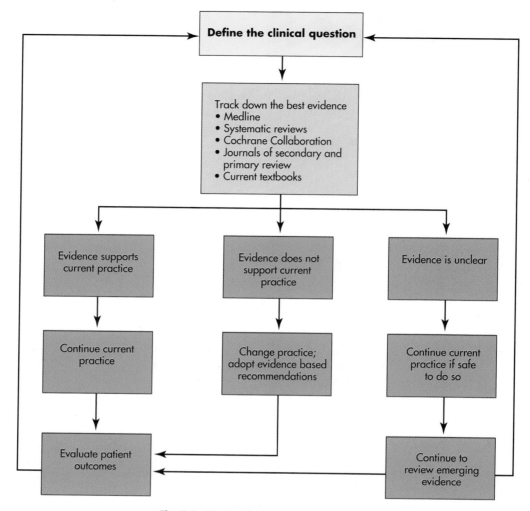

Fig. 5-1   Developing evidence based care.

tion of a precise clinical question involves defining the patient's problems, identifying the existing nursing intervention, and specifying the expected outcome. This process should be completed in partnership with the patient and family, and in collaboration with other health care providers.

Finding the evidence is the next step. Most nurses rely on textbooks, journal articles and drug booklets to help guide their practice. However each of these pose problems for the practicing psychiatric nurse who wants to stay abreast of findings in the field. For example, textbooks become outdated and nurses need to purchase the new editions of their favorite textbooks to stay current. Journal articles may produce contradictory findings and suffer from poor design, while drug booklets may be laden with promotional material. Thus finding the evidence can be challenging.

But recent advances in information technology have made it easier to search the health care literature. Access to electronic databases such as MEDLINE is now widespread. Increasingly journals offer World Wide Web pages on the Internet, displaying contents, abstracts and some full text articles. Another strategy is to use systematic reviews prepared by others. A systematic reviewer uses explicit methods of searching for and critically appraising the primary stud-

ies. If these are comparable, the reviewer may then perform a formal quantitative synthesis, called meta-analysis, of the results (Mulrow, 1994). A **meta-analysis** summarizes the findings from a number of studies in order to arrive at an objective and authoritative guide to treatment for a given condition. A particularly useful source of systematic reviews of health care interventions is the Cochrane Collaboration (1996), a regularly updated electronic library that is available on computer disk and the Internet.

Finally, there is a new type of journal available that specializes in reviewing articles that conform to rigorous methodological standards before they are subject to informed comment and summaries by seasoned clinicians. They are published in the United Kingdom and examples include *Evidence Based Nursing* and *Evidence Based Mental Heath.* No similar journal exists in the United States.

Analyzing the evidence requires that nurses develop the ability to understand and use appropriate research findings. In so doing, they will be confident that the evidence selected is of high quality and is based on rigorous and systematic study. Evidence needs to be critically evaluated for its reliability and application to the particular clinical problem. Implicit in the process of evaluating the evidence is the idea

Box 5-1

Hierarchy of Research Evidence

1. A systematic review (meta-analysis) of all relevant randomized controlled trials (RCTs)
2. At least one properly designed randomized controlled trial
3. Well designed controlled trials without randomization
4. Well designed cohort, case-controlled or other quasi-experimental study
5. Nonexperimental descriptive studies, such as comparative studies
6. Expert committee reports and opinions of respected authorities based on clinical experience

that there is a hierarchy in the quality of research evidence. A commonly used hierarchy for research designs is presented in Box 5-1.

Systematic reviews or meta-analyses of randomized controlled trials (RCTs) are the most reliable study design for the evaluation of treatments. RCTs are considered to be the "gold standard" of research design. However for many interventions, RCTs may not exist and the nurse needs to use evidence from the next level of the hierarchy. The idea being that the nurse selects the intervention that is supported by the best available evidence.

Using the evidence means that the nurse has to be able to apply research in a practical way. In fact, translating research findings into clinically usable information is one of the most challenging aspects of evidence based practice. One development in the field that can help with this process is the development of practice guidelines based on sound evidence about best practices. It is clear, however, that interpreting the evidence and translating it into health care decisions is a complex process. Evidence is helpful but not sufficient for clinical decision making. The key aspect of evidence based practice is that it ensures the best use is made of the **available** evidence.

Evaluating the outcome is the final activity of evidence based practice. Here the nurse asks whether the application of evidence leads to an improvement in care. This inquiry requires that psychiatric nursing practice incorporate ways of demonstrating effectiveness by ongoing evaluation of clearly specified outcomes. This process involves the use of outcome measurement and reevaluation.

PRACTICE GUIDELINES

Practice guidelines in psychiatric care are strategies for mental health care delivery that are developed to facilitate clinical decision making and provide patients with critical information about their treatment options. They have arisen over the past decade in direct response to the greater number of empirically validated treatments that have been identified (Nathan & Gorman, 1998). While they vary widely in format, all practice guidelines are designed to provide detailed specification of methods and procedures to ensure effective treatment for each disorder. There are more than 30 groups who have developed practice guidelines in the mental health or substance abuse field, addressing the child, adolescent, adult and geriatric populations. Experts agree that practice guidelines are valuable tools when developed, modified, and implemented in a collaborative, scientifically valid and pragmatic manner.

The goals of practice guidelines are:
- Document preferred practices
- Increase consistency in care
- Facilitate outcome research
- Enhance the quality of care
- Improve staff productivity
- Reduce costs

Practice guidelines can be developed in a variety of ways. The best mental health practice guidelines are based on a scientific review of the available clinical research literature to establish which treatments have been documented to be safe and effective for particular conditions. Guidelines have also been developed by professional associations, managed care companies, and academic centers using techniques such as expert consensus and data analysis. Regardless of how they are developed it is essential that they be updated regularly to keep up with the latest findings in the field.

Guidelines can vary in several ways:
- Clinical orientation—whether the focus is on a clinical condition, technology, or process
- Clinical purpose—whether information is presented on screening and prevention, evaluation or diagnosis, or various aspects of treatment
- Complexity—whether the guideline is relatively straightforward or presented with detail, complicated logic, or lengthy narrative
- Format—whether the guideline is presented as free text, tables, algorithms, critical pathways, or decision pathways
- Intended audience—whether the guideline is intended for practitioners, patients, regulators, or payers

There is also much variability in how guidelines are used. One of the major limitations to their use is that they may not adequately take into account all four variables that influence treatment outcome: patient characteristics, the nature of the therapeutic relationship, treatment interventions, and the placebo effect. Another limitation is that practice guidelines are often developed in isolation by only one discipline and may therefore contain treatment biases reflective of that discipline's model of practice. Other concerns are that they may be based on insufficient evidence or be too rigid or inflexible. Box 5-2 lists questions that can be helpful in judging the potential usefulness of a practice guideline.

The American College of Mental Health Administration (2000a) has created a taxonomy of building blocks for informed decision making in behavioral health assessment and treatment. This taxonomy identifies treatment options from the most general to the most specific (Figure 5-2). Those at the top of the triangle provide maximum choice and flexibility, while those at the bottom of the triangle provide for maximum accountability. Thus **best practices** are broad consensus statements of a general nature; **practice guidelines** have greater specificity; and **algorithms** or **protocols** are the most specific with the strongest evidence base. This taxonomy is a useful way of informing decision making in the practice setting. It is also unique in incorporating prevention as well as treatment options, which is an underdeveloped area in most practice guidelines. ACMHA also has identified ten characteristics of good behavioral health practice guidelines. These are listed in Box 5-3.

> *Professional associations from psychiatry and psychology have developed practice guidelines. No similar work has been done by psychiatric nursing organizations. What conclusions might you draw from this fact?*

Clinical Pathways

Many health care organizations have undertaken the creation of clinical pathways, which identify the key clinical processes and corresponding timelines to which the patient must adhere to achieve standard outcomes within a specified period of time. They provide one way to document the rationale for mental health care as well as the patient's progress and response to care (Dykes, 1999).

A clinical pathway is a written plan that serves as a map and timetable for the efficient and effective delivery of health care. Valid clinical pathways are developed over time by a multidisciplinary team. They can be constructed around DSM–IV–TR diagnoses, NANDA diagnoses, clinical conditions, treatment stages, clinical interventions, or targeted behaviors. They are most often used in inpatient settings, serve as a shortened version of the multidisciplinary plan of care for a patient, and require high levels of team cooperation

---

Box 5-2

Questions to Ask in Evaluating a Practice Guideline

- Who wrote the guideline? Is it a guild document created by one professional discipline or does it reflect an interdisciplinary point of view?
- Who sponsored the guideline? Where did the money come from that supported its creation and distribution?
- When was the guideline written? Does it reflect the latest developments in the field?
- What methodology was used? Was it based on scientific evidence? Does it differentiate between research findings and clinical opinion?
- Do the treatments recommended in the guideline respect consumer rights?
- Are the treatments recommended in the guideline affordable and accessible? Can the treatments be provided by a variety of clinicians in various settings or are they limited in some way?
- Was the guideline reviewed by a variety of groups, including nurses and consumers?
- How does the guideline compare with other guidelines in the field?

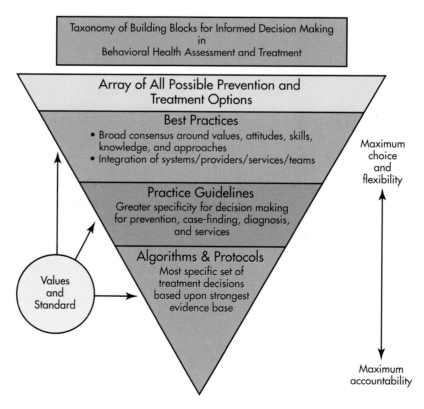

Fig. 5-2 Taxonomy of building blocks for informed decision making in behavioral health assessment and treatment.

and quality monitoring (Brown et al, 1998). Some clinical settings have computerized their paths to enhance the consistency and efficiency of care provided.

The key elements of the clinical pathway are the identification of: a target population; the expected outcome of treatment described in a measurable, realistic, and patient-centered way; specified treatment strategies and interventions; and documentation of patient care activities, variances, and goal achievement. The development of a clinical pathway includes reviewing for efficiency and necessity the events that occur when the patient enters the health care facility, and through discharge and aftercare. This review includes preadmission work-ups, tests, consultations, treatments, activities, diet, and health teaching.

Clinical pathways developed for psychiatry have received a number of criticisms. First, they often do not take into consideration the individual aspects of a patient's care. Second, they

are typically lengthy, cumbersome documents that clinicians view as unwieldy in their day to day clinical work. Finally, while they are intended to reflect an interdisciplinary team approach, they often are ignored by other members of the team and thus their implementation falls solely to nursing—defeating the purpose behind their creation (Chan & Wong, 1999).

> *Many health care providers believe that clinical pathways are more difficult to develop in psychiatry than in other specialty areas. What problems would be particularly challenging in designing clinical pathways for psychiatric treatment?*

Clinical Algorithms

Treatment or medication algorithms take practice guidelines to a greater level of specificity by providing step-by-step elaboration on issues such as treatment options, treatment sequencing, preferred dosage, and progress assessment. They thus provide clinicians with a framework that can enhance treatment planning and decision-making for individual patients.

Algorithms are rule-based deductive systems that operate with inputs, sequences, time frames, and outputs (Gilbert et al, 1998). They help the clinician select from large databases of information relevant to decision making. Algorithms are cognitive tools for the clinician. They are intended to assist and not limit clinical decision making. A clinical algorithm can be represented by a flowchart that identifies what clinical process might follow from a patient's clinical status and response to prior treatments, thereby providing a more specific statement of priority, or what to do next if the treatment is not effective, than the many options recommended by guidelines.

Algorithms in psychiatry have grown in popularity for a number of reasons. First they reduce unnecessary variation in clinical practice. They can also facilitate decision making by clinicians who cannot integrate into their daily practice all of the published data concerning new knowledge and treatments. Algorithms make explicit the "art" of diagnostic reasoning, while algorithm-based treatment should reduce symptoms and improve a patient's psychosocial functioning faster than non-algorithm-guided treatment. This approach should also reduce the cost of treatment. Finally, algorithms provide a way to compare a patient's progress and allow for important self-correcting feedback about what works best for patients and under what circumstances.

Clinical algorithms are presented in various chapters throughout this text to help the nurse integrate scientific evidence and formulate an appropriate plan of care.

> *Clinical algorithms are presented as simply drawn diagrams. What advantages does such a display have over practice guidelines that can be as many as 50 pages long?*

OUTCOME MEASUREMENT

In previous years, mental health clinicians attempted to give the best care possible to their patients. However, they did this

---

Box 5-3

Characteristics of Good Behavioral Health Practice Guidelines

1. Practice guidelines should be developed in partnership with recipients, consumers, family members, people in recovery, and a wide range of disciplines and organizations.
2. Practice guidelines should be clear, educational and fully available to recipients, consumers, families, people in recovery, all mental health providers, and all payers.
3. Practice guidelines should be a toolbox of options, and not prescriptive in nature.
4. Practice guidelines should be flexible and accommodate consumer choice as well as consumer values, goals and desired outcomes.
5. Practice guidelines should be sensitive and responsive to the individual's environment, ethnicity, culture, gender, sexual orientation, and socioeconomic status.
6. Practice guidelines should be based on scientific evidence of efficacy, effectiveness and established best practices in the field.
7. Practice guidelines should be reviewed and updated regularly.
8. A prevention framework and public health paradigm should be incorporated into every practice guideline.
9. Practice guidelines should identify process and outcome measures, including engagement in the treatment process, adherence to treatment, continuity of care, symptom reduction, enhanced quality of life, improved functional ability, integration of medical, psychiatric, and substance abuse treatment, and improved social status related to employment, housing, or school.
10. Practice guidelines should produce positive clinical outcomes that are sensitive to time for quality improvement.

From: American College of Mental Health Administration: *Moving forward practice guidelines in mental health can addiction services*, Pittsburgh, 2000, ACMHA.

Box 5-4

Categories of Outcome Indicators

CLINICAL OUTCOME INDICATORS

High-risk behaviors
Symptomatology
Coping responses
Relapse
Recurrence
Readmission
Number of treatment episodes
Medical complications
Incidence reports
Mortality

FUNCTIONAL OUTCOME INDICATORS

Functional status
Social interaction
Activities of daily living
Occupational abilities
Quality of life
Family relationships
Housing arrangement

SATISFACTION OUTCOME INDICATORS: PATIENT AND FAMILY SATISFACTION WITH:

Outcomes
Providers
Delivery system
Caregiving process
Organization

FINANCIAL OUTCOME INDICATORS

Cost per treatment episode
Revenue per treatment episode
Length of inpatient stay
Use of health care resources
Costs related to disability

most often without reliable data that compared their work with that of others in the field. Increasing emphasis is now placed on providing the most appropriate care in the most appropriate setting. To make decisions about these issues and demonstrate the effectiveness of clinical programs, outcome measurement is needed (Speer, 1998; Berman et al, 1998).

Outcomes are the extent to which services are cost-effective and have a favorable effect on the patient's symptoms, functioning, and well-being. They include all the things that happen to the patient and his or her family while they are in the health care system, such as health status, functional status, quality of life, the presence or absence of illness, type of coping response, and satisfaction with treatment. They include both positive (well-being) and negative (illness states) dimensions (Sederer & Dickey, 1996).

Outcome measurement can focus on a clinical condition, an intervention, or a caregiving process (Thornicroft & Tansella, 1996; Coughlin, 1999). It is important to measure both short-term and long-term outcomes when providing psychiatric care. These data are then used to make decisions affecting staffing levels, program development, and financial support. Outcomes that can be examined include clinical,

functional, satisfaction, and financial indicators related to the provision of psychiatric care (see Box 5-4). The specific purposes of outcome measurement are to:

- Evaluate the outcomes of care
- Suggest changes in treatment
- Analyze program effectiveness
- Profile the practice pattern of providers
- Determine the most appropriate level of care
- Predict the path of a patient's illness and recovery
- Contribute to quality improvement programs

Outcome measurement is no simple task, however. Many scientific and practical problems are involved in knowing what to measure and how to measure it. One of the most difficult aspects is selecting an appropriate scale or measurement tool. The full listing of rating scales that are commonly used in psychiatry is presented in Chapter 7. Other chapters of this text include the scales specific to the chapter content. Difficulties encountered in outcome measurement also include:

- The resistance of clinicians to complete the rating scales
- The high rates of spontaneous remission and placebo effect among psychiatric patients
- The wide variety of therapeutic approaches and interventions used by mental health clinicians
- The many interacting biological, psychological, and sociocultural factors that affect a patient's improvement
- The lack of clarity regarding when to measure outcomes (before, during, or after treatment or during long-term follow-up)
- The validity and reliability problems encountered with patient report and clinical report scales
- The lack of correlation between measures of patient satisfaction and clinical assessment of improvement
- The practical problems of administering, collecting, and analyzing the outcome data.

In spite of these problems, psychiatric nurses should routinely use rating scales to assess their patients at baseline, their progress during treatment, and the clinical progress they made at the end of treatment. In this way nurses will be able to document the effectiveness of the care they provide. Table 5-1 presents issues that should be considered in selecting outcome measures in psychiatric nursing practice.

One of your nursing colleagues complains about having to complete clinical rating scales on each new admission. She says she "doesn't have time for such busywork." How would you respond?

Patient Satisfaction

Measurement of patient satisfaction in mental health services has received increasing attention due to clinicians' and researchers' desire to measure outcomes that reflect the patient's unique perspective. The growing recognition of the importance of patient satisfaction is also reflected in the requirements of regulatory and certification agencies that mandate that treatment facilities collect and use patient satisfaction data in quality assurance activities.

However, controversy exists about the methods used to measure patient satisfaction and about the meaning and im-

Table **5-1**

Considerations in Selecting Outcome Measures in Psychiatric Nursing Practice	
Applicable	Measures should address an important aspect of the structure, process and/or outcome of care
Acceptable	Measures should be brief and easy to administer
Practical	Measures should be simple to use and interpret and inexpensive to implement
Integrity	Measures should have established reliability and validity and have been tested on the population to be assessed
Sensitive to change	Measures should be able to detect even small changes in a patient's status over time

portance of patient satisfaction data in mental health services (see Citing the Evidence). For example, patients consistently report high levels of satisfaction with services because of a variety of factors, including their relationship with the interviewing staff (Holcomb et al, 1998).

Patient satisfaction is also multidimensional. This means that patients can be satisfied with the treatment staff but not with other aspects of the treatment process such as the environment or timeliness in which the treatment was provided. Thus, while patient satisfaction is an important outcome measure in evaluating mental health services, more research is needed to understand its relation to the structure, process and outcome of psychiatric care.

Quality Report Cards

Another type of outcome measure is related not to the patient, but to the performance of the behavioral health care organization itself. Like their academic counterparts, report cards for mental health and substance abuse services are intended to provide feedback on achievements and problems. At least three dimensions must be considered when discussing report cards: content, point of view, and intended audience (Manderscheid, 1999).

Content refers to the topics that are addressed. In school, content would be the courses graded. Generally, report cards for behavioral health care services cover one or more of the following domains of care: access, appropriateness, cost and outcomes. Access and cost are most common.

Point of view refers to the perspective taken. In school, the perspective is that of the teacher. In a behavioral service setting, the perspective might be that of the payer, the managed care company, the provider, the consumer, or the family member. Most often the perspective is that of the managed care company.

Intended audience can be both explicit and implicit. In schools, the explicit audience of a report card is the parent; an implicit audience may be a future employer. In behavioral service settings, the explicit audience could be the payer, the managed care entity, the provider, the consumer or the family member. Most often, the explicit audience is the payer while the implicit audience is frequently the media.

> *Most discussions about report cards focus on their content. Why do you think the point of view and intended audience are often ignored? What are the implications of not attending to these other domains?*

Citing the Evidence on

Patient Satisfaction

BACKGROUND: Although measures of consumer satisfaction are increasingly used to supplement administrative measures in assessing quality of care, little is known about the association between these two types of indicators. This study examined that relationship.

RESULTS: Satisfaction with several aspects of service delivery was associated with fewer readmissions and fewer days readmitted. Better alliance with inpatient staff was associated with higher rates of follow-up, promptness of follow-up, and continuity of outpatient care, as well as with longer stay for the initial hospitalization.

IMPLICATIONS: The data support the idea that patient satisfaction is associated with higher quality of care and that these measures address a common underlying construct.

Druss B et al: Patient satisfaction and administrative measures as indicators of the quality of mental health care, *Psychiatr Serv* 59(8):1053, 1999.

A number of groups are developing standardized report cards on the performance of behavioral health care organizations. The Health Plan Employer Data and Information Set (HEDIS) is the most widely used system comparing health plans (Druss & Rosenheck, 1997). However, HEDIS contains relatively few measures of the quality of behavioral health care. The American Managed Behavioral Healthcare Association (AMBHA) has developed another set of measures. AMBHA represents managed behavioral health care organizations and their report card is used by patients to grade mental health services on three primary indicators: access to care, consumer satisfaction, and quality of care. The National Alliance for the Mentally Ill (NAMI) has developed a report card for the major managed behavioral health care firms and is testing a state report card. At the federal level, the Center for Mental Health Services (CMHS) has also developed a Consumer-Oriented Mental Health Report Card.

These are important aspects of outcome measurement in a managed care environment. However questions remain regarding the consistency, validity and usefulness of these various approaches. Thus, the American College of Mental Health Administration (ACMHA) is working to define a minimum set of indicators that span the entire field, and to translate the indicators into actual measures (ACHMA, 1998).

THE EVIDENCE BASE FOR PSYCHIATRIC NURSING PRACTICE

Psychiatric nurses are being asked to describe what they do and how they add value to the health care organization. They should frame their responses with sensitivity to the issues of effectiveness, cost and quality. Currently the mysteries about

mental illness are closer to being understood than ever before. New findings are emerging almost daily about their causes and most effective treatments. Nurses need to keep abreast of these developments and base their interventions on the evidence of emerging research rather than on the untested notions of tradition.

Psychiatric nurses would be wise to educate consumers, other health professionals, the business community and managed care companies on the services they can provide, including prevention and rehabilitation, and the ways in which they deliver high-quality, cost-effective care. Nurses then need to be able to support this position with data from outcome studies that reflect clinical, functional, satisfaction, and financial indicators. This research is the essence of evidence based psychiatric nursing practice (Newell & Gournay, 2000).

Current psychiatric nursing practice does not meet the ideals of evidence based care. There is much progress to be made by nurses as they move toward this goal (Lee et al, 1999). For example, many advanced practice psychiatric nurses have reported that they do not use clinical rating scales or outcome measures in their practice (Barrell et al, 1997). Yet the use of measurement or rating scales should be viewed as an essential part of psychiatric nursing practice, and nurses would benefit greatly from mastering the technology that supports this process. Furthermore it appears that much of what psychiatric nurses do is based on untested theories or cherished traditions rather than on scientifically based evidence. There is no literature describing the use of practice guidelines by psychiatric nurses, and very few studies of the clinical, functional, satisfaction or financial outcomes of psychiatric nursing care. In addition, most psychiatric nursing textbooks use secondary references instead of primary references thus creating ambiguity about the evidence base for the nursing practice. Nurses need to research the impact of their activities and control the data set related to nursing outcomes (see Citing the Evidence). They also need to know how to access, interpret, and use findings from outcome research to engage in evidence based psychiatric nursing care.

Citing the Evidence on

Nursing Outcome Research

BACKGROUND: Although there is a great deal of interest in the outcome of the nursing care of psychiatric patients, there is little empirical research about the effectiveness of nursing care. This study evaluated the medical record documentation by nurses as an important database.

RESULTS: Overall, 80% of the predicted patient outcomes were achieved by the time of discharge, with increased length of stay being a factor in increasing the likelihood of goal achievement. A positive association was found between achievement of outcomes at time of discharge and nursing interventions.

IMPLICATIONS: This study showed the importance of the nursing database in the medical records and the effectiveness of nursing interventions on predicted patient outcomes achieved by the time of discharge. More studies of this nature are needed in the field.

Poster E et al: The Johnson behavioral systems model as a framework for patient outcome evaluation, *J Am Psych Nurses Assoc* 3(3):73, 1997.

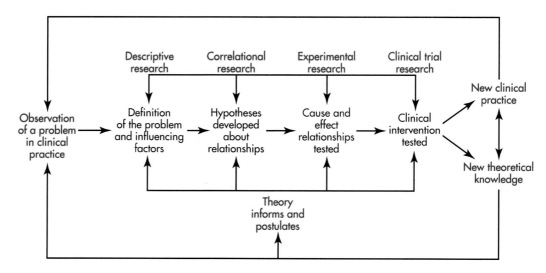

Fig. 5-3 Relationship among practice, theory, and research.

An Agenda for Psychiatric Nursing Research

The relationship between practice, theory, and research is interactive and reciprocal. For theory to be useful, it must have implications for practice, and for practice to be tested and validated, it must be based in theory. Theory that arises out of practice is validated by research, which returns to direct practice and has implications for clinical care.

This cyclical relationship is seen in Fig. 5-3. It shows how the observation of a problem in practice can lead to a more systematic observation and definition of terms, including the nature of the problem and influencing factors. Descriptive and exploratory research can further define a problem. Hypotheses may then be developed concerning relationships between identified variables, which may be tested in correlational or survey research designs. Cause-and-effect relationships between the variables might then be tested in various experiments with natural or controlled settings. Only after establishing cause and effect can specific interventions aimed at changing the clinical problem be prescribed and tested in randomized controlled clinical trials. In this way studies feed knowledge back into practice to improve health care. This progression of observing from practice, theorizing, testing in research, and subsequently modifying practice is an essential part of psychiatric nursing.

At this time psychiatric nursing research is predominantly descriptive and correlational in nature (Yonge et al, 1997). There are few outcome studies testing the effectiveness of psychiatric nursing care (Merwin & Mauck, 1995; Baradell, 1995). Most of the studies that do exist do not meet the criteria of the highest scientific evidence as represented by randomized controlled clinical trials. A current review of the psychiatric nursing journals leads one to conclude that the field has many small scale studies and theory rich insights, but little evidence necessary to direct care practices. Most studies in the field are qualitative which provide detailed experiences at an individual level. In contrast, there are relatively few quantitative studies with the rigorous methodology needed to answer questions about the efficacy and effectiveness of psychiatric nursing interventions.

Psychiatric nurse researchers need to move beyond this basic level of study and be guided by a national-international research agenda that meets the level of scientific inquiry set by the current research community. To this end it has been suggested that psychiatric nurses (Pullen et al, 1999):

- Identify the core knowledge and skills of mental health nurses to ensure the legitimacy of mental health nursing practice and safeguard nursing positions in mental health services
- Conduct evaluation research so that mental health outcomes might be established and cost effectiveness demonstrated.
- Confirm that mental health nurses make a difference in working with people with mental illness and psychiatric disabilities.

One evolving framework for measuring nursing outcomes is the Iowa Nursing Intervention Project which developed nursing intervention classification (NIC) codes (McCloskey & Bulecheck, 2000) and nursing outcome classification (NOC) codes (Johnson et al, 2000). These codes lay out a taxonomy for nursing interventions and outcomes from a biopsychosocial perspective. They are a fertile area of potential nursing research that can document the nature and outcomes of psychiatric nursing practice.

Another model identifying areas for nursing research is seen in Fig. 5-4. It proposes relationships between the different roles nurses assume in health care and outcomes expected of nursing care (Irvine et al, 1998). Psychiatric nurses can use such a model to formulate theories, test interventions and evaluate their impact on patient care outcomes, thus moving the specialty forward toward evidence based practice.

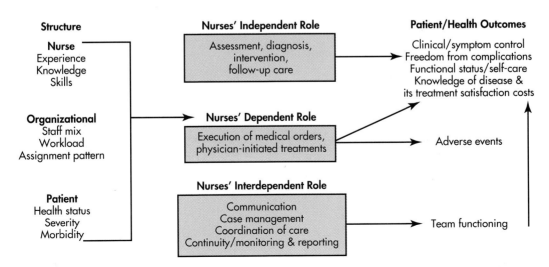

Fig. 5-4 Model for testing nursing role effectiveness.

Summary

1. Evidence based practice blends the nurse's clinical experience with the best available research evidence. It is the best basis for practice and involves defining the clinical question, finding the evidence, analyzing the evidence, using the evidence, and evaluating the outcome.

2. Practice guidelines are developed to help clinical decision making and provide patients information about their treatment options. They include best practices, clinical pathways, and algorithms or protocols. Over thirty groups have developed practice guidelines in psychiatric care.

3. Outcome measurements provide important data about the clinical program and include clinical, functional, satisfaction, and financial indicators. Patient satisfaction indicators and quality report cards are being used to measure the performance of the behavioral health care organization.

4. Current psychiatric nursing practice does not meet the ideals of evidence based practice. Nurses need to use outcome measurements, test theories and interventions through randomized controlled clinical trials, and measure the clinical, functional, satisfaction and financial outcomes of the care they provide.

 Visit MERLIN: www.mosby.com/MERLIN/Stuart to find these additional materials and student activities.

- **Worksheets**
- **"Drug of the Month" Updates**
- **"Citing the Evidence" Updates**
- **Critical Thinking Activities and Exercises**
- **Annotated Suggested Readings**
- **Web Links**
- **More!**

Chapter Review Questions

1. **Identify whether the following statements are true (T) or false (F).**

   _____ **A.** Evidence based practice is a method of self-directed, career-long learning.

   _____ **B.** Descriptive studies are the gold standard of research methodologies.

   _____ **C.** A key aspect of evidence based practice is that it ensures the best use is made of the available evidence.

   _____ **D.** Practice guidelines are similar in format and design.

   _____ **E.** Controversy exists about the methods used to measure patient satisfaction and the meaning and importance of patient satisfaction data in mental health services.

   _____ **F.** Psychiatric nurses routinely use behavioral rating scales in their practice.

2. **Fill in the blanks.**

   A. The report of the Surgeon General came to two conclusions: _____ and _____.

   B. The five steps for developing evidence based care are:
   1. _____,
   2. _____,
   3. _____,
   4. _____, and
   5. _____.

   C. A _____ summarizes the findings from a number of studies to arrive at an objective and authoritative guide to treatment.

   D. Strategies that have been developed to facilitate clinical decision making and provide patients with information about their treatment options are called _____.

   E. _____ are rule-based deductive systems that operate with inputs, sequences, time frames and outputs.

   F. Four categories of outcome indicators that can be used by nurses are _____, _____, _____, and _____.

3. **Provide short answers for the following questions.**

   A. What activities are central to the psychiatric nurse's accountability for patient care?

   B. Discuss the four bases for nursing practice. Which one is best and why?

   C. Go to the website of Best Practices - www.best4health.org. See if psychiatric nurses have submitted any of the practices.

REFERENCES

American College of Mental Health Administration (ACMHA): *Moving forward: practice guidelines in mental health care addiction services,* Pittsburgh, 2000a, ACMHA.

American College of Mental Health Administration (ACMHA): Sounding a call to action, *Behav Healthc Tomorrow* p 43 June, 2000b.

American College of Mental Health Administration (ACMHA): *The Santa Fe summit on behavioral health: preserving quality and value in the managed care equation,* Pittsburgh, 1998, ACMHA.

Baradell J: Clinical outcomes and satisfaction of patients of clinical nurse specialists in psychiatric-mental health nursing, *Arch Psychiatr Nurs* 9:240, 1995.

Barrell LM et al: Patient outcomes used by advanced practice psychiatric nurses to evaluate effectiveness of practice, *Arch Psychiatr Nurs* 11(4):184, 1997.

Benner P: *Clinical wisdom in critical care: a thinking-in-action approach,* Philadelphia, 1999, Saunders.

Berman W et al: Toto, we're not in Kansas anymore: measuring and using outcomes in behavioral health care, *Clinical psychology: science and practice* 5(1):115, 1998.

Bickman L: Our quality-assurance methods aren't so sure, *Behav Healthc Tomorrow* p 41, June 2000.

Brown S et al: Process-oriented critical pathways in inpatient psychiatry, *J Psychosoc Nurs Ment Health Serv* 36(6):31, 1998.

Chan S, Wong K: The use of critical pathways in caring for schizophrenic patients in a mental hospital, *Arch Psychiatr Nurs* 13(3):145, 1999.

Cochrane Collaboration: *The Cochrane library,* Oxford, 1996, Update Software.

Coughlin KM: *Behavioral outcomes & guidelines sourcebook: 2000 edition,* New York, 1999, Faulkner & Gray.

Druss B, Rosenheck R: Evaluation of the HEDIS measure of behavioral health care quality, *Psychiatr Serv* 48:71, 1997.

Dykes PC: *Psychiatric clinical pathways: an interdisciplinary approach,* Gaithersburg, Md, 1998, Aspen.

Gilbert D et al: Texas medication algorithm project: definitions, rationale, and methods to develop medication algorithms, *J Clin Psychiatry* 59(7):345, 1998.

Holcomb WR et al: Customer satisfaction and self-reported treatment outcomes among psychiatric patients, *Psychiatr Serv* 49(7):929, 1998.

Irvine D et al: Linking outcomes to nurses' roles in health care, *Nurs Econ* 16(2):58, 1998.

Johnson M et al: *Nursing outcomes classification (NOC),* St Louis, 2000, Mosby.

Lee JL et al: Does what nurses do affect clinical outcomes for hospitalized patients? a review of the literature, *Health Serv Res* 34(5):1011, 1999.

Manderscheid RW: Assessing performance at the millennium, In Coughlin KM, editor: *Behavioral outcomes & guidelines sourcebook: 2000 edition,* New York, 1999, Faulkner & Gray.

McCloskey J, Bulechek G: *Nursing interventions classification (NIC),* St Louis, 2000, Mosby.

Merwin E, Mauck A: Psychiatric nursing outcome research: the state of the science, *Arch Psychiatr Nurs* 9:311, 1995.

Mulrow C: Rationale for systematic reviews, *Br Med J* 309:597, 1994.

Nathan P, Gorman J: *A guide to treatments that work,* New York, 1998, Oxford University Press.

Newell R, Gournay K: *Mental health nursing: an evidence-based approach,* London, 2000, Churchhill Livingstone.

Pullen L et al: Research priorities in mental health nursing, *Issues Ment Health Nurs* 20:217, 1999.

Sackett D et al: Evidence based medicine: what it is and what it isn't, *Br Med J* 312:71,1996.

Sederer L, Dickey B: *Outcomes assessment in clinical practice,* Baltimore, Md, 1996, Williams & Wilkins.

Speer D: *Mental health outcome evaluation,* San Diego, 1998, Academic Press.

Stetler C et al: Evidence based practice and the role of nursing leadership, *J Nurs Adm* 28(7/8):45, 1998.

Thornicroft G, Tansella A, editors: *Mental health outcome measures,* Berlin Heidelberg, 1996, Springer Verlag.

U.S. Department of Health and Human Services: *Mental health: a report of the surgeon general,* Rockville, Md, 1999, National Institute of Mental Health.

Yonge O et al: Variables and designed in psychiatric/mental health nursing research articles published from 1982 to 1992, *J Psychiatr Ment Health Nurs* 4:339, 1997.

Visit **MERLIN** for *Your Internet Connection*
to websites that are related to the content in this chapter.
www.mosby.com/MERLIN/Stuart

6 Biological Context of Psychiatric Nursing Care

Michele T. Laraia

We must recollect that all our provisional ideas in psychology will some day be based on an organic substructure.
This makes it probable that special substances and special chemical processes control the operation.

SIGMUND FREUD

Although interest in the brain and human behavior has a history as old as the human race, the explosion of scientific information during the 20th century has been unprecedented. The 1990s were named by the U.S. Congress the "Decade of the Brain," and what has been learned during this time from the neurosciences has changed forever how the brain and behavior, health and illness, and thus human experience itself are understood. Research that has focused on how the brain is structured, how the nervous system functions, how these systems affect health, and how they are affected by disease has changed psychiatric nursing in significant ways. The field of neuroscience encompasses many disciplines (Fig. 6-1). They come together to provide an understanding of the human brain and its integration with the body and with the human environment. The neurosciences present new paradigms and great challenges that psychiatric nurses can embrace and thus take a significant step forward in further defining their scope of practice and in measuring the outcomes associated with psychiatric nursing care.

STRUCTURE AND FUNCTION OF THE BRAIN

The psychiatric nurse should have a working knowledge of the normal structure and function of the brain associated with mental health and neuropsychiatric illness just as the cardiac care nurse should know the structure and function of the heart. Much is known about various brain structures and how they are linked to some of the symptoms of mental illness. The reader is encouraged to review texts on basic anatomy and physiology or neurophysiology to learn more about these areas (Applegate, 2000; Nolte, 1999). A brief review of key brain regions is presented in Figs. 6-2 to 6-6 and in Box 6-1 (p. 94). This information can be used as a reference for topics discussed in this chapter.

The brain weighs about 3 pounds. It is composed of trillions of groups of cells that have formed highly specific structures and sophisticated communication pathways that have changed over millions of years of evolution. The brain continues to develop and change (**neural plasticity**) throughout the life span, and during adolescence, it refines its efficiency by eliminating unneeded circuits (**synaptic pruning**) and strengthening others. This process allows humans to have a brain that accommodates its genetic potential as well as the environmental influences surrounding it. The changing brain reacts to a variety of influences that can support health as well as illness both in utero and across the life span. There are

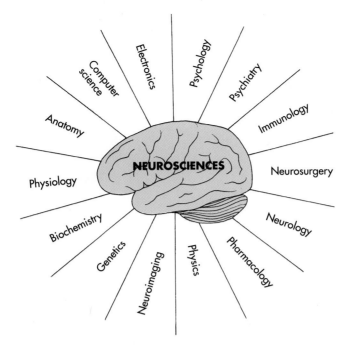

Fig. 6-1   The field of neurosciences.

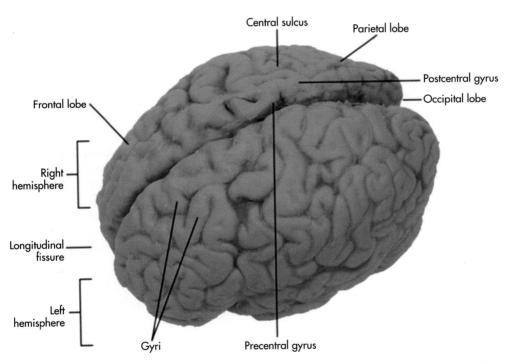

Fig. 6-2   Superior view of the brain. (From Nolte J, Angevine JB, Jr: *The human brain: in photographs and diagrams,* St Louis, 1995, Mosby.)

about 100 billion brain cells (**neurons,**) which form groups, or structures, that are highly specialized. Neurons communicate with each other through electrical impulses and chemical networks. This communication between neurons (neurotransmission) is carried out by chemical "first" messengers (neurotransmitters) and gives rise to human activity, body functions, consciousness, intelligence, creativity, memory,

dreams, and emotion. Neurotransmission is a key factor in understanding how various regions of the brain function and how interventions, such as medications and other therapies, affect brain activity and human behavior.

Neurotransmitters are manufactured in the neuron and released from the axon, or presynaptic cell, into the synapse, which is the space between neurons. From there the neuro-

Fig. 6-3 Lateral view of the left cerebral hemisphere of the brain. (From Nolte J, Angevine JB, Jr: *The human brain: in photographs and diagrams,* St Louis, 1995, Mosby.)

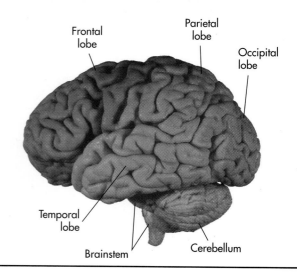

Fig. 6-4 When the brain is cut between the two hemispheres down the middle (a midsagittal section), the main divisions can be clearly seen in **A** and **C**, which are schematic representations, and **B**, a magnetic resonance imaging scan. (**A,** From Nolte J, Angevine JB, Jr: *The human brain: in photographs and diagrams,* St Louis, 1995, Mosby; **B,** from Medical University of South Carolina, Charleston, South Carolina.)

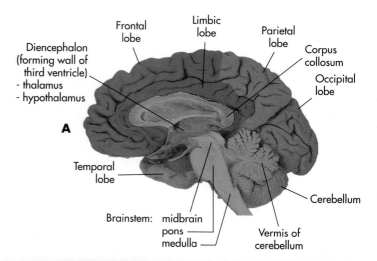

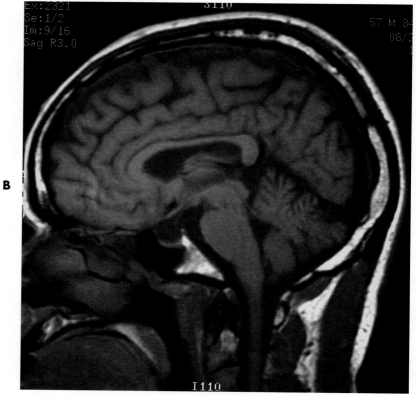

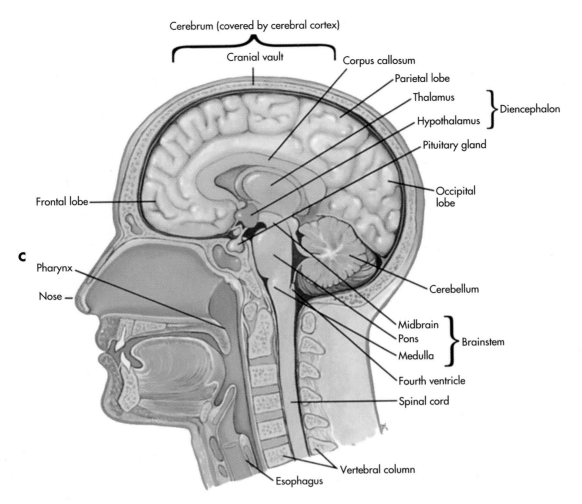

Fig. 6-4, cont'd **C,** Schematic representation of midsagittal section of the brain.

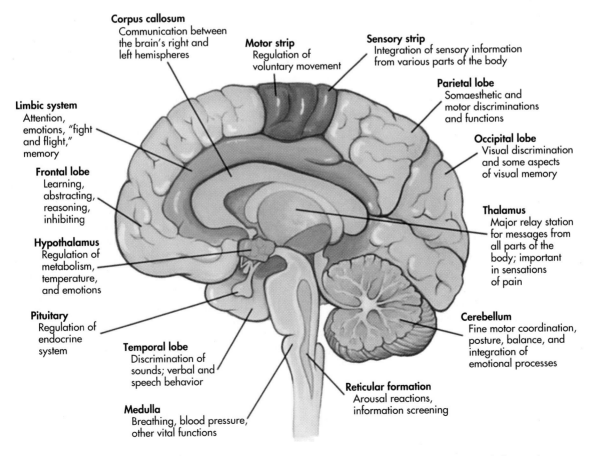

Fig. 6-5 Structure and function of the brain. (From Carson RC, Butcher JN: *Abnormal psychology and modern life,* ed 9, New York, 1992, Harper Collins.)

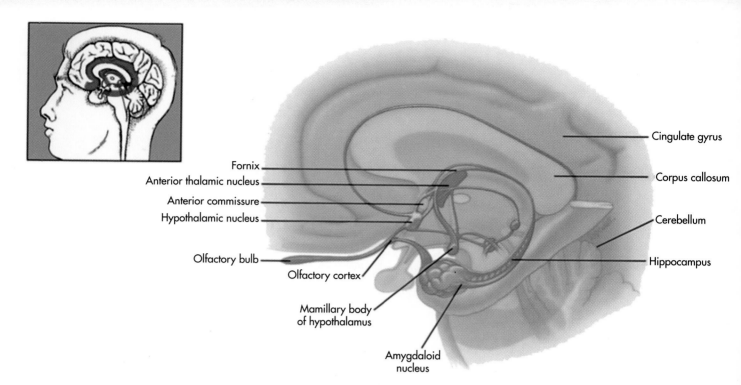

Fig. 6-6   Structures of the limbic system.   (Courtesy Scott Bodell, illustrator.)

transmitters are received by the dendrite, or postsynaptic cell, of the next neuron. This neurotransmission process makes communication between brain cells possible (Fig. 6-7). Like a key inserted into a lock, each of these chemicals fits into specific receptor cells (made of protein) embedded in the membranes of the axons and dendrites, which recognize it. These receptor cells then either open or close doors (**ion channels**) into the cell, allowing for the interchange of chemicals, such as ions like sodium (NA+), potassium (K+), and calcium (Ca+), which changes the electrical charge of the cell (**depolarization**). This then triggers a cascade of chemical and electrical processes that are caused by a variety of chemicals (**second messengers**) within the cell itself. The second messengers regulate the function of the ion channels, the production of neurotransmitters and their release into the synapse, and continue the process of neurotransmission.

Depending on the neurotransmitter, the signal it gives either excites the receiving cells, causing them to produce an action, or inhibits the receiving cells, which slows or stops an action. After release into the synapse and communication with receptor cells, the neurotransmitters are transported back from the synapse into the axon (reuptake), where they are stored for future use or are inactivated (**metabolized**) by enzymes. The nervous system cells are surrounded by myelin sheaths formed by specialized groups of cells called glial cells. These are support cells that insulate neurons, remove excess transmitters and ions from the extracellular spaces in the brain, provide glucose to some nerve cells, and direct the flow of blood and oxygen to various parts of the brain. There are several chambers (**ventricles**) within the brain that carry fluid (**cerebral spinal fluid, CSF**). The CSF cushions and protects and bathes the brain and spinal cord,

carrying chemicals, nutrients, and wastes to and from the blood stream.

From this basic explanation it is evident that neurons are very specialized, and neurotransmitters perform vital functions in the normal working brain. Their absence or excess can play a major role in brain disease and behavioral disorders. A single neurotransmitter can affect other brain chemicals as well as several different subtypes of receptor cells, each located along tracks connecting different regions of the brain. Thus the same neurotransmitter can have one effect in one part of the brain, and different effects in another part of the brain. Nearly all of the known neurotransmitters fall into one of two categories: small amine molecules (monoamines, acetylcholine, and amino acids) and peptides. These are described in Table 6-1 (p. 97).

One clinical implication of this process is that abnormalities in the structure of the brain or in its communication in specific locations can cause or contribute to neuropsychiatric disorders. For example, a communication problem in one small part of the brain can cause widespread dysfunction, since brain communication is like a chain reaction causing changes from one cell to the next, and thus from one structure to the next. The following are examples of networks of **nuclei** (groups of brain cells) that control cognitive, behavioral, and emotional functioning and thus are of particular interest in the study of psychiatric disorders:

- **Cerebral cortex:** Critical in decision making and higher-order thinking, such as abstract reasoning
- **Limbic system:** Involved in regulating emotional behavior, memory, and learning
- **Basal ganglia:** Coordinate involuntary movements and muscle tone

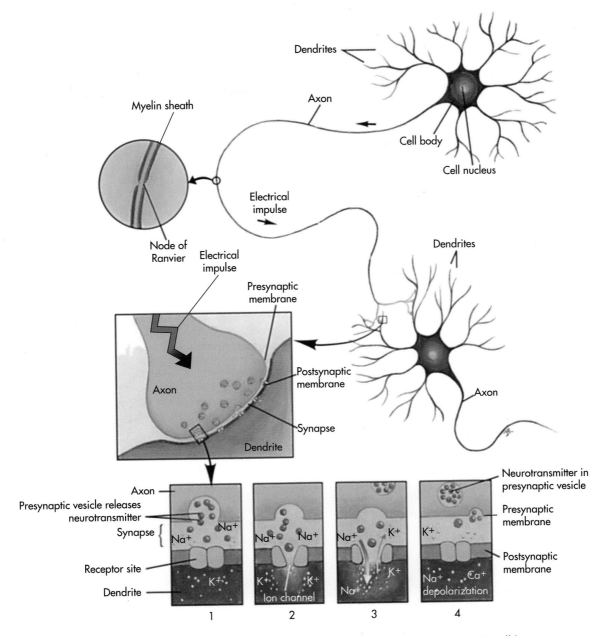

Fig. 6-7   Neurotransmission. *Bottom:* **1,** Neurotransmitter is released from presynaptic cell into synapse. **2,** Neurotransmitter, recognized by receptor cell, causes channel to open, and ions are exchanged. **3,** Exchange of ions causes impulse, which causes reaction in receptor cell. **4,** Neurotransmission has taken place, receptor channel closes, and neurotransmitter returns to presynaptic membrane (reuptake).

- **Hypothalamus:** Regulates pituitary hormones; temperature; and behaviors such as eating, drinking, and sex
- **Locus ceruleus:** Makes norepinephrine, a neurotransmitter involved in the body's response to stress
- **Raphe nuclei:** Make serotonin, a neurotransmitter involved in the regulation of sleep, behavior, and mood
- **Substantia nigra:** Makes dopamine, a neurotransmitter involved in complex movements, thinking, and emotions

A second clinical implication is related to the use of therapeutic interventions, such as psychotropic medications (see Chapter 28), electroconvulsive therapy (ECT) (see Chapter 30), cognitive therapy (see Chapter 33), and alternative therapies (see Chapter 31). All of these therapies work ultimately by regulating neurotransmission, either with a chemical,

electricity, or thoughts. The ultimate goal is to facilitate normal brain communication, thus decreasing "symptoms" of illness and enhancing "normal" behavior.

To date, many interventions effect changes too broadly, thus they lack "**specificity.**" They not only cause desired changes, but they also cause changes that are not wanted ("**side effects**"). As the understanding of the structure and function of the brain increases, research continues to provide more refined interventions, resulting in treatments that are more specific in where they go, are safer, and have fewer side effects. By understanding the neurobiological processes underlying psychiatric symptoms and the actions of interventions, the psychiatric nurse can make a correct diagnosis; select effective treatments; maximize positive effects;

Box **6-1**

Structure and Function of the Brain

CEREBRUM

Largest portion of the brain

Responsible for conscious perception, thought, and motor activity

Governs muscle coordination and the learning of rote movements

Can override most other systems

Divided into two hemispheres, each of which is divided into four lobes

Dominant Hemisphere

Left side is dominant in most people (in 95% of right-handed and more than 50% of left-handed people)

Responsible for the production and comprehension of language, mathematical ability, and the ability to solve problems in a sequential, logical fashion

Nondominant Hemisphere

Right side is nondominant in most people

Responsible for musical skills, recognition of faces, and tasks requiring comprehension of spatial relationships

Corpus Callosum

Largest fiber bundle in the brain

Connects the two cerebral hemispheres and passes information from one to the other, welding the two hemispheres together into a unitary consciousness, allowing the "right hand to know what the left hand is doing"

Cerebral Cortex

A few millimeters thick and about 2.5 square feet in area

Sheet of gray matter containing 30 billion neurons interconnected by almost 70 miles of axons and dendrites

Forms the corrugated surface of the four lobes of the cerebral hemispheres

Connected to various structures of the brain and has a great deal to do with the abilities we think of as uniquely human, such as language and abstract thinking, as well as basic aspects of perception, movement, and adaptive response to the outside world

Functional areas have been mapped by imaging technology

Damage to certain cortical areas usually results in predictable deficits, depending on the area affected

Frontal Lobes

Aid in planning for the future, motivation, control of voluntary motor function, and production of speech

Play an important part in emotional experience and expression of mood

Clinical example: Aphasia (absent or defective speech or comprehension) results from a lesion in the language areas of the cortex. The several types of aphasia depend on the site of the lesion. Damage to Broca's area, which contains the motor programs for the generation of language, results in expressive, or motor, aphasia, with difficulty producing either written or spoken words but no difficulty comprehending language.

Parietal Lobes

Reception and evaluation of most sensory informatian (excluding smell, hearing, and vision)

Concerned with the initial processing of tactile and proprioceptive (sense of position) information, complex aspects of spacial orientation and perception, and the comprehension of language (it shares Wernicke's area with the temporal lobes)

Central Sulcus

Groove or fissure on the surface of the brain that divides the frontal and parietal lobes

Temporal Lobes

Receive and processes auditory information, involved in higher order processing of visual information, involved in complex aspects of memory and learning, and is important in the comprehension of language. Associated with functions such as abstract thought and judgment.

Clinical example: Damage to Wernicke's area, which contains the mechanisms for the formulation of language, results in receptive, or sensory, aphasia, where words are produced but their sequence is defective in linguistic content, resulting in paraphasia (word substitutions), neologisms (insertion of new and meaningless words), or jargon (fluent but unintelligible speech), and there is a general deficiency in the comprehension of language. If the lesion occurs in the connection between Broca's area and Wernicke's area, conduction aphasia results, in which a person has poor repetition but good comprehension.

Lateral Fissure

Separates the temporal lobe from the rest of the cerebrum

Occipital Lobes

Reception and integration of visual input

Damage to the occipital lobes can result in blindness

DIENCEPHALON

Constitutes only 2% of the CNS by weight

Has extremely widespread and important connections; the great majority of sensory, motor, and limbic pathways involve the diencephalon

Thalamus

Composes 80% of the diencephalon

All sensory pathways and many other anatomical loops relay in the thalamus

Takes sensory information and relays it to areas throughout the cortex

Influences prefrontal cortical functions such as affect and foresight

Influences mood and general body movements associated with strong emotions, such as fear or rage

Pineal Gland

Endocrine gland involved in reproductive cycles

During darkness it secretes an antigonadotropic hormone called melatonin, which decreases during light, thus increasing gonadal function

Important in mammals with seasonal sexual cycles, its effects in humans are not yet clear, although tumors of the pineal gland affect human sexual development

May also be involved in the sleep-wake cycle

Box 6-1

Hypothalamus

Weighs only 4 g

Major control center for the pituitary gland; for maintaining homeostasis; and regulating autonomic, endocrine, emotional, and somatic functions

Controls various visceral functions and activities involved in basic drives and is very important in a number of functions that have emotional and mood relationships

Directly involved in stress-related and psychosomatic illnesses and with feelings of fear and rage

Regulates feeding and drinking behavior, temperature regulation, cardiac function, gut motility, and sexual activity

Coordinates responses for the sleep-wake cycle to other areas of the body

Contains the mamillary bodies, which are involved in olfactory reflexes and emotional responses to odors

BRAINSTEM

Connects the spinal cord to the brain

Location of cranial nerve nuclei

Controls automatic body functions such as breathing and cardiovascular activity

Midbrain

Contains ascending and descending nerve tracks

Visual cortex center

Part of auditory pathway

Regulates the reflexive movement of the eyes and head

Aids in the unconscious regulation and coordination of motor activities

Contains the part of the basal ganglia, the substantia nigra, which manufactures dopamine

Pons

Contains ascending and descending nerve tracks

Relay between cerebrum and cerebellum

Reflex center

Contains the locus ceruleus, which manufactures most of the brain's norepinephrine

Medulla Oblongata

Conduction pathway for ascending and descending nerve tracks

Conscious control of skeletal muscles

Involved in functions such as balance, coordination, and modulation of sound impulses from the inner ear

Center for several important reflexes: heart rate, breathing, swallowing, vomiting, coughing, sneezing

Reticular Formation

Central core of the brainstem

Controls cyclic activities such as the sleep-wake cycle (called the reticular activating system, or RAS)

Plays an important role in arousing and maintaining consciousness, alertness, and attention

Contributes to the motor system, respiration, cardiac rhythms, and other vital body functions

Clinical example: Damage to the RAS can result in coma. General anesthetics function by suppressing this system. It also may be the target of many tranquilizers. Ammonia (smelling salts) stimulate the RAS, resulting in arousal.

BASAL GANGLIA

Several deep gray matter structures that are related functionally and are located bilaterally in the cerebrum, diencephalon, and midbrain

Control muscle tone, activity, and posture

Coordinate large-muscle movements

Major effect is to inhibit unwanted muscular activity

Cause extrapyramidal syndromes when dysfunctional

Clinical example: Parkinson's disease (characterized by muscular rigidity; a slow, shuffling gait; and a general lack of movement) is associated with a dysfunction of the basal ganglia, probably a destruction of the dopamine-producing neurons of the substantia nigra (part of the basal ganglia but located in the midbrain).

LIMBIC SYSTEM

Forms the limbus, or border, of the temporal lobes and is intimately connected to many other structures of the brain

Concerned both with subjective emotional experiences and with changes in bodily functions associated with emotional states

Particularly involved in aggressive, submissive, and sexual behavior and with pleasure, memory, and learning

Associated with mood, motivation, and sensations, all central to preservation

Clinical example: Klüver-Bucy syndrome develops when the entire limbic system is removed or destroyed. Symptoms include fearlessness and placidity (absence of emotional reactions), an inordinate degree of attention to sensory stimuli (ceaseless and intrusive curiosity), and visual agnosia (the inability to recognize anything).

Hippocampus

Consolidates recently acquired information about facts and events, somehow turning short-term memory into long term

Contains large amounts of neurotransmitters

Clinical example: Surgical removal of the hippocampus results in the inability to form new memories of facts and events (names of new acquaintances, day-to-day events, inability to remember why a task was begun), although long-term memory, intelligence, and the ability to learn new skills are unaffected. A similar memory problem is Korsakoff's syndrome, in which patients have intact intelligence but cannot form new memories. They typically confabulate (make up answers to questions), which occurs when the hippocampus and surrounding areas are damaged by chronic alcoholism. This also is seen in Alzheimer's disease, in which the memory loss is profound, and there is extensive cellular degeneration in the hippocampus.

Amygdala

Generates emotions from perceptions and thoughts (presumably through its interactions with the hypothalamus and prefrontal cortex)

Contains many opiate receptors

Clinical example: Electrical stimulation of the amygdala in animals causes responses of defense, raging aggression, or fleeing. In humans the most common response is fear and its related autonomic responses (dilation of the pupils, increased heart rate, and release of adrenalin).

Continued

Box 6-1

Structure and Function of the Brain—cont'd

Amygdala—cont'd

Conversely, bilateral destruction of the amygdala causes a great decrease in aggression, and animals become tame and placid. This is thought to be another kind of memory dysfunction that impairs the ability to learn or remember the appropriate emotional and autonomic responses to stimuli.

Fornix

Two-way fiber system that connects the hippocampus to the hypothalamus

CEREBELLUM

"Little brain"

Full range of sensory inputs finds its way here and in turn projects to various sites in the brainstem and thalamus

Although it is extensively involved with the processing of sensory information, it also is part of the motor system and is involved in equilibrium, muscle tone, postural control, and coordination of voluntary movements

It is thought that, because of connections to other brain regions, the cerebellum may be involved in cognitive, behavioral, and affective functions

Clinical example: The malnutrition often accompanying chronic alcoholism causes a degeneration of the cerebellar cortex, resulting in the anterior lobe syndrome in which the legs are primarily affected, and the most prominent symptom is a broad-based, staggering gait and a general incoordination, or ataxia, of leg movements.

VENTRICLES

Each cerebral hemisphere contains a large cavity, the lateral ventricle

A smaller midline cavity, the third ventricle, is located in the center of the diencephalon, between the two halves of the thalamus

The fourth ventricle is in the region of the pons and medulla oblongata and connects with the central canal of the spinal cord, which extends nearly the full length of the spinal cord

Clinical example: Although the clinical significance of these findings is uncertain, imaging techniques have shown enlargement of the ventricles in many psychiatric disorders, suggesting an atrophy of the many critical structures in the brain with these illnesses.

SPINAL FLUID

Cerebral spinal fluid (CSF) is procured from the blood choroid plexuses, located in the ventricles, and fills the ventricles, subarachnoid space (between the brain and the skull), and the spinal cord

CSF bathes the brain with nutrients, cushions the brain within the skull, and exits through the bloodstream

Approximately 140 ml of spinal fluid within the central nervous system travels from its point of origin to the bloodstream at approximately 0.4 ml per minute

Clinical example: Neurotransmitters and their metabolites can be measured in the CSF, plasma, and urine and give an approximation of neurotransmitter production and metabolism in the brain. This provides clues to abnormal neurotransmission in some mental illnesses.

BLOOD-BRAIN AND BLOOD-CSF BARRIERS

Neuronal function requires a microenvironment that is protected from changes elsewhere in the body that may have an adverse effect

Blood-brain and blood-CSF barriers protect the CNS in several ways: Large molecules, such as plasma proteins, present in the blood are excluded from the CSF and nervous tissue. The brain and spinal cord are protected from neurotransmitters in the blood, such as epinephrine produced by the adrenal gland. Neurotransmitters produced in the CNS are prevented from precipitously leaking into the general circulation. Toxins are excluded either because of their molecular size (too big) or because of their solubility (only substances soluble in water and cell-membrane lipids can pass these barriers), so many drugs are not able to enter the brain and spinal cord

---

minimize unwanted effects; and predict, measure, and refine the outcomes of psychiatric nursing care.

> *How would you respond to a nursing colleague who says that psychiatric nurses do not need to know much about anatomy and physiology because what they do primarily is talk to people?*

NEUROIMAGING TECHNIQUES

Until the last few decades the only way to directly study the brain was through brain surgery, open head trauma, or autopsy. Brain imaging techniques allow direct viewing of the structure and function of the intact, living brain. These techniques not only help in diagnosing some brain disorders but also are important because they can map the regions of the brain, measure the activity or function in these regions, and correlate this activity with the effects of interventions. These

images are pictures of the working brain. Table 6-2 (p. 100) describes some of the imaging techniques used in brain research, and Fig. 6-8 (p. 99) shows positron emission tomography (PET) scans of the normal brain.

Computed tomography (CT) and magnetic resonance imaging (MRI) permit visualization of **brain structures.** They can detect structural abnormalities, changes in the volume of brain tissue, and enlargement of the cerebral ventricles. **Brain function** can be studied using other imaging techniques to determine both normal activity as well as malfunctioning in specific regions. Techniques that show brain function include brain electrical activity mapping (BEAM), which measures sensory input; PET; and single photon emission computed tomography (SPECT), which permits the study of brain metabolism and cerebral blood flow.

PET, SPECT, and the newer functional magnetic resonance imaging (fMRI) techniques can measure the use of

Table 6-1

Neurotransmitters and Neuromodulators in the Brain

Substance	Location	Function
AMINES Amines are neurotransmitters that are synthesized from amino molecules such as tyrosine, tryptophan, and histidine. Found in various regions of the brain, amines affect learning, emotions, motor control, and other activities.		
Monoamines		
Norepinephrine (NE)	Derived from tyrosine, a dietary amino acid. Located in the brainstem (particularly the locus ceruleus). *Effect:* Can be excitatory or inhibitory.	Levels fluctuate with sleep and wakefulness. Plays a role in changes in levels of attention and vigilance. Involved in attributing a rewarding value to a stimulus and in the regulation of mood. Plays a role in affective and anxiety disorders. Antidepressants block the reuptake of NE into the presynaptic cell or inhibit monoamine oxidase from metabolizing it.
Dopamine (DA)	Derived from tyrosine, a dietary amino acid. Located mostly in the brainstem (particularly the substantia nigra). *Effect:* Generally excitatory.	Involved in the control of complex movements, motivation, cognition, and regulating emotional responses. Many drugs of abuse (such as cocaine and amphetamines) cause DA release, suggesting a role in whatever makes things pleasurable. Involved in the movement disorders seen in Parkinson's disease and in many of the deficits seen in schizophrenia and other forms of psychosis. Antipsychotic drugs block dopamine receptors in the postsynaptic cell.
Serotonin (5-HT)	Derived from tryptophan, a dietary amino acid. Located only in the brain (particularly in the raphe nuclei of the brainstem). *Effect:* Mostly inhibitory.	Levels fluctuate with sleep and wakefulness, suggesting a role in arousal and modulation of the general activity levels of the CNS, particularly the onset of sleep. Plays a role in mood and probably in the delusions, hallucinations, and withdrawal of schizophrenia. Involved in temperature regulation and the pain-control system of the body. LSD (the hallucinogenic drug) acts at 5-HT receptor sites. Plays a role in affective and anxiety disorders. Antidepressants block its reuptake into the presynaptic cell.
Melatonin	A further synthesis of serotonin produced in the pineal gland. *Effect:* Implicated in seasonal affective disorder and the sleep-wake cycle.	Induces pigment lightening effects on skin cells and regulates reproductive function in animals. Role in humans is unclear.
Acetylcholine	Synthesized from choline. Located in the brain and spinal cord but is more widespread in the peripheral nervous system, particularly the neuromuscular junction of skeletal muscle. *Effect:* Can have an excitatory or inhibitory effect.	Plays a role in the sleep-wakefulness cycle. Signals muscles to become active. Alzheimer's disease is associated with a decrease in acetylcholine-secreting neurons. Myasthenia gravis (weakness of skeletal muscles) results from a reduction in acetylcholine receptors.

Continued

Table **6-1**

Neurotransmitters and Neuromodulators in the Brain—cont'd		
Substance	**Location**	**Function**
Amino Acids		
Glutamate	Found in all cells of the body, where it is used to synthesize structural and functional proteins. Also found in the CNS, where it is stored in synaptic vesicles and used as a neurotransmitter. *Effect:* Excitatory.	Implicated in schizophrenia; glutamate receptors control the opening of ion channels that allow calcium (essential to neurotransmission) to pass into nerve cells, propagating neuronal electrical impulses. Its major receptor, NMDA, helps regulate brain development. This receptor is blocked by drugs (such as PCP) that cause schizophrenic-like symptoms. Overexposure to glutamate is toxic to neurons and may cause cell death in stroke and Huntington's disease.
Gamma-aminobutyric acid (GABA)	A glutamate derivative; most neurons of the CNS have receptors. *Effect:* Major transmitter for postsynaptic inhibition on the CNS.	Drugs that increase GABA function, such as the benzodiazepines, are used to treat anxiety and to induce sleep.
PEPTIDES Peptides are chains of amino acids found throughout the body. About 50 have been identified to date, but their role as neurotransmitters is not well-understood. Although they appear in very low concentrations in the CNS, they are very potent. They also appear to play a "second messenger" role in neurotransmission; that is, they modulate the messages of the nonpeptide neurotransmitters.		
Endorphins and enkephalins	Widely distributed in the CNS. *Effect:* Generally inhibitory.	The opiates morphine and heroin bind to endorphin and enkephalin receptors on presynaptic neurons, blocking the release of neurotransmitters and thus reducing pain.
Substance P	Spinal cord, brain, and sensory neurons associated with pain. *Effect:* Generally excitatory.	Found in pain transmission pathway. Blocking the release of substance P by morphine reduces pain.

glucose (glucose utilization) and the amount of **blood flowing** in a region of the brain (regional cerebral blood flow). These are the two basic indicators of brain activity. The more active a region of the brain is, the more blood will flow through it, the more glucose it will use, and the brighter (yellow, orange, and red) the imaging scan looks.

When these techniques are coupled with neuropsychological test results, deficits in a person's performance, such as language or cognitive and sensory information processing, can be linked to the activity of the region of the brain responsible for those functions (see Fig. 6-8). The remainder of this chapter describes new developments in the understanding of the biology of the brain related to neuropsychiatric illness.

GENETICS OF MENTAL ILLNESS

The search for the genes that cause mental illness has been difficult and inconclusive to date but has stimulated signifi-

cant scientific, political, and clinical debate (see Critical Thinking about Contemporary Issues, p. 100). The history of biology was altered forever a decade ago by the launching of the Human Genome Project, a research program that is attempting to characterize the complete set of genetic instructions of the human being (Collins, 1999). The complexity of human emotions and behavior is most likely governed by a variety of genes and their interplay with each other, environmental factors, personality, and life experiences.

An example of a genetically heterogeneous (caused by more than one gene) disorder is the rare form of Alzheimer's disease (AD) that affects people before age 65. Early onset AD affects only about 10% of cases and seems to be linked to mutations in any of three specific genes responsible for amyloid-beta, causing excess deposits of this substance in the brains of persons with AD (Jorde et al, 1999). The search for the genes responsible for the more common late-onset AD and for

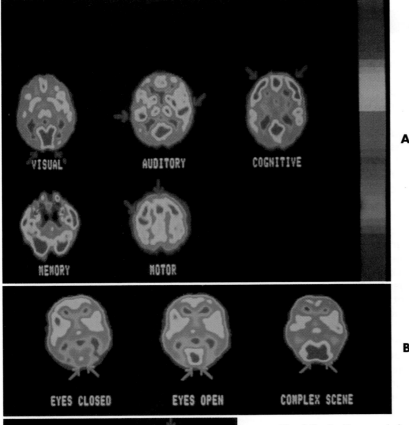

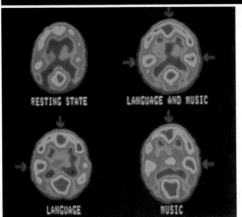

Fig. 6-8 Positron emission tomography scan shows varying patterns of glucose consumption during different tasks. The color scale ranges from 2 *(violet)* to 45 *(red)*. **A,** Different kinds of tasks cause increased glucose consumption in distinct areas of the brain. A checkerboard visual stimulus activates the occipital lobes. An auditory stimulus causes increased glucose consumption in the temporal lobes. When an individual is engaged in an active, cognitive task rather than passive perception of stimuli, glucose consumption increases in the frontal lobes. Subjects trying to remember information from a verbal stimulus (a story) show increased glucose consumption in the temporal lobes. Sequential movements of the fingers of the right hand activate motor cortex on the left and the supplementary motor arc *(vertical arrow)* **B,** Increasing complexity of a particular kind of task causes increased glucose consumption in progressively larger areas of the cortex. With the subject blindfolded ("eyes closed"), there is relatively little glucose consumption in the occipital lobes. With the eyes open, looking at a plain white light source activates the primary visual cortex of the occipital lobes. Looking at an outdoor scene ("complex scene") activates the visual association cortex in additional areas of the occipital lobes. **C,** The left hemisphere usually plays a dominant role in language functions, the right hemisphere in musical and certain other functions. When a subject listens simultaneously to a Sherlock Holmes story and a Brandenberg concerto, both superior temporal lobes and both frontal lobes are activated. Listening to just the story activates predominately the left hemisphere. Musical chords alone activate predominantly the right hemisphere. (**A** and **B,** From Phelps ME, Mazziotta JC: *Science* 228:779, 1985; **C,** Courtesy Dr. ME Phelps and Dr. JC Mazziotta, University of California School of Medicine.)

other neuropsychiatric illness is ongoing and has captured the attention of the political, scientific, and lay communities.

Several issues make research on the inheritance of mental illness difficult. These include the following:

- The psychiatric diagnostic classification system continues to change
- The psychiatric diagnostic system is organized by symptom clusters, an increasingly confusing approach

since abnormalities in different brain systems often cause similar and overlapping symptoms
- A gene that sometimes produces a psychiatric disorder may not always do so
- Several different genes may be necessary to produce psychiatric disorders
- Nongenetic factors also contribute to the development of a disorder

Continued

pacemakers located in specific areas of the brain that are subject to change by specific external cues.

Circadian rhythm is like a network of internal clocks that coordinate events in the body according to a 24-hour cycle (Fig. 6-9). This cycle corresponds to the time it takes the earth to spin on its axis, exposing all of life to daily rhythms of light, darkness, and temperature. Biological rhythms affect every aspect of health and well-being, including lifestyle, sleep, mood, eating, drinking, fertility, body temperature, and menses.

Because the body's fluids and tissues function according to circadian rhythms, physical and mental abilities and moods may vary widely from one time of day to another. To run according to the 24-hour clock, the circadian system must have a time cue from the external environment. That cue is usually sunlight, which resets the clock each day and synchronizes the body's complex set of rhythms.

Light enters the retina of the eye, which acts like an antenna of the brain. From the retina, specialized nerve cells send signals of light and dark through special pathways to the hypothalamus and other regions of the brain (Fig. 6-10). One of the most important internal timekeepers is located in the hypothalamus. It consists of two clusters of nerve cells called the **suprachiasmatic nuclei** (SCN). A direct track leads from the retina to these two clusters of cells, which in turn respond to the light signals from the retina.

The SCN is the pacemaker of circadian rhythm; it sends electrical and chemical messages to other parts of the brain, including the hypothalamus, pituitary, pineal gland, and parts of the brainstem. These brain structures send hormonal messages to other control systems in the body, such as the heart, adrenal glands, liver, kidney, and intestines, keeping them regulated to the internal clock and modulating thoughts, moods, body functions, and human activities.

Sleep

According to most surveys, people sleep between 6 to 9 hours a night, with 8 hours reported most often. Few people normally sleep fewer than 5 or more than 10 hours. Usually, people sleep in one nightly phase, although in some cultures and during some times of life, a siesta, or afternoon nap, is common. Studies show that the sleep cycle is related to the timing of circadian rhythms, changes in light and darkness, and temperature changes.

Generally, each night a person's sleep passes through a repeated sequence of five stages. The first stage is that of "falling asleep," which is called stage one sleep. A person then progresses into sleep itself (stage two), followed by deep sleep, also called delta sleep (stages three and four). After a brief return to stage two sleep the person moves into stage five, or rapid eye movement (REM), sleep. Stages two through REM repeat themselves several times a night, with deep sleep becoming briefer in the course of a night and REM sleep becoming progressively longer (see Fig. 20-3).

REM sleep occupies approximately 20% to 25% of the sleep time of adults, stage two about 50%, and stages three and four about 15%. Stages three and four occur primarily in the first half of the sleep period. The lighter stages of sleep and longer REM periods typically occur in the second half. Usually, during REM sleep the individual has vivid dreams,

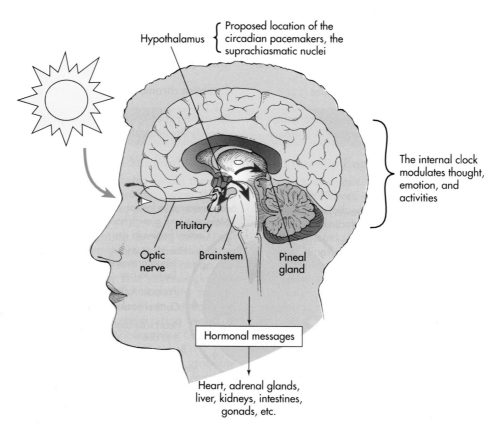

Fig. 6-10 From the sun to the brain.

and the eyes show bursts of rapid movement beneath the closed lids.

It is important for optimal health that people progress through the normal stages of sleep each night. Studies show that in depressed persons, REM sleep is excessive, the deeper stages of sleep are decreased, and dreams may be unusually intense. Thus, although they may sleep 6 to 9 hours each night, people with depression frequently report fatigue, poor concentration, and irritability associated with sleep deprivation.

PSYCHONEUROIMMUNOLOGY

Psychosocial factors can have a profound effect on a person's immune system. In particular, psychosocial stressors and the mental state associated with them may depress immune function to the point of enhancing vulnerability to almost any antigen to which the person is exposed. The central nervous system is involved in mediating any such effects.

Psychoneuroimmunology is a field that explores the interactions between the central nervous system, the endocrine system, and the immune system; the impact of behavior/stress on these interactions; and how psychological and pharmacological interventions may modulate these interactions (Glasser et al, 1999) (see Chapter 18). Communication between these systems is accomplished by a feedback loop of chemical messengers from each system: neurotransmitters produced by nerve cells, hormones secreted by endocrine glands, and cytokines and other peptides secreted by immune cells (see Fig. 18-2). Research has demonstrated the suppression of white blood cell reproduction and increased susceptibility to illness following sleep deprivation, marathon running, space flight, death of a spouse, and during the course of depression. Another example is that of natural killer cells (NK), which are believed to play a role in tumor surveillance and the control of viral infections. These cells seem to decrease with increasing levels of stress. (See Citing the Evidence on Psychoneuroimmunology.)

BIOLOGICAL ASSESSMENT OF THE PATIENT

Several steps are necessary in the assessment of psychiatric patients from a biological perspective. Brain disorders can be physical or "neurological" and can include many different diagnoses such as stroke, head and spinal cord injury, brain tumors, multiple sclerosis, Parkinson's disease, and Huntington's disease. Schizophrenia, depression, anxiety disorders, and Alzheimer's disease also are brain disorders, although they are classified as psychiatric disorders. The symptoms of psychiatric versus neurological illnesses can overlap and can even mimic each other. The treatments can be very different, and treatments for one disorder may make another disorder worse. Thus the ability to screen for both undiagnosed physical and psychiatric disorders has important implications for the psychiatric nurse in the assessment of the presenting symptoms, treatment selection, and possible need for referral to a specialist in another discipline.

Undiagnosed physical illness, particularly organic brain disorders, can be costly and dangerous if treated incorrectly. Physical illnesses such as brain tumors and endocrine disorders can cause psychiatric symptoms as well as exacerbate an

---

Citing the Evidence on

Psychoneuroimmunology

BACKGROUND: 19 spousal caregivers and 13 adult children caregivers of patients with early and middle stages of Alzheimer's disease were assessed for physical, social, and emotional health; natural killer (NK) cell number; and cytotoxicity.

RESULTS: The adult children caregivers did much worse on all measured parameters than the spousal caregivers. They were much more stressed, more depressed, had a lower quality of life, and had lower NK cell numbers and NK cytotoxicity parameters. When both groups received a relaxation intervention, both improved, but the spousal caregivers did better that the children caregivers.

IMPLICATIONS: When working with family members who are caregivers of patients with Alzheimer's disease, it is important to know that children caregivers may be significantly more stressed, more symptomatic, and at greater risk for immune system compromise than spousal caregivers, and therefore may need a more aggressive approach with interventions to avoid or modify stress-related illness.

Lewis S et al: Psychosocial and immune parameters in spousal and children caregivers of patients with Alzheimer's disease, Presented at the PsychoNeuroImmunology Research Society Meeting in Galveston Texas, July, 1999. Available at: http://www.pnirs.org/pastmeetings/99Galv/P1c.html.

existing psychiatric illness, and patients who are psychiatrically ill may be misdiagnosed in non-psychiatric settings. Thus psychiatric nurses need to include a thorough biological assessment in their evaluation of psychiatric patients. The psychiatric nurse is well-suited to screen for the major signs of physical or organic disorders that may complicate a patient's psychiatric status, to identify physical illnesses that may have been overlooked, or to refer the patient for a thorough medical diagnostic work-up if indicated. In fact, this is one of the unique areas of expertise that the psychiatric nurse brings to the mental health treatment team, and it is essential that psychiatric nurses continue to demonstrate their competence in all aspects of their biopsychosocial assessment.

A complete health care history of the patient, including lifestyle review, physical examination, analysis of laboratory values, and discussion of presenting symptoms and coping responses, is an essential element of a baseline biological assessment (Box 6-2). The nurse should be able to perform a basic physical examination to assess for gross abnormalities and be able to interpret the results of more complex physical examinations. Appearance, gait, coordination, bilateral strength, tremors and tics, speech, and symptoms such as headaches, blurred vision, dizziness, vomiting, motor weakness, disorientation, confusion, and memory problems should be assessed in detail.

Box **6-2**

Biological Assessment of the Psychiatric Patient

HEALTH CARE HISTORY
General Health Care

Regular and specialty health-care provider
Frequency of health-care visits
Date of last examination
Any unusual circumstances of birth, including mother's preterm habits and condition
Regular and speciality health-care provider
Frequency of health-care visits
Any unusual circumstances of birth, including mother's preterm habits and customs
Allergies
Immunizations
Papanicolaou smear and mammogram
Chest x-ray and ECG
TB test

Hospitalizations, Surgeries, and Medical Procedures

When, why indicated, treatments, outcome

Brain Impairment

Diagnosed brain problem
Head trauma
Details of accidents or periods of unconsciousness for any reason: blows to the head, electrical shocks, high fevers, seizures, fainting, dizziness, headaches, falls

Cancer

Full history, particularly consider metastases (lung, breast, melanoma, gastrointestinal tract, and kidney are most likely to metastasize)
Results of treatments (chemotherapy and surgeries)

Lung Problems

Details of any condition or event that restricts the flow of air to the lungs for more than 2 minutes or adversely affects oxygen absorption (the brain uses 20% of the oxygen in the body) such as with chronic obstructive pulmonary disease, near drowning, near strangulation, high-altitude oxygen deprivation, resuscitation events

Cardiac Problems

Childhood illnesses such as scarlet or rheumatic fever
History of heart attacks, strokes, or hypertension
Arteriosclerotic conditions

Diabetes

Stability of glucose levels

Endocrine Disturbances

Thyroid and adrenal function particularly

Menstrual History

Age of first menstrual period
Regularity of menstrual periods, impact on lifestyle
Date of last menstrual period, duration
Menopausal history
Assess for premenstrual syndromes

Sexual History

Assess sexual function and activity
Screen for sexual dysfunction
Safe-sex practices and sexually transmitted diseases

Reproductive History

Number of pregnancies, births, children and their ages
Assess birth control methods

LIFESTYLE
Eating

Details of unusual or unsupervised diets, appetite, weight changes, cravings, and caffeine intake

Medications

Full history of current and past psychiatric medications in self and first-degree relatives
Full history of current use of non-psychiatric prescription medicines, over-the-counter medicines, and herbal and other alternative remedies

Substance Use

Alcohol, drug, caffeine, and tobacco use

Toxins

Overcome by automobile exhaust or natural gas
Exposure to lead, mercury, insecticides, herbicides, solvents, cleaning agents, lawn chemicals
Fetal alcohol syndrome

Occupation (current and past)

Chemicals in the workplace (farming, painting)
Work-related accidents (construction, mining)
Military experiences
Stressful job circumstances

Injury

Contact sports and sports-related injuries
Exposure to violence or abuse
Rape or molestation

Impact of culture, race, ethnicity, and gender
PHYSICAL EXAMINATION

Review of Physiological Systems

Integumentary: skin, nails, hair, and scalp
Head: eyes, ears, nose, mouth, throat, and neck
Breast
Respiratory
Cardiovascular
Hematolymphatic
Gastrointestinal tract
Urinary tract
Genital
Neurological, soft signs, and cranial nerves
Musculoskeletal
Nutritive
Restorative: sleep and rest
Endocrine
Allergic and immunological
Gait, coordination, and balance

Box 6-2

Biological Assessment of the Psychiatric Patient—cont'd

LABORATORY VALUES

Hematology: CBC and sedimentation rate, screen for anemia

Chemistry, BUN, glucose, thyroid, adrenal, liver and kidney function, etc

Serology, especially syphilis screen, HIV, hepatitis

Urinalysis, screen for drugs

Stool tests for occult blood

PRESENTING SYMPTOMS AND COPING RESPONSES

Description: nature, frequency, and intensity

Threats to safety of self or others

Functional status

Quality of life

Support system

Obtaining permission from the patient to access other people and documents that will help the nurse and health care team gain a thorough view of the patient is an important step in the screening process. Particularly when brain disorders, whether physical or psychiatric, are suspected, the nurse should pay close attention to inconsistencies in the patient's account, between those of other people, and in previous health care records. Throughout the course of the screening the nurse should be alert for any indications of head trauma at any time in the patient's life, such as through accidents, fevers, surgery, or seizures.

Only after a patient has been carefully screened can the nurse determine which of the patient's problems are primarily psychiatric and amenable to psychiatric intervention and which may need the attention of a consultant in another specialty. The identified problems that are appropriate for psychiatric intervention then become the target symptoms of specific interventions, and progress toward expected outcomes can be measured throughout the course of treatment.

Why is a history of psychiatric medications taken from a patient's first-degree relatives an important part of the psychiatric nurse's biological assessment?

BIOLOGICAL COMPONENTS OF MENTAL ILLNESS

The amount of biological information about each psychiatric disorder varies considerably. In this section of the chapter, several major neuropsychiatric disorders are briefly discussed in the context of neurobiological research. These illnesses were selected because there is a great deal of biological information available about them. Implications for psychiatric nursing practice are highlighted. This discussion is intended to expose the reader to emerging knowledge and provide a model that helps the psychiatric nurse keep up-to-date with the biological context of psychiatric nursing care. In addition, an overview of biological knowledge related to specific neuropsychiatric disorders can be found in Chapters 17 through 27 and in Coleman and Kay (2000).

Schizophrenia

It is widely believed that schizophrenia, a neuropsychiatric syndrome of variable but profoundly disruptive psy-

Table 6-4

Genetic Risk of Schizophrenia

Person at Risk	Percentage of Risk
Monozygotic twin affected	50%
Dizygotic twin affected	15%
Sibling affected	10%
One parent affected	15%
Both parents affected	35%
Second-degree relative affected	2% to 3%
No affected relative	1%

chopathology, is caused by the interaction of a variety of mechanisms that are biological, environmental, and experiential. It also appears that schizophrenia affects several distinct brain regions that involve thought, perception, emotion, movement, and behavior (see Chapter 22).

Genetics. There is a 1% lifetime risk of schizophrenia in the general population, but it is higher in people with a first-degree (parents, siblings, children) or second-degree (grandparents, aunts and uncles, cousins, grandchildren) relative with the disorder (Table 6-4). The pattern of inherited vulnerability in schizophrenia most likely results from the interaction of unknown influences with several genes, probably in utero. This affects the structure and function of the brain as it continues to grow after birth. Two genetic hypothesis of particular interest are described in the following:

1. Trinucleotide repeat amplification—mutation in which a certain stretch of deoxyribonucleic acid (DNA) occurs more than once when genes are copied—could explain some of the differential rates of occurrence of schizophrenia, even among monozygotic twins, who have identical genes but only a 50% concordance rate (occurrence of the disorder in both of them) for the disease. If one child in a family carrying a gene for schizophrenia happens to have more trinucleotide repeats than the others, that child could be pushed over the threshold from health to mental illness

2. Genome screens of entire families of individuals with schizophrenia support genetic linkage for schizophrenia on chromosome 6, and possibly on 22. The aim of genetic research is to eventually map the genetic susceptibility for schizophrenia and develop genetic interventions as treatment modalities.

Biochemistry. Several brain chemicals and the balance between them in various parts of the brain have been implicated in schizophrenia. These include the following:

- An imbalance of the neurotransmitter dopamine (DA), or defects in the dopamine receptor systems. This is evidenced by drugs that change the balance of dopamine in the brain also affect schizophrenic symptoms
- An imbalance between dopamine and other neurotransmitters, particularly serotonin (5-HT). This is evidenced by atypical antipsychotic drugs that change the balance between DA and 5-HT, decreasing the symptoms of schizophrenia
- The excitatory neurotransmitter glutamate also is implicated. This is evidenced by drugs such as phencyclidine (PCP), which block glutamate's major receptor, NMDA, thus mimicking the symptoms of schizophrenia in healthy subjects and worsening them in schizophrenic subjects

New theories about the biology of schizophrenia, such as those that propose a role for glutamate, will result in new treatments. New agents, such as glycine and ampakines, decrease the symptoms of schizophrenia by actions that enhance neurotransmission at the glutamate receptors. These and other theories and treatments will keep evolving as neuroscientific research continues its focus on this severe and usually progressive disorder.

Brain Imaging. Imaging studies of schizophrenia have included various regions of the brain, but many have focused specifically on the cortex of the frontal lobes, which appears to be involved in the negative symptoms of schizophrenia, and on the limbic system within the temporal lobes, which appears to be involved in the positive symptoms of schizophrenia (see Chapter 22). A consistent group of abnormalities seem evident in the brains of people with schizophrenia, and imaging studies may continue to clarify how these functional abnormalities affect the etiology, symptoms, and treatment of schizophrenia (Fig. 6-11).

CT scans and MRI studies have demonstrated enlargement of the ventricles, implying either a lack of brain development or a loss of brain tissue. Although a clear correlation of these findings to clinical symptoms has yet to emerge, there is a trend for large ventricles to be associated with two indicators of poor prognosis: early age of onset and poor premorbid functioning. MRIs also show smaller volume in structures in the limbic region (which modulates emotional response and memory) of the temporal lobe. (See Citing the Evidence on MRI in Schizophrenia.)

PET studies have shown functional abnormalities in the way the brain utilizes glucose. For example, the Wisconsin Card Sort Test (a test of working memory and abstract thinking) has been found to activate the cerebral blood flow in the prefrontal cortex in the brains of normal controls and in the nonaffected identical twins of schizophrenics (Roberts et al, 1993). However, this same region of the brain shows lower metabolism and reduced blood flow (hypofrontality) in schizophrenics, who do worse on this test than normal controls regardless of the length of time they have been ill or whether they have been treated with antipsychotic drugs (Fig. 6-12). Imaging research continues to make significant

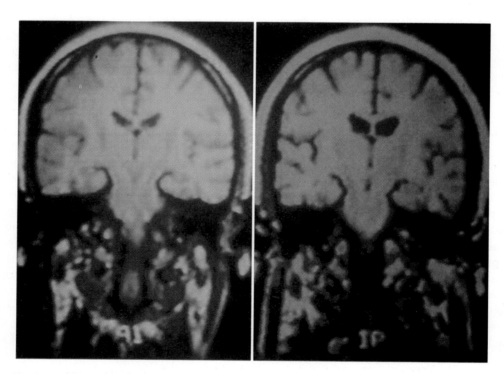

Fig. 6-11 Magnetic resonance imaging scans through the bodies of the lateral ventricles in a pair of monozygotic twins who are discordant for schizophrenia. Note the increase in the cerebrospinal fluid spaces in the twin with schizophrenia *(right)* as compared with the unaffected twin *(left)*. (From Roberts GS, Leigh PN, Weinberger DR: *Neuropsychiatric disorders,* London, 1993, Mosby-Wolfe.)

Citing the Evidence on

MRI in Schizophrenia

BACKGROUND: MRI studies in schizophrenia have brought mixed results, lending to the confusion about this disorder. These authors reviewed and compared 118 peer-reviewed and controlled MRI studies of schizophrenia done during the Decade of the Brain.

RESULTS: The researchers found (1) enlarged lateral and third ventrical sizes, implying decreased brain volume; (2) decreased volume in temporal lobe structures, which link memory and associations involving language and speech (the possible source of positive symptoms of schizophrenia); (3) mixed results in frontal lobe studies, implying that the significant frontal lobe deficits (negative symptoms) in schizophrenia may result from very subtle

volume changes; (4) decreased volume in subcortical structures such as the thalamus (relays sensory and limbic information to the cortex), corpus callosum (connects the right and left brain), basal ganglia (regulates movement); (5) these structural changes in schizophrenia seem to worsen over time.

IMPLICATIONS: The brain structures of schizophrenics differ in specific ways from those of controls, and schizophrenia appears to fit a "two-hit" model of illness: Hit No. 1: Abnormalities resulting from neurodevelopmental events (genetics, infections, etc.), and Hit No. 2: Ongoing brain changes after onset of symptoms.

McCarley R et al: MRI anatomy of schizophrenia, *Biological Psychiatry*, 45:1099, 1999.

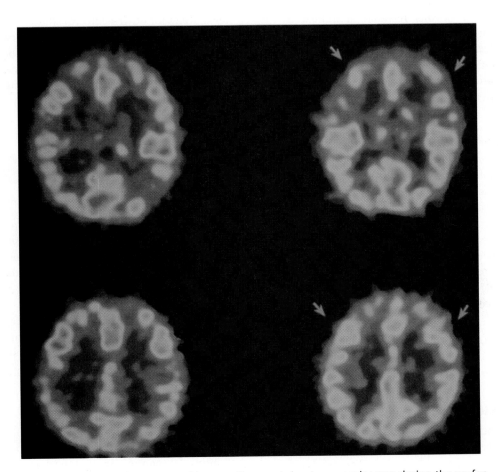

Fig. 6-12   Blood flow demonstrated by a positron emission tomography scan during the performance of the Wisconsin Card Sort Task (a task that activates prefrontal cortex in normal subjects) in a twin with schizophrenia *(right column)* and an unaffected twin *(left column)*. The arrows indicate the relatively focused failure of activation in the affected twin compared with the unaffected twin. (From Roberts GS et al: *Neuropsychiatric disorders,* London, 1993, Mosby-Wolfe.)

contributions to what is know about this neurodevelopmental disorder.

Additional Avenues of Research for Schizophrenia

Although study results vary at this time, several interesting avenues of research may eventually help identify environmental risk factors for schizophrenia. These events may increase the chances of a genetically vulnerable individual getting schizophrenia. These include the following:

Viral Pandemics and Season and Place of Birth. There is a higher rate of births of people with schizophrenia in Europe and the United States in winter and early spring and a higher incidence of schizophrenia in urban compared to rural settings. Peaks can be correlated with pandemic viral outbreaks, particularly influenza and polio virus, that occur during the second trimester. There also is a higher exposure to common infections in early childhood (Mortensen, Pedersen et al, 1999; Nicolson et al, 1999).

Obstetrical Complications and Birth Events. Many attempts have been made to study the influences of events such as placental insufficiency, prolonged labor, hemorrhage, and trauma before or at birth as possible causes of schizophrenia. Much of this research is limited by its retrospective nature because retrieving information about a complex event decades after its occurrence is very difficult. Several preliminary findings suggest an increased risk may be associated with extreme prematurity, malnutrition, during pregnancy, and oxygen deprivation at birth (Dalman et al, 1999).

CLINICAL IMPLICATIONS **Biology of Schizophrenia**
Neuroscience research has had a significant impact on helping to understand schizophrenia, viewing this illness as a neurobiological disease with documented brain, genetic, and environmental components. This research has led to the development of atypical antipsychotic drugs; to the conceptualization of new neurotransmitter hypotheses; and may soon direct the clinician to new treatments that are extremely specific and highly effective and to screening procedures and preventative strategies that may ultimately eliminate the suffering, costs, and stigma associated with the experience of schizophrenia.

What would you say to a man and woman who were trying to decide whether to have children because they both had relatives with schizophrenia?

Mood Disorders

The biological understanding of mood disorders has made significant advances in the last several decades. Neuroscientific research has identified biological markers for mood disorders, and psychopharmacological interventions have more specificity and fewer side effects and toxicities than the first-generation antidepressants of 50 years ago. In fact, the treatments for depression have better outcomes than those for many medical and other psychiatric disorders.

Genetics. Current evidence suggests a significant genetic role in the cause of recurrent depression and bipolar disorder. The lifetime risk for mood disorders in the general population is 6%. Family, twin, and adoption studies show that the lifetime risk for relatives of people with depression is 20% and 24% for relatives of people with mania. A person with an identical twin (monozygotic, or MZ) with an affective disorder is 2 to 4 times more at risk for the disorder than are fraternal twins (dizygotic, or DZ) or siblings.

No clear pattern of genetic mapping for these disorders has yet been found, but there is evidence from linkage studies that chromosome 18 may be involved in bipolar disorder. Current genetic research also points to a complex picture of genetic and environmental interactions for mood disorders. (See Citing the Evidence on Genetics and Environment.)

Biochemistry. Early biogenic amine hypotheses for mood disorders suggested norepinephrine (NE) and serotonin (5-HT) as causative biochemical factors in depression and mania. Although these theories have undergone much revision in the past few decades, the critical importance of the amounts and balance of these two neurotransmitters in the pathophysiology of mood disorders remains unquestioned. This is evidenced by the effects of antidepressant drugs in use today, all of which have their antidepressant effect by regulating the norepinephrine and/or serotonin systems. Roles for other neurotransmitters are still unclear, but a variety are under study. These include the following:

- On the basis of drug effects, it has been proposed that too little acetylcholine can cause depression and too much NE can cause mania, suggesting an imbalance between these two neurotransmitter systems

Citing the Evidence on

Genetics and Environment

BACKGROUND: Depression affects more women than men and tends to occur within families. Studying twins, these authors looked at the contributions of genetic, environmental, and gender factors to the risk of developing depression.

RESULTS: Women had a moderate family history of depression, compared with only a modest family history in men. For both men and women, individual environmental experiences played a large role in the development of depression.

IMPLICATIONS: Although both men and women are susceptible to environmental influences on mood, it appears that depression in women is more likely to be inherited than it is in men, perhaps accounting for at least part of the increased prevalence of depression in women compared with men.

Bierut L et al: Major depressive in a community-based twin sample: are there different genetic and environmental contributions for men and women? *Arch Gen Psychiatry* 56, 557-563, 1999.

- Gamma-aminobutyric acid (GABA) modulates the other neurotransmitter systems and has been found to have both an antidepressant and an antimanic effect, suggesting a role for it in mood disorders as well

Preliminary research with glutamate shows that drugs which antagonize its receptor, NMDA, may have antidepressant effects, and these drugs may eventually offer a new approach to the treatment of depression.

If depression is partly caused by disturbed biochemistry, does that mean that counseling and psychotherapy are inappropriate treatment strategies?

Brain Imaging. CT and MRI studies find various abnormalities in the structure of brains in people with mood disorders. Elevated levels of stress hormones (glucocorticoids, such as cortisol) are found in depression. MRI studies of depressed patients show a decrease in the size of the hippocampus (Bremner et al, 2000), supporting the hypothesis that increased levels of stress hormones are associated with damage to the hippocampus (a limbic structure involved in learning and memory). MRI studies show that brain structures responsible for human mood are larger in bipolar patients compared with controls (Strakowski et al, 1999). The amygdala (the limbic structure responsible for modulating feelings of aggression, anger, love, and shyness) is especially large, perhaps accounting for some of the heightened emotionality and problematic behaviors seen in manic patients.

PET studies of mood disorders consistently show decreased frontal lobe brain metabolism (hypofrontality), which is generally more pronounced on the left hemisphere in depression and on the right hemisphere in mania. This means that the frontal cortex is not using as much glucose as it should (Fig. 6-13). Also, the amygdala shows increased blood flow, which is associated with intrusive ruminations in people with severe recurrent depression and a family history of mood disorders. This finding is supported by studies which demonstrate that people with depression do poorly compared with controls on the Wisconsin Card Sort Test.

This PET abnormality is reversible with effective antidepressant therapy.

In general, studies suggest an association between mood disorders and abnormalities of large regions of the brain, especially the frontal and temporal lobes. An abnormal difference between the left (language and logical thinking) and right (spatial processing) hemispheres also is implied. Although these functions are different, they also overlap and exhibit different levels of activity that appear to be altered in mood disorders. Also, imaging studies have not always been well-correlated with neuropsychiatric testing, and results of the two techniques often conflict, suggesting that different abnormalities are detected by different methods.

Seasonality and Circadian Rhythms. A variety of studies have linked seasonal variations, such as decreases in the length of daylight hours and decreases in available sunlight in winter, to human conditions such as mood, sleeping, eating, and energy levels. Seasonal affective disorder (SAD) in particular has been shown to respond to geographical location closer to the equator or to phototherapy (light therapy) (see Chapter 30). The neurotransmitter melatonin (a synthesis of serotonin in the pineal gland), which is secreted with darkness and suppressed with bright light, is believed to regulate hypothalamic hormones involved in the generation of circadian rhythms and the synchronization of such rhythms to variations in environmental light in animals. The human sleep cycle appears to be linked to the timing of human circadian rhythms and to malfunctions in the brain's ability to follow environmental cues such as light and darkness; to unusual environmental situations such as long, dark winters in northern latitudes; or disturbances in the intensity of the circadian rhythm, such as those caused by sleep problems, body temperature changes, mood cycling, and endocrine system (hormones such as cortisol and thyrotrophin) abnormalities. Components of the internal clock system may eventually be targets of drugs to relieve jet lag, the side effects of shift work, or sleep disorders and related depressive illnesses (Young, 2000).

Biological Markers. Several biological markers have advanced the biological understanding of depression and in

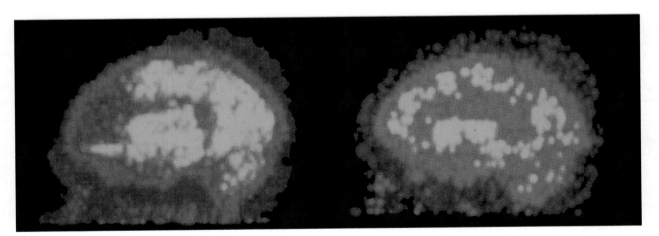

Fig. 6-13   PET scan of glucose use in a depressed subject (figure on left) showing frontal hypometabolism (left side of figure). This improves after treatment with antidepressant medication (figure on right); note increased glucose metabolism in frontal lobe (left side of figure).

some cases are useful in its diagnosis and treatment. Several examples include the following:

- Decreased REM latency: Sleep electroencephalograph (EEG) studies are abnormal in 90% of depressed patients. Normally upon falling asleep, the brain cycles through each stage of sleep for 60 to 90 minutes before it reaches stage 5, or REM (dream sleep). The time between the initiation of sleep and the occurrence of the first REM period is called REM latency. Depressed patients reach REM in 5 to 30 minutes; spend less time in the more refreshing slow wave stages of sleep (stages three and four); spend more time in REM sleep; and have increased periods of either very light sleep or awakenings during the night (see Fig. 20-3). This explains why depressed patients complain of feeling tired and unrefreshed after a night's sleep.

- Abnormal DST: Levels of the adrenal hormone cortisol are increased in some depressed people, and 60% of them have an abnormal dexamethasone suppression test (DST). Normally, there are relatively low levels of cortisol from late afternoon until 3 or 4 AM, when they begin to increase and spike at regular intervals until about noon, and then they begin to level out again. In controls, an evening dose (1 mg) of the synthetic steroid dexamethasone is enough to suppress the release of cortisol much of the day by turning down the pituitary production of adrenocorticotropic hormone (ACTH), thus blunting the adrenal production of cortisol for 24 hours. In contrast, many depressed people have erratic cortisol spikes over a 24-hour period and continue to have spikes even with the DST (Fig. 6-14). This suggests an abnormality in the hypothalamic-pituitary-adrenal (HPA) axis (see Fig. 18-2) in depression. Agents that reduce the effects of cortisol (antiglucocorticoids) are under investigation as possible treatments for depression (Pelton, 2000).

- Other evidence for hypothalamic-pituitary-endocrine dysregulation in depression includes a blunted thyroid stimulating hormone (TSH) test, a decreased growth hormone (secreted by the pituitary) response, de-

creased levels of somatostatin (a hypothalamic neuropeptide), and a blunted prolactin (secreted by the pituitary) response (see Fig. 20-4).

These and other biological markers continue to stimulate interest from a research perspective and promise to gain in their usefulness in clinical settings as the techniques are improved and their treatment implications are more fully understood.

What are the implications of being able to identify biological markers for the diagnosis and treatment of depression?

Kindling. When an animal's brain is given intermittent and repeated stimulation by low-level electrical impulses or low-dose chemicals such as cocaine, the result is an increased responsiveness to stable, low doses of the stimulation over time, resulting eventually in seizures. This phenomenon is known as kindling. Ultimately the animal becomes so sensitive that seizures continue to occur spontaneously after the stimulation is discontinued, demonstrating "behavioral sensitization." It is theorized that kindling underlies the addictive disorders and the cycling and recurrent psychiatric disorders.

Theoretically, early episodes of mania and depression in humans may be precipitated by psychosocial stressors in genetically vulnerable individuals, but later episodes can occur in the absence of any apparent external stimulus and with greater frequency and intensity over time. Additional evidence of a role for kindling in mood disorders is that many of the neurotransmitters implicated in the mood disorders inhibit kindling. Drugs used to treat bipolar disorder also affect kindling: lithium blocks behavioral sensitization and the anticonvulsants block kindling itself. Thus the effect of the environment on a vulnerable brain is the focus of continued research interest.

What environmental factors might play a role along with genetics in the increased rate of mood cycling in a bipolar patient?

CLINICAL IMPLICATIONS **Biology of Depression**
There are many different pieces to the puzzle of the biology of mood disorders, but there is not yet an all-inclusive hypothesis. It is likely, however, that mood disorders occur because integrated control systems are disrupted, as evidenced by dysregulation in neurotransmitter systems and by the fact that the brain mechanisms that control hormonal balance and biological rhythms are implicated in mood disorders. What is clear is that the etiologies are diverse, so the treatments must be both diverse and specific to the biopsychosocial context of the individual patient (see Chapter 20). Kindling and behavioral sensitization research suggest that early detection, aggressive treatment of acute episodes, and adequate long-term prophylactic treatment might inhibit or even prevent a progressively deteriorating course of illness (Bailey, 1999).

Panic and Anxiety Disorders

The biological study of anxiety has made significant advances in the past several decades. In panic disorder, in

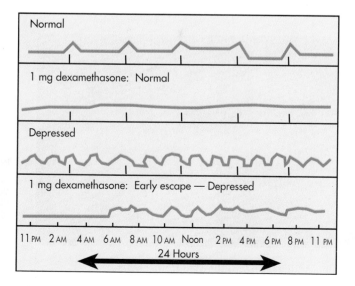

Fig. 6-14   Dexamethasone suppression test and cortisol levels.

which the human alarm system seems to be triggered independently from appropriate appraisals of environmental cues, and many of the other anxiety disorders, the results of neuroscientific exploration have been impressive and have led to promising new ideas for interventions.

Genetics. While there is little doubt from family and twin studies that abnormal genes predispose to pathological anxiety states, the heritability of these syndromes is only moderate. Thus it is clear that traumatic events and stress are as important as genetics in anxiety disorders. One early twin study remains the classic in this field and reports a significantly higher concordance for panic disorder in monozygotic than in dizygotic twins, although monozygotic twin concordance was only 31% as compared with 25% in first-degree relatives, emphasizing the importance of nongenetic factors in this disorder (Torgesen, 1990). Family studies have found that the risk for having panic disorder is between 8% to 20% among first-degree relatives of people with panic disorder compared with a risk of 2% to 4% in the general population. Many studies also distinguished between panic disorder and the other anxiety disorders, suggesting separate mechanisms for the inheritance of at least some anxiety disorders.

Gorman (2000) proposes that individuals may inherit a genetic characteristic (genotype), like a hyperactive autonomic nervous system, anxiety sensitivity, behavioral inhibition, or shyness. Then, depending on the impact of life stressors and whether or not the environment reinforces anxiety and avoidance behaviors, these traits are expressed as a specific anxiety disorder (phenotype) in these vulnerable individuals. Also, more "powerful" anxiety genes (increased "gene penetrance") would require even less environmental stress to be expressed. Thus, anxiety and panic, perhaps more than some other illnesses, provide a rich framework from which to better understand how nature and nurture interact together in health and illness.

Biochemistry. The majority of studies point to a dysfunction in multiple systems rather than isolating one particular neurotransmitter abnormality in the development of human anxiety disorders. These systems include the following:

- The GABA system: Benzodiazepines, which are potent antianxiety and antipanic drugs, increase the action of the inhibitory neurotransmitter GABA, thus turning down overly active brain cells. The areas of the brain where GABA receptors are coupled to benzodiazepine receptors include the amygdala and hippocampus, both limbic system structures that function as the center of emotions (such as rage, arousal, and fear) and memory. Patients with panic disorder may have a decreased antianxiety ability of the GABA receptors in areas of the limbic system, making them more sensitive to anxiety and panic.
- The norepinephrine (NE) system: The NE system is thought to mediate the fight-or-flight response. The part of the brain that manufactures NE (the locus ceruleus, or LC) is connected by neurotransmitter pathways to other structures of the brain implicated in anxiety, such as the amygdala, the hippocampus, and the cerebral cortex (the thinking, interpreting, and planning part of the brain). Medications that decrease the activity of the locus ceruleus (antidepressants such as

the tricyclics) effectively treat panic disorder. This suggests that panic attacks are at least partly caused by an inappropriate activation of the norepinephrine system in the locus ceruleus and an imbalance between NE and other neurotransmitter systems.

- The serotonin (5-HT) system: A dysregulation of 5-HT neurotransmission may play a role in the etiology of panic attacks, and patients experiencing panic and other anxiety disorders may have hypersensitive serotonin receptors. Drugs that regulate serotonin, such as the SSRIs (selective serotonin reuptake inhibitors), have been shown to be particularly effective in treating several of the anxiety disorders, including panic, suggesting a major role for serotonin and its balance with other neurotransmitter systems in the etiology of anxiety disorders.
- Cholecycystokinin (CCK) and the hypothalamic-pituitary-adrenal (HPA) axis: CCK is a neuropeptide found in the cerebral cortex, amygdala, and hippocampus and may have a significant effect on one's response to stress. Drugs that enhance the action of CCK (such as CCK4) activate the HPA axis, and 100% of panic disorder patients and 70% of controls experience panic when given this drug. Also, CCK receptors are highly sensitive in panic disorder patients. Benzodiazepines decrease the actions of CCK by reducing CCK-induced excitation at the CCK receptor. The promising research in this area may eventually support the development of new drugs that act directly to modify the effects of CCK and CCK receptors.

Brain Imaging. CT and MRI scans (Fig. 6-15) consistently provide evidence of brain atrophy or underdevelopment, particularly in the frontal and temporal lobes of people with panic disorder and social phobia (Davidson et al,

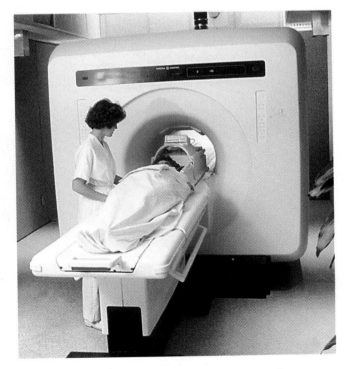

Fig. 6-15 Nurse preparing a patient for brain scanning. (Courtesy Division of Psychiatric Nursing, Medical University of South Carolina.)

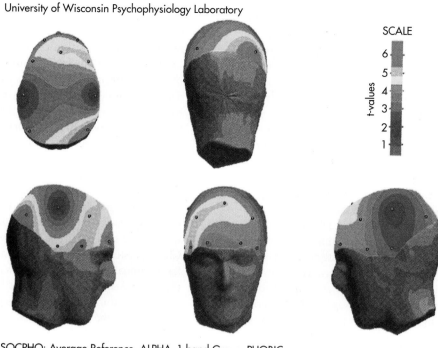

SOCPHO: Average Reference, ALPHA–1 band Group–PHOBIC
Baseline – Anticipation Change Scores

5-Jun-95 12:51:48

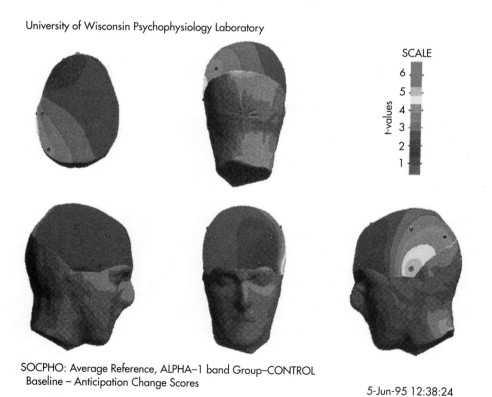

SOCPHO: Average Reference, ALPHA–1 band Group–CONTROL
Baseline – Anticipation Change Scores

5-Jun-95 12:38:24

Fig. 6-16 This study shows a marked increase *(red)* in right-sided activation in the anterior temporal and lateral prefrontal scalp regions of patients with social phobia (top half of figure) compared with controls (bottom half of figure) while waiting to make a public speech compared to after the speech was completed. These topographic maps were computer-generated using electroencephalographic recordings of six brain regions. These differences also correlated with higher levels of anxiety, heart rate, and negative affect in the phobics during anticipation of the speech. (From Davidson R et al: While a phobic waits: regional brain electrical and autonomic activity in social phobics during anticipation of public speaking, *Biol Psychiatry* 47:85, 2000.)

2000) (Fig. 6-16), although the clinical significance of these findings is unclear. Cerebral blood flow studies using PET scans show that, at rest, patients with panic disorder who have panic attacks during lactate infusions (see challenge tests in the next section) have increased cerebral blood flow to the parahippocampal gyrus, an area of the cerebral cortex that is associated with the limbic system. Normal controls and patients with panic disorder who were not sensitive to lactate did not show this effect, suggesting a role for lactate sensitivity as a marker for certain types of panic disorder. Also, there is support for the hypothesis that panic disorder patients have greater activation in the right frontal lobe, an asymmetry that is correlated with avoidance and withdrawal in negative situations (Wiedermann et al, 1999).

The brainstem reticular formation, with its widespread ascending and descending pathways and functionally specialized groups of neurons, also is associated with the mediation of arousal. Arousal refers to levels of generalized, diffuse activation of the brain and is associated with levels of consciousness and the sleep-wake cycle in humans. Blood flow to the brainstem and cerebellar regions has been correlated with various states of arousal. Reticular neurons affect activity in the regulation of norepinephrine and serotonin. This line of research promises to further explain the impact of levels of brain arousal on anxiety states.

How would you respond if a patient who is about to have an MRI scan asks you whether the procedure is painful or harmful and how it will be helpful?

Challenge Tests and Basal Physiology Studies.

Procedures that "provoke" panic in some individuals and not in others have provided a rich source of information about panic disorder for more than 30 years. Provocative challenge testing is designed to cause panic attacks under controlled laboratory conditions so that the biology of the attack can be studied. The administration of chemicals such as sodium lactate or caffeine and inhalants such as carbon dioxide cause significantly more panic attacks in panic disorder patients compared with controls. Panic disorder patients also are less likely to have another attack when challenged again after adequate treatment with antipanic medications.

Studies of basal physiology during the nonpanic state (between panic attacks) take place when the patient is still symptomatic with chronic high levels of anxiety and avoidance behavior. This strategy often leads to a better understanding of which parts of the brain may be important in triggering the panic state. For example, people with panic disorder have been shown to have blunted pituitary hormonal responses to several hypothalamic releasing hormones, suggesting either that the person cannot respond appropriately to stress, thus panic anxiety results, or the pituitary may adapt over time to repeated panic anxiety.

A final interesting physiological finding is that sleep-related panic attacks commonly occur in the transition from stage two to stage three sleep. Thus, panic attacks occur in states of apparent deep relaxation and unconsciousness, rather than during dream (REM) sleep, when it could be suggested that the panic attack was in response to a disturbing dream. This finding further supports a biological component to panic. (See Citing the Evidence on Comparing Nocturnal and Daytime Panic Attacks.)

CLINICAL IMPLICATIONS Biology of Panic and Anxiety Disorders   Although further research is needed to clarify the mechanisms for the cause of anxiety disorders, the clinical significance of current findings can be reassuring to patients. Patients can be told, for example, that panic anxiety is a dysregulation in the normal fight-or-flight response, which is important to survival. The way in which anxiety disorders present may be a combination of genetic vulnerability and a person's reactions to life's stressors. Perhaps most important, patients should be told that panic and anxiety disorders usually can be successfully treated by a variety of interventions. This information can give patients a sense of control over pathological anxiety's seemingly uncontrollable and debilitating effects. Patients can then be taught to control their responses to anxiety and to actively participate in treatment (see Chapter 17). Finally, the psychiatric nurse can assess symptoms of anxiety disorders and select the most appropriate interventions based on the brain region implicated by the symptom and the

Citing the Evidence on

Comparing Nocturnal and Daytime Panic Attacks

BACKGROUND: The purpose of this study was to determine whether nocturnal panic disorder patients have greater autonomic function than patients with daytime panic compared with controls. Panic was provoked during daytime via lactate infusion challenge. Panic was measured during nighttime via EEG sleep recordings.

RESULTS: Panic disorder patients were markedly more responsive to the lactate infusion than the controls. The panic disorder patients as a whole had lower sleep efficiency and less stage 4 sleep (deepest sleep) than controls. There were not significant differences between patients with daytime only and patients with nighttime only panic attacks.

IMPLICATIONS: Panic disorder patients have a dysregulated autonomic nervous system compared with controls that has a spontaneous component to it, since panic attacks that occur at night are not the result of dream sleep. This study underscores the biological component of the etiology of panic disorder.

Sloan E et al: Nocturnal and daytime panic attacks—Comparison of sleep architecture, heart rate variability, and response to sodium lactate challenge, *Biol Psychiatry* 45:1313, 1999.

Table **6-5**

Biological Treatment Model of Panic Disorder			
Symptom	**Brain Region**	**Function**	**Treatment**
Phobic avoidance (a learned phenomenon)	Cerebral cortex (higher brain)	Learning and complex emotion	Desensitization and cognitive restructuring (see Chapter 30)
Anticipatory anxiety (possibly sensitized by hyperventilation)	Limbic lobe (midbrain: rich in neurotransmitter receptors)	Center for human emotions	Relaxation, breathing retraining, desensitization, antipanic medications
Panic attacks	Brainstem (lower brain: includes structures that manufacture neuro-transmitters)	Primitive emotion	Antipanic medication (see Chapter 28)

Modified from Gorman JM et al: *Am J Psychiatry* 146:2, 1989.

treatments that evidence shows are most likely to affect the function of that brain region (Table 6-5).

Alzheimer's Disease

Dementia, a decline of memory and other cognitive functions, is the most disabling psychiatric disorder of adulthood. It is not caused by the normal process of aging but rather appears to have many possible causes, as described in Chapter 24. Alzheimer's disease is the fourth most common cause of death in the developed world after heart disease, cancer, and stroke and causes 100,000 deaths annually in the United States. As the baby boomers age and the proportion of people living longer increases, the number of persons afflicted with AD is expected to rise well above the 4 million Americans currently affected. A number of risk factors have been associated with AD and are listed in Box 6-3.

Because head injury is a known risk factor for the dementing syndrome, what primary prevention strategies could society take to resolve this problem?

Genetics. AD is difficult to study genetically for several reasons. First, the disease is genetically heterogeneous—more than one gene is responsible for AD. Mutations in any of three genes (on chromosomes 1, 14, and 21) have been identified in approximately half of early onset (prior to age 65) cases (accounting for 10% of cases of AD). Chromosomes 1 and 14 are involved in activities that prevent amyloid precursor protein (beta-APP) from elongating and accumulating in the brain. Chromosome 21 is the same gene that forms beta-APP, the substance from which the protein beta-amyloid is made. The normal function of this protein is not fully understood, but its production is somehow accelerated in AD, and excessive deposits form both the senile plaques clustering outside each affected neuron and amyloid deposits in the walls of cerebral blood vessels. It also is probably related to the production of the neurofibrillary tangles seen within the neurons of patients with AD. Approximately 50% of individuals in each generation of families with this genetic mutation develop AD. Interestingly, AD also is seen in the fourth and fifth decade of life in patients with Down's syndrome, who have three rather than two copies of chromosome 21. Almost all of these patients develop senile plaques, neurofibrillary tangles, and clinical signs of dementia.

Late-onset AD (after age 65) has been linked to chromosome 19 (probably a gene affecting beta-APP metabolism). A link between combinations of a fairly common cholesterol-transporting protein (Apo-E) has been found. Apparently many people with late-onset AD are born with certain combinations of Apo-E variations that attach to beta-amyloid, which may pull bits of amyloid from the bloodstream and accumulate it in the brain. Thus the development of AD may depend on which combination of Apo-E a person inherits.

The second reason that AD is difficult to study from a genetic perspective is because diagnostic accuracy for AD requires neuropathological examination at autopsy. It is only possible to assume a tentative diagnosis (80% accuracy) based on evidence from clinical symptoms and imaging studies in family members, complicating family studies of AD. Also, since the onset of AD can occur very late in life, family members carrying the gene can die from unrelated causes before developing the disease, thus will not be counted in the estimation of family risk. We do know from twin studies that the concordance rate in MZ (identical) twins is 2 to 3 times higher than in DZ (fraternal) twins. Interestingly, only 50% of twins become demented within 5 years of each other, and the rest can take as long as 16 years.

Biochemistry. Almost every neurotransmitter has been studied and implicated in AD, but cell loss and subsequent disruption in the cholinergic system is extensive in AD. The cholinergic system originates in the basal forebrain, which is positioned at the interface between the limbic system and the cerebral cortex, where it plays a role in emotion and memory. Acetylcholine (ACh) is produced in a region of the basal forebrain, which is selectively devastated in AD. It is thought that too little acetylcholine may allow a buildup of amyloid. Cholinesterase inhibitors, such as tacrine (Cognex) and donepezil (Aricept), slow the natural breakdown of acetylcholine by inhibiting the enzyme, cholinesterase, that metabolizes acetylcholine. (See Citing the Evidence on Cholinesterase Inhibitors.)

Glutamate and peptide transmitters also are affected in specific brain regions in AD. Although correlations can be drawn between transmitter deficits and pathology and clinical symptoms of AD, they seem to reflect damage specific to affected regions and specific structures of the brain rather than entire neurotransmitter systems throughout the brain. Another implication is that, unlike the neurochemistry of

Box 6-3

Risk Factors for Alzheimer's Disease

AGE

AD is a disease of old age.

The population prevalence is less than 0.01% at age 45, 2% between age 65 and 70, 5% between 70 and 80, and more than 20% at age 85.

AD affects more women than men because women tend to live longer.

An early age of onset (<65) is strongly associated with a positive family history.

FAMILY HISTORY

A positive family history in first-degree relatives is the most persistent positive association for AD.

Approximately 20% of AD cases are thought to be familial.

PARENTAL AGE

Women who bear children before 20 and after 40 years of age have an increased incidence of AD in their offspring.

This group of mothers also has increased risk of premature births, poor maternal fitness, and babies with Down syndrome.

These findings suggest that children of older parents may have a chromosomal abnormality that makes them more susceptible to AD when they reach old age.

HEAD INJURY

Descriptive reviews of case control studies often report the finding of a history of head injury in some patients with AD.

Support for head injury as a risk factor also comes from evidence that repetitive head trauma is known to cause a dementing syndrome in boxers (dementia pugilistica, or punchdrunk syndrome), which shows the same molecular pathology as AD.

POTASSIUM CHANNEL DYSFUNCTION

One study* found that patients with AD, when compared with both control groups and patients with other dementing illnesses, have a potassium (K+) channel dysfunction.

K+ channels change during acquisition of memory in studies of mammals. Thus an abnormal K+ channel may serve as a marker that would distinguish patients with AD from age-matched controls and patients with non-AD neurological and psychiatric disorders.

ENVIRONMENTAL FACTORS

Although there have been anecdotal reports of other factors as risks for AD, systematic evidence is lacking. Some of these include:

Aluminum: ingestion of foods stored in aluminum containers or use of deodorants and hairsprays with aluminum bases

Bloodborne infections: blood transfusions if the blood donor has AD and it is transmitted by an infectious agent

Chemicals: occupational exposure to chemicals

*Etcherberrigaray et al, 1993.

Parkinson's disease in which one transmitter deficit can be treated effectively by one drug intervention (L-Dopa), it seems unlikely that AD can be effectively treated by neurotransmitter replacement therapy alone.

Brain Imaging. PET scans and performance tests indicate that the brains of healthy people in their 80s are almost as active and function nearly as well (although slower) on tests of memory, perception, and language as people in early adulthood. Patients with early onset AD may show cortical atrophy, ventricular enlargement, and loss of temporal lobe volume (especially the hippocampus) with CT or MRI, as well as a marked loss in brain weight. Patients with late-onset AD who develop the disease after age 75 usually show only age-related changes. PET scans show a typical pattern of frontal, association, and temporal hypometabolism. However, these changes must be correlated with the clinical picture in order to reach a tentative diagnosis of AD in living persons (Fig. 6-17).

Neuropathological Changes. It is not known how excessive amyloid protein deposits lead to the plaques and tangles that cause extensive structural and biochemical changes in axons, dendrites, and neuronal cell bodies. These changes reduce synaptic function by as much as 40% in affected regions and reduce protein synthesis and cellular processes. However, there is no doubt that this buildup of amyloid protein, combined with the formation of neurofibrillary tangles and other structural changes in

---

Citing the Evidence on

Cholinesterase Inhibitors

BACKGROUND: Acetylcholinesterase inhibitors have recently been introduced as cognition-enhancing agents in the treatment of patients with mild to moderate Alzheimer's disease (AD). This article reviews the accumulated evidence indicating that these drugs have psychotropic properties.

RESULTS: The treatment of patients with AD with acetylcholinesterase inhibitors reduces neuropsychiatric symptoms, particularly apathy and visual hallucinations. Response profiles vary among the different drugs.

IMPLICATIONS: Acetylcholinesterase inhibitors have psychotropic effects and may play an important role in controlling neuropsychiatric and behavioral disturbances in patients with AD. These agents also may contribute to the management of other disorders with cholinergic system abnormalities and neuropsychiatric symptoms. The beneficial response is most likely mediated through limbic cholinergic structures.

Cummings JL: Cholinesterase inhibitors: A new class of psychotropic compounds, *Am J Psychiatry* 157:4, 2000.

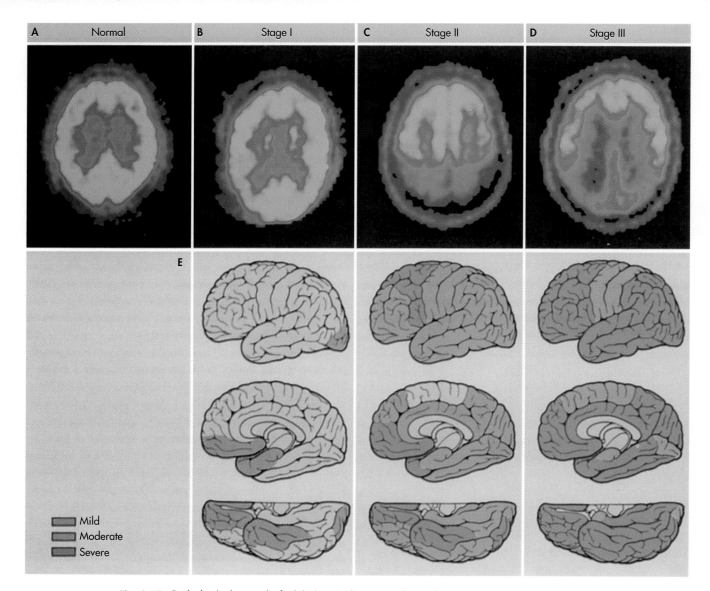

Fig. 6-17 Pathological spread of Alzheimer's disease as shown by positron emission tomography scans. **A,** Normal brain. **B,** Brain in stage I Alzheimer's disease. **C,** Brain in stage II Alzheimer's disease. **D,** Brain in stage III Alzheimer's disease. **E,** Diagrams show the spread of pathology in Alzheimer's disease. (From Roberts GS et al: *Neuropsychiatric disorders*, London, 1993, Mosby-Wolfe.)

neurons, contributes to a progressive breakdown of neuronal circuits necessary for communication in the brain. It is as if the limbic system, particularly the hippocampus, amygdala, and the association cortices (which are affected early in the AD process and are necessary to the organization of mental processes), becomes isolated and out of touch with other brain regions, hence the gradual impairment of memory, judgment, abstraction, and language. Eventually, motor and sensory regions also are affected, and the patient with AD becomes totally disabled. Table 6-6 lists some of the affected brain regions and subsequent symptoms of AD.

CLINICAL IMPLICATIONS Biology of Alzheimer's Disease Much research is being focused on understanding the molecular mechanisms underlying dementing diseases. Several new drugs (such as gamma-secretase blockers) are currently in clinical tri-

als (Vasser, Bennett, et al, 1999). These drugs are thought to block the enzymes that play key roles in the buildup of beta-amyloid, thus preventing it from entering cerebral tissue and causing the inflammatory and neurotoxic responses that result in CNS damage seen in AD. Gene therapy experiments in animals have revived degenerated brain cells linked to memory and selective attention and may be ready for experimentation in humans in the near future.

Clinical interventions are targeted at differential diagnosis, providing available drugs that may slow the disease process and provide some symptomatic relief, and managing the social and behavioral consequences of the progressive dementia of AD (see Chapters 24 and 41).

There is some evidence suggesting ways to reduce one's risk for AD. Older test subjects who regularly do aerobic exercises perform better on cognitive tests than do sedentary people in the same age group. People older than 60 are particularly sensitive to substances that interfere with the CNS, such as benzodiazepines and

Table **6-6**

Some Brain Regions Affected by Alzheimer's Disease and Resulting Symptoms		
Region Affected	Function	Symptom
Limbic system: hippocampus	Memory, learning, and emotion	First, recent memories fade and then long-standing memories are affected. Symptoms of depression may occur, probably because of damage to the locus ceruleus.
Temporal-parietal-occipital association cortex	Visual impairment, aphasia, apraxia, and agnosia	Increasing difficulty recognizing even familiar faces, places, and objects. The ability to communicate, use and understand language, write, and comprehend reading is lost. Hallucinations and delusions may occur. Seizures may occur.
Prefrontal cortex	Insight, planning, judgment, personality, behavior, and social propriety	Apathy, impaired insight, lack of judgment, concreteness, perseverance, and inefficient problem solving are seen.
Subcortical projections	Memory, learning, and behavior	More research is needed to correlate symptoms with changes seen in these areas, but it is clear that several important transmitter systems are affected: cholinergic basal forebrain, noradrenergic locus ceruleus, serotonergic raphe nuclei, and dopaminergic substantia nigra.
Motor cortex	Movement	Increasing difficulty walking, talking, and swallowing occur later in the disease process.

alcohol, and perform poorly on cognitive tests compared with younger people taking the same drugs. Nonsteroidal anti-inflammatory drugs (aspirin, indomethacin, ibuprofen, and naproxen) seem to slow the progress of AD and may even be protective against it. It remains to be seen whether early anecdotal reports of therapy with the antioxidant, vitamin E; estrogen therapy; alternative treatments such as ginko biloba; or a lifetime of balanced, low-calorie diets will have positive effects on the symptoms of AD.

The research findings for the etiology of psychiatric disorders underscore the important point that the biological understanding of psychiatric illnesses cannot stand alone. Rather, integrated biopsychosocial models and multidimensional treatment strategies are needed. Thus psychiatric nurses should continue to view each person in the context of both the environment and biology.

LEGACY OF THE DECADE OF THE BRAIN

The U.S. Congress called the 1990s the Decade of the Brain. Advances in the techniques used in the neurosciences, the scientific methodologies used in testing biological hypotheses, and the integration of nonbiological theories and findings in the clinical arena provide the biopsychosocial approach necessary for the future study of neuropsychiatric disorders in human beings.

Several well-researched lines of evidence support a biological link to mental illnesses, including the following:

- Specific mental disorders can often be differentiated from each other by studies of genetics and inheritance, neurotransmitter research, and brain imaging studies, among others.
- Exogenous chemicals can produce symptoms of mental illness or exacerbate existing symptoms, thus demonstrating that physical agents can be causative.

- A biological cause of neuropsychiatric illness is supported by in vitro simulations of some symptoms that can be replicated, such as the challenge studies in panic disorder.
- Genetic studies show that neuropsychiatric disorders are strongly influenced by inheritance.
- Many psychiatric disorders have associated biological symptoms or test results, such as altered sleep patterns and failure to suppress cortisol in the dexamethasone suppression test in depression.
- Medications can suppress symptoms associated with psychiatric disorders, thus providing chemically mediated relief for many psychiatric illnesses.

Psychiatric nurses are faced with the challenge of integrating neuroscientific information with the long-standing biopsychosocial model of psychiatric nursing care. Psychiatric nurses also need to apply this information and provide holistic, evidence-based, and individualized psychiatric nursing care.

Summary

1. Psychiatric nurses learn about the structure and function of the brain, including the neurotransmission process, to better understand the etiology, course, and most effective treatment strategies for psychiatric illnesses.
2. Brain imaging techniques such as CT, MRI, BEAM, PET, and SPECT allow direct viewing of the living brain, which helps in diagnosing some brain disorders and correlating brain structure with function.
3. The search for the gene or genes that carry mental illness has been difficult and inconclusive to date but is a promising field for future research.
4. Circadian rhythm is like a network of internal clocks that time and coordinate events within the body, including lifestyle, sleep, moods, eating, drinking, fertility, and illness according to a 24-hour cycle.

5. Psychoneuroimmunology explores the influence of psychosocial factors on the nervous system's control of immune responses.

6. Psychiatric nurses need to be able to obtain a thorough history, perform a basic physical examination, and interpret the results of laboratory tests to screen for signs of physical disorders and refer to specialists as indicated.

7. The clinical implications of neuroscientific research were discussed in relation to schizophrenia, mood disorders, panic disorder, and Alzheimer's disease.

8. Psychiatric nurses are faced with the challenge of integrating the latest neuroscientific information into the biopsychosocial model of psychiatric nursing care.

 Visit **MERLIN: www.mosby.com/MERLIN/Stuart** to find these additional materials and student activities.

- **Worksheets**
- **"Drug of the Month" Updates**
- **"Citing the Evidence" Updates**
- **Critical Thinking Activities and Exercises**
- **Annotated Suggested Readings**
- **Web Links**
- **More!**

Chapter Review Questions

1. Match the terms in Column A with the best description from Column B.

Column A	Column B
____ Basal ganglia	A. Homeostasis
____ Challenge tests	B. May underlie cyclical disorders
____ DST	C. Space between brain cells
____ Eugenics	D. Dream sleep
____ Hippocampus	E. Manufactures norepinephrine
____ Hypothalamus	F. Cause panic attacks under controlled conditions
____ Kindling	G. Neurotransmitter precursor
____ Locus ceruleus	H. Functional neuroimaging technique
____ PET	I. Movement
____ REM	J. Selective breeding
____ Synapse	K. Memory
____ Tryptophan	L. Biological marker for depression

2. Fill in the blanks.

A. The microenvironment that protects the CNS from large molecules, toxins, and peripheral chemicals is the _____ and _____ barriers.

B. Communication between neurons in the brain is called _____.

C. The scientific field made up of many disciplines that has revolutionized our understanding of mental illness is called _____.

D. The network of internal clocks that times and coordinates events within the body according to a 24-hour cycle is called _____.

E. The neurotransmitter system implicated in AD that is affected by the drugs Cognex and Aricept is the _____.

3. Identify whether the following statements are true (T) or false (F).

_____A. The gene for early onset Alzheimer's disease is currently implicated in 90% of cases.

_____B. Family, adoption, and twin studies suggest that the pattern of inherited vulnerability to mental illness probably results from the interaction of genes with the environment.

_____C. The catecholamine hypothesis is now the most recent and dominant explanation for the mood disorders.

_____D. Brain imaging techniques have generally found smaller ventricles in some people with schizophrenia, depression, and anxiety disorders than in nonaffected people.

_____E. When neurotransmission has taken place, the process by which neurotransmitters travel from the synapse back into the presynaptic axon is called reuptake.

4. Provide short answers for the following questions.

A. Briefly describe the role of each of the following components in brain communication:
Axon
Dendrite
Receptor cell
Second messengers
Reuptake
Enzymatic degradation

B. Discuss how the limbic system is involved in feelings, emotion, and self-preservation.

C. List the stages of sleep, and define REM latency and decreased REM latency.

D. How is challenge testing useful in the study of panic disorder?

REFERENCES

Applegate E: *The anatomy and physiology learning system,* ed 2, Philadelphia, 2000, WB Saunders.

Bailey K: Electrophysiological kindling and behavioral sensitization as models for bipolar illness: implications for nursing practice, *J Am Psychiatric Nurses Assoc* 5:62, 1999.

Bremner J et al: Hippocampal volume reduction in major depression, *Am J Psychiatry* 157:115, 2000.

Coleman F, Kay J: The biology of the brain. In Kay J, Tasman A, editors: *Psychiatry: behavioral science and clinical essentials,* Philadelphia, 2000, WB Saunders.

Collins F: Medical and societal consequences of the Human Genome Project, *New Engl J Med* 341:28-37, 1999.

Dalman C et al: Obstetric complications and the risk of schizophrenia, *Arch Gen Psychiatry* 56:234, 1999.

Etcheberrigaray R et al: Potassium channel dysfunction in fibroblasts identifies patients with Alzheimer's disease, *Proc Natl Acad Sci U S A* 90:8209, 1993.

Glasser R et al: Stress induced immunomodulation: Implications for infectious diseases, *JAMA* 28(24):2268-2270, 1999.

Gorman J: Anxiety disorders. In Saddock B and Saddock V, editors: *Kaplan & Saddocks comprehensive textbook of psychiatry,* ed 7, Philadelphia 2000, Lipincott Williams & Wilkins.

Jorde L et al: *Medical genetics,* ed 2, St Louis, 1999, Mosby.

Mortensen P et al: Effects of family history and place and season of birth on the risk of schizophrenia, *New Engl J Med* 340:603, 1999.

Nicholson R et al: Obstetrical complications and childhood onset schizophrenia, *Am J Psychiatry* 156:1650, 1999.

Nolte J: *The human brain: An introduction to its functional anatomy,* ed 4, St Louis, 1999, Mosby.

Pelton G: Antiglucocortcoid medication for the treatment of depression: Theory and current practice, *Psychiatric Ann* 30:139, 2000.

Roberts GW, Leigh PN, Weinberger DR: *Neuropsychiatric disorders,* London, 1993, Mosby-Wolfe.

Strakowski S et al: Brain magnetic resonance imaging of structural abnormalities in bipolar disorder, *Arch Gen Psychiatry* 56:254, 1999.

Torgesen S: Twin studies in panic disorder. In Ballenger J, editor: *Neurobiology of panic disorder,* New York, 1990, Alan R Liss.

Vassar R et al: Beta-secretase cleavage of Alzheimer's amyloid precursor protein by transmembrane aspartic protease BACE, *Science* 286:735, 1999.

Wiedermann G et al: Frontal brain asymmetry as a biological substrate of emotions in patients with panic disorders, *Arch Gen Psychiatry* 56:78, 1999.

Young M: The tick-tock of the biological clock, *Sci Am* 282:64, 2000.

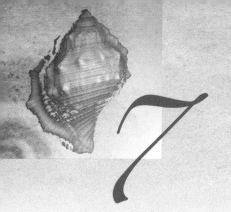

7 Psychological Context of Psychiatric Nursing Care

Gail W. Stuart

Information is of no value for its own sake, but only because of its personal significance.

ERIC BERNE

Holistic psychiatric nursing care requires the nurse to complete an assessment of the patient's biological, psychological and sociocultural health status. The assessment of the patient's psychological well-being should include a mental status examination. All nurses, regardless of the clinical setting, should be proficient in administering the mental status examination and be able to incorporate findings from it in the patient's plan of nursing care.

The mental status examination is a cornerstone in the evaluation of any patient with a medical, neurologic, or psychiatric disorder that affects thought, emotion or behavior (American Psychiatric Association, 1995; Strub, 2000). It is used to detect changes or abnormalities in a person's intellectual functioning, thought content, judgment, mood, and affect and can be used to identify possible lesions in the brain. The mental status examination is to psychiatric nursing what the physical examination is to general medical nursing.

MENTAL STATUS EXAMINATION

The mental status examination represents a cross-section of the patient's psychological life and the sum total of the nurse's observations and impressions at the moment. It also serves as a basis for future comparison to track the progress of the patient over time. The elements of the examination depend on the patient's clinical presentation as well as his or her educational and cultural background. It includes observing the patient's behavior and describing it in an objective, nonjudgmental manner.

The examination itself is usually divided into several parts. They can be arranged in different ways, as long as the nurse covers all the areas. Much of the information needed for the mental status examination can be gathered during the course of the routine nursing assessment. It should be integrated in the nurse's assessment in a smooth manner. Some parts of the mental status examination are completed through simple observation of the patient, such as by noting the patient's clothing or facial expressions. Other aspects require asking specific questions, such as those related to memory or attention span. Most of all, the nurse should remember that the mental status examination does not reflect how the patient was in the past or will be in the future; it is an evaluation of the patient's current state.

Information obtained during the mental status examination is used along with other objective and subjective data. These include findings from the physical examination, laboratory test results, patient history, description of the presenting problem, and information obtained from family, caregivers, and other health professionals. With these data the nurse is able to formulate nursing diagnoses and design the plan of care with the patient.

Do nurses on medical-surgical units routinely assess a patient's psychological status? Explain your findings given the fact that all nurses should be providing holistic, biopsychosocial nursing care.

Eliciting Clinical Information

The mental status examination requires a clinical rather than social approach to the patient. The nurse listens closely to what is said and reflects on what is not said, structuring the process in a way that allows for broad exploration of many areas for potential problems, as well as for more in-depth exploration of obvious symptoms or maladaptive coping responses. The patient is critically observed. Behaviors that the nurse might not normally attend to in more general situations must be carefully observed and described. Global and judgmental statements are not acceptable.

The skilled nurse attends to both the content and the process of the patient's communication (see Chapter 2). **Content** is the overtly communicated information. **Process** is how the communication occurs and includes feelings, intuition, and behaviors that accompany speech and thought. The content and process may not always be congruent. For example, a patient may deny feeling depressed and yet appear sad and cry. In this case, the stated message does not match the process, and the nurse should record this incongruity.

It is also important for nurses to monitor their feelings and reactions during the mental status examination. A nurse's gut reactions may reflect subtle emotions being expressed by the patient. For example, a depressed patient may make the nurse feel sad, and a hostile patient may make the nurse feel threatened and angry. The nurse's feelings are useful information for the mental status assessment.

The nurse needs to be aware of these feelings and respond in a therapeutic manner toward the patient regardless of such feelings. The nurse should remain calm throughout the interview and simply reflect observations back to the patient. These observations should be related in an objective and nonthreatening manner, as in "You are obviously quite upset about this," or "It seems like you don't feel safe here." By conveying a sense of calm, the nurse also demonstrates being in control, even if the patient is not.

The nurse should try to blend specific questions into the general flow of the interview. For example, questions about orientation, arithmetic problems, or proverbs may be introduced by soliciting patient comments about potential problems with concentration, memory, or understanding of written material. The nurse might then suggest that the patient try answering a few questions to determine whether such problems exist.

Finally, as with any other skill, nurses need to practice performing the mental status examination to gain proficiency and comfort. The nurse might start by observing a colleague conduct the examination. Videotapes of patient interviews are a particularly effective teaching-learning tool. A colleague or supervisor should then observe the nurse administering the mental status examination. The colleague can provide helpful feedback and identify ways to further enhance the nurse's competency.

CONTENT OF THE EXAMINATION

The mental status examination includes information in a number of categories (Box 7-1). It is one part of a complete psychiatric nursing assessment tool. In completing this examination it is critically important to be aware that sociocultural factors can greatly influence the outcome of the examination (Box 7-2). In addition, biologic expressions of psychiatric illness may also be evident during the interview. The content, observations, and some of the clinical implications associated with each category are now described (Trzepacz & Baker, 1993).

Appearance

In the mental status examination the nurse takes note of the patient's appearance. This part of the examination is intended to provide an accurate mental image of the patient, as in the following clinical example.

 CLINICAL EXAMPLE

Mr. W is a middle-aged white man of average weight who appears older than his stated age. He was disheveled, dressed in a torn shirt and jeans, and was unshaven. He was slightly jaundiced and had a prominent red nose and a scar on the left side of his cheek. He sat slumped in the chair and made little eye contact with the interviewer.

Box **7-1**

Categories of the Mental Status Examination

GENERAL DESCRIPTION
Appearance
Speech
Motor activity
Interaction during interview

EMOTIONAL STATE
Mood
Affect

EXPERIENCES
Perceptions

THINKING
Thought content
Thought process

SENSORIUM AND COGNITION
Level of consciousness
Memory
Level of concentration and calculation
Information and intelligence
Judgment
Insight

Box 7-2

Clinical Judgment or Sociocultural Bias?

- In completing the mental status examination clinicians need to be aware of the possibility of using subconscious and culturally determined criteria when judging a patient. Examples of potential sociocultural clinician bias include the following:
- How is the manner of dress judged (that is, what is unusual or expected dress)?
- Do all cultures accept the American norm of direct eye contact?
- What are the clinician's values about personal hygiene, and how do these values influence assessment?
- Does a person's speech and use of language vary based on social class and lifestyle?
- How does body language and use of personal space vary by ethnicity and social group?
- Given the fact that 20 to 30 million American adults lack basic educational skills, what is the expected "norm" regarding reading, writing, or problem-solving tasks?
- How familiar are common proverbs? Which interpretations of them are truly correct?

OBSERVATIONS   The following physical characteristics should be included in the assessment:

- Apparent age
- Manner of dress
- Cleanliness
- Posture
- Gait
- Facial expressions
- Eye contact
- Pupil dilation or constriction
- General state of health and nutrition

CLINICAL IMPLICATIONS   Dilated pupils are sometimes associated with drug intoxication, whereas pupil constriction may indicate narcotic addiction. Stooped posture is often seen in depression. Manic patients may dress in colorful or unusual attire.

Speech

Speech is usually described in terms of rate, volume, and characteristics. Rate is the speed of the patient's speech, and volume is how loud a patient talks.

OBSERVATIONS   Speech can be described as follows:

- Rate: rapid or slow
- Volume: loud or soft
- Amount: paucity, muteness, pressured speech
- Characteristics: stuttering, slurring of words, or unusual accents

CLINICAL IMPLICATIONS   Speech disturbances are often caused by specific brain disturbances. For example, mumbling may occur in patients with Huntington's chorea, and slurring of speech may occur in intoxicated patients. Manic patients often show pressured speech, and people suffering from depression often are reluctant to speak.

Motor Activity

Motor activity describes the patient's physical movement.

OBSERVATIONS   The nurse should record the following:

- Level of activity: lethargic, tense, restless, or agitated
- Type of activity: tics, grimaces, or tremors
- Unusual gestures or mannerisms: compulsions

CLINICAL IMPLICATIONS   Excessive body movement may be associated with anxiety, mania, or stimulant abuse. Little body activity may suggest depression, organicity, catatonic schizophrenia, or drug-induced stupor. Tics and grimaces may suggest medication side effects (see Chapter 28). Repeated motor movements or compulsions may indicate obsessive-compulsive disorder. Repeated picking of lint or dirt off clothing is sometimes associated with delirium or toxic conditions.

 Which category of psychotropic medications is most often associated with tics and grimaces?

Interaction During the Interview

Interaction describes how the patient relates to the nurse during the interview, as in this clinical example.

 ### CLINICAL EXAMPLE

The patient was interviewed in her room on the second day of hospitalization. She was a white woman slightly overweight, neatly dressed in jeans and a sweater, and appeared younger than her 36 years of age. Although she was cooperative, her guarded responses to all questions seemed excessively self-centered. She gave the interviewer the feeling that she didn't trust anyone and was preoccupied during the interview. When asked how other people treated her, she responded angrily, "I'd rather not say!"

Because this part of the examination relies heavily on nurses' emotional subjectivity, nurses must carefully examine their responses based on their personal and sociocultural biases. They must guard against overinterpreting or misinterpreting patients' behavior because of social or cultural differences (see Chapter 8).

OBSERVATIONS   Is the patient hostile, uncooperative, irritable, guarded, apathetic, defensive, suspicious, or seductive? The nurse may explore this area by asking, "You seem irritated about something. Is that an accurate observation?"

CLINICAL IMPLICATIONS   Suspiciousness may be evident in paranoia. Irritability may suggest an anxiety disorder.

Mood

Mood is the patient's self-report of the prevailing emotional state and reflects the patient's life situation.

OBSERVATIONS Mood can be evaluated by asking a simple, nonleading question such as "How are you feeling today?" Does the patient report feeling sad, fearful, hopeless, euphoric, or anxious? Asking the patient to rate his or her mood on a scale of 0 to 10 can help provide the nurse with an immediate reading. It also can be valuable for comparison of changes that occur during treatment.

If the potential for suicide is suspected, the nurse should inquire about the patient's thoughts about self-destruction (see Chapter 21). Suicidal and homicidal thoughts must be addressed directly. Has the patient felt the desire to harm him- or herself or someone else? Have any previous attempts been made, and if so, what events surrounded the attempts? To judge a patient's suicidal or homicidal risk, the nurse should assess the patient's plans, ability to carry out those plans (such as the availability of guns), the patient's attitude about death, and available support systems, as in the following clinical example.

 CLINICAL EXAMPLE

The patient responded to most of the questions in a flat, dull manner. Although he stated that he felt sad about the recent changes in his life, his lifeless posture and tone of voice did not convey any emotional response. He denied any current suicidal or homicidal plans. He related having made two suicidal gestures in the past year by "taking pills."

CLINICAL IMPLICATIONS Most people with depression describe feeling hopeless, and 25% of those with depression have suicidal ideation. Suicidal ideation is also common in anxiety disorders and schizophrenia. Elation is most common in mania.

Affect

Affect is the patient's apparent emotional tone. The patient's statements of emotions and the nurse's empathic responses provide clues to the appropriateness of the affect.

OBSERVATIONS Affect can be described in terms of the following:

- Range
- Duration
- Intensity
- Appropriateness

Does the patient report significant life events without any emotional response, indicating flat affect? Does the patient's response appear restricted or blunted in some way? Does the patient demonstrate great lability in expression by shifting from one affect to another quickly? Is the patient's response incongruent with speech content? For example, does the patient report being persecuted by the police and then laugh?

CLINICAL IMPLICATIONS Labile affect is often seen in mania, and a flat, incongruent affect is often evident in schizophrenia.

Perceptions

There are two major types of perceptual problems: hallucinations and illusions. Hallucinations are defined as false sensory impressions or experiences. Illusions are false perceptions or false responses to a sensory stimulus.

OBSERVATIONS Hallucinations may occur in any of the five major sensory modalities:

- Auditory (sound)
- Visual (sight)
- Tactile (touch)
- Gustatory (taste)
- Olfactory (smell)

Command hallucinations are those that tell the patient to do something, such as to kill oneself, harm another, or join someone in afterlife. The nurse might inquire about the patient's perceptions by asking "Do you ever see or hear things?" or "Do you have strange experiences as you fall asleep or on awakening?"

CLINICAL IMPLICATIONS Auditory hallucinations are the most common and suggest schizophrenia. Visual hallucinations suggest organicity. Tactile hallucinations suggest organic mental disorder, cocaine abuse, and delirium tremors.

 You see in the chart that a nursing order has been written placing a patient with command hallucinations on one-to-one observation. What is the rationale for this nursing intervention?

Thought Content

Thought content is the specific meaning expressed in the patient's communication. It refers to the "what" of the patient's thinking.

OBSERVATIONS Although the patient may talk about a variety of subjects during the interview, several content areas should be noted in the mental status examination (Box 7-3). They may be complicated and are often concealed by the patient, as in this clinical example.

 CLINICAL EXAMPLE

The patient's speech was rapid, and he acknowledged feeling as if his thoughts were coming too fast, saying, "My mind is racing ahead." The rapidity of his speech compounded the difficulty understanding him as he quickly moved from one topic to another in what appeared to be an unrelated manner. He denied any visual or auditory hallucinations; however, he believed that he could talk with God if he needed a consultant on his life situation. He felt this was a special blessing given to him over others.

Tactful questioning by the nurse is needed to explore these areas. Does the patient have recurring, persistent thoughts? Is the patient afraid of certain objects or situations or does

Box **7-3**

Thought Content Descriptors

Delusion: false belief that is firmly maintained even though it is not shared by others and is contradicted by social reality

Religious delusion: belief that one is favored by a higher being or is an instrument of that being

Somatic delusion: belief that one's body or parts of one's body are diseased or distorted

Grandiose delusion: belief that one possesses greatness or special powers

Paranoid delusion: excessive or irrational suspicion and distrust of others, characterized by systematized delusions that others are "out to get them" or spying on them

Thought broadcasting: delusion about thoughts being aired to the outside world

Thought insertion: delusion that thoughts are placed into the mind by outside people or influences

Depersonalization: the feeling of having lost self-identity and that things around the person are different, strange, or unreal

Hypochondriasis: somatic overconcern with and morbid attention to details of body functioning

Ideas of reference: incorrect interpretation of casual incidents and external events as having direct personal references

Magical thinking: belief that thinking equates with doing, characterized by lack of realistic relationship between cause and effect

Nihilistic ideas: thoughts of nonexistence and hopelessness

Obsession: an idea, emotion or impulse that repetitively and insistently forces itself into consciousness, although it is unwelcome

Phobia: a morbid fear associated with extreme anxiety

Box **7-4**

Thought Process Descriptors

Circumstantial: thought and speech associated with excessive and unnecessary detail that is usually relevant to a question, and an answer is ultimately given

Flight of ideas: overproductive speech characterized by rapid shifting from one topic to another and fragmenting ideas

Loose associations: lack of a logical relationship between thoughts and ideas that renders speech and thought inexact, vague, diffuse, and unfocused

Neologisms: new word or words created by the patient, often a blend of other words

Perseveration: involuntary, excessive continuation or repetition of a single response, idea or activity; may apply to speech or movement, but most often verbal

Tangential: similar to circumstantial but the person never returns to the central point and never answers the original question

Thought blocking: sudden stopping in the train of thought or in the middle of a sentence

Word salad: series of words that seem totally unrelated

OBSERVATIONS   A number of problems in a patient's thinking can be assessed (Box 7-4). The nurse might ask questions to evaluate the patient's thought process. Does the patient's thinking proceed in a systematic, organized, and logical manner? Is the patient's self-expression clear? Is it easy for the patient to move from one topic to another?

CLINICAL IMPLICATIONS   Circumstantial thinking may be a sign of defensiveness or paranoid thinking. Loose associations and neologisms suggest schizophrenia or other psychotic disorders. Flight of ideas indicates mania. Perseveration is often associated with brain damage and psychotic disorders. Word salad represents the highest level of thought disorganization.

Level of Consciousness

Mental status examinations routinely assess a patient's orientation to the current situation. Deciding whether a patient is oriented involves evaluating some basic cognitive functions.

OBSERVATIONS   A variety of terms can be used to describe a patient's level of consciousness, such as **confused, sedated,** or **stuporous.** In addition, the patient should be questioned regarding orientation to time, place, and person. Typically the nurse can determine this by the patient's answers to three simple questions:
- Person: What is your name?
- Place: Where are you today (such as in what city or in what particular building)?
- Time: What is today's date?

If the patient answers correctly the nurse can note "oriented times three." Level of orientation can be pursued in greater depth, but this area may be confounded by sociocultural factors.

the patient worry excessively about body and health issues? Does the patient ever feel that things are strange or unreal? Has the patient ever experienced being outside of his or her body? Does the patient ever feel singled out or watched or talked about by others? Does the patient think that thoughts or actions are being controlled by an outside person or force? Does the patient claim to have psychic or other special powers or believe that others can read the patient's mind? Throughout this part of the interview it is important that the nurse obtain information and not dispute the patient's beliefs.

CLINICAL IMPLICATIONS   Obsessions and phobias are symptoms associated with anxiety disorders. Delusions, depersonalization, and ideas of reference suggest schizophrenia and other psychotic disorders.

Thought Process

Thought process is the "how" of the patient's self-expression. A patient's thought process is observed through speech. The patterns or forms of verbalization rather than the content are assessed.

Box **7-5**

Questions Useful in Determining Orientation

QUESTIONS RELATED TO TIME

Have you been keeping track of the time lately?
What is the date today? (If patient claims not to recall, ask for an estimate. Estimates can help assess level of disorientation.)
What month (or year) is it?
How long have you been here?

QUESTIONS RELATED TO PLACE

There's been a lot happening these past few days (or hours); I wonder if you can describe for me where you are?
Do you recall what city we're in?
What is the name of the building we're in right now?
Do you know what part of the hospital we're in?

QUESTIONS RELATED TO PERSON

What is your name?
Where are you from?
Where do you currently live?
What kinds of activities do you engage in during your free time?
Are you employed? If so, what do you do for a living?
Are you married? If so, what is your spouse's name?
Do you have any children?

Fully functioning patients may be offended by questions about orientation, so the skilled nurse should integrate questions pertaining to this area in the course of the interview and develop other ways of assessing this category. For example, the nurse could use some of the approaches listed in Box 7-5.

CLINICAL IMPLICATIONS   Patients with organic mental disorder may give grossly inaccurate answers, with orientation to person remaining intact longer than orientation to time or place. Patients with schizophrenic disorders may say that they are someone else or somewhere else or reveal a personalized orientation to the world.

Memory

A mental status examination can provide a quick screen of potential memory problems but not a definitive answer to whether a specific impairment exists. Neuropsychological assessment is required to specify the nature and extent of memory impairment. Memory is broadly defined as the ability to recall past experiences.

OBSERVATIONS   The following areas must be tested:

- Remote memory: recall of events, information, and people from the distant past
- Recent memory: recall of events, information, and people from the past week or so
- Immediate memory: recall of information or data to which a person was just exposed

Recall of remote events involves reviewing information from the patient's history. This part of the evaluation can be woven into the history-taking portion of the nursing assessment. This involves asking the patient questions about time and place of birth, names of schools attended, date of marriage, ages of family members, and so forth. The problem with an evaluation of the patient's remote memory is that the nurse is often unable to tell whether the patient is reporting events accurately. This situation brings about the possibility of **confabulation**, when the patient makes up stories to recount situations or events that cannot be remembered. The nurse may need to call on past records or the report of family or friends to confirm this historical information.

Recent memory can be tested by asking the patient to recall the events of the past 24 hours. A reliable informant may be needed to verify this information. Another test of recent memory is asking the patient to remember three words (an object, a color, and an address) and then repeat them 15 minutes later in the interview.

Immediate recall can be tested by asking the patient to repeat a series of numbers either forward or backward within a 10-second interval. The nurse should begin with a short series of numbers and proceed to longer lists.

CLINICAL IMPLICATIONS   Loss of memory occurs with organicity, dissociative disorder, and conversion disorder. Patients with Alzheimer's disease retain remote memory longer than recent memory. Anxiety and depression can impair immediate retention and recent memory.

Level of Concentration and Calculation

Concentration is the patient's ability to pay attention during the course of the interview. Calculation is the person's ability to do simple math. These and other areas of cognitive functioning may vary in expected and unexpected ways (Box 7-6).

OBSERVATIONS   The nurse should note the patient's level of distractibility. Calculation can be assessed by asking the patient to do the following:

- Count from 1 to 20 rapidly
- Do simple calculations, such as 2×3 or $21 + 7$
- Serially subtract 7 from 100

If patients have difficulty subtracting 7 from 100, they can be asked to subtract 3 from 20 in the same way. Finally, more functional calculation skills can be assessed by asking practical questions such as "How many nickels are there in $1.35?"

CLINICAL IMPLICATIONS   The clinical implications of this part of the mental status examination must be carefully evaluated. Many psychiatric illnesses impair the ability to concentrate and complete simple calculations. It is particularly important to differentiate between organic mental disorder, anxiety, and depression.

Information and Intelligence

Information and intelligence are controversial areas of assessment, and the nurse should be cautious about judging intelligence after a brief and limited contact typical of the mental status examination (see Critical Thinking about Contemporary Issues, p. 127). The nurse should also re-

Box **7-6**

Gender Differences in the Brain

Women and men differ in physical attributes and in the way they think. The effect of sex hormones on brain organization appears to occur early in life, so the effects of the environment are secondary to the effects of biology. Behavioral, neurologic, and endocrinological studies help explain the processes giving rise to gender differences in the brain. Major gender differences in intellectual functioning seem to lie in patterns of ability rather than in the overall level of intelligence. For example, the problem-solving tasks favoring women and men are shown below.

PROBLEM-SOLVING TASKS FAVORING WOMEN

Women tend to perform better than men on tests of perceptual speed, in which subjects must rapidly identify matching items, as in pairing the house on the far left with its twin.

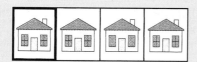

In addition, women remember whether an object or a series of objects has been displaced or rearranged.

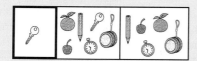

On some tests of ideational fluency, such as those in which subjects must list objects that are the same color, and on tests of verbal fluency, in which participants must list words that begin with the same letter, women also outperform men.

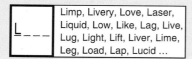

Women do better on precision manual tasks—that is, those involving fine motor coordination—such as placing the pegs in holes on a board.

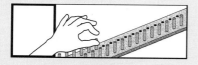

And women do better than men on mathematical calculation tests.

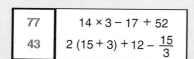

PROBLEM-SOLVING TASKS FAVORING MEN

Men tend to perform better than women on certain spatial tasks. They do well on tests that involve mentally rotating an object or manipulating it in some fashion, such as imagining turning this three-dimensional object

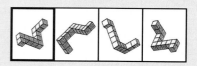

or determining where the holes punched in a folded piece of paper will fall when the paper is unfolded.

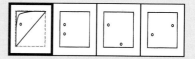

Men also are more accurate than women in target-directed motor skills, such as guiding or intercepting projectiles.

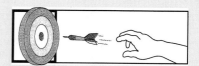

Men do better on disembedding tests, in which they have to find a simple shape, such as the one on the left, hidden within a more complex figure.

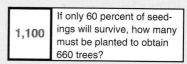

And men tend to do better than women on tests of mathematical reasoning.

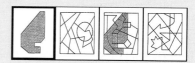

From Kimura D: *Scientific American* 267:120, 1992. (Illustrated by Jared Schneidman.)

Can a Person's Intellectual Functioning Be Validly Assessed in the Mental Status Examination?

The evaluation of a person's intellectual functioning during the mental status examination is a subject of controversy, given the brief nature of the interview and the sociocultural biases that may be brought to it. Nonetheless, knowing a patient's intellectual capacity is important to the nurse in evaluating the patient's coping resources and designing an effective treatment plan.

Furthermore, it has been suggested that there is more than one type of intelligence. Rather, there are seven different types of intelligence (Gardner, 1993).

- Linguistic intelligence
- Logical-mathematical intelligence
- Spatial intelligence
- Musical intelligence
- Bodily-kinesthetic intelligence
- Interpersonal intelligence
- Intrapersonal intelligence

The last two intelligences taken together (interpersonal and intrapersonal) can be described as forming one's personal intelligence or "emotional quotient" (Goleman 1995, 1998).

This expanded view of intelligence takes into account the talents people express in the arts, athletics, the ability to work cooperatively with people, and self-definition, as well as the more traditional verbal and mathematical skills usually assessed in standard intelligence tests. For example, a patient may have excellent spatial and mathematical intelligence but may lack formal education and interpersonal intelligence, and thus have difficulty obtaining a job. Such a person could be successful at a job that involved minimal contact with people but close work with designs and visual layouts. Nurses should take a broad approach to the assessment of intellectual functioning. This approach will allow them to identify the intellectual strengths, skills and abilities of patients that may otherwise be overlooked.

member that information in this category is highly influenced by sociocultural factors of the nurse, the patient, and the treatment setting.

OBSERVATIONS The nurse should assess the patient's last grade of school completed, general knowledge and use of vocabulary. It is also critically important to assess the patient's level of literacy. The ability to conceptualize and abstract can be tested by having the patient explain a series of proverbs. The patient can be given an example of a proverb with its interpretation and then be asked to explain what several proverbs mean. Common proverbs include the following:

- When it rains, it pours.
- A stitch in time saves nine.
- A rolling stone gathers no moss.
- The proof of the pudding is in the eating.
- People who live in glass houses shouldn't throw stones.
- A bird in the hand is worth two in the bush.

Most adults are able to interpret proverbs as symbolic of human behavior or events. However, sociocultural background should be considered when assessing a patient's information and intelligence.

If the patient's educational level is below the eighth grade, asking the patient to list similarities between a series of paired objects may better help the nurse assess the ability to abstract. The following paired objects are often used:

- Bicycle and bus
- Apple and pear
- Television and newspaper

A higher-level reply addresses function, whereas a description of structure indicates more concrete thinking. To assess a patient's general knowledge the nurse can ask the patient to name the last five presidents, the mayor, five large cities, or the occupation of a well-known person.

CLINICAL IMPLICATIONS The patient's educational level and any learning disabilities should be carefully evaluated. Mental retardation should be ruled out whenever possible. The patient's level of literacy may be part of a general assessment, but it is also an important factor in any health teaching or didactic information presented to the patient.

Judgment

Judgment involves making decisions that are constructive and adaptive. It involves the ability to understand facts and draw conclusions from relationships.

OBSERVATIONS Judgment can be evaluated by exploring the patient's involvement in activities, relationships and vocational choices. For example, is the patient regularly involved in illegal or dangerous activities or engaged in destructive relationships with others? It is also useful to determine whether the judgments are deliberate or impulsive. Finally, several hypothetical situations can be presented for the patient to evaluate:

- What would you do if you found a stamped, addressed envelope lying on the ground?
- How would you find your way out of a forest in the daytime?
- What would you do if you entered your house and smelled gas?
- If you won $10,000 what would you do with it?

CLINICAL IMPLICATIONS Judgment is impaired in organic mental disorders, schizophrenia, psychotic disorders, intoxication, and borderline or low IQ. It may also be impaired in manic patients and those with personality disorders.

? What factors would you consider in evaluating the judgment of a man who engages in bungee jumping, rock climbing and skydiving? How would this compare with a woman who has been in many relationships with abusive men?

Insight

Insight is the patient's understanding of the nature of the problem or illness.

OBSERVATIONS It is important for the nurse to determine whether the patient accepts or denies the presence of a problem or illness. In addition, the nurse should ask whether the patient blames the problem on someone else or some external factors. Several questions may help to determine the patient's degree of insight. What does the patient think about the current situation? What does the patient want others, including the nurse, to do about it? The following clinical example illustrates a patient's level of insight.

 CLINICAL EXAMPLE

The patient described several problems he was having at work. He reluctantly stated that he might have to change, but really thought his difficulties were because of his wife's drinking. He believed he could do nothing until she changed.

CLINICAL IMPLICATIONS Insight is impaired in many psychotic illnesses, including organic mental disorder, psychosis, substance abuse, eating disorders, personality disorders, and borderline or low IQ. Whether or not a patient sees the need for treatment also critically affects the therapeutic alliance, setting of mutual goals, implementation of the treatment plan, and future adherence to it.

Documenting Clinical Information

Information from the mental status examination may be recorded in various ways. Some clinicians write a descriptive report such as the one presented in the case study on p. 133. Written reports should be brief, clear, and concise and address all categories of information. Others use an outline format that is completed with short answers. Still others use a format that is compatible with computerized information systems. Regardless of the format, important findings should be documented and verbatim responses by the patient should be recorded whenever they add important information and support the nurse's assessment.

Mini-Mental State Examination

At times it is not practical or desirable to complete a full mental status examination. On these occasions, nurses may find it helpful to use the Mini-Mental State Examination (Folstein et al, 1975). It is a simplified scored form of the cognitive mental status examination. It consists of 11 questions, requires only 5 to 10 minutes to administer, and can therefore be used quickly and routinely. It is "mini" because it concentrates on only the cognitive aspects of mental functions and excludes questions concerning mood, abnormal psychological experiences, and the content or process of thinking. This examination is reproduced in Box 7-7.

PSYCHOLOGICAL TESTS

Psychological tests are of two types: those designed to evaluate intellectual and cognitive abilities and those designed to describe personality functioning. Commonly used intelligence tests are the Wechsler Adult Intelligence Scale (WAIS) and the Wechsler Intelligence Scale for Children (WISC). Although intelligence tests often are criticized as culturally biased, their ability to determine a person's strengths and weaknesses within the culture provides important therapeutic information.

Material obtained from projective tests reflects aspects of a person's personality function, including reality testing ability, impulse control, major defenses, interpersonal conflicts, and self-concept. A battery of tests is usually administered to provide comprehensive information. The Rorschach Test, Thematic Apperception Test (TAT), Bender Gestalt Test, and Minnesota Multiphasic Personality Inventory (MMPI) are commonly used by the clinical psychologist.

> *Psychological tests have typically been standardized on white, middle class populations. What implications does this have on the validity and reliability of these tests when used with individuals from other cultural backgrounds?*

BEHAVIORAL RATING SCALES

The psychological context of psychiatric nursing care goes beyond the important assessment of a patient's mental status. Neither mental health nor mental illness can be measured directly. Rather, its measurement depends on gathering a number of behavioral indicators of adaptive or maladaptive responses, which together represent the overall concept.

Many behavioral rating scales and measurement tools have been designed to help clinicians do the following:

- Measure the extent of the patient's problems
- Make an accurate diagnosis
- Track patient progress over time
- Document the efficacy of treatment

Each of these points is very important to the psychiatric nurse. The knowledge base for psychiatric care is expanding rapidly, and increased emphasis is being placed on clearly describing the nature of the patient's problems and the extent of the patient's progress toward attaining the expected outcomes of treatment (Sederer & Dickey, 1996; Faulkner & Gray, 2000). Thus nurses must be able to demonstrate in a valid and reliable way what problems they are treating and what effect their nursing care is having on attaining the treatment goals.

Nurses should become familiar with the many standardized rating scales that are available to enhance each stage of the nursing process. Many of the commonly used behavioral rating scales are listed by category in Table 7-1. Nurses with training can use any of these scales. If the scales are to be used by a group of nurses, such as nurses working together in a specific treatment program or facility, interrater reliability among the nurses should be established.

These tools do not replace required nursing documentation. Rather, they are used to complement nursing care and

Box **7-7**

Mini-Mental State Examination

MAXIMUM SCORE	SCORE	
		ORIENTATION
5	( )	What is the (year) (season) (date) (day) (month)?
5	( )	Where are we (state) (county) (town) (hospital) (floor)?
		REGISTRATION
3	( )	Name three objects: Give one second to say each. Then ask the patient to repeat all three after you have said them. Give 1 point for each correct answer. Then repeat them until the patient learns all three. Count trials and record.
		ATTENTION AND CALCULATION
5	( )	Serial sevens. Give 1 point for each correct. Stop after five answers. Alternatively, spell *world* backwards.
		RECALL
3	( )	Ask for three objects repeated above. Give 1 point for each correct.
		LANGUAGE
9	( )	Name a pencil and watch when pointed to (2 points). Repeat the following, "No ifs, ands, or buts" (1 point). Follow a three-stage command: "Take a paper in your right hand, fold it in half, and put it on the floor" (3 points). Read and obey the following: "Close your eyes" (1 point). Write a sentence (1 point). Copy design (1 point).

Total Score _____

From Folstein M, Folstein S, McHugh P: Mini-mental state: a practical method for grading the cognitive state of patients for the clinician, *J Psychiatr Res* 12:189, 1975.

provide measurable indicators of treatment outcome. For example, if the nurse is caring for a patient with depression it would be helpful to use one of the depression rating scales with the patient at the beginning of treatment to establish a baseline profile of the patient's symptoms and help confirm the diagnosis. The nurse might then administer the same scale at various times during the course of treatment to measure the patient's progress. Finally, completing the rating scale at the end of treatment would document the efficacy of the care provided.

Computer Technology

Computerized clinical information systems that provide on-line support for assessment, diagnosis, treatment planning and implementation, and outcome evaluation are becoming widely available to mental health providers (Greist, 1998; Janca & Andrews, 1999). When used with established ethical guidelines, computers offer a reliable, inexpensive,

accessible and time efficient way of assessing psychiatric symptoms.

Computer-administered versions of clinician-administered rating scales are now available for the assessment of depression, anxiety, obsessive-compulsive disorder, and social phobia (see Citing the Evidence, p. 132). Validation studies support the reliability, validity and equivalence of these scales (Kobak et al, 1996). Patient reaction has been positive, with patients being generally more honest with and often preferring the computer for assessing sensitive areas such as suicide, alcohol and drug use, sexual behavior, or HIV-related symptoms.

Use of Interactive Voice Response (IVR) technology helps with the monitoring of patients by telephone without requiring office visits to collect data. It can also increase the information available to the clinician and the quality of patient care provided through more informed decision making. It is anticipated that there will be an increase in the use of com-

Text continued on p. 133

Table **7-1**

Behavioral Rating Scales

Content Area	Scale	Content Area	Scale
GENERAL HEALTH	Clarity Health Assessment Scales Index Version		Quality of Well-Being Scale (QWB)
	Clarity Well Being Scales Comprehensive Version		Role Functioning Scale
	Freidman Quality of Life Scale		Self-Perception Profile for Adults
	Freidman Well Being Scale		Sheehan Disability Scale
	Functional Activities Questionnaire		Social Adjustment Scale II
	General Health Questionnaire (GHQ)		Social Behavior Schedule
	Katz Index of Activities of Daily Living		Social Dysfunction Rating Scale
	MOS Health Survey (SF-36)		Social Functioning Scale
	MOS Health Survey (SF-12)		Social Readjustment Scale
	OARS Social Resources Scale		Stress Response Scale (SRS)
	Sickness Impact Profile		Structured Clinical Interview for the DSM-IV
	Social Skills Inventory		Symptom Checklist-90 (SCL-90)
	Tennessee Self Concept Scale: Second Edition (TSCS:2)		Treatment Events Checklist (TEC)
			Treatment Outcome Package (TOP)
			Treatment Outcome Profile
			Young Adult Behavior Checklist
GENERAL PSYCHIATRIC	Acculturation Scale		Young Adult Self-Report (YASR)
	Assessing Coping Strategies (COPE)		
	Acuity of Psychiatric Illness, Adult Version	**AFFECTIVE DISORDERS**	Apparent Affect Rating Scale (AARS)
	Behavior and Symptom Identification Scale (BASIS-32)		Beck Depression Inventory (BDI)
	Brief Psychiatric Rating Scale (BPRS)		Beck Depression Inventory II (BDI-II)
	Behavior Rating Scale		Carroll Self-Rating Scale
	Brief Symptom Inventory (BSI)		Center for Epidemiologic Studies Depression Scale (CES-D)
	Brown Assessment of Beliefs Scale		Dementia Mood Assessment Scale (DMAS)
	Clinical Global Impression (CGI)		Depression Arkansas Scale (D-ARK Scale)
	Colorado Client Assessment Record (CCAR)		Depression Outcome Module (DOM)
	Columbia Impairment Scale (CIS)		Geriatric Depression Scale (GDS)
	Community-Oriented Programs Environmental Scale (COPES)		Hamilton Depression Scale (Ham-D)
	Compass Treatment Assessment System		Inventory for Depressive Symptomatology (IDS)
	Conners Adult ADHD Rating Scales (CAARS)		Manic-State Scale Montgomery-Asberg Depression Rating Scale (MADRS)
	Derogatis Psychiatric Rating Scale (DPRS)		Profile of Mood States
	Employee Assistance Program Index		Raskin Depression Scale
	Functional Assessment Rating Scale (FARS)		Young Mania Scale
	Functional Status Questionnaire (FSQ)		Zung Self-Rating Depression Scale (ZSRDS)
	Goal Attainment Scale		
	Global Assessment Scale (GAS)	**AGGRESSION**	Brown-Goodwin Assessment for Life History of Aggression
	Global Assessment of Functioning Scale (GAF)		Buss-Durkee Hostility Inventory
	Independent and Living Skills		Hostility and Direction of Hostility Questionnaire
	Menninger Revision of Role Functioning Scale		Overt Aggression Scale
	Million Clinical Multiaxial Inventory III (MCMI-III)	**ANXIETY DISORDERS**	Beck Anxiety Inventory (BAI)
	Multnomah Community Ability Scale		Brief Social Phobia Scale
	Neuropsychological Impairment Scale (NIS)		Covi Anxiety Scale
	Nurse Observation Scale for Inpatient Evaluation (NOSIE)		Dissociative Experience Scale
	Personal Adjustment and Role Skills (PARS)		Dissociative Disorders Interview Schedule (DDIS)
	Personal Problem Scale (PPS) and Personal Functioning Index (PFI)		Hamilton Rating Scale for Anxiety (Ham-A)
	Profile of Adaptation to Life (PAL Scale)		Maudsley Obsessional Compulsive Inventory
	PsychSentinel 3.2		Panic Disorder Outcomes Module (PDOM)
	Quality of Life Interview (QOLI)		Panic Disorder Severity Scale
	Quality of Life Inventory (QOLI)		Phobic Avoidance Rating Scale
			PTSD Inventory
			Spielberger Anxiety State-Trait

Table **7-1**

Content Area	Scale	Content Area	Scale
ANXIETY DISORDERS—CONT'D	Taylor Anxiety Scale Yale-Brown Obsessive Compulsive Scale (YBOCS) Zung Anxiety Scale		CAGE Questionnaire Chemical Use, Abuse and Dependence Scale (CUAD) Children of Alcoholics Screening Test (CAST) Clinical Institute Narcotic Assessment (CINA) Clinical Institute Withdrawal Assessment-Alcohol, Revised (CIWA-AR) Drug Abuse Screening Test (DAST) Drug Use Scale (DUS) Drug Use Screening Inventory (revised) (DUSI) Family Alcohol and Drug Survey (FADS) Follow up Drinker Profile Inventory of Drinking Situations (IDS) Michigan Alcoholism Screening Tool (MAST) Rapid Alcohol Problems Index (RAPS) Rutgers Alcohol Problem Index (RAPI) Substance Abuse Outcome Module (SAOM) Substance Abuse Subtle Screening Inventory (SASSI) Substance Abuse Treatment Schedule (SATS) Treatment Services Review (TSR)
EATING DISORDERS	Body Attitudes Test Diagnostic Survey for Eating Disorders (DSED) Eating Behaviors Diary Eating Disorders Inventory 2 (EDI-2) Eating Habits Checklist		
ORGANIC MENTAL DISORDERS	Alzheimer's Disease Assessment Scale (ADAS) Behavior Pathology in Alzheimer's Disease Blessed Dementia Scale Brief Cognitive Rating Scale Clinical Dementia Rating Scale Cognitive Abilities Screening Instrument (CASI) Cohen-Mansfield Agitation Inventory Confusion Assessment Method Cornell Scale for Depression in Dementia Delirium Index Delirium Rating Scale Delirium Symptom Interview Disruptive Behavior Scale Face-Hand Test Haycox Dementia Behavioral Scale Memory and Behavior Problems Checklist Mini-Mental Status Examination (MMSE) Multidimensional Observation Scale for Elderly Subjects NEECHAM Confusion Scale Neurobehavioral Rating Scale for Dementia (NRS) Overt Agitation Severity Scale Short Portable Mental Status Questionnaire (SPMSQ)	**SUICIDALITY**	Assessment of Suicidal Potentiality Beck Scale for Suicidal Ideation Suicide Risk Scale
		ANTIPSYCHOTIC MEDICATION SIDE EFFECTS	Abnormal Involuntary Movement Scale (AIMS) Barnes Akathesia Scale Simpson-Angus Extrapyramidal Symptoms Scale
PSYCHOTIC DISORDERS	Behavioral Observation Schedule Brief Psychiatric Rating Scale (BPRS) Life Skills Profile: Schizophrenia (LSP) Positive and Negative Syndrome Scale (PANSS) Scale for Assessment of Negative Symptoms (SANS) Scale for Assessment of Positive Symptoms (SAPS) Schizophrenia Outcomes Module (SOM) University of Washington Paranoia Scale	**CHILD**	ADHD Rating Scale - IV Ansell-Casey Life Skills Assessment 2.0 (ACLSA) Brief Psychiatric Rating Scale (BPRS) for Children Caregiver-Teacher Report Form for Ages 2-5 (C-TRF/2.5) Child and Adolescent Adjustment Profile (CAAP) Child and Adolescent Functional Assessment Scale (CAFAS) Child Assessment Schedule (CAS) Child Behavior Checklist (CBCL) Child Depression Inventory Children's Depression Rating Scale, R (CDRS-R) Children's Global Assessment Scale (CGAS) Columbia Impairment Scale Competency Skills Questionnaire (CSQ) Conners Parent and Teacher Rating Scale - Home and School Questionnaire Developmental Behavior Checklist Devereux Rating Scale School Form (DSF) Direct Observation Form and Profile for Ages 5-14 (DOF)
SUBSTANCE USE DISORDERS	Addiction Severity Index (ASI) Alcohol Dependence Scale (ADS) Alcohol/Substance Abuse Questionnaire (ASAQ) Alcohol Use Disorders Identification Test (AUDIT) Alcohol Use Inventory (AUI) Alcohol Use Scale (AUS) Brief Drug Abuse Screening Test (B-DAST)		

Continued

Table **7-1**

Behavioral Rating Scales—cont'd			
Content Area	Scale	Content Area	Scale
CHILD—CONT'D	Ohio Youth Problems, Functioning, and Satisfaction Scales		Vanderbilt Functioning Inventory (VFI)
	Revised Behavior Problem Checklist		Youth Outcome Questionnaire (YOQ)
	Severity of Psychiatric Illness: Child and Adolescent Version		Youth Self Report (YSR)
	Self-Control Rating Scale	**FAMILY**	Assessment of Strategies in Families Effectiveness Scale
	Tennessee Self Concept Scale: Second Edition (TSCS-2)		Conflict Tactics Scale
	Vanderbilt Functioning Inventory (VFI)		Family APGAR
	Yale-Brown Obsessive Compulsive Scale (YBOCS) for Children		Family Burden Interview Schedule (FBIS)
	Youth Outcome Questionnaire (YOQ)		Family Empowerment Scale
			Family Environment Scale (FES)
			Family Functioning Measures
			Zarit Burden Interview
ADOLESCENT	Adolescent Drinking Index (ADI)		
	Adolescent Treatment Outcomes Module (ATOM)	**HEALTH SERVICES**	Beginning Services Syndrome (BSS)
	Ansell-Casey Life Skills Assessment 2.0 (ACLSA)		Behavioral Healthcare Rating of Satisfaction (BHRS)
	Child and Adolescent Adjustment Profile (CAAP)		Client Experience Questionnaire (CEQ)
	Child and Adolescent Functional Assessment Scale (CAFAS)		Client Satisfaction Questionnaire (CSQ)
	Devereux Rating Scale School Form (DSF)		Client Satisfaction Survey (CSS)
	Devereux Scales of Mental Disorders (DSMD)		Consumer Satisfaction Index (CSI)
	Million Adolescent Clinical Inventory (MACI)		Inpatient Patient Satisfaction Survey System
	Million Adolescent Personality Inventory (MAPI)		Managed Care Satisfaction Survey (MCO-SS)
	Ohio Youth Problems, Functioning, and Satisfaction Scales		Older Adults Resources and Services (OARS)
	Revised Behavior Problem Index (RAPI)		Outpatient Patient Satisfaction Survey System
	Severity of Psychiatric Illness: Child and Adolescent Version		Patient Satisfaction Survey IV (PSS-IV)
	Tennessee Self Concept Scale: Second Edition (TSCS-2)		Perceptions of Care (Inpatient and Outpatient)
			Process of Care Review Form
			Satisfaction Survey (SS)
			Service Satisfaction Scale (SSS-30)
			Treatment Satisfaction Survey
			Youth Satisfaction Questionnaire

Citing the Evidence on

Computer Technology and Culture

BACKGROUND: This study was designed to test a bilingual computerized voice recognition depression-screening method to identify individuals with major depression or with a high-risk profile for depression in a women's clinic at a major public sector urban hospital.

RESULTS: Very high levels of depressive symptoms were found, and a large proportion of the women met DSM–IV–TR criteria for major depression. Depression screening with computerized voice recognition methods provided results comparable to those of live interviews in both English and Spanish.

IMPLICATIONS: Currently face-to-face interviewing is the usual way of evaluating nonliterate or non-English-speaking individuals in most treatment settings. Such interviews may place limitations on access to services for these people because of the unavailability of non-English speaking personnel, cultural miscommunications and patient suspicions of interviewer bias. Voice recognition technology and telephone-assisted interviews can be an important way to increase the access to mental health services for populations not likely or not able to seek care.

Munoz R et al: Depression screening in a women's clinic: using automated Spanish- and English-language voice recognition, *J Consult Clin Psychol* 67(4):502, 1999.

CASE STUDY

Ms. T was a stylishly dressed, neatly groomed, slender woman in apparent good physical health who appeared to be her stated 22 years of age. She was cooperative during the interview but had difficulty expressing herself in specific terms. Her vague responses left the interviewer feeling perplexed about the difficulties she was describing.

The patient was alert and awake and oriented to person, place, and time. Immediate recall and recent memory were intact, demonstrated in her ability to recall three unrelated objects immediately and again in 15 minutes. Some of the historical information given was inconsistent with historical facts reported by her father. Although the vocabulary used by Ms. T and her knowledge of general information was congruent with her twelfth-grade education and past employment, she had difficulty completing the serial sevens but performed serial threes with ease. She stated that she was "nervous," which may be a factor related to performance. She was able to abstract two of three proverbs presented.

Proverb	Interpretation
Don't cry over spilled milk.	"If something happens, then forget about it. Maybe things will get better."
A rolling stone gathers no moss.	"A good person gathers no enemies. If a person stays active, he won't get depressed."
People who live in glass houses shouldn't throw stones.	"The glass will break."

Her responses to hypothetical situations were appropriate; however, the manner in which she coped with difficulties at work and home showed impaired judgment about personal issues.

Ms. T's speech was clear, coherent, and of normal rate and tone. Except for the vague, tangential manner in which she discussed her concern for her aunt, her communication was goal directed. There were no apparent delusions, hallucinations, or illusions. She denied any obsessions, compulsions or phobias.

The central theme during the interview was her fear of being irresponsible and hurting her aunt. Her sadness and concern about her behavior in relation to the aunt pervaded the interview. She appeared nervous (looking away, fidgeting) and cried whenever she talked about her aunt. She described her mood as "low" and rated it as a 4 on a scale of 1 to 10. She denied any suicidal or homicidal ideas or plan previously or at the present time.

Her insight was questionable because she debated her need for treatment, but she agreed to return. She knew that a problem existed but was unaware of the causes of her behavior.

puterized technology because it has the advantages of structure, reliability, accessibility and low cost in the collection of clinically relevant data to support clinician decision making.

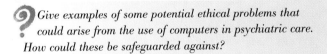
Give examples of some potential ethical problems that could arise from the use of computers in psychiatric care. How could these be safeguarded against?

Summary

1. The mental status examination represents a cross-section of the patient's psychological life at that time. It requires the nurse to observe the patient's behavior and describe it in an objective, nonjudgmental manner.

2. The categories assessed in the mental status examination include the patient's appearance, speech, motor activity, mood, affect, interaction during the interview, perceptions, thought content, thought process, level of consciousness, memory, level of concentration and calculation, information and intelligence, judgment, and insight.

3. Psychological tests evaluate intellectual and cognitive abilities and describe personality functioning.

4. Behavioral rating scales help clinicians measure the extent of the patient's problem, make an accurate diagnosis, track patient progress over time, and document the efficacy of treatment. These scales should be used by psychiatric nurses to complement nursing care and provide measurable indicators of treatment outcome. Computer technology allows these instruments to be administered more efficiently with more rapid feedback for clinical decision making.

 Visit MERLIN: www.mosby.com/MERLIN/Stuart to find these additional materials and student activities.

- **Worksheets**
- **"Drug of the Month" Updates**
- **"Citing the Evidence" Updates**
- **Critical Thinking Activities and Exercises**
- **Annotated Suggested Readings**
- **Web Links**
- **More!**

Chapter Review Questions

1. Match the terms in Column A with the correct description in Column B.

Column A

____ Affect

____ Delusion

____ Flight of ideas

____ Hallucinations

____ Illusions

____ Insight

____ Loose associations

____ Mood

Column B

A. False belief not shared by others or confirmed by reality

B. False perception or response to a sensory stimulation

C. Feeling, mood, or emotional tone

D. Lack of a logical relationship between thoughts and ideas, resulting in unfocused speech

E. Overproductive speech with rapid shifting of topics and ideas

F. Perceptual distortion arising from any of the five senses

G. Self-report by patient of his or her prevailing emotional state

H. Understanding by the patient of the nature of his or her problem or illness

2. Fill in the blanks.

A. A patient who describes the death of a younger brother without any emotional response is said to have

_____.

B. _____ are false sensory impressions that tell the patient to do something he or she would not ordinarily do.

C. The most common type of hallucination involves the sense of _____.

D. When a patient makes up stories in response to questions about situations or events that cannot be remembered it is called _____.

3. Provide short answers for the following questions.

A. What are the five major categories of information that should be included in a mental status examination?

B. What three questions have been asked when a patient is described as oriented times three?

C. Identify four reasons why psychiatric nurses should use behavioral rating scales in their practice.

D. Identify four reasons why psychiatric nurses do not use behavioral rating scales in their practice.

E. What impact do you think computer technology could have on improving mental health care for currently underserved populations?

REFERENCES

American Psychiatric Association: Practice guideline for psychiatric evaluation of adults, *Am J Psychiatry* 152(11):67, 1995 (suppl).

Faulkner, Gray: *2000 Behavioral outcomes & guidelines sourcebook,* New York, 2000, Faulkner & Gray.

Folstein M, Folstein S, McHugh P: Mini-mental state: a practical method for grading the cognitive state of patients for the clinician, *J Psychiatr Res* 12:189, 1975.

Gardner H: *Multiple intelligences,* New York, 1993, Basic Books.

Goleman D: *Emotional intelligence,* New York, 1995, Bantam.

Goleman D: *Working with emotional intelligence,* New York, 1998, Bantam.

Greist J: The computer as clinician assistant: assessment made simple, *Psychiatr Serv* 49:467, 1998.

Janca A, Andrews G: Computers in psychiatric care, *Curr Opin Psychiatr* 12:701, 1999.

Kobak K et al: Computer administered clinical rating scales: a review, *Psychpharmacology* 127(4):291, 1996.

Sederer L, Dickey B: *Outcomes assessment in clinical practice,* Baltimore, 1996, Williams & Wilkins.

Strub R: *The mental status examination in neurology,* Philadelphia, 2000, FA Davis.

Trzepacz P, Baker R: *The psychiatric mental status examination,* New York, 1993, Oxford University Press.

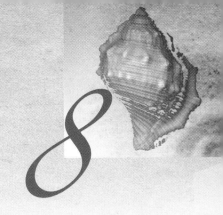

Sociocultural Context of Psychiatric Nursing Care

Linda D. Oakley

We know what we belong to, where we come from, and where we are going. We may not know it with our brains, but we know it with our roots.

NOEL COWARD, *THIS HAPPY BREED*

Holistic psychiatric nursing care includes all aspects of the individual in the assessment, diagnosis, and treatment process. An important part of this holistic perspective is the nurse's skill in recognizing the sociocultural context of care. In each interaction with the patient, the nurse is aware of the culture in which the patient lives. The nurse understands that people's perceptions of health and illness and their help seeking behavior and treatment adherence depend on their beliefs, social norms, and cultural values. Thus quality psychiatric nursing care must incorporate the unique aspects of the individual into every element of practice and be based on an understanding of the importance of culture, as outlined in Box 8-1.

CULTURAL COMPETENCE

Increasing attention has been focused on culturally relevant mental health care. Nursing expectations are also evolving from a superficial knowledge of differences in age, gender, and ethnic groups to the implementation of culturally competent nursing care.

Culturally competent nurses have the knowledge and skills to intervene successfully in the lives of patients from diverse cultures. As a practice skill, cultural competency is the ability to view each patient as a unique individual, fully considering the patient's cultural experiences within the context of the common developmental challenges faced by all people. The nurse applies this information in nursing interventions that are consistent with the life experiences and cultural values of patients (Poss, 1999; Parsons & Reiss, 1999; Bechtel & Davidhizar, 1999).

Culturally competent nurses are also in touch with their own personal and cultural experiences. These nurses provide individualized patient care and are aware of actions that may offend a patient who is not a member of the nurses' ethnic, social, or cultural group. The culturally competent nurse understands the importance of social and cultural forces, recognizes the uniqueness of each patient, respects nurse-patient differences, and incorporates sociocultural information into psychiatric nursing care.

SOCIOCULTURAL RISK FACTORS

The concept of risk factors is important to understanding how people acquire, experience, and recover from illness. Risk factors are the same as the predisposing factors that nurses assess in the Stuart Stress Adaptation Model of psy-

Box **8-1**

The Functions of Culture

Perception: Perception of reality is based on a cultural interpretation and understanding of events.
Motives: Motives for behavior are conditioned by the values assumed by a culture.
Identity: Individual and group identity is fostered by the oral, written and social constructs defining a culture.
Values: Concepts of ethics and morality are conditioned by cultural background.
Communication: Language, music and dance are the external expressions of culture.
Emotions: Emotions are significantly enabled and shaped by cultural ideas, practices and institutions.

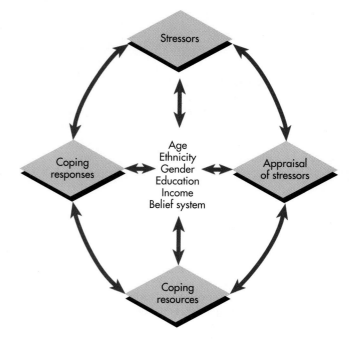

Fig. 8-1   Sociocultural context of psychiatric care.

chiatric nursing (see Chapter 4). Understanding the risk factors involved in health and illness is essential in the prevention, early detection, and effective treatment of physiological illnesses such as cardiac, pulmonary, and hepatic diseases.

Identifying risk factors is also valuable in providing psychiatric care. Risk factors for psychiatric disorders are characteristics of a person that can significantly increase the potential for developing a psychiatric disorder, decrease the potential for recovery, or both. Perhaps the most important outcome of the inclusion of risk or predisposing factors in nursing practice is the development of individualized, culturally competent, and socially relevant mental health care.

The sociocultural perspective described in this chapter focuses on age, ethnicity, gender, education, income and belief systems. No one or two of these factors alone adequately describes the sociocultural context of nursing care; however, together they provide a sociocultural profile of the patient that is essential to psychiatric nursing practice. These factors include social norms, cultural beliefs and personal values, and influence the patient's exposure to stressors, appraisal of stressors, coping resources, and coping responses, as described in the Stuart Stress Adaptation Model (Fig. 8-1).

The sociocultural factors of age, ethnicity, gender, education, income and belief system are predisposing or conditioning factors that influence the amount and type of coping resources available to a person. These factors do not cause future events. For example, being female may be a predisposing factor for the development of depression, but it does not cause depression. In fact, some of these factors may be a consequence of the illness. For example, being poor may be the result of a substance abuse disorder rather than the cause of it. These sociocultural factors are important because they influence the person's vulnerability to, development of and recovery from psychiatric disorders. Finally, it is important to realize that these factors can interact so that different ones become important at different times.

This sociocultural view does not assume that individual members of groups based on age, ethnicity, gender, education, income, or belief systems all have the same risk of developing a psychiatric disorder, nor does it assume that a person's risk of developing a psychiatric disorder is constant.

Rather, individual differences among the members of a group and contextual variations in individual risk are key principles of this perspective.

Most importantly, this view does not draw generalizations about groups based on age, ethnicity, gender, education, income, or belief system. Literature that describes and summarizes the values or beliefs of specific populations such as blacks, Hispanics, and Asians often creates new stereotypes, and these generalizations can further depersonalize nursing care. In contrast, the sociocultural view is based on the assessment of individual, social, cultural and environmental factors that change over time.

Important health-related differences do exist between various groups in society. Group differences have been reported and examined in relation to a number of physical and psychiatric illnesses. For example, researchers have noted that more females than males are diagnosed and treated for depression regardless of age, ethnicity, education or income (Robin et al, 1997). It is not known whether the different prevalence of a psychiatric disorder between groups is an indicator of clinical differences, cultural differences, or both. Specifically, it is not known whether the prevalence of depression among females is greater than that among males because the two groups are clinically different or because females are exposed more often to the social and cultural stressors that can precipitate depression. If the latter were true, it would suggest that if males were exposed to the same stressors and were taught the same coping style as females, the rate of depression for the two groups would be equal.

This example highlights the incorrect assumption that all members of a group behave, think, and feel similarly. It also shows the importance of integrating biological, psychological, and cultural contributions to fully understand the dimensions of mental health and psychiatric illness.

Much research on sociocultural risk factors for psychiatric disorders is relevant to psychiatric nursing practice. The scope of the field is beyond that of this chapter, so the reader is referred to other sources for more detailed information (Gaw, 1993; Tseng & Stretzer, 1997; Flaskerud, 2000). Some findings about each risk factor and their possible effects on holistic psychiatric nursing care are described in the following sections. Box 8-2 lists some sociocultural trends and their influences on the health-care system.

Think of a group you belong to based on one of your sociocultural characteristics. What stereotypes exist about this group? Do you fit these stereotypes?

Age

Age related variations in life stressors, support resources, and coping skills are very important. It has been reported that the frequency of seeking mental health care decreases with age and that help-seeking behavior peaks between 25 and 44 years of age and then declines. Age related increases and decreases in the use of mental health services tend to occur as a reflection of various social, cultural and developmental changes associated with aging. In terms of support resources, African American, Hispanic, and Caucasian elderly often find going to church to be an adaptive coping strategy. Additionally, among the elderly, the prevalence of depression is decreased among those with high socioeconomic status and more education (Stolley & Koenig, 1997; Goldstein & Griswold, 1998).

It has also been found that while age increases, the prevalence of depression decreases. Even when compared with younger age groups, elders tend to recover from depression more quickly and are less likely to have a recurrence. Thus younger age emerges as a risk factor for depressive illness, possibly because elders who are socioeconomically stable may also be more resilient because they may have developed effective coping strategies and have less demanding or less stressful social roles as compared with younger adults.

Ethnicity

The term ethnicity as used in this chapter includes a person's racial, national, tribal, linguistic, and cultural origin or background. Within each ethnicity or race a number of groups may be found. For example, the term Hispanic represents people united by a common language, but coming from national backgrounds as diverse as Mexico, the Caribbean islands (including Puerto Rico, Cuba and the Dominican Republic), Central and South American countries and Spain, each of which has their own unique histories, customs, beliefs, and cultural systems. Also, people known as Asian American actually represent some 40 different ethnic groups speaking 30 different languages. As a category, Native American includes Alaskan and Hawaiian natives, but for each there are hundreds of tribes with different histories, languages, and practices. Blacks living in the United States also represent diverse regional backgrounds and countries of origin. Finally, as a result of as-

Box 8-2

Sociocultural Diversity and the Health-Care System

Current U.S. data suggest that the following sociocultural trends will influence the health-care system and the way health care is provided:

- The population will increase by 60% to almost 400 million by the year 2050.
- Growth will be concentrated at the two ends of the age spectrum. By 2050 the population aged 65 and over will more than double and the population 85 years and older will be the fastest-growing age group.
- The U.S. population is becoming more diverse by race and ethnicity. By 2050 Hispanics will be about 25% of the population; African American about 14%; Asian and Pacific Islanders about 8%; American Indian, Eskimo and Aleut about 1%; and whites about 53%.
- The United States has become a predominantly urban nation, with the population occupying only 2.5% of the land mass.

These trends will have a profound impact on the health-care system for the following reasons:

- As the aging population grows, there will be an increase in chronic conditions and chronic diseases related to behavior that will exact a greater toll on the health-care system.
- A rise in the number of young people will bring new waves of problems typically committed by the young, such as murder, rape, robbery, and assault. Almost half of all violent crimes are committed by people under age 24, with those 15 to 19 years of age responsible for most. The overall crime rate has increased 500% since 1960.
- Minority populations are currently underserved, a problem that may only intensify. In addition, there is an expected increase in low–birth-weight babies among minority populations.
- Minority populations are underrepresented in all health-care professions, causing concern about whether health-care providers will understand health problems within a cultural context and be able to provide culturally sensitive care.

From: Center for Mental Health Services, *Cultural Competence Standards*, Rockville, Md, 1998, Center for Mental Health Services.

similation and intermarriage many people see themselves as multi-ethnic.

Members of minorities often have difficulty gaining access to appropriate mental health services. Many lack medical insurance or primary care clinicians who could assist with the referral process. Difficulty with language and communication or lack of knowledge in negotiating the mental health-care system also limits their ability to receive needed care. A number of studies report that members of minority groups delay seeking help until their problems are intense, chronic and difficult to treat and community and family support systems have been exhausted. Delays in entering service and early terminations create a cyclical reliance on more costly services.

Ethnicity has also been shown to influence the development of and recovery from psychiatric disorders (see Citing the Evidence). Significant differences exist in the prevalence of certain disorders among various ethnic groups and in their use of mental health services. Misdiagnosis is a problem that creates inappropriate admissions to state hospitals. For example, African Americans and Hispanics have been reported to be diagnosed on admission with severe mental illness at a rate almost twice as high as individuals from other groups. In addition, the most severe types of psychopathology tend to be diagnosed in black patients, with blacks being underrepresented in affective disorders and overdiagnosed with schizophrenia (Abreu, 1999; Baker & Bell, 1999, Trierweiler et al, 2000).

In terms of hospitalization, members of ethnic groups are admitted to psychiatric institutions three times more often than the general population. In addition, blacks, Native Americans, and Hispanics have higher rates of admission to state and county mental hospitals than to community and private psychiatric hospitals (SAMHSA, 1998). Other studies have found that blacks were more likely to use emergency mental health services and less likely to use individual or group treatment (Klinkenberg & Calsyn, 1997; Maynard et al, 1997). In contrast, Asians have extremely low admission rates to state hospitals and have low utilization of mental health services in general (Herrick & Brown, 1998; Lin & Cheung, 1999).

Studies have also examined racial differences in relation to treatment and have found that nonpsychotic black patients had shorter lengths of stay in inpatient facilities than white patients with similar disorders. White patients were more likely to be on one-to-one observational status, and clinicians were more likely to order urine drug screens for black patients with high socioeconomic status than for comparable white patients (Baker & Bell, 1999). It has also been reported that black patients coming to an emergency service were prescribed more psychiatric medication, receiving more oral doses and more injections of antipsychotic medications and higher dosages. The tendency to overmedicate black patients was lower, however, when clinicians' efforts to engage the patient in treatment were rated higher (Segal et al, 1996). These studies point to the importance of engaging patients from diverse ethnic groups in the treatment process, and the need for clinical skills and training in bridging cultural differences.

 How might ethnicity influence the coping responses and the specific symptoms expressed by a patient?

Gender

As a predisposing risk factor, gender is similar to ethnicity in that at first glance there appear to be distinctive male and female patterns of risk. However, when all psychiatric disorders are included, the prevalence of mental illness among males and females is roughly equal. The actual difference between the two groups is in the type of disorder that is most commonly diagnosed. Substance abuse and antisocial personality disorder are the most prevalent psychiatric disorders among males, whereas affective disorders and anxiety disorders are most prevalent among females. In contrast, the prevalence of schizophrenia and manic episodes for males and females is about equal.

These findings support the idea that male and female role socialization in contemporary American society is a significant determinant of the perception of health and illness and that the risk of psychiatric disorders may be sex typed by sociocultural factors. Specifically, it has been proposed that males are taught to aggressively externalize their psychological experiences, whereas females are taught to passively internalize their social experiences.

Research has also shown consistent gender differences in schizophrenia. Gender differences exist in both symptom presentation as well as course of illness. Specifically, the age of onset is later for women and they tend to have greater preillness social functioning. Men, on the other hand, are more likely to be aggressive, self-destructive, spend more time in jail, and are more likely to commit suicide. In terms of treatment, women have a better response to both pharmacological and psychosocial treatments, but they are much more vulnerable to negative psychosocial outcomes such as victimization and substance abuse (Gearon & Tamminga, 2000).

Such evidence suggests that the treatment approach for men and women with schizophrenia should be tailored to the gender differences. Specifically, women should have lower doses of medicine over shorter periods of time. They should have access to focused psychosocial treatments aimed at reducing substance abuse and the occurrence of violent sexual and physical violence. Men, in contrast, should have

---

Citing the Evidence on

Psychological Distress in Ethnic Groups

BACKGROUND: Despite the increasing number of studies that have substantiated that women who have been abused are psychologically distressed, little research has focused on women from diverse ethnic backgrounds. This correlational study examined psychological distress and psychosocial factors in a sample of 62 white and 62 Hispanic abused women.

RESULTS: White women experienced a higher prevalence of psychological distress than Hispanics. Life changes were significantly related to the severity of psychological distress, but not exposure to abuse.

IMPLICATIONS: In this study white women had more stressors related to physical abuse, such as the need to relocate, change employment status, and fear of safety, which appears to have placed them at greater risk for psychological symptoms as compared with Hispanic women. In the future, longitudinal studies can examine causative factors and provide stronger implications for appropriate treatment with abused women.

Torres S, Han H: Psychological distress in non-Hispanic White and Hispanic abused women, *Arch Psychiatr Nurs* 14(1):19, 2000.

more aggressive pharmacological treatments and psychosocial treatments aimed at improving interpersonal skills and controlling aggression.

The following clinical example demonstrates the interaction of ethnicity and gender and the way in which they can affect a person's response to stress.

 ### CLINICAL EXAMPLE

Jose Rodriguez is a 36-year-old Hispanic man. Jose planned to graduate from an MBA program in May and marry his fiancée, Lisa, in June. The couple met in class 2 years ago and have dated for 1 year. Jose visited Lisa's family for the first time during spring break. Lisa's parents are of German descent, and they were shocked when Lisa told them she planned to marry Jose in 3 months. Lisa's father informed her that if she goes through with her wedding plans he will disown her. He said that her mother and brothers agreed with him and that she had to choose between Jose and her family. When she told Jose about her father's reaction he felt they should leave immediately, but Lisa said she could not go with him if it meant going against her family.

Jose drove back to school and on the way was cited twice for speeding. When he returned to his room he spent 2 days alone drinking beer. He did not shave, shower, or change his clothes. On the third day he went out for more beer and as he walked past a group of men, one of them called him a "dirty wetback." When Jose got home he destroyed his room and everything in it, including his completed master's thesis, which he needed to hand in the next day in order to graduate in May.

 How might a psychiatric nurse's view of gender-appropriate behavior influence one's diagnosis and treatment of male and female patients?

Education

Mental status examinations are often used to determine diagnosis and treatment for various psychiatric disorders (see Chapter 7). Yet questions have been raised about the cultural context of such evaluations. It has also been noted that patients who have difficulty with English are often misdiagnosed. Therefore, programs need to adapt to the needs of people with limited English proficiency by providing either clinicians and staff members who speak native languages, or skilled translators/interpreters. Written materials and forms also need to be printed in the native languages at the literacy levels of the populations served.

Numerous studies identify the importance of education as a coping resource in protecting against the development of and promoting recovery from mental illness. For example, it has been found that education is more important than income in determining use of mental health services, with those with the highest educational level using mental health services most often.

The clinical example that follows illustrates the effect ethnicity, gender, and education can have on a person's ability to interact with others effectively.

 ### CLINICAL EXAMPLE

Ms. Wong is a 22-year-old Chinese American woman. She is employed at a university computer center and is a part-time law student. Her roommate is a second-year English major and has an active social life. Because her courses are demanding and her family expects her to be successful, Ms. Wong spends all of her free time studying. While Ms. Wong was studying one Friday afternoon, her roommate came home with several friends, including a young man from Ms. Wong's law class that she thought was very attractive. She was excited about seeing him and acted very friendly toward him until she realized that he was her roommate's date for the evening. Ms. Wong felt humiliated by her behavior and abruptly left the apartment. While she was leaving, she heard her roommate say, "Now that Miss Perfect is gone, we can party."

Ms. Wong did not know what to do or in whom to confide. She walked around town for hours. Although she was becoming exhausted, she did not stop to rest, eat, or drink. She continued to walk and smiled at the romantic couples she passed but became sad again when they did not smile back at her. Ms. Wong noticed a wig store across the street from where she stood and went in and bought a curly blonde wig that she immediately put on. She wore this wig every day and insisted that everyone call her Patty, her new American name.

Income

The negative effects of poverty on mental health are severe regardless of age, ethnicity or gender, as evidenced by many community surveys that report a relationship between lower economic status and higher level of psychiatric symptoms and inpatient admissions (Bruce et al, 1991; Muntaner et al, 1995). However, the prevalence of poverty among women, elders and ethnic minorities is significant. Some researchers believe that the difference in risk for psychiatric disorders between groups is primarily a measure of social stratification and poverty, with those at the bottom facing more daily problems than those at the top. Others suggest that the combination of poverty with other risk factors such as gender and ethnicity predicts both the onset of stress-related psychiatric disorders and the use of mental health services (Vega et al, 1999).

The following clinical example describes the effect of ethnicity and income on self-esteem.

 ### CLINICAL EXAMPLE

John Willis is a 20-year-old black man. He has been looking for work since he graduated from high school 2 years ago and has had several job interviews with local employers. Over the phone, all of these employers seemed very interested in hiring John, but he never received a job offer. Each time he called back after an interview, he was told that the position had been filled and that his application would be kept on file. Last fall, John obtained an interview for an entry-level position at a local bank. He felt that his luck had changed and this would be the perfect job for him.

He arrived early for his interview, and after waiting an hour to meet with the interviewer, John was told that the position had been filled. John was very surprised to hear this. He felt that he had not been treated fairly and that the interviewer just wanted to look him over and decided that he did not like what he saw. John asked the interviewer, "Did the position get filled before or after I got here, or don't you know that either?" The interviewer alerted security and asked John to leave. John was angry and embarrassed and asked the interviewer why he was being treated like a criminal when he came here to apply for a job. Before the interviewer could answer, John left the building. Since then, John has refused to look for work or go to another interview. He has been unemployed for 2 years and continues to live with his parents, sleeping until noon everyday and spending all of his time "hanging out" with his male friends.

> *Most single-parent households in this country are headed by women, and many of them are below the poverty level. How might this affect the mental health of the children living in these homes?*

Belief System

A person's belief system, world view, religion or spirituality can also have a positive or negative effect on mental health (see Citing the Evidence). Human beings in general need to make sense out of and explain their life experiences. This need is especially important when they are suffering or in distress. In this quest for meaning, belief systems play a vital role in determining whether a particular explanation and associated treatment plan will have meaning to the patient and others in the patient's social network (Taggart, 1994; Weaver et al, 1998). The degree of compatibility between the patient's and provider's belief systems often determines the patient's satisfaction with treatment, medication compliance, and treatment outcome (Herrick & Brown, 1999).

Adaptive belief system responses can enhance well-being, improve the quality of life, and speed recovery from illness. Maladaptive belief system responses may lead to poor adjustment to changing health status, refusal of necessary treatment or even self-injury. For example, certain religious belief systems stress avoidance of alcohol, illicit drugs, and cigarette smoking. Spiritually based intervention programs, such as 12-step programs, which encourage the individual to surrender control to an external supreme being, are commonly used treatments for addictive disorders.

> *Think about two patients you took care of last week. Did you discuss with them their belief systems about their health and current illnesses? How might this information have influenced your nursing interventions with them?*

In summary, age, ethnicity, gender, education, income, and belief system are psychiatric disorder risk factors that can increase the likelihood of psychiatric illness and decrease the likelihood of a positive treatment outcome. In particular, age, ethnicity, and gender are powerful risk fac-

Citing the Evidence on
Religiosity and Depression

BACKGROUND: The effects of religious belief and activity on remission of depression were examined in medically ill hospitalized older patients.

RESULTS: Intrinsic religiosity was significantly and independently related to time to remission, but church attendance and private religious activities were not. Depressed patients with higher intrinsic religiosity scores had more rapid remissions than patients with lower scores.

IMPLICATIONS: Religious beliefs and behaviors are commonly used by depressed older adults to cope with medical problems and may lead to faster resolution of some types of depression. Nurses should feel free to inquire about and support the healthy religious beliefs and activities of older patients with disabling health problems, realizing that these beliefs may bring comfort and promote adaptive coping.

Koenig H et al: Religiosity and remission of depression in medically ill older patients, *Am J Psychiatry* 155(4):536, 1998.

tors for psychiatric illness when combined with poverty and low education.

SOCIOCULTURAL STRESSORS

Some of the sociocultural stressors that hinder the delivery of psychiatric care are listed in Table 8-1. Disadvantagement creates profound problems in the prevention, diagnosis, and treatment of psychiatric disorders. In addition to lacking basic resources, people who are poor and poorly educated are often stereotyped in society as freeloaders or lazy. Such people are often the focus of other negative attitudes and behaviors such as intolerance, stigma, prejudice, discrimination, and racism.

For example, consider a woman who is obese. In American society thinness is highly valued and obesity is stigmatized regardless of the person's ethnicity or age. However, obese males are stigmatized less than obese females. Despite the fact that the fashion industry now markets to the "big woman," "big" has yet to become an acceptable standard of femininity in American society. In addition, although obese women and men may encounter the same amount of employment discrimination, obese women are often also viewed as asexual because of their failure to follow the social rule of thinness as a norm of female sexuality. As a result, in comparison to the overweight or obese male, obese females are more likely to be single. Because married and partnered adults consistently report less stress than adults who are single or divorced, it is evident that sociocultural attitudes and values serve as stressors and increase the risk of psychiatric disorders for some individuals.

Table **8-1**

Sociocultural Stressors

Stressor	Definition
Disadvantagement	The lack of socioeconomic resources that are basic to biopsychosocial adaptation
Stereotype	A depersonalized conception of individuals within a group
Intolerance	Unwillingness to accept different opinions or beliefs from people of different backgrounds
Stigma	An attribute or trait deemed by the person's social environment as unfavorable
Prejudice	A preconceived, unfavorable belief about individuals or groups that disregards knowledge, thought, or reason
Discrimination	Differential treatment of individuals or groups not based on actual merit
Racism	The belief that inherent differences among the races determine individual achievement and that one race is superior

IMPACT ON COPING RESPONSES

The coping responses used by individuals and the ways in which symptoms of mental illness are expressed also vary by culture (see Citing the Evidence). Coping responses and the meaning assigned to them are greatly influenced by sociocultural norms, values, beliefs and expectations. Symptoms that indicate a problem in the context of one group may be tolerated or even ignored by another group for two reasons. First, if a behavior or symptom is widespread, it may be considered normal. Second, if the behavior fits in with social values it may similarly be accepted. For example, hallucinations in Western society are considered a sign of serious illness because the social values emphasize rationality and control. In contrast, visions, hexes, and hearing voices are not necessarily considered signs of psychosis among other cultures, nor is communicating with the dead. In addition, some cultural groups would view symptoms typically associated with mental illness as signs of normality, meanness, laziness, sin, or spiritual distress.

Finally, there are many culture-specific ways of expressing distress. For example, black patients with schizophrenia have been observed to show more anger and suspicion toward others than white patients with schizophrenia. For some black patients, anger and suspicion are coping responses to chronic sociocultural stress. This coping response may be ineffective, however, in that anger and suspicion do not decrease feelings of distress, nor signal to others the need for support.

NURSING ASSESSMENT AND DIAGNOSIS

Cultural self-awareness is an essential first step for the psychiatric nurse in the delivery of culturally competent care (Lutzen et al, 1997). To prepare to be culturally responsive to a patient, the nurse should answer the following questions:

- What about the patient's appearance or behavior makes me think that what I am seeing or hearing is pathological?
- What label am I subconsciously applying to this patient and where did it come from?
- What social class am I assuming this patient comes from and what are my prejudices about that group?
- What other explanations might account for this patient's unusual behavior?

Citing the Evidence on

Coping Strategies of Korean Women

BACKGROUND: A cross-sectional survey research design was used to explore which coping strategies and demographic variables were significantly related to depression for employed Korean immigrant wives.

RESULTS: Coping strategies accounted for only 24% of the variance in depression. Specifically, wives who worked harder, as in cleaning the house and taking care of children, had more depression, while those who negotiated with their husbands were less likely to be depressed.

IMPLICATIONS: Psychiatric nurses should work within the community to foster the development of cultural and traditional norms that sanction negotiation between husbands and wives.

Um C, Dancy B: Relationship between coping strategies and depression among employed Korean immigrant wives, *Issues Ment Health Nurs* 20:485, 1999.

- What personal characteristics of the patient have I noted and what are my positive and negative reactions to those characteristics?

In effect, psychiatric nurses need to qualify their clinical assessments by offering cultural explanations for their patients' behavior and appearance.

Assessment of the patient's sociocultural risk factors and stressors greatly enhances the nurse's ability to establish a therapeutic alliance, identify the patient's problems, and develop a treatment plan that is accurate, appropriate, and culturally relevant. Box 8-3 presents questions the nurse might ask related to each of the risk factors described in this chapter.

A culturally competent psychiatric nursing diagnosis takes into account sociocultural risk factors and stressors that affect the patient's coping responses. Often, nurses exclude sociocultural information in their analysis because they want to avoid stereotyping the patient, feel that the patient's health-care problems are not related to the patient's

Box **8-3**

Questions Related to Sociocultural Risk Factors

AGE
Questions

What is the patient's current stage of development?
What are the developmental tasks of the patient?
Are those tasks age-appropriate for the patient?
What are the patient's attitudes and beliefs regarding the patient's age group?
With what age-related stressors is the patient coping?
What impact does the patient's age have on mental and physical health?

Example

Assessment. Jim is 38 years old and trying to come to terms with balancing his need for intimacy with that of finding his own identity and sense of purpose in life. He describes feelings of anxiety along with waves of hopelessness. He states, "At my age I should stop acting like I'm twenty-something and accept myself, but I just can't seem to do that."

Evaluation. Jim is worried that he will never settle down into an adult lifestyle, but he is more afraid of the high stress and loss of social attractiveness that he associates with being middle-aged.

ETHNICITY
Questions

What is the patient's ethnic background?
What is the patient's ethnic identity?
Is the patient traditional, bicultural, multicultural, or culturally alienated?
What are the patient's attitudes, beliefs, and values regarding his or her ethnic group?
With what ethnicity-related stressors is the patient coping?
What impact does the person's ethnicity have on mental and physical health?

Example

Assessment. Landa is a black woman. She strongly endorses African American values and considers herself to be culturally traditional. Landa believes that African American values are superior to Western values and that there would be less poverty and crime in black communities if all black people shared her beliefs. She spends much of her time reading about traditional African ways and has become isolated from her friends and family.

Evaluation. Landa lacks the social support she needs to feel good about her ethnicity without having to idealize or reject members of her own or other ethnic groups. She is having difficulty integrating her values with those of her family and friends.

GENDER
Questions

What is the patient's gender?
What is the patient's gender identity?
How does the patient define gender-specific roles?
What are the patient's attitudes and beliefs regarding males and females and masculinity and femininity?
With what gender-related stressors is the patient coping?
What impact does the person's gender have on mental and physical health?

Example

Assessment. Kelly is male, and enacting the male role is very important to him. As a man, he feels he must provide for his family by working hard, making money, and being smart. Kelly feels that his wife should respect how hard he works and support his plans for providing for her. Recently, he and his wife have had increasing marital conflict. He states "I am doing what is right for both of us. All my wife has to do is help me." Yet Kelly states that his wife does not want him to work 7 days a week and that she does not want to wait until he builds their house before she can go to college. He reports drinking more in the past couple of months and admits that it is difficult for him to express his emotional needs or to respond to those of his wife.

Evaluation. Kelly defines masculinity as authority, and it is extremely important to his self-image. He is unable to express feelings and is struggling to maintain a self-ideal that is in conflict with his wife's needs for her own growth as an individual as well as a spouse.

EDUCATION
Questions

What is the patient's education level?
What were the patient's educational experiences like?
What are the patient's attitudes and beliefs regarding education in general and the patient's own education in particular?
With what education-related stressors is the patient coping?
What impact does the patient's education have on mental and physical health?

Example

Assessment. Ron completed eighth grade and then dropped out of school. He learned to be a plumber by working with a family friend who owned a plumbing business. Recently the friend retired and sold the business to Ron. Ron wants his son to work with him and learn the business, but his son wants to go to college. Ron and his son have been having violent fights about this issue, and Ron has told him, "College is what you do when you don't know anything. Do you think that by going to college you'll be better than me?"

Evaluation. Ron feels bad about his lack of formal education and the negative stereotypes people hold about plumbers. His insecurity makes him unable to support his son's desire to attend college because he fears that his relationship with his son will suffer and that his son will think less of him in the future.

INCOME
Questions

What is the patient's income?
What is the source of the patient's income?
How does the patient describe his or her income group?
What are the patient's attitudes and beliefs regarding personal socioeconomic status?
With what income-related stressors is the patient coping?
What type of health insurance does the patient have, if any?
What impact does the patient's income have on mental and physical health?

Box **8-3**

Questions Related to Sociocultural Risk Factors—cont'd

INCOME—CONT'D
Example

Assessment. Amanda is unemployed. She has always believed that people who are in good health should work; however, Amanda has never been employed. She married a wealthy, older man when she was 19 years old, and for 10 years he supported her. Then with no warning, her husband left the country with a younger woman and filed for divorce. Amanda states, "He left me. I'm penniless. I'm homeless. I'm nothing." Her family is middle-income and is willing to help her if she gets a job, but she is unwilling to interview for a job because the concept of paid employment conflicts with her self-concept as a wealthy wife.

Evaluation. Amanda's self-concept and self-esteem were based on her marriage and financial status. She never imagined being without these things, and she feels unprepared and resentful of the changes she needs to make.

BELIEF SYSTEM
Questions

What are the patient's beliefs about health and illness?
What was the patient's religious or spiritual upbringing?

What are the patient's current religious or spiritual beliefs?
Who is the patient's regular health-care provider?
With what belief system-related stressors is the patient coping? What impact does the patient's belief system have on mental and physical health?

Example

Assessment. Xiao believes that illness of the mind is correct punishment. Since her mother's death 2 months ago, she has experienced insomnia, fatigue, and weight loss. She and her mother argued frequently, including the morning her mother had a fatal car accident on her way to work. Xiao now avoids her family and for the last week has been unable to go to work. Xiao states, "I did not love my mother and now I am being punished. No one can help me."

Evaluation. Xiao is unable to resolve her feelings about her mother and to grieve her loss adaptively. She feels guilt about her arguments with her mother and welcomes depression as a correct punishment. Because of this belief, seeking help is unacceptable.

---

age, ethnicity, gender, income, education or belief system, or incorrectly assume that the patient shares their world view. However, sociocultural information must be included in each phase of the nursing process because it has a significant influence on the patient's coping responses. Talking to patients about their sociocultural attitudes, feelings, beliefs, and experiences will not stereotype individuals, but not talking to patients about these important areas of their lives will.

> *Do you think it is possible that two patients displaying the same symptoms could receive two different diagnoses based on the sociocultural factors of age, ethnicity, and gender of either the patient or the clinician?*

TREATMENT IMPLICATIONS

There is growing awareness that the psychotherapeutic treatment process is influenced by the cultural and ethnic context of both the patient and the health-care provider (see Critical Thinking about Contemporary Issues). Yet there are few studies documenting successful outcomes of mental health intervention among multicultural populations. In terms of treatment planning, it is clear that the psychiatric nurse needs to be sensitive to sociocultural issues but also must transcend them. Together, the nurse and patient need to agree on the nature of the patient's coping responses, the means for solving problems, and the expected outcomes of treatment. A central responsibility of the nurse is to understand what the illness means to the patient and the way in which the patient's belief system can help to mediate the stressful events or make them easier to bear by redefining them as opportunities for personal growth.

? CRITICAL THINKING about
CONTEMPORARY ISSUES

Should Ethnic Minority Patients Be Treated by White Therapists?

The effectiveness of psychotherapy for ethnic minority patients, especially when treated by white therapists, is controversial. Some researchers and practitioners believe that ethnic minority patients are less likely to benefit from treatment. Others maintain that ethnic minority patients are just as likely as whites to show favorable outcomes from treatment and that studies of ethnic or racial matching of patients have failed to show different outcomes on the basis of the race or ethnicity of the patients and clinicians.

It is likely that ethnicity or race by itself tells very little about the values, attitudes, and experiences of patients and clinicians who engage in the treatment process (Carter, 1995). Thus ethnic matches can result in cultural mismatches, as patients and clinicians from the same ethnic group may show markedly different values. Conversely, ethnic mismatches may be cultural matches because patients and clinicians from different ethnic groups may share similar values, lifestyles, and expectations. Thus sociocultural sensitivity includes respect for individual differences regardless of one's age, ethnicity, gender, education, income, or belief system. The consideration of all of these characteristics and the ability to individualize patient care appear to be the best predictors of treatment outcome.

Service Delivery Systems

An important first consideration for effective treatment is the design of a culturally competent mental health service delivery system (Bechtel et al, 1998; Carnevale, 1999; Hanley, 1999). Mental health programs should be based on the assessment of community needs that includes representatives of minority populations in the design, implementation, analysis, and interpretation of needs assessment data.

A culturally competent mental health-care system acknowledges the importance of culture and incorporates this value into all levels of care. To do this requires the assessment of cross-cultural relations, an understanding of the dynamics of cultural differences, an expansion of knowledge about different cultures, and a commitment to adapt services to meet culturally based needs. In this way, culturally competent mental health care provides better access to more appropriate, effective care and the opportunity for improved outcomes.

Specifically, service delivery can be improved through cultural and clinical consultation by experts in the care of all populations including ethnic and cultural minorities and those with physical disabilities. Service use can be improved by the standardization of clinical assessment and treatment guidelines that address patients' cultural issues. In addition, delivery systems should be sensitive to the fact that if a mental health service operates under the auspices of a dominant ethnic, socioeconomic, or religious group, people not of that group may feel uncomfortable or unable to access that service. Staffing has also been shown to affect service use by minorities in that use of diverse staff who understand the language and culture of patients enhances service use.

Finally, an administrative environment must be created that places importance on the role of culture in understanding mental illness and treatment. Criteria should be established that holds clinicians accountable for practicing in culturally appropriate ways and provides them with the necessary tools and training. The Center for Mental Health Services funded a report (1999) urging that all public and private mental health agencies be staffed with culturally competent and appropriately qualified bicultural and bilingual personnel. Specific standards, along with 16 guiding principles form the basis of the report and are complemented by guidelines for implementation.

Counseling

Culturally responsive counseling strategies should consider ethnic identity and acculturation, family influences, sex-role socialization, religious and spiritual influences, and immigration experiences (Ruiz, 1998). In addition, sociocultural differences between the nurse and patient can be a source of misunderstanding by the nurse and resistance by the patient. Alternatively, these differences can serve as a vehicle for discussing important issues in counseling, thereby enriching the experience for both partners in the therapeutic relationship.

Family systems can be major sources of strength for people with mental illness, and nurses should view them as allies and integral components of the treatment process. Families can provide an important economic and emotional buffer against the burden imposed by the patient's illness and give the patient a supportive environment for recovery. Psychoeducational, behavioral, supportive, and family-consultation are the preferred models (see Chapters 15, 16, and 34) because they are directly responsive to families' requests for information, support, and techniques for managing their relatives' illnesses.

Religion can also be a core social and spiritual resource. Among blacks, for example, the church often provides collective support, opportunities for self-expression, and the sense of helping others, which can give meaning to life. Supernatural belief systems may also provide a natural support system for mentally ill people, as well as a culturally based way of understanding how the illness fits into the patient's life (Tuck et al, 1997).

Psychobiology

Sociocultural factors also influence various aspects of psychobiology and psychopharmacology (see Chapters 6 and 28). For example, ethnicity is one of the most important variables that contribute to variations in patients' responses to medications (Mohr, 1998; Flaskerud, 2000). Racial and ethnic differences in response to psychotropic drugs include the following:

- Extrapyramidal effects at lower dosage levels for Asians
- Lower effective dosage levels and a lower side-effect threshold for antidepressants among Hispanics
- Higher red blood cell plasma-lithium ratio in blacks

Gender differences may also result in the need for different doses of psychotropic drugs. For example, women secrete 40% less stomach acid than men, so drugs such as tricyclic antidepressants, benzodiazepines, and certain antipsychotic drugs are more likely to be absorbed before they can be neutralized by the acid, thus requiring a lower dose. In addition, over time, women accumulate more of a drug in their bodies than men do because fatty tissue stores psychotropic drugs longest.

Sociocultural characteristics, including belief systems, appear to have a significant impact on treatment compliance, and there may also be normative cultural preferences for the different ways in which medication can be taken. These findings have implications for treatment outcome and reinforce the need for sociocultural sensitivity in planning nursing care.

Equally important is the fact that indigenous systems of health beliefs and practices persist in all societies, including those exposed to modern Western medicine. The nurse should keep in mind that, despite the availability of Western medicine, traditional herbal medicines continue to be used extensively by many different cultural groups living in the United States, and some of these drugs have active pharmacologic properties that may interfere with other medications (see Chapter 30).

Summary

1. The culturally competent nurse is one who has the knowledge and skills needed to intervene successfully in the lives of patients regardless of the patient's sociocultural background.

2. Age, ethnicity, gender, education, income, and belief system are predisposing sociocultural risk factors that can increase one's potential for developing and recovering from a psychiatric disorder.

3. Disadvantagement, stereotyping, intolerance, stigma, prejudice, discrimination, and racism are common sociocultural stressors experienced by many minority groups.

4. Culturally competent psychiatric nursing care implies the ability to recognize and respond to sociocultural patient characteristics knowing that culture influences patient coping responses and symptom expression.

5. Effective assessment of predisposing sociocultural risk factors and precipitating stressors improves the nurse's ability to identify patient care needs and develop an effective psychiatric nursing treatment plan.

6. Together, the nurse and patient agree on the nature of the patient's coping responses, the means for solving problems, and the expected outcomes of treatment with a sociocultural context.

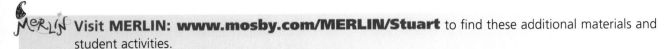

Visit **MERLIN: www.mosby.com/MERLIN/Stuart** to find these additional materials and student activities.

- **Worksheets**
- **"Drug of the Month" Updates**
- **"Citing the Evidence" Updates**
- **Critical Thinking Activities and Exercises**
- **Annotated Suggested Readings**
- **Web Links**
- **More!**

Chapter Review Questions

1. Fill in the blanks.

A. _____ are predisposing or conditioning factors that influence the amount and type of coping resources available to a patient.

B. The term _____ is used to describe a person's racial, national, tribal, linguistic, or cultural origin or background.

C. _____ and _____ disorders are the most prevalent psychiatric disorders among males.

D. _____ and _____ disorders are the most prevalent psychiatric disorders among females.

E. The prevalence of _____ and _____ disorders is about equal for males and females.

F. Risk factors are characteristics of an individual that can significantly _____ a person's potential for developing a psychiatric disorder or significantly _____ the potential for recovery, or both.

2. Match each term in Column A with the correct definition in Column B.

Column A	Column B
____ Disadvantagement	A. A depersonalized conception of individuals within a group
____ Discrimination	B. A preconceived, unfavorable belief about individuals or groups that disregards knowledge, thought, or reason
____ Intolerance	C. An attribute or trait deemed by the person's social environment as unfavorable
____ Prejudice	D. Differential treatment of individuals or groups not based on actual merit
____ Racism	E. The belief that inherent differences among the races determine individual achievement and that one race is superior
____ Stereotype	F. The lack of socioeconomic resources that are basic to biopsychosocial adaptation
____ Stigma	G. Unwillingness to accept different opinions or beliefs from people of different backgrounds

3. Provide short answers for the following questions.

A. Define cultural sensitivity.

B. Give an example of how your cultural background influences your perceptions, motives, individual identity, group identity, values, and communication.

C. Think about the facility in which you are having your psychiatric nursing experience. Evaluate whether it meets the criteria of a culturally sensitive mental health delivery system as described in this chapter.

REFERENCES

Abreu J: Conscious and nonconscious African American stereotypes: impact of first impression and diagnostic ratings by therapists, *J Consult Clin Psychol* 67(3):387, 1999.

Baker F, Bell C: Issues in the psychiatric treatment of African Americans, *Psychiatr Serv* 50(3):362, 1999.

Bechtel G, Davidhizar R: Integrating cultural diversity in patient education, *Semin Nurse Manag* 7(4):193, 1999.

Bechtel G et al: Patterns of mental health care among Mexican Americans, *J Psychosoc Nurs Ment Health Serv* 36(11):20, 1998.

Bruce M et al: Poverty and psychiatric status: longitudinal evidence from the New Haven Epidemiologic Catchment Area Study, *Arch Gen Psychiatry* 48:470, 1991.

Carnevale F: Toward a cultural conception of the self, *J Psychosoc Nurs Ment Health Serv* 37(8):26, 1999.

Carter R: *The influence of race and racial identity in psychotherapy: toward a radically inclusive model,* New York, 1995, Wiley.

Center for Mental Health Services: *Cultural competence standards,* Rockville, Md, 1998, Substance Abuse and Mental Health Services Administration.

Flaskerud J: Ethnicity, culture and neuropsychiatry, *Issues Ment Health Nurs* 21:5, 2000.

Gaw A: *Culture, ethnicity, and mental illness,* Washington, DC, 1993, American Psychiatric Press.

Gearon J, Tamminga C: Gender differences in schizophrenia, *J Calif Alliance Mentally Ill* 10(4):11, 2000.

Goldstein M, Griswold K: Cultural sensitivity and aging, *Psychiatr Serv* 49(6):769, 1998.

Hanley J: Cultural competency in the public sector, *Behav Healthc Tomorrow* 8(4):43, 1999.

Herrick C, Brown H: Mental disorders and syndromes found among Asians residing in the United States, *Issues Ment Health Nurs* 20:275, 1999.

Herrick C, Brown H: Underutilization of mental health services by Asian-Americans residing in the US, *Issues Ment Health Nurs* 19:225, 1998.

Klinkenberg W, Calsyn R: The moderating effects of race on return visits to the psychiatric emergency room, *Psychiatr Serv* 48(7):942, 1997.

Lin K, Cheung F: Mental health issues for Asian Americans, *Psychiatr Serv* 50(6):774, 1999.

Lutzen K et al: Moral sensitivity in psychiatric practice, *Nurs Ethics* 4(6):472, 1997.

Maynard C et al: Racial differences in the utilization of public mental health services in Washington state, *Admin Policy Ment Health* 24(5):411, 1997.

Mohr W: Cross-ethnic variations in the care of psychiatric patients, *J Psychosoc Nurs Ment Health Serv* 36(5):16, 1998.

Muntaner C et al: Differences in social class among psychotic patients at inpatient admission, *Psychiatr Serv* 46:176, 1995.

Parsons L, Reiss P: Promoting collaborative practice with culturally diverse populations, *Semin Nurse Manag* 7(4):160, 1999.

Poss J: Providing culturally competent care: is there a role for health promoters? *Nurs Outlook* 47(1):30, 1999.

Robin R et al: Factors influencing utilization of mental health and substance abuse services by American Indian men and women, *Psychiatr Serv* 48(6):826, 1997.

Ruiz P: New clinical perspectives in cultural psychiatry, *J Pract Psych Behav Health* 4(3):150, 1998.

SAMHSA: *Developing culturally competent systems of care for state mental health services,* Washington, DC, 1998, Western Interstate Commission for Higher Education.

Segal S et al: Race, quality of care and antipsychotic prescribing practices in psychiatric emergency services, *Psychiatr Serv* 47:282, 1996.

Stolley J, Koenig H: Religion/spirituality and health among elderly African Americans and Hispanics, *J Psychosoc Nurs Ment Health Serv* 35(11):32, 1997.

Taggart S: *Living as if: belief systems in mental health practice,* San Francisco, 1994, Jossey-Bass.

Trierweiler S et al: Clinician attributions associated with the diagnosis of schizophrenia in African American and non-African American patients, *J Consult Clin Psychol* 68(1):171, 2000.

Tseng W, Streltzer J: *Culture and psychopathology: a guide to clinical assessment,* New York, 1997, Brunner/Mazel.

Tuck I et al: Spiritual interventions provided by mental health nurses, *West J Nurs Res* 19(3):351, 1997.

Vega W et al: Gaps in service utilization by Mexican Americans with mental health problems, *Am J Psychiatry* 156(6):928, 1999.

Weaver A et al: An analysis of research on religious and spiritual variables in three major mental health nursing journals, 1991-1995, *Issues Ment Health Nurs* 19:263, 1998.

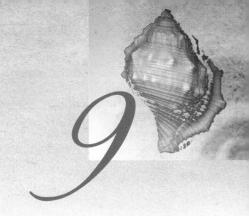

Environmental Context
of Psychiatric Nursing Care

Gail W. Stuart

9

Visit **MERLIN** for *Your Internet Connection* to websites that are related to the content in this chapter.
www.mosby.com/MERLIN/Stuart

There is a tide in the affairs of men, Which, when taken at the flood, leads on to fortune; Omitted, all the voyage of their life Is bound in shallows and in miseries. On such a full sea are we now afloat And we must take the current when it serves, Or lose our ventures.

WILLIAM SHAKESPEARE, ACT IV, SCENE III, *JULIUS CAESAR*

The environmental context of psychiatric care can be viewed from a global and national perspective. The World Bank, the World Health Organization, and several private foundations funded a major study that assessed premature death and disability from diseases and injuries around the world (Murray & Lopez, 1996). It compared a range of physical and mental disorders to determine their contribution to the burden of disease measured as disability-adjusted life years (DALYs). The data showed that depression ranked as the number one cause of disability in the world, and four other psychiatric disorders were in the top 10: alcohol use, bipolar disorder, schizophrenia, and obsessive-compulsive disorder. In terms of DALYs, depression ranked second in the United States and was projected to rank second in the world by 2020.

Two important reports in the United States also promise to impact the delivery of psychiatric care. The first is *Healthy People 2010*, which identified a list of Leading Health Indicators that reflect the major public health concerns in the United States. These include:

- Physical activity
- Overweight and obesity
- Tobacco use
- Substance abuse
- Responsible sexual behavior
- Mental health
- Injury and violence
- Environmental quality
- Immunization
- Access to health care

For each of the Leading Health Indicators, specific objectives derived from *Healthy People 2010* have been identified. The objectives related to mental health are presented in Box 9-1. This set of measures will provide a snapshot of the mental health of the United States and should have a significant impact on psychiatric care in the next decade.

The second major development was the release of *Mental Health: A Report of the Surgeon General* (USDHHS, 1999). It was the first Surgeon General's report ever issued on the topic of mental health and mental illness. The evidence based report conveys several messages. One is that mental health is fundamental to health. A second message is that mental disorders are real health conditions that have an immense impact on individuals and families throughout the United States and the world. On the strength of the findings in the report, the single, explicit recommendation is for peo-

147

Box **9-1**

Healthy People 2010 Objectives Related to Mental Health

- Reduce the suicide rate.
- Reduce the rate of suicide attempts by adolescents.
- Reduce the proportion of homeless adults who have serious mental illness.
- Increase the proportion of persons with serious mental illnesses who are employed.
- Reduce the relapse rates for persons with eating disorders including anorexia nervosa and bulimia nervosa.
- Increase the number of persons seen in primary health care who receive mental health screening and assessment.
- Increase the proportion of children with mental health problems who receive treatment.
- Increase the proportion of juvenile justice facilities that screen new admissions for mental health problems.
- Increase the proportion of adults with mental disorders who receive treatment.
- Increase the proportion of persons with co-occurring substance abuse and mental disorders who receive treatment for both disorders.
- Increase the proportion of local governments with community-based jail diversion programs for adults with serious mental illnesses.
- Increase the number of states and the District of Columbia that track consumers' satisfaction with the mental health services they receive.
- Increase the number of states, territories and the District of Columbia with an operational mental health plan that addresses cultural competence.
- Increase the number of states, territories and the District of Columbia with an operational mental health plan that addresses mental health crisis interventions, ongoing screening, and treatment services for elderly persons.

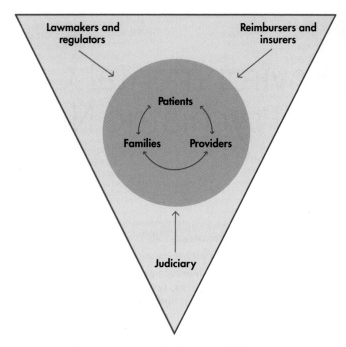

Fig. 9-1   Forces affecting psychiatric care.

ity of life, support, education, and empowerment. The provider has clinical and professional biases. If outside controls must exist, the provider wants them applied fairly, with responsibilities and liabilities clearly defined. Government organizations and other regulators want citizens to have high-quality care at the lowest cost and want providers to be accountable for their care. Reimbursers and insurance companies are concerned about paying for covered services by licensed and credentialed professionals and making a profit. Finally, the courts want to protect patients' constitutional rights regarding access to care and treatment received. The changing priorities and interactions of these six forces affect the quality, availability, and responsiveness of mental health services.

Historically, the mental health delivery system itself has been fragmented along several lines:

Private sector	*versus*	Public sector
Psychiatric illness	*versus*	Substance abuse
Inpatient care	*versus*	Outpatient care
Emotional health	*versus*	Physical health

Such divisions led to the development of many different delivery systems in different settings, using different kinds of clinicians, financed through different types of arrangements, subject to different types of regulations and standards. These dichotomies are being transformed into a more unified mental health delivery system:

Private sector	*versus*	Public sector	*into*	Managed care
Mental illness	*versus*	Substance abuse	*into*	Behavioral health
Inpatient care	*versus*	Outpatient care	*into*	Continuum of care
Emotional health	*versus*	Physical health	*into*	Integrated health care

ple to seek help if they have a mental health problem or think that they have symptoms of a mental disorder.

These studies and reports underscore the importance of mental health care and advocate for an effective and efficient mental health delivery system.

MENTAL HEALTH DELIVERY SYSTEM

The interface between mental health care and the environment has become increasingly complex in recent years. In the past, the mental health delivery system had only two parts: mental health providers and patients. Now, however, the system has grown to include six forces, each of which must be taken into account when trying to intervene with any mental health problem (Fig. 9-1).

These groups have related but slightly different interests. Patients are concerned that appropriate services are available when and where needed, and they want to be involved in establishing treatment priorities. The family wants what is best for the patient and is concerned about issues related to qual-

Table **9-1**

Comparison of Traditional and Managed Care Delivery Systems		
Characteristic	Traditional System	Managed Care System
Provider focus	Specialized care of individual patient	Total care of member population
Pricing	Separate physician and hospital fee schedules	Discounts, case rate, and capitation
Market share	Number of admissions Number of procedures Number of visits	Number of covered lives
Management focus	High inpatient occupancy rate	Low inpatient occupancy rate Correct level of care

Service line	Acute care programs as drivers: Inconsistent
	   integration
	    Physician dependent
	    Individual services
		Continuum of care:
		   Inpatient
		   Partial hospitalization
		   Outpatient
		   Residential
		Home

Cost management	Payers assume admission rate risk; provider
	   assumes length-of-stay risk
		Provider networks assume both admission
		   rate and length-of-stay risk

Costs	Cost per procedure Cost per hospitalization	Cost per life Inpatient days per 1000 Visits per 1000

Competition	Multiple hospitals for communities
	Duplicationof services and technology
		Increased consolidation and network
		   formation as occupancy declines
		Closure of beds
		   Alternative uses of hospitals

Outcomes	Qualitative measures
	   Reputation
	   Facilities
		Quantitative measures
		   Quality
		   Cost

Referral base	Focus on high-tech capabilities and separate
	   physician and hospital marketing efforts
		Ability to form primary care networks
		   Mutual goals/strategies of providers and
		   hospitals

The resulting changes are significant and affect every aspect of psychiatric nursing practice. It is essential that nurses understand the environment of mental health care to fully provide ethical, cost-effective, and high quality nursing care.

MANAGED CARE

People use the phrase **managed care** to describe a variety of systems and arrangements for planning, managing, and paying for psychiatric and mental health services. Some of these systems bring rationality and quality to the care setting. Others limit consumer choice and access without appropriate balances. In a well-functioning system of **managed care,** a defined group of people receive treatment services that are clinically necessary, medically appropriate, within defined benefit parameters, for a set amount of time, in compliance with quality standards, and with outcomes that are anticipated and measurable.

Managed care is driving changes in professional practice, the definition of mental disorders, the nature of professional accountability, the allocation of professional resources, and the relationship of mental health professionals to one another (Mechanic, 1998). Perhaps the simplest measure of change is that the term managed care, as applied to mental and substance abuse disorders, has been replaced by **managed behavioral health care,** which refers to these disorders together as one set of health problems.

> *Some people support the use of the term* behavioral health care, *believing that it helps to reduce the stigma associated with mental illness. Others oppose the term, believing that it discounts the biological basis of mental disorders. What is your position on this issue?*

Defining Characteristics. As a product of health-care reform, managed care differs in some significant ways from the traditional fee-for-service health-care delivery system. These differences are outlined in Table 9-1. Each of the characteristics on the left side of the table is described in relation to the traditional fee-for-service health delivery system and a managed care health delivery system. As can be seen from this table, managed care involves a major shift away from the **person-as-customer** to the **population-as-customer**. It also de-emphasizes high-cost, episodic inpatient admissions and procedures in favor of creating a full continuum of care and then selecting the correct level of care and treatment setting. Whereas the traditional system fostered duplication of services and technology among hospitals, managed care stimulates the consolidation of services, formation of networks, and use of primary care networks to perform referral and gatekeeping functions. Each of these characteristics reflects a major change in the delivery of health care in the United States.

A final aspect of managed care is its emphasis on value. **Value** in managed care can be defined as service that yields positive outcomes in the most efficient way. It includes the goal of controlling costs while achieving quality outcomes. Value in managed care, therefore, is represented by the equation

$$Quality/Costs = Value$$

Achieving this goal of value requires that a health-care organization track costs, measure administrative and clinical processes, measure patient outcomes and satisfaction, and integrate these data to enhance administrative policy and clinical decision making. Each of these elements poses special challenges to health-care professionals and the settings in which they work.

Finally, managed care is not a single entity. Rather, it can assume various forms. The most common are health maintenance organizations (HMOs), preferred provider organizations (PPOs), and point-of-service organizations (POSs). Each of these is described in Box 9-2. **Managed competition** is a purchasing strategy in which managed care organizations contract with several hospitals that provide cost-effective, comprehensive services. Consumers are then informed about the hospitals from which they may receive services, even though the facility may not be the patient's preferred choice.

> *One of your nursing colleagues complains that managed care is really only "managed costs." Based on the characteristics of managed care described in this chapter, how might you respond?*

Financial Aspects. One of the major forces that has moved the health-care environment to managed care is the notion that it will reduce health-care costs. It can also shift the financial risk of providing health care from the insurer to the provider. This change has implications for patients and clinicians alike. Therefore, it is important for nurses to have a clear understanding of the financial aspects of managed care so that they can base their practice on current economic realities (Mechanic, 1999).

In a managed care system there are three major payment mechanisms: discounted fee-for-service, case rate, and capitation. Under a **discounted fee-for-service** payment plan, clinicians are paid for all services that have been authorized and provided to a consumer. The payment rate is discounted or is less than the clinician's standard fee and often includes a provision for a copayment that must be collected from the consumer at the time of each visit.

Under a **case rate** system, the clinician is paid a flat fee for a predefined episode of care. The most well known typical case rate system is Medicare's Diagnostic Related Groups (DRGs). In this instance, Medicare pays a flat fee for a particular hospitalization episode regardless of how many days the person was hospitalized. This system shifts the financial risk to the provider because the provider receives a flat fee regardless of the actual cost of care.

Under a capitation system the consumer pays a fixed fee or per-member-per-month (PMPM) premium. In return, the managed care company that receives the PMPM fee agrees to provide all medically necessary health care for all covered people. In this case, most of the financial risk lies with the managed care company, which must deliver all necessary health care within the premiums received by their population pool. HMOs are the best-known examples of capitated payment systems.

Managed care exerts cost control measures through, gatekeeping, preadmission certification, utilization review, and case management.

Gatekeeping is a process that limits direct access to specialists, hospitals, and expensive procedures. Patients are expected to select a primary care provider who manages everyday care and is a gatekeeeper for referral to other health care providers. The primary care providers have incentives to be judicious in making referrals.

Preadmission certification takes into account the patient's medical and psychiatric status, level of functioning, socioenvironmental factors, and procedural issues associated with treatment. It is the role of the managed care reviewer to determine the most appropriate form of treatment and the proper treatment setting. In this way, the reviewer monitors issues of cost and quality.

Utilization review evaluates the appropriateness and necessity of services and procedures. It is a way of monitoring the care and services administered and it has the most immediate impact on patient care. The patient's treatment plan, diagnostic and therapeutic interventions, and discharge plan are continuously monitored by a third party. Determination for reimbursement of treatment is made by this third party based on current standards of care. The review and approval can be done before providing the services (precertification review), at the time the service is rendered

---

Box 9-2

Types of Managed Care Plans

HEALTH MAINTENANCE ORGANIZATIONS (HMOs):
HMOs are organized delivery systems that provide care to a defined population, usually for a predetermined fixed amount (capitation rate). Consumers enrolled in HMOs are limited to using HMO providers.

PREFERRED PROVIDER ORGANIZATIONS (PPOs):
PPOs are plans that contract with a limited number of clinicians, most often physicians, and hospitals that provide care at discounted rates. Members of these plans are given financial incentives to use the preferred providers but are not prevented from using other providers. Insurers or employers select the providers to be included in their preferred plan.

POINT-OF-SERVICE PLANS (POSs):
POSs allow consumers to choose between delivery systems at the time they seek care. In a triple-option plan, for example, people can choose among an HMO, PPO, or fee-for-service plan. Financial incentives are usually provided to encourage people to use the least expensive option.

(concurrent review), or after the service has been provided (retrospective review), which may be used to retroactively deny payment.

Case management typically is targeted to patients who have treatment complications, have high-expense episodes of care, or who need alternative, less expensive treatments or settings. This target group often includes those with serious and persistent mental illness. Case management focuses on the achievement of desirable patient outcomes, appropriate lengths of stay, efficient use of resources, and patient involvement and satisfaction.

> *Managed behavioral health-care companies often employ nurses as utilization reviewers and case managers. Identify the special skills and expertise psychiatric nurses can bring to these roles.*

Federal and State Initiatives

Today, the U.S. government is the largest buyer of health care. Through Medicaid and Medicare and numerous other public programs, it is the single most important purchaser of health care in the United States. It is here where health-care reform is taking place and where future action will continue.

Medicaid is a health-care entitlement program for Aid to Families with Dependent Children (AFDC) recipients; Supplemental Security Income (SSI) recipients; low-income, disabled, elderly people; low-income pregnant women, infants, and children; and medically needy recipients. The serious and persistently mentally ill are often recipients of Medicaid. The states and the federal government share the costs of this program. Although all states are required to provide a basic set of services, other services can be included or excluded at the discretion of the individual state.

Medicaid can give waivers to states to permit them to experiment with alternative delivery systems for the Medicaid population. These waivers can take various forms but the most important one lets the states contract with providers to provide health-care services on a managed care basis. Almost all states that have received waivers provide mental health coverage. The most common approach is to offer acute but limited treatment to all recipients through a basic plan, with a separate plan for people with greater needs. These patients are often assigned to the care of the state mental health department or a private managed care company with which the state has contracted.

These dramatic developments are bringing about major changes in public mental health care that may be as significant as the deinstitutionalization movement of the 1960s and 1970s (Emery et al, 1998). The introduction of private managed care into the public mental health system involves shifts in responsibility for mental health care, tensions about which populations receive priority for care, and significant changes in the financing and organization of services. Clearly, the prospect of fusing the public and private sectors of mental health care offers both problems and opportunities (Hoge et al, 1999; Wieman & Dorwart, 1999). If properly managed, however, it can reduce the stigma of mental health care, decrease duplicative administrative costs, and be a first step toward a truly integrated mental health delivery system.

ACCESS TO SERVICES

Access is the degree to which services and information about care are easily obtained and it is an important part of any effective mental health care delivery system. An ideal comprehensive health-care system would provide multiple points of entry for treatment, including direct access through self-referral, by a wide variety of providers.

Today, over half of the people who seek health care for mental disorders are treated by primary care practitioners. However, many who need care do not receive it, either from a primary care or specialty provider. It is also known that when access to mental health care is made difficult, the overall costs of general medical care increase because those with behavioral health care problems are frequent users of medical services. For example, people suffering from panic disorder typically are seen by 10 different health-care providers before they are properly diagnosed.

Some access problems apply to the entire health-care system, such as the lack of providers in rural areas and care for people who lack health insurance. Other problems are unique to mental health care. These include the stigma associated with seeking care, the lack of knowledge about how to find the right clinician for a highly personal problem, and the lack of general medical settings to adequately respond to mental health and substance abuse disorders. Members of the Deaf community report particular barriers to accessing mental health services (Steinberg et al, 1998).

Many controversies exist regarding managed behavioral care. One of the most common is whether patients are granted sufficient access to the care they need. Another concern is whether these systems meet the needs of those with ongoing and serious mental illnesses (Hall & Beinecke, 1998; Fletcher, 1998). Economic incentives to undertreat may result in denial of care, and managed care companies relate examples of inappropriate care demanded by patients and delivered by providers. Two important balances to offset these problems would be to adequately fund behavioral health-care benefits and services and to find ways to measure and reinforce standards for the accessibility, appropriateness, quality, and effectiveness of treatment.

Employee Assistance Programs

Employee assistance programs (EAPs) are worksite-based programs designed to help identify and resolve behavioral, health, and productivity problems that may affect employees' well-being or job performance. Their focus is wide-ranging, covering alcohol and other drug abuse, physical and emotional health, and marital, family, financial, legal, and other personal concerns. As such, they are important points of access to behavioral health care.

EAPs have developed from primarily alcoholism assessment and referral centers to specialized behavioral health programs. Many cost-effectiveness studies document the value of these programs, particularly through their prevention contributions, such as in workplace education, skill development, and policy and environmental changes. Comprehensive EAPs are defined by six major components: identification of problems based on job performance, consultation with supervisors, constructive confrontation, evaluation and referral, liaison with treatment providers, and substance abuse expertise (White et al, 1996). They thus represent a rich foundation on which other services may be added to promote access to mental health and substance abuse treatment.

Treatment Parity

An analysis of the issue of access in behavioral health care would not be complete without noting that many of the people who need treatment for mental and chemical dependency disorders do not receive it because their insurance policies deny or restrict coverage for the treatment of these illnesses (see Citing the Evidence on Health Insurance for the Mentally Ill). Historically, insurers and employers have been cautious about offering mental health and substance abuse coverage, often believing that mental disorders were not treatable or were too expensive to treat. In recent years mental health advocates and professionals have placed increased emphasis on parity in insurance coverage between physical and mental health services.

There have been some wins and losses in that struggle. A loss for the field was reflected in a new law passed by Congress in 1996. It ended the cash benefits as well as Medicare and Medicaid coverage for people whose disability is based on drug addiction or alcoholism. A win for mental health treatment was the adoption of treatment parity legislation in many states and passage of a national mental health parity bill in the United States in 1996.

In January 2000, 28 states had some degree of mental health parity, with fairness bills pending in many other state legislatures. State laws differ from each other in conditions served, specificity of parity, minimum benefits, approved providers, managed care usage, exemptions, and populations covered (Sturm & Pacula, 1999). A government sponsored study on the costs and effects of parity for mental health and substance abuse insurance benefits found that (Sing et al, 1998):

- Most state parity laws are limited in scope or application.
- State parity laws have had a small effect on premiums.
- Employers have not attempted to avoid parity laws by becoming self-insured, and they do not tend to pass on the costs of parity to employees.
- Costs for mental health and substance abuse services have not shifted from the public to the private sector.

Ideally, parity would include insurance coverage for mental and addictive disorders that is equal to that provided for any physical disease or illness in terms of service, dollar limits, deductibles, and copayments. Yet many current parity provisions are much narrower (Druss & Rosenheck, 1998).

Citing the Evidence on

Health Insurance for the Mentally Ill

BACKGROUND: This study explored the question of how insurance coverage has changed among individuals with psychiatric problems compared with the general population between 1996 and 1998.

RESULTS: The percentage of uninsured persons in the general population had not changed very much, and more respondents believed that health insurance coverage has improved rather than deteriorated over those years. However, among individuals with probable mental health disorders, more had lost insurance in those two years than had gained it and more reported decreases in health benefits. Individuals with worse mental health consistently report a deterioration of access to care compared with individuals with better mental health.

IMPLICATIONS: Substantial activity has taken place in state and federal legislation to increase the mental health benefits offered by health insurance. Although this activity could have improved health insurance especially for individuals with mental illness, such persons continue to fare significantly worse than the general population. Thus access to care remains a significant problem for the mentally ill.

Sturm R, Wells K: Health insurance may be improving - but not for individuals with mental illness, *Health Serv Res* 35(1):253, 2000.

Citing the Evidence on

The Public's Knowledge of Mental Health Benefits

BACKGROUND: This study explored knowledge of mental health benefits and preferences for providers among the general public.

RESULTS: A large proportion of the respondents were uninformed about their mental health benefits. 25% were unsure if their health plan even included mental health benefits. 43% believed that their mental health benefits were equal to those provided for general medical services. 25% of the older respondents said they would not seek care even when needed. The majority said they would initially seek care from their primary care provider for a mental health problem.

IMPLICATIONS: The general public lacks information about important mental health benefits, and this lack of information may represent a barrier in their seeking care when needed. Given the overriding preference for primary care providers to treat mental health problems, mental health issues should be given more attention at all levels of primary care education.

Mickus M et al: Knowledge of mental health benefits and preferences for type of mental health providers among the general public, *Psychiatr Serv* 51(2):199, 2000.

For example, equal coverage may be provided only for medically necessary services to people with severe mental disorders that are biologically based. Even more problematic, the federal parity law allows for the use of a wide range of cost control mechanisms for mental health services, such as higher deductibles or copayments and limits on services or hospital days that differ from those used for physical health services.

In addition, current exemptions in many state insurance regulations severely limit the number of people covered by parity laws as well as the services they may receive. Finally, parity that covers only "medical treatment" of a particular mental illness may minimize or exclude preventive services and psychosocial treatments that are necessary to maintain a person's functional capacities. Sadly, little attention is given to preventive, rehabilitative, and chronic care services. Thus although progress is being made in mandating behavioral health benefits, much additional work remains to be done (see Citing the Evidence on the Public's Knowledge of Mental Health Benefits).

> *Do you know what coverage your insurance provides for mental and chemical dependency disorders? Check your policy for inpatient, outpatient, partial hospitalization, and home care benefits. Compare these benefits with those you receive for medical and surgical illnesses. If the coverages are not similar, write a letter bringing this disparity to the attention of your insurance company and requesting a response.*

Telepsychiatry

An exciting development in the field that may have important implications for access to care issues is the emergence of telepsychiatry. Telepsychiatry connects people by audiovisual communication and is seen as one means of providing expert health-care services to patients distant from a source of care. It is suggested for the diagnosis and treatment of patients in remote locations or where psychiatric expertise is scarce. The high cost of providing the needed technology, particularly by public mental health systems with limited resources, has hampered its widespread use. Also issues of reliability of diagnosis, effectiveness of treatment and patient satisfaction all need further study.

CLINICAL APPROPRIATENESS

Clinical appropriateness is the degree to which the type, amount, and level of clinical services are delivered to promote the best clinical outcomes. A basic premise of managed behavioral health care is that more is not always better. Specifically, inappropriate hospitalizations not only incur unnecessary costs to the system, but also can harm patients by disrupting their lives through the interruption of work, family, and social functioning. In contrast, there is some evidence that restricting length of stay of in-hospital psychiatric treatment may adversely affect quality of care for some patients (Wickizer & Lessler, 1998).

In order to meet managed care's criteria of clinical appropriateness, behavioral health-care organizations are developing diversified but fully integrated continuums of care by expanding their own services, contracting with other health-care organizations, or affiliating with area providers. These continuums of care must be capable of providing services and alternative levels of care to children, adolescents, adults, and elderly people requiring psychiatric and substance abuse services. The goal is to provide "one-stop shopping" for managed behavioral care and to secure market dominance in a particular geographic area. The levels of care for each stage of treatment expected in an integrated continuum of care are listed in Table 9-2.

Medical Necessity

To comply with issues of clinical appropriateness of care, managed behavioral care companies, government agencies, professional associations, and treatment facilities have each established criteria for the medical necessity of the various

Table **9-2**

Levels of Care for Each Stage of Treatment in an Integrated Behavioral Continuum of Care				
Stages of Treatment	Crisis	Acute	Maintenance	Health Promotion
GOAL	Stabilization	Remission	Recovery	Optimal level of wellness
EXPECTED OUTCOME	No harm to self or others	Symptom relief	Improved functioning	Attain optimal quality of life
LEVEL OF CARE	• Inpatient hospitalization • 24-hour mobile emergency intervention • Crisis stabilization unit and beds • 23-hour observation beds • Outpatient detoxification • Telephone access and triage	• Partial hospitalization • Intensive remission-oriented outpatient • Assertive community treatment • Intensive in-home intervention • 23-hour respite beds • Telepsychiatry	• Rehabilitative day treatment • Multimodal recovery-oriented outpatient • Relapse prevention • Rehabilitation-oriented residential • Supported independent living	• Education • Respite care • Drop-in centers • Peer support • Social activities • School • Employment • Housing

levels of care. Criteria are strongest for hospitalization, and there is less consensus regarding outpatient therapy. General criteria for admission to psychiatric services used in one psychiatric setting are presented in Table 9-3. This setting uses additional criteria to assess suicide risk, self-injury risk, assaultiveness, acute psychosis, impaired judgment, substance detoxification, substance abuse rehabilitation, need for electroconvulsive therapy, need for medication monitoring, regulation, initiation or withdrawal, and need for diagnostic evaluation or treatment. In this way, psychiatric facilities can both document and justify the medical appropriateness of the level of psychiatric care selected for a particular patient.

Carve-Ins and Carve-Outs

Another issue debated in the field is how appropriate mental health services can best be provided (Bartels, 1999). Two systems currently exist. The first is the **carve-in**, by which consumers receive services through an integrated care system of both medical/surgical and mental health/substance abuse services. The second is the behavioral health **carve-out**, in which mental health and substance abuse benefits are accessed, provided, and otherwise managed separately from medical/surgical care.

Certain advantages and disadvantages are found in both carve-ins and carve-outs. Carve-ins allow all health care to be available at one site of service, which may enable greater access, integration, and coordination of services. The need for this integration is evident from the following facts (Strosahl, 1996):

- 50% of all mental health care is delivered solely by general practitioners.

- 67% of all psychopharmacological drugs are prescribed by general practitioners.
- 70% of all primary care visits are primarily for psychosocial concerns.

Primary care is supported in spirit and practice by carve-in arrangements, which also can promote prevention and time-efficient methods of treatment.

Carve-ins also have their disadvantages. Some have questioned whether mental health and substance abuse services receive their fair share of resources in benefits, dollars, or services offered. Primary care physicians, who often control access to mental health services, may inappropriately limit care because of their lack of training in behavioral health or because they may be given financial incentives to limit specialty services. Additionally, the quality of care given and the clinical outcomes obtained by treating psychiatric disorders in primary care settings may be inadequate. Also, payers, consumers, and providers may object to the limitations placed on their choices of mental health clinicians and facilities and to the gatekeeper role of the primary care physician.

Carve-outs also offer both advantages and disadvantages. Although carve-out service delivery models and financial arrangements vary, they generally provide for increased benefits in exchange for following a managed plan of care recommended by a defined panel of behavioral health providers. Advantages to carve-outs are that they typically allow treatment to be provided closer to a person's home or community. They also often demonstrate greater sensitivity and responsiveness to the payer and the consumer and greater expertise in treating mental and chemical depen-

Table **9-3**

General Criteria for Psychiatric Admission Across the Continuum of Care			
Level of Care			
Inpatient	Partial Hospitalization	Intensive Outpatient	Outpatient
Imminent risk for acute medical status deterioration caused by the presence of an active psychiatric or substance abuse condition Unsafe at a less intensive level of service	High risk for acute medical status deterioration caused by the presence of an active psychiatric or substance abuse condition Unsafe at a less intensive level of service Needs intensive therapeutic intervention with physician availability Adequate support system to maintain safety overnight/weekend Reasonable expectation that the patient will form a treatment alliance Unresponsive to treatment or deterioration of usual level of functioning despite participation in a less intensive level of service	Requires frequent therapeutic intervention to improve functioning Unsafe at or inappropriate for a less intensive level of service Adequate support system or coping skills to maintain stability and safety between therapeutic visits Reasonable expectation that the patient will form a treatment alliance Unresponsive to treatment, intensification of symptoms, or deterioration of usual level of functioning despite participation in a less intensive level of service	Outpatient therapy required to alleviate acute symptoms Demonstrates intent to form treatment alliance Adequate support system to maintain safety between therapeutic visits

dency disorders, and they may better address the needs of people with serious and persistent mental illness.

The disadvantage of carve-outs is the risk of limited access and undertreatment when the mental health or substance abuse services are capitated. They may also make linkages with primary care clinicians more difficult and discourage collaboration among health-care providers. Finally, consumers may encounter confusing obstacles as they seek to obtain care in two or three systems (general medical, psychiatric, and substance abuse) and among a wide array of health-care providers and sites of service. Thus the dilemma of how to best deliver behavioral health care has yet to be resolved.

One way to provide cost-effective behavioral health care in a primary care setting is to have an advanced practice registered nurse (APRN) in psychiatric and mental health care available on site to work with patients with psychiatric and substance abuse problems. What do you think would be the advantages and disadvantages of such

ACCOUNTABILITY ISSUES

Driven by the demand to demonstrate quality and reduce costs, the behavioral health-care environment is confronted by new issues of accountability. Areas of concern range from restrictions on patient autonomy in choice of treatment and service setting, to the relationship between the patient and provider, to collaborative treatment planning between patients and providers, to patient responsibility for complying with treatment recommendations, to the denial, curtail-

ment, or restriction of access to treatment (see Critical Thinking about Contemporary Issues).

Consumer Empowerment

Consumer empowerment has been an emerging movement over the past decade. The term **consumer** is one in a long list of labels that users of psychiatric services have applied to themselves. Other terms include **client, customer, patient, ex-patient,** and **survivor.** The term consumer is most often used when it applies to empowerment.

Consumer empowerment is the situation in which psychiatric patients (Geller et al, 1998):

- Form their own independent networks not dependent on professionals for support.
- Use professionals for technical assistance to make better decisions themselves in environments where they exercise full participation in decisions affecting their lives.
- Participate in treatment with professionals and paraprofessionals as collaborators, not passive people receiving treatment, where they are seen as the primary informants about what is wanted and needed from providers.
- Are respected for the legitimacy of their points of view, which are not written off as just a product of their illness.
- Are using resources from the entire community and not just the formal mental health system.
- Are operating within a health-promoting system.
- Have significant input beyond their individual treatment into decision making at program, agency, community, state, and federal levels.

CRITICAL THINKING about CONTEMPORARY ISSUES

Is Managed Care the Devil or Angel of Psychiatric and Mental Health Treatment?

Praise and blame of managed behavioral health care is common across the United States. Public reaction is mixed and the response from mental health professionals is even more conflicted. Proponents of managed care believe that the costs of health care in the United States are enormous, yet many people go without adequate treatment. They say that managed care can expand access to care, use dwindling resources more responsibly, and reduce the use of unneeded services.

Opponents of managed care raise a number of criticisms. They say that managed care adversely affects the quality of care, limits access to needed care, negatively affects the provider-patient relationship, creates problems with informed patient choice, offers unfair benefits and policy coverage, and shifts responsibility from the provider to management.

Managed care in mental health, as in general health, is neither as good nor as evil as its advocates or detractors propose. Because it is a reality of the current environment it may be more important to identify ethical principles for its implementation. The following standards have been

suggested (Surles & Fox, 1998; National Academies of Practice, 1998):

- Plans should ensure that the most intensive care goes to those with the most severe but treatable needs.
- Limits should be placed on contractual arrangements between payers and providers, discouraging powerful financial incentives and establishing that the prime concern is the professional's commitment to the patient.
- Constraints should be placed on the amount of information plans collect about enrollees, the confidentiality of patient data, and the uses to which plans put that information.
- Plans should be required to inform patients of all reasonable clinical options for care and services.
- Plans should allow for greater participation in decision making, such as through the creation of consumer and provider panels.
- Managed care is inherently neither good nor bad (Cummings, 1998). The question is how it is used, and every consumer and health-care provider shares responsibility for the answer.

- Achieve a sense of self-responsibility.
- Are sure that consumer empowerment is more than just a buzzword.

As such, empowered consumers are asking mental health delivery systems for greater accountability and responsiveness to the people they are intended to serve.

Also important are questions about the extent to which patients' rights are compromised. With managed care it is clear that limits will be placed on patients' choice of providers, service settings, and sometimes even treatment options. If only a limited number of options are available, patients may be unable to take advantage of newer treatments that could help them.

Partly in response to these concerns, a number of different groups have set forth principles for managed mental health care systems. For example, the Center for Mental Health Services has developed a set of principles that emphasizes the need for comprehensive services, continuity of care, and responsiveness to the needs of service recipients. The principles cover quality of care, consumer participation, accessibility, affordability, linkages and integration, and accountability. Also, a number of mental health organizations, including the American Psychiatric Nurses Association, have endorsed a Bill of Rights for managed care. All of these initiatives reflect a focused effort to protect patients and balance the issues of cost and quality in the current psychiatric care environment.

Provider Concerns

Providers are increasingly aware of their responsibility to provide cost-effective care in an environment of shrinking psychiatric resources. New dilemmas arise for clinicians who must balance a responsibility to both an individual patient and a population of patients. Also, the tension between patient advocacy and resource allocation has been heightened by the introduction of managed care, because providers may feel the need to serve the bottom line of the organization and, in so doing, jeopardize the interests of the patient (see Citing the Evidence above). For nurses, this focus on resource allocation can mean that staffing levels are often reduced as a cost cutting measure, while patient census and acuity levels increase.

Other problems arise when mental health clinicians move from private practice models to become part of networks or organized systems of care. In doing so, they become subject to the review of others, their activities are routinely measured, and they are held accountable for the kind and amount of care they deliver. This monitoring is viewed negatively by many mental health professionals, but others see it as a positive trend leading to an overall improvement in behavioral health-care services (Trabin, 1995).

Providers also struggle with the ambiguity of many of the rules, regulations, and expectations of this new health-care environment. They complain about the overreliance of managed care on treatment protocols that limit professional judgment and minimize individual patient or clinical factors, and they cite reduced clinician productivity because of administrative burdens and excessive documentation.

Citing the Evidence on

Impact of Managed Behavioral Health Care and Nursing

BACKGROUND: Anecdotal reports of the effects of managed care restrictions suggest an erosion of nursing and medical care. Yet little evidence exists to indicate whether patients fare better or worse. This study examined this question in a managed behavioral care population.

RESULTS: On discharge, patients showed improvement on all behavioral subsystem ratings, with significant differences in dependency, affiliative, aggressive-protective, achievement, and restorative subsystems. Patients with longer stays were significantly more impaired than patients with shorter stays on discharge Global Assessment of Functioning scores.

IMPLICATIONS: Increased research and an expansion of databases to derive meaningful conclusions about the impact of managed care on the resolution of nursing problems is needed.

Dee V et al: Managed behavioral health care patients and their nursing care problems, level of functioning, and impairment on discharge, *J Am Psych Nurses Assoc* 4(2):57, 1998.

Even the roles and functions of providers are subject to some confusion, as seen in the example of case managers. From one setting to another the activities, preparation, and expertise of case managers vary greatly. They may fill a cost-containment function, a coordination function, or a direct service delivery function. Some have college or professional degrees; others have little higher education.

Finally, the realities of the new environment often escalate conflict among disciplines rather than enhancing interdisciplinary collaboration. This heightened tension occurs because when economic resources become scarcer, disciplines revert to protecting and expanding their professional turf as a way of ensuring survival.

> *Many mental health providers and managed care companies are hotly debating which of them should decide what is best for the patient. But where is the patient in all this? Contact a managed care company in your area and ask them how they involve patients in their decision-making processes.*

Service Settings

Service settings may experience the greatest number of challenges to accountability. These challenges can occur on many fronts. For example, mental health facilities have been criticized for denying inpatient care or transferring patients to another facility for economic reasons when it is not in the patient's best interests. Another effect of managed care has been the layoffs of staff and downsizing of inpatient facilities. The resulting shortage of staff and the increased work the remaining staff must assume may adversely affect the care provided. Also, while staff size is decreasing, the severity of inpatients' problems is increasing, thus requiring an adequate number of well-trained staff to deliver quality patient care.

Another challenge arises in the area of information management. Computerization is radically changing how behavioral health-care services are managed and delivered. Computerized patient records provide standardized formats for easier data collection and analysis. Clinical, financial, and administrative information systems are being integrated so that outcomes related to quality and costs of care can be measured. Information system connections are being made between service units within an organization and among organizations, so that for many activities electronic data communication is replacing paper.

This new information technology presents both opportunities and risks. An important accountability issue is confidentiality, appropriate uses of data and protection of data, particularly in an area as sensitive as psychiatric and substance abuse disorders. Data are being shared within and among organizations, which increases the risk of problems with misrouting, mishandling, misinterpreting, and generally misusing sensitive and potentially stigmatizing data. Many technical measures are being developed to protect patients, but there is also considerable skepticism about their effectiveness. It has been noted that a comprehensive and ongoing strategy is needed to deal with the issues of confidentiality and the appropriate use of data (Ziglin, 1995). Such a strategy should address computer security, training, regulation, public information, policies and procedures, data storage and security, informed consent, planning, and locus of responsibility and structure.

Finally, some developments among accrediting organizations may provide incentives for managed care accountability. Examples of such organizations include the Utilization Review Accreditation Committee (URAC), the Joint Commission on Accreditation of Healthcare Organizations (JCAHO), and the National Committee on Quality Assurance (NCQA). The NCQA is an independent, nonprofit HMO accrediting organization composed of independent health care quality experts, employers, labor union officials, and consumers. They adopted standards that assess performance in six areas:

- Quality improvement and information
- Utilization management
- Credentialing of providers
- Members' rights and responsibilities
- Preventive health services
- Medical records

NCQA accreditation is designed for most managed care companies. It has the longest track record in managed care and is required by law in a number of states.

In order to document accountability in these areas, many service settings use standardized rating scales related to the delivery of health-care services. These are listed in Box 9-3.

Box 9-3

Behavioral Rating Scales Related to Health Services Delivery

- Beginning Services Syndrome (BSS)
- Behavioral Healthcare Rating of Satisfaction (BHRS)
- The Client Experience Questionnaire (CEQ)
- Client Satisfaction Questionnaire (CSQ)
- Client Satisfaction Survey (CSS)
- Consumer Satisfaction Index (CSI)
- Inpatient Patient Satisfaction Survey System
- Managed Care Satisfaction Survey (MCO-SS)
- Older Adults Resources and Services (OARS)
- Outpatient Patient Satisfaction Survey System
- Patient Satisfaction Survey IV (PSS-IV)
- Perceptions of Care (Inpatient and Outpatient)
- Process of Care Review Form
- Satisfaction Survey (SS)
- Service Satisfaction Scale (SSS-30)
- Treatment Satisfaction Survey
- Youth Satisfaction Questionnaire

Each night, a secretary on your surgical unit pulls up the list of psychiatric patients on his computer. When you ask him about it, he says that he wants to see whether anyone he knows is admitted so that he can visit. How would you respond to him and what actions would you take?

IMPACT ON PSYCHIATRIC NURSING

The environment in which psychiatric nurses practice is changing every day. To thrive in this environment, psychiatric nurses need to be knowledgeable about current developments and focus their talents on services, programs, and systems of care with patients and families in the center of their vision. They must continue to be patient advocates and help to create an environment that is ethical and respectful of consumers and their psychiatric and mental health needs. There are over 82,000 psychiatric nurses employed in mental health facilities in the United States (Center for Mental Health Services, 1998). Working together, they can have a significant impact on the behavioral health-care delivery system.

Roles in Managed Care

Nurses bring great value to the managed care arena through their rich blend of skills and expertise. Although there is great variability of nursing activity based on service setting and geographic location, psychiatric nurses have assumed a number of roles:

Psychiatric-mental health clinician: Nurses with various backgrounds are currently employed as direct care providers in managed care settings. They function as staff nurses in inpatient and partial hospitalization programs, nurse clinicians in home and community settings, primary care providers, and advanced practice nurses, including nurse practitioners and clinical nurse specialists.

Case manager: In this role psychiatric nurses assess patient needs, develop treatment plans, allocate resources, and supervise the care given by other providers.

Evaluation and triage nurse: Many psychiatric nurses evaluate patients, either in person or over the telephone, and are responsible for triaging the patient to the most appropriate level of care.

Utilization review nurse: Many managed care companies employ psychiatric nurses to function as utilization reviewers who review aspects of the patient's care and influence decisions about treatment assignment. In this role they serve as "gatekeepers" to mental health services.

Patient educator: Some settings hire nurses with responsibility for patient and family education. This role has grown with the growing emphasis being placed on patient compliance and disease management programs.

Risk manager: Nurses who work as risk managers are charged with the task of decreasing the probability of adverse outcomes related to patient care. They engage in identifying risk factors, individual and systemwide problems, corrective actions, and the implementation of strategies to reduce risk.

Quality improvement officer: Nurses have assumed primary responsibility for formulating and implementing quality improvement plans for managed care companies. They train other staff onsite and synthesize data related to improvement activities across the organization.

Marketing and development specialist: Some psychiatric nurses work in the managed care growth areas of marketing and development. In this role they interact with consumers, employers, providers, and regulators and make recommendations for furthering the mission and goals of the managed care organization.

Corporate managers and executives: Psychiatric nurses are also present in the boardrooms of some behavioral managed care organizations, where they influence corporate policy and strategic planning.

Threats and Opportunities

Every threat also represents an opportunity. To take advantage of the opportunities, psychiatric nurses must first accept the fact that managed care is here to stay. Nurses need to become knowledgeable about how managed care is implemented in their own communities and across the United States. This new approach includes integrating and applying the information to their practice. For example, Fig. 9-2 shows how the characteristics of managed care interact with the activities of the nursing process. Nurses must also master the computer technology and refine their business and accounting skills. In this way, they can use new developments in the environment to deliver better patient care. Finally, the current environment mandates that nurses market their skills to be included among the mental health providers of the future.

One fact remains: Throughout the environmental changes described in this chapter, individuals, families, and communities continue to experience significant emotional problems (Goldman, 1999). Thus the need for psychiatric nurses as competent and caring professionals will also continue. Nurses must be proactive in realigning their positions within the changing environment (Hiraki, 1998). As hospitals continue to downsize, more nurses are needed in the community and in home settings. Many of the programs needed by patients in the community are only beginning to be designed. Psychiatric nurses can assume a leadership role in this new frontier. They must also keep their practice current with the realities of the mental health delivery system, such as by learning new skills in brief therapy, group interventions, psychopharmacology, and disease management. Psychiatric nurses are in an ideal position to work closely with primary care providers to improve access and quality of care for patients with behavioral health problems. Finally, they should continue their commitment to working with underserved populations, the elderly, children, and the seriously mentally ill, because they have

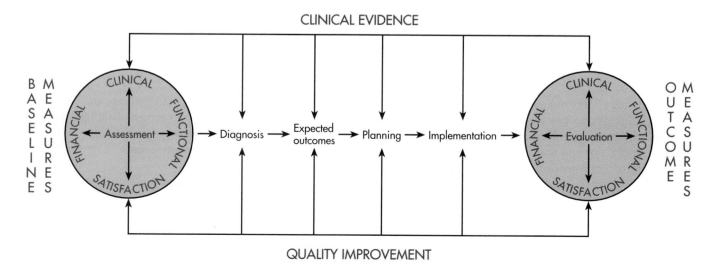

Fig. 9-2   Interaction between the elements of managed care and the nursing process.

much to offer to the care and well-being of these vulnerable groups.

Summary

1. The term managed care is used to describe a range of health-care arrangements, all focused on value, which is defined as quality divided by costs. Managed care can take a variety of forms and is different from the traditional fee-for-service system in a number of significant ways.

2. Much debate surrounds access to services under managed care. Many people who need behavioral health treatment do not receive it in the United States because their insurance policies deny or restrict coverage for these services.

3. Decisions regarding the clinical appropriateness of care are based on medical necessity and the settings in which care is provided.

4. Questions of accountability in the current environment have arisen in relation to consumer empowerment, provider concerns, and service settings. There are also national standards among accrediting organizations that may provide incentives for managed care accountability.

5. Elements of the environment directly affect psychiatric nursing practice. Nurses must keep abreast of new information and integrate it into practice to provide high-quality, cost-effective care.

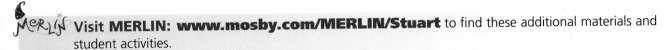

Visit **MERLIN: www.mosby.com/MERLIN/Stuart** to find these additional materials and student activities.

- **Worksheets**
- **"Drug of the Month" Updates**
- **"Citing the Evidence" Updates**
- **Critical Thinking Activities and Exercises**
- **Annotated Suggested Readings**
- **Web Links**
- **More!**

Chapter Review Questions

1. **Match each term in Column A with the correct definition in Column B.**

Column A	Column B
___ Access	A. Degree to which services and information about care are conveniently and easily obtained
___ Capitation	B. Degree to which the type, amount, and level of clinical services are delivered to promote positive outcomes for the patient
___ Case rate	C. Evaluates the appropriateness and necessity of health-care services and procedures
___ Clinical appropriateness	D. Extent to which services are cost-effective and have a favorable effect on the patient's symptoms, functioning, and well-being
___ Outcomes	E. Payment system in which the clinic is paid a flat fee regardless of the cost of care
___ Utilization review	F. Payment system in which the consumer pays a flat fee and in return receives all medically necessary health care

2. **Fill in the blanks.**

A. The term _____ is used in managed care to describe the combination of mental and substance abuse disorders.

B. Managed care involves a major shift away from the _____ as customer to the _____ as customer.

C. Value in managed care is defined as _____ divided by _____.

D. Worksite-based programs designed to help identify and facilitate the resolution of behavioral, health, and productivity problems that may adversely affect an employee's well-being or job performance are called _____.

E. The four variables that influence treatment outcome are _____, _____, _____ and _____.

F. _____ is the term used to describe audiovisual communication between people geographically apart that allows for psychiatric diagnosis and treatment.

3. **Provide short answers for the following questions.**

A. Describe the three forms of managed care organizations. If you belong to a managed care organization, identify which type of managed care plan you have.

B. Discuss how stigma associated with substance abuse may have contributed to the law passed in 1996 that ended Medicaid and Medicare coverage for people whose disability is based on drug addiction or alcoholism.

C. Some people believe that we should limit care to people with brain-based mental disorders or the major mental illnesses and not reimburse less serious or minor mental health problems. What position would you take on this issue? Compare this issue to reimbursement policies for major and minor physical illnesses.

D. Based on your experiences with patients, family, and friends, which system of care delivery for behavioral health services do you think is better: carve-ins or carve-outs?

REFERENCES

Bartels S: Community-based long-term care for older persons with severe and persistent mental illness in an era of managed care, *Psychiatr Serv* 50(9):1189, 1999.

Center for Mental Health Services: *Mental Health, United States, 1998*, Washington DC, 1998, US Government Printing Office.

Cummings N: Spectacular accomplishments and disappointing mistakes: the first decade of managed behavioral care, *Behav Healthc Tomorrow*, p 61, Aug 1998.

Druss B, Rosenheck R: Mental disorders and access to medical care in the United States, *Am J Psychiatry* 155(12):1775, 1998.

Emery B et al: The environmental trends facing state mental health agencies, *Admin Policy Ment Health* 25(3):337, 1998.

Fletcher J: Mental health nurses: guardians of ethics in managed care, *J Psychosoc Nurs Ment Health Serv* 36(7):34, 1998.

Geller J et al: A national survey of consumer empowerment at the state level, *Psychiatr Serv* 49(4):498, 1998.

Goldman H: The obligation of mental health services to the least well off, *Psychiatr Serv* 50(5):659, 1999.

Hall L, Beinecke R: Consumer and family views of managed care, *New Dir Ment Health Serv* 78:77, 1998.

Hiraki A: Corporate language and nursing practice, *Nurs Outlook* 46(3):115, 1998.

Hoge M et al: Ten dimensions of public-sector managed care, *Psychiatr Serv* 50(1):51, 1999.

Mechanic D: Emerging trends in mental health policy and practice, *Health Aff* 17(6):82, 1998.

Mechanic D: *Mental health and social policy: the emergence of managed care*, Needham Heights, Mass, 1999, Allyn and Bacon.

Murray C, Lopez A: Evidence-based health policy - lessons from the Global Burden of Disease study, *Science* 274:740, 1996.

National Academies of Practice: *Ethical guidelines for professional care and services in a managed health care environment*, Edgewood, Md, 1998, The Academies.

Sing M et al: *The costs and effects of parity for mental health and substance abuse insurance benefits*, Rockville, Md, 1998, US Department of Health and Human Services.

Steinberg A et al: Cultural and linguistic barriers to mental health service access: the deaf consumer's perspective, *Am J Psychiatry* 155(7):982, 1998.

Strosahl K: Mind and body primary mental health care: new model for integrated services, *Behav Healthc Tomorrow* 4:96, 1996.

Sturm R, Pacula R: State mental health parity laws: cause or consequence of difference in use? *Health Aff* 18(5):182, 1999.

Surles R, Fox R: Behavioral health: a view from the industry, *New Dir Ment Health Serv* 78:25, 1998.

Trabin T: Towards greater accountability in behavioral health services: more science, less art? *Behav Healthc Tomorrow* 3:1, 1995.

US Department of Health and Human Services: *Mental health: a report of the surgeon general*, Rockville, Md, 1999, National Institute of Mental Health.

White R et al: New developments in employee assistance programs, *Psychiatr Serv* 47:387, 1996.

Wickizer T, Lessler D: Do treatment restrictions imposed by utilization management increase the likelihood of readmission for psychiatric patients? *Med Care* 36:844, 1998.

Wieman D, Dorwart R: A comparison of public and privatized approaches to managed behavioral health care for persons with serious mental illness, *Ment Health Serv Res* 1(3):159, 1999.

Ziglin A: *Confidentiality and the appropriate uses of data*, Rockville, Md, 1995, Department of Health & Human Services, SAMSHA.

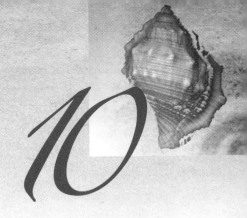

Legal-Ethical Context of Psychiatric Nursing Care

Gail W. Stuart

*P*inel immediately led Couthon to the section for the deranged, where the sight of the cells made a painful impression on him. Couthon asked to interrogate all the patients. From most, he received only insults and obscene apostrophes. It was useless to prolong the interview. Turning to Pinel, Couthon said: "Now, citizen, are you mad yourself to seek to unchain such beasts?" Pinel replied calmly: "Citizen, I am convinced that these madmen are so intractable only because they have been deprived of air and liberty."

PHILIPPE PINEL, TRAITE COMPLET DU REGIME SANITAIRE
DES ALIENES 56 (1836)

The relationship between psychiatry and the law reflects the tension between individual rights and social needs. Both psychiatry and the law deal with human behavior and the relationships and responsibilities that exist among people. Both also play a role in controlling socially undesirable behavior, and together they analyze whether the care psychiatric patients receive is therapeutic, custodial, repressive, or punitive.

Differences also exist between psychiatry and the law. For example, psychiatry is concerned with the meaning of behavior and the life satisfaction of the individual. In contrast, the law addresses the outcome of behavior and the enforcement of a system of rules to encourage orderly functioning among groups of people.

The legal context of care is important for all psychiatric nurses because it focuses concern on the rights of patients and the quality of care they receive. In the past two decades civil, criminal, and consumer rights of patients have been established and expanded through the legal system. Many of the laws vary from state to state, and psychiatric nurses must become familiar with the laws of the state in which they practice. This knowledge enhances the freedom of both the nurse and the patient and ultimately results in better care.

HOSPITALIZING THE PATIENT

Hospitalization can be either traumatic or supportive for the patient, depending on the institution, attitude of family and friends, response of the staff, and type of admission (see Citing the Evidence). There are two major types of admission: voluntary and involuntary. Table 10-1 summarizes their distinguishing characteristics.

Citing the Evidence on

Patients' Beliefs About the Need for Hospitalization

BACKGROUND: An important rationale for involuntary hospitalization is that prospective patients who refuse hospitalization at the time it is offered are likely to change their belief about the necessity of hospitalization after receiving hospital treatment. This study tested that hypothesis.

RESULTS: When reinterviewed 4 to 8 weeks after discharge, 52% of the patients who said at admission that they did not need hospitalization said that, in retrospect, they believe they had needed it. Only 5% of those who said they needed it on admission shifted on discharge to say they had not needed it. However, perceptions of coercion were stable from admission to follow-up, and patients' attitudes toward hospitalization did not become more positive. Coerced patients did not appear to be grateful for the experience of hospitalization, even if they later concluded that they needed it.

IMPLICATIONS: Patients' aversion to commitment may be a moral response to the loss of dignity and respect they experienced when deprived of their autonomy. Staff and family members need to carefully evaluate the way in which patients are pressured or forced into treatment and the long-term consequence of such actions.

Gardner W et al: Patients' revisions of their beliefs about the need for hospitalization, *Am J Psychiatry* 156(9):1385, 1999.

What were your impressions as you walked through the doors of a psychiatric hospital for the first time? How might you use your perceptions and responses to provide better nursing care for patients being admitted for inpatient treatment?

Voluntary Admission

Under voluntary admission any citizen of lawful age may apply in writing (usually on a standard admission form) for admission to a public or private psychiatric hospital. The person agrees to receive treatment and abide by hospital rules. People may seek help based on their personal decision or the advice of family or a health professional. If someone is too ill to apply but voluntarily seeks help, a parent or legal guardian may request admission. In most states children under the age of 16 years may be admitted if their parents sign the required application form.

Voluntary admission is preferred because it is similar to a medical hospitalization. It indicates that the patient acknowledges problems in living, seeks help in coping with them, and will probably actively participate in finding solutions. Most patients who enter private psychiatric units of general hospitals do so voluntarily.

When admitted in this way, the patient retains all civil rights, including the right to vote, hold a driver's license, buy and sell property, manage personal affairs, hold office, practice a profession, and engage in a business. It is a common misconception that all admissions to a mental hospital involve the loss of civil rights.

Although voluntary admission is the most desirable, it is not always possible. Sometimes a patient may be acutely disturbed, suicidal, or dangerous to self or others, yet rejects any therapeutic intervention. In these cases involuntary commitments are necessary.

Should a psychotic person be allowed to sign forms for voluntary admittance to the hospital? If not, should all voluntary patients be screened for competence before hospitalization?

Involuntary Admission (Commitment)

Involuntary commitment is based on two legal theories. First, under its **police power**, the state has the authority to protect the community from the dangerous acts of the mentally ill. Second, under its **parens patriae powers**, the state can provide care for citizens who cannot care for themselves, such as

---

Table **10-1**

Characteristics of the Two Types of Admission to Psychiatric Hospitals		
	Voluntary Admission	**Involuntary Admission**
Admission	Written application by patient	Application did not originate with patient
Discharge	Initiated by patient	Initiated by hospital or court but not by patient
Civil rights	Retained fully by patient	Patient may retain none, some, or all, depending on state law
Justification	Voluntarily seeks help	Mentally ill and one or more of the following: Dangerous to self or others Need for treatment Unable to meet own basic needs

some mentally ill people. The police power rationale for civil commitment has been emphasized over the parens patriae doctrine, using dangerousness as the standard for commitment. There has also been a trend toward strengthening the requirements for procedural due process for such commitments and the need for proof of mental illness and dangerousness by clear and convincing evidence. However, states with less stringent commitment laws still have higher admission rates to state and county hospitals (Ross et al, 1996).

Involuntary commitment means that the patient did not request hospitalization and may have opposed it or was indecisive and did not resist it. The standards for commitment vary among states and reflect the confusion in the medical, social, and legal systems of society. Most laws permit commitment of the mentally ill on the following three grounds:

- Dangerous to self or others
- Mentally ill and in need of treatment
- Unable to provide for own basic needs

The Commitment Process. State laws vary, but they try to protect the person who is not mentally ill from being detained in a psychiatric hospital against his or her will for political, economic, family, or other nonmedical reasons. Certain procedures are standard. The process begins with a sworn petition by a relative, friend, public official, physician, or any interested citizen stating that the person is mentally ill and needs treatment. Some states allow only specific people to file such a petition. One or two physicians must then examine the patient's mental status; some states require that at least one of the physicians be a psychiatrist.

The decision whether to hospitalize the patient is made next. Precisely who makes this decision determines the nature of the commitment. **Medical** certification means that

physicians make the decision. **Court** or **judicial** commitment is made by a judge or jury in a formal hearing. Most states recognize the patient's right to legal counsel, but only about half actually appoint a lawyer for patients if they do not have one. **Administrative** commitment is determined by a special tribunal of hearing officers. The Fourteenth Amendment to the U.S. Constitution protects citizens against infringements on liberty without due process of the law. For this reason medical certification is used rarely, primarily in emergencies, and administrative commitment is subject to judicial review.

If treatment is deemed necessary, the person is hospitalized. The length of hospital stay varies depending on the patient's needs. Fig. 10-1 presents a clinical algorithm of the involuntary commitment process. It identifies three types of involuntary hospitalization: emergency, short term, and long term.

> *Most states specify that any physician, not necessarily a psychiatrist, can certify a person for involuntary commitment to a psychiatric hospital. Do you agree with this? What is required by law in your state?*

Emergency Hospitalization. Almost all states permit emergency commitment for patients who are acutely ill. The goals are primarily intended to control an immediate threat to self or others. In states lacking such a law, police often jail the acutely ill person on a disorderly conduct charge, which is a criminal charge. Such a practice is inappropriate and often harmful to the patient's mental status. Most state laws limit the length of emergency commitment to 48 to 72 hours. Emergency hospitalization allows detainment in a psychiatric hospital only until proper legal steps are taken to provide for additional hospitalization.

Short-Term or Observational Hospitalization. This type of commitment is used primarily for diagnosis and short-term therapy and does not require an emergency situation. Again, the commitment is for a specified time that varies greatly from state to state. If at the end of the period the patient is still not ready for discharge, a petition can be filed for a long-term commitment.

Long-Term Hospitalization (Formal Commitment). A long-term commitment provides for hospitalization for an indefinite time or until the patient is ready for discharge. Patients in public or state hospitals more often have indefinite commitments than patients in private hospitals. Even when committed, these patients maintain their right to consult a lawyer at any time and to request a court hearing to determine whether additional hospitalization is necessary. The hospital ultimately discharges the patient, however, and a court order is not needed. Periodic reviews for long-term hospitalization may be made every 3, 6, or 12 months.

> *Do you agree with the criteria for committing patients to psychiatric hospitals? How would you assess whether a person met these criteria?*

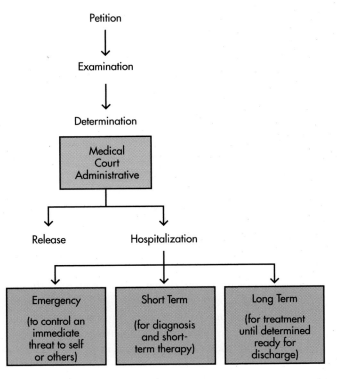

Fig. 10-1 Clinical algorithm for the involuntary commitment process.

Commitment Dilemma

Because of the many people affected by involuntary commitment and the loss of personal rights that it can entail, it becomes a matter of great legal, ethical, social, and psychiatric significance (Dickenson, 1997). In general medicine there is no equivalent loss of individual rights, except for rare cases requiring quarantine for carriers of potentially epidemic diseases.

How ill does a person need to be to merit commitment? A person's dangerousness to self or others is a pertinent consideration. Certainly psychiatric professionals consider hospitalization in this instance as a humanitarian gesture that protects both the individual and society. However, dangerousness is a vague term.

> *According to a survey commissioned by* Parade *magazine, over 57% of Americans think mentally ill people are more likely to commit acts of violence than other people. How does this compare with the facts? How do the media contribute to this impression of the mentally ill?*

Dangerousness. Interestingly, courts guard the freedom of people who are mentally healthy but dangerous. For example, after a prison sentence is served, the person is automatically released and can no longer be retained. However, someone who is mentally ill and dangerous can be confined indefinitely. The idea of preventive detention does not exist in most areas of the law because the ability to predict an action does not confer the right to control it in advance. Only illegal acts result in prolonged confinement for most citizens, except the mentally ill.

Most mentally ill people are not dangerous to themselves or others. Studies show that the vast majority of people with serious mental illness are not inherently violent and are no more dangerous than people in the general population (Bonta et al, 1998). Furthermore, violence is not associated with any specific psychiatric diagnosis. However, a subgroup of such people are more dangerous (Asnis et al, 1997; Fulwiler et al, 1997; Sreenivasan et al, 1997; Steadman et al, 1998; Swartz et al, 1998). Patients in this subgroup have a history of:

- Violent behavior
- Noncompliance with medications
- Current substance abuse
- Antisocial personality disorder

These characteristics can serve as predictors of potential violence.

It is important that patients with severe psychiatric disorders be identified and appropriately treated. It should also be remembered that violent behavior by people with serious mental illness is only one aspect of a larger problem: the failure of public psychiatric services and the deinstitutionalization of the mentally ill without adequate community support. Other aspects of this problem include the large number of mentally ill among the homeless, the large number of mentally ill in jails and prisons, and the revolving door of psychiatric readmissions.

Another issue is that there are no reliable indicators of dangerousness. Even if some mentally ill people are potentially dangerous, psychiatrists cannot predict future violence. Psychiatrists often overpredict patients' potential for dangerous acts. This may result from their medical training, which cautions that underdiagnosis is more harmful than overdiagnosis. If psychiatrists underpredict a psychiatric illness and the patient later causes harm, they are held responsible (Weinberger et al, 1998). If they overpredict illness, however, a patient is subjected to treatment unwillingly. Therefore multidisciplinary teams should be involved in determining dangerousness. Input from those familiar with the patient's home setting and sociocultural background might also improve evaluations.

Some suggest that the underlying issue is nonconformity in ways that offend others (see Citing the Evidence below). In this context, social role becomes important. For example, before the law all men and women are equal, but it is also true that most committed patients are members of the lower classes. Specifically, one study reported that the profile of a patient who has the greatest risk for involuntary admission to a psychiatric hospital is a young, unmarried black male who has schizophrenia without comorbid substance abuse (Sanguineti et al, 1996). This raises questions regarding the sociocultural context of psychiatric care (see Chapter 8) and the role of mental health professionals as enforcers of social

Citing the Evidence on

The Public's View of Persons Who Are Mentally Ill

BACKGROUND: The researchers examined American's opinions about financial and treatment competence of people with mental health problems, potential for harm to self or others, and the use of legal means to force treatment.

RESULTS: The specific nature of the problem was the most important factor shaping public opinion. Respondents viewed those with "troubles," alcohol dependence, or depression as able to make treatment decisions. Most reported that persons with alcohol or drug problems or schizophrenia cannot manage money and are likely to be violent toward others. Respondents indicated a willingness to coerce individuals into treatment.

IMPLICATIONS: Americans hold complex views of competence, dangerousness, and coercion. Study findings reflect an underlying negative attitude toward persons with mental health problems, an exaggeration of the impairment or "threat" associated with these disorders, and a negativity toward individuals with substance dependence problems. More work needs to be done to educate the public regarding the realities of mental illness.

Pescosolido B et al: The public's view of the competence, dangerousness, and need for legal coercion of persons with mental health problems, *Am J Public Health* 89(9):1339, 1999.

rules and norms (Engleman et al, 1998). Thus the behavioral standard of dangerousness can change the function of the psychiatric hospital from a place of therapy for mental illness to a place of confinement for offensive behavior.

> *How do you explain the fact that society condones certain kinds of dangerous behavior, such as race car driving, but objects to other kinds?*

Freedom of Choice. The legal and ethical question thus raised is freedom of choice. Some professionals believe that at certain times the individual cannot be self-responsible. To protect both the patient and society, it is necessary to confine the patient and make decisions for him or her. An example is the suicidal patient. In most states suicide is against the law, so law and psychiatry join to protect the person and help individuals resolve personal conflicts.

How does this compare with cancer or cardiac patients who may reject medical advice and the prescribed treatment? Should society, through law and medicine, attempt to cure these patients against their will? Some clinicians view civil commitment as basically a benevolent system that makes treatment available. They disagree with the assumption that mentally ill people are competent to exercise free will and make decisions in their own best interest, such as whether to take medications or remain outside a hospital. They contend that there are mentally ill people who may not be physically dangerous but still endanger their own prospects for a normal life. Because institutions can protect them and in many cases help them, they think it would be unethical to abolish involuntary civil commitment.

Others oppose commitment. They favor responsibility for self and the right to choose or reject treatment. If a person's actions violate criminal law, they suggest that the person be punished through the penal system. Currently a middle ground is being sought between meeting the needs of the severely mentally ill and preserving their legal rights and freedom of choice.

> *Who should decide what is in the patient's best interest if a patient is involuntarily committed? Should it be the patient, a family member, a health-care professional, or the judicial system?*

Discharge

The patient who is informally admitted to the hospital can leave at any time, limited only to reasonable hours, such as daytime hours or weekdays. The voluntarily admitted patient can be discharged by the staff when maximum benefit has been received from the treatment. Voluntary patients may also request discharge. Most states require written notice of patients' desire to leave and also that patients sign a form that states they are leaving against medical advice (AMA). This form then becomes part of the patient's permanent record.

The issue of leaving AMA presents a particular ethical dilemma for the clinician who must weigh provider accountability for the patient's safety against the patient's right to refuse treatment (see Citing the Evidence below). Two key factors in deciding to release a voluntary psychiatric patient are as follows:

- Assessment of the patient's competency
- Assessment of the patient's potential danger to self or others

Furthermore, documentation of AMA requests should include the following (McGihon, 1998):

- The mental status of the patient requesting to leave
- The patient's own description of why he or she wants to leave
- Content of discussions in which possible risks of leaving were described to the patient
- Instructions on medications and follow-up care
- Conversations with significant others who may have been present
- Destination of the patient and means of transportation

In some states voluntarily admitted patients can be released immediately; in others they can be detained 24 to 72 hours after submitting a discharge request. This allows hospital staff time to confer with the patient and family members and decide whether additional inpatient treatment is indicated. If it is and the patient will not withdraw the request for discharge, the family may begin involuntary commitment proceedings, thereby changing the patient's status.

An involuntarily committed patient has lost the right to leave the hospital when he or she wishes. Short-term and emergency commitments specify the maximum length of detainment. Long-term commitments do not, although the patient's status should be reviewed periodically. The patient may also apply for another commitment hearing. If a com-

---

Citing the Evidence on
Discharge Against Medical Advice

BACKGROUND: Discharges AMA are common for psychiatric patients, occurring in 6% to 35% of cases, but they have received little attention in the mental health literature. This study examined predictors of discharge AMA and outcomes of these patients.

RESULTS: Study results show that patients discharged AMA were more likely to live alone, have a substance abuse diagnosis, and have more previous hospitalizations. They also had higher rehospitalization rates and more severe symptoms at discharge.

IMPLICATIONS: Since patients who leave AMA have worse outcomes and are more likely to be high utilizers of inpatient resources, it is important that clinicians aggressively identify those patients and initiate early discharge planning for appropriate outpatient treatment.

Pages K et al: Predictors and outcome of discharge against medical advice from the psychiatric units of a general hospital, *Psychiatr Serv* 49(9):1187, 1998.

mitted patient leaves before discharge, the staff has the legal obligation to notify the police and committing courts. Often these patients return home or visit family or friends and can be easily located. The legal authorities then return the patient to the hospital. Additional steps are not necessary because the original commitment is still in effect.

Ethical Considerations

Nurses must analyze their beliefs regarding the voluntary and involuntary hospitalization of psychiatric patients. What should be done if the nonconformist does not wish to change behavior? Do nonconformists maintain freedom to choose even if their thinking appears to be irrational or abnormal? Is coercion fair? Can social interests be served by less restrictive methods such as outpatient therapy? Nurses are responsible for reviewing commitment procedures in their state and working for necessary clinical, ethical, and legal reforms.

The commitment dilemma exposes current practices and opens areas of controversy for the future. Studies show that more than half of the homeless population have psychiatric or substance abuse disorders. Homeless mentally ill people have a wider array of service needs than homeless people who use only social services. Many seriously mentally ill people cannot obtain or maintain access to community resources such as housing, a stable source of income, or treatment and rehabilitative services. Homeless people lack supportive social networks and underuse psychiatric, medical, and welfare programs. Many avoid the mental health system entirely, often because they are too confused to respond to offers of help. As a consequence, they are often admitted into acute psychiatric hospitals or jailed because of their lack of shelter and other resources, even though such restrictive environments may not best address their psychiatric needs.

Unfortunately, local communities often deny the problem by resisting the establishment of halfway houses or sheltered homes in their neighborhoods. Third-party insurance seldom covers extended outpatient psychiatric care. In today's mobile society, family and friends are often unable to care for the newly discharged patient, who may end up in a boarding house with little to do but watch television.

These issues must be addressed by psychiatric nurses, patients, and citizens across the United States. The value of commitment, goals of hospitalization, quality of life, and rights of patients must be preserved through the judicial, legislative, and health-care systems.

INVOLUNTARY COMMUNITY TREATMENT

There are three major ways in which involuntary community treatment can be provided for those in need: outpatient commitment, preventive commitment, and conditional release from the hospital. These initiatives arose from the mandate to offer psychiatric patients treatment in the least restrictive setting. Geller (1993) has proposed 10 guidelines to determine a patient's appropriateness for involuntary outpatient treatment (Box 10-1). They are sequential in that a patient is not evaluated for appropriateness under a guideline

unless the criteria for all preceding guidelines have been met. The guidelines also assume that the patient has a serious and persistent mental illness and a history of dangerousness to self or others.

> *How might sociocultural factors influence a nurse's interpretation of the guidelines listed in Box 10-1? How might nurses guard against potential bias based on their personal world view?*

Outpatient commitment is the process by which the courts can order patients committed to a course of outpatient treatment specified by their clinicians. This type of commitment is an alternative to inpatient treatment for people who meet the involuntary commitment criteria of dangerousness to self or others (Smith, 1995). Forty states and the District of Columbia have laws permitting outpatient commitment, but very few of them use their laws with any frequency (Kanapaux, 1999). Reasons for not using them include concerns about civil liberties, liability and financial costs, lack of information and interest, problems with enforcement and ways to deal with lack of compliance, and criteria that are too restrictive.

Like inpatient commitment, involuntary outpatient treatment is also the subject of controversy. Some believe that it is

Box 10-1

Guidelines for the Use of Outpatient Commitment

1. The patient must express an interest in living in the community.
2. The patient must have previously failed in the community.
3. The patient must have that degree of competency necessary to understand the stipulations of his or her involuntary community treatment.
4. The patient must have the capacity to comply with the involuntary community treatment plan.
5. The treatment or treatments being ordered must have demonstrated efficacy when used properly by the patient in question.
6. The ordered treatment or treatments must be such that they can be delivered by the outpatient system, are sufficient for the patient's needs, and are necessary to sustain community tenure.
7. The ordered treatment must be such that it can be monitored by outpatient treatment agencies.
8. The outpatient treatment system must be willing to deliver the ordered treatments to the patient and must be willing to participate in enforcing compliance with those treatments.
9. The public-sector inpatient support system must support the outpatient system's participation in the provision of involuntary community treatment.
10. The outpatient must not be dangerous when complying with the ordered treatment.

From Geller J: On being "committed" to treatment in the community, *Innovations Res* 2:23, 1993.

necessary to reach people who need help but don't realize it. These are people who lack insight because of their illness, refuse treatment, and wind up homeless, in jails, or in hospitals. They point to research showing that patients in outpatient commitment had fewer hospital admissions and hospital days after the court order (Geller et al, 1998b). From the consumers' perspective, they note that one study of patients' perceptions of outpatient commitment found that 75% of the respondents said that the commitment order made it more likely for them to keep their mental health appointments, take their medications, and stay out of the hospital (Borum et al, 1999). It has also been noted, however, that the use of outpatient commitment is not a substitute for intensive treatment and that it requires a substantial allocation of treatment resources to be effective (Swartz et al, 1999).

Others disagree and say this law plays into the public's fear of the dangerous mentally ill. It also undermines engaging the patient in treatment. The Bazelon Center for Mental Health Law opposes all involuntary outpatient commitment as an infringement of an individual's constitutional rights and believes that guidelines for commitment are based on speculation and are not legally permissible (Bazelon, 1999). Thus this remains a topic of controversy in the field.

Preventive commitment is a new concept found in only a few states. Preventive commitment permits commitment to outpatient treatment of people who do not yet meet the usual commitment criteria but will do so soon if intervention does not take place. The criterion used for preventive commitment is sometimes called a predicted deterioration standard, in which a person is believed to need treatment to prevent a relapse that would probably result in the person's becoming imminently dangerous.

Conditional release is the third type of involuntary community treatment. It involves continued supervision of a person who has been released from the hospital. It has been available for some time in about 40 states. Under this arrangement the hospital or court informs the conditionally released person of the conditions for release, such as reporting to a medication clinic. Violation of these conditions usually triggers rehospitalization. In contrast to outpatient commitment, which is designed as an alternative to inpatient commitment, and preventive commitment, which is anticipatory, conditional release is used primarily to see whether the person is able to function in the community under supervision.

PATIENTS' RIGHTS

In 1973 the American Hospital Association issued a Patient's Bill of Rights that many hospitals and community-based settings throughout the United States have adopted. These rights were reaffirmed in 1990 (American Hospital Association, 1990). Often they are posted for reading in a location that is easily accessible to patients. In some hospitals they may be given to patients on admission and read or explained to them.

However, the evolution of patients' rights has been uneven across the United States. Some states continue to formally acknowledge very few rights, while other states guarantee certain categories of rights while ignoring others. It is also unclear how well patients are actually informed about their rights, whether and with what frequency patients exercise their rights, and the consequences they experience when they do so (Geller et al, 1998a).

For example, one study reported that reading patients their rights on admission and giving them a copy did not necessarily result in understanding or retaining the information. Two important rights (the right to withdraw from treatment and the right to participate in the development of the treatment plan) were not understood by more than a fourth of the patients in this study (Wolpe et al, 1991). This finding suggests that a change may be needed in how psychiatric patients are informed about their rights and empowered to participate in the treatment process.

In your experience, are patients in general hospital settings granted their patient rights? How about patients in psychiatric inpatient units? What specific things could nurses do to see that these rights are honored in all hospitals?

Although there is great variation among states, psychiatric patients currently have the following rights:

- Right to communicate with people outside the hospital through correspondence, telephone, and personal visits
- Right to keep clothing and personal effects with them in the hospital
- Right to religious freedom
- Right to be employed if possible
- Right to manage and dispose of property
- Right to execute wills
- Right to enter into contractual relationships
- Right to make purchases
- Right to education
- Right to habeas corpus
- Right to independent psychiatric examination
- Right to civil service status
- Right to retain licenses, privileges, or permits established by law, such as a driver's or professional license
- Right to sue or be sued
- Right to marry and divorce
- Right not to be subject to unnecessary mechanical restraints
- Right to periodic review of status
- Right to legal representation
- Right to privacy
- Right to informed consent
- Right to treatment
- Right to refuse treatment
- Right to treatment in the least restrictive setting

Some of these rights deserve more discussion.

Did you know that 44 states still have laws on the books that restrict the right of some people with treatable psychiatric illnesses to vote? How do you think such laws perpetuate stigma, prejudice, and discrimination against people with mental illness? Does your state have such laws?

Right to Communicate with People Outside the Hospital

This right allows patients to visit and hold telephone conversations in privacy and send unopened letters to anyone of their choice, including judges, lawyers, families, and staff. Although the patient has the right to communicate in an uncensored manner, the staff may limit access to the telephone or visitors when it could harm the patient or be a source of harassment for the staff. The hospital can also limit the times when telephone calls are made and received and when visitors can enter the facility.

Right to Keep Personal Effects

The patient may bring clothing and personal items to the hospital, taking into consideration the amount of storage space available. The hospital is not responsible for their safety, and valuable items should be left at home. If the patient brings something of value to the hospital, the staff should place it in the hospital safe or otherwise provide for safekeeping. The hospital staff is also responsible for maintaining a safe environment and should take dangerous objects away from the patient if necessary.

How are patients informed of their rights on your psychiatric unit? Talk to some of the patients and see whether they can recall any of the rights that were explained to them.

Right to Execute Wills

A person's competency to make a will is known as testamentary capacity. Patients can make a valid will if the following conditions are met:

- They know they are making a will.
- They know the nature and extent of their property.
- They know who their friends and relatives are and what the relationships mean.

Each of these criteria must be documented for the will to be considered valid. This means that patients must not be mentally confused at the time they sign their will. It does not imply that they must know exact details of their property holdings or specific bank account figures, but they cannot attempt to give away more than they possess. Furthermore, the law requires that patients know who their relatives are but does not require them to bequeath anything to them.

Right to Enter into Contractual Relationships

The court considers contracts valid if the person understands the circumstances of the contract and its consequences. Once again, a psychiatric illness does not invalidate a contract, although the nature of the contract and degree of judgment needed to understand it are influencing factors.

Incompetency. Related to this right is the issue of mental incompetency. Every adult is assumed to be mentally competent, mentally able to carry out personal affairs. To prove otherwise requires a special court hearing to declare an individual incompetent. This is a legal term without a precise medical meaning. To prove incompetence, it must be shown that:

- The person has a mental disorder
- This disorder causes a defect in judgment
- This defect makes the person incapable of handling personal affairs

All three elements must be present, and the exact diagnostic label is not important in this case. If a person is declared incompetent, the court will appoint a legal guardian to manage his or her affairs. This often is a family member, friend, or bank executive. Incompetency rulings are most often filed for people with senile dementia, cerebral arteriosclerosis, chronic schizophrenia, and mental retardation.

The legislative trend is to separate the concepts of incompetency and involuntary commitment because the reasons for each are essentially different. Incompetency arises from society's desire to guard its citizens' assets from their inability to understand and transact business. Involuntary commitments are intended to protect patients from themselves (in the case of suicide), protect others from dangerous patients (as in homicide), and administer treatment. However, many states still consider the two equivalent.

If ruled incompetent, a person cannot vote, marry, drive, or make contracts. A release from the hospital does not necessarily restore competency. Another court hearing is required to reverse the previous ruling before the person can once again manage private affairs.

How is education provided for emotionally ill children living in your community? Are they mainstreamed in the school system, given special educational resources, or both?

Right to Education

Many parents exercise this right on behalf of their emotionally ill or mentally retarded children. The U.S. Constitution guarantees this right to everyone, although many states have not provided adequate education to all citizens and are now required to do so.

How is the right to education honored in a children's psychiatric inpatient setting? How does this compare with the education provided children in a pediatric hospital?

Right to Habeas Corpus

Habeas corpus is an important constitutional right patients retain in all states even if they have been involuntarily hospitalized. Its goal is the speedy release of any person who claims being detained illegally. A committed patient may file a writ at any time on the grounds of being sane and eligible for release. The hearing takes place in court, where those who wish to restrain the patient must defend their actions. Patients are discharged if they are judged as sane.

Right to Independent Psychiatric Examination

Under the Emergency Admission Statute, the patient has the right to demand a psychiatric examination by a physician of choice. If this physician determines that the patient is not mentally ill, the patient must be released.

Right to Privacy

The right to privacy implies the person's right to keep some personal information completely secret. Confidentiality involves the disclosure of certain information to another person. Every psychiatric professional is responsible for protecting a patient's right to confidentiality, including even the knowledge that a person is in treatment or in a hospital. Revealing such information might damage the patient's reputation or the ability to get or keep a job. The protection of the law applies to all patients. This can create ethical and professional dilemmas, such as the one experienced by the nurse described in this clinical example.

 CLINICAL EXAMPLE

On a Wednesday morning in Springfield, Illinois, a man walked into Lauterbach's Cottage Hardware Store, grabbed an ax, and began swinging. When he left, one person was dead and two others were critically injured. Ten days later, police received a call from Mr. K, who was a patient in the 49-bed psychiatric unit at St. John's Hospital. Mr. K told the police that his roommate at the hospital confessed the crime. However, he didn't know his roommate's name. He asked Nurse M to identify him but she refused to do so because she believed that his name was shielded by a state law guaranteeing the privacy of mental health records. Hospital administrators supported her decision even after she was fined $250 by a county judge for refusing to give the man's name to a grand jury. Nurse M did tell the police that the suspect was not a patient in St. John's at the time of the murder and that he resembled their composite sketch.

The issue of confidentiality is becoming increasingly important. Various agencies require information about a patient's history, diagnosis, treatment, and prognosis, and sophisticated methods for obtaining information through computer systems have been developed. These methods threaten the individual's right to privacy (Appelbaum, 1998a; Shellow, 1998).

Clinicians are free from legal responsibility if they release information with the patient's written and signed request. Written consent is desirable for two reasons: It makes clear to both parties that consent has been given, and if questions arise about the consent, a documentary record of it exists. Therefore it should be made a part of the patient's permanent chart. As a rule, it is best to reveal as little information as possible and discuss with the patient what will be released.

Confidentiality builds on the element of trust necessary in a patient-clinician relationship. Patients place themselves in the care of others and reveal vulnerable aspects of their personal life. In return they expect high-quality care and the protection of their interests. Thus the patient-clinician relationship is an intimate one that demands trust, loyalty, and privacy.

> *One of the adolescent girls on your unit runs away while going to the hospital cafeteria. When you speak to the girl's mother to let her know what has happened, the mother asks you to call the radio and television stations and have them announce it so that the girl can be found. How would you respond to this request?*

Privileged Communication. The legal term **privilege** or, more accurately, testimonial privilege, applies only in court-related proceedings. It includes communications between husband and wife, attorney and client, and clergy and church member. The right to reveal information belongs to the person who spoke, and the listener cannot disclose the information unless the speaker gives permission. This right protects the patient, who could sue the listener for disclosing privileged information. It also gives the patient the confidence necessary to make a full account of symptoms and conditions so that treatment can be administered.

Testimonial privilege between health professionals and patients exists only if established by law. It varies greatly among professions, even within the same state. A minority of the states allow privilege between nurses and patients. Nurses may also be covered in states that have adopted privileges between psychotherapists and patients. The psychotherapist-patient privilege is usually limited. It applies only when a therapist-patient relationship exists, and only communications of a professional nature are protected. Third persons present during the communication between the therapist and the patient may be required to testify and are not included in privilege.

> *What is the law in your state regarding testimonial privilege between nurses and patients? How would you change the law if it does not include nurses?*

Circle of Confidentiality. This discussion is summarized in Fig. 10-2. Within the circle, patient information may be shared. Those outside the circle require the patient's permission to receive information. Within the circle are treatment team members, staff supervisors, health-care students and their faculty working with the patient, and consultants who actually see the patient. All of these people must be informed about the patient's clinical condition to be able to help. The patient is also inside the circle (an obvious point but one that is often overlooked). The patient can reveal any aspect of his or her life, problems, treatments, and experiences to anyone. This is an important point for the nurse to remember in situations where the requirements of confidentiality are uncertain.

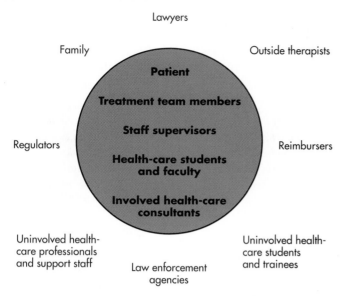

Fig. 10-2 The circle of confidentiality.

Many people are outside the circle, and these relationships must be carefully considered by the nurse. For example, family members of adult patients are not automatically entitled to clinical information about the patient. Although nurses may wish to engage the family in a therapeutic alliance, it is equally important to remember that information about the patient belongs to the patient. It is essential, therefore, that the nurse first discuss with the patient the benefits of involving the family in the treatment process and obtain clear consent from the patient before doing so. A specific form for release of information to families indicating the types of information that may be released has been found useful (Bogart & Solomon, 1999). This may create uncomfortable situations for the nurse who is pressured by a family to reveal patient information, but it is a critical aspect of patient confidentiality and the nurse-patient relationship.

Legal representatives, outside or previous therapists, reimbursers or insurance companies, students, health-care professionals and support staff not directly involved in the care of the patient, and the police or other law enforcement or regulatory agencies are outside the circle of patient confidentiality. A signed written consent from the patient is required to release information to any of these parties. However, in some situations breaching confidentiality and testimonial privilege is both ethical and legal. These exceptions are listed in Box 10-2.

Patient Records. Most treatment facilities keep psychiatric records separately so that they are less accessible than medical records. The law and psychiatric professionals view them as more sensitive than medical records. Many states allow or require that patients have access to their own records. If a patient makes such a request, the clinician should explore the reasons for the request, determine the laws that apply in the particular state, prepare the patient for the review, and be present with the patient to discuss any questions the

patient might have. The clinician must not release material from any other sources and must not alter or destroy any part of the record before the patient sees it.

Finally, it is important for the nurse to realize that the physical record itself is the property of the treatment facility or therapist, but the information contained in the record belongs to the patient. Thus the original record should never be given to the patient; only a copy of it should be provided. A patient's record or chart can be brought into court and its contents used in a lawsuit because privilege does not apply to records or charts.

> *The parents of one of your patients ask for information about their adult son. The patient has been very specific about not wanting to see his family and not wanting them to know anything about his treatment. How would you respond?*

Protecting a Third Party. Another aspect of confidentiality and privilege stems from the case of *Tarasoff v. Regents of the University of California et al* (1974). In this case the psychotherapist did not warn Tatiana Tarasoff or her parents that his client had stated he intended to kill Tatiana when she returned from summer vacation. In the lawsuit that followed Tatiana Tarasoff's death, California's Supreme Court decided that the treating therapist has a duty to warn the intended victim of a patient's violence. When a therapist is reasonably certain that a patient is going to harm someone, the therapist has the responsibility to breach the confidentiality of the relationship and warn or protect the potential victim (Beck, 1998; Mason, 1998).

Most states now recognize some variation of the duty to warn. This duty obliges the clinician to do the following:

- Assess the threat of violence to another
- Identify the person being threatened
- Implement some affirmative, preventive act

A clinical algorithm to assist clinicians in decisions regarding protective measures is presented in Fig. 10-3. Four

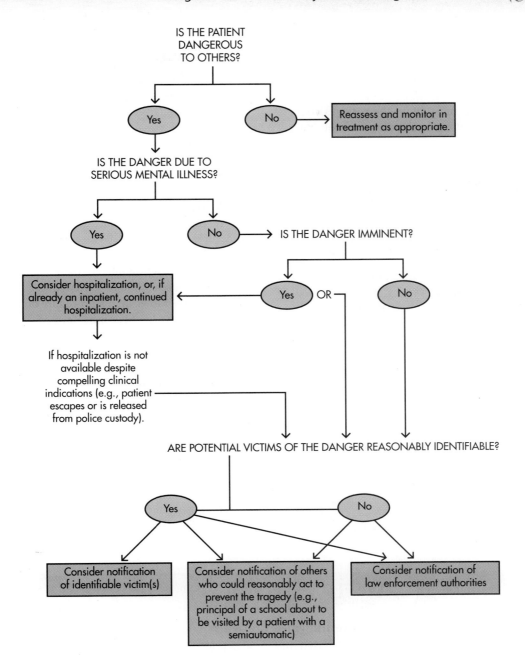

Fig. 10-3 Clinical algorithm to protect third parties. (From Felthous A: The clinician's duty to protect third parties, *Psychiatr Clin North Am* 22[1]:52, 1999.)

important questions for the clinician to consider are (Felthous, 1999):

1. Is the patient dangerous to self or others?
2. Is the danger due to serious mental illness?
3. Is the danger imminent?
4. Is the danger targeted at identifiable victims?

More recently, courts have extended the *Tarasoff* duty to include mental health paraprofessionals and a duty to protect property, as well as persons. Current controversy also exists about how long following treatment therapists can be held liable for the actions of their patients, as well as whether after issuing a *Tarasoff* warning, therapists can find themselves as prosecution witnesses in cases against patients arrested for serious violent crimes (Curry & Beck, 1997).

One study examined the effects of such warnings on the warned person and the therapeutic relationship. It found that most warnings were issued for patients in inpatient units and emergency rooms. In almost half of the cases the intended victim could not be contacted but the threat was reported to a law enforcement agency. In about three fourths of the cases in which the intended victim was contacted, the person knew of the threat. The most common reaction among those warned was gratitude, and most said that they would take steps to increase their safety. The second most common reaction was denial that the patient would ever hurt them. Clinicians reported that in most cases issuing the warning to an intended victim had a minimal or a positive effect on the psychotherapeutic relationship (Binder & McNiel, 1996).

Right to Informed Consent

The goal of informed consent is to help patients make better decisions. Informed consent means that a physician must give the patient a certain amount of information about the proposed treatment and must attain the patient's consent, which must be **competent, understanding,** and **voluntary.**

Box 10-3

Obtaining Informed Consent

INFORMATION TO DISCLOSE

Diagnosis: description of the patient's problem
Treatment: nature and purpose of the proposed treatment
Consequences: risks and benefits of the proposed treatment including physical and psychological effects, costs, and potential resulting problems
Alternatives: viable alternatives to the proposed treatment and their risks and benefits
Prognosis: expected outcome with treatment, with alternative treatments, and without treatment

PRINCIPLES OF INFORMING

Assess the patient's ability to give informed consent.
Simplify the language so that a layperson can understand.
Offer opportunities for the patient and family to ask questions.
Test the patient's understanding after the explanation. Reeducate as often as needed.
Document all relevant factors, including what was disclosed, the patient's understanding, competency, voluntary agreement to treatment, and the actual consent.

The physician should explain the treatment and possible complications and risks. The information to be disclosed in obtaining informed consent is listed in Box 10-3. The patient must be able to consent and not be a minor or judged legally incompetent. Even if a patient is psychotic, the physician is not relieved from attempting to obtain informed consent for treatment. Psychosis does not necessarily mean that a person is unable to consent to treatment, and many psychotic patients are capable of giving informed consent. For patients who are not able to consent and for minors, informed consent should be obtained from a substitute decision maker.

The doctrine of informed consent is consistent with the provision of good clinical care. It allows patients and clinicians to become partners in the treatment process and respects patients' autonomy, needs, and values. Furthermore, informed consent should be viewed as a continuing educational process rather than a procedure done merely to comply with the law. In obtaining informed consent the clinician should adhere to the principles listed in Box 10-3. Consent forms usually require the signature of the patient, a family member, and two witnesses. Nurses are often called on to be witnesses. The form then becomes part of the patient's permanent record.

Informed consent should be obtained for all psychiatric treatments, including medication, particularly neuroleptics because of the risk of tardive dyskinesia; somatic therapies, such as electroconvulsive therapy (ECT); and experimental treatments. Whether consent should be obtained for psychotherapy is unclear at present, and other aspects related to obtaining informed consent remain controversial (Appelbaum, 1997) (see Critical Thinking about Contemporary Issues).

? CRITICAL THINKING about CONTEMPORARY ISSUES

Can Patients with Mental Disorders Give Informed Consent?

Informed consent is a critical variable in the self-determination of consumers receiving health and mental health services. Obtaining informed consent from psychiatric patients has received recent attention as questions have been raised regarding the capacity of these patients to understand the risks and benefits of consenting both to treatment and to participation in clinical research trials. Immense controversy specifically surrounds the question of whether it is unethical for individuals with mental illness to participate in research.

Empirical studies indicate that (Roberts, 1998; Roberts et al, 2000):

- Psychiatric symptoms significantly affect informed consent
- Psychiatric patients may possess certain strengths with respect to research involvement
- Proxy decision-making is problematic
- Informed consent is also difficult to attain with the medically ill and others
- Patients are motivated to participate in research by the hope of personal benefit

- Ethical aspects of research are poorly documented
- Institutional review processes may not be adequate to protect vulnerable subjects.

The National Bioethics Advisory Commission (1998) has thus issued a series of recommendations designed to protect psychiatric patients who participate in medical research. Their 21 recommendations cover six areas: review bodies, research design, informed consent and capacity, categories of surrogate decision making, and education, research, and support.

Patient-focused studies have identified a clinical tool, the MacCAT-T that offers a flexible yet structured method to assess, rate, and report patients' capacities to make treatment decisions (Grisso et al, 1997). Studies also show that patients with schizophrenia who were research subjects were able to understand and retain critical components of informed consent information when adequate procedures are followed (Wirshing et al, 1998). Thus the real issue may not be related as much to a patient's capacity as it is to the procedures and process used to obtain informed consent by health-care providers.

How is informed consent obtained in your psychiatric treatment setting? Ask to observe this process and evaluate it based on the criteria listed in Box 10-3.

Right to Treatment

Early court cases extended the right to treatment to all mentally ill and mentally retarded people who were involuntarily hospitalized. The courts defined three criteria for adequate treatment:

- A humane psychological and physical environment
- A qualified staff with a sufficient number of members to administer adequate treatment
- Individualized treatment plans

Most important is the requirement for an individualized treatment plan. Failure to provide it means that the patient must be discharged unless he or she agrees to stay voluntarily.

The right to treatment is not a guarantee of treatment for all patients. It applies only to involuntary or committed patients. In addition, the right to treatment identifies minimal treatment standards, not optimal treatment; it does not guarantee that adequate treatment occurs and it does not require that a range of treatments be available (one treatment choice is adequate). Thus, although much has been gained through this legislation, much remains to be done.

Right to Refuse Treatment

The relationship between the right to treatment and the right to refuse treatment is complex (Winick, 1997). The right to refuse treatment includes the right to refuse involuntary hospitalization. It has been called the right to be left alone. Some people believe that therapy can control a person's mind, regulate thoughts, and change personality, and the right to refuse treatment protects the patient. This argument states that involuntary therapy conflicts with two basic legal rights: freedom of thought and the right to control one's life and actions as long as they do not interfere with the rights of others.

A group of patients with serious mental illness were surveyed about their experiences and attitudes toward forced psychiatric treatment. The results indicated that at some time during the course of their illness, 57% reported being pressured or forced into hospitalization. In the year before the survey, 30% reported being pressured or forced into taking medication and 26% into attending a therapy or rehabilitation program. The most common type of pressure or force was verbal persuasion. Generally, respondents reported negative effects from forced treatment but about half retrospectively felt that the forced treatment was in their best interest (Lucksted & Coursey, 1995).

This finding suggests that treatment can be successful in a variety of coerced situations and that issues such as degree and source of coercion must be considered. In addition, dialogue in decision making is important to patients, not because it necessarily changes the outcome, but for its symbolic and expressive value. On a day-to-day basis between staff and patients, dialogue such as the nurses' use of tact and polite talking has been found to produce a sense of fairness in hospitalized psychiatric patients (Susman, 1998).

The following patient factors can also predict a positive outcome (Group for the Advancement of Psychiatry, 1994):

- Patients who have the ability to understand the immediate consequences of refusing to comply with treatment even though they may not appreciate the effects of the illness itself.
- Patients who value what will be lost if the treatment is refused.
- Patients who trust that compliance with treatment will help them avoid negative consequences.
- Patients who are able to cooperate at least minimally.
- Patients whose problems are psychiatrically treatable.

Forcing Medications. There are many reasons why patients refuse medication. Symptoms such as delusions and denial may cause the refusal, and patients who refuse medication are generally sicker than those who comply. Staff members faced with a patient who refuses medication have several options. First, they can offer the patient a lower dosage or no medication at all. A second option would be to discharge the patient against medical advice if no other staff action can relieve the patient's symptoms and the patient does not meet the criteria for commitment. Another approach would be to have the patient declared incompetent and seek a court order permitting the medication. A guardian can also consent to medication when the patient's refusal can be shown to result from inability to make a rational decision.

Nurses should judge each situation on a case-by-case basis. Three criteria that may justify coerced treatment are as follows:

- The patient must be judged to be dangerous to self or others.
- It must be believed by those administering treatment that it has a reasonable chance of benefiting the patient.
- The patient must be judged to be incompetent to evaluate the necessity of the treatment.

Even if these three conditions are met, the patient should not be deceived but should be informed regarding what will be done, the reasons for it, and its probable effects.

Is the refusal of treatment the same as noncompliance? If not, how would you distinguish between them and what nursing intervention would be most appropriate for each?

Nurses are often on the front line in dealing with patients who refuse treatments and medications. It is clear that voluntary patients have the right to refuse any treatment and should not be forcibly medicated except in exceptional situations when the patient is actively violent to self or others and when all less restrictive means have been unsuccessful. The behavior of the patient should be clearly documented and all interventions recorded.

Nurses must know the guidelines identified by the courts and the legislature in the state in which they practice in order to administer medication properly to involuntarily committed patients. Some questions that can help guide the nurse's decision are:

- Has the patient been given a psychiatric diagnosis?
- Is the treatment consistent with the diagnosis?
- Is there a set of defined target symptoms?
- Has the patient been informed about the treatment outcome and side effects?
- Have medical and nursing assessments been completed?
- Are therapeutic effects of treatment being monitored?
- Are side effects being monitored?
- Is the patient overmedicated or undermedicated?
- Is drug therapy being changed too quickly?
- Are pro re nata (PRN) and stat doses being used too often?
- Is drug therapy being prescribed for an indefinite period of time?

Finally, it is important for the nurse to remember that a therapeutic nurse-patient relationship is critical in working with a patient who refuses to take medication. A positive, caring relationship between the nurse and patient can play a vital role in reversing treatment refusal.

Imagine that your mother was admitted to a psychiatric hospital in need of treatment. Once there, however, she refused to take any medication. How would you feel if the staff forced medication on her? How would you feel if they honored her right to refuse treatment? What could you do to help your mother get the treatment she needed?

Right to Treatment in the Least Restrictive Setting

The right to treatment in the least restrictive setting is closely related to the right to adequate treatment. Its goal is evaluating the needs of each patient and maintaining the greatest amount of personal freedom, autonomy, dignity, and integrity in determining treatment. This right applies to both hospital-based and community programs. Another consideration in the right to the least restrictive alternative is that it applies not only to when a person should be hospitalized but also to how a person is cared for. It requires that a patient's progress be carefully monitored so that treatment plans are changed based on the patient's current condition.

Issues related to the use of seclusion and restraints are of particular concern. There must be adequate rationale for the use of these practices. Documentation should include a description of the event that led to seclusion or restraint, alternatives attempted or considered, the patient's behavior while secluded or restrained, nursing interventions, and ongoing evaluation of the patient. It is important to remember that seclusion and restraint must be therapeutically indicated and justified (see Chapter 31).

Restriction has two aspects: (1) the nature of the choices being restricted and (2) the method by which choices are restricted. Box 10-4 presents a hierarchy of restrictiveness in which each item is a more stringent limitation of choice and thus a greater denial of liberty (Olsen, 1998). The list thus proceeds from the most restrictive to the least.

Box 10-4

Hierarchy of Restrictiveness

1. Body movement, for example, four-point restraint (hands and feet)
2. Movement in space, for example, seclusion rooms, restriction to the unit
3. Decisions of daily life, for example, selection of food or a television program, the choice of when or where to smoke or with whom to socialize
4. Meaningful activities, for example, participation in treatment, access to work
5. Treatment choice, for example, court-mandated treatment, unwanted social interventions
6. Control of resources, for example, use of money
7. Emotional or verbal expression, for example, censorship, discouraging personal expression

From Olsen D: Toward an ethical standard for coerced mental health treatment: least restrictive or most therapeutic? *J Clin Ethics* 9(3):235, 1998.

Which do you think is more restrictive—to be living in the community while actively psychotic or to be involuntarily committed to a psychiatric hospital for treatment?

Role of Nursing

The National League for Nursing (1977) issued a statement on the nurse's role in patients' rights. It identified respect and concern for patients and competent care as basic rights, along with patients receiving the necessary information to understand their illness and make decisions about their care. The League urged nurses to get involved in ensuring patients' human and legal rights.

The League identified many of the previously mentioned rights, plus the following:

- Right to health care that is accessible and meets professional standards, regardless of the setting
- Right to courteous and individualized health care that is equitable, humane, and given without discrimination based on race, color, creed, sex, national origin, source of payment, or ethical or political beliefs
- Right to information about their diagnosis, prognosis, and treatment, including alternatives to care and risks involved
- Right to information about the qualifications, names, and titles of health-care personnel
- Right to refuse observation by those not directly involved in their care
- Right to coordination and continuity of health care
- Right to information on the charges for services, including the right to challenge these charges
- Above all, the right to be fully informed about all their rights in all health-care settings

Perhaps the single most important factor is the attitude of mental health professionals. Sensitivity to patients' rights cannot be imposed by the court, the legislature, administrative agencies, or professional groups. If nurses ignore them, implement them casually, or are outwardly hostile about honoring them, patients' rights are an empty legal concept. But if professionals are sensitive to patients' needs in all aspects of their relationships with them, they will secure these human and legal rights.

Ethical Considerations

Ensuring patients' rights is often complicated by ethical considerations. For example, consider the crucial element of power. In the psychiatric setting the nurse can function in many roles, from a custodial keeper of the keys to a skilled therapist. Each of these roles includes a certain amount of power because all nurses have the ability to influence the patient's treatment and serve as the major source of information regarding a patient's behavior. This is particularly true in inpatient settings, in which a nurse and patient spend more time together and the nursing staff is the only group to work a 24-hour day. Nurses also participate in team meetings, individual and group psychotherapy, and behavior modification programs. Finally, nurses can greatly influence decisions about patient medications, such as type, dosage, and frequency.

Many ethical dilemmas arise from health-care professionals' paternalistic attitude toward patients (Breeze, 1998; Horsfall, 1998). Paternalism can be defined as deciding what is best for another person without consideration of the person's thoughts or feelings. It occurs when something is done "for the patient's own good" even though the patient would probably disagree with the action. This attitude reduces adult patients to the status of children and interferes with their freedom of action.

The right to treatment also poses several ethical questions. One involves the appropriateness of treatment and whether confinement itself can be therapeutic. A second question deals with the untreatable patient. Should such a patient be released after a certain time? Another problem is the unwilling patient. Might a person refuse treatment and then seek release, claiming that the right to adequate treatment was denied?

Ethical dilemmas also arise in considering the right to refuse treatment. Does the right apply to all treatments, including medications, or only to those that are hazardous, intrusive, or severe? How can staff meet their obligation for the right to treatment when a patient refuses to be treated? How can refusal, resisting treatment, and noncompliance be differentiated, and does each of these require a different response? There are no solutions to these complex issues, but they concern nurses, who are often responsible for delivering prescribed treatments such as medications.

Finally, the right to treatment in the least restrictive setting raises a number of difficult questions. How do mental health professionals balance human rights with the human needs of patients? Are sufficient funds available to provide adequate supportive care in the community? Can community centers provide better care than institutions? How can one counter community resistance to local placement of mentally ill patients? And most important, given economic constraints, how can limited resources be used wisely to provide a full range of needed mental health services?

Ethical Dilemmas

An ethical dilemma exists when moral claims conflict with one another (see Chapter 12). It can be defined as:

- A difficult problem that seems to have no satisfactory solution
- A choice between equally unsatisfactory alternatives

Ethical dilemmas pose such questions as "What should I do?" and "What is the right thing to do?" They can occur both at the nurse-patient-family level of daily nursing care and at the policymaking level of institutions and communities. Although ethical dilemmas arise in all areas of nursing practice, some are unique to psychiatric and mental health nursing. Many of these dilemmas fall under the umbrella issue of behavior control.

At first glance, behavior control may seem a simple issue: Behavior is a personal choice, and any behavior that does not impose on the rights of others is acceptable. Unfortunately, this does not help to address complex situations. For example, a severely depressed person may choose suicide as an alternative to an intolerable existence. On one level, this is an individual choice not directly harming others, yet suicide is forbidden in American society. In many states it is a crime that can be prosecuted. As another example, in some states it is illegal for consenting adults of the same sex to have sexual relations, although it is not illegal for a man to rape his wife. These examples raise difficult questions: When is it appropriate for society to regulate personal behavior? Who will make this decision? Is its goal personal adjustment, personal growth, or adaptation to social norms? And finally, how do we measure the costs and benefits of attempting to control personal freedom in a free society?

One of the most fundamental problems is the blurry line between science and ethics in the field of psychiatry. Theoretically, science and ethics are separate entities. Science is descriptive, deals with what is, and rests on validation; ethics is predictive, deals with what ought to be, and relies on judgment. However, psychiatry is neither purely scientific nor value-free.

Despite these ambiguities, nurses must identify their professional commitment. Are they committed to the happiness of the individual or the smooth functioning of society? Ideally, these values should not conflict, but in reality they sometimes do. The patient's rights to treatment, to refuse treatment, and to informed consent highlight this conflict-of-interest question. Nurses must consider whether they are forcing patients to be socially or politically acceptable at the expense of patients' personal happiness. Nurses may not be working for either the patient's best interests or their own; they may be acting as agents of society and not be aware of it.

All nurses participate in some therapeutic psychiatric regimens whose scientific and ethical bases are ambiguous. The American health-care system continues to apply a medical model of wellness and illness to human behavior. Wellness is socially acceptable behavior, and illness is socially unacceptable. It becomes critically important for each nurse to analyze such ethical dilemmas as freedom of choice versus coercion, helping versus imposing values, and focusing on cure versus prevention. The nurse must also become active in defining adequate treatment and deciding important resource allocations.

LEGISLATIVE INITIATIVES

The connection between psychiatry and the law is becoming increasingly complex. Mental health professionals are concerned about the quantity and quality of psychiatric care. Legal reformers are indignant about perceived violations of patients' rights. Judges are angry that in the day-to-day implementation of the commitment law, their only option is to prosecute the mentally ill defendant. Psychiatric hospitals are understaffed, underfunded, and attacked on all sides for their inability to care for and cure psychiatric patients. Community programs are few and poorly supported, often resulting in deinstitutionalized patients living without treatment in urban ghettos or being treated as criminals. The public is frightened at the thought of psychiatric patients in their neighborhoods. Concerned citizens demand that mental health programs exercise greater control over this population, whom they perceive as dangerous.

Clearly, mechanisms are needed by which patients, families, mental health professionals, attorneys, and concerned citizens can work together to advance mental health care and the rights of all patients. The mentally ill need protection not only of their legal rights but also of their clinical needs and general welfare. No one profession can fulfill all these needs, but increased cooperation among mental health advocates can achieve this goal.

Federal Budget Acts

Legislation has changed the nature of psychiatric care and service delivery in the United States. One major event was passage of the Omnibus Budget Reconciliation Act (OBRA) in 1981. It placed mental health service programs formerly administered by the federal government into alcohol and drug abuse and mental health service block grants to be administered by the states. Overall, this had a negative impact on the quality of mental health services provided throughout the United States because each state was able to allocate resources to mental health based on its own priorities and political climate. Although some states made significant progress in developing community-based systems, in most state governments mental health funding was not given high priority.

In 1985 the Consolidated OBRA (COBRA) prohibited the transfer of indigent patients with acute medical conditions from general medical hospitals or emergency departments to public psychiatric hospitals that are ill equipped to provide medical care. The OBRA passed in 1987 established criteria for Medicaid- or Medicare-certified nursing homes to use in admitting or retaining mentally ill patients. The effect of this law was to reduce the use of antipsychotic medications and physical restraints in nursing homes (Snowden & Roy-Byrne, 1998).

The federal Balanced Budget Act of 1997 (Public Law 105-33) led to further restrictions in mental health services, especially for the severely mentally ill. Programs such as Medicare as well as Medicaid and disability benefits have been decreased or are being phased out.

Protection and Advocacy Act

Under the Protection and Advocacy for Mentally Ill Individuals Act of 1986, all states must designate an agency that is responsible for protecting the rights of the mentally ill. The following three areas of advocacy help to maximize the fulfillment of patients' rights:

- To educate the mental health staff and implement policies and procedures that recognize and protect patients' rights
- To establish an additional procedure to permit the speedy resolution of problems, questions, or disagreements that occur based on legal rights
- To provide access to legal services when patients' rights have been denied

In addition to representing individuals, protection and advocacy programs agencies provide referral and information services, public education, outreach, training, and class-action representation (Olley & Ogloff, 1995; Sundram, 1995). As mental health systems change and more patients are treated in outpatient settings, access to protection and advocacy services for people living in the community is becoming increasingly important and psychiatric nurses have the opportunity to participate in these initiatives (Spratlen, 1997).

Americans with Disabilities Act

The Americans with Disabilities Act (ADA), passed in 1990, protects over 43 million Americans with physical or mental disabilities from discrimination in jobs, public services, and accommodations. It prohibits discrimination against people with physical and mental disabilities in hiring, firing, training, compensation, and advancement in employment. Employers are prohibited from asking job applicants whether they have a disability, and medical examinations and questions about disability may be required only if the concerns are job related and necessary (Wasserbauer, 1997).

Each of these prohibitions has major implications for people with psychiatric disabilities. However, because the disability is often not obvious, and because of widespread stigma and discrimination, or simply as a statement of self-sufficiency, many people choose not to identify themselves as disabled. If they do, there is concern that employers and co-workers will assume that any work or personal difficulties the person has are related to the psychiatric disability. Thus discrimination and unintended negative consequences in psychiatric disability coverage has been one outcome of the ADA (Appelbaum, 1998b; Campbell & Kaufmann, 1997).

Although the act has produced some encouraging advances in job placement, education, and training, the majority of people with psychiatric disabilities remain unemployed or continue to work in sheltered settings (see Citing the Evidence on p. 177). Between 1992 and 1996, almost 13% of ADA claims were based on "emotional" or "psychi-

Citing the Evidence on

The ADA and Employment Practices

BACKGROUND: Little is known about the impact the ADA has had on employment practices, or on employers' efforts to provide a supportive work environment. This study reports on the response of the business community to the ADA with a specific focus on the employment of those with mental disabilities.

RESULTS: Of the businesses that reported complying with ADA, 15% had specific policies for hiring those with mental disabilities, and 38% had hired such individuals. These companies were more likely to be large and to have specific policies for the hiring of minorities and those with physical disabilities. Employers did not believe that hiring those with mental disabilities was their responsibility and supported increased efforts by the rehabilitation community to improve employment opportunities for individuals with mental disabilities.

IMPLICATIONS: Mental health providers need to work more closely with employers in their regions and educate them about the capabilities of people with mental disabilities. They also need to inform employers that the types of accommodations necessary are neither costly nor difficult to implement.

Scheid T: The Americans with Disabilities Act, Mental Disability, and Employment Practices, *J Behav Health Serv Res* 25(3):312, 1998.

atric" impairments, with the greatest number of those based on depressive illness. This figure excludes mental retardation. The ADA disability most often reported was back problems, which accounted for nearly 20% of claims.

Partly because of the ambiguity of the wording of the act, instructions were issued in 1995 to eliminate pregnancy, physical characteristics, common personality traits, cultural and economic disadvantages, a range of sexual disorders, and current illegal drug use. In 1997 the Equal Employment Opportunity Commission (EEOC) issued guidelines on how the ADA applies to psychiatric disabilities. The user-friendly question-and-answer format and examples contained in the guidelines will be helpful to consumers, families, and advocates seeking better understanding of the specific requirements of this important law (EEOC, 1997).

Unfortunately, a study reported that the majority of psychiatric nurses surveyed did not have the knowledge necessary to act as advocates with respect to the ADA. Moreover, few psychiatric nurses in the study had provided patients with ADA information (Wasserbauer, 1996). Nonetheless, the act does constitute a cultural as well as legal mandate to include people with disabilities in the social and economic mainstream. It is not likely to totally eliminate the myths,

fears, and discrimination faced by people with disabilities, but it does contribute to the educational effort needed to combat widespread biases and misperceptions about people with disabilities, including mental illness.

> *Early in the semester, one of your friends shared with you that she has been diagnosed with bipolar disorder and has been successfully stabilized with treatment. One day she arrives in class very agitated and verbal. How might you interpret this behavior? Would your interpretation be different if she had not shared her psychiatric history with you?*

Advanced Directives

Advanced directives came about as a result of the Patient Self-Determination Act (PSDA) of 1990. They are documents, written while a person is competent, that specify how decisions about treatment should be made if the person becomes incompetent. The Bazelon Center for Mental Health Law (1998) has sample forms or templates that can be used to prepare such a directive.

Use of advanced directives is particularly appropriate for people with mental illness who may alternate between periods of competence and incompetence. For example, they could formalize a patient's wishes about forced medication, treatment approach, treatment setting, methods to handle emergencies, persons who should be notified, and willingness to participate in research studies.

Some states are encouraging patients to fill out advanced directive forms (Backlar & McFarland, 1996). In addition, federal regulations require all facilities that receive Medicare or Medicaid to inform patients, including psychiatric patients, at admission about their rights under state law to sign advanced directives. To date, advanced directives have not had a major impact on psychiatric treatment, but that may change. Potential effects of mental health advanced directives include enhanced consumer empowerment; improved functioning; better communication among consumers, family members, and providers; increased tolerance for consumer autonomy in community mental health agencies; and reduced use of hospital services and court proceedings (Srebnik & La Fond, 1999).

> *Does your psychiatric setting comply with federal law that requires having patients sign advanced directives? If so, talk with some patients and ask them what this document means to them.*

PSYCHIATRY AND CRIMINAL RESPONSIBILITY

The determination of criminal responsibility concerns the accused person's condition when the crime was committed. It has received much public attention as the "insanity defense." It proposes that a person who has committed an act usually considered criminal is not guilty by reason of "insanity." This is a difficult decision to make (Gutheil, 1999;

Reid, 1998). Defense attorneys often call on psychiatrists to testify (Slovenko, 1995). Nurses are seldom directly involved, but they should understand the law in this area as both citizens and psychiatric professionals.

This defense is based on the humanitarian rationale that people should not be blamed for crimes if they did not know what they were doing or could not help themselves. With the complexity of today's society and judicial system, however, many believe that this defense is being abused, but this belief is not supported by evidence (Janofsky, 1996). One more recent change is the movement away from using the defense "not guilty by reason of insanity" (NGBI) to the more recent "guilty but mentally ill" (GBMI). In addition, three states—Montana, Idaho, and Utah—have abolished the insanity defense completely.

Three sets of criteria are used in the United States to determine the criminal responsibility of an offender who is mentally ill: the M'Naghten Test, the Irresistible Impulse Test, and the American Law Institute's Test (Table 10-2). The American Law Institute's Test is the one most often used.

> *In the 1994 case of Lorena Bobbitt, who was found not guilty by reason of insanity, the jury concluded that she could not resist the impulse to sever her husband's penis. Mrs. Bobbitt was committed to a psychiatric hospital for observation and was released when she was found not to be psychiatrically ill. Do you agree with the court's decision? Defend your position.*

Disposition of Mentally Ill Offenders

Those found not guilty by reason of insanity (NGBI) are rarely set free. In some states they may be committed at the court's discretion, and in almost a third of the states they are automatically hospitalized. Some offenders are treated in special hospitals, others are sent to state mental hospitals, and still others go to prison treatment facilities. Those found guilty but mentally ill (GBMI) are never freed. Because the insanity defense is used most often in capital offenses, it is usually better to have good security, and penal institutions or maximum security forensic psychiatric hospitals are the best option.

After hospitalization and recovery the patient may be discharged by the court that ordered the commitment. In other states the governor may discharge the patient. Still others al-

low the mental institution to make that decision. The major criteria for discharge are that the patient is not likely to repeat the offense and that it is safe to release the patient to the community.

> *Do you believe in the legal defenses of NGBI and GBMI? What are the pros and cons of each insanity defense?*

LEGAL ROLE OF THE NURSE

Professional nursing practice is not determined by simply following patients' rights. Rather, it is an interplay between the rights of patients, the legal role of the nurse, and concern for quality psychiatric care (Fig.10-4). The psychiatric nurse performs three roles while completing professional and personal responsibilities: provider of services, employee or contractor of services, and private citizen. These roles are simultaneous, and each carries certain rights and responsibilities.

Nurse as Provider

Malpractice. All psychiatric professionals have legally defined duties of care and are responsible for their own work. If these duties are violated, malpractice exists. Malpractice involves the failure of professionals to provide the

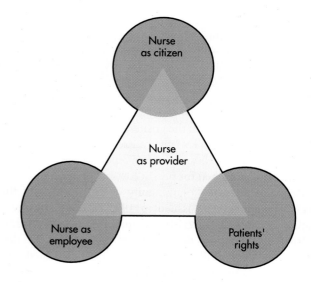

Fig. 10-4 Legal influences on psychiatric nursing practice.

Table **10-2**

Three Sets of Criteria Used to Determine the Criminal Responsibility of a Mentally Ill Offender	
Name of Test	Criteria
M'Naghten Test	The person did not know the nature and quality of the act. The person did not know that the act was wrong.
Irresistible Impulse Test	A person is impulsively driven to commit the criminal act with lack of premeditation and a strong urge to do so. This test is usually used with the M'Naghten test.
American Law Institute's Test	A person lacks the capacity to appreciate the wrongfulness of an act or to conform conduct to the requirements of the law. It excludes the sociopath and is the most common criterion for determining criminal responsibility.

proper and competent care that is given by members of their profession, resulting in harm to the patient. Nurses are held to national standards of care.

Most malpractice claims are filed under the law of negligent tort. A tort is a civil wrong for which the injured party is entitled to compensation. Under the law, individuals are responsible for their own torts, so each nurse can be held responsible in malpractice claims. For this reason, all nurses should carry malpractice liability insurance. Under the law of negligent tort the plaintiff must prove the following:

- A legal duty of care existed.
- The nurse performed the duty negligently.
- Damages were suffered by the plaintiff as a result.
- The damages were substantial.

When patients are admitted to a psychiatric hospital, the problems of litigation in connection with their care are many and varied.

Box 10-5

Common Areas of Liability in Psychiatric Services

- Sexual contact with a patient
- Patient suicide
- Failure to diagnose
- Problems related to electroconvulsive therapy
- Misuse of psychoactive prescription drugs
- Breach of confidentiality
- Failure to refer a patient
- False imprisonment in civil commitment
- Failure to obtain informed consent
- Inadequate supervision of trainees and employees
- Failure to warn potential victims
- Failure to report abuse

Litigation. Lawsuits alleging malpractice in psychiatric diagnosis or treatment are increasing. Some of the more common sources of malpractice suits are listed in Box 10-5. Lawsuits against nurses are uncommon. However, they can occur when the nurse errs while acting either dependently or independently. The most common causes of malpractice suits against psychiatric nurses are negligence in suicide precautions and while assisting in ETC. Other causes for malpractice suits against nurses include patient falls; failing to follow physician orders or established protocols; medication errors; improper use of equipment; failure to remove foreign objects; failure to provide sufficient monitoring; and failure to communicate (Eskreis, 1998; Fiesta, 1998). Box 10-6 describes three recent cases involving psychiatric nurses.

Legal Responsibilities. The nurse is responsible for reporting pertinent information to co-workers involved in the patient's care. The degree of nursing care depends on the patient's condition, with the seriously ill demanding a higher degree of care to protect them from injury and self-destruction.

Reporting information includes written as well as oral communication, and accurate records are crucial. Box 10-7 lists characteristics of good nursing records. For example, notes that record specific suicidal precautions clarify the nurse's actions. The nurse should also record all patient and family education such as explaining the food precautions needed when taking monoamine oxidase inhibitor (MAOI) medication. Such a note would provide a good defense against a possible lawsuit should the patient violate dietary restrictions and become ill.

Unlike patients' charts, some hospital records, such as incident reports, are not admissible in court to prove facts but they can cast doubt on the credibility of the involved parties. Currently, many insurance companies are requiring hospitals to keep incident reports, and more state and federal

Box 10-6

Selected Litigation Involving Psychiatric Nurses

CASE 1: VALENTINE V. STRANGE (597 F. SUPP. 1316 VA.)

Problem: Nurses were sued when psychiatric patient set self on fire. **Facts:** Despite two previous attempts to burn herself, the health-care providers permitted the patient to keep her cigarettes and lighter. Patient subsequently set fire to her clothing and suffered third-degree burns.

Legal lesson: The failure of health-care professionals to take precautions in the face of imminent danger to the life of an involuntarily committed patient constitutes a violation of liberty interests protected by the due process clause of the Fourteenth Amendment.

CASE 2: DELICATA V. BOURLESSES (404 N.E. 2ND 667-MASS.)

Problem: Nursing psychiatric assessment disagreed with the psychologist's assessment. **Facts:** A nursing assessment indicated that a depressed patient should be closely supervised as potentially suicidal. An evaluation by the staff psychologist advised that suicidal precautions were not necessary. The patient subsequently killed herself in a locked bathroom.

Legal lesson: Medical orders by a staff psychiatrist or an evaluation by a staff psychologist must be questioned when there is a change or deterioration in a patient's condition. Nursing assessments should include the evaluation of such changes in the patient's apparent physical and psychological condition. The responsibility of nursing assessment includes the necessity for making appropriate nursing judgments and implementing nursing actions based on these nursing assessments.

CASE 3: VATTIMO V. LOWER BUCKS HOSPITAL (428 A. 2ND 765-PA.)

Problem: Patient required restraint and supervision by psychiatric nurses. **Facts:** A patient with a psychotic fascination with fire set fire to his hospital room, resulting in the death of the other occupant. The patient had been diagnosed as a paranoid schizophrenic, and staff had been warned of his preoccupation with fire.

Legal lesson: The hospital was required to exercise reasonable care under the circumstances to restrain, supervise, and protect mentally deficient patients.

Box 10-7

Characteristics of Good Nursing Records

- Accurate
- Clear
- Complete
- Concise
- Descriptive
- Factual
- Legible
- Objective
- Relevant
- Timely

agencies are demanding the right to review them. Because they can be seen and used by so many people, what a nurse writes on an incident report should be carefully considered, and unfounded statements, opinions, interpretations, and vague descriptions should be avoided.

In summary, a psychiatric nurse can follow these preventive measures to avoid possible lawsuits:

- Implement nursing care that meets the *Scope and Standards of Psychiatric–Mental Health Clinical Nursing Practice* as described by the American Nurses' Association (2000) (see Chapters 11 and 12).
- Know the laws of the specific state, including the rights and duties of the nurse as well as the rights of the patients.
- Stay current with advances and new knowledge in the field.
- Keep accurate and concise nursing records.
- Maintain the confidentiality of patient information.
- Maintain current malpractice liability insurance coverage.
- Consult a lawyer if any questions arise.

Nurse as Employee

The role of the employee, or contractor of service, is less often studied but also very important. It involves the practitioner's rights and responsibilities in relation to employers, partners, consultants, and other professional colleagues. Professionals often do not know the rights and responsibilities of employees and contractors of service. However, these are the basis of the practitioner's economic security, professional future, and peer relationships.

As employees, nurses have the responsibility to supervise and evaluate those under their authority for the quality of care given. They must also observe their employer's rights and responsibilities to clients and other employees, fulfill the obligations of the contracted service, inform the employer of circumstances and conditions that impair the quality of care, and report negligent care by others. This includes the legal duty to communicate any concerns about other nurses and other mental health professionals (DeMarco, 1998).

You have seen a colleague sexually touching a patient on the unit. What should you do based on your legal and professional obligations?

In return, nurses can expect certain rights from their employer. These include consideration for service, adequate working conditions, adequate and qualified assistance when necessary, documented grievance procedures, and the right to respect all of their other rights and responsibilities.

You arrive for work one morning and are told that you and an aide are the only staff assigned to work the day shift on a 25-bed closed acute psychiatric unit. Based on your legal roles, rights, and responsibilities, how should you respond?

Nurse as Citizen

The third role that the nurse plays is that of citizen. This role is significant because all other roles, rights, responsibilities, and privileges are based on the inherent rights of citizenship. The U.S. government grants these as inherent: civil rights, property rights, right to protection from harm, right to a good name, and right to due process. These form the foundation for the nurse's other legal relationships. Unfortunately, the best interests of the patient, nurse, and employer do not always coincide. Conflict can occur when, for example, the nurse's right to live and work without threat to personal security is violated by a patient who harms the nurse, as is evident in the following clinical example.

 CLINICAL EXAMPLE

A psychotic patient who has hallucinations that are adequately controlled with psychotropic medications but who refuses to take them was recently admitted to a locked psychiatric unit. Before intervening, the staff considered the following possibilities:

- Failing to medicate may deny the patient's right to treatment.
- Failing to medicate the patient could have harmful side effects, such as the unnecessary and possibly irreversible continuation of illness.
- Failing to medicate the patient may lead to a psychotic episode and result in injury to self, other patients, or the staff.
- Failing to medicate the patient may lead to a psychotic episode but no violence.
- Medicating the patient in the absence of an emergency situation and without a clear threat of violence violates the patient's right to refuse treatment.

The staff decided not to medicate the patient. When the night nurse checked on the patient in his room that evening, he struck the nurse in the face, resulting in severe bruises and the loss of several teeth. This development leads to new questions:

- Was the patient competent and legally liable for his actions?
- What were the circumstances of the incident?
- Was the nurse sufficiently aware of the potential hazard and, if so, was she responsible for assuming the risk?
- Was staffing adequate to discourage, respond to, and control a potentially violent situation?
- Was there a provision in the unit for potentially violent patients and, if so, why wasn't it used for this patient?
- Was the nurse able to sue the patient for assault and battery?

Obviously, there are no simple or perhaps even equitable solutions to such clinical dilemmas, yet they are real and ever present. All mental health professionals must focus on prevention. This requires a knowledge of legislation, rights, responsibilities, and potential conflicts. In addition, professional nursing judgment requires examining the context of nursing care, the possible consequences of nurses' actions, and practical alternatives. Only then do rights and responsibilities become meaningful.

Summary

1. There are two types of admission to a psychiatric hospital: voluntary and involuntary commitment. Involuntary commitment poses many legal and ethical issues for patients, the law, and psychiatric professionals.

2. Involuntary community treatment mandates a course of outpatient treatment. It can be provided in three ways: outpatient commitment, preventive commitment, and conditional release.

3. Psychiatric patients have a wide variety of personal and civil rights. They should be informed of these rights, and hospitals must honor them. Some of these rights are controversial and create dilemmas for psychiatric nurses.

4. Current legislative initiatives that affect ethical psychiatric care provided in the United States include Budget Acts, the Protection and Advocacy Act, the Americans with Disabilities Act, and Advanced Directives.

5. Three sets of criteria are used in the United States to determine the criminal responsibility of an offender who is mentally ill: the M'Naghten Test, the Irresistible Impulse Test, and the American Law Institute's Test, which is the one most often used.

6. The psychiatric nurse has three roles in performing professional and personal duties: provider of services, employee or contractor of services, and private citizen.

 Visit MERLIN: www.mosby.com/MERLIN/Stuart to find these additional materials and student activities.

- **Worksheets**
- **"Drug of the Month" Updates**
- **"Citing the Evidence" Updates**
- **Critical Thinking Activities and Exercises**
- **Annotated Suggested Readings**
- **Web Links**
- **More!**

Chapter Review Questions

1. **Identify whether the following statements are true (T) or false (F).**

___ A. Patients who are voluntarily admitted to a psychiatric hospital retain all civil rights.

___ B. The parens patriae doctrine for civil commitment is currently emphasized over the police power rationale.

___ C. The profile of the patient at greatest risk for involuntary admission is that of a white, middle-aged woman with depression.

___ D. People with mental illness are more likely to commit acts of violence than other people.

___ E. Involuntary community treatment is underused in the current mental health-care system.

___ F. *Incompetent* is a legal term without precise medical meaning.

___ G. Police and lawyers are always entitled to information about committed psychiatric patients.

___ H. Information can be released without a patient's consent when it is related to child custody disputes.

___ I. Patients are allowed to keep their records when they are discharged from treatment.

___ J. Mental illness is the most commonly reported disability reported under the American Disabilities Act.

___ K. None of the states in the United States have abolished the insanity defense.

2. **Fill in the blanks.**

A. Emergency commitment is usually limited to _____ hours.

B. Psychiatric patients who appear to be prone to violence display a _____, _____, and _____.

C. _____ is the process by which courts can order patients committed to a course of outpatient treatment specified by their clinicians.

D. Informed consent must be _____, _____, and _____.

E. The _____ act mandates that all states designate an agency that is responsible for protecting the rights of the mentally ill.

F. Documents, written while a person is competent, that specify how decisions about treatment should be made if the person becomes incompetent are called

_____.

G. The most commonly used criterion to determine the criminal responsibility of an offender in the United States is the _____.

3. Provide short answers for the following questions.

A. List the three grounds that permit commitment or involuntary hospitalization of the mentally ill. Do you believe these are justifiable? Defend your answer.

B. How is confidentiality different from privilege or testimonial privilege? If you were seeing a therapist, would the concept of privileged communication be important to you? Why or why not?

C. What is the duty to warn and how might it affect you first as a nurse and then as a citizen?

D. Describe an ethical dilemma you have experienced in relation to your psychiatric nursing experience and the process you used to choose a course of action.

REFERENCES

American Hospital Association: *A patient's bill of rights,* Chicago, 1990, The Association.

American Nurses' Association: *Scope and standards of psychiatric—mental health nursing practice,* Washington, DC, 2000, The Association.

Applebaum P: A "health information infrastructure" and the threat to confidentiality of health records, *Psychiatr Serv* 49(1):27, 1998a.

Appelbaum P: Discrimination in psychiatric disability coverage and the Americans with Disabilities Act, *Psychiatr Serv* 49(7):875, 1998b.

Appelbaum P: Informed consent to psychotherapy: recent developments, *Psychiatr Serv* 48(4):445, 1997.

Asnis G et al: Violence and homicidal behaviors in psychiatric disorders, *Psychiatr Clin North Am* 20(2):405, 1997.

Backlar P, McFarland B: A survey on use of advance directives for mental health treatment in Oregon, *Psychiatr Serv* 47:1387, 1996.

Bazelon Center for Mental Health Law: *Psychiatric advance directive,* Washington, DC, 1998, Bazelon Center.

Bazelon Center for Mental Health Law: *Position statement on involuntary commitment,* Washington, DC, 1999, Bazelon Center.

Beck J: Legal and ethical duties of the clinician treating a patient who is liable to be impulsively violent, *Behav Sci Law,* 16:375, 1998.

Binder R, McNiel D: Application of the Tarasoff ruling and its effect on the victim and the therapeutic relationship, *Psychiatr Serv* 47:1212, 1996.

Bogart T, Solomon P: Procedures to share treatment information among mental health providers, consumers and families, *Psychiatr Serv* 50(10):1321, 1999.

Bonta J et al: The prediction of criminal and violent recidivism among mentally disordered offenders: a meta analysis, *Psychol Bull* 123(2):123, 1998.

Borum R et al: Consumer perceptions of involuntary outpatient commitment, *Psychiatr Serv* 50(11):1489, 1999.

Breeze J: Can paternalism be justified in mental health care? *J Adv Nurs* 28(2):260, 1998.

Campbell J, Kaufmann C: Equality and difference in the ADA: unintended consequences for employment of people with mental health disabilities. In Bonnie R, Monahan J, editors: *Mental disorder, work disability, and the law,* Chicago, 1997, The University of Chicago.

Curry J, Beck J: The legal evolution of the Tarasoff doctrine: implications and applications for the practicing clinician, *J Pract Psychiatry Behav Health* 3:203, 1997.

DeMarco R: Caring to confront in the workplace: an ethical perspective for nurses, *Nurs Outlook* 46(3):130, 1998.

Dickenson D: Ethical issues in long term psychiatric management, *J Med Ethics* 23:300, 1997.

Equal Opportunity Employment Commission: *EEOC enforcement guidelines on the American with disabilities act and psychiatric disabilities,* Washington, DC, 1997, Publications Distribution Center.

Engleman N et al: Clinicians' decision making about involuntary commitment, *Psychiatr Serv* 49(7):941, 1998.

Eskreis T: Seven common legal pitfalls in nursing, *Am J Nurs* 9(4):34, 1998.

Felthous A: The clinician's duty to protect third parties, *Psychiatr Clin North Am* 22(1):49, 1999.

Fiesta J: Psychiatric liability: parts 1, 2 and 3, *Nurs Manage* 27(7,8,9):10,18,16, 1998.

Fulwiler C et al: Early-onset substance abuse and community violence by outpatients with chronic mental illness, *Psychiatr Serv* 48(9):1181, 1997.

Geller J: On being "committed" to treatment in the community, *Innovations Res* 2:23, 1993.

Geller J et al: The rights of state hospital patients: from state hospitals to their alternatives, *Admin Policy Ment Health* 25(4):387, 1998a.

Geller J et al: The efficacy of involuntary outpatient treatment in Massachusetts, *Admin Policy Ment Health* 25(3):271, 1998b.

Grisso T et al: The MacCAT-T: a clinical tool to assess patients' capacities to make treatment decisions, *Psychiatr Serv* 48(11):1415, 1997.

Group for the Advancement of Psychiatry: *Forced into treatment: the role of coercion in clinical practice,* Washington, DC, 1994, American Psychiatric Press.

Gutheil T: A confusion of tongues: competence, insanity, psychiatry, and the law, *Psychiatr Serv* 50(6):767, 1999.

Horsfall J: Structural impediments to effective communication, *Aust N Z J Ment Health Nurs* 7:74, 1998.

Janofsky J et al: Insanity defense pleas in Baltimore City: an analysis of outcome, *Am J Psychiatry* 153:1464, 1996.

Kanapaux W: Outpatient commitment builds momentum, *Behav Healthcare Tomorrow* 8:12, 1999.

Lucksted A, Coursey R: Consumer perceptions of pressure and force in psychiatric treatments, *Psychiatr Serv* 46:146, 1995.

Mason T: Tarasoff liability: its impact for working with patients who threaten others, *Internat J Nurs Stud* 35:109, 1998.

McGihon N: Discharges against medical advice: provider accountability and psychiatric patients' rights, *J Psychosoc Nurs* 36(1):22, 1998.

National Bioethics Advisory Commission: *Research involving persons with mental disorders that may affect decisionmaking capacity,* Washington, DC, 1998, The Commission.

National League for Nursing: *Nursing's role in patient's rights,* Pub No 11-1671, New York, 1977, The League.

Olley M, Ogloff J: Patients' rights advocacy: implications for program design and implementation, *J Ment Health Admin* 22:368, 1995.

Olsen D: Toward an ethical standard for coerced mental health treatment: least restrictive or most therapeutic? *J Clin Ethics* 9(3):235, 1998.

Reid W: Evaluating criminal defendants: responsibility and competence to stand trial, *J Pract Psychiatry Behav Health* 4:373, 1998.

Roberts L: The ethical basis of psychiatric research: conceptual issues and empirical findings, *Comp Psychiatry* 39(3):99, 1998.

Roberts L et al: Perspectives of patients with schizophrenia and psychiatrists regarding ethically important aspects of research participation, *Am J Psychiatry* 157(1):67, 2000.

Ross R et al: A framework for classifying state involuntary commitment statutes, *Admin Policy Ment Health* 23:341, 1996.

Sanguineti V et al: Retrospective study of 2200 involuntary psychiatric admissions and readmissions, *Am J Psychiatry* 153:392, 1996.

Shellow R: Maintaining privacy, *J Pract Psychiatry Behav Health* 4:377, 1998.

Slovenko R: *Psychiatry and criminal culpability,* New York, 1995, Wiley.

Smith C: Use of involuntary outpatient commitment in community care of the seriously and persistently mentally ill patient, *Issues Ment Health Nurs* 16:275, 1995.

Snowden M, Roy-Byrne P: Mental illness and nursing home reform: OBRA-87 ten years later, *Psychiatr Serv* 49(2):229, 1998.

Spratlen L: Ombudsman: a new role for advanced practice nurses in psychiatric-mental health care, *Perspect Psychiatr Care* 33(3):5, 1997.

Srebnik D, La Fond J: Advance directives for mental health treatment, *Psychiatr Serv* 50(7):919, 1999.

Sreenivasan S et al: Predictors of recidivistic violence in criminally insane and civilly committed psychiatric inpatients, *Internat J Law Psych* 20(2):279, 1997.

Steadman H et al: Violence by people discharged from acute psychiatric inpatient facilities and by others in the same neighborhood, *Arch Gen Psychiatry* 55:393, 1998.

Sundram C: Implementation and activities of protection and advocacy programs for persons with mental illness, *Psychiatr Serv* 46:702, 1995.

Susman J: The role of nurses in decision making and violence prevention, *J Psychosoc Nurs* 36:18, 1998.

Swartz M et al: Violence and severe mental illness: the effects of substance abuse and nonadherence to medication, *Am J Psychiatry* 155(2):226, 1998.

Swartz M et al: Can involuntary outpatient commitment reduce hospital recidivism?: findings from a randomized trial with severely mentally ill individuals, *Am J Psychiatry* 156(12):1968, 1999.

Tarasoff v Regents of the University of California et al, 1974, 529 p 2d 553.

Wasserbauer L: Psychiatric nurses' knowledge of the Americans with Disabilities Act, *Arch Psychiatr Nurs* 10:328, 1996.

Wasserbauer L: Mental illness and the Americans with Disabilities Act: understanding the fundamentals, *J Psychosoc Nurs* 35:22, 1997.

Weinberger L et al: Extended civil commitment for dangerous psychiatric patients, *J Am Acad Psychiatr Law* 26(1):75, 1998.

Winick B: *The right to refuse mental health treatment,* Washington, DC, 1997, American Psychological Association.

Wirshing D et al: Informed consent: assessment of comprehension, *Am J Psychiatry* 155(11):1508, 1998.

Wolpe P et al: Psychiatric inpatients' knowledge of their rights, *Hosp Commun Psychiatry* 42:1168, 1991.

11 Implementing the Nursing Process: Standards of Care

Gail W. Stuart

To be what we are, and to become what we are capable of becoming, is the only end of life.

ROBERT L. STEVENSON, *FAMILIAR STUDIES OF MEN AND BOOKS*

The nurse-patient relationship is the vehicle for applying the nursing process. The goal of nursing care is to maximize the patient's positive interactions with the environment, promote a level of wellness, and enhance self-actualization. By establishing a therapeutic nurse-patient relationship and using the nursing process, the nurse strives to promote and maintain patient behavior that contributes to integrated functioning. This is the essence of the nursing therapeutic process and the framework on which this text is based.

In 1980 *Nursing: A Social Policy Statement* defined nursing as "the diagnosis and treatment of human responses to actual or potential health problems" (American Nurses' Association [ANA]). The 1995 update, *Nursing's Social Policy Statement* (ANA) added to this definition by acknowledging the following features of contemporary nursing practice:

- Attention to the full range of human experiences and responses to health and illness without restriction to a problem-focused orientation

- Integration of objective data with knowledge gained from an understanding of the patient or group's subjective experience
- Application of scientific knowledge to the processes of diagnosis and treatment
- Provision of a caring relationship that facilitates health and healing

Four defining characteristics of nursing are phenomena, theory, actions, and effects. These characteristics reflect the integration of education, practice, and research (Fig. 11-1). **Phenomena** refers to the need to understand the full range of human experiences and responses to health and illness. **Theory** is the conceptual model and research bases for psychiatric-mental health nursing practice. **Action** includes the nursing interventions used in the nursing process. **Effects** indicates the need to evaluate the outcomes of care provided.

This chapter discusses each component of the therapeutic nursing process as described in the newest version of the ANA *Scope and Standards of Psychiatric-Mental Health Clinical Nursing Practice* (ANA, 2000). The standards of professional performance are described in Chapter 12.

THE NURSING PROCESS

The nursing process is an interactive, problem-solving process. It is a systematic and individualized way to achieve the outcomes of nursing care. The nursing process respects the individual's autonomy and freedom to make decisions and be involved in nursing care. The nurse and patient emerge as partners in a relationship built on trust and directed toward maximizing the patient's strengths, maintaining integrity, and promoting adaptive responses to stress.

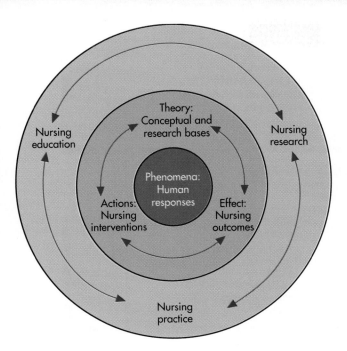

Fig. 11-1 Elements of nursing as an applied science.

❓ *Some psychotic patients are discouraged and dispirited by their illness. As a result, it may be difficult to engage them in the treatment process. What strategies might you use to connect with these patients and develop a therapeutic alliance with them?*

ASSESSMENT

STANDARD I: ASSESSMENT
The psychiatric-mental health nurse collects patient health data.

▼ *Rationale*

The assessment interview—which requires linguistically and culturally effective communication skills, interviewing, behavioral observation, record review, and comprehensive assessment of the patient and relevant systems—enables the psychiatric-mental health nurse to make sound clinical judgments and plan appropriate interventions with the patient.

▼ *Nursing conditions*
Self-awareness
Accurate observations
Therapeutic communication
Responsive dimensions of care

▼ *Nursing behaviors*
Establish nursing contract
Obtain information from patient and family
Validate data with patient
Organize data

▼ *Key elements*
Identify the patient's reason for seeking help
Assess for risk factors related to the patient's safety including potential for:
  Suicide or self-harm
  Assault or violence
  Substance abuse withdrawal
  Allergic reaction or adverse drug reaction
  Seizure
  Falls or accidents
  Elopement (if hospitalized)
  Physiological instability
Complete a biopsychosocial assessment of patient needs related to this treatment encounter including:
  Patient and family appraisal of health and illness
  Previous episodes of psychiatric care in self and family
  Current medications
  Physiological coping responses
  Mental status coping responses
  Coping resources, including motivation for treatment and functional supportive relationships
  Adaptive and maladaptive coping mechanisms
  Psychosocial and environmental problems
  Global assessment of functioning
  Knowledge, strengths, and deficits

In dealing with psychiatric patients, the nursing process can present unique challenges. Emotional problems may be vague and elusive, not tangible or visible like many physiological disruptions. Emotional problems also can show different symptoms and arise from a number of causes. Similar past events may lead to very different forms of present behavior. Many psychiatric patients are initially unable to describe their problems. They may be withdrawn, highly anxious, or out of touch with reality. Their ability to participate in the problem-solving process may also be limited if they see themselves as powerless victims or if their illness impairs them from fully engaging in the treatment process.

It is essential that the nurse and the patient become partners in the problem-solving process (Wilson & Hobbs, 1995). Nurses may be tempted to exclude patients, particularly if they resist becoming involved, but this should be avoided for two reasons. First, learning is most effective when patients participate in the learning experience. Second, by including patients as active participants in the nursing process, the nurse helps restore their sense of control over life and their responsibility for action. They reinforce the message that patients, whether they have an acute crisis or a serious and persistent mental illness, can choose either adaptive or maladaptive coping responses.

The phases of the nursing process as described by the *Scope and Standards of Psychiatric-Mental Health Clinical Nursing Practice* are assessment, diagnosis, outcome identification, planning, implementation, and evaluation. Validation is part of each step, and all phases may overlap or occur simultaneously. The nursing conditions and nursing behaviors related to each of these phases are shown in Fig. 11-2. Each of these phases as it applies to psychiatric nursing practice is now described.

In the assessment phase, information is obtained from the patient in a direct and structured manner through observations, interviews, and examinations. An assessment tool or nursing history form can provide a systematic format that becomes part of the patient's written record. This format enables the nurse to assess the patient's level of functioning and serves as a basis for diagnosis, outcome identification,

ASSESSMENT

NURSING CONDITIONS
Self-awareness
Accurate observations
Therapeutic communication
Responsive dimensions of care

NURSING BEHAVIORS
Establish nursing contract
Obtain information from patient and family
Validate data with patient
Organize data

DIAGNOSIS

NURSING CONDITIONS
Logical decision making
Knowledge of normal parameters
Inductive and deductive reasoning
Sociocultural sensitivity

NURSING BEHAVIORS
Identify patterns in data
Compare data with norms
Analyze and synthesize data
Problems and strengths identified
Validate problems with patient
Formulate nursing diagnosis
Set priorities of problems

OUTCOME IDENTIFICATION

NURSING CONDITIONS
Critical thinking skills
Partnership with patient
and family

NURSING BEHAVIORS
Hypothesizing
Specify expected outcomes
Validate goals with patient

PLANNING

NURSING CONDITIONS
Application of theory
Respect for patient and family

NURSING BEHAVIORS
Prioritize goals
Identify nursing activities
Validate plan with patient

IMPLEMENTATION

NURSING CONDITIONS
Past clinical experiences
Knowledge of research
Responsive and action
dimensions of care

NURSING BEHAVIORS
Consider available resources
Implement nursing activities
Generate alternatives
Coordinate with other team members

EVALUATION

NURSING CONDITIONS
Supervision
Self-analysis
Peer review
Patient and family participation

NURSING BEHAVIORS
Compare patient's responses and expected
outcome
Review nursing process
Modify nursing process as needed
Participate in quality improvement activities

Fig. 11-2 Nursing conditions and behaviors related to psychiatric nursing standards of care.

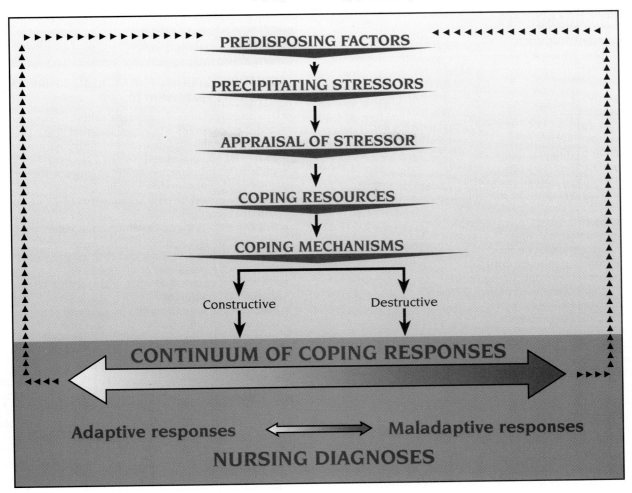

Fig. 11-3 The Stuart Stress Adaptation Model of psychiatric nursing care.

planning, implementation, and evaluation of nursing care. Using a specified data collection format helps ensure that the necessary information is obtained. It also reduces repetition of the patient's medical history and provides a source of information available to all health-care team members.

The nurse should also use the most appropriate psychological assessment tools and behavioral rating scales (see Chapter 7). These can help define current pretreatment aspects of the patient's problems, document the patient's progress over time and the efficacy of the treatment plan, and compare the patient's responses to those of groups of people with the same illness. This information can help formulate diagnoses and treatment plans, as well as document clinical outcomes of care.

The patient data identified in Standard I relate to all of the components of the Stuart Stress Adaptation Model (Fig. 11-3) used in this text: predisposing factors, precipitating stressors, appraisal of stressor, coping resources, coping mechanisms, and coping responses as described in Chapter 4.

The baseline data should reflect both content and process, and the patient is the ideal source of validation. The nurse should select a private place, free from noise and distraction, in which to interview the patient. Interviewing is a goal-directed method of communication that is required in a formal admission procedure. It should be focused but open ended, progressing from general to specific and allowing spontaneous patient self-expression. The nurse's role is to maintain the flow of the interview and to listen to the verbal and nonverbal messages conveyed by the patient. Nurses must also be aware of their responses to the patient.

Although the patient should be regarded as a source of validation, the nurse should also be prepared to consult with family members or other people knowledgeable about the patient. This is particularly important when the patient is unable to provide reliable information because of the symptoms of the psychiatric illness. The nurse might also consider using a variety of other information sources, including the patient's health-care record, nursing rounds, change-of-shift reports, nursing care plan, and evaluation by other health professionals such as psychologists, social workers, or psychiatrists. In using secondary sources, nurses should not simply accept the assessment of another health-care team member. Rather, they should apply the information they obtain to their nursing framework for data collection and formulate their own impressions and diagnoses. This brings another perspective to the work of the health-care team and an unbiased receptivity to patients and their problems.

NURSING DIAGNOSIS

STANDARD II: DIAGNOSIS

The psychiatric-mental health nurse analyzes the assessment data in determining diagnoses.

▼ *Rationale*

The basis for providing psychiatric-mental health nursing care is the recognition and identification of patterns of response to actual or potential psychiatric illnesses and mental health problems.

▼ *Nursing conditions*

Logical decision making
Knowledge of normal parameters
Inductive and deductive reasoning
Sociocultural sensitivity

▼ *Nursing behaviors*

Identify patterns in data
Compare data with norms
Analyze and synthesize data
Identify problems and strengths
Validate problems with patient
Formulate nursing diagnoses
Set priorities of problems

▼ *Key elements*

Diagnoses should reflect adaptive and maladaptive coping responses based on nursing frameworks such as those of the North American Nursing Diagnosis Association (NANDA).

Diagnoses should incorporate health problems or disease states such as those identified in the *Diagnostic and Statistical Manual of Mental Disorders* (*DSM–IV–TR*) (American Psychiatric Association, 2000) and the *International Classification Diseases and Statistical Manual of Mental Diseases* (WHO, 1993).

Diagnoses should focus on the phenomena of concern to psychiatric-mental health nurses as described in Box 11-1.

Box **11-1**

Psychiatric-Mental Health Nursing's Phenomena of Concern

ACTUAL OR POTENTIAL MENTAL HEALTH PROBLEMS OF PATIENTS PERTAINING TO:

- The maintenance of optimal health and well-being and the prevention of psychobiological illness
- Self-care limitations or impaired functioning related to mental and emotional distress
- Deficits in the functioning of significant biological, emotional, and cognitive systems
- Emotional stress or crisis components of illness, pain, and disability
- Self-concept changes, developmental issues, and life process changes
- Problems related to emotions such as anxiety, anger, sadness, loneliness, and grief
- Physical symptoms that occur along with altered psychological functioning
- Psychological symptoms that occur along with altered physiological functioning
- Alterations in thinking, perceiving, symbolizing, communicating, and decision making
- Difficulties in relating to others
- Behaviors and mental states that indicate that the patient is a danger to self or others or has a severe disability
- Symptom management, side effects/toxicities associated with psychopharmacological intervention, and other aspects of the treatment regimen
- Interpersonal, systemic, sociocultural, spiritual, or environmental circumstances or events that affect the mental and emotional well-being of the individual, family, or community

From American Nurses' Association: *Scope and standards of psychiatric-mental health clinical nursing practice*, Washington, DC, 2000, The Association.

NANDA diagnoses were first developed in 1973, while the DSM was first published in 1952. What impact do you think that this time difference has had on the use and acceptance of each classification system?

After collecting all data, the nurse compares the information to documented norms of health and adaptation. Because standards of behavior are culturally determined, the nurse should allow for both the patient's individual characteristics and the larger social group to which the patient belongs.

The nurse then analyzes the data and derives a nursing diagnosis. **A nursing diagnosis is a clinical judgment about individual, family, or community responses to actual or potential health problems/life processes. A nursing diagnosis provides the basis for selection of nursing interventions to achieve outcomes for which the nurse is accountable** (NANDA, 1999). The subject of nursing diagnoses is the patient's behavioral response to stress. This response, as represented in Fig. 11-3, may lie anywhere on the coping continuum from adaptive to maladaptive.

According to NANDA, the components of a nursing diagnosis are the label or name of the diagnosis; its definition; the defining characteristics of the diagnosis; related factors; and risk factors. The defining characteristics are particularly helpful because they reflect the behaviors that are the target of nursing intervention. They also provide specific indicators for evaluating the outcomes of psychiatric nursing interventions.

Relationship to Medical Diagnosis

The relationship between medicine and nursing includes sharing information, ideas, and analyses and developing appropriate care plans for the patient. Interventions are based on the nursing assessment as well as the medical evaluation and ensure a thorough and coordinated plan of treatment. Therefore, while formulating nursing diagnoses and using the nursing process, nurses should also be familiar with medical diagnoses and treatment plans.

A medical diagnosis is the health problem or disease state of the patient. In the medical model of psychiatry the health problems are mental disorders or mental illnesses. These are classified in the *DSM–IV–TR* (American Psychiatric Association, 2000) which comprehensively describes the symptoms of mental disorders but does not attempt to discuss cause or how the disturbances come about. However, specific diagnostic criteria are provided for each mental disorder. Chapters 3 and 4 of this text discuss the medical model and the *DSM–IV–TR* in greater detail.

If nurses are to be familiar with DSM–IV–TR medical diagnoses, should physicians be similarly knowledgeable about NANDA diagnoses?

OUTCOME IDENTIFICATION

STANDARD III: OUTCOME IDENTIFICATION
The psychiatric-mental health nurse identifies expected outcomes individualized to the patient.
▼ *Rationale*
Within the context of providing nursing care, the ultimate goal is to influence health outcomes and improve the patient's health issues.
▼ *Nursing conditions*
  Critical thinking skills
  Partnership with patient and family
▼ *Nursing behaviors*
  Hypothesizing
  Specifying expected outcomes
  Validating goals with patient
▼ *Key elements*
  Outcomes should be mutually identified with the patient.
  Outcomes should be identified as clearly and objectively as possible.
  Well-written outcomes help nurses determine the effectiveness and efficiency of their interventions.
  Before defining expected outcomes the nurse must realize that patients often seek treatment with goals of their own.

These goals may be expressed as relieving symptoms or improving functional ability. Sometimes a patient cannot identify specific goals or may describe them in general terms. Translating nonspecific concerns into specific goal statements is not easy. The nurse must understand the patient's coping responses and the factors that influence them. Some of the difficulties in defining goals are as follows (Krumboltz & Thorensen, 1969).

The patient may view a personal problem as someone else's behavior. This may be the case of a father who brings his adolescent son in for counseling. The father may view the son as the problem, whereas the adolescent may feel his only problem is his father. One approach to this situation is to focus help on the person who brought the problem into treatment because he "owns" the problem at that moment. The nurse might suggest, "Let's talk about how I could help you deal with your son. A change in your response might lead to a change in his behavior also."

The patient may express a problem as a feeling, such as, "I'm lonely," or "I'm so unhappy." Besides trying to help the patient clarify the feeling, the nurse might ask, "What could you do to make yourself feel less alone and more loved by others?" This helps patients see the connection between actions and feelings and increase their sense of responsibility for themselves.

The patient's problem may be one of lacking a goal or an idea of exactly what is desired out of life. In this case it might be helpful for the nurse to point out that values and goals are not magically discovered but must be created by people for themselves. The patient can then actively explore ways to construct goals or adopt the objectives of a social, service, religious, or political group with whom the patient identifies.

The patient's goals may be inappropriate, undesirable, or unclear. However, the solution is not for the nurse to impose goals on the patient. Even if the patient's desires seem to be against self-interests, the most the nurse can do is reflect the patient's behavior and its consequences. If the patient then asks for help in setting new goals, the nurse can help.

The patient's problem may be a choice conflict. This is especially common if all the choices are unpleasant, unacceptable, or unrealistic. An example is a couple who want to divorce but do not want to see their child hurt or suffer the financial hardship that would result. Although undesirable choices cannot be made desirable, the nurse can help patients use the problem-solving process to identify the full range of alternatives available to them.

The patient may have no real problem but may just want to talk. Nurses must then decide what role to play and carefully distinguish between a social and a therapeutic relationship.

Clarifying goals is an essential step in the therapeutic process. Out of this clarification emerges the mutually agreed on goals on which the patient-nurse relationship is based. A well-intentioned nurse sometimes overlooks the patient's goals and devises a treatment plan leading to an outcome that the nurse believes is better. However, this approach may be a conflict-producing situation that the patient has already experienced. Therefore the experience of working cooperatively with the nurse to evolve mutually acceptable goals is extremely valuable (Henson, 1997). If the patient does not share one of the nurse's goals, it may be best to defer it until the patient agrees on its importance.

Expected Outcomes

Once overall goals are agreed on, the nurse must state them explicitly. Box 11-2 lists qualities of well-written outcome criteria. Expected outcomes are derived from the diagnoses, guide later nursing actions, and enhance the evaluation of care. Expected outcomes can be documented using standardized classification systems, such as the Nursing Outcomes Classification (NOC) (Johnson et al, 2000).

Box **11-2**

Qualities of Well-Written Outcome Criteria

- Specific rather than general
- Measurable rather than subjective
- Attainable rather than unrealistic
- Current rather than outdated
- Adequate in number rather than too few or too many
- Mutual rather than one-sided

Review some of the treatment plans in your clinical setting. Are the expected outcomes and long- and short-term goals well written given the qualities listed in Box 11-2?

Long- and short-term goals should contribute to the expected outcomes. Following is a sample expected outcome and long- and short-term goals:

Expected outcome: Social involvement will improve with treatment from limited to substantial

Long-term goal:

- The patient will travel about the community independently within 2 months.

Short-term goals:

- At the end of 1 week the patient will sit on the front steps at home.
- At the end of 2 weeks the patient will walk to the corner and back home.
- At the end of 3 weeks the patient, accompanied by the nurse, will walk in the neighborhood.
- At the end of 4 weeks the patient will walk in the neighborhood alone.
- At the end of 6 weeks the patients will drive her car in the neighborhood
- At the end of 8 weeks that patient will drive to the mall and meet a friend for dinner.

Each goal is stated in terms of an observable behavior and includes a period of time in which it is to be accomplished. It also includes any other relevant conditions, such as whether the patient is to be alone or accompanied by the nurse. In writing goals, psychiatric nurses should remember that they can be classified into three domains: cognitive, affective, and psychomotor. Correctly identifying the domain of the expected outcome is very important in planning nursing interventions. Some psychiatric nurses assume that the only outcomes necessary are those related to learning new information (cognitive). They forget about the equally important needs of patients to acquire new values (affective) or master new motor skills (psychomotor).

For example, it would be of limited help to teach a patient about medication if the patient did not value taking medications based on a personal belief system or previous life experiences. It would be equally unsuccessful to engage in medication education if the patient did not know how to take public transportation to fill the prescription.

Finally, it is important to explore with the patient the cost/benefit effect of all identified goals, that is, what is being given up (cost) versus what is being gained (benefit) from attaining the goal. This can be thought of as exploring advantages, or positive effects, and disadvantages or negative effects. Patients are not likely to commit themselves to a goal or to work toward attaining a goal if the stakes are too high and the payoffs too low. Exploring advantages and disadvantages helps the patient anticipate what price will be paid to achieve the goal and then decide if the change is worth the cost to oneself or significant others. Sometimes it is helpful to write these down in the form of two columns (advantages and disadvantages) that can be added to or changed at any time.

PLANNING

STANDARD IV: PLANNING
The psychiatric-mental health nurse develops a plan of care that prescribes interventions to attain expected outcomes.

▼ *Rationale*
A plan of care is used to guide therapeutic interventions systematically, document progress, and achieve the expected patient outcomes.

▼ *Nursing conditions*
Application of theory
Respect for patient and family

▼ *Nursing behaviors*
Prioritize goals
Identify nursing activities
Validate plan with patient

▼ *Key elements*
The plan of nursing care must always be individualized for the patient.
Planned interventions should be based on current knowledge in the field and contemporary clinical psychiatric-mental health nursing practice.
Planning is done in collaboration with the patient, the family, and the health-care team.
Documentation of the plan of care is an essential nursing activity.

One of the most important tasks facing the nurse and patient is to assign priorities to the goals. Often several goals can be pursued simultaneously. Those related to protecting the patient from self-destructive impulses always receive top priority. When identifying expected outcomes and long- and short-term goals, the nurse must keep the proposed time sequence firmly in mind.

Because the nursing care plan is dynamic and should adapt to the patient's coping responses throughout contact with the health-care system, priorities are constantly changing. If the focus is always on the patient's behavioral responses, priorities can be set and modified as the patient changes. This personalizes nursing care, and the patient participates in its planning and implementation.

Once the goals are chosen, the next task is to outline the plan for achieving them. The nursing care plan applies theory and research from nursing and related biological, behavioral, and social sciences to the unique responses of the individual patient. This assumes that as the nurse identifies patient needs, appropriate resources will be consulted. Skilled psychiatric nursing requires a commitment to the ongoing pursuit of knowledge that will enhance professional growth.

The patient's active involvement leads to a more successful care plan. After writing a tentative care plan, the nurse must validate this plan with the patient. This saves time and effort for them both as they continue to work together. It also communicates to the patient a sense of self-responsibility in getting well. The patient can tell the nurse that a proposed plan is unrealistic regarding financial status, lifestyle, value system, or, perhaps, personal preference. Usually there are several possible approaches to a patient's problem. Choosing the one most acceptable to the patient improves the chances for success.

If a goal answers the question of **what**, the plan of care answers the questions **how** and **why**. The plan chosen obviously depends on the nursing diagnosis, the nurse's theoretical orientation, the evidence supporting the intended intervention, and the nature of the outcomes pursued. Failure to reach a goal through one plan can lead to the decision to adopt a new approach or reevaluate the goal. These activities commonly occur in the working phase of the relationship.

Documentation

The Joint Commission on Accreditation of Healthcare Organizations (JCAHO) standards specify that the nursing plan of care must contain the six elements listed in Box 11-3 and that the primary place to document the nursing process is in the patient's health care record (see Citing the Evidence).

Box 11-3
Essential Elements of the Nursing Plan of Care

- Initial assessment and reassessment
- Nursing diagnoses or patient care needs
- Interventions identified to meet the patient's nursing care needs
- Nursing care provided
- Patient's response to and the outcomes of the nursing care provided
- Ability of the patient or significant other to manage continuing care needs after discharge

Citing the Evidence on

Documentation

BACKGROUND: The purpose of this study was to examine the language by which psychiatric nursing staff describe patients in their medical records. Charts of former psychiatric patient were studied for the quality of the words used to communicate about patient behaviors.

RESULTS: Nurses' entries most often focused on patients in judgmental and unflattering ways. The word "manipulative" was the perjorative descriptor used most often, followed by argumentative, controlling, defensive, defiant, inappropriate, and noncompliant. Nonperjorative adjectives included quiet, pleasant, cooperative, compliant and appropriate.

IMPLICATIONS: The values and assumptions of nurses should be clarified before approaching patients, and assessments should not focus solely on handicaps or areas of patients' weakness. The evaluation of patients should be removed from labeling and be operationalized to reflect the range of patient competencies and behaviors that are evaluated objectively within the context of space and time.

Mohr W, Noone M: Deconstructing progress notes in psychiatric settings, *Arch Psychiatr Nurs* 11:325, 1997.

Psychiatric nurses are beginning to use a variety of formats that often differ from the traditional nursing care plan. Many of these changes have been prompted by changes in the treatment settings and by the advanced computer technology available.

For example, computerized programs have been developed that can provide rapid entry of patient data, retrieve psychiatric treatment plans, and produce a finished document that is clinically useful and highly readable. Another advantage of a computerized information system is its ability to store clinical data that can also be used for outcome research, quality improvement activities, and resource management. In addition to computerized plans of care, psychiatric nurses use clinical practice guidelines, clinical protocols, flow sheets, clinical pathways, and treatment algorithms in their practice settings.

> *What are the potential problems in using computerized patient information systems in psychiatric health-care facilities?*

IMPLEMENTATION

STANDARD V: IMPLEMENTATION
The psychiatric-mental health nurse implements the interventions identified in the plan of care.

▼ *Rationale*
In implementing the plan of care, psychiatric-mental health nurses use a wide range of interventions designed to prevent mental and physical illness and to promote, maintain, and restore mental and physical health. Psychiatric-mental health nurses select interventions according to their level of practice. At the basic level, nurses may select counseling, milieu therapy, promotion of self-care activities, intake screening and evaluation, psychobiological interventions, health teaching, case management, health promotion and health maintenance, crisis intervention, community-based care, psychiatric home health-care, telehealth, and a variety of other approaches to meet the mental health needs of patients. In addition to the intervention options available to the basic-level psychiatric-mental health nurse, at the advanced level the APRN-PMH may provide consultation, engage in psychotherapy, and prescribe pharmacological agents where permitted by state statutes or regulations.

▼ *Nursing conditions*
Past clinical experiences
Knowledge of research
Responsive and action dimensions of care

▼ *Nursing behaviors*
Consider available resources
Implement nursing activities
Generate alternatives
Coordinate with other team members

▼ *Key elements*
Nursing interventions should reflect a holistic, biopsychosocial approach to patient care.
Nursing interventions are implemented in a safe, efficient, and caring manner.
The level at which a nurse functions and the interventions implemented are based on the nursing practice acts in one's state, the nurse's qualifications (including

education, experience, and certification), the caregiving setting, and the nurse's initiative.

STANDARD VA: COUNSELING

The psychiatric-mental health nurse uses counseling interventions to help patients in improving or regaining their previous coping abilities, fostering mental health, and preventing mental illness and disability.

STANDARD VB: MILIEU THERAPY

The psychiatric-mental health nurse provides, structures, and maintains a therapeutic environment in collaboration with the patient and other health-care providers.

STANDARD VC: SELF-CARE ACTIVITIES

The psychiatric-mental health nurse structures interventions around the patient's activities of daily living to foster self-care and mental and physical well-being.

STANDARD VD: PSYCHOBIOLOGICAL INTERVENTIONS

The psychiatric-mental health nurse uses knowledge of psychobiological interventions and applies clinical skills to restore the patient's health and prevent further disability.

STANDARD VE: HEALTH TEACHING

The psychiatric-mental health nurse, through health teaching, assists patients in achieving satisfying, productive, and healthy patterns of living.

STANDARD VF: CASE MANAGEMENT

The psychiatric-mental health nurse provides case management to coordinate comprehensive health services and ensure continuity of care.

STANDARD VG: HEALTH PROMOTION AND HEALTH MAINTENANCE

The psychiatric-mental health nurse employs strategies and interventions to promote and maintain health and prevent mental illness.

ADVANCED PRACTICE INTERVENTIONS VH-VJ

The following interventions (VH-VJ) may be performed only by the Advanced Practice Registered Nurse in psychiatric-mental health nursing (APRN-PMH).

STANDARD VH: PSYCHOTHERAPY

The APRN-PMH uses individual, group, and family psychotherapy, and other therapeutic treatments to assist patients in preventing mental illness and disability and in improving mental health status and functional abilities.

STANDARD VI: PRESCRIPTION OF PHARMACOLOGICAL AGENTS

The APRN-PMH uses prescriptive authority, procedures, and treatments in accordance with state and federal laws and regulations to treat symptoms of psychiatric illness and improve functional health status.

STANDARD VJ: CONSULTATION

The APRN-PMH provides consultation to enhance the abilities of others to provide services for patients and effect change in the system.

Implementation is the actual delivery of nursing care to the patient and his or her response to that care. Nursing interventions should be based on existing evidence of the efficacy of the intended treatment. The use of a standardized classification system of interventions that nurses perform, such as the Nursing Interventions Classification (NIC) (McCloskey & Bulchek, 2000) is useful for clinical documentation, communication of care across settings, integration of data across systems, effectiveness research, productivity measurement, competency evaluation, and reimbursement.

Good planning increases the chances of successful implementation. Such factors as available people, equipment, resources, time, and money must be considered as nursing actions are planned. It is helpful when planning care to identify alternative nursing actions that are also appropriate to the goal. If this is done, the nurse is not left floundering if the first approach fails. Considering several alternatives makes the implementation phase of the nursing process highly flexible.

In implementing psychotherapeutic interventions, the nurse helps the psychiatric patient do two things: **develop insight** and **change behavior**. These two areas for nursing intervention correspond with the responsive and action dimensions of the nurse-patient relationship described in Chapter 2. Insight is the patient's development of new emotional and cognitive understandings (Baier et al, 1998). Often the patient becomes more anxious as defense mechanisms are broken down. This is the time when resistance commonly occurs. But knowing something on an intellectual level does *not* inevitably lead to a change in behavior. Nurses who terminate their interventions at this point are not fully carrying out the therapeutic process to the patient's benefit. An additional step is needed. Patients must decide whether they will revert to maladaptive coping mechanisms, remain in a resisting, immobilized state, or adopt new, adaptive, and constructive approaches to life.

The first step in helping a patient translate insight into action is to build adequate incentives to abandon old patterns of behavior. The nurse should help the patient see the consequences of actions and that old patterns do more harm than good. The patient will not learn new patterns until the motivation to acquire them is greater than the motivation to retain old ones. The nurse should encourage the patient's desires for mental health, emotional growth, and freedom from suffering. The nurse also should continue to motivate and support patients as they test new behaviors and coping mechanisms.

Within the nurse-patient relationship the patient can actively work toward adaptive goals. It is important to allow sufficient time for change. Many of the patient's maladaptive patterns have built up over years; the nurse cannot expect the patient to change them in a matter of days or weeks. Finally, the nurse must help the patient evaluate these new patterns, integrate them into life experiences, and practice problem solving to prepare for future experiences. In this way secondary-prevention nursing interventions also fulfill primary and tertiary prevention goals.

The standards of care for implementation are detailed and explicit. The standards identify the range of activities psychiatric nurses use. Information related to each of these implementation standards appears in various chapters throughout this text.

Psychiatric nurses need to be skilled in biological, psychological, and sociocultural skills to implement these nursing interventions. The current psychiatric population has a higher level of acuity, increased mortality rates, and more complex problems than in the past. Specifically, 50% of people with mental illness are estimated to have a known co-morbid medical disorder; another 35% are estimated to suffer from undiagnosed and untreated medical disorders; and, on average, people with mental illness die 10 to 15 years earlier than the general population (Farnam et al, 1999; Harris & Barraclough, 1998). Thus it is essential that psychiatric nurses stay current with their biomedical as well as psychosocial skills.

Graduating nursing students are sometimes advised to work in a medical-surgical setting before going into psychiatry so that they can learn "basic nursing skills." Why is this suggestion no longer valid given contemporary psychiatric patients and the range of treatment settings?

Treatment Stages

A final issue for the psychiatric nurse to consider in the implementation process is that there are four possible treatment stages:

- Health promotion
- Maintenance
- Acute
- Crisis

These stages reflect the range of adaptive/maladaptive coping responses, and patients can move between these stages at any time. The goal, assessment, intervention, and expected outcome vary with each stage, as seen in Fig. 11-4. It is critically important for psychiatric nurses to determine the patient's stage of treatment and then implement nursing activities that target the treatment goal in the most cost-effective and efficient manner.

EVALUATION

STANDARD VI: EVALUATION
The psychiatric-mental health nurse evaluates the patient's progress in attaining expected outcomes.

▼ *Rationale*
Nursing care is a dynamic process involving change in the patient's health status over time, giving rise to the need for data, different diagnoses, and modifications in the plan of care. Therefore evaluation is a continuous process of appraising the effect of nursing and the treatment regimen on the patient's health status and expected outcomes.

▼ *Nursing conditions*
Supervision
Self-analysis
Peer review
Patient and family participation

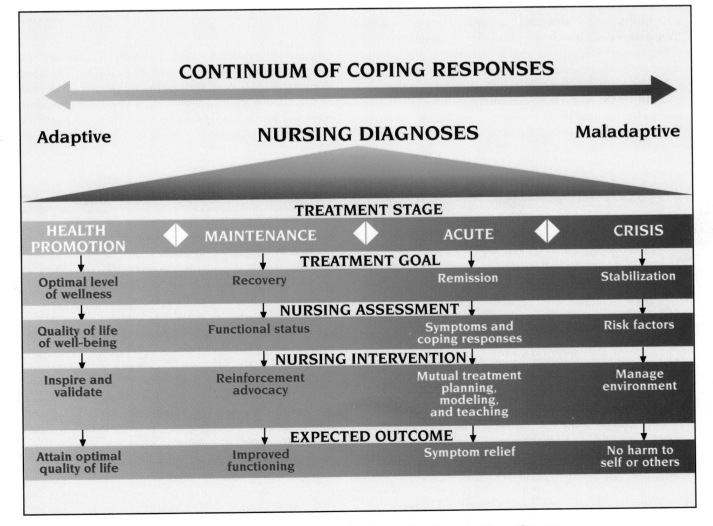

Fig. 11-4 Treatment stages related to implementation of psychiatric nursing care.

▼ *Nursing behaviors*
   Compare patient's responses and expected outcome
   Review nursing process
   Modify nursing process as needed
   Participate in quality improvement activities
▼ *Key elements*
   Evaluation is an ongoing process.
   Patient and family participation in evaluation is essential.
   Goal achievement should be documented and revisions in
   the plan of care should be implemented as appropriate.

When evaluating care the nurse should review all previous phases of the nursing process and determine whether the expected outcomes for the patient have been met. Key words for the evaluation phase of the nursing process are **mutual, competent, accessible, effective, appropriate, efficient,** and **flexible.** Often, progress with psychiatric patients is slow and occurs in small steps rather than dramatic leaps. Realizing that progress has been made can produce growth and inspire new enthusiasm in both the patient and the nurse.

Above all, evaluation is a mutual process based on the patient's and family's previously identified goals and level of satisfaction (Druss et al, 1999). Patients, families, and psychiatric nurses often have different views of treatment and the effectiveness of care. It is therefore critical that psychiatric nurses have a systematic and objective way to learn from patients and families which aspects of the nursing care provided were helpful and what additional nursing actions may have further enhanced their well-being.

Finally, evaluation is a continuous, active process that begins early in the relationship and continues throughout. It is an activity that must be documented by psychiatric nurses so that they can demonstrate the value of psychiatric nursing

services to consumers, administrators, reimbursers, and other health-care providers (see Critical Thinking about Contemporary Issues). Perhaps more than any other phase of the nursing process, evaluation and outcome measurement will be the key aspects of psychiatric nursing activities in the decade to come.

? CRITICAL THINKING about CONTEMPORARY ISSUES

Does Psychiatric Nursing Care Really Make a Difference?

Most nurses reading this question would automatically and emphatically say, "Yes, of course it does!" But does it really? More specifically, what evidence exists that the care provided by psychiatric nurses actually results in a decrease in patients' symptoms, improvement in patients' functional status, or improved quality of life? What evidence would you provide a hospital administrator who was proposing that all but one of the psychiatric nursing positions on the units be replaced with counselors? How would you convince the director of a community mental health program for the seriously mentally ill that, as a nurse, you should be hired to work with this population rather than the social worker who is also being interviewed?

In fact, very few well-designed psychiatric nursing studies have demonstrated the effectiveness of psychiatric nursing care (Merwin, 1995). Of the hundreds of articles cited in recent reviews, very few psychiatric nursing studies are mentioned. It is clear that psychiatric nurses believe they make a valuable contribution to the health-care of patients. However, providing the evidence of this contribution remains a challenge for the field.

))) CASE STUDY

This case study describes the use of the nursing process with a psychiatric patient. It illustrates the interrelationship of the phases of the nurse-patient relationship, the therapeutic dimensions, and the various activities as the nurse works with the patient to foster adaptive coping behavior and more integrated functioning.

ASSESSMENT

Ms. G came to the psychiatric outpatient department of the local hospital requesting treatment with a female therapist. The psychiatric nurse specialist agreed to perform the initial screening and evaluation and consider serving as her primary therapist.

To collect the initial data the nurse followed the admission format required by the department. A description of the presenting problem revealed that Ms. G was a 29-year-old single woman who was neat in appearance and markedly overweight. She reported feelings of "confusion and depression" and said that superficially she appeared "outgoing and friendly and

played the role of a clown." In reality, however, she said she had few close friends, felt insecure about herself, felt unsuccessful in her job, and believed she "overanalyzed her problems." She said she had feelings of worthlessness and loss of pleasure in her daily activities on and off for the past 2 years.

Additional information was obtained in other significant areas of her life. Her psychosocial history revealed a disrupted family situation. Her mother died of tuberculosis when she was 11 years of age. Her father, age 73, was alive but had been an alcoholic for as long as Ms. G could remember. She had one sister, age 20, who married at age 16 and was now divorced. She also had one stepsister, age 45, who was married, had two adopted sons, and lived out of state. In giving this family information, Ms. G revealed that her stepsister was her natural mother, but she had continued to call her father's wife "mother." After her "mother" died, her stepsister took over the house. Two years later, however, this stepsister married and moved out of state. Ms. G reported feeling closest to this stepsister and felt

Continued from previous page

abandoned when she left. Ms. G then took charge of the house until age 14, when her father placed her and her younger sister in a group home, where she had difficulty making friends.

She completed high school and college. In college she had four good friends who were all married now. Her only close heterosexual relationship was in high school, and this boyfriend eventually married her best friend. Since that time she had never dated and stated she had no desire to marry.

After college she obtained a job as a "girl Friday" for a law firm and expressed much pleasure with it. She then saw the opportunity to make more money as a waitress and switched jobs. She currently worked at a restaurant, and her schedule involved day and night rotations as well as weekend shifts. She expressed dissatisfaction with many aspects of her job but was unable to identify alternatives. Her goal in life was to have a fulfilling career.

She lived alone. Her best friend was her immediate supervisor at work. She currently had no male friends and only two other female acquaintances.

Pertinent medical history revealed a major weight problem. She was 36 kg (80 pounds) overweight and extremely conscious of it. She viewed her body negatively and believed others were also "repulsed" by her weight. She also recently recovered from infectious hepatitis. She drank an occasional beer when out with friends (once or twice a month), denied any drug use, and smoked three fourths of a pack of cigarettes a day.

Diagnosis

After consultation the psychiatric nurse agreed to work with Ms. G as primary therapist. In the following session they established a contract for working together, and a fee was set. At this time they explored her expressed guilt over seeking help, the reason for her request for a female therapist, their mutual roles, and the confidential nature of the relationship. The nurse also shared with Ms. G the maladaptive coping responses she had noted and the inferences she had made. They discussed these areas, and the following nursing diagnoses were identified:

1. *Self-esteem disturbance related to childhood rejection and unrealistic self-ideals, as evidenced by feelings of worthlessness*
2. *Social isolation related to ambivalence regarding male-female relationships and lack of socialization skills, as evidenced by lack of close friends*
3. *Altered role performance related to job dissatisfaction with working hours and nature of the work, as evidenced by feeling unsuccessful in her job*
4. *Body image disturbance related to weight control problem, as evidenced by negative feelings*

   Ms. G's DSM–IV–TR diagnosis was identified as dysthymia, a mood disorder.

Outcome Identification

They mutually agreed to work on her problem areas in weekly therapy sessions. After 3 months they would evaluate the achievement of the following expected outcomes: consistently positive self-esteem; substantial social involvement; substantially adequate role performance; and consistently positive body

image. These expected outcomes would be met through the attainment of the following goals:

1. *Ms. G will describe her expectations of the therapeutic process and her commitment to it.*
2. *Aspects of Ms. G's self-ideal will be identified and realistically evaluated.*
3. *Cognitive distortions influencing her self-concept and negative, stereotyped self-perceptions will be analyzed.*
4. *Interpersonal relationships will be examined to include her patterns of relating, her expectations of others, and specific areas of difficulty.*
5. *Alternative employment opportunities will be identified.*
6. *The advantages and disadvantages of a job change will be compared.*

Planning

In discussing these areas they agreed that nursing diagnosis 1 was a central one and problems 2, 3, and 4 directly contributed to it. Her coping mechanisms included intellectualization and denial, and she compensated for her self-doubts by an outward appearance that was social, joking, and friendly, yet superficial. The strengths Ms. G brought to the therapy process included her introspective nature and ability to analyze events, her openness to new ideas, the resource people available to her in her immediate environment, and a genuine sense of humor.

Implementation

Because they were in the introductory phase of the relationship, many of the goals involved areas needing further assessment. During this phase of treatment Ms. G displayed much anxiety, testing behavior, and ambivalence, and the nursing actions were focused on promoting respect, openness, and acceptance and minimizing her anxiety. Through the nurse's use of empathic understanding, Ms. G became less jovial and superficial and began to attain some intellectual insight into her behavior. With guidance she began to appraise her own abilities and became more open in expressing feelings.

She feared intimate personal involvement and could not tolerate physical closeness. The nurse incorporated this into nursing actions by initially minimizing confrontation, setting limits on anxiety-producing topics, and arranging the office seating to allow the patient to select her proximity to the nurse.

As they discussed the patient's relationships, the nurse confronted her with the dependent role Ms. G played and the unrealistic expectations she placed on others in the exclusiveness and amount of time she demanded from them. Her pattern of relating was also manipulative in that she elicited a sympathetic response and then used it to meet her own needs. She had great difficulty with mutuality and autonomy in relating to others. She was inexperienced in heterosexual relationships and missed many of the normal adolescent growth experiences in this area. Finally, she had much emotion and fear vested in her family of origin. The only trusting relationship Ms. G could recall was with her stepsister-mother. When this stepsister abruptly left home to marry, Ms. G perceived this as a personal rejection. She had since isolated herself from her family and continued to

Continued

Continued from previous page

blame herself for her rejection by others, thus lowering her self-esteem and ability to trust others.

At the end of 2 months Ms. G was being considered for a promotion at work to hostess but, on the basis of an evaluation by her best friend and supervisor, was rejected for it. This precipitated a suicide attempt, which Ms. G revealed at her next regular session. At this point the issue of trust within the relationship became critical, as well as her inability to express anger because she feared rejection. The nurse now began more actively confronting Ms. G in her areas of ambivalence and inconsistency, setting limits on her self-destructive behavior, and suggesting alternatives. Ms. G then revealed that her relationship with her friend-supervisor was also a sexual one, and she expressed fears of homosexuality and loss of identity.

In later sessions Ms. G's relationship with this friend became a critical therapeutic issue because it reflected many of her conflicts. The therapy process presented a threat to the unhealthy parts of this relationship, and during the course of therapy Ms. G decided she needed to choose between maladaptive behaviors and more growth-producing options.

The nurse-patient relationship had now moved into the working phase, where focus was placed on specifics, and problem-solving activities began. After 3 months the nursing diagnoses were reevaluated to include the following:

1. Potential for self-directed violence related to perceived rejection by friend, as evidenced by suicide attempt
2. Personal identity disturbance related to childhood rejection and unrealistic self-ideals, as evidenced by self-statements
3. Social isolation related to inability to trust, lack of socialization skills, and feelings of inadequacy, as evidenced by relationship patterns
4. Powerlessness related to fear of rejection by others, as evidenced by perceived lack of control over life events
5. Altered role performance related to job dissatisfaction with working hours and nature of the work, as evidenced by feeling unsuccessful in her job

At this time the nurse sought consultation as she further evolved her plan of care. Neither medication nor hospitalization was indicated. These formulations were shared with Ms. G, who contracted for safety with the nurse, and together they collaborated about her future progress. They agreed to focus on changing Ms. G's maladaptive behavior by exploring past events and conflicts and helping her learn more productive patterns of living. Ms. G was now ready to commit herself to the work of therapy and interpersonal change, and she began to assume increased responsibility for this therapeutic work.

Because her self-ideal was unrealistically high, specific short-term goals became essential. The nurse's theoretical orientation incorporated the dynamics of Sullivan's and Peplau's interpersonal theories, Beck's cognitive framework, and Glasser's reality therapy. The relationship was focused on through the use of immediacy and became a model for examining many of her conflicts. This proved to be an excellent learning opportunity as Ms. G and the nurse dealt with resistance, transference, and countertransference reactions. During

the next couple of months Ms. G made much progress, including the following changes:

1. She moved into an apartment with another girlfriend.
2. She left her previous job and resumed working in an office, where she received more personal satisfaction and a work schedule that allowed her to increase her social activities.
3. She began a diet regimen.
4. She participated in additional activities, such as a dancing class and a health spa.
5. She learned to verbalize her anger more freely with the nurse, friends, and others at work. This included discussing the many relationships in her past that were terminated without her agreement and in which she had internalized her anger.
6. She contacted her stepsister-mother and visited her. This was an important therapeutic goal because it allowed her to review her early experiences and provided her with actual feedback from those involved. Consequently, many of her misperceptions became evident and open to exploration in therapy.
7. She was able to admit her ambivalent feeling about her friend-supervisor and discuss the negative aspects of the relationship.
8. She stopped further sexual contact with her because she felt exploited. Over time, the nature of this relationship changed, and it eventually became a casual acquaintance.
9. She learned about the variety of sexual feelings and responses and saw her needs in this area as appropriate developmental tasks. She became open to evaluating both heterosexual and homosexual expressions of her own sexual feelings.
10. Her perception of personal space changed, and her tolerance for physical closeness increased.
11. She developed new male and female friends and socialized frequently with them.

EVALUATION

The terminating phase of the relationship began after about 6 months. At this time Ms. G was independently solving problems and, in therapy, the nurse primarily validated and supported her thinking. She was now receiving and accepting much positive feedback from others, had lost 15 kg (40 pounds), was continuing to diet, was planning future career goals, and had achieved more satisfactory interpersonal relationships with both men and women. The mutual goals for therapy had been met.

Terminating was difficult because of the close, trusting bond that had developed between them. The nurse had feelings of pleasure in Ms. G's growth, as well as personal satisfaction in her effectiveness as therapist. Ms. G openly described her feelings about terminating and raised the question of a possible social relationship between them. Over the course of the sessions she came to realize that the premise of the relationship was therapy and changing individual perceptions or patterns of relating would not be feasible or desirable. Most important, she had control over terminating this relationship and the opportunity to work it through in a positive way.

Summary

1. The nursing process is an interactive, problem-solving process used by the nurse as a systematic and individualized way to fulfill the goal of nursing care.
2. Assessment should reflect content, process, and information about the patient's biopsychosocial world.
3. The nursing diagnosis should include the patient's adaptive or maladaptive health response, defining characteristics of that response, and contributing stressors. Knowledge of both NANDA and *DSM* diagnoses is needed.
4. Outcome identification involves setting goals that are mutual, congruent, realistic, and appropriately timed.
5. The plan of care should include prioritized nursing diagnoses and expected outcomes, as well as prescribed nursing strategies to achieve those outcomes.
6. Nursing interventions should be based on existing evidence and directed toward helping the patient develop insight and resolve problems through carrying out a positive plan of action. Psychiatric nursing practice includes both basic and advanced activities.
7. Evaluation involves reviewing all previous phases of the nursing process and determining the degree to which expected outcomes were attained.

MERLIN Visit **MERLIN: www.mosby.com/MERLIN/Stuart** to find these additional materials and student activities.

- **Worksheets**
- **"Drug of the Month" Updates**
- **"Citing the Evidence" Updates**
- **Critical Thinking Activities and Exercises**
- **Annotated Suggested Readings**
- **Web Links**
- **More!**

Chapter Review Questions

1. **Match the phase of the nursing process identified in Column A with the appropriate nursing behavior in Column B.**

Column A	Column B
___ Data collection	A. Comparing responses and expected outcome, making modifications as needed
___ Evaluation	B. Considering available resources, generating alternatives, and coordinating with other team members
___ Implementation	C. Establishing a contract and collecting, validating, and organizing data
___ Nursing diagnosis	D. Hypothesizing and validating goals with the patient
___ Outcome identification	E. Identifying patterns, analyzing, and synthesizing data.
___ Planning	F. Prioritizing goals and identifying nursing activities

2. **Fill in the blanks.**

Well-written outcome criteria or goals are:
A. _____ rather that general.
B. _____ rather than subjective.
C. _____ rather than unrealistic.
D. _____ rather than outdated.
E. _____ rather than too few or too many.
F. _____ rather than one-sided.

G. The three advanced practice interventions for psychiatric nurses are _____, _____, and _____.
H. The four stages of psychiatric treatment are _____, _____, _____, and _____.
I. In implementing psychotherapeutic interventions, the nurse helps the patient do two things: _____ and _____.
J. The _____ is the ideal source of validation of data.
K. It is important to explore with the patient the _____ versus the _____ of all identified goals.

3. **Provide short answers for the following questions.**

A. Identify the four defining characteristics of nursing and relate these to psychiatric nursing.
B. Why is it important for the psychiatric nurse to be knowledgeable about *DSM–IV–TR* diagnoses?
C. Discuss the special problems that can arise in establishing mutual goals when caring for psychiatric patients. How would you deal with them?
D. Do you think that the use of computers in health care dehumanizes it? Explain your position.

REFERENCES

American Nurses' Association: *Nursing: a social policy statement,* Kansas City, Mo, 1980, The Association.

American Nurses' Association: *Nursing's social policy statement,* Kansas City, Mo, 1995, The Association.

American Nurses' Association: *Scope and standards of psychiatric-mental health clinical nursing practice,* Washington, DC, 2000, The Association.

American Psychiatric Association: *Diagnostic and statistical manual of mental disorders,* Fourth Edition, Text Revision, Washington, DC, American Psychiatric Association, 2000.

Baier M et al: Conceptualization and measurement of insight, *Arch Psychiatr Nurs* 12:32, 1998.

Druss B et al: Patient satisfaction and administrative measures as indicators of the quality of mental health care, *Psychiatr Serv* 50:1053, 1999.

Farnam C et al: Health status risk factors of people with severe and persistent mental illness, *J Psychsoc Nurs* 37:16, 1999.

Harris E, Barraclough B: Excess mortality of mental disorder, *Br J Psychiatry* 173:11, 1998.

Henson R: Analysis of the concept of mutuality, *Image* 29:77, 1997.

Johnson M et al: *Nursing outcomes classification (NOC),* St Louis, 2000, Mosby.

Krumboltz J, Thorensen C: *Behavioral counseling: cases and techniques,* New York, 1969, Holt, Rinehart & Winston.

McCloskey J, Bulechek G: *Nursing interventions classifications (NIC),* St Louis, 2000, Mosby.

Merwin E, Mauck A: Psychiatric nursing outcome research: the state of the science, *Arch Psychiatr Nurs* 9:311, 1995.

North American Nursing Diagnosis Association: *Nursing diagnoses: definitions and classification 1999-2000,* Philadelphia, 1999, The Association.

Wilson J, Hobbs H: Therapeutic partnership: a model for clinical practice, *J Psychosoc Nurs* 33:27, 1995.

World Health Organization: *International classification of diseases,* ed 10, Geneva, 1993, The Organization.

Actualizing the Psychiatric Nursing Role: Professional Performance Standards

12

Gail W. Stuart

LEARNING OBJECTIVES

After studying this chapter the student should be able to:

- Describe how accountability and autonomy relate to the psychiatric nurse's professional role responsibilities
- Analyze the conditions and behaviors of the psychiatric nurse related to the quality of care activities
- Analyze the conditions and behaviors of the psychiatric nurse related to performance appraisal
- Analyze the conditions and behaviors of the psychiatric nurse related to education
- Analyze the conditions and behaviors of the psychiatric nurse related to collegiality
- Analyze the conditions and behaviors of the psychiatric nurse related to ethics
- Analyze the conditions and behaviors of the psychiatric nurse related to collaboration
- Analyze the conditions and behaviors of the psychiatric nurse related to research
- Analyze the conditions and behaviors of the psychiatric nurse related to resource use

The professional motive is the desire and perpetual effort to do the thing as well as it can be done, which exists just as much in the Nurse, as in the Astronomer in search of a new star, or in the Artist completing a picture.

FLORENCE NIGHTINGALE

The standards of care from the American Nurses' Association (2000) *Scope and Standards of Psychiatric–Mental Health Clinical Nursing Practice,* as presented in Chapter 11, describe what the psychiatric nurse does; the standards of professional performance from the same document presented in this chapter describe the context in which the psychiatric nurse performs these activities. Neither set of standards can be taken in isolation; together they complete the picture of contemporary psychiatric nursing practice.

ACCOUNTABILITY AND AUTONOMY

Psychiatric nursing is characterized by rules of competency and service. The standards of professional performance ap-ply to self-regulation and accountability for practice by psychiatric nurses, both individually and as a group. They also address issues of professional autonomy and self-definition. As such, the standards of performance are critical.

Accountability means to be answerable to someone for something. It focuses responsibility on the individual nurse for personal actions, or perhaps lack of action. The preconditions of accountability include ability, responsibility, and authority. Accountability also includes formal review processes and an attitude of integrity and vigilance.

Autonomy implies self-determination, independence, and shared power. It is the condition that allows for definition of and control over a work domain. For psychiatric nursing, attaining autonomy means being able to define the domain of nursing and being able to exercise control over psychiatric nursing practice. This idea of shaping destiny, rather than letting outside forces be in control, views power as a positive force that allows nurses to attain goals. It involves a conscious decision to identify objectives, plan strategy, assume responsibility, exercise authority, and be held accountable.

Autonomy has two major interrelated components. The first is **control over nursing tasks**, which means:

- Having the opportunity for independent thought and action
- Having use of time, skills, and ability by being able to eliminate, refuse, or delegate nonnursing tasks
- Having the authority and responsibility for implementing goals related to the quality of care
- Being able to initiate changes and innovations in practice

The second component of autonomy is **participation in decision making**. It requires the nurse's participation in the following:

- Determining and implementing quality standards
- Making decisions affecting each nurse's job context, including salary, staffing, and professional growth
- Setting institutional policies, procedures, and goals

This second component of participation in decision making is particularly problematic for nursing. Most nurses are employed in health-care organizations in which authority rests primarily with administrators, physicians, and board members. Furthermore, nurses often are expected to do tasks they are overqualified for, which results in underuse of their many important skills.

Nurses are thus caught in the crossfire. They staff clinical areas around the clock, make important decisions, and shoulder major responsibility for coordinating and managing patient care, but they often lack decision-making authority as to the allocation of resources. Because nurses are usually not compensated on a fee-for-service basis, they are often not seen as a source of revenue by administrators and therefore lack a critical base for power. It is not surprising that if nurses do not have a role in organizational decision making, they will have limited ability to exercise control of their practice.

The full realization of nursing's potential will be obtained through a negotiated process with other health professionals, consumers, and society at large. It requires increased access to resources, demonstration of expertise, and acknowledgment of the skills of nurses by other professionals. Psychiatric nursing is practiced largely in collaboration, coordination, and cooperation with a variety of other professionals working with and on behalf of the patient. As nurses see themselves in a positive way, they will increase their ability to assert themselves, articulate the contributions they make, and function effectively. The conditions and behaviors related to each standard of professional performance are shown in Fig. 12-1. Each of these standards is now discussed.

QUALITY OF CARE

STANDARD I: QUALITY OF CARE
The psychiatric-mental health nurse systematically evaluates the quality of care and effectiveness of psychiatric-mental health nursing practice.

▼ *Rationale*
The dynamic nature of the mental health care environment and the growing body of psychiatric nursing knowledge and research provide both the impetus and the means for the psychiatric-mental health nurse to be competent in clinical practice, to continue to develop professionally, and to improve the quality of patient care.

▼ *Nursing conditions*
Personal and professional integrity
Openness to inquiry
Critical thinking skills

▼ *Nursing behaviors*
Identify improvement opportunities
Collect and analyze relevant data
Formulate a planned approach for improvement
Implement suggested changes

▼ *Key elements*
The nurse should be open to critically analyzing the caregiving process.
The patient and family should be partners with the nurse in the evaluation of care activities.
Improving the quality of care provided goes beyond discussion and analysis to actually implementing actions that will improve practice.

Psychiatric nurses actively participate in the formal organizational evaluation of overall patterns of care through a variety of quality improvement or process improvement activities (Baker et al, 2000; Williams, 1998). In these activities the focus is not on the nurse clinician but on the patient, the overall program of care, and health-related outcomes of care. The current commitment to critically reviewing health care stems from several sources: consumer demand for high-quality but reasonably priced health-care, third-party payer demand for controlled health care costs, increased professional accountability, and regulatory and federal groups that monitor the quality of care.

The purpose of quality or process improvement programs is to design, implement, evaluate, guide, and modify a process for improving the performance of a health-care organization and to initiate improvement activities. Specific objectives include the following:

- Continuous improvement of customer satisfaction
- Continuous improvement of patient outcomes
- Efficient use of resources
- Adherence to professional and regulatory standards

Continuous monitoring of performance indicators and feedback from patients and staff allows the organization to identify opportunities for improvement. Because of the complexity of patient care and work processes, an interdisciplinary team is formed to collect information and analyze the systems and processes that influence the outcomes achieved, incorporating the unique perspectives of the various team members. The team then designs and implements new processes and collects data to evaluate the effectiveness of the new activities.

Psychiatric nurses play essential roles in identifying opportunities for improvement, collecting data for analysis of the current process, evaluating the effectiveness of the new processes, and representing nursing's perspective in the improvement team's deliberations. Fig. 12-2 is a representation of the quality improvement process, which really is the problem-solving process or nursing process applied to making health-care processes and outcomes better.

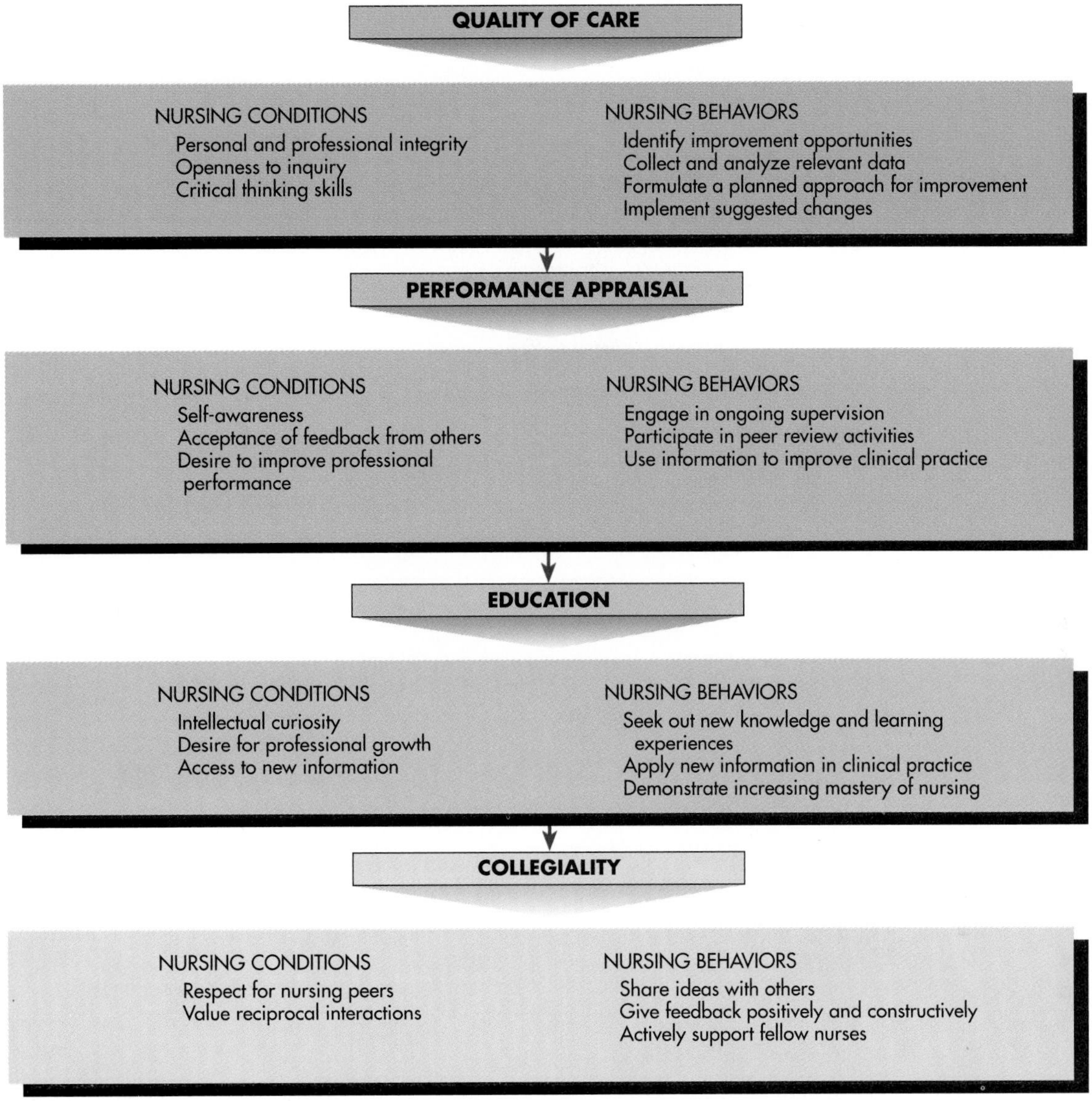

QUALITY OF CARE

NURSING CONDITIONS	NURSING BEHAVIORS
Personal and professional integrity	Identify improvement opportunities
Openness to inquiry	Collect and analyze relevant data
Critical thinking skills	Formulate a planned approach for improvement
	Implement suggested changes

PERFORMANCE APPRAISAL

NURSING CONDITIONS	NURSING BEHAVIORS
Self-awareness	Engage in ongoing supervision
Acceptance of feedback from others	Participate in peer review activities
Desire to improve professional performance	Use information to improve clinical practice

EDUCATION

NURSING CONDITIONS	NURSING BEHAVIORS
Intellectual curiosity	Seek out new knowledge and learning experiences
Desire for professional growth	Apply new information in clinical practice
Access to new information	Demonstrate increasing mastery of nursing

COLLEGIALITY

NURSING CONDITIONS	NURSING BEHAVIORS
Respect for nursing peers	Share ideas with others
Value reciprocal interactions	Give feedback positively and constructively
	Actively support fellow nurses

Fig. 12-1 Nursing conditions and behaviors related to the psychiatric nursing standards of professional performance.

Continued

Find out about a quality improvement project that is currently underway in your clinical facility. Does it relate to customer satisfaction, patient health outcomes, use of resources, or adherence to standards?

PERFORMANCE APPRAISAL

STANDARD II: PERFORMANCE APPRAISAL
The psychiatric-mental health nurse evaluates one's own practice in relation to professional practice standards and relevant statutes and regulations.
▼ *Rationale*
The psychiatric-mental health nurse is accountable to the public for providing competent clinical care and has inherent responsibility as a professional to evaluate the role and performance of psychiatric-mental health nursing practice according to standards established by the profession and licensing bodies.

▼ *Nursing conditions*
Self-awareness
Acceptance of feedback from others
Desire to improve professional performance
▼ *Nursing behaviors*
Engage in ongoing supervision
Participate in peer review activities
Use information to improve clinical practice
▼ *Key elements*
Supervision should be viewed as an essential and ongoing aspect of one's professional life.
The nurse should strive to grow and develop professional knowledge, skills, and expertise.

Performance appraisal for the psychiatric nurse is generally provided in two ways: administrative and clinical. Administrative performance appraisal involves the review, management, and regulation of competent psychiatric nursing

ETHICS

NURSING CONDITIONS	NURSING BEHAVIORS
Ability to engage in introspection Sensitivity to social and moral issues Commitment to the value clarification process	Guide practice by the *Code for Nurses* Practice with legal and ethical responsibility Act as patient and family advocate

COLLABORATION

NURSING CONDITIONS	NURSING BEHAVIORS
Positive self-concept Clear sense of professional identity and accountability Ability to work with others in a cooperative manner	Assertively contribute one's professional expertise Share planning and decision making with others Make referrals when appropriate

RESEARCH

NURSING CONDITIONS	NURSING BEHAVIORS
Quest for new knowledge or answers to questions Acute observational and analytical skills Persistence and attention to detail	Review reports of nursing research Generate questions and identify clinical problems Implement research findings in practice

RESOURCE USE

NURSING CONDITIONS	NURSING BEHAVIORS
Knowledge of the political and economic environment Ability to evaluate costs and benefits of treatment Skill in negotiating and accessing resources	Fact-based decision making Cost-effective allocation of resources Patient advocacy on an individual and collective basis

Fig. 12-1, cont'd

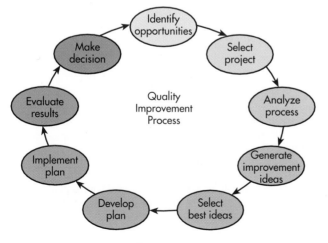

Fig. 12-2 Quality improvement process.

practice. It involves a supervisory relationship in which a nurse's work performance is compared with role expectations in a formal way, such as in a nurse's annual performance evaluation. Administrative performance evaluations should identify areas of competency and areas for improvement. There should also be a method for recognizing quality performance (see Critical Thinking about Contemporary Issues).

Many nursing departments have adopted clinical advancement programs or other formal mechanisms to recognize nursing excellence. Clinical advancement programs have been established to formally validate nurses for increasing mastery in practice. They allow the nurse to be promoted and economically rewarded for providing direct patient care. Such programs identify levels of professional development in nursing based on increased critical thinking and advanced application of nursing skills (Fig. 12-3). These characteristics result in better care provided by psychiatric nurses throughout their professional career.

What Kind of Recognition Do Staff Nurses Value?

It is well known that recognition is central to nurses' morale. However, it is less clear what type of recognition is valued and why it is given. A survey asked 239 staff nurses about this issue (Goode et al, 1993). They found that verbal feedback was identified as the most meaningful type of recognition. This was followed by letters of praise for performance or achievement, organizational awards, honors or public announcements of outstanding performance, promotion or a prestigious assignment with increased responsibility, being personally thanked and praised during an evaluation, and finally monetary bonuses, salary increases, or gifts.

The main reasons given for receiving recognition included outstanding performance in patient care and positive attitude, followed by demonstrated expertise, willingness to assume extra work, involvement in professional activities, completion of a certification or degree program, and years of service in an organization. Finally, recognition came most often from the head nurse, followed by the nurse administrator, patients and families, coworkers, physicians, and hospital administrators. Studies such as this help to clarify meaningful aspects of administrative performance appraisals and ways to commend nurses for a job well done.

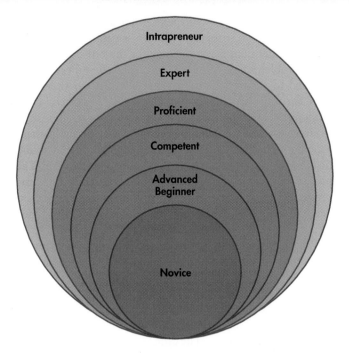

Fig. 12-3   Levels of differentiated nursing practice.

One of your nursing colleagues tells you that she thinks nurses' pay should be based on their experience, not their education. After all, she argues, if two nurses do the same job, what does it matter if they have different educational degrees? How would you respond?

Clinical Supervision

Clinical performance appraisal is guidance provided through a mentoring relationship with a more experienced, skilled, and educated nurse. The professional psychiatric nurse is aware of the need for ongoing mentorship to achieve increasing levels of mastery of psychiatric nursing practice. Clinical supervision not only reviews one's clinical care but can also be used as a support system for the nurse because nurses must care about themselves before being able to care for others (Billings, 1998).

In many ways the process of supervision parallels the nurse-patient relationship. Both involve a learning process that takes place in the context of a meaningful relationship that facilitates positive change. Self-exploration is a critical element of both. The supervisor should provide the same responsive and action dimensions present in the nurse-patient relationship to help supervised nurses live effectively with themselves and others.

There are four common forms of supervision:

- The dyadic, or one-on-one, relationship, in which the supervisor meets the one being supervised in a face-to-face encounter
- The triadic relationship, in which a supervisor and two nurses of similar experience and training meet for supervision
- Group supervision, in which several supervised nurses meet for a shared session with the supervisory nurse
- Peer review, in which nurses meet without a supervisor to evaluate their clinical practice

All four forms have a similar purpose: exploring the problem areas and maximizing the strengths of the ones being supervised.

Process of Supervision. The process of supervision requires the nurse to record the interactions with the patient. Both written notes and audio recordings have been used for this purpose, but neither yields as accurate and complete information as that provided by videotape recordings. Videotaped sessions minimize distortion of data. The supervised nurse then analyzes the data, extracts themes, and identifies problems relevant to nursing care. The nurse reviews the literature, draws inferences, evaluates effectiveness, and formulates plans for the next session. In the supervision conference the nurse shares this analysis and receives feedback from the supervisor or peers, if it is a group or peer conference.

Supervision can be seen as a didactic process in which the theory and concepts related to nursing practice are reviewed, or it can be a quasitherapeutic process that explores countertransference problems, attitudes, values, and the nurse's emotional needs and personal biases. A third approach is a process-centered model of supervision that is neither personal therapy nor simply a didactic process of conveying information on theory and technique. In this model the supervisor is an active participant in an affectively charged learning process, the focus of which is learning and personal growth rather than psychotherapy for the one being supervised. Problems between the clinician and the supervisor are believed to shed light on problems that exist between the clinician and patient. The very problems experienced in one relationship affect and are reflected in the other relationship.

However, the goal of supervision is not to eliminate these problems, but to use them to achieve greater understanding of the ongoing dynamic processes at work in therapy. The problems become the vehicles through which therapeutic progress may be made. Thus the most effective supervision depends on active insight into the many forces in the parallel processes of therapy and supervision (Dombeck & Brody, 1995). Finally, it is important to remember that tension in the supervisory relationship is inevitable, but when understood and handled skillfully, it can be very helpful to the clinician's growth.

Purpose and Goals. Despite its intensity, supervision is not therapy. The essential difference between the two is a difference of purpose. The aim of supervision is to teach psychotherapeutic skills, whereas the goal of therapy is to alter a person's characteristic patterns of coping to function more effectively in all areas of life. The problems of the one being supervised in the supervisory and therapeutic relationships are dealt with only to the extent that they affect the nurse's ability to learn from the supervisor and be effective with patients. Therefore the problems are limited in scope and depth; they do not include all other aspects of the life of the one being supervised. With the resolution of the particular problem, the focus of supervision returns to the teaching of psychotherapeutic skills and their implementation by the nurse. The therapeutic implications for the supervisee are therefore related to the primary goal of supervision: the teaching of psychotherapeutic skills.

Supervision or consultation is necessary for the practicing psychiatric nurse. Although it is crucial for novices, it is equally important for experienced practitioners (Farkas-Cameron, 1995). Personal limitations create a need for assistance in remaining objective throughout the therapeutic process and the "normal" stresses it presents. Obviously, supervision is only as helpful as the skill of the supervisor, the openness of the supervised nurse, and the motivation of both to learn and grow.

EDUCATION

STANDARD III: EDUCATION
The psychiatric-mental health nurse acquires and maintains current knowledge in nursing practice.
▼ *Rationale*
The rapid expansion of knowledge pertaining to basic and behavioral sciences, technology, information systems, and research requires a commitment to learning throughout the psychiatric-mental health nurse's professional career. Formal education, continuing education, independent learning activities, experiential and other learning activities are some of the means the psychiatric-mental health

nurse uses to enhance nursing expertise and advance the profession.
▼ *Nursing conditions*
Intellectual curiosity
Desire for professional growth
Access to new information
▼ *Nursing behaviors*
Seek out new knowledge and learning experiences
Apply new information in clinical practice
Demonstrate increasing mastery of nursing
▼ *Key elements*
Professional learning should be regarded as a lifelong process.
The nurse should pursue a variety of educational opportunities.
New knowledge should be translated into professional nursing practice.

The nature of psychiatric care, the mental health delivery system, and the boundaries of nursing are changing rapidly. In addition, the scientific basis for practice is expanding rapidly, and psychiatric nurses need to keep up with this knowledge.

Psychiatric nurses are expected to engage in a continuous learning process to maintain currency with the latest information in the field (Macklin & Matthews, 1998). They may do this in the following ways:

- Formal educational programs
- Continuing education programs
- Independent learning activities
- Lectures, conferences, and workshops
- Credentialing
- Certification

Reading journals and textbooks and collaborating with colleagues are other important ways to remain current with expanding areas of knowledge. Fig. 12-4 lists journals that relate to psychiatric nursing practice and are good sources of new information.

The Internet

The most exciting new resource for psychiatric nurses is the Internet. This technology allows nurses access to information

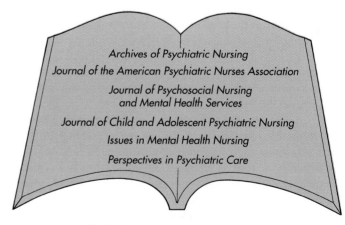

Archives of Psychiatric Nursing

Journal of the American Psychiatric Nurses Association

Journal of Psychosocial Nursing and Mental Health Services

Journal of Child and Adolescent Psychiatric Nursing

Issues in Mental Health Nursing

Perspectives in Psychiatric Care

Fig. 12-4 Psychiatric nursing journals.

from around the globe using a desktop or laptop computer, a telephone line, and a modem. Using browser software such as Netscape and Internet Explorer, nurses can receive textual information complemented by sound, video, and graphics on the World Wide Web, a subset of the Internet that allows the use of multimedia (Huang &Alessi, 1999; Sparks & Rizzolo, 1998). In addition, the Internet can help nurses communicate through e-mail and network with other nurses through discussion groups or newsgroups (see Citing the Evidence).

The number of Web home pages is growing rapidly. These sites offer a wide range of information, from updates on current psychiatric medications, to information on various mental disorders, to resources on mental health organizations and delivery systems, to teaching modules for clinical training (Clark, 2000; Galanter et al, 1997; Gound et al, 1998). The amount of information available through this technology is revolutionizing the way in which psychiatric nurses acquire and maintain current knowledge in nursing practice.

With its access to the MERLIN website, this text facilitates the use of the Internet by providing web links to home pages on the World Wide Web that are relevant to the content of each chapter. Nurses are encouraged to access these resources to further their knowledge and professional growth.

COLLEGIALITY

STANDARD IV: COLLEGIALITY
The psychiatric-mental health nurse interacts with and contributes to the professional development of peers, healthcare providers, and others, as colleagues.
 ▼ *Rationale*
The psychiatric-mental health nurse is responsible for sharing knowledge, research, and clinical information with colleagues, through formal and informal teaching methods, to enhance professional growth.
 ▼ *Nursing conditions*
   Respect for nursing peers
   Value reciprocal interactions
 ▼ *Nursing behaviors*
   Share ideas with others
   Give feedback positively and constructively
   Actively support fellow nurses
 ▼ *Key elements*
The nurse should regard other nurses as colleagues and partners in caregiving. Mentorship within nursing is important both to nurses as individuals and to the nursing profession as a whole.

Collegiality requires that nurses view their nurse peers as collaborators in the caregiving process who are valued and respected for their unique contributions, regardless of educational, experiential, or specialty background. It suggests that nurses view themselves as members of an organized professional group or unit and that nurses trust, remain loyal, and demonstrate commitment to other nurses.

Many have observed that nursing, as a profession, has sometimes struggled with this concept. For example, nurses have voiced complaints about "ivory-tower" nurse educators, "nonsupportive" nurse administrators, "nonintellectual" nurse clinicians, and "irrelevant" nurse researchers in the past. Also, psychiatric nurses in various institutions or organizations have had difficulty joining forces and working together on a common psychiatric nursing agenda. However, this intradisciplinary conflict is not consistent with professional performance standards. It has also prevented the profession from acting as a united group in pursuing health-care initiatives at local, regional, and national levels.

Nurses need to work together as colleagues to blend their various skills and abilities in creating a better health-care system and enhancing the quality and quantity of psychiatric nursing services provided. One specific way to do this is for psychiatric nurses to join a professional nursing organization. The largest psychiatric nursing organization that is open to nursing students and psychiatric nurses of all educational and experiential backgrounds is

Citing the Evidence on

The Internet

BACKGROUND: This study attempted to learn how psychiatric nurses use the Internet, how those that do have learned the skills needed to make themselves understood, and what nurses project the impact of the Internet will be on psychiatric nursing culture.

RESULTS: Respondents came from the United Kingdom, United States, New Zealand, Australia, Finland, Holland, Hong Kong, and Japan. They identified communicating and networking, researching, obtaining software, recreation, and keeping abreast of developments in the field as the main ways in which they used the Internet. Communication was the dominant use, while e-mail, chat rooms, World Wide Web, and telenet were the most common applications described. Respondents viewed the Internet as having the potential to affect nursing culture in three areas: (1) help to build an international community of psychiatric nurses; (2) enhance interdisciplinary and intradisciplinary communication; and (3) facilitate educational opportunities.

IMPLICATIONS: The Internet has the potential to shape new roles for psychiatric nurses such as on-line consulting and counseling, health education, and clinical supervision. In education the Internet is providing a virtual classroom. The challenge to psychiatric nurses is to use the technology in a way that facilitates a global psychiatric nursing culture and enhances the well-being of those for whom they care.

Lakeman R: The Internet: facilitating an international nursing culture for psychiatric nurses, *Computers Nurs* 16(2):87, 1998.

the American Psychiatric Nurses Association (APNA). The mission and goals of this organization are described in Box 12-1.

> **?** *You approach a colleague about joining the APNA but she tells you that she does not have the money to join a nursing organization. You know that membership in APNA costs about $2 a week and it includes a subscription to the Journal of the American Psychiatric Nurses Association. How would you respond?*

ETHICS

STANDARD V: ETHICS

The psychiatric-mental health nurse's assessments, actions, and recommendations on behalf of patients are determined and implemented in an ethical manner.

▼ *Rationale*

The public's trust and its right to humane psychiatric-mental health care are upheld by professional nursing practice. Ethical Standards describe a code of behaviors to guide professional practice. People with psychiatric-mental health needs are an especially vulnerable population. The foundation of psychiatric-mental health nursing practice is the development of a therapeutic relationship with the patient. Boundaries need to be established to safeguard the patient's well-being.

▼ *Nursing conditions*

Ability to engage in introspection
Sensitivity to social and moral issues
Commitment to the values clarification process

▼ *Nursing behaviors*

Guide practice by the code for nurses
Practice with legal and ethical responsibility
Act as a patient and family advocate

▼ *Key elements*

Nurses should be sensitive to the social, moral, and ethical environment in which they practice.
Patient and family advocacy is a core aspect of nursing practice.
Ethical conduct is essential to the nurse-patient relationship.

Box 12-1

Overview of the American Psychiatric Nurses Association (APNA)

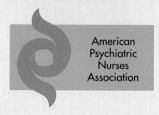

American Psychiatric Nurses Association

MISSION

To provide leadership to advance psychiatric-mental health nursing practice, improve mental health care for culturally diverse individuals, families, groups, and communities, and shape health policy for the delivery of mental health services.

GOALS

- Facilitate the professional development of psychiatric-mental health nurses through programs and services related to the creation, exchange, and engineering of new knowledge and skills
- Enhance the quality of care provided by psychiatric-mental health nurses through the promotion of established standards of clinical practice and professional performance
- Participate as partners and leaders in the formulation of policies and the design, implementation, and evaluation of delivery systems in psychiatric-mental health care
- Represent psychiatric-mental health nursing as a diverse but integrated specialty in the professional and public forum of the health-care community
- Refine the association's infrastructure to facilitate the successful achievement of the strategic plan

DUES

Regular membership: $110
Student membership: $66

INTERNET

http://www.apna.org

Ethical considerations combine with legal and therapeutic issues to affect all aspects of psychiatric nursing practice. The legal-ethical context of psychiatric nursing care is discussed in Chapter 10. Boundary violations related to the nurse-patient relationship are described in Chapter 2.

Ethical Standards

An ethic is a standard of behavior or a belief valued by an individual or group. It describes what ought to be, rather than what is—a goal to which an individual aspires. These standards are learned through socialization, growth, and experience. As such, they are not static but evolve to reflect social change.

Groups, such as professions, can also hold a code of ethics. Such a code guides the profession in serving and protecting consumers. It also provides a framework for decision mak-

ing for members of the profession. Two major purposes for a code of ethics are structuring and sensitizing. Structuring is preventive and aims to restrain impulsive and unethical behavior. Sensitizing is educative, with the goal of raising members' ethical consciousness.

The American Nurses' Association (1985) published a code of ethics for nurses (Box 12-2). It emphasizes nurses' accountability for the quality of care they give and their duty to act as patient advocates in ensuring the quality of care given by others.

Ethical Decision Making

Ethical decision making involves trying to distinguish right from wrong in situations without clear guidelines (Artnak &

Box **12-2**

American Nurses' Association Code for Nurses

- The nurse provides services with respect for human dignity and the uniqueness of the client unrestricted by considerations of social or economic status, personal attributes, or the nature of health problems.
- The nurse safeguards the client's right to privacy by judiciously protecting information of a confidential nature.
- The nurse acts to safeguard the client and public when health care and safety are affected by the incompetent, unethical, or illegal practice of any person.
- The nurse assumes responsibility and accountability for individual nursing judgments and actions.
- The nurse maintains competence in nursing.
- The nurse exercises informed judgment and uses individual competence and qualification as criteria in seeking consultation, accepting responsibilities, and delegating nursing activities to others.
- The nurse participates in activities that contribute to the ongoing development of the profession's body of knowledge.
- The nurse participates in the profession's efforts to implement and improve standards of nursing.
- The nurse participates in the profession's efforts to establish and maintain conditions of employment conducive to high-quality nursing care.
- The nurse participates in the profession's effort to protect the public from misinformation and misrepresentation and to maintain the integrity of nursing.
- The nurse collaborates with members of the health professions and other citizens in promoting community and national efforts to meet public health needs.

From American Nurses' Association: *Code for nurses with interpretive statements*, Kansas City, Mo, 1985, The Association.

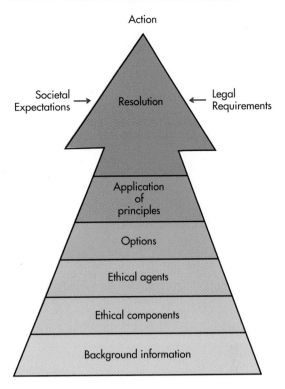

Fig. 12-5 Model for ethical decision making. Societal expectations and legal requirements may sway the resolution of the conflict one way or another. However, the notions of what is legal (or expected) may or may not coincide with what is good, right, or proper. (From Curtin L: A proposed model for critical ethical analysis, *Nurs Forum* 17:12, 1978.)

Dimmitt, 1996). A decision-making model can help identify factors and principles that affect a decision.

Curtin (1978) proposed a model for critical ethical analysis (Fig. 12-5) that describes steps or factors that the nurse should consider in resolving an ethical dilemma. The first step is **gathering background information** to obtain a clear picture of the problem. This includes finding available information to clarify the underlying issues. The next factor is **identifying the ethical components** or the nature of the dilemma, such as freedom versus coercion or treating versus accepting the right to refuse treatment. The next step is the **clarification of the rights and responsibilities of all ethical agents,** or those involved in the decision making. This can include the patient, the nurse, and possibly many others, including the patient's family, physician, health-care institution, clergy, social worker, and perhaps even the courts. Those involved may not agree on how to handle the situation, but their rights and duties can be clarified. **All possible options must then be explored** in light of everyone's responsibilities, as well as the purpose and potential result of each option. This step eliminates alternatives that violate rights or seem harmful. The nurse then engages in the **application of principles,** which stem from the nurse's philosophy of life and nursing, scientific knowledge, and ethical theory (Duldt, 1995). Ethical theories suggest ways to structure ethical dilemmas and judge potential solutions. Four possible approaches include the following:

Utilitarianism which focuses on the consequences of actions. It seeks the greatest amount of happiness or the least amount of harm for the greatest number, or "the greatest good for the greatest number."

Egoism is a position in which the individual seeks the solution that is best personally. The self is most important, and others are secondary.

Formalism considers the nature of the act itself and the principles involved. It involves the universal application of a basic rule, such as "do unto others as you would have them do unto you."

Fairness is based on the concept of justice, and benefit to the least advantaged in society becomes the norm for decision making.

The final step is **resolution into action.** Within the context of social expectations and legal requirements, the nurse decides on the goals and methods of implementation. Table 12-1 summarizes these steps and suggests questions nurses can ask themselves in making complex ethical choices in psychiatric nursing practice.

Table **12-1**

Steps and Questions in Ethical Decision Making	
Steps	**Relevant Questions**
Gathering background information	Does an ethical dilemma exist?
	What information is known?
	What information is needed?
	What is the context of the dilemma?
Identifying ethical components	What is the underlying issue?
	Who is affected by this dilemma?
Clarification of agents	What are the rights of each involved party?
	What are the obligations of each involved party?
	Who should be involved in the decision making?
	For whom is the decision being made?
	What degree of consent is needed by the patient?
Exploration of options	What alternatives exist?
	What is the purpose or intent of each alternative?
	What are the potential consequences of each alternative?
Application of principles	What criteria should be used?
	What ethical theories are subscribed to?
	What scientific facts are relevant?
	What is the nurse's philosophy of life and nursing?
Resolution into action	What are the social and legal constraints and ramifications?
	What is the goal of the nurse's decision?
	How can the resulting ethical choice be implemented?
	How can the resulting ethical choice be evaluated?

? *Think of an ethical problem you have encountered in caring for a psychiatric patient and family. Use the model for ethical decision making to decide on the best course of action.*

COLLABORATION

STANDARD VI: COLLABORATION
The psychiatric-mental health nurse collaborates with the patient, significant others, and health-care providers in providing care.
▼ *Rationale*
Psychiatric-mental health nursing practice requires a coordinated, ongoing interaction between consumers and providers to deliver comprehensive services to the patient and the community. Through the collaborative process, different abilities of health-care providers are used to identify problems, communicate, and plan; implement interventions; and evaluate mental health services.
▼ *Nursing conditions*
Positive self-concept
Clear sense of professional identity and accountability
Ability to work with others in a cooperative manner
▼ *Nursing behaviors*
Assertively contribute one's professional expertise
Share planning and decision making with others
Make referrals when appropriate
▼ *Key elements*
Respect for others grows out of respect for self.
The nurse should be able to clearly articulate his or her professional abilities and areas of expertise to others.
Collaboration involves the ability to negotiate and formulate new solutions with others.

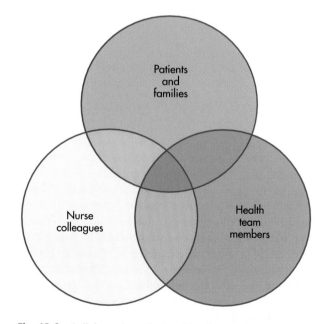

Fig. 12-6   Collaborative relationships for psychiatric nurses.

Collaboration is the shared planning, decision making, problem solving, goal setting, and assumption of responsibilities by individuals who work together cooperatively and with open communication. Three key ingredients are needed for collaboration:
- Active and assertive contributions from each person
- Receptivity and respect for each person's contribution

Table **12-2**

Mental Health Personnel, Training, and Roles		
Personnel	Training	Role
Psychiatric nurse	Registered nurse (RN) with specialized training in the care and treatment of psychiatric patients. May have an AD, BS, MS, or PhD degree	Accountable for the biopsychosocial nursing care of patients and their milieu
Psychiatrist	Medical doctor with internship and residency training in psychiatry	Accountable for the medical diagnosis and treatment of patients
Social worker	BS, MSW, or PhD degree with specialized training in mental health settings	Accountable for family casework and community placement of patients
Psychologist	PhD or PsyD degree with research and clinical training in mental health	Accountable for psychological assessments, testing, and treatments
Activity therapist	May have a BS degree with training in mental health settings	Accountable for recreational, occupational, and activity programs
Case worker	Varying degrees of training and usually works under supervision	Accountable for helping patients to be maintained in the community and receive needed services
Substance abuse counselor	Varying degrees of training in alcohol and substance use disorders	Accountable for evaluating and treating patients with substance use problems

- Negotiations that build on the contributions of each person to form a new way of conceptualizing the problem

Psychiatric nurses have many potential collaborators, including patients and families, interdisciplinary colleagues, and nursing peers (Fig. 12-6). Each of these groups allows the psychiatric nurse an opportunity to solve problems in new ways and thus better plan and implement nursing care.

Interdisciplinary Mental Health Teams

An essential part of contemporary practice is working with other health-care providers (Akhavain et al, 1999; Gianakos, 1997). Nurses may be members of three different types of teams: unidisciplinary, having all team members of the same discipline; multidisciplinary, having members of different disciplines who provide specific services to the patient; and interdisciplinary, having members of different disciplines involved in a formal arrangement to provide patient services while maximizing educational interchange. Most organized mental health settings use an interdisciplinary team approach, which requires highly coordinated and often interdependent planning based on the separate and distinct roles of each team member (Table 12-2).

It has been said that nurses seek mutual colleagiality, while physicians encourage teamwork with subordinates. How would these different views affect the process of collaboration?

Interdisciplinary collaboration does not always proceed smoothly. There are many barriers to interdisciplinary collaboration, including inappropriate education and training

Box **12-3**

Steps for Interdisciplinary Team Building
- Develop and agree on a team philosophy of care
- Understand and respect the contributions of each discipline
- Establish new professional interaction patterns
- Define disciplinary and individual roles and responsibilities
- Accept personal and professional changes in authority and status
- Specify lines of authority and decision making and conflict resolution procedures
- Accept shared authority and responsibility
- Communicate regularly, openly, and clearly
- Use multidisciplinary treatment plans and consolidated charting
- Strive for consistent leadership and low staff turnover
- Encourage constant review and exchange of ideas

of mental health team members, traditional organizational structures, goal and role conflict, competitive and accommodating interpersonal interactions, power and status inequities, and personal qualities of individuals that do not promote shared problem solving. If roles, functions, and channels of communication among the various team members are not clarified and agreed on, confusion, resentment, crossing of boundaries, and inappropriate use of psychiatric team members are likely to result. Steps that can be taken to facilitate the formation of interdisciplinary teams are listed in Box 12-3.

It is also important for nurses to maintain their professional integrity in the midst of interdisciplinary collaboration. Nurses must not abandon the nursing perspective when they participate in an interdisciplinary team (Lindeke

& Block, 1998; McCloskey & Maas, 1998). Finally, psychiatric nurses must determine whether they as a group are ready to engage in collaborative practice. Questions that should be considered include the following:

- Can psychiatric nurses define, describe, and appropriately defend psychiatric nursing roles and functions?
- Is the psychiatric nursing leadership ready for collegial practice?
- Are psychiatric nursing roles and functions appropriate for nurses' education, experience, and expertise?
- Is nurse staffing appropriate in numbers, patterns, and ratios?
- Are the other disciplines prepared for and supportive of collaboration?
- Is the organizational climate conducive to collaboration?

With positive answers to these questions, psychiatric nurses should be able to move forward in implementing collaborative practice.

> *Most people think that there are more collaborative interdisciplinary relationships in psychiatry than in other specialty areas because of the nature of the work. Others believe that there is more interdisciplinary conflict in psychiatry because roles overlap and boundaries are often unclear. What position would you take on this issue based on your observation of the mental health-care team?*

RESEARCH

STANDARD VII: RESEARCH
The psychiatric-mental health nurse contributes to nursing and mental health through the use of research methods and findings.
▼ *Rationale*
Nurses in psychiatric-mental health nursing are responsible for contributing to the further development of the field of mental health by participating in research. At the basic level of practice the psychiatric-mental health nurse uses research findings to improve clinical care and identifies clinical problems for research study. At the advanced level the psychiatric-mental health nurse engages and/or collaborates with others in the research process to discover, examine, and test knowledge, theories, and creative approaches to practice.
▼ *Nursing conditions*
  Quest for new knowledge or answers to questions
  Acute observational and analytical skills
  Persistence and attention to detail
▼ *Nursing behaviors*
  Review reports of nursing research
  Generate questions and identify clinical problems
  Implement research findings in practice
▼ *Key elements*
  Research links nursing theory and practice and is essential to the development of a profession.
  Outcome research helps to establish the value of nursing in an era of health-care reform.

The progression of observing from practice, theorizing, testing in research, and subsequently modifying practice is an essential part of psychiatric nursing. The clinical problems are numerous, and as nurses gain the skills and experience to validate their work scientifically, they can make a significant contribution to psychiatric theory and practice (see Citing the Evidence on the next page). The nature and process of outcomes research and evidence-based practice are discussed in detail in Chapter 5.

It is important to encourage close collaboration between nurse researchers and nurse clinicians to ensure that the right questions are asked and the right variables are tested. It is also necessary to clearly define how nurses with different educational backgrounds can participate in research. Table 12-3 summarizes the research expectations for nurses based on educational preparation. Finally, one research study on psychiatric nurses' attitudes toward involvement in nursing research found that the three major blocks to clinical nursing research were lack of time, lack of knowledge, and lack of administrative support (Poster et al, 1992). It found that positive attitudes toward nursing research were related to nurses' advanced levels of education, although the authors suggested that research skills could be fostered through inservice education classes and individualized learning experiences.

RESOURCE USE

STANDARD VIII: RESOURCE USE
The psychiatric-mental health nurse considers factors related to safety, effectiveness, and cost in planning and delivering patient care.
▼ *Rationale*
The patient is entitled to psychiatric-mental health care that is safe, effective, and affordable. As the cost of health-care increases, treatment decisions must be made in such a way as to maximize resources and maintain quality of care. The psychiatric-mental health nurse seeks to provide cost-effective, high-quality care by using the most appropriate resources and delegating care to the most appropriate, qualified health-care provider.
▼ *Nursing conditions*
  Knowledge of the political and economic environment
  Ability to evaluate costs and benefits of treatment
  Skill in negotiating and accessing resources
▼ *Nursing behaviors*
  Fact-based decision making
  Cost-effective allocation of resources
  Patient advocacy on an individual and collective basis
▼ *Key elements*
  Nurses play a critical role in integrating and coordinating health-care services.
  Nurses should be fiscally accountable for the care they provide.
  Resources should be allocated based on cost/benefit analyses and documented expected outcomes.

Resource use is one of the most important aspects of psychiatric nursing practice. Discussing the costs and benefits of treatment options with patients, families, providers, and reimbursers is an essential part of the professional psychiatric nursing role. To fulfill this performance standard, psychiatric nurses need to request and obtain both cost and outcome information related to tests, consultations, evaluations, therapies, and continuum of care alternatives. Nurses need to assume an active role in questioning, advising, and advocating for the most cost-effective use of resources.

One of the most critical resources in the mental health field is that of psychiatric labor (Merwin & Fox, 1992). Because each team member has different competencies, a challenge for the mental health system is to use the best that each discipline has to offer and to develop an integrated set of clinical services that will offer the highest quality care (Stuart et al, 2000).

Citing the Evidence on

Psychiatric Nursing Research

BACKGROUND: Through a collaborative research project, nurse clinicians and nurse academics identified and prioritized the most important research questions arising from the current and future practice of mental health nurses in an eastern Canadian region.

RESULTS: Nine categories of research questions arose. The top four categories were preparation of helpers, the service system, caregiver needs, and patients with major behavior problems. Other categories included abuse, assaultive behavior, helping relationships, community integration, and medication use.

IMPLICATIONS: The partnership of nurse clinicians and nurse academicians is valuable in identifying issues embedded in the everyday practice of psychiatric nursing most in need of research attention. There is an urgent need for research that explores what it is that nurses need to know to achieve and maintain standards of practice and to improve patient care outcomes.

Davidson et al: Voices from practice: mental health nurses identify research priorities, *Arch Psychiatr Nurs* 11(6):340, 1997.

Psychiatric nurses must become increasingly cost and outcome conscious. Identify three commonly ordered tests for psychiatric patients. Find out how much they cost and analyze how helpful they are in planning treatment.

Summary

1. The standards of professional performance apply to self-regulation and accountability for practice that must be demonstrated by psychiatric nurses both individually and as a group. The standards also relate to professional autonomy and self-definition.
2. Psychiatric nurses need to participate actively in the formal organizational evaluation of overall patterns of care through a variety of quality improvement activities, including systems, consumer, and clinical evaluation.
3. Performance appraisal involves administrative review of work performance and clinical supervision of nursing care.
4. Psychiatric nurses are expected to engage in a continual learning process to maintain currency with the latest information in the field.
5. Collegiality requires that psychiatric nurses view their nurse peers as collaborators in the caregiving process who are valued and respected for their unique contributions.
6. Ethical considerations combine with legal and therapeutic issues to affect all aspects of psychiatric nursing practice and require the use of ethical decision making in caring for patients.
7. Collaboration is the shared planning, decision making, problem solving, goal setting, and assumption of responsibilities by people who work together cooperatively and with open communication. Psychiatric nurses collaborate with patients, families, nurse colleagues, and members of the health-care team.
8. Research is an essential professional activity for psychiatric nurses, and additional research is needed on the outcomes of psychiatric nursing intervention to determine its effectiveness.
9. Psychiatric nurses must evaluate the most appropriate use of resources in the delivery of care. Issues of costs, benefits, outcomes, treatment setting, and appropriate use of mental health-care providers must be considered.

Table 12-3

Nursing Research Participation Based on Education	
Educational Preparation	**Research Involvement**
Associate degree in nursing	Help identify clinical problems in nursing practice, assist in data collection within a structured format, use research findings in practice with supervision
Baccalaureate degree in nursing	Identify clinical problems in need of research, help experienced investigators gain access to clinical sites, influence the selection of appropriate methods of data collection, participate in data collection and implementation of research findings
Master's degree in nursing	Collaborate in proposal development, data collection, data analysis, and interpretation; appraise the clinical relevance of research findings; provide leadership for integrating findings into practice
Doctoral education	Develop nursing knowledge through research and theory development, conduct funded independent research projects, develop and coordinate funded research projects, disseminate research findings to the scientific community

MERLIN Visit MERLIN: www.mosby.com/MERLIN/Stuart to find these additional materials and student activities.

- **Worksheets**
- **"Drug of the Month" Updates**
- **"Citing the Evidence" Updates**
- **Critical Thinking Activities and Exercises**
- **Annotated Suggested Readings**
- **Web Links**
- **More!**

Chapter Review Questions

1. **Identify whether the following statements are true (T) or false (F).**
   ___ A. Adherence to professional and regulatory standards is one of the areas of quality improvement.
   ___ B. An associate degree in nursing qualifies one to become a certified generalist in psychiatric nursing.
   ___ C. The American Psychiatric Nurses Association is the largest specialty organization for psychiatric nurses.
   ___ D. Fairness is the ethical theory that seeks the greatest good for the greatest number.
   ___ E. All nurses, regardless of educational background, can participate in research activities.

2. **Fill in the blanks.**
   A. _____ focuses responsibility on the individual nurse for personal and professional actions.
   B. The condition that allows for definition and control of a work domain and that implies self-determination, independence, and shared power is _____.

   C. In many ways the supervision process parallels the _____.
   D. The _____ is technology that allows nurses access to information from around the globe using a computer.
   E. An _____ is a standard of behavior or a belief valued by an individual or group that describes what ought to be rather than what is.
   F. An _____ team is one in which members of different disciplines are involved in a formal arrangement to provide patient services while maximizing educational exchange.

3. **Provide short answers for the following questions.**
   A. Describe how the nursing process is similar to the quality improvement process used in health-care organizations.
   B. Discuss the differences between clinical supervision and therapy.
   C. Identify an ethical problem you have experienced. Describe how you would use the model in Fig. 12-5 to decide on a course of action.

REFERENCES

Akhavain P et al: Collaborative practice: a nursing perspective of the psychiatric interdisciplinary treatment team, *Holistic Nurs Pract* 13(2):1, 1999.

American Nurses' Association: *Code for nurses with interpretive statements*, Kansas City, Mo, 1985, The Association.

American Nurses' Association: *Scope and standards of psychiatric-mental health clinical nursing practice*, Washington, DC, 2000, The Association.

Artnak K, Dimmitt J: Choosing a framework for ethical analysis in advanced practice settings: the case for casuistry, *Arch Psychiatr Nurs* 10:16, 1996.

Baker J et al: Using quality improvement teams to improve documentation in records at a community mental health center, *Psychiatr Serv* 51(2):239, 2000.

Billings C: Professional insights: on peer feedback, *J Am Psychiatr Nurs Assoc* 4(3):103, 1998.

Clarke B: Testing the cyber-couch, *Behavioral Healthcare Tomorrow* 9:10, 2000.

Curtin L: A proposed model for critical ethical analysis, *Nurs Forum* 17:12, 1978.

Dombeck M, Brody S: Clinical supervision: a three-way mirror, *Arch Psychiatr Nurs* 9:3, 1995.

Duldt B: Integrating nursing theory and ethics, *Perspect Psychiatr Care* 31:4, 1995.

Farkas-Cameron M: Clinical supervision in psychiatric nursing, *J Psychosoc Nurs* 33:31, 1995.

Galanter M et al: Using the Internet for clinical training: a course on network therapy for substance abuse, *Psychiatr Serv* 48(8):999, 1997.

Gianakos D: Physicians, nurses and collegiality, *Nurs Outlook* 45(2):57, 1997.

Goode C et al: What kind of recognition do staff nurses want? *Am J Nurs* 1993:64, 1993.

Gound P et al: A computerized learning tool, *Am J Nurs* 98(11):56, 1998.

Huang M, Alessi N: Developing trends of the world wide web, *Psychiatr Serv* 50(1):31, 1999.

Lindeke L, Block D: Maintaining professional integrity in the midst of interdisciplinary collaboration, *Nurs Outlook* 46(5):213, 1998.

Macklin N, Matthews J: Ensuring quality in continuing education, *Am J Nurs* 98(4):60, 1998.

McCloskey J, Maas M: Interdisciplinary team: the nursing perspective is essential, 46(4): 157, 1998.

Merwin E, Fox J: Cost-effective integration of mental health professions, *Issues Ment Health Nurs* 13:139, 1992.

Poster E et al: Psychiatric nurses' attitudes toward and involvement in nursing research, *J Psychosoc Nurs Ment Health Serv* 30:26, 1992.

Sparks S, Rizzolo M: World wide web search tools: *Image: J Nurs Scholarship* 30(2):167, 1998.

Stuart G et al: Role utilization of nurses in public psychiatry, *Admin Policy Ment Health* 27(6):423, 2000.

Williams R: Nurse leaders' perceptions of quality nursing: an analysis from academe, *Nurs Outlook* 46(6):262, 1998.

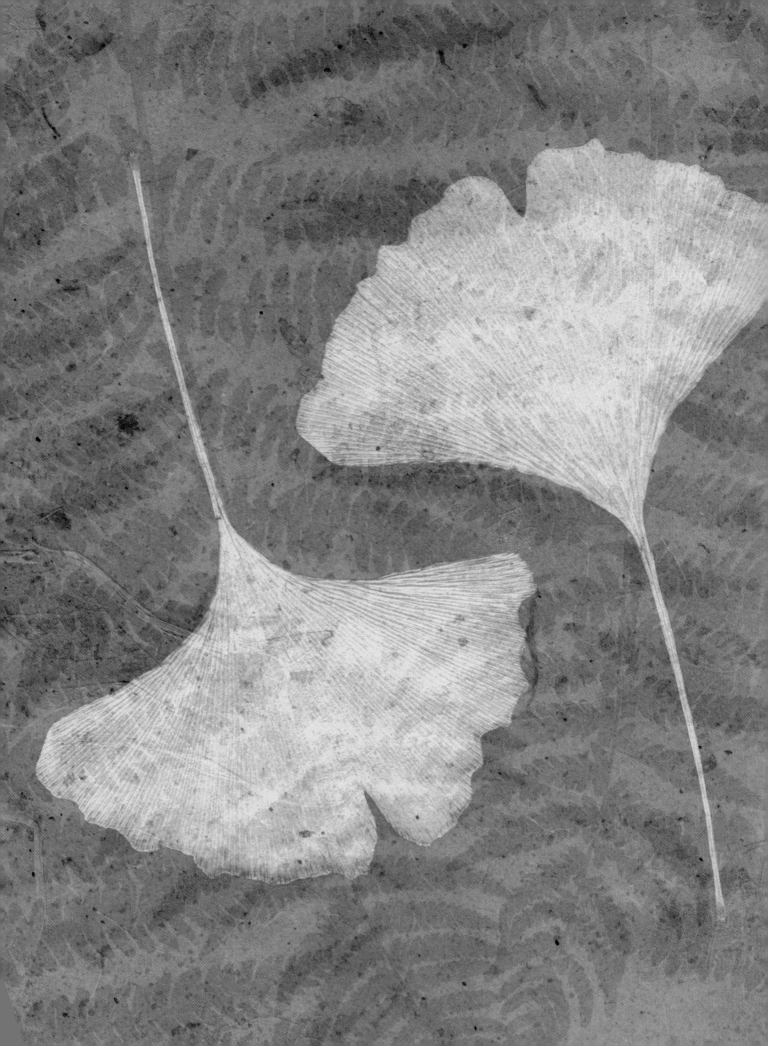

Unit 2
Continuum of Care

Continuum. What an interesting word. It means "a series of variations, or a sequence of things in regular order." As such, it is the perfect descriptor of the levels of contemporary psychiatric treatment. The continuum of psychiatric care allows nurses to use the full range of their skills and talents, often in new settings and innovative programs. Perhaps best of all, it provides patients, families, and communities with the healing ability to build competence, resilience, and health rather than merely to treat disability, illness, and disease. It therefore includes working with patients in crisis, acute, maintenance, and health promotion stages of treatment. Such is the brave new world of psychiatric and mental health nursing.

In this unit you will learn about intervening with primary, secondary, and tertiary prevention activities. You will also hear from family members about their role in the continuum of care. All nurses, regardless of their specialty area, need to know how to promote mental health, intervene with patients and families in crisis, and build rehabilitative functioning in those who are ill. In the future you will use these skills more often than you might ever have imagined, and you will think back to this unit and the information it imparted with greater appreciation for the caregiving continuum.

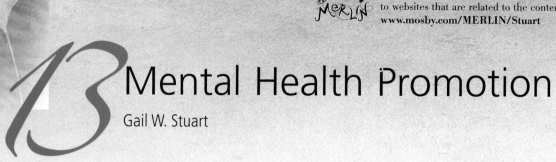

13 Mental Health Promotion

Gail W. Stuart

What is this thing called health? Simply a state in which the individual happens transiently to be perfectly adapted to his environment. Obviously, such states cannot be common, for the environment is in constant flux.

        H. L. MENCKEN, *THE AMERICAN MERCURY,* **MARCH 1930**

Mental health promotion and mental illness prevention are important parts of psychiatric nursing care. In the classic work, *Principles of Preventive Psychiatry,* Caplan (1964) applied the three levels of preventive intervention from the public health model to mental illness and emotional disturbance.

Primary prevention is lowering the **incidence** of a mental disorder or reducing the rate at which new cases of a disorder develop.

Secondary prevention involves reducing the **prevalence** of a mental disorder by reducing the number of existing cases. Secondary prevention activities include early case finding, screening, and prompt effective treatment.

Tertiary prevention activities attempt to reduce the severity of a mental disorder and associated disability through rehabilitative activities.

Each of these has implications for nursing practice. Primary prevention is the focus of this chapter; secondary prevention is addressed in Chapter 14 on Crisis Intervention; and tertiary prevention is described in Chapter 15 on Psychiatric Rehabilitation.

CONCEPTUALIZING PRIMARY PREVENTION

Primary prevention is often described with such slogans as "An ounce of prevention is worth a pound of cure" or "Curing is costly; prevention is priceless." However, the major emphasis in the United States has been on secondary prevention activities or the treatment of mental disorders. Only recently is primary prevention emerging as a substantial force in the mental health movement. One of the reasons it is gaining momentum is because of changes in the health-care system. As health and mental health-care move toward capitated payment and managed care, there is a greater economic incentive to prevent illness rather than treat it.

This change is evident in three recent reports. The first report, prepared by the National Mental Health Association (1998), presented a risk and evidence-based framework for maintaining and measuring prevention services in managed care. It recommended a strategic plan that would take advantage of existing knowledge by targeting prevention strategies for major depression across the life span, low birthweight and child maltreatment, alcohol and drug use in children who have an alcohol-or drug-abusing parent, mental health problems in the physically ill, and conduct disorders in children.

The second report by the National Advisory Mental Health Council Workgroup on Mental Disorders Prevention Research (1998) made recommendations to the National Institute of Mental Health on prevention research. This report noted that the field is ready to initiate a third generation of prevention research building on prior research accomplishments and integrating these with advances in the biomedical, behavioral, and cognitive sciences.

The third document is the *Report of the Surgeon General on Mental Health* (U.S. Department of Health and Human Services, 1999), which states that mental health is fundamental to health and that qualities of mental health are essential to leading a healthy life. This report urges Americans to assign priority to the task of promoting mental health and preventing mental disorders.

The idea of promoting mental health in general is attractive. Promotion sounds optimistic and positive. It is consistent with the idea of self-help and being self-responsible for health. It implies changing human behavior and draws on a holistic approach to health. Also, the ability to prevent the development of a psychiatric illness would reap many benefits for individuals, families, communities, and society. Thus primary prevention activities in psychiatric care have two basic aims (Tudor, 1996):

- To help people to avoid stressors or to cope with them more adaptively
- To change the resources, policies, or agents of the environment so that they no longer cause stress but rather enhance people's functioning

These are both important functions of contemporary psychiatric nursing practice.

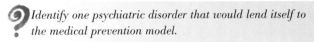

The terms **health promotion** *and* **illness prevention** *are often used interchangeably. In what ways do they overlap and how are they different?*

Medical Prevention Model

The medical prevention model focuses on genetic counseling and on biochemical and brain research to discover the specific causes of mental illness. It suggests that primary prevention activities are best focused on illness prevention. This model consists of the following steps:

1. Identify a disease that warrants the development of a preventive intervention program. Develop reliable methods for its diagnosis so that people can be divided into groups according to whether they do or do not have the disease.
2. By a series of epidemiological and laboratory studies, identify the most likely cause of the disease.
3. Launch and evaluate an experimental preventive intervention program based on the results of those studies.

This model has been effective for a broad array of communicable diseases such as smallpox, typhus, malaria, diphtheria, tuberculosis, rubella, and polio and nutritional diseases such as scurvy, pellagra, rickets, kwashiorkor, and endemic goiter. It has also proved useful in a variety of mental disorders caused by poisons, chemicals, licit or illicit drugs, electrolyte imbalances, and nutritional deficiencies.

All these diseases have one thing in common: a known necessary, but not always sufficient, causative factor.

Identify one psychiatric disorder that would lend itself to the medical prevention model.

Nursing Prevention Model

The nursing prevention model stresses that mental disorders do not have a single identified precondition, but are caused by many factors that are interactive, situational, and sociocultural. They thus require that mental illness prevention be thought of in a more behavioral way as the prevention of problems or maladaptive responses. By doing so, many of the services already available in the community can be identified and publicly acknowledged as prevention efforts.

Problems defined in this way can include both single-episode events such as a divorce and long-standing conditions such as marital conflict. They can also reflect either an acute health problem or a chronic health problem. For example, the following categories of problems can arise from alcohol abuse:

- Acute health problems such as overdose or delirium tremens
- Chronic health problems such as cirrhosis of the liver
- Casualties, such as accidents on the road, in the home, or elsewhere, and suicide
- Violent crime and family abuse
- Problems of demeanor such as public drunkenness and use of alcohol by teenagers
- Default of major social roles (work or school and family roles)
- Problems of feeling state (demoralization and depression and experienced loss of control)

The nursing prevention model assumes that problems are multicausal, that everyone is vulnerable to stressful life events, and that any disability or problem may arise as a consequence. For example, four vulnerable people can face a stressful life event, such as the collapse of a marriage or the loss of a job. One person may become severely depressed, the second may be involved in an automobile accident, the third may head down the road to alcoholism, and the fourth may develop coronary artery disease. The nursing prevention model does not search for a cause for each problem. Rather, it involves the following steps:

1. Identify a biopsychosocial stressor that appears to have undesirable consequences in a significant proportion of the population. Develop procedures for reliably identifying people who have undergone or are undergoing that stressful experience.
2. By epidemiological and laboratory methods, study the consequences of that stressor and develop hypotheses related to how its negative consequences might be reduced or eliminated.
3. Launch and evaluate experimental preventive intervention programs based on these hypotheses.

The nursing model also includes application of the nursing process, with a focus on the primary prevention of maladaptive coping responses associated with an identified stressor. It thus incorporates the following aspects:

Assessment: Identifying a stressor that precipitates maladaptive responses and a target or population group that is vulnerable or at risk for it

Planning: Formulating specific prevention strategies and social institutions and situations through which the strategies may be applied

Implementation: Applying selected nursing interventions aimed at decreasing maladaptive responses to the identified stressor and enhancing adaptation

Evaluation: Determining the effectiveness of the nursing interventions with regard to short- and long-term outcomes, use of resources, and comparison with other prevention strategies

The nursing process can thus be used in a goal-directed way to decrease the incidence of mental illness and promote mental health.

 Analyze the problem of child abuse from the nursing prevention perspective.

ASSESSMENT

Risk Factors and Protective Factors

The concepts of risk and protective factors are central to evidence-based prevention programs.

Risk factors are those predisposing characteristics that, if present for a person, make it more likely that he or she will develop a disorder. Some risk factors are fixed, such as gender and family history, while others can be changed, such as social support and inability to read. Current research is focusing on the interplay between biological, psychosocial, and environmental risk factors and how they can be modified to eventually prevent a biological risk factor, such as the genes that may contribute to developing a mental illness, from being expressed.

Protective factors are the coping resources and coping mechanisms that can improve a person's response to stress, resulting in adaptive behavior. These factors exist in the individual, family, and community. They can have a powerful effect on the influence of risk factors, and the potential for altering these factors is great.

Target Populations

Three types of preventive interventions based on target populations have been identified (Mrazek & Haggerty, 1994):

- **Universal:** targeted to the general population group without consideration of risk factors
- **Selective:** targeted to individuals or groups with a significantly higher risk of developing a particular disorder
- **Indicated:** targeted to high-risk individuals identified as having symptoms foreshadowing a specific mental disorder or biological markers indicating predisposition for the disorder

A knowledge of normal growth and development is essential for assessing a person's functioning and for intervening with preventive nursing interventions. The nurse should be familiar with normative stages, tasks, and parameters to know what issues the person has faced in the past and what challenges lie ahead. In addition to understanding the person's development, the nurse must know about the family cycle because many nursing interventions are directed at the family, from mobilizing their support of a patient to modifying dysfunctional family patterns.

Assessment in primary prevention therefore involves identifying individuals and groups of people who are vulnerable to developing mental disorders or who may display maladaptive coping responses to specific stressors or risk factors. To complete such an assessment, the nurse needs to draw on information generated from theory, research, and clinical practice.

It is also important for the nurse to realize that not all people in these groups are at equal risk. What these groups share is the experience of a life event, stressor, or risk factor that represents a loss of some kind or places an excessive demand on one's ability to cope. The more clearly the subgroup can be defined, the more specifically the prevention strategies can be researched, identified, and implemented.

Behavioral rating scales that can be used by the nurse to assess a person's general health status are listed in Box 13-1.

 Identify three groups of people vulnerable to the development of psychiatric illness, one based on biological factors, one based on psychological factors, and one based on sociocultural factors.

PLANNING AND IMPLEMENTATION

The Stuart Stress Adaptation Model presented in Chapter 4 and represented in Fig. 13-1 is useful for the nurse in planning strategies for primary prevention. If the overall nursing goal is to promote constructive coping mechanisms and maximize adaptive coping responses, then the model suggests that prevention strategies should be directed toward in-

Box **13-1**

Behavioral Rating Scales Related to General Health

- Clarity Health Assessment Scales Index Version
- Clarity Well Being Scales Comprehensive Version
- Freidman Quality of Life Scale
- Freidman Well Being Scale
- Functional Activities Questionnaire
- General Health Questionnaire (GHQ)
- Katz Index of Activities of Daily Living
- MOS Health Survey (SF-36)
- MOS Health Survey-Short Version (SF-12)
- OARS Social Resources Scale
- Sickness Impact Profile
- Social Skills Inventory
- Tennessee Self Concept Scale: Second Edition (TSCS:2)

fluencing predisposing factors, precipitating stressors, appraisal of stressors, coping resources, and coping mechanisms through the following interventions:

- Health education
- Environmental change
- Social support

In each of these areas the nurse can focus on decreasing risk factors or increasing protective factors. Furthermore, a single intervention can affect many parts of a person's life. For example, an environmental change, such as changing jobs, can affect an individual's predisposition to stress, decrease the amount of stress, change the appraisal of the threat, and perhaps increase financial or social coping resources. This interactive effect can thus justify the use of these prevention strategies for vulnerable groups.

Health Education

The health education strategy of primary prevention in mental health involves the strengthening of individuals and groups through competence building. It is based on the assumption that many maladaptive responses are the result of a lack of competence, that is, a lack of perceived control over one's own life and the lowered self-esteem that results. Competence building is also referred to as **resiliency**. It may be the single most important preventive strategy. A competent individual or community is aware of resources and alternatives, can make reasoned decisions about issues, and can cope adaptively with problems.

Self-Efficacy. Self-efficacy is a belief in one's personal capabilities. It is the notion that a person has control over the events in his or her life and that his or her actions will be effective. A high level of self-efficacy has been shown to positively affect one's thoughts, motivation, mood, and physical health (Bandura, 1997). People with a low sense of efficacy tend to avoid difficult tasks. They have low aspirations and weak commitment to their goals. They turn inward on their self-doubts instead of thinking about how to perform successfully. When faced with stress, they dwell on obstacles and their personal deficiencies. They give up in the face of difficulty, recover slowly from setbacks, and easily fall victim to depression.

In contrast, people with high self-efficacy approach difficult tasks as challenges to be mastered rather than threats to be avoided. They are deeply interested in what they do, set high goals, and maintain strong commitments. This outlook sustains motivation, reduces stress, and lowers any vulnerability to depression. Preventive interventions related to health education can equip people to take control of their lives and start a process of self-regulated change guided by a sense of resiliency and personal efficacy.

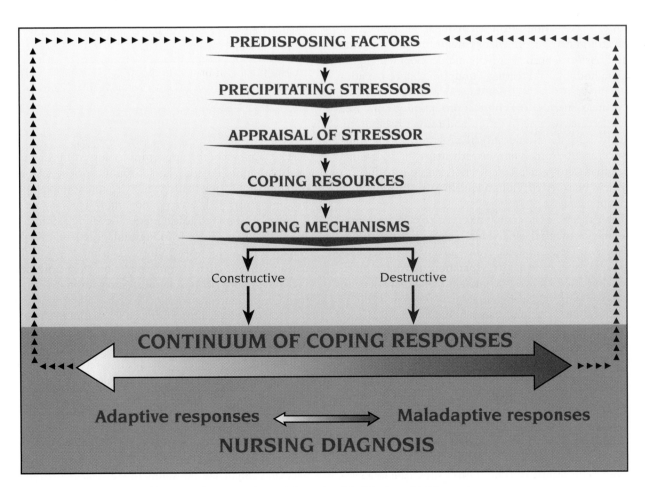

Fig. 13-1 The Stuart Stress Adaptation Model of psychiatric nursing care.

How is the concept of competency similar to the concept of positive mental health?

Levels of Intervention.

Health education related to competence building or increasing self-efficacy has four aspects:

- Increasing awareness of issues and events related to health and illness. Awareness of normal developmental tasks and potential problems is fundamental.
- Increasing understanding of potential stressors, possible outcomes (both adaptive and maladaptive), and alternative coping responses.
- Increasing knowledge of where and how to acquire the needed resources. Many health professionals assume that this is common knowledge, but for many people it is not.
- Increasing the actual abilities of the individual or group. This means improving or maximizing coping skills such as problem-solving, communication skills, tolerance of stress and frustration, motivation, hope, anger management, and self-esteem.

Programs and Activities.

Mental health education can take place in any setting, can have a formal or informal structure, can be directed toward individuals or groups, and can be related to predisposing factors or potential stressors (Redman, 1997; Stubblefield, 1997). Health education directed toward strengthening an individual's predisposition to stress can take various forms (Rankin & Stallings, 1996). Growth groups may be formed for parents that focus on parent-child relations, normal growth and development, or effective methods of child rearing. Groups of children or adolescents can discuss peer relationships, sexuality, or potential problem areas, such as drug abuse or promiscuity. Employee groups can discuss career burnout and related issues. Or a more activity-centered educational program can be initiated, such as Outward Bound, which helps the individual discover that step-by-step competence can be expanded to master new, unexpected, and potentially stressful situations in an adaptive way.

Probably the most common type of health education program is one that helps the individual cope with a specific potential stressor (see Citing the Evidence). For example, families about to experience marital separation are vulnerable to emotional problems, physical complaints, and increased use of health-care services. Such families may be offered educational and supportive group intervention aimed at enhancing their ability to cope. Education groups can similarly be offered to those experiencing retirement, bereavement, or any other stressful event (see Critical Thinking about Contemporary Issues).

Parent education classes are a well-known example of anticipatory guidance that can be offered to high-risk groups (Nardi, 1999). Although raising children is considered an important responsibility, until recently little attention has been directed to the belief that effective parenting is not an innate ability. Whether nurses subscribe to a specific set of beliefs and strategies for parenting or choose an

Citing the Evidence on

Preventing Conduct Problems

BACKGROUND: Fast Track is a multisite, multicomponent preventive intervention for young children at high risk for long-term antisocial behavior. Based on a comprehensive developmental model, intervention included a universal-level classroom program plus social skills training, academic tutoring, parent training, and home visiting to improve competencies and reduce problems in a high-risk group of children selected in kindergarten.

RESULTS: At the end of grade 1 there were moderate positive effects on children's social, emotional, and academic skills; peer interactions and social status; and conduct problems and special education use. Parents reported less physical discipline and greater parenting satisfaction and engaged in more appropriate and consistent discipline, positive involvement, and involvement with the school.

IMPLICATIONS: This study documents support for the early effectiveness of the Fast Track intervention program. One focus of future research will be to assess the extent to which changes in these risk factors may account for changes in child antisocial behavior and may contribute over time to more adaptive child developmental trajectories.

Conduct Problems Prevention Research Group: Initial impact of the Fast Track prevention trial for conduct problems: I. The high-risk sample, *J Consult Clin Psychol* 67(5):631, 1999.

eclectic approach, the opportunities for promoting mental health abound. Possibly one of the most beneficial results of parent education is the acknowledgment that all parents become frustrated, angry, and ambivalent toward their children. Parent education goes beyond acknowledging feelings and includes learning and practicing alternative ways of interacting with children. During these classes, situations are anticipated, and discussions focus on identifying potential crisis situations and dealing with them through simulated encounters such as role playing. Education for mental health can thus address the needs of both children and parents as family roles shift and respond to societal change.

Stigma.

Finally, health education activities can be directed to the larger community. One way to do this is by changing the attitudes and behavior of health-care providers and consumers. This may involve activities related to dispelling myths and stereotypes associated with vulnerable groups, providing knowledge of normal parameters, increasing sensitivity to psychosocial factors affecting health and illness, and enhancing the ability to give sensitive, supportive, and humanistic health care (see Box 13-2). Misperceptions

CRITICAL THINKING about CONTEMPORARY ISSUES

What Is the Future for Children with Mentally Ill Parents?

Living with a mentally ill parent does not necessarily mean that the child will develop the disorder, but it can make growing up more difficult. Although the mechanisms for transmitting psychiatric illness across generations are controversial, many studies support the fact that parental illness affects children. For example, it has been noted that coping with a mentally ill parent may be more difficult than coping with parental loss. These children also feel psychologically vulnerable and fear becoming ill themselves. The major research findings on this topic are as follows:

- Children of mentally ill parents are at greater risk for psychiatric and developmental disorders than are children of well parents.
- The risk to children is greater if the mother rather than the father is the ill parent.
- In studies of depressed versus nondepressed groups, differences in the mother-child interaction are evident as early as 3 months postpartum.
- Many children with emotionally disturbed parents do not become disordered themselves. The nature of the parent's illness, the child's genetic and constitutional make-up, the family's functional ability, and the availability of healthy attachment figures all play an important role in the mental health of the child.

The evidence suggests that psychiatric nurses need to focus more attention on the children of mentally ill parents. They should assess parenting problems whenever parents with children at home are hospitalized for psychiatric care (Mohit, 1996). They can also implement psychoeducational, preventive nursing interventions that will enhance mental health in high-risk children and families.

Box **13-2**

Anti-Stigma: Do You Know the Facts?

- Do you know that an estimated 50 million Americans experience a mental disorder in any given year?
- Do you know that stigma is about disrespect and that stigma is about the use of negative labels to identify a person living with a mental illness?
- Do you know that many people would rather tell employers that they have committed a petty crime and were in jail than admit to being in a psychiatric hospital?
- Do you know that stigma results in inadequate insurance coverage for mental health services?
- Do you know that stigma results in fear, mistrust, and violence against people living with mental illness?
- Do you know that stigma results in families and friends turning their backs on people with mental illness?
- Do you know that stigma keeps people from getting needed mental health services?

From SAMHSA's Center for Mental Health Services, 1999.

The stigma, misunderstanding, and fear surrounding mental illness are related to both the agencies providing mental health services and the people receiving these services, who are often elderly, poor, or members of social minority groups. Unlike physical illness, which tends to evoke sympathy and the desire to help, mental disorders tend to disturb and repel people. Yet everyone encounters stress, and all people are subject to maladaptive coping responses. Mental health professionals can educate the public that health is a continuum and illness is caused by a complex combination of factors. Consumers must begin to understand that no one is immune from mental illness or emotional problems and that the fear, anxiety, and even anger we feel about people who suffer these problems may reflect some of our own deepest fears and anxieties.

Have you observed the stigma associated with psychiatric illness in your personal or professional life? If so, what steps have you taken or could you take to overcome it?

Environmental Change

Activities in primary prevention involving environmental change have a social setting focus. They require the modification of an individual's or group's immediate environment or the larger social system. They are particularly appropriate actions when the environment has placed new demands on the person, when it is not responding to the person's developmental needs, and when it provides a diminished level of positive reinforcement.

Various environmental changes may prove to promote mental health, including changes in economic, work, housing, or family situations. Economically, resources for financial aid or assistance in budgeting and money management may be obtained. Work changes may include vocational testing, guidance, education, or retraining that can result in a change of

---

about vulnerable subgroups of the population must be corrected. They are the result, in part, of the cultural stigma against mental illness that is prevalent in contemporary society. A community-level strategy, therefore, would be to provide public education on mental health issues and community resources.

Stigma, in its original definition, meant a "scar left by a hot iron on the face of an evil doer." Stigma is now defined as a mark of disgrace that is used to identify and separate out people whom society sees as deviant, sinful, or dangerous. For the psychiatrically ill, stigma is a barrier that separates them from society and keeps them apart from others. Patients and their families often report that the diagnosis of a mental illness is followed by increasing isolation and loneliness as family and friends withdraw (see Chapter 16). Patients feel rejected and feared by others, and their families are met by blame (Wahl, 1999). Stigma against mental illness is a reflection of the cultural biases of contemporary American society that are shared by consumers and health-care providers alike.

jobs or careers. It may also mean that an adolescent, a homemaker, or an older adult may be placed in a new career. Changes in housing can involve moving to new quarters, which may mean leaving family and friends or returning to them, improvements in existing housing, or the addition or subtraction of coinhabitants, whether they are family, friends, or roommates. Environmental changes that may benefit the family include attaining child care facilities, enrolling in a nursery school, grade school, or camp, or obtaining access to recreational, social, religious, or community facilities.

The potential benefit of all of these changes should not be minimized or overlooked by psychiatric nurses. They can promote mental health by increasing coping resources, modifying the nature of stressors, and increasing positive, rewarding, and self-enhancing experiences.

Organizations and Politics. Nurses can also effect environmental changes at a larger organizational and political level. One way is by influencing health-care structures and procedures (Cohen et al, 1996). Nurses might become involved in training community, nonprofessional caregivers to increase the social supports available to vulnerable groups. Another approach would be to stimulate support for women's issues related to mental health, such as through studying the psychology of women; dispelling sex-role stereotypes; promoting feminist therapy; sponsoring programs, conferences, and workshops on women's issues; and recruiting more women into the mental health field (Cowan, 1996).

Obviously, if nurses believe that their profession makes a valuable contribution to health promotion, they should document the cost-effectiveness and quality of nursing care, lobby for greater patient access by nurses, and seek adequate compensation and reimbursement for nursing services. Many of these goals can be obtained if nursing has greater participation in the decision-making structures of healthcare institutions, such as hospital boards, advisory groups, health system agencies, and legislative bodies.

Within organizations, environmental change can be achieved through program consultation. Such consultation with a large corporation, for example, may lead to the formulation of more flexible retirement plans or a preretirement counseling program. Involvement in community planning and development can have an impact in many different areas. For instance, a community may be helped to meet the needs of the elderly for educational opportunities, recreational programs, and access to social support networks through telephone or transportation services. Also, the stress associated with environmental pollutants, such as chemicals and radiation, can be addressed.

Some environmental changes require involvement at the national level that may be directed toward the media's portrayal of violence, laws on drunk driving, gun control legislation, access to family planning services, and advocating changes in child-rearing practices, including the provision of day-care centers, flex time, and paternity leave.

Of course, many aspects of the broader social system are in need of change, including racism, sexism, ageism, poverty, and inadequate housing and education. The dilemma is that global problems such as these are too broad, pervasive, and diffuse to be adequately addressed, let alone resolved. For any prevention strategies to be successful in the future, it will be necessary to document the ways in which a particular group is vulnerable to a specific stressor, how the proposed prevention program will be beneficial and cost-effective, and the degree to which it succeeds or fails.

What legislation in your state is being considered that pertains to mental health care? What is your position on it and how can you influence its chances for passage?

Social Support

As a primary prevention strategy, supporting social systems does not mean removing or minimizing the stressor or risk factor. Rather, it is an attempt to strengthen social supports as a protective factor, buffering or cushioning the effects of a potentially stressful event (Box 13-3). Social support systems can be helpful in emphasizing the strengths of individuals and families and focusing on health rather than illness. It is an important concept for all levels of prevention—primary, secondary, and tertiary—and it has implications for the following:

- Encouraging health promotion behavior
- Helping people seek assistance earlier
- Improving the functioning of the immune system or other biological processes
- Reducing the occurrence of potentially stressful events
- Fostering the ability to cope with stressful events
- Helping one to deal with chronic mental and physical illness

Box 13-3

Support System Enhancement

DEFINITION
Facilitation of support to patient by family, friends, and community

ACTIVITIES
Assess psychological response to situation and availability of support system
Determine adequacy of existing social networks
Identify degree of family support
Identify degree of family financial support
Determine support systems currently used
Determine barriers to using support systems
Monitor current family situation
Encourage the patient to participate in social and community activities
Encourage relationships with people who have common interests and goals
Refer to a self-help group as appropriate
Assess community resource adequacy to identify strengths and weaknesses
Refer to a community-based promotion, prevention, treatment, or rehabilitation program as appropriate
Provide services in a caring and supportive manner
Involve family, significant others, and friends in the care and planning
Explain to concerned others how they can help

From McCloskey J, Bulechek G: *Nursing interventions classification*, ed 3, St Louis, 2000, Mosby.

People with poor social support—whether it is defined by the number of social contacts, the satisfaction derived from them, or a combination of the two—have a higher risk of dying from all causes. The effects of isolation are even more dramatic in chronic illnesses. People with coronary artery disease who lack both a spouse and a confidant have a 50% death rate over a 5-year period. For those less isolated, the death rate is under 20% (Williams, 1999).

How can the goal of maximizing social support systems be achieved? First, the amount of social support needed by a high-risk group must be determined and compared with the amount of social support available. Although the question is straightforward, it is complicated by the fact that there are many determinants of each element.

The need for social support is influenced by predisposing factors, the nature of the stressors, and the availability of other coping resources such as economic assets, individual abilities and skills, and defensive techniques. The availability of social supports is also influenced by age, gender, socioeconomic status, the nature of the stressor, and the characteristics of the environment. Acute episodic stressors tend to elicit more intense support, while support resources for chronic problems tend to fade away. Also, changes or stressors viewed in a positive way by the individual's social network, such as the birth of a baby or a promotion, may generate a great deal of support, whereas a negative event, such as a divorce, might stimulate little support. Finally, the quantity and type of social support that meets one need may not meet another.

Types of Interventions. Even though many variables related to social support need further study, social support can still be used to design and implement interventions in primary prevention. Four particular types of interventions are possible.

First, social support patterns can be used to assess communities and neighborhoods to identify problem areas and high-risk groups. Not only will information about the quality of life be gained, but the social isolation of a particular group might become apparent, as well as central individuals who may be enlisted to help develop community-based programs.

A second preventive intervention would be to improve links between community support systems and formal mental health services. Often mental health professionals are not aware of or comfortable with the existence or functioning of community support systems. They should be taught how to use and mobilize community resources and social support systems. All health-care providers need to recognize when patients need social support and to provide them with access to appropriate community support systems.

The third type of intervention is to strengthen natural, existing caregiving networks. Health professionals can provide information and support to informal caregivers in the community, who serve a very important and somewhat different function than more formalized and organized support systems. Informal support systems provide:

- A natural training ground for the development of problem-solving skills
- A medium in which people grow and develop by learning to direct the process of change for themselves

- A supportive milieu that capitalizes on the strength of existing ties among people in communities, rather than fragmenting intact social units on the basis of diagnosed needs or specialized services

A fourth possible intervention may be to help the person or group develop, maintain, and use a network. The person may also be encouraged to consider expanding one's network. On the other hand, the network can be influenced more directly. Network therapy involves bringing together all the important members of the family's kin and friendship network. The focus is then on tightening bonds within the network and breaking dysfunctional patterns. For families who are isolated and whose networks are depleted, network members may not be available for such a strategy. In this case, arranging for the use of mutual support groups may be effective.

Informal Support Groups. There are many informal support groups. They may include church groups, civic organizations, clubs, women's groups, or work and neighborhood supports. Self-help groups are becoming more common as members organize themselves to solve their own problems. The members all share a common experience, work together toward a common goal, and use their strengths to gain control over their lives (Murray, 1996). The processes involved in self-help groups are social affiliation, learning self-control, modeling methods to cope with stress, and acting to change the social environment. Characteristics of self-help groups are listed in Box 13-4.

Self-help groups such as Alcoholics Anonymous, Weight Watchers, Parents Without Partners, Recovery, and Parents Anonymous are familiar to the public. They have shown their ability to help people experiencing psychiatric problems and grief reactions, such as widows and parents of children who died of sudden infant death syndrome. Because self-help groups use a variety of methods and membership criteria, each group should be assessed individually for its general effectiveness and appropriateness for particular individuals and families. Some areas for the nurse to assess before recommending involvement in a self-help group are presented in Box 13-5.

Working with natural, informal support systems should be done cautiously, however, to minimize undesirable consequences. The nurse should attempt to create the least

---

Box 13-4

Characteristics of Self-Help Groups

- Supportive and educational in nature rather than therapeutic
- Based on shared experiences and the fact that the individual is not alone
- Focus on a single life-disrupting event
- Purpose is to support personal responsibility and change
- Anonymous and confidential in nature
- Voluntary membership
- Members lead the group and implement principles of self-governance
- Nonprofit orientation

amount of disruption possible and not to suppress the natural repertoire of helping behaviors of informal caregivers. Finally, although supporting social supports is an effective intervention, it is not limited to primary prevention activities. Rather, all nurses in all settings can use this strategy as a way of providing holistic care to maximize the health of individuals, families, and groups.

> ❓ *Attend one of the self-help groups in your community. Describe the specific ways in which it helped those who attended.*

EVALUATION

When talking about primary prevention, there is a tendency to think in terms of the total elimination of mental illness and stress. Yet these are not realistic goals, and maintaining them can only discourage any possible action. Perhaps it is possible to set goals of reducing suffering and enhancing the capacity to cope, but even these may be unattainable, given that the environment is constantly changing and adaptation is an ongoing challenge. Rather, if the focus is directed toward specific problems of a vulnerable group in society, nursing activity becomes more concentrated and the chance of success increases.

Clearly a need exists for the evaluation of programs in primary prevention. In a world of shrinking resources, only programs with proven effectiveness are likely to be supported in the future. It must be demonstrated that the prevention strategy used has both short-term and long-term effects that benefited the individual and society. Also, it is necessary to determine whether the specific strategy implemented was the most effective, appropriate, and efficient. Considering alternative approaches and comparing clinical and financial outcomes are essential aspects of the evaluation process.

Although preventing all illness is not possible, preventing some particular problems is. But a number of barriers exist that make expansion of primary prevention activities difficult. When faced with a choice, the needs of the ill consistently take precedence over prevention. This holds true for nurses as well as for the larger society. Yet by being more visionary, both groups could benefit greatly.

Box 13-5

Assessment Guidelines for Self-Help Groups

QUESTIONS FOR THE GROUP
What is its purpose?
Who are the group members and leaders?
What are the beneficial aspects of the group?
For whom would the group not be suitable?
What problems are inherent in the group?
Is the group effective in preventing further emotional distress?

QUESTIONS FOR THE POTENTIAL MEMBER
How does the person feel about attending a self-help group?
How compatible is the group with the individual's approach to the problem?
How accessible is the group to the potential member?

Summary

1. Caplan's three levels of preventive intervention were described. The major thrust in current psychiatric care is secondary prevention, although primary prevention is beginning to evolve as a major force in the mental health movement.

2. A nursing model for primary prevention was presented that attempts to reduce the incidence of particular stressful life events for vulnerable groups, and it was applied to the nursing process.

3. Assessment in primary prevention was presented as the identification of groups of people who are vulnerable to developing mental disorders or maladaptive coping responses to specific stressors or risk factors.

4. Prevention strategies include health education, environmental change, and social support.

5. In evaluating preventive strategies, one needs to consider specific criteria and use a systematic rating scale of scientific evidence.

Competent Caring **A Clinical Exemplar of a Psychiatric Nurse**
PENELOPE CHASE, MSN, MEd, RN, CS

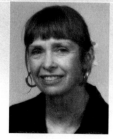

I was changing planes, having just left an inspiring psychiatric clinical nurse specialist conference in Florida, and was on my way to Boston to attend the reunion of my diploma nursing school. I was traveling alone and feeling safe from social interruptions. I was looking forward to some anonymity and a time to reflect and rest.

As I approached the check-in counter of the airport, I saw a young woman sitting nearby in the waiting area. The seats on either side of her were empty except for a soft knapsack on her left. She was wearing the loose-fitting cotton clothing and the nylon-strap sandals that college students often wear. She looked as if she were about to burst into tears or change her mind about being here and dash for the exit. I stopped in my tracks to observe her without being aware of deciding to do so. She turned her head with stiff, slightly jerky movements.

"Responding to internal stimuli," "seizure disorder," "hasn't taken her psychotropic medication" went through my professional mind, while "don't get involved" went through my personal mind, along with, "You're on vacation. Don't mess it up. Relax, you're not the only one who can help." So I went ahead

Competent Caring   A Clinical Exemplar of a Psychiatric Nurse—cont'd

and checked in. I chose to wait in a seat in the row behind the young woman. "She may not be able to ask for help. I should assess further," my professional self reasoned. "Maybe she's not alone. Maybe someone is traveling with her and will be back in a minute."

She compared her ticket information with the boarding announcement and sat back in her seat. A moment later, she shifted in her seat and put her hands over her face. It was then that I noticed that a man, somewhat older than she, seated two rows away and facing her was watching her intensely. My private self was afraid he might be a lonely traveler sizing up a vulnerable young woman that he could take advantage of. I intensified my vigil. I would be her advocate and protector.

I read a bit in my novel, keeping my peripheral vision and ears attuned in her direction. I had difficulty concentrating on my reading because I was constantly interrupted by imposing, opposing thoughts of "Do something" and "Let it be." At one point a uniformed airline employee passed near me on his way out the boarding door. I approached him and said, "I think there's a young lady in trouble here." "I'm a pilot," he replied. "The person you need to talk with is that gentleman at the counter." I wondered what I should do. If I were to say something, the young woman might be embarrassed, delayed, or asked to answer questions that might destroy whatever composure and dignity she was able to preserve. She had not indicated she needed any help . . . yet.

I was still deliberating when my flight was called. The young woman looked at her ticket, got up, and joined the line. I sat and waited until my row number was called. As the flight attendant checked the young woman's boarding pass, she looked carefully at the anguished face, then asked, "Are you okay?" The girl nodded. "Are you sure?" Another nod, but the flight attendant paused in her checking and turned briefly to watch as the girl began down the boarding ramp. It was then that I decided how to resolve my professional-helper's dilemma. I identified myself to the flight attendant as a psychiatric nurse and said that if there were an emergency, they could call on me. "Oh, you noticed her, too," the woman smiled. "Thank you."

I had just gotten settled in my seat when the flight attendant approached me. "I pulled her up in the computer. It's an emergency flight—a death in the family." "Oh," I ventured, the underlying cause of the scenario suddenly becoming clearer in my mind. "Loss and grief are one of my specialties. I'd be happy to sit with her if she'd like, but only if she says she'd like someone with her." I suddenly remembered traveling 450 miles, mostly alone, to my younger brother's funeral.

Within a few minutes the flight attendant returned saying, "She said she'd like that." So I took my purse and moved toward the back of the plane. As I approached her seat, the young woman looked up at me. I smiled, introduced myself by name, and said I was the person who would sit with her if that would be all right. She nodded assent, managed a wan smile, and said, "Thank you." I was trying to decide what my role would be. This was all happening rather quickly, yet somewhere in my gut or heart I knew it would be okay. I knew I wanted to stay in my role of a psychiatric nurse and a representative of my profession, and I was also aware that in a couple of hours our relationship would be ending. The time limit helped me focus on my goal of simply being available to her as a support.

Realizing that my seat partner was probably in the initial stage of shock in the grief process and thus lacked her usual coping skills, I decided to do a bit of framing for her. "The flight attendant told me you had a death in your family. I'm sorry," I said. "I'm a nurse who works with people who are going through losses. You could talk about it if you want to, or I could just sit here and read my book. It's up to you." I offered her two simple choices.

She sat silently, but with slightly changing facial expressions, and I thought she was getting ready to speak. I focused my attention softly on her and waited. "He wasn't supposed to die. He was going to have chemotherapy," she began. As her story unfolded, I listened, asked clarifying questions occasionally, and acknowledged her words and anguish. In between bits of content, I learned that she was being met by friends of the family and her sister at the airport with a subsequent 45-minute drive until she was in her hometown. At one point she said sadly, "Now he'll never see his grandchildren," and buried her head on my shoulder and sobbed for a little while. After a bit she said, "I think I need to sleep." That sounded like a good idea to me. As she slept, I evaluated what had unfolded and thought about where to go from here. I needed a plan for closure, for termination of the intervention.

I thought of how long she would have to stand in the aisle waiting to get off this big plane. I asked the flight attendant if there were some way the young woman could be one of the first passengers off the plane. We were moved to the first-class section near the door after she awoke. We talked briefly of how she wanted to depart. I let her know I was available to walk off the plane with her if she wanted and that I thought she could manage "just fine" without me, as well. "I'll be all right," she said, giving me a hug as we stood up to disembark. "You don't know how much we appreciate this," the flight attendant said to me with sincere eye contact. I acknowledged her thanks. I motioned for my seat-mate to go ahead of me. As we approached the waiting area, I looked questioningly at her to see how she was managing. "I've got it," she said, and gave me the thumbs-up sign. I smiled and walked on. I was met by two classmates and felt clear, reflective, and exhilarated. I felt that my clinical skills had positively influenced the outcome. I felt I had acted in a professionally responsible and caring manner. I felt good about being a psychiatric nurse.

MERLIN Visit MERLIN: **www.mosby.com/MERLIN/Stuart** to find these additional materials and student activities.

- **Worksheets**
- **"Drug of the Month" Updates**
- **"Citing the Evidence" Updates**
- **Critical Thinking Activities and Exercises**
- **Annotated Suggested Readings**
- **Web Links**
- **More!**

Chapter Review Questions

1. Match each term in Column A with the activity associated with it from Column B.

Column A   Column B
____ Primary prevention   A. Incidence
____ Secondary prevention   B. Prevalence
____ Tertiary prevention   C. Severity

2. Fill in the blanks.

A. The two goals of primary prevention activities are to
_____ and
_____.

B. The health education strategy of
_____ is based on increasing perceived control over one's life, effective coping strategies, and self-esteem.

C. The government document that describes a national incentive to promote health and prevent disease in the United States is called _____.

D. The term used to describe a mark of disgrace that separates out those people that society sees as deviant, sinful, or dangerous is called _____.

E. Becoming involved in health-care organizations and political processes is a nursing intervention related to
_____.

F. Social support has important implications for
_____ levels of prevention.

3. Provide short answers for the following questions.

A. How do the medical and nursing prevention models differ?

B. Identify and describe three types of primary prevention interventions based on the assessment of targeted populations.

C. Describe the four aspects of health education and give an example of each.

D. Select one specific psychiatric disorder and research the impact of social support on its expression and resolution.

E. Relate one environmental change that would promote the mental health of people living in your community.

REFERENCES

Bandura A: *Self-efficacy: the exercise of control,* New York, 1997, Freeman.

Caplan G: *Principles of preventive psychiatry,* New York, 1964, Basic Books.

Cohen S et al: Stages of nursing's political development: where we've been and where we ought to go, *Nurs Outlook* 44:259, 1996.

Cowan P: Women's mental health issues: reflections on past attitudes and present practices, *J Psychosoc Nurs* 34:20, 1996.

Mrazek P, Haggerty R: *Reducing risks for mental disorders,* Washington, DC, 1994, National Academy Press.

Murray P: Recovery, Inc., as an adjunct to treatment in an era of managed care, *Psychiatr Serv* 47:1378, 1996.

Nardi D: Parenting education as family support, *J Psychosoc Nurs* 37(7):11, 1999.

National Advisory Mental Health Council Workgroup on Mental Disorders Prevention Research: *Priorities for Prevention Research at NIMH,* Rockville, Md, 1998, National Institute of Mental Health.

National Mental Health Association: *Preventing mental health and substance abuse problems in managed health care settings,* Alexandria, Va, 1998, NMHA.

Rankin S, Stallings K: *Patient education: issues, principles, practices.* Philadelphia, 1996, Lippincott.

Redman B: *The practice of patient education,* ed 8, St Louis, 1997, Mosby.

Stubblefield C: Persuasive communication: marketing health promotion, *Nurs Outlook* 45(4):173, 1997.

Tudor K: *Mental health promotion,* London, 1996, Routledge.

U.S. Department of Health and Human Services: *Mental health: a report of the surgeon general,* Rockville, Md, 1999, U.S. Department of Health and Human Services, Substance Abuse and Mental Health Services Administration, Center for Mental Health Services, National Institutes of Health, National Institute of Mental Health.

Wahl O: *Telling is risky business,* New Brunswick, NJ, 1999, Rutgers University Press.

Williams R: Social ties and health, *Harvard Ment Health Lett* April 1999.

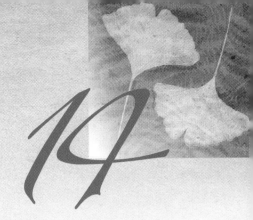

Crisis Intervention

Sandra E. Benter

Visit **MERLIN** for *Your Internet Connection* to websites that are related to the content in this chapter.
www.mosby.com/MERLIN/Stuart

LEARNING OBJECTIVES

After studying this chapter the student should be able to:

- Define crisis, the continuum of adaptive and maladaptive crisis responses, and three types of crises
- Discuss the goals, phases, and balancing factors in crisis intervention
- Analyze aspects of the nursing assessment related to crisis responses, including behaviors, precipitating events, perception of events, coping resources, and coping mechanisms
- Plan and implement nursing interventions for patients related to their crisis responses
- Develop a patient education plan to cope with crisis
- Evaluate nursing care for patients related to their crisis responses
- Describe the settings in which crisis intervention may be practiced
- Discuss modalities of crisis intervention

TOPICAL OUTLINE

Continuum of Crisis Responses
  Adaptive and Maladaptive Crisis Responses
  Types of Crises
  Crisis Intervention
Assessment
  Behaviors
  Precipitating Event
  Perception of the Event
  Support Systems and Coping Resources
  Coping Mechanisms
Planning and Implementation
  Environmental Manipulation
  General Support
  Generic Approach
  Individual Approach
  Techniques
Evaluation
Settings for Crisis Intervention
Modalities of Crisis Intervention
  Mobile Crisis Programs
  Group Work
  Telephone Contacts
  Disaster Response
  Victim Outreach Programs
  Health Education

He knows not his own strength that hath not met adversity.
FRANCIS BACON, OF FORTUNE

Stressful events, or crises, are a common part of life. They may be social, psychological, or biological in nature, and there is often little that a person can do to prevent them. Nurses, as the largest group of health-care providers, are in an excellent position to help people in times of crisis and promote healthy outcomes. Crisis intervention is a brief, focused, and time-limited treatment strategy that has been shown to be effective in helping people adaptively cope with stressful events. Knowledge of crisis intervention techniques is an important clinical skill of all nurses, regardless of clinical setting or practice specialty.

CONTINUUM OF CRISIS RESPONSES
Adaptive and Maladaptive Crisis Responses

A crisis is a disturbance caused by a stressful event or a perceived threat. The person's usual way of coping becomes ineffective in dealing with the threat, causing anxiety. The threat, or precipitating event, can usually be identified. It may have occurred weeks or days ago, and it may or may not be linked in the individual's mind to the crisis state. Precipitating events are perceived losses, threats of losses, or challenges.

After the precipitating event the person's anxiety rises and four phases of a crisis emerge. In the first phase the anxiety activates the person's usual methods of coping. If these do not bring relief and there is inadequate support, the person moves to the second phase, which involves more anxiety because coping mechanisms have failed. In the third phase new coping mechanisms are tried or the threat is redefined so that old ones can work. Resolution of the problem can occur in this phase. However, if resolution does not occur, the person goes on to the fourth phase, in which the continuation of severe or panic levels of anxiety may lead to psychological disorganization. This is discussed in detail in Chapter 17.

In describing the phases of a crisis, it is important to consider the balancing factors shown in Fig. 14-1. These include the individual's perception of the event, situational supports, and coping mechanisms. Successful resolution of the crisis is more likely if the person has a realistic view of the event, if situational supports are available to help solve the problem, and if effective coping mechanisms are present (Aguilera, 1998).

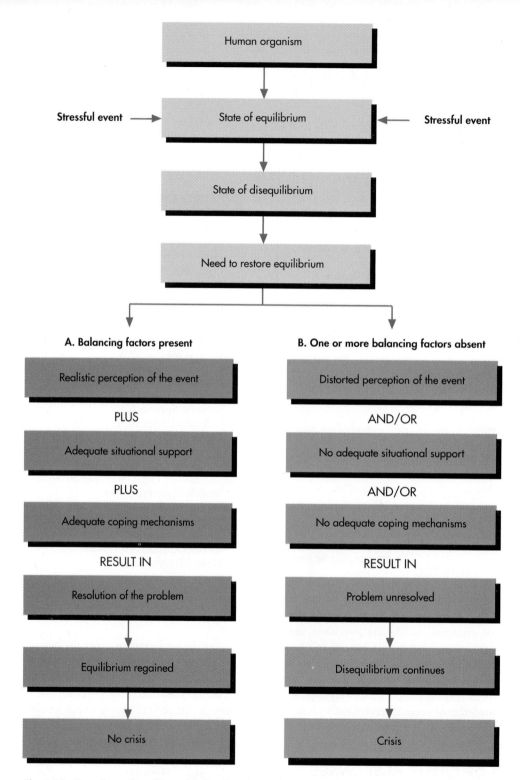

Fig. 14-1 Paradigm: the effect of balancing factors in a stressful event. (From Aguilera DC: *Crisis intervention: theory and methodology,* ed 8, St Louis, 1998, Mosby.)

The phases of a crisis and the impact of balancing factors are similar to the components of the Stuart Stress Adaptation Model described in Chapter 4. However, by definition, crises are self-limiting. People in crisis are too upset to function at such a high level of anxiety indefinitely. The time needed for resolution, whether it be a positive solution or a state of disorganization, may be 6 weeks or even longer.

It is also important to recognize that periods of intense conflict can result in increased growth, as seen in the continuum of crisis responses (Fig. 14-2). How the crisis is handled determines whether growth or disorganization will result. Growth comes from learning in new situations. People in crisis feel uncomfortable, often reach out for help, and accept help until they feel that their lives are back to normal.

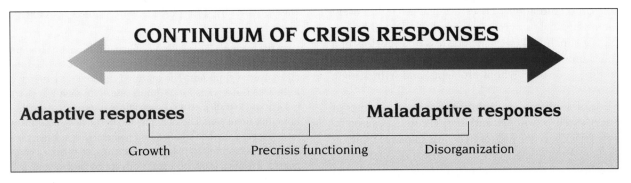

Fig. 14-2 Continuum of crisis responses.

The fact that crises can lead to personal growth is important to remember when working with patients in crisis.

 Think of a crisis you have experienced. Do you feel that the way you handled it made you a better person in some way? If so, how?

Types of Crises

There are two types of crises: maturational and situational. Sometimes these crises can occur simultaneously. For example, an adolescent who is having difficulty adjusting to a change in role and body image (maturational crisis) may at the same time undergo the stress related to the death of a parent (situational crisis).

Maturational. Maturational crises are developmental events requiring role changes. For example, successfully moving from early childhood to middle childhood requires the child to become socially involved with people outside the family. With the move from adolescence to adulthood, financial responsibility is expected. Both social and biological pressures to change can precipitate a crisis.

The nature and extent of the maturational crisis can be influenced by role models, interpersonal resources, and the ease of others in accepting the new role. Positive role models show the person how to act in the new role. Interpersonal resources encourage the trying out of new behaviors to achieve role changes. Other people's acceptance of the new role is also important. The greater the resistance of others, the more stress the person faces in making the changes.

Transitional periods during adolescence, parenthood, marriage, midlife, and retirement are key times for the onset of maturational crises. Some conflicts related to maturational crises are seen in the clinical examples that follow.

 CLINICAL EXAMPLE

Ms. J was a 19-year-old black, single, unemployed woman who came to the mental health clinic a month after the birth of her first child. Ms. J complained of feeling depressed. Her symptoms included difficulty falling asleep, early morning awakening, crying spells, a poor appetite, and difficulty in caring for the baby because of fatigue and apathy. The patient lived with her parents and siblings and had never lived on her own. She had always depended on her mother to take care of her. Her mother worked, however, and the patient was totally responsible for her daughter's care each day. Also, Ms. J's mother was angry that she had a child and often refused to care for the baby. The patient's boyfriend, who was the baby's father, had promised to marry her, but he had recently decided he was too young to handle the responsibility of a wife and child. In summary, the young woman who had unmet dependency needs of her own was now a parent and had to meet the dependency needs of her infant. This precipitated a crisis for her.

Selected Nursing Diagnoses

- Ineffective individual coping related to birth of a child, as evidenced by feelings of depression
- Altered family processes related to birth of a grandchild, as evidenced by lack of family support
- Altered parenting related to being a single mother, as evidenced by difficulty caring for her baby

CLINICAL EXAMPLE

Mr. R was a 67-year-old white, married pharmacist who came to the mental health clinic complaining of anxiety, depression, and insomnia. His symptoms had begun 2 weeks ago when his wife decided that they should move to a retirement community in Florida. He described his wife as a strong, willful woman who was also outgoing and charming and made friends easily. He considered himself a quiet, nervous person who was comfortable only with old friends and his two sons and their families. Mr. R, although at retirement age, had continued to work as a pharmacist, doing relief work for a drugstore chain when the regular pharmacists were absent. In moving to Florida, he would lose his pharmacist's license, which was valid only in his state of residence. He expressed difficulty in making the transition from work to retirement. He had fears of becoming directionless and useless. He was anxious about leaving his sons and his friends. The prospect of complete retirement and moving to another state precipitated his distress.

Selected Nursing Diagnoses

- Relocation stress syndrome related to pending retirement, as evidenced by feelings of anxiety
- Altered family processes related to conflict about lifestyle changes, as evidenced by inability to plan future

Situational. Situational crises occur when a life event upsets an individual's or group's psychological equilibrium. Examples of situational crises include loss of a job, loss of a loved one, unwanted pregnancy, onset or worsening of a medical illness, divorce, school problems, and witnessing a crime.

The loss of a job can result in financial stress, feelings of inadequacy as a breadwinner, and marital conflict caused by a spouse's anger over the lost job. The loss of a loved one results in bereavement and can also cause financial stress, change in roles of family members, and loss of emotional support. Homelessness is another possible outcome of the loss of a job or a loved one. The onset or worsening of a medical illness causes anticipatory grief and fear of the loss of a loved one. Again, financial stress and change in roles of family members often occur. Divorce is similar to the stress of the loss of a loved one, except that the crisis can recur with the stress of dealing with the ex-spouse. An unwanted pregnancy is stressful because it requires decisions to be made about whether to complete the pregnancy or to abort it, and whether to keep the baby or place it for adoption. If the pregnancy is aborted or adoption occurs, there can be the need to deal with feelings of grief or anger. If the baby is to be kept, changes in lifestyle are required. Finally, being the victim of or witnessing a crime can cause feelings of helplessness, distrust of others, fear, nightmares, and guilt about causing or not stopping the crime.

Situational crises can also be accidental, uncommon, and unexpected events. For example, fires, tornadoes, earthquakes, hurricanes, or floods, which disrupt entire communities, are situational crises. Recent mass tragedies, which have become all too common, are also examples of situational crises and include group kidnappings (the taking of hostages), group killings in the workplace or at schools, airplane crashes, riots in cities, and the explosion of bombs in crowded areas.

Disaster-precipitated emotional problems often surface weeks or even months after the disaster. The symptoms usually occur in roughly four phases, which are described in Table 14-1. If the reconstruction phase does not begin within 6 months after the disaster, the likelihood of lasting psychological problems is greatly increased. The severe psychological stress resulting from adventitious crises is described in a classic work by Terr (1981), who studied 23 child kidnap victims:

> In the town of Chowchilla, California, a school bus containing 26 children and a bus driver was stopped by three masked men and taken over at gunpoint. The captured children were driven around in boarded-over vans for 11 hours and were then transferred to a buried truck trailer. After 16 additional hours, two of the oldest boys dug them out. The children suffered from initial misperceptions, fears of further trauma, and hallucinations. Later they experienced posttraumatic play reenactment, personality changes, repeated dreams, fears of being kidnapped again, and a fear of common mundane experiences.

> *Some crises, such as obtaining a divorce, develop over time and are of longer duration. Other crises, such as an earthquake, are sudden and unexpected. How do you think the element of time affects the response to crisis?*

Crisis Intervention

Crisis intervention can offer the immediate help a person in crisis needs. It is an inexpensive, short-term therapy focused on solving the immediate problem, and it is usually limited to 6 weeks. The goal of crisis intervention is for the individual to return to a precrisis level of functioning. Often the person advances to a level of growth that is higher than the precrisis level because new ways of problem solving have been learned.

It is important for the nurse to remember that cultural attitudes strongly influence the communication and response style of the crisis worker. These attitudes are deeply ingrained in the processes of asking for, giving, and receiving help. They also affect the victimization experience, so it is essential to understand and respect the cultural values of the victims. Specific cultural factors to be considered in crisis intervention include the following:

- Migration and citizenship status
- Gender and family roles
- Religious belief systems
- Child-rearing practices
- Use of extended family and support systems

The age of the survivors is also important for the nurse to consider when providing crisis intervention (Adams et al,

Table **14-1**

Four Phases of Disaster Response	
Phase	**Response**
Heroic	Begins at time of impact. A cooperative spirit exists among survivors as they perform acts to save lives.
Honeymoon	Begins to appear 2 weeks to 6 months after the disaster. Massive relief efforts are begun. The community works together, with the help of donated resources, to begin community life again. Survivors feel a sense of security.
Disillusionment	Lasts from several months to a year. Begins when supportive agencies and services withdraw. A time of anger, resentment, and disappointment. Survivors feel a sense of abandonment.
Reconstruction	Lasts for several years. Problem solving improves. Survivors rebuild their community.

From U.S. Department of Health and Human Services: *Training manual for human service workers in major disasters*, Washington, DC, 1996, Government Printing Office.

1999). Responses to stressor events differ across the life span. Therefore age-appropriate interventions are most effective in helping survivors return to their previous level of functioning. For example, 4-year-old children may best express themselves through play, while adolescents may best work through crisis issues in peer group discussions.

 Describe how sociocultural factors might affect a woman's decision to seek help after being raped.

ASSESSMENT

The first step of crisis intervention is assessment. At this time data about the nature of the crisis and its effect on the patient must be collected. From these data, an intervention plan will be developed.

Although the crisis situation is the focus of the assessment, more significant and long-standing problems may be identified by the nurse. It is important, therefore, to identify which areas can be helped by crisis intervention and which problems must be referred for further treatment.

During this phase the nurse begins to establish a positive working relationship with the patient. A number of specific areas should be assessed. These balancing factors are impor-

tant in the development and resolution of a crisis and include the following:

- Precipitating event or stressor
- Patient's perception of the event or stressor
- Nature and strength of the patient's support systems and coping resources
- Patient's previous strengths and coping mechanisms

The components of the Stuart Stress Adaptation Model that parallel the balancing factors in crisis intervention are highlighted in Fig. 14-3.

Behaviors

People in crisis experience many symptoms, including those listed in Box 14-1. Sometimes these symptoms can cause further problems. For example, problems at work may lead to loss of a job, financial stress, and lowered self-esteem. Crises can also be complicated by old conflicts that are brought out by the current problem, making crisis resolution more difficult.

Precipitating Event

To help identify the precipitating event, the nurse should explore the patient's needs, the events that threaten those needs, and the time at which symptoms appear. Four kinds

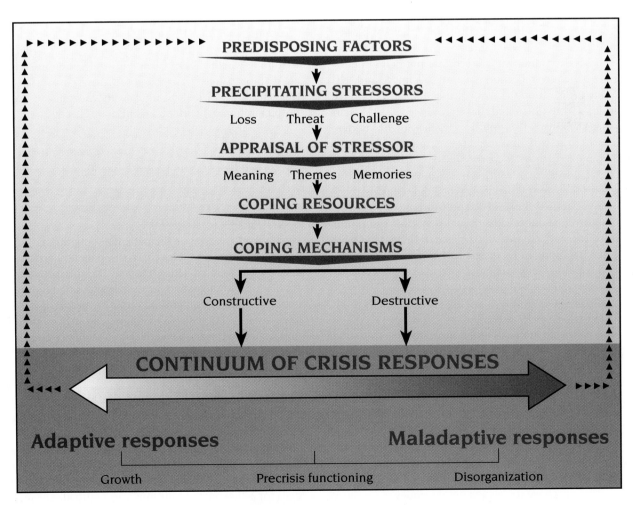

Fig. 14-3 The Stuart Stress Adaptation Model related to crisis responses.

Box 14-1

Behaviors Commonly Exhibited after a Crisis

Anger	Nightmares
Apathy	Numbness
Backaches	Overeating or undereating
Boredom	
Crying spells	Poor concentration
Diminished sexual drive	Sadness
Disbelief	School problems
Fatigue	Self-doubt
Flashbacks	Shock
Forgetfulness	Social withdrawal
Headaches	Substance abuse
Helplessness	Suicidal thoughts
Hopelessness	Survivor guilt
Insomnia	Work difficulties
Intrusive thoughts	
Irritability	
Lability	

of needs that have been identified are related to self-esteem, role mastery, dependency, and biological function. **Self-esteem** is achieved when the person attains successful social role experience. **Role mastery** is achieved when the person attains work, sexual, and family role successes. **Dependency** is achieved when a satisfying interdependent relationship with others is attained. **Biological function** is achieved when a person is safe and life is not threatened.

The nurse determines which needs are not being met by asking the patient to reflect on issues of self-image and self-esteem, the areas of life that are considered a success, one's relationships with others, and the degree of safety and security in life. The nurse looks for obstacles that might interfere with meeting the patient's needs. What recent experiences have been upsetting? What areas of life have had changes?

Coping patterns become ineffective and symptoms appear usually after the stressful incident. When did the patient begin to feel anxious? When did sleep disturbances begin? At what point in time did suicidal thoughts start? If symptoms began last Tuesday, ask what took place in the patient's life on Tuesday or Monday. As the patient connects life events with the breakdown in coping mechanisms, an understanding of the precipitating event can emerge.

Perception of the Event

The patient's perception or appraisal of the precipitating event is very important. What may seem trivial to the nurse may have great meaning to the patient. An overweight adolescent girl may have been the only girl in the class not invited to a dance. This may have threatened her self-esteem. A man with two unsuccessful marriages may have just been told by a girlfriend that she wants to end their relationship; this may have threatened his need for sexual role mastery. An emotionally isolated, friendless woman may have had car trouble and been unable to find someone to give her a ride to work. This may have threatened her dependency needs. A

chronically ill man who has had a recent relapse of his illness may have had his need for biological function threatened.

Themes and surfacing memories of the patient give further clues to the precipitating event. Current issues of concern are often connected to past issues. For example, a female patient who talks about the death of her father, which occurred 3 years ago, may, on questioning, reveal a recent loss of a relationship with a male. A patient who talks about feelings of inadequacy he had as a child because of poor school performance may, on questioning, reveal a recent experience in which his feelings of adequacy on his job were threatened. Because most crises involve losses or threats of losses, the theme of loss is a common one. In assessment the nurse looks for a recent event that may be connected to an underlying theme.

Support Systems and Coping Resources

The patient's living situation and supports in the environment must be assessed. Does the patient live alone or with family or friends? With whom is the patient close, and who offers understanding and strength? Is there a supportive clergyman or friend? Assessing the patient's support system is important in determining who should come for the crisis therapy sessions. It may be decided that certain family members should come with the patient so that the family members' support can be strengthened. If the patient has few supports, participation in a crisis therapy group may be recommended.

Assessing the patient's coping resources is also vital in determining whether hospitalization would be more appropriate than outpatient crisis therapy. If there is a high degree of suicidal and homicidal risk along with weak outside resources, hospitalization may be a safer and more effective treatment.

Identify people in your social system that you would turn to in a time of crisis. Compare your list with that of a friend.

Coping Mechanisms

Next, the nurse assesses the patient's strengths and previous coping mechanisms. How has the patient handled other crises? How were anxieties relieved? Did the patient talk out problems? Did the patient leave the usual surroundings for a period of time to think things out from another perspective? Was physical activity used to relieve tension? Did the patient find relief in crying? Besides exploring previous coping mechanisms, the nurse should also note the absence of other possible successful mechanisms.

PLANNING AND IMPLEMENTATION

The next step of crisis intervention is planning; the previously collected data are analyzed and specific interventions are proposed. Dynamics underlying the present crisis are formulated from the information about the precipitating event. Alternative solutions to the problem are explored, and steps for achieving the solutions are identified. The nurse de-

PATIENT EDUCATION PLAN *Coping with Crisis*

CONTENT	INSTRUCTIONAL ACTIVITIES	EVALUATION
Describe the crisis event	Ask about the details of the crisis including: 　A timeline of the crisis 　Who was affected 　The events of the crisis 　Any precipitating events	Patient describes the crisis event in detail
Explore feelings, thoughts, and behaviors related to the crisis event	Determine precrisis level of functioning Discuss patient's perception of the crisis event Determine acute and long-term needs, threats, and challenges	Patient discusses precrisis level of functioning and perceptions crisis event Patient's needs are identified
Identify coping mechanisms	Ask how stressful events have been handled in the past Analyze whether these are adaptive or maladaptive for the current crisis event Suggest additional coping strategies	Patient identifies adaptive coping mechanisms for the current crisis event
Develop a plan for coping adaptively with the crisis event	Reinforce adaptive coping mechanisms and healthy defenses With the patient, construct a coping plan for the aftermath of the crisis event	Patient develops a plan for coping with the crisis event
Assign the patient activities from coping plan	Review implementation of the coping plan Help patient generalize coping strategies for use in future crisis events	Patient reports satisfaction with coping abilities and level of functioning

cides which environmental supports to engage or strengthen and how to do this, as well as which of the patient's coping mechanisms to develop and which to strengthen.

This process is outlined in the Patient Education Plan for coping with crisis above The expected outcome of nursing care is that the patient will recover from the crisis event and return to a precrisis level of functioning. A more ambitious expected outcome would be for the patient to recover from the crisis event to a higher than precrisis level of functioning and improved quality of life.

Nursing interventions can take place on many levels using a variety of techniques. In a classic model, Shields (1975) described four levels of crisis intervention that represent a hierarchy from the most basic to the most complex (Fig. 14-4). Each level includes the interventions of the previous level, and the progressive order indicates that the nurse needs additional knowledge and skill for high-level interventions. It is often helpful to consult with others when deciding which approach to use.

Environmental Manipulation

Environmental manipulation includes interventions that directly change the patient's physical or interpersonal situation. These interventions provide situational support or remove stress. Important elements of this intervention are mobilizing the patient's supporting social systems (see Chapter 13) and serving as a liaison between the patient and social support agencies.

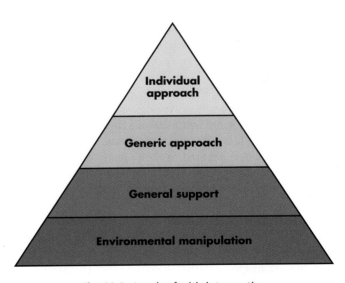

Fig. 14-4 Levels of crisis intervention.

For example, a patient who is having trouble coping with her six children may temporarily send several of the children to their grandparents' house. In this situation some stress is reduced. Similarly, a patient having difficulty on his or her job may take a week of sick leave to be removed temporarily from that stress. A patient who lives alone may move in with his or her closest sibling for several days. Likewise, involving the patient in family or group crisis therapy provides environmental manipulation for the purpose of providing support.

General Support

General support includes interventions that convey the feeling that the nurse is on the patient's side and will be a helping person. The nurse uses warmth, acceptance, empathy, caring, and reassurance to provide this type of support.

Generic Approach

The generic approach is designed to reach high-risk individuals and large groups as quickly as possible. It applies a specific method to all people faced with a similar type of crisis. The expected course of the particular type of crisis is studied and mapped out. The intervention is then set up to ensure that the course of the crisis results in an adaptive response.

Grief is an example of a crisis with a known pattern that can be treated by the generic approach. Helping the patient to overcome ties to the deceased and find new patterns of rewarding interaction may effectively resolve the grief. Applying this intervention to people experiencing grief, especially with a high-risk group such as families of disaster victims, is an example of the generic approach.

Another example of the generic approach is the use of debriefing. Originally a military concept, debriefing can be used as a therapeutic intervention to help people recall events and clarify traumatic experiences. It attempts to place the traumatic event in perspective, allows the individual to relive the event in a factual way, encourages group support, and provides information on normal reaction to critical events (Dyregrol, 1997). The goal of debriefing is to help prevent the maladaptive responses that may result if the trauma is suppressed (see Citing the Evidence on Debriefing).

Individual Approach

The individual approach is a type of crisis intervention similar to the diagnosis and treatment of a specific problem in a specific patient. The nurse must understand the specific patient characteristics that led to the present crisis and must use the intervention that is most likely to help the patient develop an adaptive response to the crisis.

This type of crisis intervention can be effective with all types of crises. It is particularly useful in combined situational and maturational crises. The individual approach is also helpful when symptoms include homicidal and suicidal risk. In these instances the nurse should make a formal safety contract in which the patient agrees not to harm himself or herself or others (see Chapter 21). The individual approach should also be applied if the course of the crisis cannot be determined and to crises that have not responded to the generic approach.

Interventions are aimed at facilitating cognitive and emotional processing of the traumatic event and at improving coping. Five core interventions to assist survivors of acute stress are (Osterman & Chemtob, 1999):

- Restore psychological safety
- Provide information
- Correct misattributions

Citing the Evidence on

Debriefing

BACKGROUND: Following a catastrophic natural disaster, the investigators evaluated whether brief psychological intervention (debriefing 6 months later) reduced disaster-related psychological distress as measured by the Impact of Event Scale.

RESULTS: Two groups of subjects who had been exposed to Hurricane Iniki in Hawaii were assessed. The intervention was aimed to provide ventilation of feelings, normalization of responses, and education about common psychological reactions to the disaster in the context of group support. The measured distress scores were reduced in both intervention groups.

IMPLICATIONS: This study provides preliminary evidence to support the effectiveness of postdisaster psychological intervention and for the feasibility of treatment research in postdisaster environments.

Chemtob C et al: Postdisaster psychosocial intervention: a field study of the impact of debriefing on psychological distress, *Am J Psychiatry* 154(3):415, 1997.

- Restore and support effective coping
- Ensure social support

How might each level of crisis intervention be used in a high school after a star player of the football team commits suicide?

Techniques

The nurse uses techniques that are active, focused, and explorative to carry out the interventions. The intervention must be aimed at achieving quick resolution. The nurse also must be active in guiding the crisis intervention through its various steps. A passive approach is not appropriate because of the time limitations of the crisis situation.

The nurse should be creative and flexible, trying many different techniques. Some of these include catharsis, clarification, suggestion, reinforcement of behavior, support of defenses, raising self-esteem, and exploration of solutions. A brief description of these techniques is presented.

Catharsis is the release of feelings that takes place as the patient talks about emotionally charged areas. As feelings about the events are realized, tension is reduced. Catharsis is often used in crisis intervention. The nurse solicits the patient's feelings about the specific situation, recent events, and significant people involved in the particular crisis. The nurse asks open-ended questions and repeats the patient's words so that more feelings are expressed. The nurse does not discourage crying or angry outbursts but rather sees them as a positive release of feelings. Only when feelings seem out of control, such as in extreme rage or despondency, should the nurse discourage catharsis and help the patient concentrate on thinking rather than feeling. For example, if a patient angrily talks of wanting to kill a specific person, it is better to shift the focus to a discussion of the consequences of carrying out the act rather than to encourage free expression of the angry feelings.

Clarification is used when the nurse helps the patient to identify the relationship between events, behaviors, and feelings. For example, helping a patient see that it was after being passed over for a promotion that he or she felt too sick to go to work is clarification. Clarification helps the patient gain a better understanding of feelings and how they lead to the development of a crisis.

Suggestion is influencing a person to accept an idea or belief. In crisis intervention the patient is influenced to see the nurse as a confident, calm, hopeful, empathic person who can help. By believing the nurse can help, the patient may feel more optimistic and less anxious and may want to please the nurse by getting better. It is a technique in which the nurse engages patients' emotions, wishes, or values to their benefit in the therapeutic process. Suggestion is a way of influencing the patient by pointing out alternatives or new ways of looking at things.. For example, the nurse may want to point out to the patient who takes pride in independence that he or she is responsible for much of the work of solving his or her problem.

Reinforcement of behavior occurs when healthy, adaptive behavior of the patient is reinforced by the nurse, who strengthens positive responses made by the patient by agreeing with or complimenting those responses. For example, when a patient who has passively allowed himself or herself to be criticized by the boss reports asserting himself or herself in a discussion with the boss, the nurse can compliment the patient on this assertiveness.

Support of defenses occurs when the nurse encourages the use of healthy defenses and discourages those that are maladaptive. Defense mechanisms are used to cope with stressful situations and to maintain self-esteem and ego integrity. When defenses deny, falsify, or distort reality to the point that the person cannot deal effectively with reality, they are maladaptive. The nurse should encourage the patient to use adaptive defenses and discourage those that are maladaptive. For example, when a patient denies the fact that her husband wants a separation despite the fact that he has told her so, the nurse can point out that she is not facing facts and dealing realistically with the problem. This is an example of discouraging the maladaptive use of the defense mechanism of denial. If a patient who is furious with his boss writes a letter to his boss's supervisor rather than assaulting his boss, the nurse should encourage the adaptive use of the defense mechanism of sublimation.

In crisis intervention, defenses are not attacked but rather are more gently encouraged or discouraged. When defenses are attacked, the patient cannot maintain self-esteem and ego integrity. There is also not enough time in crisis intervention to replace the attacked defenses with new ones. Returning the patient to a prior level of functioning is the goal of crisis intervention, not the restructuring of defenses.

Raising self-esteem is a particularly important technique. The patient in a crisis feels helpless and may be overwhelmed with feelings of inadequacy. The fact that the patient has found it necessary to seek outside help may further increase feelings of inadequacy. The nurse should help the patient regain feelings of self-worth by communicating confidence that the patient can find solutions to problems. The nurse should also convey that the patient is a worthwhile person by listening to and accepting the patient's feelings, being respectful, and praising help-seeking efforts.

Exploration of solutions is essential because crisis intervention is geared toward solving the immediate crisis. The nurse and patient actively explore solutions to the crisis. Answers that the patient had not thought of before may become apparent during conversations with the nurse as anxiety decreases. For example, a patient who has lost her job and has not been able to find a new one may become aware of the fact that she knows many people in her field of work whom she could contact to get information regarding the job market and possible openings.

These crisis intervention techniques are summarized in Box 14-2. In addition to using these techniques, there are other attitudes that the crisis worker should have. The crisis worker should see this work as the treatment of choice with people in crisis rather than a second-best treatment. Assessment of the present problem should be viewed as necessary for treatment, but complete diagnostic assessment is unnecessary. The goal and time limitations of crisis intervention should be kept in mind constantly, and unrelated material should not be explored. An active directive role must be taken, and flexibility of approach is essential. If more complex problems are identified that are not suitable for crisis intervention, the patient should be referred for further treatment. Table 14-2 describes interventions for helping individuals and families cope with stress resulting from crisis.

EVALUATION

The last phase of crisis intervention is evaluation, when the nurse and patient evaluate whether the intervention resulted in a positive resolution of the crisis. Specific questions the nurse might ask include the following:

- Has the expected outcome been achieved, and has the patient returned to the precrisis level of functioning?
- Have the needs of the patient that were threatened by the event been met?
- Have the patient's symptoms decreased or been resolved?
- Does the patient have adequate support systems and coping resources on which to rely?
- Is the patient using constructive coping mechanisms?
- Is the patient demonstrating adaptive crisis responses?
- Does the patient need to be referred for additional treatment?

The nurse and patient should also review the changes that have occurred. The nurse should give patients credit for suc-

Box 14-2

Techniques of Crisis Intervention

Technique: **Catharsis**
Definition: The release of feelings that takes place as the patient talks about emotionally charged areas
Example: "Tell me about how you have been feeling since you lost your job."

Technique: **Clarification**
Definition: Encouraging the patient to express more clearly the relationship between certain events
Example: "I've noticed that after you have an argument with your husband you become sick and can't leave your bed."

Technique: **Suggestion**
Definition: Influencing a person to accept an idea or belief, particularly the belief that the nurse can help and that the person will feel better
Example: "Many other people have found it helpful to talk about this and I think you will, too."

Technique: **Reinforcement of behavior**
Definition: Giving the patient positive responses to adaptive behavior
Example: "That's the first time you were able to defend yourself with your boss and it went very well. I'm so pleased that you were able to do it."

Technique: **Support of defenses**
Definition: Encouraging the use of healthy, adaptive defenses and discouraging those that are unhealthy or maladaptive
Example: "Going for a bicycle ride when you were so angry was very helpful because when you returned you and your wife were able to talk things through."

Technique: **Raising self-esteem**
Definition: Helping the patient to regain feelings of self-worth
Example: "You are a very strong person to be able to manage the family all this time. I think you will be able to handle this situation, too."

Technique: **Exploration of solutions**
Definition: Examining alternative ways of solving the immediate problem
Example: "You seem to know many people in the computer field. Could you contact some of them to see whether they might know of available jobs?"

Table 14-2

Nursing Interventions for Crisis Events

Target Areas	Nursing Interventions
Basic needs	Provide liaison to social agencies
Physical deficits	Attend to physical emergencies
	Refer to other health-care providers as necessary
PSYCHOLOGICAL EFFECTS	
Shock	Attentive listening to the crisis details
Confusion	Give nurturing support, permit regression
Denial	Permit intermittent denial; identify patient's primary concern
Anxiety	Provide structure, enact antianxiety interventions
Lethargy/heroics	Encourage sublimation and constructive activity
PROTECTIVE FACTORS	
Coping	Encourage patient's favored, adaptive coping mechanisms; emphasize rationalization, humor, sublimation
Self-efficacy	Support patient's previous successes and belief in own abilities, dilute irrational self-doubts, emphasize power of expectations to produce results
Support	Add social supports to the patient's world, provide professional support, refer for counseling when necessary, help patient develop new coping strategies

Modified from Hardin SB: Catastrophic stress. In McBride AB, Austin JK, editors: *Psychiatric-mental health nursing*, Philadelphia, 1996, WB Saunders.

cessful changes so that they can realize their effectiveness and understand that what they learned from a crisis may help in coping with future crises. If the goals have not been met, the patient and nurse can return to the first step, assessment, and continue through the phases again. At the end of the evaluation process, if the nurse and patient believe referral for additional professional help would be useful, the referral should be made as quickly as possible (see Critical Thinking about Contemporary Issues).

All of the phases of crisis intervention are presented in the Case Study on p. 238.

SETTINGS FOR CRISIS INTERVENTION

Nurses work in many settings in which they see people in crisis. Hospitalizations are often stressful for patients and their families and are precipitating causes of crises. The patient who becomes demanding or withdrawn or the spouse who becomes bothersome to the nursing staff is a possible candidate for crisis intervention. The diagnosis of an illness, the limitations imposed on activities, and the changes in body image because of surgery can all be viewed as losses or threats that may precipitate a situational crisis. Simply the stress of being dependent on nurses for care can precipitate a crisis for the hospitalized patient.

Nurses who work in obstetric, pediatric, geriatric, or adolescent settings often observe patients or family members undergoing maturational crises. The anxious new mother, the acting-out adolescent, and the newly retired depressed patient are all possible candidates for crisis therapy. If physical illness is an added stress during maturational turning points, the patient is at an even greater risk. Emergency room and critical care settings are also flooded with crisis cases. People who attempt suicide, psychosomatic patients, survivors of sudden cardiac arrest, and crime and accident victims are all possible candidates for crisis intervention (see Citing the Ev-

CRITICAL THINKING about **CONTEMPORARY ISSUES**

Should Medication Be Included as a Crisis Intervention Treatment for Acute Traumatic Stress?

Although people who are suffering from traumatic stress may experience a range of mental health symptoms in the acute phase of the trauma, it is unclear whether all problems share the same biological characteristics. It is also unclear in the initial phases of assessment which symptoms may quickly resolve with crisis intervention and which may last and ultimately meet criteria for a psychiatric disorder amenable to medication. Should psychopharmacological agents be offered to victims in the early stages of traumatic stress, which ones would be appropriate, and when in the process of crisis intervention would this be most helpful? Also, are there contraindications for biological interventions under some circumstances?

One might begin this decision-making process by assessing precrisis symptoms (and treatments, if any), history of substance use, family history of psychiatric disorders, and the person's belief system regarding psychiatric medications. Is the symptom already of long duration and, if so, how was it treated in the past? Does the person use substances such as alcohol that could complicate his or her reaction to the crisis or assessment of the crisis impact? If there is a family history of a psychiatric disorder, the person may be at greater risk for developing that or a similar disorder. Psychopharmacological interventions may be inap-

propriate if many of the symptoms will be short-lived (given the fact that some medications take several weeks to work), if many of the symptoms are natural reactions to trauma rather than symptoms of psychiatric disorders, or if the medications will lead to adverse side effects and possibly stigmatize an already traumatized person.

Some may argue that medications might blunt a person's cognitive abilities at a time when concentration and problem solving are important, but an important question is whether withholding a treatment from a person who may benefit from it is an ethical decision. Could medication given immediately after exposure to a traumatic event avert a chronic posttraumatic illness? There are no clear-cut answers to these questions, but crisis clinicians are best guided by a few clinical principles (Kudler & Davidson, 1995):

- What bothers this person the most?
- Can this problem be controlled through psychotherapeutic, environmental, or psychopharmacological interventions?
- What treatment is most likely to make this person feel or function better?
- Is there a reason **not** to prescribe this treatment?

Answers will be governed by a careful assessment of each person's circumstances and a holistic view of care provided.

---

idence). If the nurse is not in a position to work with the patient on an ongoing basis, a referral should be made.

Community and home health nurses work with patients in their own environments and can often spot and intervene in family crises. The child who refuses to go to school, the man who refuses to learn how to give himself an insulin injection, and the family with a member dying at home are possible candidates for crisis intervention. Community health nurses are also in an ideal position to evaluate high-risk families such as those with new babies, ill members, recent deaths, and a history of difficulty coping (England, 1995).

Finally, nurses in community mental health centers, departments of psychiatry, managed care clinics, schools, occupational health centers, and home health agencies also may see patients in crisis, such as those experiencing depression, anxiety, marital conflict, suicidal thoughts, illicit drug use, and traumatic responses. Crisis intervention can be implemented in any setting and should be a competency skill of all nurses, regardless of specialty area.

MODALITIES OF CRISIS INTERVENTION

Crisis intervention modalities are based on the philosophy that the health-care team must be aggressive and go out to the patients rather than wait for the patients to come to them. Nurses working in these modalities intervene in a variety of community settings, ranging from patients' homes to street corners.

Citing the Evidence on

The Cardiac Arrest Experience

BACKGROUND: Progress in resuscitation medicine allows an increasing proportion of patients to survive an out-of-hospital cardiac arrest. However, little is known about long-term adaptation of these individuals. This study assessed the emotional disability of cardiac arrest survivors.

RESULTS: Cardiac arrest survivors had levels of psychological adjustment similar to those cardiac patients whose clinical course was not complicated by cardiac arrest. However, the diagnosis of psychotraumatic symptoms in cardiac arrest survivors led to a sharp separation between favorable and unfavorable outcome in affective regulation and level of functioning. Those with high scores of intrusion and avoidance reported a higher sense of demoralization and more somatic complaints, depression, anxiety, lack of confidence in the future, and narrowing of social activities.

IMPLICATIONS: This study provides the first empirical evidence that the application of the posttraumatic stress disorder paradigm in the long-term evaluation of cardiac arrest survivors significantly contributes to defining a patient population at high risk for serious emotional disability.

Ladwig K et al: Long-acting psychotraumatic properties of a cardiac arrest experience, *Am J Psychiatry* 156(6):912, 1999.

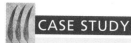
CASE STUDY

ASSESSMENT

Mr. A was a 39-year-old, medium-built, casually dressed black man who was referred to the mental health clinic by his primary care provider. The patient came to the center alone. The nurse working with Mr. A collected the following data.

The patient worked in a large naval shipyard that was recently scheduled for closing. It was laying off many workers and reassigning others. One month earlier Mr. A was assigned to an area where he had difficulty 2 years ago. The foreman, the patient believed, was harassing him, as he had done previously. Two weeks ago the patient got angry at the foreman and had thoughts of killing him. Instead, Mr. A became dizzy and his head ached. He requested medical attention but was refused. He then passed out and was taken by ambulance to the dispensary. Since that time Mr. A had a comprehensive physical examination and was found to be in excellent health. He was prescribed diazepam (Valium) on an as-needed basis, which was only slightly helpful. He returned to work for 2 days this week but again felt sick.

Mr. A complained of being depressed, nervous, and tense. He was not sleeping well, was irritable with his wife and children, and was preoccupied with angry feelings toward his foreman. He denied suicidal thoughts but admitted that he felt like killing the foreman. He quickly added that he would really never do anything like that.

He appeared to have good comprehension, above-average intelligence, adequate memory, and some paranoid ideation related to the foreman at work. His thought processes were organized, and there was no evidence of a perceptual disorder. Ego boundary disturbance was evident in the patient's paranoid thoughts. It seemed that the foreman was a difficult man to get along with, but the description of personal harassment seemed distorted.

Mr. A was raised by his parents. His father beat him and his siblings often. His mother was quiet and always agreed with his father. The patient had a younger brother and sister and an older sister. The patient and his brother had always been close. The two of them had stopped their father's beatings by ganging up on him and "psyching him out." As a child, Mr. A hung around with a tough crowd and fought frequently. He believed that he could physically overpower others but tried to keep out of trouble by talking to people rather than fighting.

Mr. A had no psychiatric history. His physical health was excellent, and he was taking no medication other than the prescribed Valium. He had a tenth-grade education, and his work record up to this time was good. His interests included bowling and other sports. He had been married for 17 years and had three daughters, ages 16, 13, and 9. Mr. A stated that he had a good relationship with his wife and daughters and that both his wife and his brother were strong supports for him.

His usual means of coping were talking calmly with the threatening party and working hard on his job, at home, and in leisure activities. These coping mechanisms failed to work for him at this time but they had been successful in the past. He

had no arrest record and was able to think through his actions rather than act impulsively. Mr. A showed strong motivation for working on his problem. He was reaching out for help and was able to form a therapeutic relationship with the nurse. Although his wife and brother were supportive, he felt a need for outside support because his previous coping skills were not working.

NURSING DIAGNOSIS

Mr. A was in a situational crisis. The threat or precipitating stress was his transfer to a former boss, whom he felt was harassing him. The patient's need for role mastery was not being met because he was not feeling successful at his job. Soon after the transfer, Mr. A's usual means of coping became ineffective and he experienced increased anxiety.

His nursing diagnosis was ineffective individual coping related to changes at work, as evidenced by physical complaints of dizziness and tension. His DSM–IV–TR diagnosis was adjustment disorder with mixed anxiety and depressed mood.

OUTCOME IDENTIFICATION AND PLANNING

The expected outcome of treatment was for Mr. A to return to his precrisis level of functioning. If possible, he could reach a higher level, having learned new methods of problem solving. The patient showed good potential for growth, and the nurse made a contract with him for crisis intervention. Mutually identified short-term goals included the following:

- Mr. A will explore his thoughts and feelings about recent work events.
- Mr. A will not harm his boss.
- Mr. A will describe coping mechanisms that have been successful for him in the past.
- Mr. A will identify three new ways of coping with work stress.
- Mr. A will implement two of the new coping strategies.
- Mr. A will be free of symptoms and function well at work.

IMPLEMENTATION

The level of intervention used by the nurse was the **individual approach**, which includes the generic approach, general support, and environmental manipulation.

Environmental manipulation involved having the patient remain home from work temporarily. Letters were written by the nurse to his employer explaining Mr. A's absence in general terms. Mr. A was encouraged to talk to his wife about his difficulties so that she could understand his anxiety and provide emotional support.

General support was given by the nurse, who provided an atmosphere of reassurance, nonjudgmental caring, warmth, empathy, and optimism. Mr. A was encouraged to talk freely about the problem, and the nurse assured him that his problem could be solved and that he would be feeling better soon.

The **generic approach** was used to decrease the patient's anxiety and guide him through the steps of problem solving. Levels of anxiety were assessed and ways of reducing anxiety

Continued from previous page

and helping the patient tolerate moderate anxiety were identified. The patient was encouraged to use his anxiety constructively to solve his problem and develop new coping mechanisms.

*The **individual approach** was used in assessing and treating the specific problems of Mr. A, who was strongly sensitive to mistreatment as a result of early childhood experiences. His emotional response was to strike out physically, as his father had struck out at him. Intellectually, Mr. A knew this would be disastrous, and his conflict was solved by becoming sick and passing out so that he could not assault his boss. Mr. A's intense anger was recognized, and a high priority was placed on channeling the anger in a positive direction. As a way of formalizing this intervention, Mr. A signed a safety contract with the nurse agreeing not to harm himself or others.*

*The first two meetings were used for data gathering and establishing a positive therapeutic relationship. Through the use of catharsis the patient vented angry feelings but did not concentrate on wanting to kill his boss. The nurse used **clarification** to help the patient begin to understand the precipitating event and its effect on him. **Suggestion** was used to allow the patient to see the nurse as one who could help. The nurse told the patient the problem could be worked out by the two of them and that he would soon be feeling better. Mr. A decided to contact several people at work to obtain information about transferring to another department and filing a formal complaint against the foreman. The patient and nurse therefore were **exploring solutions**. The nurse **reinforced** the patient's use of problem solving by telling him that his ideas about alternative solutions were good ones. Throughout these and other sessions the nurse **raised his self-esteem** by communicating her confidence that he could find solutions to his problems. She listened to and accepted his feelings and treated him with respect. By contacting others at work, the patient also found some supportive people.*

*During the third session the patient described an incident in which he became furious at a worker in an automobile repair shop. The repairs on the patient's car were never right, and the patient kept returning the car there. The patient shoved the worker but limited his physical assault to that. He then felt nervous and jittery. The patient had previously expressed pride in his ability to control his angry feelings and not physically strike out at others. **Suggestion** was used by telling the patient that he showed control in stopping the assault before it had become a full-blown fight and he could continue to do so. Mr. A's ability to honor the safety contract he made with the nurse was also reinforced. During this session the patient spoke of old, angry feelings toward his father. Some of this venting was allowed, but soon thereafter the focus was guided back to the present crisis.*

*In the fourth session the patient reported no episodes of uncontrollable anger. However, he still put much emphasis on being harassed by others. The nurse questioned the notion that others were out to intentionally harass the patient. Mr. A's defenses were not attacked, but his gross use of projection was discouraged. In the fifth session the patient reported that a car tried to run him off the road. At a red traffic light the patient spoke calmly to the driver and the driver apologized. The nurse **reinforced this behavior** and **supported his use of sublimation** as a defense. Discussion of termination of the therapy was begun.*

In the sixth session Mr. A said that things were going well at work and that he would soon be going to a different department. He also talked about a course he had begun at a community college. He showed no evidence of anxiety, depression, or paranoia and thought he didn't need to come back to the mental health clinic.

EVALUATION

The interventions resulted in an adaptive resolution of the crisis. The patient's need for role mastery was being met. He was once again comfortable and successful at work. His symptoms of anxiety, paranoia, dizziness, headaches, passing out, and homicidal thoughts had ended. He no longer felt harassed. His original coping mechanisms were again effective. He was talking calmly to people he was having difficulty with, and he was again working hard in a goal-oriented way (his college course). He had learned new methods of coping, which included talking about his feelings to significant others, following administrative or official avenues of protest, and seeking support. The patient and nurse discussed how Mr. A could use the methods of problem solving he had learned from the experience to help cope with future problems. The expected outcome, return to the precrisis level of functioning, had been attained.

It was also recommended to the patient that he engage in psychotherapy so that he could deal with the old angers that continued to interfere with his life. Mr. A refused the recommendation at that time and stated he would contact the clinic if he changed his mind.

Mobile Crisis Programs

Mobile crisis teams provide front-line interdisciplinary crisis intervention to individuals, families, and communities. The nurse who is a member of a mobile crisis team may respond to a desperate person threatening to jump off a bridge in a suicide attempt, an angry person who is becoming violent toward family members at home, or a frightened person who has barricaded himself in an office building. By defusing the immediate crisis situation, lives can be saved, incarcerations and hospitalizations can be avoided, and people can be stabilized (Lamb et al, 1995; Zealberg et al, 1996, 1998).

Mobile crisis programs throughout the country vary in the services they provide and the procedures they use. However, they are usually able to provide on-site assessment, crisis management, treatment, referral, and educational services to patients, families, law enforcement officers, and the community at large (Hoff & Adamowski, 1998) (see Citing the Evidence).

A survey of mobile crisis services found that 39 states have implemented mobile crisis services, dispatching teams to a range of settings (Geller et al, 1995). Although these services provide favorable outcomes for patients and families and lower hospitalization rates, the survey found that few service systems evaluate the efficiency or cost-effectiveness of these services. Carefully designed studies are needed that specify the target populations, clinical team composition, nature of the mobile intervention, goal of the intervention, cost comparisons with other modalities, and follow-up outcomes.

Group Work

Crisis groups follow the same steps that individual intervention follows. The nurse and group help the patient solve the problem and reinforce the patient's new problem-solving behavior. The nurse's role in the group is active, focal, and present oriented. The group follows the nurse's example and uses similar therapeutic techniques. The group acts as a support system for the patient and is therefore of particular benefit to socially isolated people. Often the way the patient functions in the group suggests the faulty coping pattern that is responsible for the patient's current problem. For example, a patient's interaction with group members may show that he does not appear to listen to anything said by others. This same patient may be in a crisis because his girlfriend left him because she thought he did not care about her thoughts and feelings. The nurse can comment on the faulty coping behavior seen in the group and encourage group discussion about it.

Most crisis groups focus on people who have common traits or stressors. For example, Grosz et al (2000) established groups for children and parents to decrease traumatic distress when children were victims of extrafamilial sexual abuse. While Leske (1998) described how nurses working in a critical care unit organized crisis groups for families who had one of their members critically injured. The groups provided the opportunity for members to express common concerns and experiences, foster hope, and build mutual support.

Nurses practicing on acute psychiatric units can use crisis intervention in working with patients and families to prepare for discharge and prevent rehospitalization. With the shortened lengths of hospital stays, crisis intervention is often the treatment of choice. The hospitalization itself may be viewed as an environmental manipulation and part of the crisis intervention.

Telephone Contacts

Crisis intervention is sometimes practiced by telephone rather than through face-to-face contacts. When individuals in crisis use the telephone, it is usually when they are at the peak of their distress. Nurses working for hotlines or those who answer emergency telephone calls may find themselves practicing crisis intervention without visual cues. Referrals for face-to-face contact should be made, but often, because of the patient's unwillingness or inability to cooperate, the

Citing the Evidence on

Police Responses to the Mentally Ill in Crisis

BACKGROUND: Relatively little is known about police perceptions of responding to the mentally ill in crisis. This study sampled police officers from three law enforcement agencies, each of which had different system responses to the mentally ill. One department relied on field assistance from a mobile crisis team; the second had a team of officers specially trained in crisis intervention with the mentally ill; and the third had a team of in-house social workers to assist in responding to calls.

RESULTS: Calls involving mentally ill people in crisis were frequent and were perceived by most of the officers to be a significant problem. However, most officers reported feeling prepared to handle these calls. Officers from the department with a specialized team of trained officers rated their program as being highly effective in meeting the needs of the mentally ill in crisis, keeping the mentally ill out of jail, minimizing the amount of time officers spent on these calls, and maintaining community safety. Officers from the other two departments rated their programs as moderately effective.

IMPLICATIONS: Focused training of police officers in crisis intervention techniques to use with the mentally ill in crisis may be more effective and yield better outcomes for both the mentally ill and the community than mobile crisis teams or the addition of a health professional.

Borum R et al: Police perspectives on responding to mentally ill people in crisis: perceptions of program effectiveness, *Behav Science Law* 16(4):393, 1998.

telephone remains the only contact. Listening skills must therefore be emphasized in the nurse's role. Most emergency telephone services have extensive training programs to teach this specialized type of crisis intervention. Manuals written for the crisis worker include content such as suicide-potential rating scales, community resources, drug information, guidelines for helping the caller discuss concerns, and advice on understanding the limitations of the crisis worker's role.

Disaster Response

As part of the community, nurses are called on when adventitious crises strike the community. Floods, earthquakes, airplane crashes, fires, nuclear accidents, and other natural and unnatural disasters precipitate large numbers of crises (Weaver, 1995). It is important that nurses in the immediate postdisaster period go to places where victims are likely to gather, such as morgues, hospitals, and shelters. Nursing response after tornadoes devastated communities in central

Tennessee is a good example of such intervention. Later, if Federal Disaster Assistance Centers are established, nurses may assist in the centers. This was a critically important part of nursing intervention in the aftermath of the Oklahoma City bombing (Flynn, 1995). Rather than waiting for people to publicly identify themselves as being unable to cope with stress, it is suggested that nurses work with the American Red Cross, talk to people waiting in lines to apply for assistance, go door-to-door, or, at a relocation site, ask people how they are managing their affairs and explore their reactions to stress.

> *Nurses are often called on to help out in times of disaster. What special needs might nurses have in situations where they are both victims and caregivers?*

Experts in the field of disaster response suggest that organized plans for crisis response be developed and practiced during nondisaster times. Disaster plans are needed for large and small communities so that multiple complex needs can be met. The combination of services used during a disaster depends on the type of event and the specific groups identified to be at high risk for crisis (Young et al, 1999).

Common psychiatric responses to disaster should be considered when developing plans. These are listed in Table 14-3. Examples of agencies, organizations, and individuals to be included in disaster planning include hospitals, mental health programs, substance abuse agencies, departments of health, employee assistance programs, housing programs, university-affiliated nurses, and school district nurses (Anteau & Williams, 1997; Franklin et al, 2000; Wilhite et al, 1997).

Nurses providing crisis therapy during large disasters use the generic approach to crisis intervention so that as many people as possible can receive help in a short amount of time. Tragedies such as group kidnappings and group killings in communities may affect fewer people and may at times require the individual approach. The nurse may choose to work with families or groups rather than individuals during adventitious crises so that people can gain support from others in their family or community who are undergoing stresses similar to theirs.

A good example of mental health professionals helping victims of an adventitious crisis occurred in Kansas City, Missouri, in the days and weeks following the collapse of the overhead walkways at the Hyatt Hotel. Eight mental health centers in the Kansas City metropolitan area joined to help care for the emotional sufferings of the people involved. The centers formed an unofficial coalition and prepared a joint press release describing the many aspects of the grieving process and publicizing the services they would offer to the survivors of those killed at the hotel, the injured, the observers, and the rescue workers. The services were of three kinds. First, all centers offered phone counseling and support groups free of charge. Second, special services were planned, such as a grief workshop that was attended by about 200 people who had been at the scene. Other related

Table 14-3

Common Psychiatric Responses to Disaster
PSYCHIATRIC DIAGNOSES
Organic mental disorders secondary to head injury, toxic exposure, illness, and dehydration
Acute stress disorder
Adjustment disorder
Substance use disorders
Posttraumatic stress disorder
GENERALIZED ANXIETY DISORDER
Psychological factors affecting physical disease (in the injured)
PSYCHOLOGICAL/BEHAVIORAL RESPONSES
Grief reactions and other normal responses to an abnormal event
Family violence

From Ursano R et al: Psychiatric dimensions of disaster: patient care, community consultation, and preventive medicine. APA Online: http://www.psych.org/psych/pract_of_psych/disaster_psych.html.

seminars were also held. Third, the centers and media worked together to let the public know about other resources and services as these became available and to reassure people that their strong reactions to the tragedy were normal.

Recently, attention has been focused on offering support and help to the helpers in disasters (Lesaca, 1996; Turnbull, 1998). Health and mental health professionals who are victims of disasters as well as providers of care during disasters often feel overwhelmed with stress. These care providers describe feelings of concern for both their patients and their own families as well as themselves. Crisis intervention strategies for the caregivers are essential. For example, Stuart and Huggins (1990) described the actions that psychiatric nurse administrators used to care for their psychiatric nursing staff, and Stanley (1990) reported on a hospital-wide crisis stabilization program that provided large-group debriefing and small-group follow-up sessions for all nursing staff after Hurricane Hugo devastated South Carolina in 1989. Similarly, Tucker et al (1998) described debriefing services for firefighters, law enforcement officers, medical examiner personnel, and medical and mental health workers following the Oklahoma City bombing.

Victim Outreach Programs

Violent crime has become a global issue, concerning people in every walk of life and in every country. Many victim outreach programs use crisis intervention techniques to identify the needs of victims and then to connect them with appropriate referrals and other resources. Patient concerns such as the personal meaning of the crime, who to tell, and the reaction of others should be discussed. A victim advocate can contact employers regarding the need for temporary time off, can mobilize community resources for food and shelter if necessary, and can arrange for grace periods with debtors to delay payment of bills without penalty until the victim recovers. Although crisis intervention is not considered the appropriate treatment for serious consequences of victimization, such as posttraumatic stress disorder (PTSD) or depression, it is very useful as a community support for victims in the immediate aftermath of crime and may provide an important link for referral for more comprehensive services when needed (Falsetti & Resnick, 1995).

Crisis intervention is successful in the acute phase of rape. It uses an integrated framework of outreach, emergency care, and advocacy assistance. Nurses often work in rape crisis centers, where victims are often seen immediately after the rape. These victims need thorough evaluation, empathic support, information, and help with the legal system. The objectives of crisis intervention are to validate the crisis and criminal nature of the rape, carefully review the details of the rape, identify a supportive social network and self-enhancing ways of solving problems related to the rape and any subsequent events, and identify referral for follow-up of the often prolonged aftermath (Burgess & Hartman, 1996). Chapter 41 presents more information regarding care of survivors of violence.

Another important issue is that of abusive relationships. Whether the victim is a spouse, a child, or an elder, abusive relationships are experienced by people of both genders and of all racial, ethnic, economic, educational, and religious backgrounds. The widespread incidence and complex nature of abusive adult intimate relationships has been well documented. Nurses are often in ideal situations to identify and intervene with these people, most of whom are women. The nurse's validation of and response to people in abusive relationships is one component of a unified community-wide response that is headed by local domestic violence programs in many communities and is needed in all communities to prevent violence and abuse in the home (Fishwick, 1995).

Health Education

Although health education can take place during the entire crisis intervention process, it is emphasized during the evaluation phase. At this time the patient's anxiety has decreased, so better use can be made of cognitive abilities. The nurse and patient summarize the course of the crisis, and the intervention is to teach the patient how to avoid other similar crises. For example, the nurse helps the patient to identify the feelings, thoughts, and behaviors experienced following the stressful event. The nurse explains that if these feelings, thoughts, and behaviors are again experienced, the patient should immediately become aware of being stressed and take steps to prevent the anxiety from increasing. The nurse then teaches the patient ways to use these newly learned coping mechanisms in future situations.

Nurses are also involved in identifying people who are at high risk for developing crises and in teaching coping strategies to avoid the development of the crises. For example, coping strategies that can be taught include how to request information, access resources, and obtain support.

The public also needs education so that they can identify those needing crisis services, be aware of available services, change their attitudes so that people will feel free to seek ser-

vices, and obtain information about how others deal with potential crisis-producing problems. For example, a mother who learns about reactions to rape may identify her daughter as a rape victim. She then may take her daughter to the nearest rape crisis center. The mother, in encouraging her daughter to go to the crisis center, tells her daughter that rape is not the fault of the victim, thus enabling her to change her attitude about the rape and feel positive about obtaining outside help. At the center the mother may be given a pamphlet that describes how to help rape victims, which she shares with friends so that they can cope quickly and effectively if their loved ones are raped.

> *Explain how conducting a group on stress management for critical care nurses is an example of health education as crisis intervention.*

The nurse educates the public by participating in programs in the media, by leading or participating in educational groups in the community, and by taking every opportunity to advertise crisis services. For instance, if a nurse is a member of a church group that has developed crisis services, the availability of these services should be shared with school staff members and parent-teacher associations. Nurses, as health-care professionals, have a great opportunity to provide health education and crisis intervention, thus preventing mental illness and promoting mental health.

Summary

1. A crisis is a disturbance resulting from a perceived threat that challenges the person's usual coping mechanisms. Crises are a time of increased vulnerability, but they can also stimulate growth. There are two types of crises: maturational and situational.
2. Crisis intervention is a brief, active therapy with the goal of returning the individual to a precrisis level of functioning.
3. In assessing a patient the nurse should identify the patient's behaviors, precipitating event, perception of the event, support systems and coping resources, and previous strengths and coping mechanisms.
4. The expected outcome of nursing care is that the patient will recover from the crisis event and return to a precrisis level of functioning. Levels of crisis intervention include environmental manipulation, general support, generic approach, and individual approach.
5. The nurse and patient should consider the following factors in evaluating nursing care: the patient's level of functioning, symptoms, coping resources, coping mechanisms, evidence of adaptive coping responses, and need for referral for further treatment.
6. Crisis intervention can be implemented in any setting, including hospitals, clinics, community health centers, and the home. It should be a competency skill of all nurses.
7. Modalities of crisis intervention include mobile crisis programs, group work, telephone contacts, disaster response, victim outreach programs, and health education.

Competent Caring   A Clinical Exemplar of a Psychiatric Nurse

BETH MAREE, MSN, RN, CS

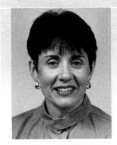

The mental health center setting presents many challenges, but few are broader in scope and higher in intensity than what I experienced while working there. My patient, S, was a 28-year-old, married, unemployed woman with a 4-year-old son. The marriage was interracial, and her husband, 32 years her senior, was terminally ill with cancer. His disease had progressed to the point that he was unable to provide for the family either financially or emotionally. S found herself, for the first time, responsible for the family but without the necessary skills or resources.

At our first meeting, S was an emergency walk-in patient with complaints of anxiety, sadness, tearfulness, lack of appetite, poor impulse control, ambivalent feelings, helplessness, and hopelessness. Upon initial assessment, it was identified that her father was an alcoholic who had been physically abusive to her, her mother, and her siblings. Her mother had fled the home, leaving the children with the father. Both parents later remarried, and S lived with her mother and stepfather, who also was an alcoholic. She experienced much emotional trauma during her youth and reported having difficulty in dealing with the eventual deaths of her parents and her stepfather. She had been only minimally involved with her siblings, since they were unhappy with the choices she had made in her life. Her identified source of support was her husband, who had promised "to always care for her." S spoke haltingly and was obviously in great distress. During the assessment, she shared that she had abused her own child when he was 6 months old, and she feared losing control again under such extreme stress. This was the precipitating factor for seeking help. S expressed a need to be cared for herself and an inability to cope with the demands of her son and her terminally ill husband. I knew that much care would be needed for this patient and her family system. I decided that crisis intervention would be my primary strategy to ensure the family's safety.

This first meeting was critical for obtaining an accurate assessment, establishing a sound rapport, and developing a plan of action. From here on it would be important for me to maintain a nonjudgmental approach, display empathy, validate concerns, and gain cooperation in establishing safety and ensuring her ongoing involvement in treatment. This could be difficult given the circumstances.

I offered positive reinforcement to S for her courage in admitting past abusive behavior and her recognition of its possible recurrence. The responsibility for reporting information related to abuse was explained to her and framed in a nonpunitive, protective manner. Her reaction of anger and fear was expected and accepted. She was encouraged to vent these feelings. In addition, her expectations of help were discussed and consequences of inadequate actions were explored.

S was able to accept the need to mobilize all available forms of assistance for her and her family as quickly as possible. The Department of Social Services was notified during the first meeting, and a caseworker was assigned to assess the home situation. With help, S was able to identify behavioral cues and situations that evoked her feelings of rage and hopelessness that often led to impulsive acts. She was able to contract for safety until her follow-up appointment and was provided with verbal and written instructions for emergency contacts via the mental health center and Department of Social Services' 24-hour phone line.

S also agreed to ongoing treatment. The targeted problem areas were grief reaction associated with the progressive loss of her husband, combined with few effective coping and parenting skills, dependency issues, and low self-esteem. She had a poor social support network and required mobilization and coordination of many agencies, programs, and professionals to meet her needs and those of her family. In addition to the protective services offered by the Department of Social Services, I enlisted help from the following agencies and professionals:

The mental health center psychiatrist for psychiatric evaluation and follow-up

The patient's medical doctor, with her permission

Family services for formalized parenting classes providing both information and a supportive peer group

Hospice for provision of daily nursing care visits to the husband and teaching S about his case

The youth division of the mental health center to provide evaluation and treatment for her son

Vocational rehabilitation for skill development and exploration of employment opportunities

I also continued as her nurse clinician for crisis intervention and follow-up care. The care I provided during our sessions remained largely supportive and educative. S, with a safety net of resources, began to work on grief and loss issues and related these to feelings of rejection and abandonment from her family of origin. She was allowed to progress through the phases of grief and to develop insight and personal growth at her own pace. Slowly, S began to identify her strengths and set goals. Together we formed a partnership to accomplish these goals with collaboration from the many services now involved in her treatment. My role as coordinator, facilitator, educator, and advocate was to assist S in meeting her goals and improving her self-esteem. In this case the importance of the patient as a human being with dignity and worth was reinforced, and the relationship of the individual to the family and the community was never more apparent.

Termination was the last critical task of our relationship; in this case the termination was twofold. First, her husband died with S at his bedside. She notified me, and support was offered at her request with my quiet presence at his funeral. A home visit was arranged shortly afterward to evaluate her adjustment to her husband's death. Second, due to a change in position, I was no longer able to serve as her clinician. Before I was transferred, S was able to meet her new clinician and establish some rapport with her. This transition went very smoothly, and S became an active, participating member in a strong therapy group. Months later I received a follow-up letter from her in which she expressed a new vision for herself that included assuming responsibility for providing a future for herself and her son. My goal of providing S with a sense of hope and a framework that would support her was accomplished. Looking back on it, I still feel good about what I was able to accomplish as a psychiatric nurse.

Merlin Visit MERLIN: **www.mosby.com/MERLIN/Stuart** to find these additional materials and student activities.

- **Worksheets**
- **"Drug of the Month" Updates**
- **"Citing the Evidence" Updates**
- **Critical Thinking Activities and Exercises**
- **Annotated Suggested Readings**
- **Web Links**
- **More!**

Chapter Review Questions

1. Match each term in Column A with the correct definition in Column B.

Column A

___ Catharsis

___ Clarification between certain events

___ Reinforcement of behavior

___ Exploration of solutions

___ Raising self-esteem

___ Suggestion

___ Support of defenses

Column B

A. Encourage the patient to express more clearly the relationship

B. Encourage the use of healthy, adaptive defenses and discourage those that are unhealthy or manipulative

C. Examining alternative ways of solving the immediate problem

D. Giving the patient positive responses to adaptive behavior

E. Helping the patient to regain feelings of self-worth

F. Influencing an individual to accept an idea or belief (for example, that the nurse can help and the patient will feel better)

G. The release of feelings that takes place as the patient talks about emotionally charged areas

2. Fill in the blanks.

A. A disturbance caused by a stressful event or perceived threat to self that challenges the individual's usual coping mechanisms is a _____ .

B. In crisis theory, perceived losses, threats of loss, or challenges that precede the stressor or threat are called _____ .

C. Crisis intervention is an active therapy, usually limited in time, with the goal of returning the patient to a _____ level of functioning.

D. The first step of crisis intervention is _____ .

E. When the nurse teaches the patient or the public principles of crisis intervention and healthy coping mechanisms in times of crisis, he or she is acting in the role of _____ .

3. Identify whether the following statements are true (T) or false (F).

___ A. When a person's usual way of coping becomes ineffective in dealing with a threat, the result is usually anxiety.

___ B. A crisis, by definition, is a chronic, long-term event requiring 12 or more months of treatment.

___ C. The fact that crises can lead to personal growth is important to remember when working with patients in crisis.

___ D. The patient's perception or appraisal of the precipitating events of a crisis is a relatively unimportant factor in crisis intervention.

___ E. The level of crisis intervention designed to reach high-risk individuals and large groups quickly, and that applies specific methods to similar types of crises, is the individual approach.

4. Provide short answers for the following questions.

A. List the two types of crisis and briefly describe each one.

B. Briefly describe cultural factors to be considered in crisis intervention.

C. Think of a crisis you have experienced in the past year. Identify which of the balancing factors of crisis intervention helped you cope positively with the event and which ones could have helped you even more.

REFERENCES

Adams S et al: Mental health disaster response: nursing interventions across the life span, *J Psychosoc Nurs* 37:11, 1999.

Aguilera DC: *Crisis intervention: theory and methodology,* ed 8, St Louis, 1998, Mosby.

Anteau C, Williams L: The Oklahoma bombing: lessons learned, *Crit Care Nurs Clin North Am* 9(2):231, 1997.

Burgess AW, Hartman CR: Rape trauma and posttraumatic stress disorder. In McBride AB, Austin JK, editors: *Psychiatric-mental health nursing,* Philadelphia, 1996, WB Saunders.

Dyregrol A: The process in critical incident stress debriefing, *J Traumatic Stress* 10(4):589, 1997.

England M: Crisis and the filial caregiving situation of African American adult offspring, *Issues Ment Health Nurs* 16:143, 1995.

Falsetti SA, Resnick HS: Helping victims of violent crime. In Freedy JR, Hobfoll SE, editors: *Traumatic stress: from theory to practice,* New York, 1995, Plenum Press.

Fishwick N: Getting to the heart of the matter: nursing assessment and intervention with battered women in psychiatric mental health settings, *J Am Psychiatr Nurs Assoc* 1:48, 1995.

Flynn BW: Thoughts and reflections after the bombing of the Alfred P Murrah Federal Building in Oklahoma City, *J Am Psychiatr Nurs Assoc* 1:166, 1995.

Franklin J et al: Hurricane Floyd: response of the Pitt County medical community, *NC Med J* 61(1):384, 2000.

Geller J et al: A national survey of mobile crisis services and their evaluation, *Psychiatr Serv* 46:893, 1995.

Grosz C et al: Extrafamilial sexual abuse: treatment for child victims and their families, *Child Abuse Neglect* 24(1):9, 2000.

Hoff L, Adamowski K: *Creating excellence in crisis care: a guide to effective training and program designs,* San Fransisco, 1998, Jossey-Bass.

Kudler H, Davidson JRT: General principles of biological intervention following trauma. In Freedy JR, Hobfoll SE, editors: *Traumatic stress: from theory to practice,* New York, 1995, Plenum Press.

Lamb H et al: Outcome for psychiatric emergency patients seen by an outreach police-mental health team, *Psychiatr Serv* 46:1267, 1995.

Lesaca T: Symptoms of stress disorder and depression among trauma counselors after an airline disaster, *Psychiatr Serv* 47:424, 1996.

Leske JS: Treatment for family members in crisis after critical injury, *AACN Clin Issues* 9(1):129, 1998.

Osterman J, Chemtob C: Emergency intervention for acute traumatic stress, *Psychiatr Serv* 50(6):739, 1999.

Shields L: Crisis intervention: implications for the nurse, *J Psychiatr Nurs* 13:37, 1975.

Stanley SR: When the disaster is over: helping the healers to mend, *J Psychosoc Nurs Ment Health Serv* 28:13, 1990.

Stuart G, Huggins E: Caring for the caretakers in times of disaster, *J Child Adolesc Psychiatr Nurs* 3:144, 1990.

Terr LC: Psychic trauma in children: observations following the Chowchilla school bus kidnapping, *Am J Psychiatry* 138:14, 1981.

Tucker P et al: Oklahoma City:disaster challenges mental health and medical administrators, *J Behav Health Serv Res* 25(1):93, 1998.

Turnbull G: A review of post-traumatic stress disorder. Part II: treatment, *Internat J Care Injured* 29(3):169, 1998.

Weaver JD: *Disasters: mental health interventions,* Sarasota, Fla, 1995, Professional Resource Press.

Wilhite M et al: Responding to disaster: flood in North Dakota, *J Am Psychiatr Nurs Assoc* 3(5):157, 1997.

Young B et al: Disaster mental health: current status and future directions. *New Dir Ment Health Serv* 82:53, 1999.

Zealberg J et al: *Comprehensive emergency mental health care,* Dunmore, Penn, 1996, WW Norton.

Zealberg J et al: Mental health clinicians role in responding to critical incidents in the community, *Psychiatr Serv* 49(3):301, 1998.

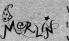

Visit **MERLIN** for *Your Internet Connection*
to websites that are related to the content in this chapter.
www.mosby.com/MERLIN/Stuart

15 Psychiatric Rehabilitation

Sandra J. Sundeen

Of equality—as if it harm'd me giving others the same chances and rights as myself—as if it were not indispensable to my own rights that others possess the same.

WALT WHITMAN, *THOUGHT*

The public health model of prevention identifies tertiary prevention as the limitation of disability related to an episode of illness. The *Report of the Surgeon General on Mental Health* addressed the need for a comprehensive array of mental health services.

"The fundamental components of effective service delivery, which include integrated community-based services, continuity of providers and treatments, family support services (including psychoeducation), and culturally sensitive services are broadly agreed upon, yet certain of these and other mental health services are inconsistently short supply, both regionally and, in some instances, nationally. Because the service system as a whole, as opposed to treatment services considered in isolation, dictates the outcome of recovery-oriented mental health care, it is imperative to expand the supply of effective, evidence-based services throughout the Nation" (U.S. Department Health and Human Services, 1999).

Any episode of illness may involve lasting change in a person's level of functioning. A person who has been seriously ill is more likely to have problems living productively in the community. Hospitalization is especially disruptive, and it is often difficult to adjust after discharge. Nurses must be aware of the total range of patient care needs both during and after hospitalization.

The goal of tertiary prevention is to reduce the rate of maladaptive functioning related to mental disorders in a community. Although concepts of tertiary prevention can be applied to anyone who has experienced an episode of illness, they are particularly relevant to those with serious and persistent mental illnesses, sometimes called chronic mental illness. Because of the stigma associated with the term **chronic**, the term **serious mental illness** is used in this chapter.

It is estimated that 5.4% of adults in the United States have a serious mental illness. Nurses care for these people in a variety of settings: private and public psychiatric hospitals, psychiatric and medical-surgical units in general hospitals, emergency rooms, community-based treatment and rehabilitation programs, and patients' homes. As patients alternate between community-based and hospital-based care, nurses in all settings share responsibility for their care. Knowledge of the special needs and characteristics of this population is important for all nurses.

REHABILITATION

Tertiary prevention is carried out through activities identified as rehabilitation. This is the process of helping the person return to the highest possible level of functioning. Psychosocial rehabilitation is the range of social, educational, occupational, behavioral, and cognitive interventions for increasing the role performance of persons with serious and persistent mental illness and enhancing their recovery (Barton, 1999).

Psychiatric rehabilitation grew out of a need to create opportunities for people diagnosed with severe mental illness to live, learn, and work in their own communities. It proposes that mental illness should be perceived as a disability. Like people with physical disabilities, people with psychiatric disabilities need a wide range of services, often for extended periods of time. Psychiatric rehabilitation uses a person-centered, people-to-people approach that differs from the traditional medical model of care (Table 15-1). It is supported by the following research findings related to people with long-term mental illness (Palmer-Erbs & Anthony, 1995):

- They can function in the community with minimal use of inpatient services.
- They can be helped to function more successfully in the community with interventions to enhance skills and support.
- Measures of skills and support, more than psychiatric diagnoses and symptom patterns, determine how well they function in the community.
- Improved functioning in one area of a person's life does not indicate that the other life areas have been similarly improved.
- Interventions to develop skills and supports may take time to have an effect on their functioning in the community.
- Their typical prognosis may not be increasing deterioration between episodes, but rather stable functioning between episodes and often gradual improvement over the long term.

Principles of psychosocial rehabilitation are listed in Box 15-1.

Compare the principles of psychiatric rehabilitation with your knowledge of physical rehabilitation. How do the principles affect nursing intervention?

Rehabilitative psychiatric nursing must be studied in the contexts of the patient and social system. This requires the nurse to focus on three elements: the individual, the family, and the community. The nursing care of people with serious mental illnesses is related to these three elements and the activities of assessment, intervention, and evaluation.

ASSESSMENT
The Individual

Assessment of the need for rehabilitation begins with the initial contact between the nurse and the patient. A comprehensive psychiatric nursing assessment, as described in Chapters 6 to 8, provides information that enables the nurse to help the patient achieve maximum possible functioning. Behavioral rating scales related to general psychiatric care are presented in Box 15-2. In addition to identifying deficits, nurses are expected to identify and reinforce strengths as one means of helping the patient to cope. This is basic to the concept of rehabilitation. Thus good nursing care is really rehabilitative nursing care.

The Stuart Stress Adaptation Model (Fig. 15-1) can be applied within the context of rehabilitative nursing practice. It is important for the nurse to identify stressors that may interfere with the patient's adjustment to a health-promoting lifestyle. Nurses need to be aware of patients' perceptions of

Box **15-1**

Principles of Psychosocial Rehabilitation

- Believe in the recovery process from psychiatric disability
- Engender hope and the possibility of change
- Maintain a person-centered focus that promotes individual choices and empowerment
- Facilitate collaborative consumer/family participation in developing rehabilitation goals and plans
- Use holistic assessment of physical, emotional, intellectual, social, and spiritual dimensions
- Develop educational opportunities that build life skills and knowledge to maximize independence in life roles and daily functioning
- Build and strengthen community and social support systems that consumers learn to access easily
- Educate health-care providers, legislators, and the public about psychiatric disabilities to reduce stigma and foster understanding

From Palmer-Erbs V et al: Nursing perspectives on disability and rehabilitation. In Anchor K, editor: *Disability analysis handbook,* Dubuque, Iowa, 1996, Kendall/Hunt Publishing Co.

Table **15-1**

Comparison of Psychiatric Rehabilitation and Traditional Medical Models of Care

Aspect of Care	Psychiatric Rehabilitation	Traditional Medical Rehabilitation
Focus	Focus on wellness and health, not symptoms	Focus on disease, illness, and symptoms
Basis	Based on person's abilities and functional behavior	Based on person's disabilities and intrapsychic functioning
Setting	Caregiving in natural settings	Treatment in institutional settings
Relationship	Adult-to-adult relationship	Expert-to-patient relationship
Medication	Medicate as appropriate and tolerate some illness symptoms	Medicate until symptoms are controlled
Decision making	Case management in partnership with patient	Physician makes decisions and prescribes treatment
Emphasis	Emphasis on strengths, self-help, and interdependence	Emphasis on dependence and compliance

Box **15-2**

Behavioral Rating Scales Related to General Psychiatric Care

- Acculturation Scale
- Assessing Coping Strategies (COPE)
- Acuity of Psychiatric Illness, Adult Version
- Behavior and Symptom Identification Scale (BASIS-32)
- Behavior Rating Scale
- Brief Psychiatric Rating Scale (BPRS)
- Brief Symptom Inventory (BSI)
- Brown Assessment of Beliefs Scale
- Clinical Global Impression (CGI)
- Colorado Client Assessment Record (CCAR)
- Columbia Impairment Scale (CIS)
- Community-Oriented Programs Environmental Scale (COPES)
- Compass Treatment Assessment System
- Conners' Adult ADHD Rating Scales (CAARS)
- Derogatis Psychiatric Rating Scale (DPRS)
- Employee Assistance Program Index
- Functional Assessment Rating Scale (FARS)
- Functional Status Questionnaire (FSQ)
- Goal Attainment Scale
- Global Assessment Scale (GAS)
- Global Assessment of Functioning Scale (GAF)
- Independent and Living Skills
- Menninger Revision of Role Functioning Scale
- Million Clinical Multiaxial Inventory III (MCMI-III)
- Multnomah Community Ability Scale
- Neuropsychological Impairment Scale (NIS)
- Nurse Observation Scale for Inpatient Evaluation (NOSIE)
- Personal Adjustment and Role Skills (PARS)
- Personal Problem Scale (PPS) and Personal Functioning Index (PFI)
- Profile of Adaptation to Life (PAL Scale)
- Profile of Mood States
- PsychSentinel 3.2
- Quality of Life Interview (QOLI)
- Quality of Life Inventory (QOLI)
- Quality of Well-Being Scale (QWB)
- Role Functioning Scale
- Self-Perception Profile for Adults
- Sheehan Disability Scale
- Social Adjustment Scale II
- Social Readjustment Scale
- Social Behavior Schedule
- Social Functioning Scale
- Stress Response Scale (SRS)
- Structured Clinical Interview for the DSM-IV
- Symptom Checklist-90 (SCL-90)
- Treatment Events Checklist (TEC)
- Treatment Outcome Package (TOP)
- Treatment Outcome Profile
- Young Adult Behavior Checklist
- Young Adult Self-Report (YASR)

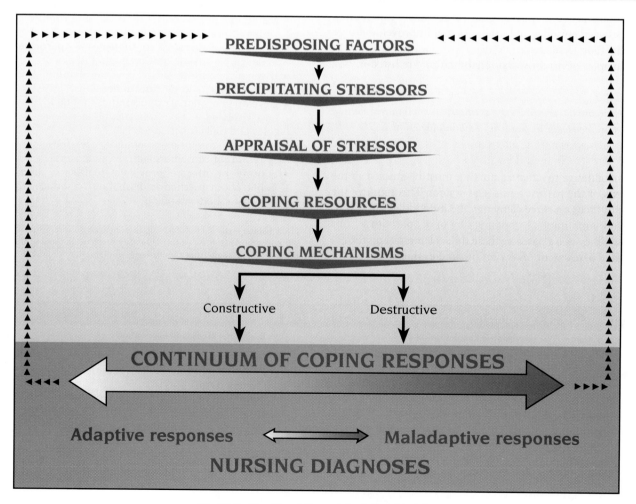

Fig. 15-1 The Stuart Stress Adaptation Model.

their experiences. It is also essential to validate each person's response to significant life changes.

When conducting an initial assessment the nurse needs to think beyond the limits of the patient care setting and try to anticipate the patient's other contacts with the health-care system. In hospitals this process is provided through discharge planning. Nurses in community settings should also expect patients to progress to other levels of care. Although some people will need long-term outpatient care, others will be discharged from psychiatric care.

Characteristics of Serious Mental Illness.

People who have serious mental illnesses are likely to have both primary and secondary symptoms. **Primary symptoms** are directly caused by the illness. For example, hallucinations and delusions are primary symptoms of schizophrenia, and elation and hyperactivity are primary symptoms of bipolar disorder. **Secondary symptoms** such as loneliness and social isolation are caused by the person's response to the illness or its treatment.

Behaviors related to primary symptoms may violate social norms and be considered deviant. Society then tries to protect itself from the person's norm violation. An example of this is community opposition to the establishment of group homes. As behavior problems become more serious, people increasingly identify themselves as mentally ill. They begin to relate to society in terms of this identity rather than others, such as wife, mother, husband, father, or worker.

The person's acceptance of mentally ill status and adjustment to society in terms of this role are accompanied by the secondary symptoms of serious mental illness. A nursing study of the perceptions of people with serious mental illness identified the following themes related to secondary symptoms (Vellenga & Christenson, 1994):

- **Stigmatization**, or the sense of being discredited or shamed because of their illness
- **Alienation** caused by the outcome of being stigmatized and ostracized
- **Loss** of relationships and vocational opportunities
- **Distress** caused by the effects of the illness and one's related suffering
- **Acceptance** of oneself as having a mental illness and the need for acceptance by others

Behaviors Related to Serious Mental Illness.

People with serious mental illnesses are generally unemployed, less educated, less likely to be involved in close relationships, and more likely to live in poverty than their peers. The exact causes of these characteristics have not been identified. Some could be related to primary and secondary symptoms or disabilities of the illness and others to society's reaction to the person with mental illness. Attitudes that could contribute to this reaction are illustrated by the list of myths about people with mental illness compiled by the National Institutes of Mental Health (Table 15-2). None of these myths is true, but they are commonly believed and stigmatize people with mental illness. This often prevents people with mental illness from gaining access to needed services and opportunities.

> ❓ *Copy the list of myths about mental illness and discuss them with a group of people who have little personal experience with mental illness. Then discuss the list with a small group of people who have a serious mental illness. Compare the responses of the two groups.*

Activities of daily living.

Activities of daily living (ADL) are the skills that are necessary to live independently, such as housekeeping, shopping, food preparation, money management, and personal hygiene. A major goal of psychosocial rehabilitation is to help the person to develop independent living skills.

Interpersonal relations.

People who have serious mental illnesses are often described as apathetic, withdrawn, and socially isolated. Previously, it was assumed that relationship problems were a result of prolonged institutional life, which did not encourage close friendships. As more is learned about the nature of neurobiological disorders, it is becoming apparent that these difficulties are more closely related to the primary symptoms of the illness (see Citing the Evidence below). For instance, depression causes apathy and withdrawal and schizophrenia leads to problems in perceiving and processing communications from others. These behaviors create serious problems in establishing close relationships.

Citing the Evidence on

Interpersonal Relationships and the Seriously Mentally Ill

BACKGROUND: Women with severe mental illness were surveyed to explore issues in living with mental illness, personal relationships, and professional relationships and health care. The women's responses were compared to a survey of men to see if the issues affected women and men similarly.

RESULTS: A larger proportion of women than men cited personal relationships as their most formative experiences, while men identified mental illness as the most influential factor. Most women reported normal concerns rather than illness-related ones, and most were relatively satisfied with their lives. Women reported both more and better quality personal relationships than men, including those with their providers. About one quarter to one third of women reported not receiving proper care for birth control and menopause and not receiving pelvic or breast examinations.

IMPLICATIONS: The survey results suggest that personal relationships are central in women's lives, that women with severe mental illness do not see their illness as the main features of their identities, and that women's experience of living with severe mental illness is considerably different from that of men.

Ritsher E et al: A survey on issues in the lives of women with severe mental illness, *Psychiatr Serv* 48:1273, 1997.

Table **15-2**

Myths and Facts about People with Mental Illness	
Myths	Facts
A person who has been mentally ill can never be normal	Mental illness is often temporary or episodic. Former mentally ill patients deserve to be judged on their own merits.
Even if some mentally ill people return to normal, chronically mentally ill people remain different—in fact, crazy.	Many people who have chronic mental illnesses have been hospitalized for a long time. After discharge, they must continue to take medication. The combination of the illness and medication side effects may cause them to look or act strange, but the longer they are in the community, the more they look like everyone else.
If people who recover from other illnesses can cope on their own, recovered mental patients should be able to do so, too.	Most people who have been through a disabling illness, mental or physical, need rehabilitation. For mentally ill people this is focused on social support.
People with mental illness are unpredictable.	Although some mentally ill people are impulsive and unpredictable when they are actively ill, most are consistent in their behavior when recovered.
Those with schizophrenia or other severe mental disorders must be really crazy.	With appropriate treatment, people who have severe mental disorders tend to be calm and reliable.
Mentally ill people are dangerous.	Patients who have come through mental illness and have returned to the community are more apt to be anxious, timid, and passive. They rarely present a danger to the public.
Recovered mentally ill patients are surely potentially dangerous. They could go berserk at any time.	Most people who are mentally ill never went "berserk" in the first place. Mentally ill patients are more likely to be depressed and withdrawn than wild and aggressive. Most relapses develop gradually.
Anyone who has had shock treatment must really be sick.	Electroconvulsive therapy (ECT) is an effective treatment for serious depression. There is no reason to assume that someone who has received this therapy is sicker than others.
When you learn a person has been mentally ill, you have learned the most important thing about his or her personality.	Every type of disturbance is different in every patient. A recovered patient needs to be viewed as an individual rather than as an anonymous member of a stereotyped group.
You can't talk to someone who has been mentally ill.	Most recovered people who have had mental illnesses are rational and intelligent. Even people with current illnesses are likely to be rational in many ways.
If a former mentally ill patient has a really bad history, there isn't much hope.	Some people may be ill for many years before they receive effective treatment or their condition improves for other reasons. Once recovered, they may remain well for the rest of their lives.
A former mentally ill patient is bound to make a second-rate employee.	Many recovered patients make excellent employees. Some people who are subject to relapses may need to work in a flexible situation.
Perhaps recovered mentally ill patients can work successfully at low-level jobs, but they aren't suited for really important or responsible positions.	The career potentials of recovered mentally ill patients, as with anyone else, depend on the person's talents, abilities, experience, motivation, and health status.
Recovered mentally ill patients have a tough row to hoe, but there's not much that can be done about it.	The way we act toward former mentally ill patients can make all the difference.

From the National Institutes of Mental Health: *The 14 worst myths about recovered mental patients*, DHHS Pub No (ADM) 88-1391, Washington, DC, 1988, DHHS.

Nonetheless, formal and informal networks are needed by the seriously mentally ill (Pickens, 1999).

Low self-esteem. Self-esteem is the feeling of self-worth or regard for oneself. It is difficult to maintain high self-esteem when a person is aware of low achievement compared to cultural expectations. Lack of ability to maintain employment, live independently, marry, and have children contributes to low self-esteem. People who have serious mental illnesses often feel cheated of the life experiences they expected to enjoy before they became ill. They feel inadequate, especially if they believe that their illness is the result of a personality flaw rather than a biological disorder.

One mental health professional who also has a serious mental illness describes her experience of being diagnosed with schizophrenia during adolescence (Deegan, 1993):

I was told I had a disease that was like diabetes, and if I continued to take neuroleptic medications for the rest of my life and avoided stress, I might be able to cope. I remember that as these words were spoken to me by my psychiatrist it felt as if my whole teenage world—in which I aspired to dreams of being a valued person in valued roles, of playing lacrosse for the U.S. Women's Team or maybe joining the Peace Corps—began to crumble and shatter. It felt as if these parts of my identity were being stripped from me. I was beginning to undergo that radically dehumanizing and devaluing transformation from being a person to being an illness; from being Pat Deegan to being a schizophrenic.

Motivation. For many people with serious mental illness, success and greater competence result in increased anxiety, causing regression, rather than in pride and continued progress. Patients attribute their uneasiness with success to fear that it will lead to higher expectations by others that they may not be able to attain. Fear of failure often results in reluctance to try new experiences. This may be perceived by others as lack of motivation. Apparent lack of motivation may also be caused by low energy. This can be related to the biological effect of the illness or to medication. In this case the person may want to be more active but is physically unable.

Strengths. Rehabilitation depends on the control of illness, as well as on the development of health potential by mobilizing strengths. A strength is an ability, skill, or interest that a person has used before. An emphasis on strengths provides hope that improved functioning is possible. Strengths may be related to recreational and leisure activities, work skills, educational accomplishments, self-care skills, special interests, talents and abilities, and positive interpersonal relationships. People with serious mental illness often need help in defining their skills, abilities, and interests as strengths. Low self-esteem may lead them to believe that they have only problems, not strengths.

Nonadherence. Lack of adherence to prescribed treatment is often cited as a behavior of people who have serious mental illnesses. Some states have attempted to ensure that people with mental illness comply with treatment by enacting involuntary outpatient commitment laws. The individual is brought before a court and ordered to comply with treatment. If he does not comply, the person may be subject to involuntary hospitalization. Critics of these laws say that the real problem is a lack of adequate and acceptable community services for people who have serious mental illness. The issue of outpatient commitment is discussed in Chapter 10.

Failure to take medication is a common cause of rehospitalization (see Citing the Evidence). It is important to assess the reasons for nonadherence. There may be a denial of the illness or a lack of understanding of the reason for the treatment regimen. Sometimes the person wants to comply but needs help such as transportation to a pharmacy or advice about obtaining a medical assistance card. Some patients do not like the side effects of their medication. They may not be assertive enough to tell the prescriber about their discomfort. The nurse can help patients by rehearsing what to say before the appointment or accompanying them to provide support. Teaching patients to write notes about care providers' instructions and to keep lists of questions for the provider may also increase adherence.

Living Skills Assessment. The nursing assessment of a patient who has a serious mental illness should include an analysis of the person's community living skills. Some of the rating scales presented in Box 15-2 are specifically related to

Citing the Evidence on

Medication Compliance and Rehabilitation

BACKGROUND: Noncompliance with psychotropic medications is a primary reason for inpatient hospitalization. A 6-month study compared the effectiveness of treatment modalities in persons with schizophrenia. The patients were divided into a clubhouse group or traditional group and then subgrouped based on their taking of oral or depot medications.

RESULTS: The clubhouse patients had fewer inpatient hospital days than patients in the traditional group. Patients on oral psychotropic medications were more compliant than those on injectable neuroleptics if they attended the clubhouse program.

IMPLICATIONS: This study suggests that the clubhouse atmosphere might "normalize" the routine of taking psychotropic medications and enhance compliance. The supportive, vocational, and educational functions of clubhouses appear to improve the quality of life and functioning of patients.

Delaney C: Reducing recidivism: medication versus psychosocial rehabilitation, *J Psychosoc Nurs* 36(11):28, 1998.

cognitive functioning and activities of daily living. Table 15-3 presents a matrix of the skills required for successful functioning in the community. It lists the physical, emotional, and intellectual components of the skills needed for living, learning, and working. The nurse may use these examples in working with the patient to identify strengths, establish goals, and set priorities for skill development. Such a model provides a rational basis for assessing the patient's readiness to function productively in the community. It also provides objective information on quality of life that can be shared with other mental health-care providers (Skinner et al, 1999).

The Family

The image of isolated people with serious mental illness who return to a community where they have no connections has been widely publicized. However, most people with mental illness are involved with their families and have frequent contact with family members while they are in the community. Approximately 65% of people who have mental illnesses live with their families. Therefore family resources must be assessed when a rehabilitation plan is being developed.

A survey of families of people with mental illness found that professionals did not actively involve caregivers in the treatment of their family member with mental illness, and caregivers ranked more communication with professionals as their greatest need (Biegel et al, 1995). Although issues of confidentiality and respect for the patient's wishes regarding disclosure of treatment information must always be primary,

Table **15-3**

Potential Skilled Activities Needed to Achieve the Goal of Psychiatric Rehabilitation		
Physical	**Emotional**	**Intellectual**
LIVING SKILLS		
Personal hygiene	Human relations	Money management
Physical fitness	Self-control	Use of community resources
Use of public transportation	Selective reward	Goal setting
Cooking	Stigma reduction	Problem development
Shopping	Problem solving	
Cleaning	Conversational skills	
Sports participation		
Using recreational facilities		
LEARNING SKILLS		
Being quiet	Speech making	Reading
Paying attention	Question asking	Writing
Staying seated	Volunteering answers	Arithmetic
Observing	Following directions	Study skills
Punctuality	Asking for directions	Hobby activities
	Listening	Typing
WORKING SKILLS		
Punctuality	Job interviewing	Job qualifying
Use of job tools	Job decision making	Job seeking
Job strength	Human relations	Specific job tasks
Job transportation	Self-control	
Specific job tasks	Job keeping	
	Specific job tasks	

From Anthony WA: *Principles of psychiatric rehabilitation*, Baltimore, 1980, University Park Press.

nurses should strive as much as possible to include family members as partners in the treatment process. Family members can help by identifying potential problem areas and enhancing the patient's compliance with the treatment plan.

Incorporating the family in the continuum of care is the focus of Chapter 16. Family interventions are discussed in Chapter 34.

Components of Family Assessment. The nurse who assesses the family as part of a rehabilitation plan should include the following areas:

- Family structure, including developmental stage, roles, responsibilities, norms, and values
- Family attitudes toward the mentally ill member
- The emotional climate of the family (fearful, angry, depressed, anxious, calm)
- The social supports that are available to the family, including extended family, friends, financial support, religious involvement, and community contacts
- Past family experiences with mental health services
- The family's understanding of the patient's problem and the plan of care

Some of this information may be obtained from the social worker. However, it is the nurse's responsibility to be available to the family. This includes regular planned contacts with the family and inclusion of the family as part of the treatment team.

Family Burden. The mental illness of a family member affects the entire family (Saunders, 1999). This impact is of-

ten called family burden. A survey was conducted of behaviors that family members found most disturbing, broken out by diagnosis. The most disturbing behaviors associated with schizophrenia were poor grooming and personal care, suspiciousness, and talking to oneself. For bipolar illness the most disturbing behaviors were lack of consideration of others, excessive arguing, upsetting neighbors and friends, unusual religious beliefs, and inappropriate sexual behavior. Depressed people had more problematic eating and sleeping behaviors and suicide attempts. It is also important to note that on nine other behaviors, such as lack of motivation, poor handling of money, difficulty in completing tasks, and noncompliance with medication, there were no differences among diagnostic groups (Hatfield et al, 1994).

Mental illness can have a negative impact on the rest of the family as well. Problems identified by family members include the following (Doornbos, 1997):

- Increased family stress and conflict
- Members blaming each other for the illness
- Difficulty understanding or accepting the illness
- Tension during family gatherings
- Disproportionate amount of family time, energy, or money given to the ill member

Burden may be objective or subjective. Objective burden is related to the patient's behavior, role performance, adverse effects on the family, need for support, and financial costs of the illness. Subjective burden is the person's own feeling of being burdened; it is individual and not consistently related to the elements of objective burden. For instance, a patient may lack ambition and remain in a dependent role well into adulthood. Family members who value success and upward mobility would be likely to feel more subjective burden related to this situation than members who are comfortable with nurturing and supporting someone.

By assessing family burden the nurse can work with the family to identify concerns with which they would like help. Several responses are frequently noted in families who have members with serious mental illness. It is helpful to consider these when assessing subjective burden.

Grief is common and is related to the loss of the person they knew before the illness, as well as loss of the future that they expected to share with the ill family member. Because serious mental illness is usually cyclical, grief tends to be recurrent; it subsides during remissions and returns during exacerbations. This is especially difficult for families to handle. In addition, social support systems may not recognize or respond to their need because of discomfort with the situation or the related stigma.

Family members may feel guilty about their relative's illness. It is also common for those who are close to a person with any serious illness to wonder whether they could have done something to prevent it. For instance, the wife of a heart attack victim may think she could have prevented it if she had not encouraged him to shovel snow. Similarly, parents of a depressed woman may believe that they could have prevented her depression if they had not shared their own worries with her. In neither of these situations did relatives cause the illnesses, but they feel guilt because of their interpretation of the situation. Another source of guilt for relatives of people with mental illness is the need to set limits on the patient's behavior at times. For instance, the family of a patient who is physically abusive may need to arrange involuntary hospitalization if the patient becomes dangerous. In these situations, grief therapy for relatives of persons with serious mental illness may be a helpful intervention (Miller, 1996).

Anger may be directed toward the patient, but it is more often felt toward other family members, mental health care providers, or the entire system. Anger within the family relates to differing perceptions of the patient and varied ideas about how to manage the illness. Prolonged stress results in irritability that is often taken out on those to whom one is closest. Anger at the system often is justified because it is related to deficiencies in the accessibility or acceptability of services.

Powerlessness and fear often result from families' realization that they are dealing with a long-term recurrent illness. Most people believe that the health-care system should cure illnesses. When this is impossible, they feel powerless and frustrated. This understanding can also result in fear about the future of the ill family member and for themselves. Powerlessness and fear are especially troublesome for parents who are aging and worried about care arrangements for their mentally ill child when they can no longer provide care. Some families also fear ill members who may be dangerous because of the symptoms of the illness.

Social Support Needs. Families who are providing care for members who have serious mental illnesses often feel iso-

---

Citing the Evidence on

Services to Families of the Seriously Mentally Ill

BACKGROUND: A survey of state mental health programs was conducted to determine the extent to which states are facilitating the delivery of services to families with severe and persistent mental illness.

RESULTS: Of the 44 responding states, 73% did not have a policy about the types of services delivered to families, but 80% reported that they funded family support intervention. The majority of these were family-to-family programs such as those sponsored by NAMI.

IMPLICATIONS: This study draws attention to the gap in services by mental health professionals and underscores the importance of the advocacy movement in obtaining funding and support for services to families.

Dixon L et al: State policy and funding of services to families of adults with serious and persistent mental illness, *Psychiatr Serv* 50(4):551, 1999.

---

lated and alone in dealing with the challenges of caregiving. Previous sources of social support may be lost or limited because of the demands of attending to the mentally ill family member. Caregivers may be embarrassed about the illness or fear that the person with mental illness will behave inappropriately in the presence of others. Sometimes a family member may decide to stop working to be available at home. All of the aspects of the subjective burden of the illness may also limit access to social support systems. These families will need assistance in rebuilding their social supports (see Citing the Evidence on Services to Families of the Seriously Mentally Ill).

Support may also be found within the family. Even though a mental illness can be stressful for all family members, many families meet this challenge with a great deal of resilience. The person who has the mental illness can contribute to the family, helping to ease the stress on other members. Persons with serious mental illness can contribute to the family in the following ways (Hamera et al, 1998):

- Helping with household tasks
- Showing concern and support for other family members and expressing gratitude for their help
- Sharing positive personal characteristics, such as a sense of humor
- Contributing to family solidarity
- Caring for self by such activities as taking medication or following the treatment plan
- Giving peace of mind by communicating how one is feeling

Nurses can play an important role in offering family members opportunities to discuss their concerns and taking action to meet their needs whenever possible. Table 15-4 lists support needs expressed by family caregivers.

Table **15-4**

Support Needs Expressed by Family Caregivers	
EMOTIONAL SUPPORT	
Acceptance	Absence of stigmatization; acceptance of the caregiver despite his or her relationship to a mentally ill patient
Commitment	Demonstrating to the caregiver a commitment to the well-being of the patient, or sharing the burden of caregiving, if only through contact with the caregiver
Social involvement	Social contacts and companionship for the caregiver
Affective	Showing love and caring for the caregiver, including concern for his or her well-being (with qualities of sympathy, compassion, and occasionally true empathy)
Mutuality	Reciprocity in supportive exchanges
FEEDBACK SUPPORT	
Affirmation	Validation of the actions, feelings, and decisions associated with the caregiving role
Listening	Active listening by the support person, provision of a sounding board, and allowing for unburdening by the caregiver
Talking	The opportunity to talk with another person (without the quality of active listening, emotional presence, or the feeling of unburdening)
INFORMATIONAL OR COGNITIVE SUPPORT	
Illness information	Information about the patient's illness, care, or supervision
Behavior management	Information about behavior management strategies
Coping	Advice about personal coping strategies for the caregiver
Decision	Help in the decision-making process around caregiving issues and offering solutions
Perspective	Supportive interactions that give the caregiver a new perspective about caregiving or about the caregiving situation
INSTRUMENTAL SUPPORT	
Resources	Help in locating resources, negotiating systems, or advocating for needs
Respite	Provision of time off for the caregiver and support for the caregiver's own needs
Care help	Provision of help with the actual tasks of caregiving, including physical care assistance and monitoring activities (watching the patient and setting limits)
Backup	Help is available when needed, including financial help
Household	Help with such home activities as repairs, grocery shopping, and housecleaning

From Norbeck J et al: Social support needs of family caregivers of psychiatric patients from three age groups, *Nurs Res* 40:208, 1991.

❓ You are approached by the parent of a hospitalized young adult patient who has a serious mental illness. The family is upset because the discharge plan is to refer the patient to a community program that has not been helpful in the past. What nursing interventions would you suggest in this case?

The Community

The community greatly influences rehabilitation of its mentally ill members. Mental health professionals have a unique role in the community because they are community members and advocates for people with mental illness and their families at the same time. Care providers, including nurses, should assume a leadership role in assessing the adequacy and effectiveness of community resources and in recommending changes.

Nurses in all settings must be familiar with the community agencies that provide services to people with mental illnesses. Most communities have a social and medical services directory that can be consulted for basic information such as location, type, and cost of the services provided. Most agencies serve people who come from a particular geographical area such as one part of a city or, in a rural area, one or several counties. As nurses gain experience, they will become familiar with other agencies that provide services for the same people. Nurses should pay attention to patients' evaluations of the agencies from which they receive services. This information helps to identify agencies that are responsive and helpful as opposed to those that are difficult for patients to approach.

Personal contact with community agencies can be very useful as part of a community assessment. This may be done by making an appointment with an agency staff member. However, a more realistic picture of an agency's services can be obtained by going to the agency with someone who is requesting services. The nurse will see how the agency responds to the patient and how the patient handles personal affairs in the community. The nurse can also provide emotional support if the patient is insecure in a new situation. Nurses should introduce themselves to the staff of the agency and explain that they, as well as the patient, would like to learn more about the services. Collaborative relationships between mental health-care providers and community agencies are essential if rehabilitation is to succeed.

A wide range of community services must be available to patients. Those that are directed toward basic needs include provisions for shelter, food, and clothing; household management; income and financial support; meaningful activities; and mobility and transportation. Other services provide for special needs that may differ from one person to the next, such as general medical services, mental health services, habilitation and rehabilitation programs, vocational services, and social services. A third group of services coordinates the system. These include patient identification and outreach, individual assessment and service planning, case management, advocacy and community organization, community information, and education and support.

PLANNING AND IMPLEMENTATION

The Individual

Treatment planning and intervention in rehabilitative psychiatric nursing focus on fostering independence by maximizing the person's strengths. This is directly parallel to the nurse's role in physical rehabilitation. It differs from nursing care that is given to patients when they are acutely ill. During acute illness, people require nurturing. The nurse must provide for all of the basic life functions that the person is unable to manage. However, the relationship becomes less dependent as patients grow stronger and are able to care for themselves. Residual functional deficits may remain. The nurse and patient must work together to find ways for the patient to overcome any remaining impaired areas of functioning.

Three basic interventions are used in psychiatric rehabilitation to help people:

- Develop their strengths and potential
- Learn living skills
- Access environmental supports

The nursing treatment plan should be organized around very specific behavioral goals that are based on a comprehensive assessment of the person's living skills. These goals should build on those that are developed during the acute phase of the illness. This part of the nursing care plan may be called the discharge plan in an inpatient treatment setting. Discharge plans should also be developed in community settings. This will remind the nurse and patient that the expected outcome of nursing care is independent functioning. Even patients who need long-term medication can usually receive maintenance prescriptions from their family physician as part of their general health care program. This helps to put the mental illness into perspective as a chronic health problem that is not so different from other chronic problems the person might have.

The nurse and patient must decide together on the desired level of functioning. If the patient is unwilling to take on activities that the nurse thinks would be helpful, it is important to discover why. Sometimes nurses try to push a patient ahead too rapidly. Behavior that has developed gradually over time cannot be changed quickly. Learning new behavior patterns and giving up old ones is frightening and causes anxiety. The nurse must be sure that the patient's coping skills are adequate to deal with the stress of growth. Feedback must be requested to be sure that the rehabilitation plan continues to address the patient's needs. Sometimes the plan assumes greater importance than the patient. The nurse must prevent this from happening.

Developing Strengths and Potentials. The development of the patient's strengths and potentials is important. Nursing interventions that develop strengths and potentials can help patients develop independent living skills, interpersonal relationships, and coping resources and thus help meet their special needs. Ultimately, the expected outcome of such interventions is change in the patient's self-concept and an increase in self-esteem, as described in Chapter 19. The negative self-concept and low self-esteem that characterize people who have serious mental illnesses interfere with their ability to see themselves as individuals with strengths and potentials.

Through experiences of adequacy, self-concept can be altered and self-esteem increased. One intervention that helps patients alter their negative self-perceptions is for nurses to describe their perception of patients' strengths. Nursing interventions in which patients become aware of their strengths fall into two categories: those that occur spontaneously and those that are planned. The following clinical example illustrates a nurse's use of spontaneously occurring situations to increase awareness of strengths.

 ## CLINICAL EXAMPLE

Theresa, a woman in her fifties, had been in and out of psychiatric hospitals for 30 years and had been living in a supervised apartment in the community for 1 year. Theresa shared the apartment with two roommates. She was a talented musician and had her own baby grand piano. Despite her love for classical music, she played only the "oldies and goodies" her roommates preferred. She said that she didn't want to upset her roommates by practicing classical music. She was afraid that if she brought the issue out in the open she might get so upset she would hurt someone. She offered as evidence the numerous times she'd been placed in seclusion rooms for violent behavior. Clearly, keeping peace was her priority.

The nurse and Theresa discussed her strengths as a peacemaker, as well as ways in which she might calmly express her own needs to her roommates. The nurse offered to be with Theresa during the discussion. Declining the nurse's offer, Theresa said that even though she was somewhat anxious, she had a clearer understanding of the abilities she had to use in the situation, and she wanted to try to "pick up" for herself in a situation of interpersonal conflict. She carried out her plan and expressed surprise that her roommates accepted her need and quickly arranged 2 hours a day for her to practice. As she told of her success, Theresa smiled, saying she wondered what would have happened if she had tried expressing her needs many months earlier.

Cindy, in her early twenties, had recently moved into the supervised apartment with Theresa and one other roommate. Cindy arrived at the day treatment program crying because she had fainted while at her nursing home job the evening before. She felt that in addition to having been embarrassed, she had failed to live up to the trust invested in her by the director of the nursing home. She had decided to quit her job.

The nurse explored with Cindy the meaning of these events in terms of her many strengths in caring for others. Her sensitivity to anticipated criticism and rejection from the director was related to the same sensitivity that allowed her to respond creatively to others' needs. At this point, Cindy firmly stated that the job was important to her sense of being needed. The nurse encouraged her to call the nursing home, express both her embarrassment and sense of failure, yet state that she wanted to continue working there. Cindy made the phone call with the nurse present for support. Her pleasure at finding out the job was still hers, that she was not viewed unfavorably by the director of nursing, and her sense of personal achievement at having taken a risk and won were so visible and contagious that the other patients staged an impromptu celebration.

Selected Nursing Diagnoses

- Theresa: Impaired social interaction related to fear of aggressive impulses, as evidenced by social inhibition
- Cindy: Chronic low self-esteem related to fear of rejection, as evidenced by feelings of inadequacy

Learning Living Skills. Social skills training uses cognitive and behavioral techniques, as described in Chapter 32, to help people gain the knowledge and skills they need to live in the community. The patient is taught a structured way of examining and modifying his or her own thoughts and behavior that can be continued with decreasing clinician involvement as the patient becomes more skillful at managing difficult situations. These include holding conversations, establishing and maintaining friendships, dating, managing medications, grooming, and the numerous other activities listed in Table 15-5. Social skills training programs typically use videotapes, role-playing, practice, and homework assignments centered around practical problems. They are an evidence-based psychiatric rehabilitation intervention.

Another important aspect of psychiatric rehabilitation relates to promoting the physical well-being of those with serious mental illness. Problems such as high tobacco use, low exercise level, poor oral health, high-risk sexual behavior, and limited contact with physicians and dentists are common among the seriously mentally ill. Thus psychiatric nurses need to intervene in a holistic way in all health-care settings with patients who experience serious and long-term psychiatric illness.

Psychoeducation is an approach that supports the rehabilitation process by teaching the patient and family about the mental illness and the coping skills that will help with successful community living. Psychoeducation is defined as the process of imparting illness management information in a way that maximizes the receptivity and capability of the individual for appropriate illness management (Bauer & McBride, 1997). The increased use of educational approaches to treatment is related to the increased focus on prevention and outpatient intervention, as well as to the ris-

---

Box 15-3

Elements of a Psychoeducation Plan

- Signs and symptoms
- Natural course of the illness
- Possible etiologies
- Diagnostic tests and measures
- Indicated lifestyle changes
- Treatment options
- Expected treatment outcomes
- Medication effects and side effects
- Therapeutic strategies
- Adaptive coping responses
- Potential compliance problems
- Early warning signs of relapse
- Balancing needs and taking care of oneself

Table 15-5

Consumers' Need for Help and Receipt of Help in 17 Areas

Area of Need	Perceived Need (%)	Receiving Help (%)	Want More Help (%)
Keeping busy to avoid getting bored or lonely	51	25	37
Recognizing and controlling symptoms	46	37	35
Finding or getting along with boyfriend, girlfriend, or spouse	53	16	33
Making or getting along with friends	51	19	30
Controlling anger or temper	48	30	27
Getting or keeping a job	61	29	19
Managing money	50	27	19
Housing problems	28	18	19
Maintaining a home	36	18	18
Obtaining Social Security Disability Insurance, Supplemental Security Income, or other benefits	29	20	18
Getting around town	26	14	16
Shopping for groceries, preparing meals	27	14	12
Keeping aftercare appointments	26	15	10
Personal care and grooming	20	7	8
Taking medications	87	88	5

From Uttaro T, Mechanic D: The NAMI consumer survey analysis of unmet needs, *Hosp Community Psychiatry* 45:372, 1994.

ing expectations of managed care organizations. Thus it is important that nurses be able to apply concepts of adult education, cognitive behavioral theory, and empowerment in implementing patient and family education (Blair & Ramones, 1997; Schofield, 1998).

Adult learners require an individualized approach to education that focuses on their self-identified needs and engages them as active participants in the teaching-learning process. Psychoeducational curricula and materials should be individualized based on the characteristics of the learner. Techniques vary but the information conveyed to the patient and family usually covers all aspects of the illness and its treatment, as shown in Box 15-3.

Behaviors related to the mental illness may affect the person's ability to learn. It is particularly important to assess memory and attention span when preparing to implement psychoeducation (Silverstein et al, 1998). Cognitive behavioral interventions such as a token economy approach may then be used to improved impaired functioning in these ar-

eas. This type of intervention is especially helpful for individuals who have a serious mental illness and difficulty learning from a social skills training curriculum.

The interests of the learner should also be considered. Studies have found differences in patient and staff identification of patient learning needs (Pollio et al, 1998; Payson et al, 1998). If staff planned a psychoeducation program based on their ideas about patient needs, it would be likely to be unsuccessful. This would be frustrating for the patients and staff members alike.

Consumers are growing to expect health teaching to be a part of the health-care services they receive. Nurses are well prepared to offer this important intervention to patients, families, and communities. A more general Patient Education Plan for coping with psychiatric illness is presented below.

Accessing Environmental Supports. Supporting people who have serious mental illnesses in community settings requires the development of a wide array of commu-

PATIENT EDUCATION PLAN *Coping with Psychiatric Illness*

CONTENT	INSTRUCTIONAL ACTIVITIES	EVALUATION
Identify and describe common psychiatric diagnoses	Provide handouts outlining behaviors Discuss coping behaviors Assign homework from lay literature Compare mental illness to physical illness	Patient recognizes characteristics of the diagnosis Patient distinguishes between cure and coping
Describe the role of stress in contributing to psychiatric disorders	Sensitize the patient to signs of increased stress Define stress as a test of coping skills Teach relaxation exercises	Patient verbalizes level of stress Patient performs relaxation exercises and describes a reduction in perceived stress
Help to gain a sense of control by recognizing personal pattern of signs and symptoms	Provide feedback when symptomatic behavior occurs Instruct patient to keep a diary of behavior and to identify symptoms	Patient consistently labels symptoms and seeks professional help when necessary
Enhance social and living skills to enable full participation in vocational and recreational activities	Role play social interaction in a variety of situations Review vocational preparation and current level of functioning Assess recreational activities and opportunities for future growth	Patient participates in progressively more rewarding social and work activities
Identify and describe community support systems	Provide a list of community support programs, including self-help groups, mental health-care agencies, and social agencies Invite representatives of programs to speak to patient group Escort to first agency contact	Patient selects community programs that offer needed resources Patient becomes able to access agency independently
Describe and discuss psychoactive medications	Instruct about actions, side effects, and contraindications to common psychoactive medications Distribute handouts describing the patient's medications Suggest systems to help patient remember when to take medication and how much	Patient describes characteristics of prescribed medications Patient reports effects of prescribed medications Patient takes medication as prescribed

nity support programs. Some of these are rehabilitation centers, housing services, employment opportunities, education, crisis intervention and outreach, and case management. When these services are provided, it has been demonstrated that people who would have spent much of their time in the hospital can live successfully in the community.

Rehabilitation programs. Psychiatric rehabilitation programs (also called psychosocial rehabilitation) were developed in response to the plight of people who had been discharged from state mental hospitals lacking the skills and resources needed to live independently. Several models are presented here as an overview of some of the psychiatric rehabilitation approaches that have evidence supporting their effectiveness.

Fountain House. Fountain House, in New York City, was established in the late 1940s by a group of former state mental hospital patients. It began as a consumer-operated program, but a decade later employed a professional staff. Many of the current psychiatric rehabilitation programs are built on the Fountain House (1999) model.

Fountain House functions as a club in which patients are members. The usual hierarchical distinctions between staff (the healthy) and patients (the ill) do not exist. It is a place where members care about each other and pool their resources and abilities as they work toward increasing independence. Thus Fountain House combats loneliness and isolation while providing a variety of living and work situations that require differing levels of functional ability.

The first month at Fountain House is a residential phase, and members are taught skills necessary for apartment living. Fountain House owns and leases apartments that have staff on call, although not in residence. These supervised apartments allow people to make a gradual transition to independent living in the community.

Fountain House runs several businesses, providing a protected environment in which members can develop self-confidence and job skills. Progressing to a more complex work situation, Fountain House has creatively arranged for transitional employment placements (TEPs). Recognizing that job interviews are tremendously stressful, staff, rather than members, seek out and contract with businesses for jobs. The jobs are assigned to Fountain House rather than to individuals. Staff assign a member to a transitional employment position for as long as needed. The employer is promised that if members are unable to manage the job or do not show up, Fountain House staff will work in their place. Fountain House members, who share responsibility for a job with staff, can assume increasing responsibility as they are able to handle it. A TEP can easily be transferred from a member who is ready for a more complex work experience to a member who needs a TEP. Furthermore, employers are satisfied because the quality of work is guaranteed.

Ronald Peterson, a veteran of 10 years of residence in a state hospital, speaks poignantly of the loneliness and isolation he felt when he left the state hospital to live alone in a small hotel room. Because he had no job, knew no one, and lived on welfare, it never occurred to him that things could be any different. He said, "You take what you can get. There is no choice." Eventually becoming a staff member of Fountain House, Peterson (1978) spoke for many people trying to adjust to community living when he described the wish for a place where one belongs and is needed.

I think the greatest need is to have a place to go where you are expected each day, a place where you can be with people like yourself and do things that mean something to yourself and others . . . places to go and be with people who need us to contribute, to take part, to help, and who notice when we're not present and do something about it (Peterson, 1978).

Assertive community treatment (ACT). Assertive community treatment (ACT) programs are based on the Program of Assertive Community Treatment (PACT) that was developed in the 1970s by Stein and Test in Madison, Wisconsin. They are designed to provide intensive community supports to individuals who have serious mental illnesses. The goal is to prevent hospitalization and support the individual in achieving the highest possible level of functioning. A multidisciplinary team is used, including nurses, social workers, case managers, employment counselors, addictions counselors, and a psychiatrist. Some programs also employ peer counselors, people who have mental illnesses. These staff members are often effective in reaching individuals who are reluctant to participate in treatment, such as homeless people, and engaging them in treatment. ACT is characterized by 24-hour, 7-days-a-week staff coverage; comprehensive treatment planning; ongoing responsibility; continuity of staff; and small caseloads. ACT programs are discussed in detail in Chapter 36.

Consumer-run services. Many of the former mental hospital patients (consumers) who founded Fountain House became dissatisfied with the program after it came under the control of professionals and left. There continues to be a strong feeling among some consumers that psychosocial rehabilitation programs are not truly responsive to their needs unless they are consumer controlled. In recent years there has been slow but steady growth of new consumer-run programs in many communities. Some of these are drop-in centers that provide peer support and a safe place to be, whereas others offer a full range of rehabilitative services.

Successful consumer-run programs include specific elements. They should address needs identified by the members, and participation in all or part of the total program should be voluntary. Help is provided either by members or by others whom the member selects. Consumers are responsible for the administrative direction of the program, and they determine criteria for membership. Finally, the program is mainly accountable to the members and strict confidentiality is maintained.

What is your response to the idea that consumers should run alternative treatment programs? Discuss positive and negative implications.

Residential services. Housing is consistently identified as a critical element of successful psychiatric rehabilitation services. Appropriate housing must be safe, affordable, and acceptable to the consumer. Early housing programs tended to focus on existing supervised living situations, such as foster care. There was little oversight of these programs, and exploitation of patients was not uncommon. More recently, an array of housing options has been developed under the leadership of consumers and psychiatric rehabilitation professionals.

Group homes and supervised apartments are the predominant types of housing for people with serious mental illness. Most incorporate some form of rehabilitation program along with housing. Staff supervision ranges from intensive 24-hour awake staffing to telephone consultation, based on the consumer's level of need. Although these programs are a distinct improvement on foster care, there are also drawbacks. Most housing programs focus on providing a "normal" community living experience but fall short of this goal. Supervision needs may lead to organization of housing around levels of care, sometimes requiring consumers to move if their needs become more or less intensive. This can be very disruptive. Consumers rarely have a choice of housemates and they hardly ever lease or own the house in their own names. This type of housing program structure also leads to clustering of group homes or supervised apartments, reinforcing stigmatization and triggering community apprehension (see Critical Thinking about Contemporary Issues).

Some traditional residential programs are evolving into supported housing programs where housing is thought of as a basic service that should mirror the housing choices of others in the community. As such, it is permanent and under the control of the resident. Housing program staff help consumers to find affordable housing of their choice. If people decide to live together it is also their choice. Staff may introduce consumers to each other, but they decide whether to establish a household. Mental health and rehabilitative services are flexible and designed to help the person to live successfully in the community.

Some supported housing programs are part of comprehensive psychiatric rehabilitation programs and are an element of a broader supportive living approach. In this case staff intervention is directed not only at maintaining the person in housing but also at asserting the consumer to become fully involved in community life. A personal future planning process helps the consumer to identify goals, preferences, and the important people who can help in accomplishing these.

Although the supported housing approach works well for some consumers, it is still important to provide a choice of living arrangements. Many patients and families prefer a range of choices from 24-hour supervised group residences to completely independent living (Friedrich et al, 1999; Holley et al, 1998).

Vocational services. Psychiatric rehabilitation programs often provide vocational rehabilitation services. Prevocational training usually begins within the program itself. Members may be organized into work teams around the activities needed to keep the program running, usually clerical, food service, and maintenance tasks. Aside from the devel-

CRITICAL THINKING about CONTEMPORARY ISSUES

Housing the Seriously Mentally Ill—Not In My Neighborhood?

One of the major problems providing residential housing to the seriously mentally ill is the opposition some communities have raised under the cry of "not in my neighborhood." Neighbors often object to proposed group homes or other housing arrangements because of the presumed negative effect it will have on their neighborhood. They cite potential problems of resident safety, declining property values, changes in the residential character of the neighborhood, traffic problems, and noise (Cook, 1997). These concerns lead to neighborhoods residents' opposition to the development of group homes through the use of restrictive local ordinances, bureaucratic obstacles, political pressure on elected officials, and occasional violence.

Neighbors' opposition to group homes has many negative effects. For example, as a result of such protests, group homes are often found in neighborhoods characterized by low socioeconomic status, high crime, low property values, and low voting frequency. Yet despite the opposition, many people are unaware that group homes even exist in their neighborhoods, and it has been noted that resistance tends to diminish over time. In addition, neighbors can and do provide significant support to group homes. Research in this area indicates that potential neighbors of group homes respond well to information, including letters, community meetings, video presentations, or visits to other group homes (Cook, 1998). Nurses can be active in providing community members with opportunities to learn about programs that may be entering their neighborhood and in this way combat the "not in my neighborhood" phenomenon.

opment of marketable work skills, the goal of these programs is to foster good work habits. Some members continue indefinitely in prevocational services. Others may move into temporary employment placements such as those developed at Fountain House. The final stage of vocational rehabilitation is finding competitive employment. Some consumers use vocational services to achieve this goal (Donegan & Palmer-Erbs, 1998). Models of vocational rehabilitation services are presented in Box 15-4.

It has been shown that over a short period of time, targeted vocational programs can help people with severe mental illness develop the skills and attitudes necessary to attain employment or entry into the vocational rehabilitation system (Blankertz & Robinson, 1996). In addition, helping people with severe mental illness obtain competitive jobs that correspond with their explicit job preferences increases their job satisfaction and tenure in the job (Becker et al, 1996).

Although mental health service providers support the idea of vocational rehabilitation, they are reluctant and sometimes actively opposed to hiring consumers to work in mental health settings. If they do, it is often as a janitor, housekeeper, or groundskeeper. Consumers have begun to assert their unique qualifications as counselors and case managers. They

Box **15-4**

Models of Vocational Rehabilitation in Psychiatric Care

SUPPORTED EMPLOYMENT PROGRAMS (SEP)

This model is individualized and provides on-site, one-on-one support, job-coaching services, and occurs in competitive, "real work" settings; job-coach services are gradually faded and removed.

TRANSITIONAL EMPLOYMENT PROGRAMS (TEP)

This model offers a temporary work experience to individuals, having the same supports and services as SEP. They must move on to competitive employment within an agreed-upon length of time. Staff often cover contract positions, working in the job for a day in cases of illness or with changes in participants' schedules.

CLUBHOUSES

Programs are "member directed" with members defined as individuals with serious mental illness. Members have individual daily responsibilities and schedules to fulfill as preparation for entry or re-entry into the world of work. Membership in a clubhouse is lifelong, and members provide each other ongoing support.

JOB CLUBS

There are two main types: in-house clubs and postprogram graduate clubs. In-house clubs provide practical guidance in resume writing, work exploration, opportunities to practice interviewing skills and, in some cases, vocational assessment and interest identification. Postprogram graduate clubs provide essential offsite support services, such as working with new co-workers, adjusting to job requirements, handling issues of stigma, and disclosure and feelings of isolation.

PEER AND NATURAL SUPPORTS

These circles of support are central to the continued success of individuals with serious psychiatric conditions who are attaining and maintaining employment. Circles include wider community links to religious organizations, recreational and activity groups, public libraries, volunteer activities, and peer support activities.

Modified from Donegan K et al: Promoting the importance of work for persons with psychiatric disabilities–the role of the psychiatric nurse, *J Psychosoc Nurs* 36(4):13, 1998.

have been successfully employed in this role and have achieved good outcomes for themselves and those to whom they provide services.

For example, an analysis was conducted on the benefits and limitations of a vocational program called Project WINS (Work Incentives and Needs Study) (Mowbray et al, 1998). This project employed consumers in the role of peer support specialists (PSSs). These staff members were responsible for such duties as helping consumers prepare resumes, open bank accounts, select clothing for interviews, work, or learn the bus system. The PSSs were surveyed on the benefits and problems of the project for them. Benefits to the PSS that were identified included earning money; sat-

isfaction in having a job; skill development; having a work routine; learning interpersonal skills and ways to manage anger and frustration; feeling safe at work; positive attitudes from others; job security; positive feedback; finding a career direction; personal growth; and involvement with other PSSs. Problems for the PSSs included dealing with difficult clients; personal stress related to disappointment with one's performance; lack of understanding about how to do the job; lack of administrative support; having too much responsibility; lack of a career path; and boundary issues. In such programs it is very important to be aware of issues related to role change as experienced by the consumer-employees as well as by other staff in the program, especially if the consumer-employees have been members of the program. If these issues are not identified and discussed openly, they can interfere with the ability of the consumer-employees to be successful.

Educational services. Many people with serious mental illnesses have not completed formal education through high school or beyond because of the effects of the illness. Rehabilitation programs often offer remedial education related to vocational services. Education that is offered in a supportive environment can increase self-esteem, improve job qualifications, and encourage some consumers to pursue higher education.

Review a book intended for mental health consumers. Critique it in terms of accuracy, practical advice, and emotional tone. Ask a consumer or a family member of a consumer to review the book. Compare your critiques.

The Family

Family support is very important to the successful rehabilitation of a person with mental illness. The mental illness of a member is often a shock and a source of great stress to the family. Nurses are in a favorable position to help families cope with the stress and adapt to changes in the family structure. Three categories of programs for families of people with serious mental illnesses include empowerment, treatment, and education. These interventions are also discussed in Chapter 34.

Empowerment. Several common trouble spots in family life can be anticipated. Learning ways to handle these troublesome areas empowers the family by giving them a sense of control over their lives. The problem areas include the following:

- Disrupted communications
- Mechanics of everyday life, including the need for privacy and control over personal space, keeping a regular schedule, television usage, money management, and grooming
- Responding to hallucinations, delusions, and odd behavior, particularly coping with violent or suicidal threats
- Alcohol and drug use
- Need for relatives to remember to take care of themselves

This last area of concern is often ignored by family members and professionals alike. However, it can be accomplished by the following:

- Accepting the fact that a family member has a mental illness.
- Planning a self-care program.
- Continuing to pursue personal activities and interests.
- Getting involved with organizations such as self-help groups or churches.
- Avoiding the advice and opinions of those who have not lived with a person with mental illness.
- Remembering that happiness is possible.
- Avoiding blaming oneself.

Reviewing this list gives the nurse some understanding of the pain and stress experienced by the family of a person with mental illness.

Families and mental health-care providers sometimes become engaged in power struggles related to the care of the mentally ill family member. This interferes with their ability to work as a team. Nurses should strive to understand the family's fears and concerns and help members to develop effective coping mechanisms.

Identifying feelings related to the illness is the first step toward coping. Sharing feelings with each other can be a great relief to people who feel isolated. When feelings are revealed, family members can be supportive of each other, including the ill person. Coping with feelings also allows the person to be receptive to information about the illness and mental health services. The combination of coping and education empowers the family and facilitates their involvement in the recovery process. Because nurses are usually viewed as supportive and helpful, they are in a good position to address the needs of families.

Family Education. Family education has become a primary nursing intervention in providing rehabilitative services to relatives of people with serious mental illness. Nurses have established workshops for family members that have been well received and have helped families cope with the challenges presented by the mental illness. Programming for these workshops can include information and skill-building exercises (Wilson & Hobbs, 1999). The experiences of the more seasoned family members can be particularly helpful because they can share their successes and failures in using various coping strategies and provide needed social support (see Citing the Evidence on Family Support Groups).

A study of the educational and support needs of family members of hospitalized patients found that 75% identified the following learning and support needs: advocacy in communicating with professionals, hospital treatment and rehabilitation, medication compliance, and side effects of medications. The lowest ranked needs were for informal and formal support groups. This may be related to the fact that their family members were hospitalized at the time of the survey (Gasque-Carter & Curlee, 1999). Other family members may find that the opportunity to meet one another for mutual support is especially important. These opportunities may be formal, such as support groups or local chapters of the National Alliance of the Men-

Citing the Evidence on

Family Support Groups

BACKGROUND: Support groups often help families cope more effectively with relatives' mental illnesses. This study examined the differences between support groups led by professionals and those led by family members, focusing specifically on group participation benefits and group content.

RESULTS: Participants of both professional and family-led groups reported that the groups provided them with needed information about mental illness and its treatment, and that the groups improved their relationships with their ill relatives. Professional-led groups placed a greater emphasis on the relatives' problems and coping with emotions, and family-led groups placed a greater emphasis on advocacy.

IMPLICATIONS: Families are diverse and may benefit from various types of groups. Professionals and family leaders who work together for the good of the group may provide even greater benefits to participants.

Pickett S et al: Professional-led versus family-led support groups: exploring the differences, *J Behav Health Serv Res* 25(4):437, 1998

tally Ill (NAMI), or informal, such as family recreational gatherings.

If you were responsible for developing a nursing program for psychiatric rehabilitation, what would it be like? Describe the setting, the program, its goals, and the roles of staff and patients.

The Community

There are several ways nurses can intervene in the community to encourage the establishment of tertiary prevention programs. Among these are health education, membership in advocacy groups, networking, and political action. It has been noted that stigma decreases with increased formal education. Most nurses have a strong background and a firm belief in health education. Mental health education in the community can have a real impact on the experience of patients in the community. Greater understanding of the behaviors and needs of people with mental illness could increase community acceptance, leading to the development of better services. Thus nurses should take advantage of opportunities to speak to community groups about mental health.

Psychiatric nurses can also perform a valuable service by educating their co-workers and professional colleagues about current research related to serious mental illnesses. Although they are seldom discussed, stigmatizing attitudes toward mental illness exist among health-care workers. These attitudes are transmitted to the general public. Professionals have even taken the lead in opposing the establishment of group homes in their neighborhoods. Well-informed nurses can make health-care workers aware of their prejudices and assist them to change their behavior.

Membership by nurses in community advocacy groups can also be helpful. Nurses can join forces with other professional and lay people who share concerns about the care of the mentally ill. The National Mental Health Association is the largest advocacy group that addresses mental health issues. Members of this organization have been influential in drawing attention to the needs of people with mental illness and in supporting positive legislation at the federal and state levels. They monitor the effectiveness of the mental health-care system.

Nurses can also promote working relationships among advocacy groups, professional organizations, self-help groups, and concerned citizens. With limited funding available and health-care costs escalating, the formation of coalitions is essential to lobby for the allocation of resources to mental health care. Psychiatric nurses have taken a leadership role in coalitions to influence reforms in the American health-care system.

The activities of community-wide networks are often directed toward the political system. Aside from allocation of money and other resources, the nature of mental health-care in a community is strongly influenced by the political structure of that community. As described in Chapters 9 and 10, environmental and legal issues have a great effect on mental health-care delivery. Nurses need to be aware of and involved in the political process. They should communicate directly with legislators at all levels, sharing their interests and concerns. Politicians are well aware of the need to respond to the priorities of their constituents.

Nurses can also become more directly involved in the political system. They can run for office and support other nurses who are legislators. Nurses are often invaluable members of appointed boards and commissions on health-care. Their knowledge can be shared with others who are planning community health-care systems. These voluntary activities are time-consuming, but they can have great impact on the health-care system. Community-level policies can either inhibit or facilitate direct care efforts. Active involvement in professional organizations often leads to productive and rewarding community activities. There is a great sense of satisfaction to be derived from selling a community on a new idea and seeing it become a reality.

> *Obtain a copy of a bill considered by your state legislature that is relevant to psychiatric rehabilitation. Explain the effect this legislation would have on the mental health care system, including the potential effect on nursing practice.*

EVALUATION

Evaluation of psychiatric rehabilitation services usually covers the impact on the patient and family and the effectiveness of the community service system.

Patient Evaluation

Evaluation of the services provided to patients and family members must focus on the achievement of the expected outcomes of the intervention. Most psychiatric rehabilitation programs rely on both objective and subjective measures of outcome. Objective measures are generally related to the following questions:

- Is the person living in housing of personal choice?
- Have days of hospitalization in the last year decreased?
- How many emergency room visits has the person made?
- How many days in the last year have been spent in a transitional employment placement? In competitive employment?
- How often does the person have contact with family members? Who are they?
- Can the person identify people to provide support in a crisis?
- Is the person involved in community activities?
- Is the person enrolled in an adult education course? In an academic education program?

The answers to such questions are compared with the individual rehabilitation plans, providing a picture of the success of the services. They should be discussed with program participants and their families as a basis for further planning.

Subjective measures of effectiveness include periodic discussions with patients and families about the progress of rehabilitation. Staff members share their observations about the person's response to the program and invite feedback from the consumers. Many programs also conduct regular consumer satisfaction surveys. More recently, consumers have been employed as advocates to seek information about consumer dissatisfaction and present complaints to program administrators.

Program Evaluation

Program evaluation is conducted to inform administrators about the relevance and cost effectiveness of the services they offer. It is often required by funding, regulatory, and licensure agencies to confirm that public mental health dollars are being spent wisely.

Program evaluation is evolving as program funders and the public demand greater accountability from service providers. Community advisory boards, legislators, and consumer advocates are all recognizing the importance of reviewing the effectiveness of individual programs and service systems. As comprehensive community-based service systems for people with serious mental illnesses continue to grow, evaluation approaches will provide direction.

Summary

1. Psychiatric rehabilitation is the tertiary prevention process of helping the person who has a serious mental illness return to the highest possible level of functioning.
2. Assessment related to rehabilitative psychiatric nursing focuses on the individual, the family, and the community. Behaviors that are assessed include activities of daily living, interpersonal relations, self-esteem, motivation, strengths,

and compliance. Family assessment focuses on family burden and social support needs.

3. Planning and implementation of rehabilitative psychiatric nursing care consist of developing strengths and potentials, learning living skills, and accessing environmental supports. Family intervention is built on empowerment and education. Nurses intervene at the community level by serving as advocates for mental health services and fighting stigma.

4. Evaluation takes place at the patient and program levels.

Competent Caring A Clinical Exemplar of a Psychiatric Nurse

IONA BRADLEY, RN, C

Ms. C was one of the first patients in my mobile treatment caseload. She had had multiple admissions to the state hospital. Her psychiatric diagnosis was bipolar disorder. The referral to this new program was made in an attempt to help her to spend more time in the community. We have now been working together for 6 years. Soon after I met her I realized that there were several nursing problems that I would need to address. She had a history of poor compliance with her medications. She was also diabetic and not good about following her prescribed diet. Because of her diabetes, she had a neurogenic bladder for which an indwelling catheter had been inserted. She was not managing her catheter care very well. She had been living with an abusive alcoholic boyfriend. Although she knew that this was not a good situation for her, she was unable to break away from him. Her conditional release from the hospital required her to live in supervised housing. This forced her to distance herself from him. A stable living situation also enabled me to observe her behavior over time.

I discovered that her bipolar cycle involved manic episodes every 21 days. Knowing this, I could work with her to schedule her life to accommodate her cycle. For instance, she is not pressured to attend her daytime psychosocial rehabilitation program during the manic phase. I also observed a relationship between the manic phase of her bipolar disorder and her diabetes. While manic, she craves sweets and is unable to control her carbohydrate intake. I have worked with the residential staff to remove as many sweets as possible from the house when her manic phase is due to happen. If she does eat sweets she becomes irritable and agitated. Because all of her caregivers are aware of this, she is supported until she regains her stable state.

It took a long time to gain Ms. C's trust. I had to demonstrate over and over that I really cared about her. Once she was able to trust me, I was able to focus on some of her physical nursing care needs. Her urinary catheter was a major inconvenience. She didn't always secure the collection bag well and sometimes it would be found around her ankle. In the past, her boyfriend had pulled it out. With a great deal of support, she agreed to the insertion of a suprapubic catheter. This was easier for her to care for and she has even regained some bladder tone. Her diabetes is becoming more fragile. It is expected that she will need to take insulin in the near future. I have found that pharmacy students are available to monitor medication use in the home for patients who are having problems with self-administration or compliance. I have referred Ms. C to that program. I am also teaching the residential staff about meal planning and nutritious diets.

A long-term relationship like this is rewarding but also challenging. Ms. C and I have shared important life experiences. This has led to a closeness that is not a friendship, but is deeper than I have experienced with patients in other settings. I have become a part of her life. I have participated in the realization by her and her boyfriend that they cannot live together. I have had the opportunity to help both of them recognize and deal with their feelings. I feel good that they were able to remain friends while gaining a realistic view of their relationship. I have learned that working in the community means that the psychiatric nurse has to attend to all of the patient's needs, not just the psychiatric needs. In fact, sometimes the psychiatric needs are not the most important. I have dealt with medical needs, financial needs, needs for housing, and relationship needs. It has been a growth experience for me to be Ms. C's nurse as she has begun to cope with her many problems. It has been very satisfying to be a part of her progress and her road to health.

 Visit MERLIN: www.mosby.com/MERLIN/Stuart to find these additional materials and student activities.

- **Worksheets**
- **"Drug of the Month" Updates**
- **"Citing the Evidence" Updates**
- **Critical Thinking Activities and Exercises**
- **Annotated Suggested Readings**
- **Web Links**
- **More!**

Chapter Review Questions

1. **Identify whether the following statements are true (T) or false (F).**

____ **A.** People who have serious mental illnesses and their families experience grief over the loss of potential life achievements.

____ **B.** Serious mental illness prevents a person from being successful at work or school.

____ **C.** Families of people with mental illness generally want and need to be involved with their ill family member.

____ **D.** Consumers of mental health services should not be hired as providers of mental health services.

____ **E.** Measures of skills and support, more than psychiatric diagnoses and symptom patterns, determine how well a person with a serious mental illness can function in the community.

2. **Fill in the blanks.**

A. Tertiary prevention is carried out by the performance of activities identified as _____.

B. The impact on the family of a member's mental illness is often called _____.

C. The process of moving long-term hospital patients to the community is called _____.

D. _____ is the use of cognitive and behavioral techniques to help people gain the knowledge and skills they need to live in the community.

E. The approach that supports the rehabilitation process by teaching the patient and family about the mental illness and the coping skills that will help with successful community living is called _____.

3. **Provide short answers for the following questions.**

A. Identify four common responses families have to the mental illness of a member.

B. Describe the three basic interventions used in psychiatric rehabilitation.

C. Think about someone you know who has a psychiatric illness. Relate three ways in which you, as a nurse, can help to empower this person and his or her family.

REFERENCES

Barton R: Psychosocial rehabilitation services in community support systems: a review of outcomes and policy recommendations, *Psychiatric Serv* 50:525, 1999.

Bauer M, McBride L: Psychoeducation: conceptual framework and practical considerations, *J Pract Psychiatr Behav Health* 3(1):18, 1997.

Becker D et al: Job preferences of clients with severe psychiatric disorders participating in supported employment programs, *Psychiatr Serv* 47:1223, 1996.

Biegel et al: A comprehensive analysis of family caregivers' perceived relationships with mental health professionals, *Psychiatr Serv* 46:477, 1995.

Blair D, Ramones V: Education as psychiatric intervention: the cognitive-behavioral context, *J Psychosoc Nurs Ment Health Serv* 35:30, 1997.

Blankertz L, Robinson S: Adding a vocational focus to mental health rehabilitation, *Psychiatr Serv* 47:1216, 1996.

Cook J: Neighbors' perceptions of group homes, *Commun Ment Health J* 33:287, 1997.

Cook J: Interactions between group homes and neighbors: neighbor preferences, *J Behavioral Health Serv Res* 25:425, 1998.

Deegan P: Recovering our sense of value after being labeled mentally ill, *J Psychosoc Nurs Ment Health Serv* 31:7, 1993.

Donegan K, Palmer-Erbs V: Promoting the importance of work for persons with psychiatric disabilities—the role of the psychiatric nurse, *J Psychosoc Nurs Ment Health Serv* 36:13, 1998.

Doornbos M: The problems and coping methods of caregivers of young adults with mental illness, *J Psychosoc Nurs Ment Health Serv* 35:22, 1997.

Fountain House: The wellspring of the clubhouse model for social and vocational adjustment of persons with serious mental illness, *Psychiatr Serv* 50(11):1473, 1999.

Friedrich R et al: Family and client perspectives on alternative residential settings for persons with severe mental illness, *Psychiatr Serv* 50:509, 1999.

Gasque-Carter K, Curlee M: The educational needs of families of mentally ill adults: the South Carolina experience, *Psychiatr Serv* 50:520, 1999.

Hamera E, et al: Reciprocity between individuals with severe and persistent mental illness and their family members, *J Am Psychiatr Nurs Assoc* 4:182, 1998.

Hatfield A, et al: Family responses to behavior manifestations of mental illness, *Innovations Res* 3:41, 1994.

Holley H et al: Moving psychiatric patients from hospital to community: views of patients, providers ad families, *Psychiatr Serv* 49(4):513, 1998.

Miller F: Grief therapy for relatives of persons with serious mental illness, *Psychiatr Serv* 47(6):633, 1996.

Mowbray C et al: Consumers as mental health providers: first-person accounts of benefits and limitations, *J Behav Health Serv Res* 25:397, 1998.

Palmer-Erbs V, Anthony W: Incorporating psychiatric rehabilitation principles into mental health nursing, *J Psychosoc Nurs* 33:36, 1995.

Payson A, et al: Health teaching needs of clients with serious and persistent mental illness: client and provider perspectives, *J Psychosoc Nurs Ment Health Serv* 36:32, 1998.

Peterson R: What are the needs of chronic mental patients? In Talbott J, editor: *The chronic mental patient: problems, solutions, and recommendations for a public policy,* Washington, DC, 1978, The American Psychiatric Association.

Pickens J: Social networks for women with serious mental illness, *J Psychosoc Nurs* 37(5):30, 1999.

Pollio D et al: Content and curriculum in psychoeducation groups for families of persons with severe mental illness, *Psychiatr Serv* 49(6):816, 1998.

Saunders J: Family functioning in families providing care for a family member with schizophrenia, *Issues Ment Health Nurs* 20:95, 1999.

Schofield R: Empowerment education for individuals with serious mental illness, *J Psychosoc Nurs* 36(11):35, 1998.

Silverstein S, et al: Identifying and addressing cognitive barriers to rehabilitation readiness, *Psychiatr Serv* 49:34, 1998.

Skinner E et al: Met and unmet needs for assistance and quality of life for people with severe and persistent mental disorders, *Ment Health Serv Res* 1(2):109, 1999.

U.S. Department of Health and Human Services: *Mental health: a report of the Surgeon General,* Rockville, MD, 1999, U.S. DHHS, SAMHSA, CMHS, NIH, NIMH.

Vellenga B, Christenson J: Persistent and severely mentally ill clients' perceptions of their mental illness, *Issues Ment Health Nurs* 15:359, 1994.

Wilson J, Hobbs H: The family educator: a professional resource for families, *J Psychosoc Nurs Ment Health Serv* 37:22, 1999.

Visit **MERLIN** for *Your Internet Connection*
to websites that are related to the content in this chapter.
www.mosby.com/MERLIN/Stuart

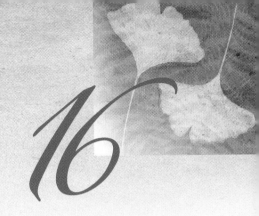

Incorporating the Family in the Continuum of Care

Victoria Conn

16

To multiply the harbors does not reduce the sea.

EMILY DICKINSON

Ever since Florence Nightingale, nurses have involved family members in the care of patients with heart disease, cancer, diabetes and similar disorders. In contrast, the families of patients with mental illnesses were for many years considered to be part of the problem, not part of the solution. Consequently, psychiatric nurses and other mental health professionals tended to distance themselves from families or even to treat them as adversaries. However, during the l990s, professional perceptions of families changed dramatically. This chapter is intended to encourage psychiatric nurses to involve families as partners in care while simultaneously providing them with preventive services to reduce family burden.

BENEFITS TO FAMILY INVOLVEMENT

The benefits of family involvement in the care of their loved ones with mental illness are well-documented. Research has shown that the benefits are maximized when families are appropriately supported and educated for partnership roles. For example, there are 22 controlled studies of psychoeducational family work integrated with optimal drug therapy and case management that have shown substantial additional benefits for people with schizophrenic disorders. Specifically, major exacerbations of psychotic symptoms and admissions to hospitals were more than halved; social disability was reduced with increased employment rates; and burden for family caregivers was lowered while their health improved (Falloon, 1999). Family interventions using psychoeducation, problem-solving, and support although not widely employed, have a strong body of evidence favoring

their efficacy for reducing relapse (McFarlane, 1997). In spite of these findings, barriers to their adoption still need to be overcome (Lehman et al, 1995).

The provision of education for patients' families is now a criterion for accreditation by the Joint Commission of Health Care Organizations (JCHCO). The advantages of family involvement in care are recognized both by professional organizations and by advocacy groups. For example, family involvement is called for in the American Psychiatric Association's *Treatment Guidelines for Schizophrenia and for Bipolar Disorder*, in the American Psychiatric Nurses' Association's *Position Paper on Collaboration*, and in the policy statements of the National Alliance of the Mentally Ill (NAMI) and the World Fellowship of Schizophrenia and Allied Disorders.

Unfortunately, the good intentions promoted at the policy level have not translated well into practice. According to the landmark Schizophrenia Patient Outcomes Research Team (PORT) study, fewer than one in 10 families receives needed education and support services, and overall a significant gap exists between best practices and usual practices for families of persons with schizophrenia (Dixon et al, 1999).

Is a family psychoeducation program offered at your clinical facility? If so, attend a session. If not, ask if they have considered starting one.

BARRIERS TO FAMILY INVOLVEMENT

The following barriers to family involvement are often found in treatment settings:

- Professional bias against families based on past exposure to family systems courses that suggested families in some way caused the illness.
- Family attitudes that equate all family interventions with past, unwelcome experiences with family therapy.

- Professional fears that an alliance with the family will endanger confidentiality and threaten the therapeutic alliance with the patient.
- Administrative restraints in a managed-cost environment, where services to families (as non-patients) receive the lowest priority.

These barriers are gradually disappearing, but only when the parameters of treatment and prevention are drawn around the family unit (as opposed to the individual) will they disappear completely. To the extent that professional caregivers truly understand the impact of long-term mental illness on the family, the more they will work to involve family members as treatment partners and provide them with preventive interventions.

There is now extensive family literature to help nurses understand family burden (see Chapter 15), as well as a national network of NAMI affiliates that welcome nurses as members. In addition, more nurse researchers are studying the family experience and identifying theoretical models that help professionals empathize with caregivers. A case in point is symbolic interactionism, which explains family attitudes, beliefs, and behaviors toward the ill person in terms of the symbolic meaning that the experience of living with the ill person has for each family member. It has been suggested that nurses learn to "walk in the shoes" of family members by asking questions such as, "What situations create stress in your family? How do you feel about your family member's dependency, social interactions, or response to treatment? How much support do you receive from mental health professionals, the community or your extended family?" (Saunders, 1997).

Other nurse researchers, after examining international data sets about the family experience of mental illness, concluded that there is a moral imperative for family education to be part of every treatment plan. It has been proposed that nurses assume educator roles and suggest that curriculum content be tailored to the specific needs of spouses, siblings, parents or children, as well as adapted for different cultural and geographical groups (Yamashita & Forsyth, 1998).

> *Find out if a NAMI group meets in your community. Attend a meeting and share your experience with your peers and instructor.*

Nurses who take the time to question family caregivers about the history of the illness typically learn that family members were the first to notice that something was not right. During the prodromal stages, families are likely to notice changes in sleep and appetite patterns, loss of interest in favorite pastimes, and unexpected interest in religion or philosophy. However, they rarely connect these changes with mental illness.

We thought at first he was just having a difficult adolescence. Then we thought he might be into drugs. But mental illness? Not in our family!

When our daughter started sending hundred dollar contributions to TV evangelists, we assumed she was just another born again Christian.

When a crisis precipitates a hospital admission, families are shocked into the realization that they are dealing with something very serious. At this point, if asked, they are often able to provide important diagnostic clues otherwise not available to the admission team.

But families have other roles and needs in addition to that of informant. Family members who witness a psychiatric emergency need to unwind by verbally replaying the events that led up to the crisis. They need to be told they have done the right thing by bringing their loved one in and appraised of what is happening to him if he is no longer in their presence. These needs are superimposed on basic needs that may have gone unmet during the emergency, such as the need for rest, food and drink.

When I brought my husband to the emergency room for a psychiatric evaluation, the nurse heeded my request to stay near him. She listened to my story, kept me informed and brought me coffee. In other words, she helped me through the worst night in my life.

When the immediate crisis has settled down, nurses should complete their assessment of the mental and physical status of family members. At minimum, families will need an explanation of the likely diagnosis, the proposed treatment and a referral to a family support group. Some families may opt for a continuing program of family consultation, and psychotherapy may also be an option (see Chapter 34). In response to the need for continuing support and/or education, some hospitals have established a Family Resource Center staffed by volunteers and stocked with books, journal articles, videos and access to mental health websites.

I had two sons, one with multiple sclerosis and one with schizophrenia. The one with multiple sclerosis became totally dependent on us for dressing, bathing and everything else, but he earned a doctoral degree. He was given every kind of assistance: a van to transport his wheelchair, student aides and a computer. When he was awarded his degree, the whole audience stood up and cheered. Our son with schizophrenia was just as intelligent, but he dropped out of college. No medication helped him, and he began wandering. He got arrested for causing a disturbance in a public place and died under mysterious circumstances in jail.

Informed family members who see the patient on a daily basis can provide professionals with information to supplement their own observations, and sometimes they may be more reliable informants than the patient.

My brother who lives with us was seeing a therapist once a week, and we couldn't figure out why his only treatment was talking to the therapist and reading books the therapist recommended. He really wasn't even reading the books because he couldn't concentrate. He was hearing voices almost all the time. Finally, I called the therapist and told her what was going on. She was surprised, because my brother hadn't told her he was still hearing voices.

My daughter stayed up all night cutting pictures out of magazines to make collages on the outside of manila envelopes. She told me excitedly that she had invented "self-mailing Valentines." I telephoned her doctor, who had recently reduced the dosage of her lithium. Before I could explain, he expressed displeasure that it was I who had made the call and asked to talk to his patient. When she got on the phone, she managed to sound completely normal. Afterwards, she told me, "My doctor thinks you exaggerate because you're a nurse and you need me to be your little patient." He didn't increase the lithium, and a week later she was rehospitalized.

Of all the barriers to collaboration, confidentiality issues may well be the most problematic because the perception that professionals are caught between the patient's right to a confidential therapeutic relationship and the family caregiver's right to information (see Chapter 10). However, professionals who believe in the merits of collaboration can usually find ways to obtain the patient's permission to communicate with the family (Solomon, 1996; Bogart & Solomon, 1999). Failure to include family caregivers in treatment planning which directly involves them is not only unfair but may precipitate or perpetuate troubled family relationships, as was the case in the following scenario.

The treatment plan for a 35-year-old, single, pregnant woman who was suffering from depression and addiction to cocaine called for her and the future baby to live in the parents' home after her discharge from the hospital. When the father and mother came in to visit, they were stunned to learn that the discharge date had been moved up, and their daughter would be coming home the following day. They wondered aloud if their efforts to hide their resentment at being excluded from the discharge planning would be successful.

Even when a treatment objective involves increasing the patient's autonomy and separation from the family, there are advantages to family involvement. Such a plan is more likely to be carried out if the parents and other relatives understand the goal, agree with it, and contribute their ideas as to how it can be achieved. Obviously, not all patients with serious mental illness have family members who are willing or able to provide care. The point is that family involvement (and its corollary, family support and education) should become the rule, not the exception.

How would you respond to a colleague who says, "We have no time to work with families. They just slow us down and we can't get reimbursed for the time we spend meeting with them."

FAMILIES AS A POPULATION AT RISK

Parents, children, and siblings are at risk for mental illness and other stress related disorders on two counts: heredity and environment. Spouses escape the heredity factor, but are very much affected by living in a stressful environment. Psychoanalysts used to call the intraspousal transfer of symptoms "folie a deux." Currently, members of support groups for spouses facetiously refer to their spouses' symptoms as "contagious." A social worker who has a son with schizophrenia has compared the ripple effect of mental illness on the family to a large stone skipping across water (Wasow, 1995). The response of family members is movingly described in Box 16-1.

In the wake of the Oklahoma City bombing by terrorists, nurses were deployed to care for the victims and to minister to their shocked and grieving families. Serious mental illness can be a comparable catastrophe, and the victims' families suffer similar trauma. The impact of mental illness is a shattering, traumatic event in the life of a family and, as such, family members are ideal candidates for secondary intervention strategies.

Aging parents who expected an empty nest find themselves in their fifties, sixties and seventies, sharing the nest with adult children being treated for mental illness. In addition to accepting that their dreams for their children must be dramatically revised, these parents must learn to coexist with loved ones whose moods and behaviors are often baffling and sometimes dangerous. It is not surprising when NAMI chapter newsletters report heart attacks or strokes suffered in apparent response to a relative's relapse, suicide attempt or encounter with the law. Less dramatic but also unfortunate, are the family members who suffer from depression, separate or divorce, or become alcoholics or drug users. The subjective and objective burden of living with a loved one for whom effective treatment has not been found has been called "mourning without end" (Willick, 1994; Cuijpers & Stam, 2000). At the same time, some families say their lives have been strengthened by the experience.

We have this terrible feeling of loss and grieve for the son we knew. We feel cheated out of watching him mature and flower the way adolescents do as they grow into young adults. When I meet his former classmates who are now working, finishing graduate degrees or married, I am always aware that these things are not possible for him, just the same as someone would feel had their son died. Yet this mourning is strange, because our son is not dead at all. He is very much still with us, seemingly eternally 13 years old, needing care and attention.

In the dark soul of the night, I grieve for all of us–for the anguish of the past and the present, and the uncertainty of the future. Most of all, I grieve for my daughter, for her lost hopes and expectations. At the same time, we have emerged from this emotional holocaust as better, stronger and more tolerant people.

Well siblings attracted the attention of early researchers primarily because they had escaped the illness. The question was, "How did the schizophrenic mother manage to raise well children?" Some theorized that the siblings were only superficially normal; others surmised that they escaped major pathology by detaching themselves from the family, or because they were neglected by their mothers.

Contemporary researchers have made similar observations, but different interpretations, about the status of siblings (see Citing the Evidence on p. 269). Many surveys have revealed that siblings suffer problems in living (Friedrich et al, 1999). The reality is that when the emotional and financial resources are devoted disproportionally to the son or daughter with the illness, there is less available for the siblings. They may be resentful, but are unable to express their resentment because of survivor's guilt. Consequently, some siblings detach from the family. Others remain involved, often at the expense of career and marriage options. Many become members of helping professions.

The 37-year-old sister of a woman diagnosed with schizophrenia graduated from a hospital school of nursing instead of a more expensive college program. She lives in the family home and divides her time between work and being a liaison between her sister's professional caregivers and her parents. Weekends are devoted to her sister, who comes home from the hospital on pass. Of the few men she has dated, none has survived the sister test.

Siblings and offspring are likely to have problems as adults because they had less parental attention than they needed as children and adolescents. It is ironic that professional caregivers who are very knowledgeable about the effects of child-

Box **16-1**

The Meaning of Mental Illness to the Family

When a loved one is stricken with mental illness, every member of the family feels pain. Whether the patient is your mother, father, son, daughter, sister, brother, grandchild or grandparent, you share in the suffering. But you have other feelings that confuse and frighten you.

Before the doctors gave you a diagnosis, you probably went through a long period of uncertainty–trying to make sense of what was happening. You were stunned and bewildered. You hoped that the odd behavior and scary talk would stop, that soon things would be back to normal. Maybe a crisis occurred.

In one way or another, your family member was brought to treatment. Once the diagnosis was made, you began asking questions: "Will my loved one get better and lead a normal life again?" "What have I done wrong?" "Why did this happen to me, to us?"

Your questions and your feelings are quite natural. Your grief, shame, and anger, your sense of helplessness, your hours of anxiety: All are shared by others going through similar experiences. But depending on your relationship to the mentally ill family member, you also have feelings that are not shared by others.

Perhaps it is your child who has fallen ill. Suddenly a promising young person, on the threshold of becoming an adult, takes a sharp turn. Now there is a stranger in your midst. Your once happy and content son or daughter becomes withdrawn, unkempt, and unable to function. He argues, destroys possessions, says, and does things that make no sense. You, like other parents, want to protect and nurture your child. When your desire is thwarted, you feel that you have failed. Perhaps you blame him. Such feelings are not unique to parents of mentally ill persons. Parents of children with severe physical illnesses such as cancer or heart disease also tend to blame themselves, to harbor feelings of resentment toward the victim. Because mental illness affects such intensely personal aspects of our being, it is not surprising that parents of mental patients do likewise. Professionals—often unwittingly—may augment your guilt by blaming you for the tragedy.

When it is your spouse who becomes mentally ill you have special problems. This is, after all, the person you chose to marry: your mate, companion, and lover. Not only do once-shared responsibilities fall solely on you, but you must also try to find help for your spouse. Perhaps help is not welcomed. Without diminishing your partner's status, you must juggle the roles of mother, father, homemaker and breadwinner all at once.

Other family members may escape the responsibilities that fall to a parent or spouse of the mentally ill person, but they share equally painful feelings. Brothers and sisters are bewildered, hurt and sometimes ashamed and angry. Grandparents are perplexed and saddened. Adult children find it difficult to assume the role of caretaker when a parent becomes incompetent.

One out of four families has a close relative who is mentally ill. They, like you, typically go through a period of intense searching. Patients, family members, and doctors alike tend to place blame to identify an event or a person responsible for the breakdown. "Why me?" is an understandable cry.

In time, most families come to accept the illness. Somehow, they find resources to sustain themselves over the rocky period. Many become stronger in the process. When they look back over years of living with chronic mental illness, they almost invariably remember the earliest period as the hardest. They may have been surprised by the amount of energy, resourcefulness and courage they were able to muster. They come to feel pride in their capacity to face tragedy and conquer defeat.

While no cure is now known for the more severe, chronic mental illnesses, almost everyone can be helped to live worthwhile and meaningful lives. Caring relatives must continue to hope for improvement, set reasonable expectations, and maintain faith in the patient's recuperative and restorative powers. Realities change. What may have been impossible at one time may become quite possible. There will be regressions, plateaus when all anyone can expect to do is "hang on," without forward movement.

A short time ago families who had known mental illness for a long time were asked how it affected them. As might be expected, many reported the negative consequences. But many also saw positive changes in their lives. One mother said she no longer takes life for granted. "I've learned to appreciate the little things in life," she said. "I make it a point to find something to enjoy each day." Other family members reported that they were more compassionate, less judgmental and more understanding of others. Most had made what they considered a more mature reevaluation of their lives, thereby achieving a truer vision of what really counts. They believed that their lives had become more significant, more basic and more meaningful.

Most families, in short, found they had wellsprings of strength they never knew they had until they met the great challenge of mental illness.

From Hatfield A: *Coping with mental illness in the family: a family guide*, Arlington, Va, 1986, The National Alliance for the Mentally Ill.

---

hood trauma in general terms are often unaware of the specific difficulties faced by children growing up in families preoccupied by mental illness.

Despite the known genetic risks for the offspring of parents with schizophrenia, and the even greater risk for those who have parents with bipolar disorder or major depression, these children are underserved in the mental health system. This lack of service results in part from the fact that women in treatment for serious mental illnesses often do not reveal that they have children, for fear that they will be removed from their care. Consequently, offspring and siblings may present for treatment years later, exhibiting problems with

identity, self-esteem, and dependence on the approval of others. There may be difficulties with trust and intimacy, an excessive need for perfectionism and control, and developmental delays with respect to marriage and careers. On the other hand, children raised in the shadow of mental illness can achieve success in life and even become prominent public figures. A case in point is the actress, Marilyn Monroe, whose mother suffered from schizophrenia and whose grandmother (also afflicted) tried to suffocate her with a pillow when she was 13 months old (Marshall, 1996).

In keeping with the theme that siblings and offspring gravitate toward the helping professions, a number of nurses

Citing the Evidence on

Siblings of Adults with Mental Illness

BACKGROUND: Little is known about the intentions of adult siblings to assume the caregiving role. This study examined the factors associated with the involvement of siblings in the life of a brother or sister who has mental illness or mental retardation.

RESULTS: The two groups of siblings show striking differences in their expectations about the responsibility for future caregiving. Almost 60% of the siblings of adults with mental retardation expected to assume primary caregiving responsibility in the future, but only 33% of the siblings of adults with mental illness held this expectation. For both groups, competing family responsibilities limited the involvement of siblings, whereas closeness to the family of origin led to greater sibling involvement.

IMPLICATIONS: The findings highlight the importance of clinicians' work to support and strengthen family relationships, which loom large in determining the extent to which siblings are involved in the care of a brother or sister with disabilities.

Greenberg J et al: Siblings of adults with mental illness or mental retardation: current involvement and expectation of future caregiving, *Psychiatr Serv* 50(9):1214, 1999.

and social workers contributed their personal accounts to the Journal of the California Alliance for the Mentally Ill.

I had to grow up fast as a child. I recognize that my mother's illness deprived me of having any sort of a carefree, normal childhood. Periodically, I have been angry at one or both of my parents for the atmosphere at home (Bruge, 1996).

As a child it was often difficult to know which of my mother's behaviors were normal and which were due to the illness (List, 1996).

Daddy always had to tell us, "Don't step off the curb" before we left for school. I was so used to it; it was such a part of my daily routine, that I never realized the absurdity of it (Poe, 1996).

The professor had just finished a compressed overview on what was known about schizophrenia. "Oh, my God!" I gasped, to myself. "That's what my father has" (Steinert, 1996).

The following have been suggested as ways in which professionals can help young people living in families with mental illness (Marsh & Johnson, 1997):

- Become informed about the family experience of mental illness.
- Strengthen and support the family system.
- Reach out as early as possible and assure them they are not to blame.
- Address the needs of young family members in an age-appropriate manner.
- Enlist the help of teachers, principals, guidance counselors and school psychologists.

Box 16-2

NAMI Family to Family Curriculum

Class 1. Introduction. Special features of the course, emotional reactions to the trauma of mental illness; your goals for your family member with mental illness

Class 2. Schizophrenia, Major Depression, Mania, Schizoaffective Disorder. Diagnostic criteria; characteristic features of psychotic illnesses; keeping a Crisis File

Class 3. Mood Disorders and Anxiety Disorders. Types and sub-types of depression and bipolar disorder; causes of mood disorders; diagnostic criteria for panic disorder and obsessive-compulsive disorder

Class 4. Basics about the Brain. Functions of key brain areas; research on functional and structural brain abnormalities; chemical messengers in the brain; genetic research; the biology of recovery; NAMI Science and Treatment Video

Class 5. Problem Solving Skills Workshop. How to define a problem; sharing our problem statements; solving the problem; setting limits

Class 6. Medication Review. How medications work; basic psychopharmacology of mood disorders, anxiety disorders, and schizophrenia; side effects; key treatment issues; stages of adherence to medications; early warning signs of relapse

Class 7. Inside Mental Illness. The subjective experience of coping with a brain disorder; maintaining self-esteem and positive identity; gaining empathy for your relative's psychological struggle to protect one's integrity despite mental illness

Class 8. Communication Skills Workshop. How illness interferes with the capacity to communicate; learning to be clear; how to respond when the topic is loaded; talking to the person behind the symptoms

Class 9. Self-Care. Learning about family burden; handling feelings of anger, entrapment, guilt, and grief; how to balance our lives

Class 10. The Vision and Potential of Recovery. Learning about key principles of rehabilitation and model programs of community support; a first hand account of recovery

Class 11. Advocacy. Challenging the power of stigma in our lives; learning how to change the system; the NAMI Campaign to End Discrimination; meet a NAMI advocate

Class 12. Review, Sharing and Evaluation. Certification ceremony. Celebration!

- Assure them that their needs matter and support their goals.
- Offer counseling for those who are experiencing particular difficulty.

 What personal and social impact do you think stigma has on the siblings of those who are mentally ill?

BUILDING BRIDGES

In the late 1980s, NAMI's Curriculum and Training Network offered a program to train two persons from each state affiliate as "family education specialists." Later, a 30-hour curriculum known as the NAMI Family to Family Education Program was written (Box 16-2). By the end of 1999, this

Box 16-3

Family Involvement Competencies for Mental Health Professionals

DEVELOPING A COLLABORATION WITH THE FAMILY

Make a positive first contact
Identify family's needs
Address confidentiality

OFFERING INFORMATION ON MENTAL ILLNESS

Diagnosis, etiology, prognosis, treatments
Long-term course of serious mental illness
Educational sessions

ENHANCING FAMILY COMMUNICATION AND PROBLEM SOLVING

Teach principles of effective communication
Teach problem-solving strategies

HELPING WITH SERVICE SYSTEM USE

Help access entitlements, support, and rehabilitation
Explain the roles of different mental health providers
Establish needed linkages
Translate the language of mental health services
Help access crisis services
Help access housing

HELPING FAMILY MEMBERS MEET OWN NEEDS

Help family members access support services
Understand burden and grief
Assess for stress-related disorders
Offer services or referrals
Encourage self-care
Encourage advocacy

ADDRESSING SPECIAL ISSUES CONCERNING THE PATIENT

Treatment is not working
Illness is of recent onset
Patient has multiple diagnoses
Patient is in jail
Patient refuses treatment

ADDRESSING SPECIAL ISSUES CONCERNING THE FAMILY

The family does not speak English
The family is very important or of high status in the community
The family belongs to an ethnic minority
The family is missing
The family is disinterested

Modified from Glynn S et al: *Involving families in mental health services: competencies for mental health workers,* Los Angeles, 1997, Human Interaction Research Institute.

peer-taught program had been presented free of charge to over 40,000 families across the nation. It is no coincidence that many of the family members trained to teach the course have a nursing background. In order to make this unique referral resource better known to mental health professionals, a Clinician's Guide to the NAMI Family-to-Family Education Program was written (Weiden, 1999).

In 1990, NAMI and the Human Interaction Research Institute of Los Angeles collaborated on a Center for Mental Health Services funded project which identified seven competencies that professionals need in order to involve families as partners in treatment. Psychiatric nurses should assess the extent to which they practice these skills (see Box 16-3).

More recently, the American Psychiatric Nursing Association (APNA) formed a working alliance with NAMI for the purpose of jointly promoting public policy pertaining to mental health/illness issues. APNA also testified before Congress on behalf of NAMI's policy on the limitations on restraints and seclusion (see Chapter 31). As a result, legislation protecting patients from the inappropriate use of seclusion and restraints has been enacted in several states. This is but one example of the potential impact that joint advocacy between nursing and family organizations can have on the field.

Summary

1. Research indicates that involving family members of patients with serious mental illness as partners in treatment benefits both patients and families. Therefore, psychiatric nurses should endeavor to overcome any barriers and involve patients' families as standard nursing practice.

2. Parents, children, and siblings of those with serious mental illness have a demonstrated need for education and support to reduce family burden, prevent problems, and promote adaptive coping skills.

3. Collaboration between psychiatric nurses and families (and psychiatric nursing organizations and family advocacy groups) can reap rich rewards in terms of advancing prevention, treatment, and recovery in the field.

MERLIN Visit MERLIN: **www.mosby.com/MERLIN/Stuart** to find these additional materials and student activities.

- **Worksheets**
- **"Drug of the Month" Updates**
- **"Citing the Evidence" Updates**
- **Critical Thinking Activities and Exercises**
- **Annotated Suggested Readings**
- **Web Links**
- **More!**

Chapter Review Questions

1. What preventive strategies from Chapter 13 can you use with the siblings of a patient who is mentally ill?
2. How can families serve as balancing factors, as described in Chapter 14, in helping a person with mental illness who is in crisis?
3. In what ways can the rehabilitative interventions detailed in Chapter 15 be enhanced by including family members?
4. Talk with the family of a psychiatric patient. Listen to their story of how psychiatric illness has affected their lives.

REFERENCES

Bogart T, Solomon P: Procedures to share treatment information among mental health providers, consumers and families, *Psychiatr Serv* 50(10):1321, 1999.

Bruge D: Thoughts about my mother, *J Calif Alliance Mentally Ill* 7:15, 1996.

Cuijpers P, Stam H: Burnout among relatives of psychiatric patients attending psychoeducational support groups, *Psychiatr Serv* 51(3):375, 2000.

Dixon L et al: Services to families of adults with schizophrenia: from treatment recommendations to dissemination, *Psychiatr Serv* 50(2):233, 1999.

Falloon I: Newsletter of the World Fellowship of Schizophrenia and Allied Disorders, Toronto, Canada, 1999.

Friedrich R et al: Well siblings living with schizophrenia, *J Psychosoc Nurs Ment Health Serv* 37(8):11, 1999.

Lehman A et al: Schizophrenia treatment outcomes research, *Schizophr Bull* 21(4):585, 1995.

List A: On becoming authentic: a daughter's story, *J Calif Alliance Mentally Ill* 7:37, 1996.

Marsh D, Johnson D: The family experience of mental illness: implications for interventions, *Professional Psychology: Research and Practice* 28(3):232, 1997.

Marshall L: Marilyn Monroe: a child of mental illness, *J Calif Alliance Mentally Ill* 7:31, 1996.

McFarlane W: Integrating family psychoeducation and assertive community treatment, *Admin Policy Ment Health* 25(2):191, 1997.

Poe S: Sailing similar seas, *J Calif Alliance Mentally Ill* 7:16, 1996.

Solomon P: Moving from psychoeducation to family education for families of adults with serious mental illness, *Psychiatr Serv* 47:1364, 1996.

Saunders J: Walking a mile in their shoes: symbolic interactionism for families living with severe mental illness, *J Psychosoc Nurs Ment Health Serv* 35(6):10, 1997.

Steinert P: Why didn't you tell me? *J Calif Alliance Mentally Ill* 7:22, 1996.

Wasow M: *The skipping stone: ripple effects of mental illness in the family,* Palo Alto, Calif, 1995, Science and Behavior Books.

Weiden P: The road back: working with those with severe mental illness, *J Pract Psych Behav Health* 4:354, 1999.

Willick M: Mourning without end. In Andreasen N, editor: *Schizophrenia: mind to molecule,* Washington, DC, 1994, American Psychiatric Press.

Yamashita M, Forsyth D: Family coping with mental illness: an aggregate from two studies, Canada and United States, *J Am Psych Nurses Assoc* 4(1):1, 1998.

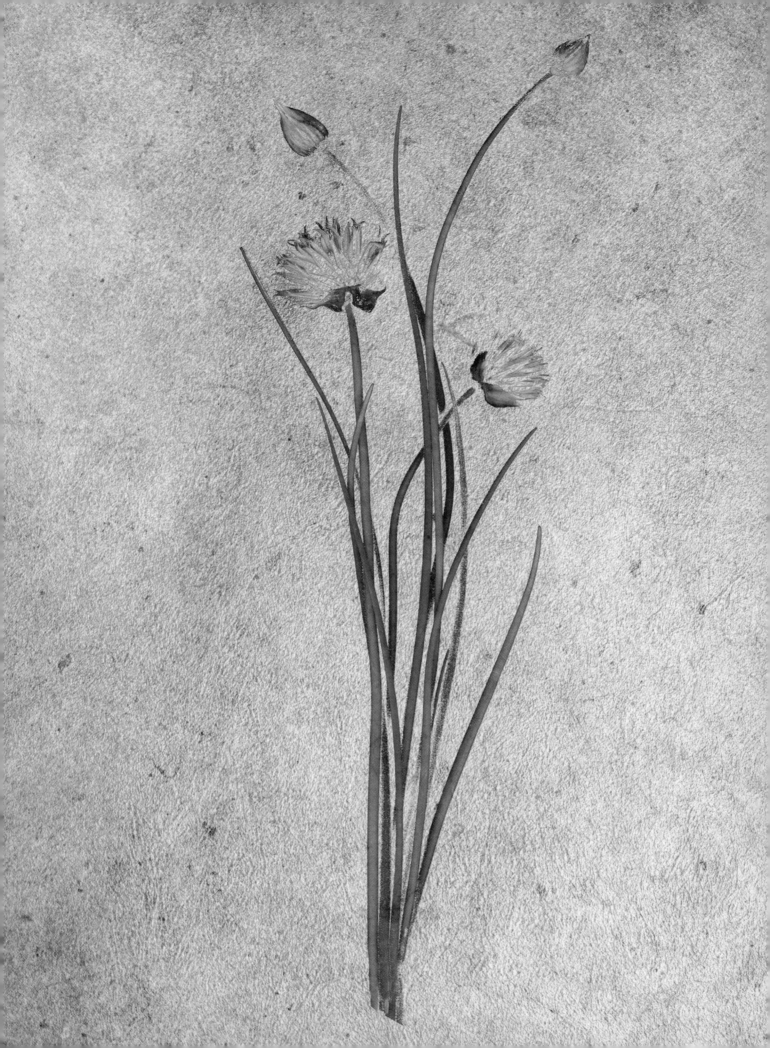

Applying Principles in Nursing Practice

Have you thought that most people with psychiatric problems were suffering from schizophrenia? Did you ever suspect that one of your friends or family members had an emotional or psychiatric problem but dismissed the idea as impossible? Have you ever worried about the barometer of your own mental health but felt embarrassed to discuss it? If you have answered "yes" to any of these questions, you are in for an awakening. The fact is that almost half of all Americans experience some type of psychiatric problem in their lifetime. Most of these problems are not what nurses commonly think of as a psychiatric illness, but anxiety disorders, mood disorders and substance use disorders are by far the most common psychiatric disorders, and they are experienced by people more often than many physical illnesses. They are disabling disorders that cause people significant distress, yet they are often underdiagnosed and undertreated. These facts are more than interesting. They suggest that health-care professionals need a wide variety of educational and treatment strategies to address these issues.

In this unit you will explore the adaptive and maladaptive coping responses used by people experiencing stress. Some of what you read will surprise you, some of it will concern you, and it is hoped that most of it will intrigue you. It is important that you understand, however, that these psychiatric problems are a common part of the human experience. As such, they merit careful study and consideration by nurses like yourself.

17

Anxiety Responses and Anxiety Disorders

Gail W. Stuart

LEARNING OBJECTIVES

After studying this chapter the student should be able to:

- Describe the continuum of adaptive and maladaptive anxiety responses
- Identify behaviors associated with anxiety responses
- Analyze predisposing factors, precipitating stressors, and appraisal of stressors related to anxiety responses
- Describe coping resources and coping mechanisms related to anxiety responses
- Formulate nursing diagnoses for patients related to anxiety responses
- Examine the relationship between nursing diagnoses and medical diagnoses related to anxiety responses
- Identify expected outcomes and short-term nursing goals related to anxiety responses
- Develop a patient education plan to promote the relaxation response
- Analyze nursing interventions related to anxiety responses
- Evaluate nursing care related to anxiety responses

TOPICAL OUTLINE

Continuum of Anxiety Responses
   Defining Characteristics
   Levels of Anxiety
Assessment
   Behaviors
   Predisposing Factors
   Precipitating Stressors
   Appraisal of Stressors
   Coping Resources
   Coping Mechanisms
Nursing Diagnosis
   Related Medical Diagnoses
Outcome Identification
Planning
Implementation
   Severe and Panic Levels of Anxiety
   Moderate Level of Anxiety
Evaluation

The fears we know are of not knowing. . . . It is getting late. Shall we ever be asked for? Are we simply not wanted at all?
        WH AUDEN, *THE AGE OF ANXIETY*

Anxiety is a pervasive aspect of contemporary life. Between 10% and 25% of the population of the United States suffers from an anxiety disorder (Box 17-1). Anxiety has always existed and belongs to no particular era or culture. It derives from the Greek root meaning "to press tight." **Anxious** is related to the Latin word **angere**, which means "to strangle" and "to distress." It resembles the word **anger**, when defined as "grief" or "trouble." It is also related to **anguish**, which is described as "acute pain, suffering, or distress." It involves one's body, perceptions of self and relationships with others, making it a foundational concept in the study of psychiatric nursing and human behavior.

CONTINUUM OF ANXIETY RESPONSES

Anxiety as is a diffuse apprehension that is vague in nature and associated with feelings of uncertainty and helplessness. Feelings of isolation, alienation and insecurity are also present. The person perceives that the core of his or her personality is being threatened. Experiences provoking anxiety begin in infancy and continue throughout life. They end with the fear of the greatest unknown, death.

Defining Characteristics

Anxiety is an emotion and a subjective individual experience. It is an energy and cannot be observed directly. A nurse infers that a patient is anxious based on certain behaviors. The nurse needs to validate this inference with the patient. Also, anxiety is an emotion without a specific object. It is provoked by the unknown and precedes all new experiences such as entering school, starting a new job, or giving birth to a child.

This characteristic of anxiety differentiates it from fear. **Fear** has a specific source or object that the person can identify and describe. Fear involves the **intellectual appraisal** of a threatening stimulus; anxiety is the **emotional response** to that appraisal. A fear is caused by physical or psychological exposure to a threatening situation. Fear produces anxiety. The two emotions are differentiated in speech; we speak of **having** a fear but of **being** anxious.

Anxiety is communicated interpersonally. If a nurse is talking with a patient who is anxious, within a short time the

Box **17-1**

The Prevalence of Anxiety Disorders

Anxiety disorders are the most common psychiatric disorders in America.

- More than 23 million people are afflicted by these debilitating illnesses each year (approximately one out of every four individuals).
- Anxiety disorders cost the United States $46.6 billion in 1990 in direct and indirect costs, nearly one third of the nation's total mental health bill of $148 billion.
- People with panic disorder spend heavily on health services. One survey found that a patient with panic attacks made an average of 37 medical visits a year, as compared with 5 visits in the general population.
- Fewer than 25% of panic disorder sufferers seek help—mainly because they do not realize their physical symptoms, such as heart palpitations, chest pains and shortness of breath, are caused by a psychiatric problem.

From: NIMH, 1996, Anxiety Education Program.

nurse will also experience feelings of anxiety. Similarly, if a nurse is anxious in a particular situation, this anxiety will be communicated to the patient. The contagious nature of anxiety can therefore have positive and negative effects on the therapeutic relationship. The nurse must carefully monitor these effects. It is also important to remember that anxiety is part of everyday life. It is basic to the human condition and provides a valuable warning. In fact, the capacity to be anxious is necessary for survival.

The crux of anxiety is self-preservation. Anxiety occurs as a result of a threat to a person's selfhood, self-esteem, or identity. It results from a threat to something central to one's personality and essential to one's existence and security. It may be connected with the fear of punishment, disapproval, withdrawal of love, disruption of a relationship, isolation, or loss of body functioning.

Culture is related to anxiety because culture can influence the values one considers most important. Underlying every fear is the anxiety of losing one's own being. This anxiety is the frightening element, but a person can meet the anxiety and grow from it to the extent that the person confronts, moves through, and overcomes anxiety-creating experiences.

 Name two situations that provoke anxiety in you. Compare these to two situations that stimulate fear in you.

Levels of Anxiety

Peplau (1963) identified four levels of anxiety and described their effects:

- **Mild anxiety** is associated with the tension of day-to-day living. During this stage the person is alert and the perceptual field is increased. The person sees, hears, and grasps more than before. This kind of anxiety can motivate learning and produce growth and creativity.

- **Moderate anxiety**, in which the person focuses only on immediate concerns, involves the narrowing of the perceptual field as the person sees, hears, and grasps less. The person blocks selected areas but can attend to more if directed to do so.

- **Severe anxiety** is marked by a significant reduction in the perceptual field. The person tends to focus on a specific detail and not think about anything else. All behavior is aimed at relieving anxiety, and much direction is needed to focus on another area.

- Panic is associated with awe, dread, and terror. At this stage details are blown out of proportion. Because of a complete loss of control, the person is unable to do things even with direction. Panic involves the disorganization of the personality. There is increased motor activity, decreased ability to relate to others, distorted perceptions and loss of rational thought. Panic is a frightening and paralyzing experience. The person in panic is unable to communicate or function effectively. This level of anxiety cannot persist indefinitely because it is incompatible with life. A prolonged period of panic would result in exhaustion and death. It is a common and debilitating phenomenon that can be safely and effectively treated (Beck, 1996; Laraia, 1995; Stuart & Laraia, 1996).

The nurse needs to be able to identify which level of anxiety a patient is experiencing by the behaviors observed. Fig. 17-1 shows the range of anxiety responses from the most adaptive response of anticipation to the most maladaptive response of panic. The patient's level of anxiety and its position on the continuum of coping responses is relevant to the nursing diagnosis and influences the type of intervention the nurse implements.

ASSESSMENT
Behaviors

Anxiety can be expressed directly through physiological and behavioral changes or indirectly through the formation of symptoms or coping mechanisms developed as a defense against anxiety. The nature of the behaviors displayed depends on the level of anxiety. The intensity of the behaviors increases with increasing anxiety. Box 17-2 lists behavioral rating scales commonly used to measure anxiety and anxiety disorders.

In describing anxiety's effects on physiological responses, mild and moderate anxiety heighten the person's capacities. Conversely, severe and panic levels paralyze or overwork capacities. The physiological responses associated with anxiety are modulated primarily by the brain through the autonomic nervous system (Fig. 17-2). The body adjusts internally without a conscious or voluntary effort. Two types of autonomic responses exist:

- Parasympathetic responses, which conserve body responses
- Sympathetic responses, which activate body processes

Studies support the predominance of the sympathetic reaction. This reaction prepares the body to deal with an

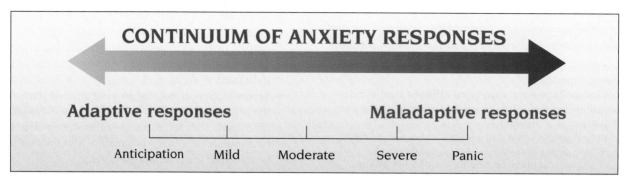

Fig. 17-1   Continuum of anxiety responses.

Box **17-2**

Behavioral Rating Scales Related to Anxiety and Anxiety Disorders

- Beck Anxiety Inventory (BAI)
- Brief Social Phobia Scale
- Covi Anxiety Scale
- Dissociative Experience Scale
- Dissociative Disorders Interview Schedule (DDIS)
- Hamilton Rating Scale for Anxiety (Ham-A)
- Maudsley Obsessional Compulsive Inventory
- Panic Disorder Outcomes Module (PDOM)
- Panic Disorder Severity Scale
- Phobic Avoidance Rating Scale
- PTSD Inventory
- Spielberger Anxiety State-Trait
- Taylor Anxiety Scale
- Yale-Brown Obsessive Compulsive Scale (YBOCS)
- Zung Anxiety Scale

emergency situation by a fight or flight reaction. It can also trigger the general adaptation syndrome, as described by Selye (see Chapter 18). When the cortex of the brain perceives a threat, it sends a stimulus down the sympathetic branch of the autonomic nervous system to the adrenal glands. Because of a release of epinephrine, respiration deepens, the heart beats more rapidly and arterial pressure rises. Blood is shifted away from the stomach and intestines to the heart, central nervous system, and muscles. Glycogenolysis is accelerated and the blood glucose level rises. For some people, however, the parasympathetic reaction may coexist or predominate and produce opposite effects. Other physiological reactions may also be evident. The variety of physiological responses to anxiety that the nurse may observe in patients is summarized in Box 17-3.

Psychomotor manifestations, or behavioral responses, are also observed in the anxious patient. Their effects have both personal and interpersonal aspects. High levels of anxiety affect coordination, involuntary movements, and responsiveness and can also disrupt human relationships. In an interpersonal situation anxiety can warn a person to withdraw from a situation where discomfort is antici-

pated. The anxious patient typically withdraws and decreases interpersonal involvement. The possible behavioral responses the nurse might observe are presented in Box 17-3.

Mental or intellectual functioning is also affected by anxiety. Cognitive responses the patient might display when experiencing anxiety are described in Box 17-3.

Finally, the nurse can assess a patient's emotional reactions, or affective responses, to anxiety by the subjective description of the patient's personal experience. Often, patients describe themselves as tense, jittery, on edge, jumpy, worried or restless. One patient described feelings in the following way: "I'm expecting something terribly bad to happen, but I don't know what. I'm afraid, but I don't know why. I guess you can call it a generalized bad feeling." All these phrases are expressions of apprehension and overalertness. It seems clear that the person interprets his or her anxiety as a kind of warning sign. Additional affective responses are listed in Box 17-3.

Anxiety is an unpleasant and uncomfortable experience that most people try to avoid. They often try to replace anxiety with a more tolerable feeling. Pure anxiety is rarely seen. Anxiety is usually observed in combination with other emotions. Patients might describe feelings of anger, boredom, contempt, depression, irritation, worthlessness, jealousy, self-depreciation, suspicion, sadness, or helplessness. This combination of emotions makes it difficult for the nurse to discriminate between anxiety and depression, for instance, because the patient's descriptions may be similar.

Close ties exist between anxiety, depression, guilt, and hostility. These emotions often function reciprocally; one feeling acts to generate and reinforce the others. The relationship between anxiety and hostility is particularly close. The pain experienced with anxiety often causes anger and resentment toward those thought to be responsible. These feelings of hostility in turn increase anxiety.

This cycle was evident in the case of a dependent and insecure wife who was very attached to her husband. She expressed numerous vague fears. In exploring her feelings, she also expressed great hostility toward him and their relationship. This hostility symbolized her helplessness and increased her feelings of weakness. Verbalizing these angry feelings further increased her anxiety and unresolved con-

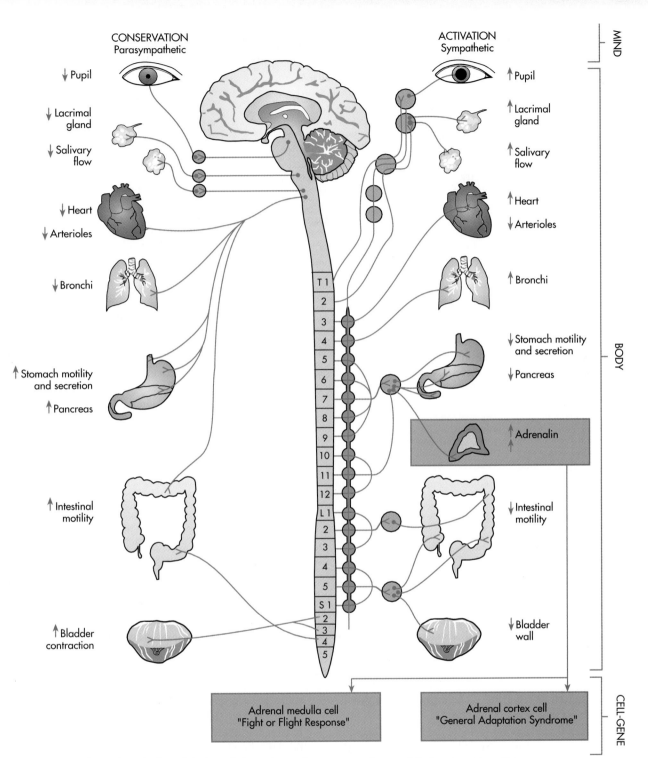

Fig. 17-2 Mind modulation of the autonomic nervous system and its two branches, the parasympathetic (conserving) and the sympathetic (activating), down to the cellular level.

flict. Thus anxiety is often expressed through anger, and a tense and anxious person is more likely to become angry.

Think of a patient you cared for recently who appeared to be angry or critical. Could this have been the patient's way of dealing with anxiety? If so, how would your nursing interventions have been different?

Predisposing Factors

Anxiety is a prime factor in the development of the personality and formation of individual character traits. Because of its importance, various theories of the origin of anxiety have been developed.

Psychoanalytic View. Freud (1969) identified two types of anxiety: primary and subsequent. Primary anxiety, the traumatic state, begins in the infant as a result of the sud-

Box **17-3**

Physiological, Behavioral, Cognitive, and Affective Responses to Anxiety

PHYSIOLOGICAL		BEHAVIORAL	COGNITIVE	AFFECTIVE
Cardiovascular	**Neuromuscular**	Restlessness	Impaired attention	Edginess
Palpitations	Increased reflexes	Physical tension	Poor concentration	Impatience
Racing heart	Startle reaction	Tremors	Forgetfulness	Uneasiness
Increased blood	Eyelid twitching	Startle reaction	Errors in judgment	Tension
pressure	Insomnia	Hypervigilance	Preoccupation	Nervousness
Faintness*	Tremors	Rapid speech	Blocking of thoughts	Fear
Actual fainting*	Rigidity	Lack of coordination	Decreased	Fright
Decreased blood	Fidgeting	Accident proneness	perceptual field	Frustration
pressure*	Pacing	Interpersonal withdrawal	Reduced creativity	Helplessness
Decreased pulse	Strained face	Inhibition	Diminished	Alarm
rate*	Generalized weakness	Flight	productivity	Terror
	Wobbly legs	Avoidance	Confusion	Jitteriness
Respiratory	Clumsy movement	Hyperventilation	Self-consciousness	Jumpiness
Rapid breathing			Loss of objectivity	Numbing
Shortness of breath	**Urinary Tract**		Fear of losing	Guilt
Pressure on chest	Pressure to urinate*		control	Shame
Shallow breathing	Frequent urination*		Frightening visual	Frustration
Lump in throat			images	Helplessness
Choking sensation	**Skin**		Fear of injury or	
Gasping	Flushed face		death	
	Localized sweating		Flashbacks	
Gastrointestinal	(palms)		Nightmares	
Loss of appetite	Itching			
Revulsion toward	Hot and cold spells			
food	Pale face			
Abdominal	Generalized sweating			
discomfort				
Abdominal pain*				
Nausea*				
Heartburn*				
Diarrhea*				

*Parasympathetic response.

den stimulation and trauma of birth. Anxiety continues with the possibility that hunger and thirst might not be satisfied. Primary anxiety therefore is a state of tension or a drive produced by external causes. The environment is capable of threatening as well as satisfying. This implicit threat predisposes the person to anxiety in later life.

With increased age and ego development, a new kind of anxiety arises. Freud viewed this subsequent anxiety as the emotional conflict between two elements of the personality: the id and the superego. The id represents instinctual drives and primitive impulses. The superego reflects conscience and culturally acquired restrictions. The ego, or I, tries to mediate the demands of these two clashing elements. Freud therefore suggested that one major function of anxiety was to warn the person that the ego was in danger of being overtaken.

Interpersonal View. Sullivan (1953) disagreed with Freud. He believed that anxiety could not arise until the organism had some awareness of its environment. He believed that anxiety is first conveyed by the mother to the infant. The

infant responds as if he and his mother were one unit. As the child grows older, he sees this discomfort as a result of his own actions. He believes that his mother either approves or disapproves of his behavior. In addition, developmental traumas such as separations and losses can lead to specific vulnerabilities (Shear, 1996). Sullivan believed that anxiety in later life arises when a person perceives that he or she will be viewed unfavorably or will lose the love of a person he or she values.

A person's level of self-esteem is also an important factor related to anxiety. A person who is easily threatened or has a low level of self-esteem is more susceptible to anxiety. This is evident in students with test anxiety. Anxiety is high because they doubt they can succeed. This anxiety may have nothing to do with their actual abilities or how much they studied. The anxiety is caused only by their perception of their ability, which reflects their self-concept. They may be well prepared for the examination, but their severe level of anxiety reduces their perceptual field significantly. They may omit, misinterpret, or distort the meaning of the test items. They may even block out all their previous studying. The result will be a poor grade, which reinforces their poor perception of self.

Behavioral View. Some behavioral theorists propose that anxiety is a product of frustration caused by anything that interferes with attaining a desired goal. An example of an external frustration might be the loss of a job. Many goals may thus be blocked, such as financial security, pride in work, and perception of self as family provider. An internal frustration is evidenced by young college graduates who set unrealistically high career goals and are frustrated by entry-level job offers. In this case their view of self is threatened by their unrealistic goals. They are likely to experience feelings of failure, insignificance and mounting anxiety.

Other experimental psychologists believe that anxiety begins with the attachment of pain to a particular stimulus. If the reaction is strong enough, it may become generalized to similar objects and situations. Learning theorists believe that people who have been exposed in early life to intense fears are more likely to be anxious in later life. In this respect, parental influences are important. Children who see their parents respond with anxiety to every minor stress soon develop a similar pattern. Paradoxically, if parents are completely unmoved by potentially stressful situations, children feel alone and lack emotional support from their families. The appropriate emotional response of parents gives children security and helps them learn constructive coping methods.

Anxiety may also arise through conflict that occurs when the person experiences two competing drives and must choose between them. A reciprocal relationship exists between conflict and anxiety. Conflict produces anxiety, and anxiety increases the perception of conflict by producing feelings of helplessness. In this view, conflict derives from two tendencies: approach and avoidance. Approach is the tendency to do something or move toward something. Avoidance is the opposite tendency: not to do something or not to move toward something. There are four kinds of conflict:

- **Approach-approach,** in which the person wants to pursue two equally desirable but incompatible goals. This type of conflict seldom produces anxiety.
- **Approach-avoidance,** in which the person wishes to both pursue and avoid the same goal. The patient who wants to express anger but feels great anxiety and fear in doing so experiences this type of conflict. Another example is the ambitious business executive who must compromise values of honesty and loyalty to be promoted.
- **Avoidance-avoidance,** in which the person must choose between two undesirable goals. Because neither alternative seems beneficial, this is a difficult choice usually accompanied by much anxiety.
- **Double approach-avoidance,** in which the person can see both desirable and undesirable aspects of both al-

Citing the Evidence on

Use of Health Care

BACKGROUND: Patients with panic symptoms are heavy users of the health-care system, although many do not seek care specifically for those symptoms. This study documents the use of various sources of health care for those patients.

RESULTS: Subjects with panic symptoms had higher utilization rates for the services of psychiatrists and psychologists and for ambulance services than control subjects. The two groups did not differ in barriers to access, but the control group reported that their medical insurance covered more types of services.

IMPLICATIONS: This study supports the findings of heavy use of the health-care system by people with panic. This use is primarily to get help for panic symptoms. This heavy use occurs despite barriers to access to care and limitations in health insurance coverage.

Katerndahl D, Realini J: Use of health care services by persons with panic symptoms, *Psychiatr Serv* 48(8):1027, 1997.

ternatives. This kind of conflict is experienced by a person living with the pain of one's social and emotional life and destructive coping patterns. The alternative is to seek psychiatric help and expose oneself to the threat and potential pain of the therapy process. Double approach-avoidance conflict feelings are often described as ambivalence.

 Think of an example of each of the four kinds of conflict you have experienced in your life.

Family Studies. Epidemiological and family studies show that anxiety disorders run in families and that they are common and of different types. Anxiety disorders can overlap, as do anxiety disorders and depression. People with one anxiety disorder are more likely to develop another or to experience a major depression within their lifetime. It has been estimated that only about a quarter of those with anxiety disorders receive treatment. However, these people are high users of health-care facilities, as they seek treatment for the various symptoms caused by anxiety such as chest pain, palpitations, dizziness, and shortness of breath (see Citing the Evidence on Use of Health Care).

Biological Basis. There have been considerable advances in the understanding and treatment of anxiety disorders in the past 20 years (Antai-Otong, 2000). Some of the most recent developments are described in Chapter 6. For example, investigators have learned that the brain contains specific receptors for benzodiazepines and that these receptors help to regulate anxiety. This regulation of anxiety is related to the activity of the neurotransmitter gamma-aminobutyric acid (GABA), which controls the activity, or firing rates, of neurons in the parts of the brain responsible for producing anxiety. GABA is the most common inhibitory neurotransmitter in the brain. When it crosses the synapse and attaches or binds to the GABA receptor on the postsynaptic membrane, the receptor channel opens, allowing for the exchange of ions. This exchange results in an inhibition or reduction of cell excitability, and thus a slowing of cell activity. The theory is that people who have an excess of anxiety have a problem with the efficiency of this neurotransmission process.

When a person with anxiety takes a benzodiazepine (BZ) medication, which is from the antianxiety class of drugs, it binds to a place on the GABA receptor next to GABA. This makes the postsynaptic receptor more sensitive to the effects of GABA, enhancing neurotransmission and causing even more inhibition of cell activity (Fig. 17-3).

The GABA receptors to which BZs bind are concentrated in two areas of the brain: the limbic system, an area thought to be of central importance for emotional behavior; and the locus ceruleus, the primary manufacturing center of norepinephrine, which is an excitatory neurotransmitter. The effect of GABA and BZ at the GABA receptor in various parts of the brain is a reduced firing rate of cells in areas implicated in anxiety disorders. The clinical result is that the person becomes less anxious.

In the case of a person with one of the anxiety disorders, both BZs and antidepressant drugs are effective, indicating that these disorders may involve additional alterations in synaptic functioning in the norepinephrine and serotonin pathways in the brain and indicating that these two neurotransmitters have an effect on each other. Rigorous studies of drugs that relieve or produce anxiety should help provide additional information regarding the biological basis for anxiety disorders.

It has also been shown that a person's general health has a great effect on predisposition to anxiety. Anxiety may accompany some physical disorders such as those listed in Box 17-4. Coping mechanisms may also be impaired by toxic influences, dietary deficiencies, reduced blood supply, hormonal changes, and other physical causes. In addition, symptoms from some physical disorders may mimic or exacerbate anxiety.

Similarly, fatigue increases irritability and feelings of anxiety. It appears that fatigue caused by nervous factors predisposes the person to a greater degree of anxiety than does fatigue caused by purely physical causes. Thus fatigue may actually be an early symptom of anxiety. Patients complaining of nervous fatigue may already be suffering from moderate anxiety and be more susceptible to future stress situations.

Precipitating Stressors

Given these theories about the origin of anxiety, what kinds of events might precipitate feelings of anxiety? Clearly, experiencing or witnessing a source of trauma of any kind has been associated with a variety of anxiety disorders, particularly posttraumatic stress disorder (PTSD). Maturational and situational crises, as described in Chapter 14, can all precipitate a maladaptive anxiety response. These precipitating stressors can be grouped into two categories: threats to physical integrity and threats to self-system.

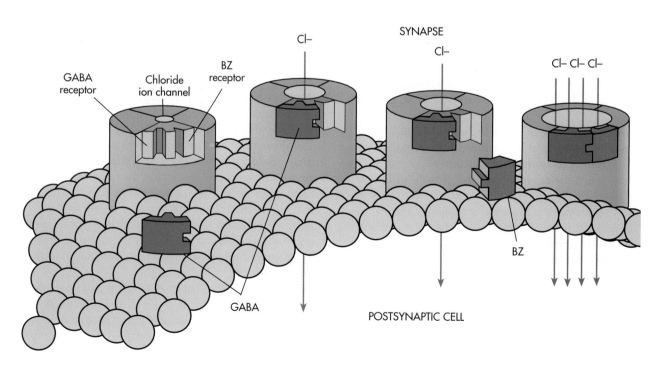

Fig. 17-3 Effects of GABA at the cellular level. *BZ,* Benzodiazepine drug; *Cl-,* chloride ion; *GABA,* gamma-aminobutyric acid.

Threats to Physical Integrity. These threats suggest impending physiological disability or decreased ability to perform the activities of daily living. They may include both internal and external sources. External sources may include exposure to viral and bacterial infection, environmental pollutants, safety hazards, lack of adequate housing, food, or clothing, and traumatic injury. Internal sources may include the failure of physiological mechanisms such as the heart, immune system, or temperature regulation. The normal biological changes that can occur with pregnancy and failure to participate in preventive health practices are other internal sources. Pain is often the first indication that physical integrity is being threatened. It creates anxiety that often motivates the person to seek health care.

Threats to Self-System. Threats in this second category imply harm to a person's identity, self-esteem and integrated social functioning. Both external and internal sources can threaten self-esteem. External sources may include the loss of a valued person through death, divorce or relocation, a change in job status, an ethical dilemma, and social or cultural group pressures. Internal sources may include interpersonal difficulties at home or at work or assuming a new role, such as parent, student or employee. In addition, many threats to physical integrity also threaten self-esteem because the mind-body relationship is an overlapping one.

This distinction of categories is only theoretical. The person responds to all stressors, whatever their nature and origin, as an integrated whole. No specific event is equally stressful to all people or even to the same person at different times.

Appraisal of Stressors

A true understanding of anxiety requires integration of knowledge from all the various points of view. The Stuart Stress Adaptation Model integrates data from psychoanalytical, interpersonal, behavioral, genetic, and biological perspectives. It suggests a variety of causative factors and emphasizes the relationship among them in explaining present behavior as described in Box 17-5.

Coping Resources

The person can cope with stress and anxiety by mobilizing coping resources in the environment. Such resources as economic assets, problem-solving abilities, social supports, and cultural beliefs can help the person integrate stressful experiences and adopt successful coping strategies. They can also help the person find meaning in the experience and suggest alternative strategies for mediating stressful events.

Box 17-4

Medical Disorders Associated with Anxiety

CARDIOVASCULAR/RESPIRATORY

Asthma
Cardiac arrhythmias
Chronic obstructive pulmonary disease
Congestive heart failure
Coronary insufficiency
Hyperdynamic beta-adrenergic state
Hypertension
Hyperventilation syndrome
Hypoxia, embolus, infections

ENDOCRINOLOGICAL

Carcinoid
Cushing's syndrome
Hyperthyroidism
Hypoglycemia
Hypoparathyroidism
Hypothyroidism
Menopause
Pheochromocytoma
Premenstrual syndrome

NEUROLOGICAL

Collagen vascular disease
Epilepsy
Huntington's disease
Multiple sclerosis
Organic brain syndrome
Vestibular dysfunction
Wilson's disease

SUBSTANCE RELATED
Intoxications

Anticholinergic drugs
Aspirin
Caffeine
Cocaine
Hallucinogens including phencyclidine ("angel dust")
Steroids
Sympathomimetics
THC

Withdrawal Syndromes

Alcohol
Narcotics
Sedative-hypnotics

Box 17-5

Causative Factors in Anxiety Disorders

- There is a built-in neurobiological substance that prepares the person to cope with danger.
- Evolution has affected this substance in such a way that stimuli threatening to survival are selectively avoided.
- People may be born with a central nervous system that is overly sensitive to stimuli that are generally harmless.
- Childhood and adult learning experiences may determine the extent, severity, and nature of the situations that will evoke anxiety.
- Chronic inability to cope with dangerous situations adaptively could increase the tendency to respond with anxiety.
- The cognitive functions might permit continual focusing on anxiety reactions, so the mere anticipation of aversive stimuli would provoke anxiety.
- Such a person might be more vulnerable to insecurities, especially if intelligent and introspective.

How might a person's religious or spiritual belief system serve as a resource in coping with a moderate level of anxiety?

Coping Mechanisms

As anxiety increases to the severe and panic levels, the behaviors displayed become more intense and potentially injurious, and quality of life decreases (see Citing the Evidence). People seek to avoid anxiety and the circumstances that produce it. When experiencing anxiety, people use various coping mechanisms to try to relieve it (see A Patient Speaks).

The inability to cope with anxiety constructively is a primary cause of pathological behavior. To neutralize, deny or counteract anxiety, the person develops patterns of coping. The pattern used to cope with mild anxiety dominates when anxiety becomes more intense. Anxiety plays a major role in the psychogenesis of emotional illness because many symptoms of illness develop as attempted defenses against anxiety.

The nurse needs to be familiar with the coping mechanisms people use when experiencing the various levels of anxiety. For **mild anxiety**, caused by the tension of day-to-day living, there are several coping mechanisms including crying, sleeping, eating, yawning, laughing, cursing, physical exercise, and daydreaming. Oral behavior, such as smoking and drinking, is another means of coping with mild anxiety. When dealing with other people, the individual copes with low levels of anxiety through superficiality, lack of eye contact, use of clichés, and limited self-disclosure. People can also protect themselves from anxiety by assuming comfortable roles and limiting close relationships to those with values similar to their own.

Citing the Evidence on

Quality of Life

BACKGROUND: This was an integrated review of studies that have investigated quality of life in patients with panic disorder, social phobia, posttraumatic stress disorder, generalized anxiety disorder, and obsessive-compulsive disorder.

RESULTS: The studies show a uniform picture of anxiety disorders as illnesses that markedly compromise quality of life and psychosocial functioning. Effective pharmacological or psychotherapeutic treatment has been shown to improve the quality of life for these patients.

IMPLICATIONS: A more thorough understanding of the impact of quality of life may lead to increased public awareness of anxiety disorders as serious mental illnesses worthy of further investment in research, prevention, and treatment.

Mendlowicz M, Stein M: Quality of life in individuals with anxiety disorders, *Am J Psychiatry* 157(5):669, 2000.

Moderate, severe, and panic levels of anxiety pose greater threats to the ego. They require more energy to cope with the threat. These coping mechanisms can be categorized as task-oriented and ego-oriented reactions.

Task-Oriented Reactions. Task-oriented reactions are thoughtful, deliberate attempts to solve problems, resolve conflicts, and gratify needs. They are aimed at realistically meeting the demands of a stress situation that has been objectively appraised. They are consciously directed and action oriented. These reactions can include attack, withdrawal, and compromise.

In **attack behavior** a person attempts to remove or overcome obstacles to satisfy a need. There are many possible ways of attacking problems, and this type of reaction may be destructive or constructive. Destructive patterns are usually accompanied by great feelings of anger and hostility. These feelings may be expressed by negative or aggressive behavior that violates the rights, property, and well-being of others. Constructive patterns reflect a problem-solving approach. They are evident in self-assertive behaviors that respect the rights of others.

Withdrawal behavior may be expressed physically or psychologically. Physically, withdrawal involves removing oneself from the source of the threat. This reaction can apply to biological stressors, such as smoke-filled rooms, exposure to irradiation, or contact with contagious diseases. A person

A Patient Speaks

It's hard to describe what it feels like. You know something isn't right. Most people don't have to check their doors five or six times before they go to bed. Most people aren't afraid to be near children or feel like they have to count their money over and over again before they can put it back in their wallet. But that's the way my life has been ever since I was a little girl.

Of course I realized I needed help, so I saw a number of different professionals. With one psychologist we discussed every aspect of my childhood and my earliest memories of life. Unfortunately, I finished that therapy still counting everything around me. Next I went to a physician, but he told me that I was just nervous about getting married and things would get better with time. They didn't. Then my mother suggested I go to the university and see someone. That's where I met the psychiatric nurse who did a number of things I'll always remember. First she put me at ease and clearly told me that I wasn't crazy. Then she told me that what I had was obsessive-compulsive disorder and gave me lots of great books and information to read. Finally, she told me that it was a treatable illness and together we devised a treatment plan. It included both medication and behavioral therapy and wow, what a difference! I'm sure glad I was persistent, but I'm even more glad that there are caring professionals out there who can really help.

can also withdraw in various psychological ways, such as by admitting defeat, becoming apathetic, or lowering aspirations. As with attack, this type of reaction may be constructive or destructive. When it isolates the person from others and interferes with the ability to work, the reaction creates additional problems.

Compromise is necessary in situations that cannot be resolved through attack or withdrawal. This reaction involves changing usual ways of operating, substituting goals, or sacrificing aspects of personal needs. Compromise reactions are usually constructive and are often used in approach-approach and avoidance-avoidance situations. Occasionally, however, the person realizes with time that the compromise is not acceptable; a solution must then be renegotiated or a different coping mechanism adopted.

The capacity for task-oriented reactions and effective problem solving is influenced by the person's expectation of at least partial success. This prediction in turn depends on remembering past successes in similar situations. On this basis it is possible to go forward and deal with the current stressful situation. Perseverance in problem solving also depends on the person's expectation of a certain level of pain and discomfort and on the belief in being capable of tolerating the problem. Here lies the balance between courage and anxiety.

> *What coping mechanisms do you use when you are mildly, moderately, and severely anxious? How adaptive or maladaptive are they?*

Ego-Oriented Reactions. Task-oriented reactions are not always successful in coping with stressful situations. Consequently, ego-oriented reactions are often used to protect the self. These reactions, also called ego defense mechanisms, are the first line of psychic defense. Everyone uses defense mechanisms, and they often help people cope successfully with mild and moderate levels of anxiety. They protect the person from feelings of inadequacy and worthlessness and prevent awareness of anxiety. However, they can be used to such an extreme degree that they distort reality, interfere with interpersonal relationships, and limit the ability to work productively.

As coping mechanisms, they have certain drawbacks. First, ego-oriented reactions operate on unconscious levels. The person has little awareness of what is happening and little control over events. Second, they involve a degree of self-deception and reality distortion. Therefore, they usually do not help the person to cope with the problem realistically. Table 17-1 lists some of the more common ego defense mechanisms with an example of each.

The evaluation of whether the patient's use of certain defense mechanisms is adaptive or maladaptive involves four issues:

- The accurate recognition of the patient's use of the defense mechanism by the nurse.
- The degree to which the defense mechanism is used. Does it imply a high degree of personality disorganization? Is the person unresponsive to facts about his or her life situation?
- The degree to which use of the defense mechanism interferes with the patient's functioning and his or her progress toward health.
- The reason the patient used the ego defense mechanism.

The nurse will better understand the patient and plan more effective nursing care after considering these areas.

Many coping mechanisms can be used to minimize anxiety. Some of them are essential for emotional stability. The exact nature and number of the defenses used strongly influence the personality pattern. When these defenses are overused or used unsuccessfully, they cause many physiological and psychological symptoms commonly associated with emotional illness.

NURSING DIAGNOSIS

The nurse who has adequately assessed a patient and uses the Stuart Stress Adaptation Model can formulate a nursing diagnosis based on the patient's position on the continuum of anxiety responses (Fig. 17-4).

Initially the nurse needs to determine the quality and quantity of the anxiety experienced by the patient. In considering the quality of the anxiety, the nurse might question the appropriateness of the patient's response to the perceived threat. Is it adaptive or irrational? A problem may exist if the response is out of proportion to the threat. This disproportionate response would indicate that the patient's cognitive appraisal of the threat is unrealistic. The quantity of the reaction is the next consideration. When anxiety reaches the severe and panic levels, it indicates that the conflict is increasingly problematic for the patient.

The nurse also needs to explore how the patient is coping with the anxiety. Constructive coping mechanisms are protective responses that consciously confront the threat. Destructive coping mechanisms involve repression into the unconscious. They tend to be ineffective, inadequate, disorganized, inappropriate, and exaggerated. They may be evident in bizarre behavior or symptom formation.

Finally, the nurse needs to determine the overall effect of the anxiety. Is it stimulating growth? Or is it interfering with effective living and life satisfaction? Is it enhancing one's sense of self? Or is it depersonalizing? Whenever possible, the patient should be included in identifying problem areas. This involvement may not always be feasible, however, particularly if the patient's anxiety is at the severe or panic level.

There are three primary NANDA nursing diagnoses concerned with anxiety responses: **anxiety, ineffective coping,** and **fear.** Many additional nursing problems may be identified from the way the patient's anxiety reciprocally influences interpersonal relationships, self-concept, cognitive functioning, physiological status, and other aspects of life.

Nursing diagnoses related to the range of possible maladaptive responses and related medical diagnoses are identified in the Medical and Nursing Diagnoses box on p. 285. The primary NANDA nursing diagnoses and examples of complete nursing diagnoses are presented in the Detailed Diagnoses box on p. 286.

Table **17-1**

Ego Defense Mechanisms

Defense Mechanism	Example
Compensation: Process by which a person makes up for a perceived deficiency by strongly emphasizing a feature that he or she regards as an asset.	A businessman perceives his small physical stature negatively. He tries to overcome this by being aggressive, forceful, and controlling in business dealings.
Denial: Avoidance of disagreeable realities by ignoring or refusing to recognize them; the simplest and most primitive of all defense mechanisms.	Mrs. P has just been told that her breast biopsy indicates a malignancy. When her husband visits her that evening, she tells him that no one has discussed the laboratory results with her.
Displacement: Shift of emotion from a person or object to another, usually neutral or less dangerous person or object.	A 4-year-old boy is angry because he has just been punished by his mother for drawing on his bedroom walls. He begins to play war with his soldier toys and has them fight with each other.
Dissociation: The separation of a group of mental or behavioral processes from the rest of the person's consciousness or identity.	A man is brought to the emergency room by the police and is unable to explain who he is and where he lives or works.
Identification: Process by which a person tries to become like someone he or she admires by taking on thoughts, mannerisms, or tastes of that person.	Sally, 15 years old, has her hair styled like that of her young English teacher, whom she admires.
Intellectualization: Excessive reasoning or logic is used to avoid experiencing disturbing feelings.	A woman avoids dealing with her anxiety in shopping malls by explaining that shopping is a frivolous waste of time and money.
Introjection: Intense identification in which a person incorporates qualities or values of another person or group into his or her own ego structure. It is one of the earliest mechanisms of the child, important in formation of conscience.	Eight-year-old Jimmy tells his 3-year-old sister, "Don't scribble in your book of nursery rhymes. Just look at the pretty pictures," thus expressing his parents' values.
Isolation: Splitting off of emotional components of a thought, which may be temporary or long term.	A second-year medical student dissects a cadaver for her anatomy course without being disturbed by thoughts of death.
Projection: Attributing one's thoughts or impulses to another person. Through this process one can attribute intolerable wishes, emotional feelings, or motivations to another person.	A young woman who denies she has sexual feelings about a co-worker accuses him without basis of trying to seduce her.
Rationalization: Offering a socially acceptable or apparently logical explanation to justify or make acceptable otherwise unacceptable impulses, feelings, behaviors, and motives.	John fails an examination and complains that the lectures were not well organized or clearly presented.
Reaction formation: Development of conscious attitudes and behavior patterns that are opposite to what one really feels or would like to do.	A married woman who feels attracted to one of her husband's friends treats him rudely.
Regression: Retreat to behavior characteristic of an earlier level of development.	Four-year-old Nicole, who has been toilet trained for over a year, begins to wet her pants again when her new baby brother is brought home from the hospital.
Repression: Involuntary exclusion of a painful or conflictual thought, impulse, or memory from awareness. It is the primary ego defense, and other mechanisms tend to reinforce it.	Mr. R does not recall hitting his wife when she was pregnant.
Splitting: Viewing people and situations as either all good or all bad. Failure to integrate the positive and negative qualities of oneself.	A friend tells you that you are the most wonderful person in the world one day, and how much she hates you the next day.
Sublimation: Acceptance of a socially approved substitute goal for a drive whose normal channel of expression is blocked.	Ed has an impulsive and physically aggressive nature. He tries out for the football team and becomes a star tackle.
Suppression: A process often listed as a defense mechanism but really a conscious counterpart of repression. It is intentional exclusion of material from consciousness. At times, it may lead to repression.	A young man at work finds he is thinking so much about his date that evening that it is interfering with his work. He decides to put it out of his mind until he leaves the office for the day.
Undoing: Act or communication that partially negates a previous one; a primitive defense mechanism.	Larry makes a passionate declaration of love to Sue on a date. On their next meeting he treats her formally and distantly.

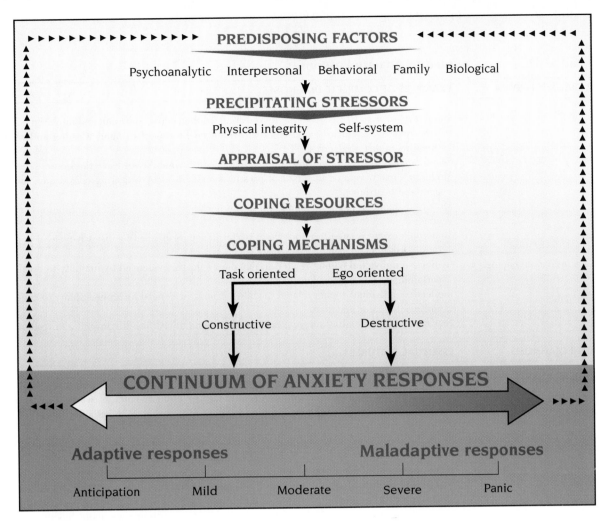

Fig. 17-4 The Stuart Stress Adaptation Model related to anxiety responses.

Medical and Nursing Diagnoses *related to* Anxiety Responses

RELATED MEDICAL DIAGNOSES (*DSM–IV–TR*)*	RELATED NURSING DIAGNOSES (NANDA)†
Panic disorder without agoraphobia	Adjustment, impaired
Panic disorder with agoraphobia	**Anxiety‡**
Agoraphobia without panic attacks	Breathing pattern, ineffective
Specific phobia	Communication, impaired verbal
Social phobia	Community coping, ineffective
Obsessive-compulsive disorder	Confusion, acute
Posttraumatic stress disorder	**Coping, ineffective individual‡**
Acute stress disorder	Diarrhea
Generalized anxiety disorder	**Fear‡**
	Health maintenance, altered
	Injury, risk for
	Memory, impaired
	Nutrition, altered
	Posttrauma syndrome
	Powerlessness
	Self-esteem disturbance
	Sensory/perceptual alterations
	Sleep pattern disturbance
	Social interaction, impaired
	Thought processes, altered
	Urinary elimination, altered patterns

*Reprinted with permission from *Diagnostic and statistical manual of mental disorders*, Fourth Edition, Text Revision, Copyright 2000, the American Psychiatric Association.
†From North American Nursing Diagnosis Association: *NANDA nursing diagnoses: definitions and classifications 1999-2000*, Philadelphia, 1999, The Association.
‡Primary nursing diagnosis for anxiety.

Detailed Diagnoses *related to* Anxiety Responses

NANDA DIAGNOSIS STEM	EXAMPLES OF COMPLETE DIAGNOSES
Anxiety	Panic level of anxiety related to family rejection, evidenced by confusion and impaired judgment.
	Severe anxiety related to sexual conflict, evidenced by repetitive hand washing and recurrent thoughts of dirt and germs.
	Severe anxiety related to marital conflict, evidenced by inability to leave the house.
	Moderate anxiety related to financial pressures, evidenced by recurring episodes of abdominal pain and heartburn.
	Moderate anxiety related to assumption of motherhood role, evidenced by inhibition and avoidance.
	Moderate anxiety related to poor school performance, evidenced by excessive use of denial and rationalization.
Ineffective individual coping	Ineffective individual coping related to daughter's death, evidenced by inability to recall events pertaining to the car accident.
	Ineffective individual coping related to child's illness, evidenced by limited ability to concentrate and psychomotor agitation.
Fear	Fear related to impending surgery, evidenced by generalized hostility to staff and restlessness.

DSM–IV–TR DIAGNOSIS	ESSENTIAL FEATURES*
Panic disorder without agoraphobia	Recurrent unexpected panic attacks (Box 17-6), with at least one of the attacks followed by a month (or more) of persistent concern about having additional attacks, worry about the implications of the attack or its consequences, or a significant change in behavior related to the attacks. Also the absence of agoraphobia.
Panic disorder with agoraphobia	Meets the above criteria. In addition, the presence of agoraphobia, which is anxiety about being in places or situations from which escape might be difficult or embarrassing or in which help may not be available in the event of a panic attack. Agoraphobic fears typically involve characteristic clusters of situations that include being outside the home alone, being in a crowd or standing in a line, being on a bridge, and traveling in a bus, train, or car. Agoraphobic situations are avoided, or endured with marked distress or with anxiety about having a panic attack, or require the presence of a companion.
Agoraphobia without history of panic disorder	The presence of agoraphobia without meeting criteria for panic disorder.
Specific phobia	Marked and persistent fear that is excessive or unreasonable, cued by the presence or anticipation of a specific object or situation (such as flying, heights, animals, receiving an injection, or seeing blood). Exposure to the phobic stimulus almost invariably provokes an immediate anxiety response. The person recognizes the fear is excessive, and the distress or avoidance interferes with the person's normal routine.
Social phobia	A marked and persistent fear of social or performance situations in which the person is exposed to unfamiliar people or to possible scrutiny by others. The person fears that he or she will act in a way (or show anxiety symptoms) that will be humiliating or embarrassing. Exposure to the feared situation almost invariably provokes anxiety. The person recognizes the fear is excessive, and the distress or avoidance interferes with the person's normal routine.
Obsessive-compulsive disorder	Either obsessions or compulsions (Box 17-7) are recognized as excessive and interfere with the person's normal routine.
Posttraumatic stress disorder	The person has been exposed to a traumatic event in which both of the following were present: The person has experienced, witnessed, or been confronted with an event that involved actual or threatened death or serious injury, or a threat to the physical integrity of oneself or others. The person's response involved intense fear, helplessness, or horror. The traumatic event is re-experienced, and there is an avoidance of stimuli associated with the trauma and a numbing of general responsiveness.
Acute stress disorder	Meets the criteria for exposure to a traumatic event and experiences three of the following symptoms: sense of detachment, reduced awareness of one's surroundings, derealization, depersonalization, and dissociated amnesia
Generalized anxiety disorder	Excessive anxiety and worry, occurring more days than not for at least 6 months, about a number of events or activities. The person finds it difficult to control the worry and experiences at least three of the following symptoms: restlessness or feeling keyed up or on edge, fatigue, difficulty concentrating or mind going blank, irritability, muscle tension, sleep disturbance.

*Reprinted with permission from the *Diagnostic and statistical manual of mental disorders*, Fourth Edition, Text Revision, Copyright 2000, American Psychiatric Association.

Box **17-6**

Panic Attack Criteria

A panic attack is a discrete period of intense fear or discomfort in which at least four of the following symptoms develop abruptly and reach a peak within 10 minutes:

- Palpitations, pounding heart, or accelerated heart rate
- Sweating
- Trembling or shaking
- Sensations of shortness of breath or smothering
- Feeling of choking
- Chest pain or discomfort
- Nausea or abdominal distress
- Feeling dizzy, unsteady, lightheaded or faint
- Derealization (feelings of unreality) or depersonalization (being detached from oneself)
- Fear of losing control or going crazy
- Fear of dying
- Paresthesias (numbness or tingling sensations)
- Chills or hot flushes

Box **17-7**

Obsession and Compulsion Criteria

OBSESSION

Recurrent and persistent thoughts, impulses, or images are experienced during the disturbance as intrusive and inappropriate and cause marked anxiety or distress.

The thoughts, impulses, or images are not simply excessive worries about real-life problems.

The person attempts to ignore or suppress such thoughts or impulses or to neutralize them with some other thought or action.

The person recognizes that the obsessional thought, impulses, or images are a product of one's own mind.

COMPULSION

The person feels driven to perform repetitive behaviors (such as hand washing, ordering, checking) or mental acts (such as praying, counting, repeating words silently) in response to an obsession or according to rules that must be applied rigidly.

The behaviors or mental acts are aimed at preventing or reducing distress or preventing some dreaded event or situation; however, these behaviors or mental acts either are not connected in a realistic way with what they are designed to neutralize or prevent or are clearly excessive.

Related Medical Diagnoses

Many patients with mild or moderate anxiety have no medically diagnosed health problem. However, patients with more severe levels of anxiety usually have neurotic disorders that fall under the category of anxiety disorders in the *DSM-IV–TR* (American Psychiatric Association, 2000). A neurosis is a mental disorder characterized by anxiety that involves no distortion of reality. Neurotic disorders are maladaptive anxiety responses associated with moderate and severe levels of anxiety.

Psychosis is disintegrative and involves a significant distortion of reality. It can emerge with the panic level of anxiety. Psychotic people feel they are "breaking into pieces." They fear they are failing in the process of living and in the process of being (see Chapter 22).

The nurse must also discriminate between anxiety and other disorders. For example, a relationship has been established between anxiety disorders and alcohol use disorders (Kushner et al, 1999). So too, anxiety and depression often overlap because anxious patients are often depressed and depressed patients are often anxious. For example, both anxious and depressed patients share the following symptoms: sleep disturbances, appetite changes, nonspecific cardiopulmonary and gastrointestinal complaints, difficulty concentrating, irritability, and fatigue or lack of energy. Yet there are often discrete (if subtle) differences between the two groups. These are described in Box 17-8.

Also, posttraumatic stress disorder (PTSD) is rarely a patient's only psychiatric diagnosis and it is sometimes difficult to distinguish overlapping independent symptoms from effects of the trauma. Nearly half of all people with PTSD also suffer from major depression, and more than a third from phobias and alcoholism (Harvard Mental Health Letter, 1996). Behavior that results from child abuse may also take the form of a personality disorder, and the symptoms of PTSD are occasionally mistaken for psychotic illness or an organic brain syndrome. This similarity among these disorders has raised questions regarding the diagnosis of PTSD and how prevalent it is (see Critical Thinking about Contemporary Issues).

Finally, about 25% of people will experience an anxiety disorder sometime in their life. These are the most common psychiatric disorders in American society. Specifically, obsessive-compulsive disorder (OCD) affects about 2% of the U.S. population; generalized anxiety disorder (GAD) about 3% to 4%; phobias between 13% to 15%; panic disorder about 1% to 2%; and posttraumatic stress disorder (PTSD) about 8% of the population.

Anxiety disorders occur twice as often in women as in men, and obsessive-compulsive disorder is about equally prevalent in women and men. No outstanding differences in the prevalence of anxiety disorders have been found on the basis of race, income, education, or rural versus urban dwelling.

The essential features of the medical diagnoses related to anxiety responses are presented in the Detailed Diagnoses box on p. 286.

OUTCOME IDENTIFICATION

Goals such as "decrease anxiety" and "minimize anxiety" lack specific behaviors and evaluation criteria. Therefore, these goals are not particularly useful in guiding nursing care and evaluating its effectiveness. The expected outcome for patients with maladaptive anxiety responses is as follows:

The patient will demonstrate adaptive ways of coping with stress.

Short-term goals can break this down into readily attainable steps. This identification of steps allows the patient and nurse to see progress even if the ultimate goal still appears distant.

Box **17-8**

Differences between Anxiety and Depression

ANXIETY

Predominantly fear or apprehension
Difficulty falling asleep (initial insomnia)
Phobic avoidance behavior
Rapid pulse and psychomotor hyperactivity
Breathing disturbances
Tremors and palpitations
Sweating and hot or cold spells
Faintness, lightheadedness, dizziness
Depersonalization (feeling detached from one's body)
Derealization (feeling that one's environment is strange, unreal, or unfamiliar)
Selective and specific negative appraisals that do not include all areas of life
Sees some prospects for the future
Does not regard defects or mistakes as irrevocable
Uncertain in negative evaluations
Predicts that only certain events may go badly

DEPRESSION

Predominantly sad or hopeless with feelings of despair
Early morning awakening (late insomnia) or hypersomnia
Diurnal variation (feels worse in the morning)
Slowed speech and thought processes
Delayed response time
Psychomotor retardation (agitation may also occur)
Loss of interest in usual activities
Inability to experience pleasure
Thoughts of death or suicide
Negative appraisals are pervasive, global, and exclusive
Sees the future as blank and has given up all hope
Regards mistakes as beyond redemption
Absolute in negative evaluations
Global view that nothing will turn out right

CRITICAL THINKING about CONTEMPORARY ISSUES

Is PTSD in Danger of Becoming Merely a Fashionable Diagnosis That Removes Responsibility for Personal Behavior by Projecting Blame onto Common Traumatic Events?

Epidemiological data show that PTSD is more unusual than usual following exposure to a variety of traumatic events. Research also shows the existence of risk factors other than trauma as predictors of PTSD, and questions have been raised about the differences between people who experience traumatic events and cope adaptively and those who develop PTSD (Classen et al, 1998). Other issues have been raised related to the symptoms of PTSD because they may appear immediately after the event or years later. They can remain for less than a month or for many months, or sometimes even years. Other areas of controversy include whether one has to experience the event directly or whether indirect exposure is sufficient, and whether it needs to be an extreme form of trauma and how **extreme** is defined. These questions have led to complaints that PTSD is simply an excuse to obtain disability benefits, win personal injury lawsuits, or evade responsibility for crimes (Resnick, 1998).

The decision to establish PTSD as a diagnosis 15 years ago recognized the rights and needs of victims who were stigmatized, misunderstood, or ignored by the mental health field and it helped to make sense of their suffering. There is considerable evidence that traumatic experiences are associated with PTSD symptoms and that the related symptoms can be very disabling. Current research is revealing interesting findings about the neurobiology of PTSD and the fact that it does not follow the stress response described by Selye, but may be a progressive sensitization of biological systems that leave the person hyperresponsive to a variety of stimuli (Yehuda & McFarlane, 1995).

Clearly, PTSD is an evolving concept. But the controversy surrounding this diagnosis is likely to continue as long as there are questions about what kinds of events are traumatic, how they are perceived and interpreted, and how personal coping resources and coping responses differ.

When the nursing diagnosis describes the patient's anxiety at the severe or panic levels, the highest-priority short-term goals should address lowering the anxiety level. Only after this decreased anxiety has been achieved can additional progress be made. The reduced level of anxiety should be evident in a reduction of behaviors associated with severe or panic levels. Following are examples of short-term goals for a particular patient.

After 4 days Mr. Jones will:

- Attend and remain seated during all meetings
- Participate at least three times during each meeting
- Discuss one topic for a minimum of 10 minutes when meeting with his nurse

- Attend all occupational therapy sessions
- Sleep a minimum of 6 hours a night

When these goals are met, the nurse can assume that the patient's level of anxiety has been reduced. The nurse may then develop new short-term goals directed toward insight or relaxation therapy. In addition, since anxiety is a subjective response, a useful measure would be to ask the patient to rate his level of anxiety from 1 to 10. Obtaining a rating of 2 or 3 might be another expected outcome.

PLANNING

The main goal of the nurse working with anxious patients is not to free them totally from anxiety. Patients need to develop the capacity to tolerate mild anxiety and to use it consciously and constructively. In this way the self will become stronger and more integrated. As they learn from these experiences, they will move on in their development.

Anxiety can be considered a war between the threat and the values people identify with their existence. Maladaptive behavior means that the struggle has been lost. The constructive approach to anxiety means that the struggle is won by the person's values. Thus a general nursing goal is to help patients develop sound values. This approach does not mean that patients assume the nurse's values. Rather, the nurse helps the patient to sort out his or her own values.

Anxiety can also be an important factor in the patient's decision to seek treatment. Because anxiety is undesirable, the patient will seek ways to reduce it. If the patient's coping mechanism or symptom does not minimize anxiety, the motivation for treatment increases. Conversely, anxiety about the therapeutic process can delay or prevent the person from seeking treatment.

The patient should actively participate in planning treatment strategies. If the patient is actively involved in identifying relevant stressors and planning possible solutions, the success of the implementation phase will be maximized. A patient in extreme anxiety initially will not be able to participate in the problem-solving process. However, as soon as anxiety is reduced, the nurse should encourage patient involvement. This participation reinforces that patients are responsible for their own growth and personal development.

IMPLEMENTATION

Practice guidelines have been developed to treat a variety of anxiety disorders (American Psychiatric Association, 1998; March et al, 1998). Empirically validated treatments for some of the medical diagnoses related to anxiety disorders are summarized in Table 17-2.

Severe and Panic Levels of Anxiety

Establishing a Trusting Relationship. The patient with severe or panic levels of anxiety may need inpatient treatment or partial hospitalization (Bystrisky et al, 1996). To reduce the patient's level of anxiety, most nursing actions are supportive and protective. Initially nurses need to establish an open, trusting relationship. Nurses should actively listen to patients and encourage them to discuss their feelings of anxiety, hostility, guilt, and frustration. Nurses should answer patients' questions directly and offer unconditional acceptance. Their verbal and nonverbal communications should convey awareness and acceptance of patients' feelings. Nurses should remain available and respect the patient's personal space. A 6-foot distance in a small room may create the optimum condition for openness and discussion of fears. The more this distance is increased or decreased, the more anxious the patient may become (Brown & Yantis, 1996).

Nurses' Self-Awareness. Nurses' feelings are particularly important in working with highly anxious patients.

They may find themselves being unsympathetic, impatient, and frustrated. These are common feelings of reciprocal anxiety. If nurses are alert to the development of anxiety in themselves, they can learn from it and use it therapeutically. Nurses should be alert to the signs of anxiety in themselves, accept them, and attempt to explore their cause. The nurse may ask the following questions:

- What is threatening me?
- Have I failed to live up to what I imagine to be the patient's ideal?
- Am I comparing myself to a peer or another health professional?
- Is the patient's area of conflict one that I have not resolved in myself?
- Is my anxiety related to something that will or may happen in the future? Is my patient's conflict really one of my own that I am projecting?

If nurses deny their own anxiety, it can have detrimental effects on the nurse-patient relationship. Because of their own anxiety, nurses may be unable to differentiate between levels of anxiety in others. They may also transfer their fears and frustrations to patients, thus compounding their problem. Finally, nurses who are anxious arouse defenses in patients and other staff that interfere with their therapeutic usefulness. Nurses should strive to accept their patients' anxiety without reciprocal anxiety by continually clarifying their own feelings and role, as indicated in the following clinical example.

 CLINICAL EXAMPLE

Ms. R was a 35-year-old married woman and mother of three children, ages 4, 6, and 9. She was a full-time homemaker and mother. Her husband was a salesperson and spent about 2 nights each week out of town. She came to the clinic complaining of severe headaches that "come upon me very suddenly and are so terrible that I have to go to bed. The only thing that helps is for me to lie down in a dark and absolutely quiet room." She said that these headaches were becoming a real problem for everyone in the family, and her husband told her that she "just had to get over them and get things back to normal."

Mr. W, a psychiatric nurse, offered to see Ms. R in therapy once a week. After 3 weeks, he was asked to present his evaluation, treatment plans and progress report to the clinic staff at their weekly team conference. Mr. W began his presentation by stating, "This case is really a tough nut to crack. I'll start with the progress report and say that there is none because I can't seem to get past all the complaining this patient does!" He then went on to discuss his evaluation and treatment plan in depth. It became obvious to the other members of the staff that Mr. W saw his patient as a woman who was not living up to her roles and responsibilities. He defended Ms. R's husband even though the husband refused to come to the sessions with his wife. When the psychiatrist asked about the possibility of a medication evaluation for Ms. R, the nurse replied, "Everyone gets headaches. I don't think we should reward or reinforce this woman's complaints."

In reviewing this case the staff noted that Mr. W appeared to have problems relating empathetically to his patient because of her

Table **17-2**

Summarizing the Evidence on Anxiety Disorders

DISORDER:	Generalized anxiety disorder
TREATMENT:	■ Most treatment outcome studies have shown active treatments to be superior to nondirective approaches, and uniformly superior to no treatment; however, most of these studies failed to demonstrate differential rates of efficacy among active treatments ■ Recent studies suggested cognitive-behavioral therapy (combining relaxation exercises and cognitive therapy), with the goal of bringing the worry process under control, to be most efficacious ■ The benzodiazepines reduced the anxiety and worry symptoms of GAD ■ Buspirone appeared comparable to the benzodiazepines in alleviating GAD symptoms ■ The tricyclic antidepressants have been useful in the treatment of GAD
DISORDER:	Obsessive compulsive disorder (OCD)
TREATMENT:	■ Cognitive-behavioral therapy involving exposure and ritual prevention methods reduced or eliminated the obsessions and behavioral and mental rituals of OCD ■ Approximately 40% to 60% of OCD patients respond to serotonergic reuptake inhibitors (SRIs), including clomipramine, fluvoxamine, paroxetine, fluoxetine and sertraline, with mean improvement in obsessions and compulsions of approximately 20% to 40%
DISORDER:	Panic disorder with and without agoraphobia
TREATMENT:	■ Situational in vivo exposure substantially reduced symptoms of panic disorder with agoraphobia ■ Cognitive-behavioral treatments that focused on education about the nature of anxiety and panic and provided some form of exposure and coping skills acquisition significantly reduced symptoms of panic disorder without agoraphobia ■ Tricyclic antidepressants and monoamine oxidase inhibitors reduced the number of panic attacks and also reduced anticipatory anxiety and phobic avoidance, although side effects caused some patients to drop from clinical trials ■ The benzodiazepines (e.g., Alprazolam) eliminated panic attacks in 55% to 75% of patients ■ More recently, serotonin reuptake inhibitors (SRIs), and selective serotonin reuptake inhibitors (SSRIs), have produced reductions in panic frequency, generalized anxiety, disability and phobic avoidance
DISORDER:	Posttraumatic stress disorder (PTSD)
TREATMENT:	■ Monoamine oxidase inhibitors (MAOIs) reduced intrusive thoughts, improved sleep, and moderated anxiety and depression in PTSD patients ■ Tricyclic antidepressants reduced intrusive thoughts and obsessions and moderated depression in these patients ■ Selective serotonin reuptake inhibitors (SSRIs) markedly reduced intrusive thoughts, avoidance, and sleep problems ■ Exposure therapies (systematic desensitization, flooding, prolonged exposure and implosive therapy) and, to a lesser extent, anxiety management techniques (using cognitive-behavioral strategies) reduced PTSD symptoms, including anxiety and depression, and increased social functioning

From: Nathan P, Gorman J: *A guide to treatments that work*, New York, 1998, Oxford University Press.

particular set of problems and some of his own values and perceptions. Mr. W agreed with this and said he had thought of asking someone else to work with Ms. R. Mr. W's supervisor observed that the nurse had problems with this type of patient in the past, and a more constructive approach would be to increase his supervision on this case, focusing on the dynamics between the patient and nurse that were blocking learning and growth for both of them. Mr. W and his supervisor set a time when they could begin to meet for this purpose.

What clinical situations or patient problems raise your anxiety?

Protecting the Patient. Another major area of intervention is protecting and reassuring the patient of his or her safety. One way to decrease anxiety is by allowing the patient to determine the amount of stress he or she can handle at the time. Nurses should not force severely anxious patients into situations they are not able to handle. They should also not attack their coping mechanisms or try to strip them of these. Rather, nurses should attempt to protect patients' defenses.

The coping mechanism or symptom is attempting to deal with an unconscious conflict. Usually patients do not understand why the symptom has developed or what they are gaining from it. They know only that the symptom relieves some of the intolerable anxiety and tension. If they are unable to release this anxiety, their tension mounts to the panic level and they could lose control. It is also important to remember that the severely anxious patient has not worked through the area of conflict and therefore has no alternatives or substitutes for present coping mechanisms.

This principle also applies to severe levels of anxiety, such as obsessive-compulsive reactions, phobias, and panic attacks. Nurses should not initially interfere with the repetitive act or force patients to confront the avoided situation or phobic object. They should not ridicule the nature of the defense. Also, nurses should not attempt to argue with patients about it or reason them out of it. Patients need their coping mechanisms to keep anxiety within tolerable limits. Neither should nurses reinforce the phobia, ritual, avoidance, or physical complaint by focusing attention on it and talking about it a great deal. With time, however, nurses can place some limits on patients' behavior and attempt to help them find satisfaction with other aspects of life.

Modifying the Environment. The nurse can consult with others to identify anxiety-producing situations and attempt to reduce them. The nurse can set limits by assuming a quiet, calm manner and decreasing environmental stimulation. Limiting the patient's interaction with other patients will minimize the contagious aspects of anxiety. Supportive physical measures such as warm baths, massages or whirlpool baths may also be helpful in decreasing a patient's anxiety.

Encouraging Activity. The nurse needs to encourage the patient's interest in activities. This involvement limits the time available for destructive coping mechanisms and increases participation in and enjoyment of other aspects of life. The nurse might suggest physical activities such as walking, a sport or an active hobby. This form of physical exercise helps to relieve anxiety because it provides an emotional release and directs the patient's attention outward. Family members should be involved in the planning because they can be very supportive in setting limits and stimulating outside activity (see A Family Speaks).

Some nursing interventions can increase anxiety in severely anxious patients. These include pressuring the patient to change prematurely, being judgmental, verbally disapproving of the patient's behaviors, and asking the patient a direct question that brings on defensiveness. Focusing in a critical way on the patient's anxious feelings with others present, lacking awareness of one's own behaviors and feelings, and withdrawing from the patient can also be harmful.

Medication. Nursing intervention may include the administration of medications to the highly anxious patient (Table 17-3). Because anxiety is a pervasive problem, large portions of the population take antianxiety drugs. Americans are now spending more than $500 million each year for drugs to relieve anxiety. Among these drugs, the benzodiazepines are often the medication of choice and are the most widely prescribed drugs in the world. They have almost replaced the barbiturates in the treatment of anxiety because of their effectiveness and wide margin of

A Family Speaks

My daughter has obsessive-compulsive disorder (OCD). I didn't always know that, and I've spent many years of my life wondering what was wrong with her and if I were to blame. It's not easy living with someone who has an illness like that. At times it is just annoying. At other times it really makes you mad, and still other times you want to burst out laughing, but all that only makes it worse.

I think the one thing the family needs from the mental health-care system is for health-care professionals to talk with them. The nurse who sees my daughter told me that I can call her with questions, and she explained all about OCD to my husband and me in great detail. Families want to help and support their members who are suffering, but how can we help if we don't know what to do? I used to try to physically stop my daughter from checking things. Then I told her how ridiculous it was. I even tried ignoring it for a while. How was I supposed to know what to do? Things are different now. We've all learned about this illness and how we can best help our daughter. After all, that's all we ever really wanted.

safety. Use of these drugs in combination with alcohol, however, may result in a serious or even fatal sedative reaction. Antidepressants have gained popularity in the treatment of anxiety disorders in light of studies documenting their effectiveness and the low side effect profile of some of them. Antipsychotic drugs are often prescribed for patients experiencing a panic level of anxiety of psychotic proportions.

Although some patients may need to take antianxiety drugs for extended periods, these drugs should always be used together with psychosocial treatments. Potential dangers of benzodiazepines include withdrawal syndrome side effects and addiction (see Chapter 25). It should be emphasized that medication is not a substitute for an ongoing therapeutic relationship but it can enhance the therapeutic alliance. Chemical control of painful symptoms allows the patient to direct attention to the conflicts underlying the anxiety. More detailed information on medications is presented in Chapter 28.

The Nursing Treatment Plan Summary on p. 293 reviews interventions related to severe and panic levels of anxiety.

Moderate Level of Anxiety

The nursing interventions previously mentioned are supportive and directed toward the short-term goal of reducing severe or panic-level anxiety. When the patient's anxiety is reduced to a moderate level, the nurse can begin helping with problem-solving efforts to cope with the stress. Long-term goals focus on helping the patient understand the cause of the anxiety and learn new ways of controlling it.

Table **17-3**

Antianxiety Drugs	
Chemical Class Generic Name (Trade Name)	Usual Dosage Range (mg/day)
ANTIANXIETY DRUGS	
Benzodiazepines	
Alprazolam (Xanax)	0.5-10
Chlordiazepoxide (Librium)	10-150
Clorazepate (Tranxene)	7.5-60
Clonazepam (Klonopin)	0.5-10
Diazepam (Valium)	2-40
Halazepam (Paxipam)	60-160
Lorazepam (Ativan)	1-6
Oxazepam (Serax)	15-120
Prazepam (Centrax)	10-60
Antihistamines	
Diphenhydramine (Benadryl)	50
Hydroxyzine (Atarax)	100
Beta-Adrenergic Blocker	
Propranolol (Inderal)	10
Anxiolytic	
Buspirone (BuSpar)	10-40
ANTIDEPRESSANT/ANTIANXIETY DRUGS	
Selective Serotonin Reuptake Inhibitors	
Citalopram (Celexa)	20-50
Fluoxetine (Prozac)	20-80
Fluvoxamine (Luvox)	50-300
Paroxetine (Paxil)	20-50
Sertraline (Zoloft)	25-200
Other Newer Antidepressants	
Mirtazepine (Remerom)	15-45
Nefazodone (Serzone)	200-600
Reboxetine (Vestra)	4-10
Trazodone (Desyrel)	50-600
Venlafaxine (Effexor)	25-375
Tricyclics	
Amitriptyline (Elavil)	50-300
Desipramine (Norpramin)	50-300
Clomipramine (Anafranil)	50-250
Imipramine (Tofranil)	50-300
Nortriptyline (Pamelor)	50-150
MAOI	
Phenelzine (Nardil)	45-90

Education is an important aspect of promoting the patient's adaptive responses to anxiety. The nurse can identify the health teaching needs of each patient and then formulate a plan to meet those needs. Plans should be designed to increase patients' knowledge of their own predisposing and precipitating stressors, coping resources, and adaptive and maladaptive responses. Alternative coping strategies can be identified and explored. Health teaching should also address the beneficial aspects of mild levels of anxiety in motivating learning and producing growth and creativity.

Goals include recognition of anxiety, insight into the anxiety, and coping with the threat. They incorporate principles and techniques of cognitive behavioral therapy (see Chapter 32) and can be implemented in any setting: psychiatric, community, home, or general hospital.

Recognition of Anxiety. After analyzing the patient's behaviors and determining the level of anxiety, the nurse helps the patient to recognize anxiety by helping him or her explore underlying feelings with such questions as "Are you feeling anxious now?" or "Are you uncomfortable?" It is also helpful for the nurse to identify the patient's behavior and link it to the feeling of anxiety (for example, "I noticed you smoked three cigarettes since we started talking about your sister. Are you feeling anxious?"). In this way the nurse acknowledges the patient's feeling, attempts to label it, encourages the patient to describe it further, and relates it to a specific behavioral pattern. The nurse is also validating inferences and assumptions with the patient.

However, the patient's goal is often to avoid or deny anxiety and he or she may use any of the resistive approaches described in Box 17-9. All these approaches may create feelings of frustration, irritation, or reciprocal anxiety in the nurse, who must recognize personal feelings and identify the patient's behavior pattern that might be causing them.

At this time, a trusting relationship is very important. If nurses establish themselves as warm, responsive listeners, give patients adequate time to respond, and support the patient's self-expression, they will become less threatening. In helping patients recognize their anxiety, nurses should use open questions that move from nonthreatening topics to central issues of conflict. In time, supportive confrontation may be used to address a particularly resistive pattern. However, if the patient's level of anxiety begins to rise rapidly, the nurse might choose to refocus the discussion to another topic.

Insight into the Anxiety. Once the patient is able to recognize anxiety, subsequent nursing interventions strive to expand the present context of the patient. The patient may be asked to describe the situations and interactions that immediately precede the increase in anxiety. Together the nurse and patient make inferences about the precipitating causes or biopsychosocial stressors.

The nurse then helps the patient see which values are being threatened by linking the threat with underlying causes, analyzing how the conflict developed, and relating the patient's present experiences to past ones. It is also important to explore how the patient reduced anxiety in the past and what kinds of actions produced relief.

Coping with the Threat. If previous coping responses have been adaptive and constructive, the patient should be encouraged to use them (Albucher et al, 1998). If not, the nurse can point out their maladaptive effects and help the patient see that the present way of life appears unsatisfactory and distressing and that the patient is not attempting to improve the situation. The patient needs to assume responsibility for actions and realize that limitations have been self-imposed. Other people must not be blamed.

In this phase of intervention the nurse assumes an active role by interpreting, analyzing, confronting, and correlating

NURSING TREATMENT PLAN *Summary* *Severe and Panic Anxiety Responses*

NURSING DIAGNOSIS: Severe/panic level anxiety
EXPECTED OUTCOME: The patient will reduce anxiety to a moderate or mild level.

SHORT-TERM GOAL	INTERVENTION	RATIONALE
The patient will be protected from harm.	Initially accept and support, rather than attack, the patient's defenses. Acknowledge the reality of the pain associated with the patient's present coping mechanisms. Do not focus on the phobia, ritual, or physical complaint itself. Give feedback to the patient about behavior, stressors, appraisal of stressors, and coping resources. Reinforce the idea that physical health is related to emotional health and that this is an area that will need exploration. In time, begin to place limits on the patient's maladaptive behavior in a supportive way.	Severe and panic levels of anxiety can be reduced by initially allowing the patient to determine the amount of stress that can be handled. If the patient is unable to release anxiety, tension may mount to the panic level and the patient may lose control. At this time the patient has no alternative coping mechanisms.
The patient will experience fewer anxiety-provoking situations.	Assume a calm manner with the patient. Decrease environmental stimulation. Limit the patient's interaction with other patients to minimize the contagious aspects of anxiety. Identify and modify anxiety-provoking situations for the patient. Administer supportive physical measures such as warm baths and massages.	The patient's behavior may be modified by altering the environment and the patient's interaction with it.
The patient will engage in a daily schedule of activities.	Initially share an activity with the patient to provide support and reinforce socially productive behavior. Provide for physical exercise of some type. Plan a schedule or list of activities that can be carried out daily. Involve family members and other support systems as much as possible.	By encouraging outside activities, the nurse limits the time the patient has available for destructive coping mechanisms while increasing participation in and enjoyment of other aspects of life.
The patient will experience relief from the symptoms of severe anxiety.	Administer medications that help reduce the patient's discomfort. Observe for medication side effects and initiate relevant health teaching.	The effect of a therapeutic relationship may be enhanced if the chemical control of symptoms allows the patient to direct attention to underlying conflicts.

Box **17-9**

Patient Resistances to Recognizing Anxiety

Screen symptoms. The patient focuses attention on minor physical ailments to avoid acknowledging anxiety and conflict areas.

Superior status position. The patient attempts to control the interview by questioning the nurse's abilities or asserting the superiority of the patient's knowledge or experiences. The nurse should not respond emotionally to this approach or accept the patient's challenge and compete because this would only further avoid the issue of anxiety.

Emotional seduction. The patient attempts to manipulate the nurse and elicit pity or sympathy.

Superficiality. The patient relates on a surface level and resists the nurse's attempts to explore underlying feelings or analyze issues.

Circumlocution. The patient gives the pretense of answering questions, but actually talks around the topic to avoid it.

Amnesia. This is a type of purposeful forgetting of an incident to avoid confronting and exploring it with the nurse.

Denial. The patient may use this approach only when discussing significant issues with the nurse or may generalize denial to all others, including self. The purpose is often to avoid humiliation.

Intellectualization. Patients who use this technique usually have some knowledge of psychology or medicine. They are able to express appropriate insights and analysis yet lack personal involvement in the problem they describe. They are not actually participating in the problem-solving process.

Hostility. The patient believes that offense is the best defense and therefore relates to others in an aggressive, defiant manner. The greatest danger in this situation is that the nurse will take this behavior personally and respond with anger. This reinforces the patient's avoidance of his or her anxiety.

Withdrawal. The patient may resist the nurse by replying in vague, diffuse, indefinite, and remote ways.

Box 17-10

Cognitive Behavioral Treatment Strategies for Anxiety Disorders

ANXIETY REDUCTION
Relaxation training
Biofeedback
Systematic desensitization
Interoceptive exposure
Flooding
Vestibular desensitization training
Response prevention
Eye movement desensitization and reprocessing (EMDR)

COGNITIVE RESTRUCTURING
Monitoring thoughts and feelings
Questioning the evidence
Examining alternatives
Decatastrophizing
Reframing
Thought stopping

LEARNING NEW BEHAVIOR
Modeling
Shaping
Token economy
Role playing
Social skills training
Aversion therapy
Contingency contracting

cause-and-effect relationships. The nurse should proceed clearly so that the patient can follow while keeping anxiety within appropriate limits. If the patient's anxiety becomes too severe, the nurse may change topics temporarily.

The nurse can help the patient in problem-solving efforts in various cognitive and behavioral ways. Specifically, cognitive behavioral therapy has been shown to be very effective in treating many anxiety disorders across age groups (Simpson & Kozak, 2000; Bryant et al, 1999; Wells, 1997; Clark et al, 1999). These treatments include a number of therapeutic strategies, which can be divided into three groups: anxiety reduction, cognitive restructuring, and learning new behavior. The specific strategies are listed in Box 17-10 and are explained in detail in Chapter 32.

One way of helping the patient cope is to reevaluate the nature of the threat or stressor. Is it as bad as the patient perceives it? Is the cognitive appraisal realistic? Together the nurse and patient might discuss fears and feelings of inadequacy. Does the patient fear that others are as critical, perfectionistic and rejecting as the patient is of others? Is the conflict based in reality, or is it the result of unvalidated, isolated, and distorted thinking? By sharing fears with family members, peers and staff, the patient often gains insight into such misperceptions.

Another approach is to help the patient modify behavior and learn new ways of coping with stress. The nurse may act as a role model in this regard or engage the patient in role playing. This activity can decrease anxiety about new responses to problem situations. One nursing function therefore is to teach the patient how aspects of mild anxiety can be constructive and produce growth. Physical activity should be encouraged as

 PATIENT EDUCATION PLAN   *The Relaxation Response*

CONTENT	INSTRUCTIONAL ACTIVITIES	EVALUATION
Describe the characteristics and benefits of relaxation	Discuss physiological changes associated with relaxation and contrast these with the behaviors of anxiety	Patient identifies own responses to anxiety Patient describes elements of a relaxed state
Teach deep muscle relaxation through a sequence of tension-relaxation exercises	Engage the patient in the progressive procedure of tensing and relaxing voluntary muscles until the body as a whole is relaxed	Patient is able to tense and relax all muscle groups Patient identifies muscles that become particularly tense
Discuss the relaxation procedure of meditation and its components	Describe the elements of meditation and help the patient use this technique	Patient selects a word or scene with pleasant connotations and engages in relaxed meditation
Help patient overcome anxiety-provoking situations through systematic desensitization	With patient, construct a hierarchy of anxiety-provoking situations or scenes Through imagination or reality, work through these scenes using relaxation techniques	Patient identifies and ranks anxiety-provoking situations Patient exposes self to these situations while remaining in a relaxed state
Allow the rehearsing and practical use of relaxation in a safe environment	Role play stressful situations with the nurse or other patients	Patient becomes more comfortable with new behavior in a safe, supportive setting
Encourage patient to use relaxation techniques in life	Assign homework of using the relaxation response in everyday experiences	Support success of patient Patient uses relaxation response in life situations Patient is able to regulate anxiety response through use of relaxation techniques

a way to discharge anxiety. Interpersonal resources such as family members or close friends should be incorporated into the nursing plan of care to provide the patient with support.

Often the cause for anxiety arises from an interpersonal conflict. In this case it is constructive to include the people involved when analyzing the situation with the patient. In this way, cause-and-effect relationships are more open to examination. Coping patterns can be examined in light of their effect on others, as well as on the patient.

Working through this problem-solving or reeducative process with the patient takes time because it has to be accepted both intellectually and emotionally. Breaking previous behavioral patterns can be difficult. Nurses need to be patient and consistent and continually reappraise their own anxiety.

Promote the Relaxation Response. In addition to problem solving, one can also cope with stress by regulating the emotional distress associated with it. Long-term goals directed toward helping the patient regulate emotional distress are supportive.

Relaxation can be taught individually, in small groups, or in large-group settings. A Patient Education Plan for teaching the relaxation response is presented on the opposite page. It is within the scope of nursing practice, requires no special equipment, and does not need a physician's supervision. As a group of interventions, relaxation can be implemented in various settings. A major benefit for patients is that after several training sessions, they can practice the techniques on their own. This puts the control in their hands and increases their self-reliance. Relaxation training is described in detail in Chapter 32. The Nursing Treatment Plan Summary for patients with moderate anxiety is presented below.

NURSING TREATMENT PLAN *Summary* *Moderate Anxiety Responses*

NURSING DIAGNOSIS: Moderate level of anxiety
EXPECTED OUTCOME: The patient will demonstrate adaptive ways of coping with stress.

SHORT-TERM GOAL	INTERVENTION	RATIONALE
The patient will identify and describe feelings of anxiety	Help the patient identify and describe underlying feelings Link the patient's behavior with such feelings Validate all inferences and assumptions with the patient Use open questions to move from nonthreatening topics to issues of conflict Vary the amount of anxiety to enhance the patient's motivation In time, supportive confrontation may be used judiciously	To adopt new coping responses, the patient first needs to be aware of feelings and to overcome conscious or unconscious denial and resistance
The patient will identify antecedents of anxiety	Help the patient describe the situations and interactions that immediately precede anxiety Review the patient's appraisal of the stressor, values being threatened, and the way in which the conflict developed Relate the patient's present experiences with relevant ones from the past	Once feelings of anxiety are recognized, the patient needs to understand their development, including precipitating stressors, appraisal of the stressor, and available resources
The patient will describe adaptive and maladaptive coping responses	Explore how the patient reduced anxiety in the past and what kinds of actions produced relief Point out the maladaptive and destructive effects of present coping responses Encourage the patient to use adaptive coping responses that were effective in the past Focus responsibility for change on the patient Actively help the patient correlate cause-and-effect relationships while maintaining anxiety within appropriate limits Help the patient reappraise the value, nature, and meaning of the stressor when appropriate	New adaptive coping responses can be learned through analyzing coping mechanisms used in the past, reappraising the stressor, using available resources, and accepting responsibility for change
The patient will implement two adaptive responses for coping with anxiety	Help the patient identify ways to restructure thoughts, modify behavior, use resources, and test new coping responses Encourage physical activity to discharge energy supports Include significant others as resources and social in helping the patient learn new coping responses Teach the patient relaxation exercises to increase control and self-reliance and reduce stress	One can also cope with stress by regulating the emotional distress that accompanies it through the use of stress management techniques

EVALUATION

Even before beginning to formulate the nursing diagnosis, the nurse should ask, "Did I critically observe my patient's physiological and psychomotor behaviors? Did I listen to my patient's subjective description of anxiety? Did I fail to see the relationships between my patient's expressed hostility or guilt and underlying anxiety? Did I assess intellectual and social functioning?"

After collecting the data, the nurse should analyze it: "Was I able to identify the precipitating stressor for the patient? What was the patient's perception of the threat? How was this influenced by physical health, past experiences, and present feelings and needs? Did I correctly identify the patient's level of anxiety and validate it?"

When using the criteria of adequacy, effectiveness, appropriateness, efficiency, and flexibility in evaluating the nursing goals and actions, the following questions can be raised:

- Were the planning, implementation and evaluation mutual?
- Were goals and actions adequate in number and sufficiently specific to minimize the patient's level of anxiety?
- Were maladaptive responses reduced?
- Were new adaptive coping responses learned?
- Was the nurse accepting of the patient and able to monitor personal anxiety throughout the relationship?

The nurse will also identify personal strengths and limitations in working with the anxious patient. Plans may then be made for overcoming the areas of limitation and further improving nursing care.

Summary

1. Anxiety is diffuse apprehension that is vague and associated with feelings of uncertainty and helplessness. It is an emotion without an object that is subjective and communicated interpersonally. Levels of anxiety include mild, moderate, severe, and panic.
2. Patient behaviors related to anxiety include physiological, behavioral, cognitive, and affective responses.
3. Predisposing factors for anxiety responses are described from psychoanalytical, interpersonal, behavioral, family, and biological perspectives. Precipitating stressors include threats to physical integrity and self-system.
4. Coping mechanisms can be categorized as task-oriented reactions such as attack, withdrawal, and compromise, or ego-oriented reactions also known as defense mechanisms.
5. Primary NANDA diagnoses related to anxiety responses are anxiety, ineffective coping, and fear.
6. Primary *DSM–IV–TR* diagnoses are categorized as anxiety disorders.
7. The expected outcome of nursing care for patients with maladaptive anxiety responses is that the patient will demonstrate adaptive ways of coping with stress.
8. Interventions include establishing a trusting relationship, self-awareness, protecting the patient, modifying the environment, encouraging activity, medication and learning new ways to cope with stress.
9. The nurse should use the criteria of adequacy, effectiveness, appropriateness, efficiency and flexibility in evaluating nursing care.

Competent Caring A Clinical Exemplar of a Psychiatric Nurse

Madelyn Myers, BS, RN

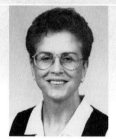

As the night shift charge nurse on an adult psychiatric unit, I learned that the graveyard shift was anything but routine. On return to the unit after my days off, I was told that Mr. B's behavior had deteriorated in the last few days. Mr. B was a 68-year-old man with a diagnosis of organic brain syndrome secondary to alcohol abuse. He was unable to stay in bed for more than a few minutes at a time and he was at risk for falls because of his confusion and as a side effect of his tranquilizing medication. The previous nights the staff had found it necessary to contain Mr. B with soft restraints to keep him in bed and reduce the risk of his falling.

After shift report I made my nursing rounds, accounting for all patients and assessing the situation of the unit. Mr. B was obviously distraught and anxious. His first question to me was, "You're not going to rope me, are you?" I sat down to talk with Mr. B to reassure him and explain that it was time for him to get ready for bed. He refused to change his clothing, stating that he just needed to walk around a little longer. I asked the

therapeutic assistants if they would walk him around a while longer to try calming him down. I went to the office to start verifying the day's orders, but found it impossible to get much done as Mr. B was calling me and coming to the nursing office to ask questions very frequently. The staff were also getting frustrated because he seemed very tired but would sit down for only a few minutes before he would jump up again. After I did a few more tasks, I relieved the staff member sitting with Mr. B. I was able to get Mr. B to lie down on his bed only after he saw me take the posey off the bed and out of the room. I watched him as he lay down and he seemed to doze off to sleep almost immediately. Then again just as quickly he awoke and started out of bed. He said, "Something is very wrong with me–I'm afraid I might die." We discussed his anxiety, and I reassured him that one of the staff would sit with him if that would make him feel more secure. He nodded in affirmation. I sat by his bedside. He fell asleep immediately and again repeated his previous pattern of awakening with a start, but this time he just looked over, saw me, and returned to sleep.

A short while later, one of the other staff came to relieve me. I shared with her my concern that Mr. B had been quite anxious and my plan was to sit at his bedside and gradually move

Competent Caring A Clinical Exemplar of a Psychiatric Nurse—cont'd

the chair back until we were sitting just outside his room but still in his line of sight. This way, he would be reassured that staff were still close by and we could observe him if he tried to get out of bed. That night he actually slept 4 hours with only two brief awakenings. The previous nights he had only dozed for minutes at a time.

The next morning I spoke with the nurse on his team about his fear of dying and of being "roped" with the posey. I shared with her the strategy we used of sitting with him and how he was able to sleep. The new plan of care was placed in his Kardex for all to follow. The next few nights we continued with our plan and each night Mr. B slept a little longer. He would even change into his pajamas before bed. He no longer started to "escalate" at bedtime. As he was sleeping better, Mr. B was

also feeling better physically and his anxiety level decreased dramatically. He required less medication for his anxiety; thus he was much more stable on his feet, no longer at risk for falls. Mr. B's ability to perform his activities of daily living (ADLs) increased over the next week and he was able to return to his previous living situation.

Many of his symptoms seemed to have been from sleep deprivation, high levels of anxiety, and the untoward effects of tranquilizers. This rewarding experience was not an isolated event on the night shift. It seems many people sleep through the night and see only the shadows of the staff making rounds, but there are others for whom the care they receive during these darkened hours makes a critical difference.

MeRLiN Visit MERLIN: www.mosby.com/MERLIN/Stuart to find these additional materials and student activities.

- **Worksheets**
- **"Drug of the Month" Updates**
- **"Citing the Evidence" Updates**
- **Critical Thinking Activities and Exercises**
- **Annotated Suggested Readings**
- **Web Links**
- **More!**

Chapter Review Questions

1. Match each term in Column A with the correct definition in Column B.

Column A

____ Affective responses

____ Anxiety

____ Cognitive responses

____ Ego-oriented reactions

____ Fear

____ Moderate anxiety

____ Neurosis

____ Panic

____ Psychosis

____ Task-oriented reactions

Column B

A. Diffuse, vague, subjective apprehension with feelings of uncertainty and helplessness

B. Attack behavior, withdrawal behavior, compromise

C. Forgetfulness, confusion, hypervigilance, fear of injury or death, poor concentration and judgment

D. Awe, dread, terror, loss of control, disorganization of the personality

E. A mental disorder characterized by anxiety that involves no distortion of reality

F. An individual ideation with a specific identifiable source

G. Edginess, impatience, uneasiness, tension, nervousness, fright, fear, alarm

H. A mental disorder that involves a disintegration of self, a fear of defeat in the process of being

I. Repression, splitting, denial, dissociation, projection, intellectualization, rationalization

J. Focus is only on immediate concerns, with a narrowing of the perceptual field

2. Fill in the blanks.

A. Difficulty in falling asleep, psychomotor hyperactivity, and selective negative appraisals are characteristic of _____. Early morning wakening, psychomotor retardation or agitation, and absolute negative evaluations characterize _____.

B. Recurrent and persistent thoughts, impulses, or images that are intrusive and inappropriate, and cause marked anxiety or distress, are called _____.

C. When the patient resists recognizing anxiety and attempts to manipulate the nurse and elicit sympathy or pity, it is called _____.

D. Precipitating stressors that threaten the patient and cause anxiety fall into two categories: threats to _____ and _____.

E. The two main categories of medications to treat anxiety disorders are the _____ and _____.

3. Provide short answers for the following questions.

A. Explain the behavioral view that anxiety arises from conflict.

B. Consider the nursing intervention categories for working with the anxious patient. What are some principles you can follow to protect the patient with an anxiety disorder?

C. Describe the criterion of flexibility when evaluating nursing care. How could you have been more flexible last time you worked with an anxious patient?

REFERENCES

Albucher R et al: Defense mechanism changes in successfully treated patients with obsessive-compulsive disorder, *Am J Psychiatry* 155(4):558, 1998.

American Psychiatric Association: *Diagnostic and statistical manual of mental disorders,* Fourth Edition, Text Revision. Washington, DC, American Psychiatric Association, 2000.

American Psychiatric Association: Practice guidelines for the treatment of patients with panic disorder, *Am J Psychiatry* 155(5):1, 1998.

Antai-Otong D: The neurobiology of anxiety disorders: implications for psychiatric nursing practice, *Issues Ment Health Nurs* 21:71, 2000.

Beck C: A concept analysis of panic, *Arch Psychiatr Nurs* 5:265, 1996.

Brown P, Yantis J: Personal space intrusion and PTSD, *J Psychosoc Nurs Ment Health Serv* 24:23, 1996.

Bryant R et al: Treating acute stress disorder: an evaluation of cognitive behavior therapy and supportive counseling techniques, *Am J Psychiatry* 156(11):1780, 1999.

Bystritsky A et al: A preliminary study of partial hospital management of severe obsessive-compulsive disorder, *Psychiatr Serv* 47:170, 1996.

Clark D et al: Brief cognitive therapy for panic disorder: a randomized controlled trial, *J Consult Clin Psychol* 67(4):583, 1999.

Classen C et al: Acute stress disorder as a predictor of posttraumatic stress symptoms, *Am J Psychiatry* 155(5):620, 1998.

Freud S: *A general introduction to psychoanalysis,* New York, 1969, Pocket Books.

Harvard Mental Health Letter, *Post-traumatic stress disorder,* Parts I & II, 12:1, and 13:1, 1996.

Kushner M et al: Prospective analysis of the relation between DSM-III anxiety disorders and alcohol use disorders, *Am J Psychiatry* 156(5):723, 1999.

Laraia M: Panic disorder: understanding and education are key to treatment, *Adv Nurse Practitioners* 3:5, 1995.

March J et al: The expert consensus guidelines series: treatment of obsessive-compulsive disorder, *Expert Knowledge Systems,* 1998.

Peplau H: A working definition of anxiety. In Burd S, Marshall M, editors: *Some clinical approaches to psychiatric nursing,* New York, 1963, Macmillan.

Resnick P: Malingering of posttraumatic psychiatric disorders, *J Pract Psych Behav Health* 4:329, 1998.

Shear M: Factors in the etiology and pathogenesis of panic disorder: revisiting the attachment-separation paradigm, *Am J Psychiatry* 153:125, 1996.

Simpson H, Kozak M: Cognitive-behavioral therapy for obsessive-compulsive disorder, *J Psych Practice* 6:59, 2000.

Stuart G, Laraia M: Panic disorder with agoraphobia. In McBride AB, Austin JK, editors: *Psychiatric-mental health nursing: integrating the behavioral and biological sciences,* Philadelphia, 1996, WB Saunders.

Sullivan H: *The interpersonal theory of psychiatry,* New York, 1953, WW Norton.

Wells A: *Cognitive therapy of anxiety disorders: a practice manual and conceptual guide,* New York, 1997, John Wiley.

Yehuda R, McFarlane A: Conflict between current knowledge about posttraumatic stress disorder and its original conceptual basis, *Am J Psychiatry* 152:1705, 1995.

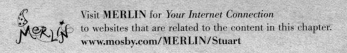
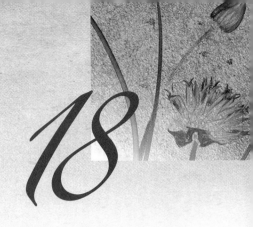

Psychophysiological Responses and Somatoform and Sleep Disorders

Gail W. Stuart

The cure of many diseases is unknown to the physicians of Hellas, because they disregard the whole, which ought to be studied also, for the part can never be well unless the whole is well.

PLATO

Throughout history, philosophers and scientists have debated the nature of the relationship between the mind (**psyche**) and body (**soma**). Recently there has been a renewed interest in holistic health practices, based on the idea that mental processes influence physical well-being and vice versa. Research is identifying the links between thoughts, feelings, and body functioning. Many now believe that all illness has a psychophysiological component: Physical disorders have a psychological component and mental disorders a physical one.

CONTINUUM OF PSYCHOPHYSIOLOGICAL RESPONSES

Current thinking about psychophysiological responses is related to an increased understanding of the role of stress in human life. Stress theory was significantly advanced when Hans Selye published *The Stress of Life* in 1956. Selye described the stress response in detail, creating a greater understanding of the effect of stressful experiences on physical functioning. He identified a three-stage process of response to stress. This generalized response is called the general adaptation syndrome (GAS). These levels of response are:

- The alarm reaction. This reaction is the immediate response to a stressor in a localized area. Adrenocortical mechanisms respond, resulting in behaviors associated with the fight-or-flight response.
- Stage of resistance. There is some resistance to the stressor. The body adapts and functions at a lower than optimal level. This requires a greater than usual expenditure of energy for survival.

- Stage of exhaustion. The adaptive mechanisms become worn out and fail. The negative effect of the stressor spreads to the entire organism. If the stressor is not removed or counteracted, death will result.

Any experience believed by the individual to be stressful may stimulate a psychophysiological response. The stress does not have to be recognized consciously, and often it is not. If people recognize that they are under stress, they are often unable to connect the cognitive understanding of stress with the physical symptoms of the psychophysiological disorder. Fig. 18-1 illustrates the range of possible psychophysiological responses to stress, based on Selye's theory.

ASSESSMENT

Behaviors

Many behaviors are associated with psychophysiological disorders. Careful assessment is needed so that organic problems are defined and treated. This type of illness should never be dismissed as "only psychosomatic" or "all in one's head." Serious psychophysiological disorders can be fatal if not treated properly.

Physiological. The primary behaviors observed with psychophysiological responses are the physical symptoms. These symptoms lead the person to seek health care. Psychological factors affecting the physical condition may involve any body part. The most common organ systems involved are listed in Box 18-1. In addition, longer general hospital stays have been reported to be associated with greater psychological comorbidity, particularly depression, anxiety, and organicity. Such research underscores the importance of linking physiological and psychological assessments.

People are often reluctant to believe that a physical problem may be related to psychological factors. In part, this is because being physically ill is more socially acceptable than having psychological problems. The situation is compounded because the patient has physical symptoms.

Denial of the psychological component of the illness may lead to "doctor shopping." The patient searches for someone who will find an organic cause for the illness. This tendency to experience and communicate psychological distress in the form of physical symptoms and to seek help for them in general medical settings is a widespread phenomenon. The following clinical example illustrates this problem.

 CLINICAL EXAMPLE

Mr. R was a successful 42-year-old executive who had risen quickly to the top of his company. He worked long hours and had difficulty delegating any of his responsibilities. He set high standards for his employees and was believed to be insensitive to human concerns. He viewed himself as tough, but fair. However, he had little sympathy for a worker who requested extra time off for personal business.

Mr. R was married but saw little of his family. He expected his wife and children to do their part to maintain his standing in the community by associating with "the right people." He seldom interacted with his children except to reprimand them if they disturbed him while he was working. His wife reported that their sexual relationship was unsatisfying to her. Mr. R used it for physical release for himself but was not concerned about meeting her

Box **18-1**

Physical Conditions Affected by Psychological Factors

CARDIOVASCULAR	**SKIN**
Migraine	Neurodermatitis
Essential hypertension	Eczema
Angina	Psoriasis
Tension headaches	Pruritus

MUSCULOSKELETAL	**GENITOURINARY**
Rheumatoid arthritis	Impotence
Low back pain	Frigidity
(idiopathic)	Premenstrual syndrome

RESPIRATORY	**ENDOCRINOLOGICAL**
Hyperventilation	Hyperthyroidism
Asthma	Diabetes

GASTROINTESTINAL
Anorexia nervosa
Peptic ulcer
Irritable bowel syndrome
Colitis
Obesity

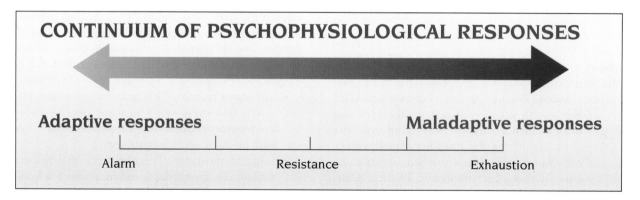

CONTINUUM OF PSYCHOPHYSIOLOGICAL RESPONSES

Adaptive responses   **Maladaptive responses**

Alarm   Resistance   Exhaustion

Fig. 18-1   Continuum of psychophysiological responses.

needs. She suspected that he was involved in an extramarital affair but did not want to endanger the marriage by confronting him.

Mr. R was expecting to be named to the board of directors of a prestigious philanthropic foundation. He expected that this would add to his social prominence in the community. Shortly before the announcement was to be made, his 14-year-old son was arrested in a drug raid in the lower-middle-class part of town. Mr. R did not get the appointment. He was furious with his son but dealt with his anger by withdrawing still more. One day at work, he experienced an episode of dizziness, followed by a severe headache. He attributed it to tension, took some aspirin, and continued to work. However, after several similar episodes, he decided to consult his family doctor. The physician arrived at a diagnosis of essential hypertension. He tried to discuss work, family, and social behavior with Mr. R but received only superficial responses. Although concerned about Mr. R's condition and stress level, the doctor gave in to Mr. R's demand for medication to lower his blood pressure. He also advised Mr. R to exercise and to find a relaxing activity.

Selected Nursing Diagnoses

- Impaired adjustment related to family and work stress, as evidenced by denial and development of physical symptoms
- Altered family processes related to rigid role expectations, as evidenced by withdrawal and lack of communication

---

Mr. R is typical of many people with stress-related psychophysiological disorders. He is reluctant to admit to a lack of control over his mind and body. He expects a magical cure that will let him follow his usual lifestyle without interruption. He will probably stop taking his medication as soon as he feels better. Distance from the stressor may allow him to function for a while without noticeable symptoms of his hypertension. Sooner or later, however, new stressors will lead to another dizzy spell, headaches, or possibly myocardial infarction or cerebrovascular accident.

Psychological. Some people have physical symptoms without any organic impairment, and these are called somatoform disorders. They include somatization disorder, in which the person has many physical complaints; conversion disorder, in which a loss or alteration of physical functioning occurs; hypochondriasis, the fear of or belief that one has an illness; body dysmorphic disorder, in which a person with a normal appearance is concerned about having a physical defect; and pain disorder, in which psychological factors play an important role in the onset, severity, or maintenance of the pain. The next clinical example is a case history of a person with a medical diagnosis of somatization disorder.

 CLINICAL EXAMPLE

Ms. O, a 28-year-old single woman, was admitted to the medical unit of a general hospital for a complete medical work-up. When asked about her main problem during the nursing assessment, she replied, "I've never been very well. Even when I was a child I was sick a lot." Ms. O listed multiple complaints during the physical assessment. These included palpitations, dizzy spells, menstrual irregularity, painful menses, blurred vision, dysphagia, backache,

pain in her knees and feet, and a variety of gastrointestinal symptoms including stomach pain, nausea, vomiting, diarrhea, flatulence, and intolerance to seafood, vegetables of the cabbage family, carbonated beverages, and eggs. Except for the food intolerances, none of the symptoms was constant. They occurred at random, making her fearful of going out of her home.

The psychosocial assessment revealed that Ms. O lived with her parents. She was the youngest of three children. Her siblings were living away from the parental home. She had graduated from high school but had poor grades because of her frequent absences. She had tried to work as a clerk in a retail store but was fired because of absenteeism. She did not seem particularly bothered by the loss of her job. She had never tried to find other work, although she had been unemployed for 8 years. When asked how she spent her time, she said that she did some gardening and some housework when she felt well enough. However, she spent most of her time watching television.

Ms. O's parents visited her most of every day. Her mother asked whether she could spend the night in her daughter's room and was displeased when told no. The family had many complaints about the quality of the nursing care, mostly about failures to anticipate the patient's needs. Extensive diagnostic studies failed to reveal any organic basis for Ms. O's physical complaints. When informed that the problem was most likely psychological and advised to obtain psychotherapy, the family protested angrily and refused a referral to a psychiatric clinic. Ms. O was discharged and returned to her parents' home.

Selected Nursing Diagnoses

- Ineffective denial related to physical and emotional health status, as evidenced by repeated medical care visits and refusal to obtain psychiatric treatment
- Altered family processes related to mother-daughter dependency issues, as evidenced by excessive caretaking by mother and passivity of daughter

---

Ms. O shows the dependent behavior that is typical of people with somatization disorder. Her many symptoms allowed her to be taken care of and to avoid the demands of adult responsibility. Her need to be cared for fit with her mother's need to nurture. Therefore, she had little incentive to give up her symptoms. A periodic hospital stay reinforced the seriousness of her problem.

Secondary gain related to the gratification of dependency needs is a powerful deterrent to change in many patients. Secondary gain is an indirect benefit, usually obtained through an illness or disability. Such benefits may include personal attention, release from unpleasant situations and responsibilities, or monetary and disability benefits.

Another type of somatoform disorder is conversion disorder. Symptoms of some physical illnesses appear without any underlying organic cause. The organic symptom reduces the patient's anxiety and usually gives a clue to the conflict. For example, a patient who has an impulse to harm his domineering father may develop paralysis of his arms and hands. The primary gain is that the patient is unable to carry out his impulses. He also may experience secondary gain in the form of attention, manipulation of others, freedom from responsibilities, and economic benefits. Conversion symptoms might include the following:

- Sensory symptoms such as numbness, blindness, or deafness
- Motor symptoms such as paralysis, tremors or mutism
- Visceral symptoms such as urinary retention, headaches, or difficulty breathing

It is often difficult to diagnose this reaction. Other patient behaviors may be helpful. Patients often display little anxiety or concern about the conversion symptom and its resulting disability. The classic term for this lack of concern is **la belle indifference**. The patient also tends to seek attention in ways not limited to the actual symptom.

Hypochondriasis is another type of somatoform disorder. These people have an exaggerated concern with physical health that is not based on any real organic disorders. They fear presumed diseases and are not helped by reassurance. They also tend to seek out and use information about diseases to convince themselves that they are ill or about to become ill. Unlike the conversion reaction, no actual loss or distortion of function occurs. Patients appear worried and anxious about their symptoms. This concern may be based on physical sensations overlooked by most people or on symptoms of a minor physical illness that the patient magnifies. This is often a chronic behavior pattern accompanied by a history of visits to numerous practitioners (Wise, 1997).

Hypochondriacal behavior is not related to a conscious decision. If a person decides to fake an illness, the behavior is called malingering. This behavior is usually done to avoid responsibilities the person views as burdensome. Many otherwise healthy people malinger at one time or another. For instance, a person involved in an automobile accident may feign neck pain to receive insurance money. Often, the person exaggerates symptoms, is evasive, and tells contradictory stories about the illness.

Pain. Pain is increasingly recognized as more than simply a sensory phenomenon, but as a complex sensory and emotional experience underlying potential disease. Pain is influenced by behavioral, cognitive and motivational processes requiring sophisticated assessments and multifaceted treatments for its control (Keefe & Goli, 1996).

Acute pain is a reflex biological response to injury. By definition, chronic pain is pain of a minimum of 6 months duration. **Somatoform pain disorder** is a preoccupation with pain in the absence of physical disease to account for its intensity. It does not follow a neuroanatomical distribution. There may also be a close correlation between stress and conflict and the initiation or exacerbation of the pain.

The experience, expression and treatment of pain are subject to cultural norms and biases. For example, in Western cultures, being female is often a predictor of poor pain management because male expressions of pain are typically taken more seriously by health-care practitioners (Vallerand, 1995). Also, members of minority groups who seek health care in culturally insensitive settings may have their requests for support in coping with pain misunderstood because support is culturally defined and varies across ethnic and racial groups (Oakley & Patten, 1997).

Sleep. Sleep disorders are common in the general population and among people with psychiatric disorders (Nowell et al, 1997). Most importantly, sleep disturbances can influence the development and course of mental illnesses and addictive disorders and can also affect treatment and recovery.

Insomnia is the most prevalent sleep disorder. Up to 30% of the population have insomnia and seek help for it. Other sleep disturbances include excessive daytime sleepiness, difficulty sleeping during desired sleep time, and unusual nocturnal events such as nightmares and sleepwalking. Sleep disorders are more common in the elderly.

Sleep disorders are classified by the Association of Sleep Disorders Centers (ASDC) into four major groupings with considerable overlap (Lilie & Lahmeyer, 1991):

- Disorders of initiating or maintaining sleep, also known as insomnia. Anxiety and depression are major causes of insomnia.
- Disorders of excessive somnolence, also known as hypersomnia. This category includes narcolepsy, sleep apnea, and nocturnal movement disorders such as restless legs.
- Disorders of the **sleep-wake schedule**, characterized by normal sleep but at the wrong time. These are transient disturbances associated with jet lag and work shift changes. They are usually self-limited and resolve as the body readjusts to a new sleep-wake schedule.
- Disorders associated with sleep stages, also known as parasomnia. This category includes conditions such as sleepwalking, night terrors, nightmares, restless legs syndrome, and enuresis. These sleep problems are often experienced by children and can have a significant effect on functioning and well-being.

Approximately 40 million Americans suffer from chronic disorders of sleep and wakefulness, such as narcolepsy, sleep apnea, and the insomnias. The majority of those affected are undiagnosed and untreated (see Citing the Evidence on Insomnia). An additional 20 to 30 million people experience intermittent sleep-related problems. In addition, millions of other people get inadequate sleep because of demanding work schedules, school and other lifestyle issues.

The consequences of sleep disorders, sleep deprivation, and sleepiness are significant and include reduced productivity, lowered cognitive performance, increased likelihood of accidents, higher morbidity and mortality risk, depression, and decreased quality of life (National Center on Sleep Disorders, 1999; Yantis, 1999). Furthermore, the consequences span all aspects of modern society, including health care, education, and family and social life (Wake Up America, 1993).

The assessment of patients with sleep problems is multifaceted, involving a detailed history and medical and psychiatric examinations, extensive questionnaires, the use of sleep diaries or logs, and often psychological testing. Many patients are referred for formal sleep studies, which include all night polysomnography and physiological measures of daytime sleepiness (Buysse & Perlis, 1996). Many members of

Citing the Evidence on

Insomnia

BACKGROUND: This study explored the following unanswered questions: 1) What are the prevalence and clinical patterns of insomnia among primary care patients? 2) What functional impairment and health-care utilization is associated with insomnia? 3) How is insomnia currently treated?

RESULTS: About 10% of the primary care patients reported current major insomnia (taking at least two hours to fall asleep almost every night). Current insomnia was associated with greater functional impairment, more days of disability and greater health-care utilization. Of patients with current insomnia, 14% received benzodiazepines and 19% received antidepressants.

IMPLICATIONS: Insomnia is a significant if underappreciated health-care problem. Clinicians should attempt to detect and treat it to avoid negative sequelae.

Simon G, VonKorff M: Prevalence, burden, and treatment of insomnia in primary care, *Am J Psychiatr* 154(10):1417, 1997.

the health-care team collaborate within sleep centers to deliver multidisciplinary care.

Have you ever had a problem sleeping? Which ASDC grouping would your problem have fit into, and what did you do to relieve it?

Predisposing Factors

A number of biopsychosocial factors influence psychophysiological responses to stress. Most of the relationships between physical and psychological processes are still not well described. Thus it is important for the nurse to consider all possibilities when assessing factors that might predispose the patient to a particular disorder.

Biological. Biological factors may predispose a person to psychophysiological illness. Research has linked emotions to arousal of the neuroendocrine system through release of corticosteroids by the hypothalamic-pituitary-adrenal (HPA) axis, as well as to the actions of neurotransmitter systems, particularly norepinephrine and serotonin. Research measuring changes in postsynaptic receptors in response to stress and the effect on neurotransmission (and thus human behavior) is producing interesting results. By understanding the effects of stress and coping strategies at the level of the synapse, clinicians can design effective treatment strategies (Lowery & Houldin, 1996).

Genetic factors are also important. A biological tendency for particular psychophysiological responses may be inherited. For instance, epidemiological studies have shown that the lifetime prevalence for somatization disorder in the general population is 0.1% to 0.5%, and is more common in women. In the mothers and sisters of affected patients, however, it increases to 10% to 20%. The rate in monozygotic (identical) twins is 29%, and in dizygotic (fraternal) twins it is 10%. Thus there is clearly an inherited tendency for this disorder.

The genetic theory suggests that any prolonged stress can cause physiological changes, which result in a physical disorder. Each person has a "shock organ" that is genetically vulnerable to stress. Thus some patients may be prone to cardiac illness, whereas others may react with gastrointestinal distress or skin rashes. People who are chronically anxious or depressed are believed to have a greater vulnerability to psychophysiological illness.

Psychoneuroimmunology. Psychoneuroimmunology is the scientific field that explores the relationship between psychological states and the immune system. Research on the ways in which the brain protects itself from cells damaged by trauma, disease or stress has emerged (Streit & Kincaid-Colton, 1995). This field is based on the mind-body connection that extends to the cellular level (Fig. 18-2).

For example, glial cells are found throughout the central nervous system. As numerous as neurons, they form an extensive defensive network in the brain, monitoring and even enhancing normal brain function, and migrating to trouble spots to ingest microbes, dying cells and other debris. Research has also shown that these cells can lose control and, in some people, exacerbate or even cause several disabling conditions such as stroke, Alzheimer's disease, multiple sclerosis, Parkinson's disease, dementia associated with HIV, and other neurodegenerative disorders.

The immune response can be modified by behavior modification techniques. Researchers are now investigating the possibility of modifying the immune response in the treatment of autoimmune illnesses such as rheumatoid arthritis, systemic lupus erythematosus, myasthenia gravis, and pernicious anemia. Other research is exploring the relationship between the immune system, stress, and cancer. It is suspected that high stress, especially if prolonged, can decrease the immune system's ability to destroy neoplastic growths.

Psychological. Philosophers and scientists have long speculated about the roles of personality and stress in the development of illness. In the 1930s and 1940s personality profiles were developed of those prone to several diseases, including hypertension, coronary artery disease (CAD), cancer, ulcers, and rheumatoid arthritis.

Research suggests that a negative affective style marked by depression, anxiety, and hostility may be associated with the development or recovery from such diseases as asthma, headaches, ulcers, arthritis, and cancer (see Citing the Evidence on Survival in Breast Cancer). The clearest evidence to date relates to the negative effects of chronic hostility on cardiovascular disease.

Type A behavior, which has been characterized by competitive drive, impatience, hostility, irritability, and aggressiveness, has been shown to predict both the physiological changes that are associated with CAD and the development of CAD itself. Type A people are also more likely to have ac-

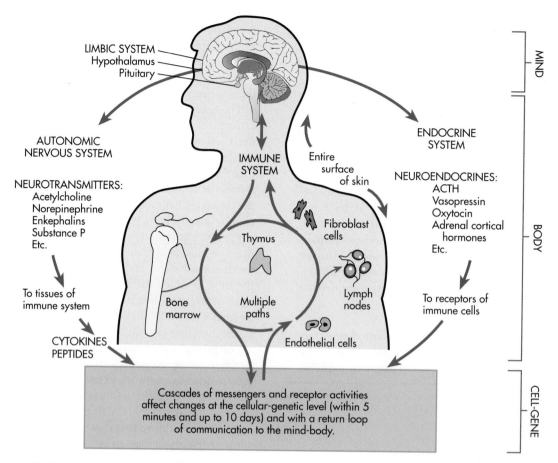

Fig. 18-2   Updated view of Selye's general adaptation syndrome emphasizing the mind-body-cell/gene communication loop of the immune system.

Citing the Evidence on

Survival in Breast Cancer

BACKGROUND: The psychological response to breast cancer has been suggested as a prognostic factor with an influence on survival. This study investigated the effect of psychological response on disease outcome in a large cohort of women with early-stage breast cancer.

RESULTS: There was a significantly increased risk of death from all causes by 5 years in women who scored high on the depression scales, and a significantly increased risk of relapse or death on those who scored high on the helplessness and hopelessness scales. There were no significant results found for the category of "fighting spirit."

IMPLICATIONS: The results reinforce the need to detect a response of helplessness or hopelessness and serious depression, and treat these responses vigorously to help women improve the quality of their lives and optimize their length of survival.

Watson M et al: Influence of psychological response on survival in breast cancer, *The Lancet* 354:1331, Oct 16, 1999.

cidents, to die as a result of accidents or violence, to have migraine headaches, to smoke more, and to have higher levels of serum cholesterol. Thus Type A behavior appears to be a risk factor not only for cardiovascular disease but also for an array of other disorders.

Although such research suggests the possibility of a disease-prone personality, the exact nature of the relationship between personality and susceptibility is unknown. For example, a negative emotional state may:

- Produce pathological physiological changes
- Lead people to practice faulty health behaviors
- Produce illness behavior but no underlying pathology
- Be associated with illness through other unknown factors

Complementing the research on negative emotional states and disease is the increasing focus on the protective role of positive emotional states. One idea regarding these traits is that of a self-healing personality, which is characterized by enthusiasm (Friedman, 1991). Self-healing, emotionally balanced people are believed to be alert, responsive, and energetic, although they may also be calm and conscientious. They are curious, secure, and constructive. Self-healing personalities also have a sense of continuous growth and resilience and an extra margin of emotional stability that they can call on when their capacities are challenged.

Two other positive traits are optimism and perceived control. Optimists appear to have fewer physical symptoms and

Box 18-2

Somatoform Syndromes of Various Cultures

Ataque de nervios: Distress recognized by many Latin American groups with common symptoms of uncontrollable crying, trembling, heat in the chest rising to the head, fainting, and a sense of having lost control. They frequently follow a stressful event affecting the individual or one's family.

Brain fag: A West African term used to describe symptoms experienced by young people related to the stress of study including difficulties in concentration, memory, and thinking.

Dhat: A folk term used by men in India relating to sexual dysfunction and signs of weakness and exhaustion.

Hwa-byung: A Korean folk syndrome attributed to the suppression of anger with symptoms of insomnia, fatigue, indigestion, anorexia, and generalized aches and pains.

Shenjing shuairuo (neurasthenia): In China, a condition characterized by physical and mental fatigue, dizziness, headaches, concentration, and sleep difficulties.

Susto ("fright" or "soul loss"): A Latin American folk illness that follows a frightening experience. Symptoms include appetite and sleep disturbance, lack of motivation, muscle pains, headaches, and abdominal pain and diarrhea.

CRITICAL THINKING about CONTEMPORARY ISSUES

Is Chronic Fatigue Syndrome a Culturally Sanctioned Form of Illness Behavior?

There is much interest in the recently defined chronic fatigue syndrome, which is characterized by exhaustion or fatigue and marked reduction in activity and correlated with a high prevalence of psychiatric disorders and psychophysiological symptoms secondary to stress (Wessely et al, 1996). This interest results from reports of its growing frequency, substantial morbidity and unclear pathogenesis. This interest is also fueled by debates about emotional factors related to the illness and questions as to whether it is a discrete disorder (Demitrack, 1998).

Currently the diagnosis of chronic fatigue syndrome is more common among women. It has been proposed that it is related to the struggle of American culture with the expanding role of women and the mismatch between women's ambitions and social possibilities. Today, illness and the sick role are the only socially legitimate excuses for abandoning work and the pursuit of achievement. Thus a diagnosis of chronic fatigue syndrome may provide a legitimate "medical" reason for a variety of psychophysiological responses, allowing the person to withdraw from situations that are intolerable. This example of the cultural shaping of illness and disease underscores society's greater understanding of physical illness and the continued stigmatization of psychiatric illness and emotional distress.

---

may show faster recoveries from illness. Belief in personal control, or **self-efficacy**, affects the likelihood of developing illness by directly influencing the practice of health behaviors and by buffering people against the adverse effects of stress (Bandura, 1997).

> *Think of people you know who always seem to be ill. What personality characteristics do they share? How do they compare with people you know who are hardly ever ill?*

Sociocultural. It has been proposed that health, illness and suffering are patterned by culture and realized as personal worlds of experience. Box 18-2 presents some unique somatoform syndromes of various cultures (American Psychiatric Association, 2000). In this view psychophysiological illness derives from the relationships between body, psyche and society. Illness is not seen as simply the natural unfolding of an exclusively biological process. Rather, its course is also influenced by sociocultural factors (see Critical Thinking about Contemporary Issues).

The social course of illness has at least two meanings. The first is that the severity of the person's symptoms is influenced by aspects of the social environment. This means that subjectively experienced distress can be increased or decreased by the nature and number of problems in the person's world, changes in the emotional climate of that world, and by the ill person's social life.

In the second meaning the symptoms shape and structure the person's social world, as the illness causes a series of changes in the person's environment. The resulting chain of illness-related interpersonal events thus becomes a part of

the social course of the person's illness. This can be seen in the concept of the **sick role**, first described in the 1950s by Parsons. It proposes that being sick is a social role as well as a condition and that society places certain beliefs and expectations on the person who falls ill (Parsons, 1951). These include the following:

- The sick are allowed to be exempt from their usual social responsibilities.
- The sick are not seen as being responsible for being ill.
- The sick are expected to want to get well.
- The sick are expected to seek competent help and cooperate with the helper in trying to get well.

Although the premises of the sick role have been questioned, they do show the impact of sociocultural factors on the expression and resolution of psychophysiological responses.

> *Compare this society's beliefs and expectations about the sick role for people with multiple sclerosis, alcoholism, lung cancer, and depression. Do they differ based on each diagnosis and, if so, how and why?*

Precipitating Stressors

Any experience that the person interprets as stressful may lead to a psychophysiological response. Some of these responses are mild and short-lived. Examples include diarrhea before an examination or a dry mouth when speaking before a large group of people. Sometimes the response is more serious and indicates a higher level of anxiety. For instance, a person might feel panicky and experience tachycardia when boarding an airplane. Because the psychophysiological disorder is an attempt to deal with anxiety, information on stressors related to anxiety (Chapter 17) should be reviewed.

One type of stressor that has been shown to cause physical illness and even death is the loss of a significant interpersonal relationship. An increased mortality rate has been found among recently widowed people. Similar observations have been made about people admitted to institutions such as nursing homes, who are separated from significant others. Children who have been separated from their mothers, especially if placed in an impersonal environment, also show a decline in physical health. The effect of a loss may cause both physical and psychological symptoms for an extended period of time. Illnesses and deaths related to loss of a loved person seem to represent the exhaustion phase of the general adaptation syndrome.

Sometimes a psychophysiological problem is a response to an accumulation of rather small stressors. A patient may find it difficult to identify one specific stressor that preceded a particular problem. Careful assessment may reveal a pattern of overwork and overcommitment or a series of seemingly minor events that all required extra effort. Most of the psychophysiological disorders come and go. This pattern of occurrence may be related to changes in the person's stress level. When the cumulative stress gets too high, the body "calls time out" by developing physical symptoms.

Appraisal of Stressors

The complex interaction between mind and body is perhaps most evident in psychophysiological responses to stress. These responses reinforce the need for an integrated approach to etiology and great sensitivity by the nurse to a person's appraisal of stress and its effects. Social and cultural factors play a particularly important role in the expression of adaptive and maladaptive behaviors. They also must be considered in planning effective, individualized treatment strategies.

Coping Resources

One of the most important parts of promoting adaptive psychophysiological responses involves changing health habits. People who adopt positive health practices and good health measures can prevent biopsychosocial illnesses (see Chapter 13). Patient Education Plans that include coping skills training, such as the one below, can increase a person's knowledge about the effect of stress, reduce anxiety, increase a person's feelings of purpose and meaning in life, reduce pain and suffering, and improve coping abilities.

Social support from family, friends and caregivers is also an important resource for adaptive psychophysiological responses (see A Family Speaks). It may lower the likelihood of developing maladaptive responses, speed the recovery from illness, and reduce the distress and suffering that accompany illness. Social support groups are another coping resource that can satisfy needs that are unmet by family members and caregivers.

A Family Speaks

I worry about my husband. He drives himself so hard. I also feel guilty at times because I know he's doing it for me and the children. But I sure would like for him to slow down. Here's a good example of how things go in our house. Every year in the weeks before Christmas he works overtime to give us a little extra money. But then on Christmas Eve, without fail, his ulcer kicks up and we wind up spending part of each holiday in the hospital visiting him.

I know every family has problems and maybe ours aren't so bad. But then again, maybe they are. This last Christmas our doctor recommended that we see a family therapist to discuss the situation. I want to go, but my husband says it's silly. Maybe this year for Christmas I'll ask him to give me that as my present and we'll finally have a really happy New Year.

PATIENT EDUCATION PLAN *Coping with Stress*

CONTENT	INSTRUCTIONAL ACTIVITIES	EVALUATION
Define and describe stress	List feelings that indicate stress Discuss behaviors associated with elevated stress	Patient identifies general behaviors associated with stressful situations
Recognize stressful situations	Ask patient to describe situations personally experienced as stressful Role play the situation(with videotape if possible) Discuss stress-relatedbehaviors observed and feelings experienced	Patient identifies stressful experiences Patient describes own behaviors when stressed
Review common life stressors	Discuss common elements of stressful experiences	Patient identifies stressful aspects of life
Identify adaptive and maladaptive coping mechanisms	Review the role-played stressful situations Discuss alternative ways to cope with the stressors Role play at least one adaptive coping mechanism	Patient identifies and practices adaptive coping mechanisms
Assign use of adaptive strategy to cope with stress	Provide feedback about the effectiveness of the selected coping mechanism	Patient selects an adaptive coping strategy when experiencing stress

Coping Mechanisms

Psychophysiological disorders may be attempts to cope with the anxiety associated with overwhelming stress. Unconsciously the person links the anxiety to the physical illness. Secondary gain then adds to the psychological relief experienced.

Several of the defense mechanisms described in Chapter 17 may be seen in psychophysiological disorders. Repression of feelings, conflicts and unacceptable impulses often leads to physical symptoms. The maintenance of repression over long periods of time requires a great deal of psychic energy. As the system approaches a state of exhaustion, physical symptoms occur. When a psychological basis for illness is suggested, the patient denies it. This denial indicates the inability to handle the anxiety that would otherwise be released if the person admitted the psychic conflicts being repressed. The need for this defense should be respected.

Some people respond to psychophysiological illness with compensation. They attempt to prove that they are actually healthy by being more active and exerting themselves physically even if told to rest. This coping style is typical of Type A people, who need desperately to prove that they are in control of their bodies, not controlled by them. The opposite of this reaction is the person who uses regression as a coping mechanism. This person becomes dependent and embraces the sick role to avoid responsibility and conflict.

Common to each of these coping mechanisms is the need not to confront the basic conflict that is leading to stress and anxiety. This need is so strong that premature attempts to convince the person of psychological conflicts may result in the use of a less adaptive coping mechanism. In extreme cases, if the person is stripped of all efforts to cope and not provided with a substitute, death can result, either from worsening of the organic disorder or from suicide.

NURSING DIAGNOSIS

The nursing diagnosis must reflect the complex biopsychosocial interaction that is the hallmark of psychophysiological disorders. The patient's effort to cope with stress-related anxiety may result in many somatic and emotional disorders. All possible disruptions must be considered when formulating a nursing diagnosis.

The Stuart Stress Adaptation Model (Fig. 18-3) may help in the diagnostic process. A thorough interview will reveal many of the predisposing factors and precipitating stressors present. The nurse must use good communication skills

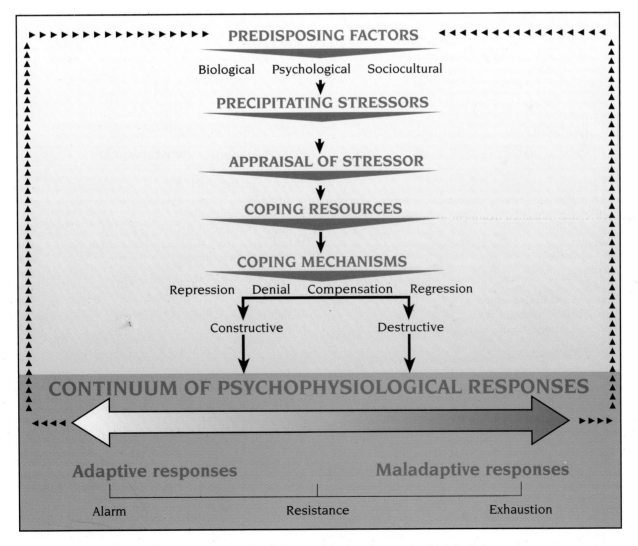

Fig. 18-3   The Stuart Stress Adaptation Model related to psychophysiological responses.

during the interview to enable the patient to share his or her experience as completely as possible. Areas of resistance and gaps in information should be noted as possible indicators of a conflict. These may be explored more completely as trust is established in the nurse-patient relationship.

Questions related to lifestyle and activities may help identify precipitating stressors and coping behaviors. It is particularly important to elicit the patient's view of what is happening. This response will provide valuable information about the patient's awareness of the relationship between mind and body. Nonverbal behaviors also give clues about the patient's concerns. Apparent lack of concern may reveal the use of denial suggestive of a conversion disorder.

As the diagnosis is formulated, the nurse must consider the patient's coping in the context of the stress response. Is the patient in a stage of alarm with many coping resources at hand? Or is the patient in the stage of resistance, using coping mechanisms but depleting personal energy resources? Has the patient reached the stage of exhaustion, needing intensive intervention? Determination of the level of stress and coping being used influences the interventions chosen.

There are three primary nursing diagnoses for maladaptive psychophysiological responses. The first is **impaired adjustment**, a state in which the patient is unable to modify his or her lifestyle in order to improve health status. The second is **chronic pain**, a state that continues for more than 6 months. The third is **sleep pattern disturbance**, which is a disruption of sleep time that causes discomfort or interferes

with desired lifestyle. Nursing diagnoses related to the range of possible maladaptive responses and related medical diagnoses are identified in the Medical and Nursing Diagnoses box below. The primary NANDA diagnoses and examples of complete nursing diagnoses are presented in the Detailed Diagnoses box on the opposite page.

Related Medical Diagnoses

Medical disorders related to maladaptive psychophysiological responses are classified under the general categories of somatoform disorders, sleep disorders, and psychological factors affecting medical condition (American Psychiatric Association, 2000). The specific medical diagnoses and essential features in each of these diagnostic classes in the *DSM–IV–TR* are described in the Detailed Diagnoses box.

OUTCOME IDENTIFICATION

The expected outcome when working with a patient with maladaptive psychophysiological responses is as follows: *The patient will express feelings verbally rather than through the development of physical symptoms.*

This expectation is a long-term goal, and some may never reach it. However, an increased level of self-awareness is beneficial and should be achievable by all patients. An improved ability to deal with conflict will reduce the patient's need to use repression and denial. This in turn will decrease stress and allow the patient to function with fewer episodes of

---

 Medical and Nursing Diagnoses *related to* **Psychophysiological Responses**

RELATED MEDICAL DIAGNOSES (*DSM–IV–TR*)*	RELATED NURSING DIAGNOSES (NANDA)†
Somatization disorder	**Adjustment, impaired‡**
Conversion disorder	Anxiety
Hypochondriasis	Body image disturbance
Body dysmorphic disorder	Coping, individual, ineffective
Pain disorder	Denial, ineffective
Primary insomnia	Family processes, altered
Primary hypersomnia	Fear
Narcolepsy	Health maintenance, altered
Breathing-related sleep disorder	Hopelessness
Circadian rhythm sleep disorder	Mobility, impaired physical
Psychological factors affecting medical conditions	Nutrition, altered: less than body requirements
	Pain, chronic‡
	Powerlessness
	Self-care deficits
	Self-esteem disturbance
	Skin integrity, impaired
	Sleep pattern disturbance‡
	Social interaction, impaired
	Social isolation
	Spiritual distress

*Reprinted with permission from the *Diagnostic and statistical manual of mental disorders*, Fourth Edition, Text Revision. Copyright 2000, American Psychiatric Association.
†From North American Nursing Diagnosis Association: *NANDA nursing diagnoses: definitions and classifications 1999-2000*, Philadelphia, 1999, The Association.
‡Primary nursing diagnosis for maladaptive psychophysiological responses.

physical illness. In addition, specific goals can be set to address problems related to pain and sleep.

The establishment of goals with these patients is often a problem. The patient's primary goal is to ease the physical symptoms of the illness, often through medical or surgical treatment. Exploration of psychological conflicts is likely to be seen as unnecessary. This resistance is related to the need to maintain defenses against the extreme anxiety that has led to the illness. The nurse must identify common treatment goals.

Detailed Diagnoses *related to* Psychophysiological Responses

NANDA DIAGNOSIS STEM	EXAMPLES OF COMPLETE DIAGNOSIS
Impaired adjustment	Impaired adjustment related to fear of assuming adult responsibilities, evidenced by multiple somatic complaints.
	Impaired adjustment related to inability to express hostile and competitive feelings, evidenced by labile hypertension.
Chronic pain	Chronic pain related to marital conflict, evidenced by back problems and protected gait.
	Chronic pain related to work pressures, evidenced by reports of headaches and facial mask.
Sleep pattern disturbance	Sleep pattern disturbance related to financial and familial concerns, evidenced by difficulty falling asleep and frequent awakening during the night.

DSM–IV–TR DIAGNOSIS	ESSENTIAL FEATURES*
Somatization disorder	A history of many physical complaints beginning before the age of 30, occurring over a period of several years, and resulting in treatment being sought or significant impairment in social or occupational functioning. The patient must display at least four pain symptoms, two gastrointestinal symptoms, one sexual symptom and one symptom suggesting a neurological disorder.
Conversion disorder	One or more symptoms or deficits affecting voluntary motor or sensory function, suggesting a neurological or general medical condition. Psychological factors are judged to be associated with the symptom or deficit because the initiation or exacerbation of the symptom or deficit is preceded by conflicts or other stressors. The symptom or deficit cannot be fully explained by a neurological or general medical condition and is not a culturally sanctioned behavior or experience.
Hypochondriasis	Preoccupation with fears of having, or ideas that one has, a serious disease based on the person's misinterpretation of bodily symptoms. The preoccupation persists despite appropriate medical evaluation and reassurance and has existed for at least 6 months. It causes clinically significant distress or impairment in functioning.
Body dysmorphic disorder	Preoccupation with an imagined or exaggerated defect in appearance that causes clinically significant distress or impairment in functioning.
Pain disorder	Pain in one or more anatomical sites is the predominant focus of the clinical presentation. It is of sufficient severity to warrant clinical attention and causes clinically significant distress or impairment in functioning. Psychological factors are judged to have an important role in the onset, severity, exacerbation, or maintenance of the pain.
Primary insomnia	Difficulty initiating or maintaining sleep, or nonrestorative sleep, for at least 1 month that causes clinically significant distress or impairment in functioning.
Primary hypersomnia	Excessive sleepiness for at least 1 month, as evidenced by prolonged sleep episodes or daytime sleep episodes occurring almost daily that cause clinically significant distress or impairment in functioning.
Narcolepsy	Irresistible attacks of refreshing sleep occurring daily over at least 3 months with cataplexy (brief episodes of sudden bilateral loss of muscle tone) and hallucinations or sleep paralysis at the beginning or end of sleep episodes.
Breathing-related sleep disorder	Sleep disruption leading to excessive sleepiness or insomnia judged to be caused by sleep apnea or central alveolar hypoventilation syndrome.
Circadian rhythm sleep disorder	Persistent or recurrent pattern of sleep disruption leading to excessive sleepiness or insomnia that is caused by a mismatch between the sleep-wake schedule required by a person's environment and one's circadian sleep-wake pattern that causes clinically significant distress or impairment in functioning.
Psychological factors affecting medical condition	Presence of a medical condition in which psychological factors influence its cause, interfere with its treatment, constitute additional health risks, or elicit stress-related physiological responses that precipitate or exacerbate its symptoms.

*Reprinted with permission from the *Diagnostic and statistical manual of mental disorders*, Fourth Edition, Text Revision. Copyright 2000, American Psychiatric Association.

The nurse also wants the patient to obtain relief from physical symptoms. Many patients undergo medical or surgical treatment and related nursing care. At the same time, the nurse should try to build a trusting relationship so that the patient can feel safe in exploring interpersonal conflicts and feelings.

Significant others must also be considered in developing the plan of care. It is important to explore their understanding of the patient's problem. They can be valuable allies in encouraging the patient to make a lifestyle change, if this is necessary. At the same time, the nurse must recognize that a change in one family member requires a change in all the others. The family may be active participants in the patient's maladaptive behavioral style. In this case, goals should include addressing the family relationships with the patient.

PLANNING

Treatment plans for these patients may be lengthy. The nurse must attend to all of the patient's biopsychosocial needs. Most patients, while having needs in all areas, have their most urgent needs in a limited area of functioning. Physical disorders are usually disabling and may be life threatening. Psychosocial problems will hinder recovery from the physical illness and must also be given immediate attention.

How would you plan care with a patient who denies that problems with his ulcerative colitis are related to work stress and marital conflict, as reported by his wife?

IMPLEMENTATION

Patients with psychophysiological illnesses are most often seen in general hospital and outpatient settings. They usually seek health care because of symptoms related to physiological functioning. Only after a thorough medical examination can the role of psychosocial stressors in the disorder be evaluated.

In some cases a pathophysiological disruption requires physical nursing intervention. If the physical condition is life threatening, this intervention is given highest priority. For instance, a person with a bleeding ulcer needs intensive care to maintain life. However, once the physical crisis is past, the nurse can help the patient avoid similar problems in the future.

Physical illnesses with psychosocial etiologies require psychiatric nursing care. Skilled and compassionate nursing care directed to the patient's physical needs is the first step in establishing the trusting relationship. A person who is in pain, bleeding, or covered with a rash is unable to discuss emotions or interpersonal relationships. The most important principle for patients with psychophysical disorders is to assess the patient's stress level and, whenever possible, act to reduce it. Stress and anxiety are at the root of the patient's problem. The nurse must care for immediate needs before addressing less obvious ones.

Empirically validated treatments for some of the medical diagnoses related to psychophysiological responses are summarized in Table 18-1.

Psychological Approaches

The psychophysiological symptom defends the person from overwhelming anxiety. It provides a way to receive help and nurturance without admitting the need for it. Others are protected from expressing frightening aggressive or sexual impulses. Recognizing the defensive nature of the symptom, the nurse should never try to convince the patient that the problem is entirely psychological. Likewise, the attitude that the

Table **18-1**

Summarizing the Evidence on Psychological Responses
DISORDER: Body dysmorphic disorder
TREATMENT: ■ Cognitive-behavior therapy helped patients identify and challenge distorted body perceptions and interrupted self-critical thoughts, especially when used in conjunction with guided exposure and response prevention.
DISORDER: Hypochondriasis
TREATMENT: ■ Cognitive-behavior therapy has proven helpful in correcting the misinformation and exaggerated beliefs as well as pointing out the cognitive processes maintaining disease fears in hypochondriasis.
DISORDER: Pain disorder
TREATMENT: ■ Individual and group cognitive-behavior therapy reduced pain-related distress and disability. ■ Antidepressants decreased pain intensity.
DISORDER: Sleep disorders
TREATMENT: ■ The benzodiazepines and zolpidem typically reduced sleep onset by 15 to 30 minutes, decreased the number of awakenings to an absolute level of 1to 3 per night, and increased total sleep time by about 15 to 45 minutes. These pharmacological agents act more reliably than behavioral interventions in the short-term. ■ Over the long-term, behavioral interventions, including stimulus control, sleep restriction, relaxation strategies and cognitive-behavioral therapy reduced sleep onset, decreased awakenings and increased total sleep time. These behavioral interventions produced more sustained effects than pharmacological agents.

Nathan P, Gorman J: *A guide to treatments that work,* New York, 1998, Oxford University Press.

patient needs only to get his or her life under control to get better is not therapeutic. The patient has not made a conscious choice to be hypertensive or to develop a conversion disorder.

The dilemma of these disorders is that the patient consciously would like nothing more than to be cured but is unconsciously unable to give up the symptom. Conscious recognition of the psychological role of the symptom defeats its purpose and is therefore vigorously resisted. An example of this resistance is illustrated in the following clinical example.

 ## CLINICAL EXAMPLE

Ms. W was a 20-year-old woman admitted to the general hospital after the sudden onset of blindness. There was no evidence of any pathophysiological process affecting her eyes. Assessment revealed that she had witnessed her father's suicide by gunshot at the age of 5, although she claimed to have no memory of this. Her boyfriend had recently been expressing suicidal thoughts to her.

It appeared that the blindness was a conversion reaction. To confirm the diagnosis, the physician decided to interview Ms. W while she was sedated with amobarbital sodium. The interview was videotaped. During the interview, Ms. W was able to see. She read the day's menu and told the time by looking at a clock across the room. She also described her father's suicide. However, when the sedation wore off, Ms. W was again blind. The decision was made to play the videotape for her so that she would recognize the psychogenic nature of her blindness. As the tape was played, she re-

gained the ability to see. However, when it reached the part in which she described her father's suicide, she became deaf.

Selected Nursing Diagnoses

- Ineffective denial related to early life events, as evidenced by symptoms affecting sight and hearing
- Impaired social interaction related to boyfriend's depressive thoughts, as evidenced by development of physical symptoms

It is not unusual for a person with a conversion disorder to substitute another symptom if the original one is taken away. This substitution happens because the basic conflict remains. The ego still needs to be defended from experiencing repressed anxiety. The patient really needs assistance in dealing with the conflict. When this is resolved, the symptom will disappear because there is no longer a need for it.

Great skill is needed to intervene therapeutically with patients with maladaptive psychophysiological responses. Psychological approaches include supportive therapy, insight therapy, group therapy, cognitive behavioral strategies, stress reduction, relaxation training and psychopharmacology (see Citing the Evidence). The nurse should be supportive and available to talk with the patient and provide physical care (see A Patient Speaks). Alternative and complementary therapies can also be helpful (see Chapter 30).

The process of insight-oriented therapy for patients with psychophysiological disorders requires that the patient's underlying feelings be recognized and confronted in a supportive manner. As the patient becomes aware of anger, appropriate expression of it may be difficult. The nurse should accept the patient's attempts to express anger and provide feedback. Sometimes patients in this phase of therapy are labeled as hostile or demanding and avoided by nursing staff. This reaction only reinforces their conviction that angry feelings are unacceptable.

Citing the Evidence on

Cognitive Behavior Therapy for Chronic Fatigue Syndrome

BACKGROUND: No definitive treatment or etiology has been established for chronic fatigue syndrome. The purpose of this study was to test whether cognitive behavior therapy was significantly superior to relaxation, controlling for such treatment factors as support, therapist time and attention, expectations, and homework practice.

RESULTS: Functional impairment and fatigue improved more in the group that received cognitive behavior therapy. At 6 month follow up, 70% of those who completed the cognitive behavior therapy group achieved good outcomes compared with 19% of those in the relaxation group.

IMPLICATIONS: As chronic fatigue syndrome is heterogeneous, effective clinical practice will probably require the pragmatic, flexible use of a range of behavioral and cognitive techniques closely tailored to the individual. The issues of who benefits from specific aspects of treatment and how the response rate can be maximized deserves further study.

Deale A et al: Cognitive behavior therapy for chronic fatigue syndrome: a randomized controlled trial, *Am J Psychiatr* 154(3):408, 1997.

 ### A Patient Speaks

All I want to do is to feel better. My husband tells me that I make up all these complaints, but who would want to be sick? It isn't any fun missing out on family and church events because you don't feel good. It isn't fun going to bed with a headache and waking up with back pain day after day after day. On the other hand, my doctors tell me that they can't find anything wrong. Where does that leave me?

Right now I'm working with a nurse who is helping me to learn new habits that may help my physical condition. She has taught me how I can relax myself when I am tense and in pain. She has suggested some activities that I can start doing right now and is also reviewing with me situations and events that seem to trigger my physical problems. Will it help? I don't know, because we're just starting out, but I do know that she is at least one person I can talk to who supports me in my fight to feel like my old self again.

The next step in therapy is to identify and explore the patient's defenses. The therapist proceeds very carefully, helping the patient discover and test new, more adaptive coping mechanisms as the dysfunctional ones are given up. The nurse should support the patient in using new behaviors. Spending time with the patient and appreciating the patient's positive qualities will help the patient build self-esteem and confidence. The nurse should be alert to signs of increased anxiety and report these immediately. The physical disorder may worsen if the therapy moves too rapidly. The therapist may recommend changes in the environment to help the patient function more comfortably. If the patient must consider a job change or another lifestyle change, the nurse can offer time to talk about alternatives.

Patients may also need help in explaining lifestyle change or changes in themselves to significant others. The family is a system, and a change in one component of the system requires adjustment in the other parts. For instance, a man who was very involved in his job and out several nights a week agreed to limit himself to 8-hour work days. This change affected the rest of the family. Although his wife had protested for years that he spent too much time away from home, she built her life around his schedule. She spent several evenings a week in other activities. If he were to be at home every evening, she would have to reevaluate her activities and decide whether she should go out or be with him. These are not easy decisions for family members to make.

It is important that any underlying feelings of resentment be revealed and discussed to prevent indirect expression, which would create a new stressor for the patient. Family therapy may be necessary if family members have been supporting the patient's disorder. For instance, families sometimes become adjusted to having a dependent member and unwittingly sabotage efforts to foster independence.

Because social support systems may help patients cope with their illnesses, the nurse may need to look for alternatives when the family is not supportive. Self-help groups often provide the needed social support. Group interventions are also helpful in decreasing overuse of health-care services by patients with somatoform disorders.

Nurses must be aware that countertransference often occurs with these patients (see Chapter 2). It is easy to become impatient with a demanding patient who is not acutely ill when sicker patients also need nursing care. Reacting to this behavior by avoidance or anger only adds to the patient's anxiety. Clinical supervision by an experienced psychiatric nurse is highly recommended for nurses who work with these difficult patients. Frequent nursing care conferences are also helpful. If possible, a limited number of staff members should be assigned to the care of these patients. This consistent care fosters the development of a trusting relationship.

Patient Education

Health education is important in caring for the patient with a psychophysiological disorder. Such patients usually need instruction about medications, treatments and lifestyle changes. The patient and family will need information about mental health promotion (see Chapter 13), follow-up care, and crisis management (see Chapter 14), and education about ways to cope with anxiety and stress (see Chapter 17). Group classes on stress management may be productive. They may enable patients to share experiences and make suggestions to each other about coping behaviors. Former patients who have made successful life adjustments can also be effective teachers of coping strategies.

Do you think that patients with maladaptive psychophysiological responses will be more or less likely to comply with their treatment plans? How might you enhance their adherence?

Physiological Support

A variety of physiological treatments can also be implemented by the nurse. Relaxation training, described in Chapter 32, can be very helpful in promoting adaptive psychophysiological responses. Encouraging physical activity is also a positive way of promoting stress reduction. Ideally, it should be an activity that the patient enjoys and can share with others. Diet counseling may be helpful in building the person's resistance to stress and illness. Patients under stress should not overuse dietary stimulants such as caffeine. They may need education about the elements of a healthful diet and help in planning balanced meals. A patient who has been relying on alcohol or drugs to cope with stress should be encouraged to find more adaptive coping mechanisms (see Chapter 25). Antidepressant medication is useful if there is a comorbid depression.

Box 18-3

Sleep Hygiene Strategies

- Set a regular bedtime and wake-up time 7 days a week.
- Exercise daily to aid sleep initiation and maintenance; however, vigorous exercise too close to bedtime may make falling asleep difficult.
- Schedule time to wind down and relax before bed.
- Avoid worrying when trying to fall asleep.
- Guard against nighttime interruptions. Earplugs may help with a noisy partner. Heavy window shades help to screen out light. Create a comfortable bed.
- Maintain a cool temperature in the room. A warm bath or warm drink before bed helps some people fall asleep.
- Excessive hunger or fullness may interfere with sleep. Avoid large meals before bed. If hungry, a light carbohydrate snack may be helpful.
- Avoid caffeine, excessive fluid intake, stimulating drugs, and excessive alcohol in the evening and before bed.
- Excessive napping may make it difficult for some people to fall asleep at night.
- Do not eat, read, work, or watch television in bed. The bed and bedroom should be used only for sleep and sex.
- Maintain a reasonable weight. Excessive weight may result in daytime fatigue and sleep apnea.
- Get out of bed and engage in other activities if not able to fall asleep.

Finally, the effective treatment of sleep disorders requires that the underlying cause of the sleep problem be identified. Drugs and alcohol often produce fragmented sleep, as does caffeine (Blumenthal & Fine, 1996). Poor sleep hygiene habits may also be a problem, and the patient can be encouraged to develop good sleep hygiene habits (Box 18-3). Sedative medications (Table 18-2) can also be used to help induce sleep, but these drugs should be used for only a limited time because of the risk of dependence (see Chapter 28). Melatonin may be helpful when insomnia is related to shift work and jet lag; however, its use is controversial (Rajput & Bromley, 1999). Although prescription medications and sleep hygiene behavior therapy have similar short-term efficacy, behavioral interventions are recommended as the first line treatment because of their greater safety and long-term efficacy (Eddy & Walbroehl, 1999).

The Nursing Treatment Plan Summary for patients with maladaptive psychophysiological responses is presented below.

EVALUATION

The evaluation of the nursing care of the patient with psychophysiological illness is based on the identified patient care goals. If goal achievement is not attained, the nurse must ask the following questions:

- Was the assessment complete enough to correctly identify the problem?
- Did the patient agree with the goal?
- Was enough time allowed for goal achievement?

- Was I skilled enough to carry out the desired intervention?
- Were there environmental constraints that affected goal accomplishment?
- Did additional stressors change the patient's ability to cope?
- Was the goal achievable for this patient?
- What alternative approaches should be tried?

It is very important that neither the patient nor the nurse interpret the lack of goal achievement as a failure. The nurse should look at it as a challenge and convey that attitude to the patient. It is not helpful to add failure to achieve a goal to the patient's collection of stressors. The care of these patients is very complex. The nurse may need to modify the treatment plan several times before finding a successful approach. The most important thing is to keep trying and to encourage the patient to persist in the effort to find health.

Table **18-2**

Sedative-Hypnotic Medications and Doses	
Sedative-Hypnotic Drugs	Usual Dose (mg/night)
Flurazepam (Dalmane)	1-2
Temazepam (Restoril)	15-30
Triazolam (Halcion)	0.25-0.5
Zolpidem (Ambien)	10
Secobarbital (Seconal)	100-200
Pentobarbital (Nembutal)	100-200
Chloral hydrate (Noctec)	500-2000
Zaleplon (Sonata)	5-10

NURSING TREATMENT PLAN Summary *Maladaptive Psychophysiological Responses*

NURSING DIAGNOSIS: Impaired adjustment
EXPECTED OUTCOME: The patient will express feelings verbally rather than through the development of physical symptoms.

SHORT-TERM GOAL	INTERVENTION	RATIONALE
The patient will identify areas of stress and conflict and relate feelings, thoughts, and behaviors to them.	Assist patient in identifying stressful situations by reviewing events surrounding the development of physical symptoms. Facilitate the association among cognitions, feelings and behaviors.	Inability to deal with intrapsychic conflict leads to anxiety and stress, resulting in physiological dysfunction.
The patient will describe present defenses and evaluate whether they are adaptive or maladaptive.	Proceed slowly in analyzing defenses. Explore alternative coping behaviors with the patient. Teach the patient stress management techniques such as relaxation and imagery.	Defenses should not be attacked; rather, the nurse should support positive exploration by the patient and suggest alternative responses.
The patient will adopt two new coping mechanisms to deal with stress.	Give patient positive feedback for new adaptive behaviors. Actively support patient in testing new coping mechanisms. Enlist the support of family and significant others to reinforce change.	Change requires time and positive reinforcement from others. Family members can be important in promoting adaptive responses.
The patient will display a decrease in physical symptoms and greater biological integrity.	Encourage physical activity to reduce stress. Counsel the patient on diet and nutrition needs. Review the patient's sleep habits and promote good sleep hygiene practices.	Wellness requires a balance between biological and psychosocial needs. Interventions focused on the patient's physiological needs can help the patient restore biological integrity.

Summary

1. The continuum of possible psychophysiological responses to stress based on Selye's theory includes the stages of alarm, resistance and exhaustion.

2. Patient behaviors related to psychophysiological responses include physical conditions affected by psychological factors, psychological symptoms such as somatization, conversion, body dysmorphic and pain disorders, hypochondriasis, and sleep problems.

3. Predisposing factors are described from biological, psychological and sociocultural perspectives. Precipitating stressors include any experience the patient interprets as stressful.

4. A variety of coping mechanisms are used in psychophysiological response such as repression, denial, compensation, and regression.

5. Primary NANDA nursing diagnoses for psychophysiological responses are impaired adjustment, chronic pain and sleep pattern disturbance.

6. Primary *DSM–IV–TR* diagnoses are categorized as somatoform disorders, sleep disorders and psychological factors affecting medical condition.

7. The expected outcome of nursing care is that the patient will express feelings verbally rather than through the development of physical symptoms.

8. Interventions include psychological approaches, patient education and physiological support.

9. The care of these patients is complex, and the nurse may need to modify the treatment plan several times before finding a successful approach.

Competent Caring A Clinical Exemplar of a Psychiatric Nurse

AUDREY JOSEPH, MSN, RN

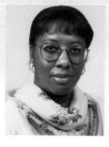

Often it is difficult for health-care professionals to communicate with their patients about psychosomatic illness. Also, the patient's denial or rejection of this diagnosis does not make the communication process any easier. Psychiatric staff and family members can get caught in the middle when primary care physicians fail to tell their patients that they need a psychiatric evaluation to rule out a psychosomatic illness. I know this from an experience I had that taught me much about psychiatric care.

I was working the evening shift as a staff nurse on an inpatient unit when Mrs. O, an elderly woman, presented herself on the unit for voluntary admission. She was well dressed and quite cheerful. Her medical history revealed that she had visited her family doctor and the emergency room weekly for the last 2 months. She had many diagnostic studies, the results of which were all negative. Mrs. O reported that she was referred by her family doctor for a diagnostic work-up. A psychosocial assessment revealed that her husband had recently died and that she lived alone. The patient was allowed to become acclimated to the unit. Then, as the staff explained to her why she was admitted, she became angry and left against medical advice.

About 3 weeks later Mrs. O's son arranged for her to be readmitted because she was constantly going to the emergency room and to her family doctor. She was angry with her son for having her admitted. To keep her in the hospital, he told her that he would have her committed if necessary. On this admission, Mrs. O was neatly dressed but looked tired. Her chief complaint was choking and a general infection throughout her body that was causing a vaginal discharge. Her family doctor still did not tell her that he could not find anything physically wrong with her. She was started on a regimen of antidepressant medication. During the 2 weeks she was in the hospital, she spent most of her time socializing with other patients. She was not interested in psychotherapy and did not develop a therapeutic alliance with the staff.

On her third admission, approximately 2 months later, Mrs. O's family doctor still had not told her that he thought she had a psychosomatic illness. At this time she was disheveled and looked physically ill. Mrs. O spent most of the day in bed. She constantly complained of choking and a vaginal discharge. She admitted that she stopped taking the antidepressant medication right after discharge from the hospital. At this point she was angry with all her children and thought they were all against her. She could not understand why they would not accept the fact that she was physically ill. After 3 weeks of treatment Mrs. O was discharged home. Two years later I met Mrs. O in another psychiatric hospital where she was again admitted for treatment.

Clearly this is not a success story. In fact, it taught me much about the problems of nonintegrated physical and psychiatric systems of care in which patients are treated as parts rather than wholes. I also realized that I shared responsibility for not providing better care for Mrs. O. To this day, she is often in my thoughts, and I now advocate for treating patients broadly within the context of their world view rather than within the narrow realm our society defines as medical care.

Chapter Review Questions

1. Match each term in Column A with the correct definition in Column B.

Column A

___ Body dysmorphic disorder

___ Conversion disorder

___ Hypersomnia

___ Hypochondriasis

___ Insomnia

___ Pain disorder

___ Parasomnia

___ Sleep pattern disturbance

___ Somatization disorder

___ Somatoform disorders

Column B

A. Physical symptoms without organic impairment

B. A history of many physical complaints

C. Loss or alteration of voluntary motor or sensory function that cannot be explained by a medical condition

D. Preoccupation with fears of having a serious disease

E. An imagined or exaggerated defect in appearance

F. A disorder in which psychological factors have an important role in the onset, severity, exacerbation or maintenance

G. Sleepwalking, night terrors, nightmares, enuresis

H. Narcolepsy, sleep apnea, nocturnal movement disorders

I. Disorders of initiating or maintaining sleep

J. Difficulty falling asleep and frequent awakening during the night

2. Fill in the blanks.

A. The continuum of possible psychophysiological responses to stress, based on Selye's theory, include the stages of _____, _____, _____.

B. A variety of coping mechanisms are used in psychophysiological response such as _____, _____, and _____.

C. The expected outcome of nursing care is that the patient will express feelings _____ rather than through the development of _____ symptoms.

D. It is not unusual for a person with _____ to substitute another symptom if the original one is taken away without attention to the underlying stressor.

E. _____ is the scientific field that explores the relationship between psychological states and the immune response.

3. Provide short answers for the following questions.

A. Describe four psychological interventions the nurse might use in the treatment of the patient with a maladaptive psychophysiological response to stress.

B. Define secondary gain. Give several examples from your personal experience.

C. Research indicates that people with clinical depression who smoke are at higher risk for lung cancer than people without depression who smoke. Based on this information, how would you differ in your educational approach to patients with and without depression who smoke?

REFERENCES

American Psychiatric Association: *Diagnostic and statistical manual of mental disorders,* Fourth Edition, Text Revision. Washington, DC, American Psychiatric Association, 2000.

Bandura A: *Self-efficacy: the exercise of control,* New York, 1997, WH Freeman.

Blumenthal SJ, Fine T: Sleep abnormalities associated with mental and addictive disorders: implications for research and clinical practice, *J Pract Psychiatry Behav Health* 3:67, 1996.

Buysse DJ, Perlis ME: The evaluation and treatment of insomnia, *J Pract Psych Behav Health* 3:80, 1996.

Demitrack M: Chronic fatigue syndrome and fibromyalgia: dilemmas in diagnosis and clinical management, *Psychiatr Clin North Am* 21(3):671, 1998.

Eddy M, Walbroehl G: Insomnia, *Am Fam Physician* April 1, 1999.

Friedman H: *The self-healing personality: why some people achieve health while others succumb to illness,* New York, 1991, Holt.

Keefe FJ, Goli V: A practical guide to behavioral assessment and treatment of chronic pain, *J Pract Psych Behav Health* 5:151, 1996.

Lilie J, Lahmeyer H: Psychiatric management of sleep disorders, *Psychiatr Med* 9:245, 1991.

Lowery BJ, Houldin AD: From stressor to illness: the psychobiological-biological connection. In McBride AB, Austin JK, editors: *Psychiatric-mental health nursing: integrating the behavioral and biological sciences,* Philadelphia, 1996, WB Saunders.

National Center on Sleep Disorders Research Working Group: Recognizing problem sleepiness in your patients, *Am Fam Physician,* Feb 15, 1999.

Nowell P et al: Clinical factors contributing to the differential diagnosis of primary insomnia and insomnia related to mental disorders, *Am J Psychiatry* 154(10):1412, 1997.

Oakley LD, Potter C: *Psychiatric primary care,* St Louis, 1997, Mosby.

Parsons T: *The social system,* New York, 1951, The Free Press.

Rajput V, Bromley S: Chronic insomnia: a practical review, *Am Fam Physician* Oct 1, 1999.

Selye H: *The stress of life,* New York, 1956, McGraw-Hill.

Streit WJ, Kincaid-Colton CA: The brain's immune system, *Sci Am* 11:54, 1995.

Vallerand A: Gender differences in pain, *J Nurs Scholarsh* 27:235, 1995.

Wake up America: a national sleep alert, Report of the National Commission on Sleep Disorders Research, Washington, DC, 1993, US Department of Health and Human Services.

Wessely S et al: Psychological symptoms, somatic symptoms, and psychiatric disorder in chronic fatigue and chronic fatigue syndrome: a prospective study in the primary care setting, *Am J Psychiatry* 153:1050, 1996.

Wise T: The worried patient: clinical management of the patient with hypochondriasis, *J Pract Psych Behav Health* 3:223, 1997.

Yantis M: Identifying depression as a symptom of sleep apnea, *J Psychosoc Nurs Ment Health Serv* 37(10):28, 1999.

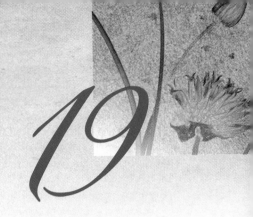

Self-Concept Responses and Dissociative Disorders

Gail W. Stuart

To venture causes anxiety, but not to venture is to lose one's-self. And to venture in the highest sense is precisely to be conscious of one's self.

SØREN KIERKEGAARD

Of all human attributes the self is the most complex and intangible. It is the frame of reference through which one perceives, conceives, and evaluates one's world. Self-concept is defined as all the notions, beliefs, and convictions that constitute a person's self-knowledge and that influence relationships with others. It includes one's perceptions of personal characteristics and abilities, interactions with other people and the environment, values associated with experiences and objects, and goals and ideals.

The self-concept is critical to the understanding of people and their behavior. No two people have identical self-concepts. The self-concept emerges or is learned through each person's internal experiences, relationships with other people, and interactions with the outer world. Because it is the frame of reference through which the person interacts with the world, it has a powerful influence on human behavior. It is impossible to understand a person fully or to predict behavior accurately without understanding the person's internal frame of reference. This involves sharing the person's perceptual world and view of the self. Thus understanding a patient's self-concept is a necessary part of all nursing care.

CONTINUUM OF SELF-CONCEPT RESPONSES
Self-Concept

Developmental Influences. From birth the self develops gradually as the infant recognizes and distinguishes others and begins to gain a sense of differentiation from others. The boundaries of the self are defined as the result of exploratory activity and experience with one's own body. At first self-differentiation is slow, but with the development of language it accelerates. Use of the child's own name helps with the identification and perception of individuality—of being someone special, unique, and independent. Human language allows clear distinctions to be made between the self and the rest of the world and the ability to symbolize and understand experiences. The continued process of self-concept development is greatly aided by the following:

- Interpersonal and cultural experiences that generate positive feelings and a sense of worth
- Perceived competence in areas valued by the individual and society
- Self-actualization, or the implementation and realization of a person's true potential

Significant Others. The self-concept is learned in part through accumulated social contacts and experiences with other people. Sullivan (1963) called this development "learning about self from the mirror of other people." What a person believes about himself is a function of his interpretation of how others see him, as inferred from their behavior toward him. His concept of self therefore rests partly on what he thinks others think of him.

For a young child the most significant others are his parents, who help him grow and react to his experiences. The family provides the person with his earliest experiences of:

- Feelings of adequacy or inadequacy
- Feelings of acceptance or rejection
- Opportunities for identification
- Expectations concerning acceptable goals, values, and behaviors

Research indicates that parental influence is strongest during early childhood and continues to have a significant impact through adolescence and young adulthood. Over time, however, the power and influence of friends and other adults increase, and they become significant others to the person. Culture and socialization practices also affect self-concept and personality development. General cultural patterns and cultural subdivisions, such as social class, have formative influences on one's view of self.

What sociocultural factors had an impact on your self-concept as you were growing up? Which ones currently influence your self-concept?

Self-Perceptions. Each person can observe his or her own behavior the same way that others do and form opinions about oneself. One's perception of reality is selective, however, according to whether the experience is consistent with one's current concept of self. The way a person behaves is a result of how he or she perceives the situation, and it is not the event itself that elicits a specific response but rather the individual's subjective experience of the event.

One's needs, values, and beliefs strongly influence perceptions. People are more likely to perceive what is meaningful and consistent with present needs and personal values. Similarly, people behave in a manner consistent with what they believe to be true. In this case a fact is not what is but what one believes to be true. Once perceptions are acquired and incorporated into one's self-system, they can be difficult to change. Ways exist to change perceptions, however, including modifying cognitive processes, taking drugs, sensory deprivation, and biochemical changes within the body.

A person with a weak or negative self-concept who is unsure of himself is likely to have narrowed or distorted perceptions. Because he feels easily threatened, his anxiety level will rise quickly and he will become preoccupied with defending himself. In contrast, a person with a strong or positive self-concept can explore his world openly and honestly because he has a background of acceptance and success. Positive self-concepts result from positive experiences leading to perceived competence.

In conclusion, people with positive self-concepts function more effectively. Negative self-concept is correlated with personal and social maladjustment (Horowitz et al, 1996). Fig. 19-1 describes the continuum of self-concept responses from the most adaptive state of self-actualization to the most maladaptive response of depersonalization.

The nurse therefore needs an understanding of various components of the self, including body image, self-ideal, self-esteem, role, and identity, which are briefly discussed here.

Body Image

The concept of one's body is central to the concept of self. The body is the most material and visible part of the self, and, although it does not account for one's entire sense of

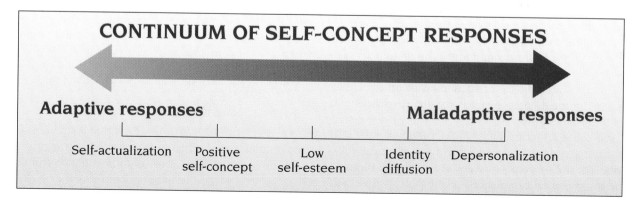

Fig. 19-1 Continuum of self-concept responses.

self, it remains a lifelong anchor for self-awareness. A person's attitude toward the body may mirror important aspects of identity. A person's feelings that his or her body is big or small, attractive or unattractive, or weak or strong also reveal something about the self-concept. Numerous research studies have documented the close positive relationship between self-concept and body image. This association appears to exist in all cultures.

Body image is the sum of the conscious and unconscious attitudes the person has toward his or her own body. It includes present and past perceptions as well as feelings about size, function, appearance, and potential. Body image is dynamic because it is constantly changing with new perceptions and experiences. It is a target or screen on which the person projects significant personal feelings, anxieties, and values.

As one's body image develops, extensions of the body become important. Clothes become identified closely with the body, and in the same way toys, tools, money, and possessions also serve as extensions of the body. Body image, appearance, and positive self-concept are related. Studies indicate that the more a person accepts and likes his or her own body, the more secure and free from anxiety he or she feels. It has also been shown that people who accept their bodies are more likely to have high self-esteem than people who dislike their bodies. Problems related to body image are discussed in more detail in Chapter 26.

 What does it mean when one says that "a child lives in his body but an adult lives in his mind"?

Self-Ideal

The self-ideal is the person's perception of how to behave, based on certain personal standards. The standard may be either a carefully constructed image of the type of person he or she would like to be or merely a number of aspirations, goals, or values that he or she would like to achieve. The self-ideal creates self-expectations based in part on society's norms, to which the person tries to conform.

Formation of the self-ideal begins in childhood and is influenced by significant others, who place certain demands or expectations on the child. With time the child internalizes these expectations, and they form the basis of the child's own self-ideal. New self-ideals are taken on during adolescence, formed from identification with parents, teachers, and peers. In old age additional adjustments must be made that reflect diminishing physical strength and changing roles and responsibilities.

Various factors influence self-ideal. First, a person tends to set goals within a range determined by personal abilities. A person does not ordinarily set a goal that is accomplished without any effort or that is entirely beyond his or her abilities. Self-ideals are also influenced by cultural factors as the person compares self-standards with those of peers. Other influencing factors include ambitions and the desire to excel and succeed, the need to be realistic, the desire to avoid failure, and feelings of anxiety and inferiority.

Based on these factors, one's self-ideal may be clear and realistic and thus facilitate personal growth and relations with others, or it may be vague, unrealistic, and demanding. The adequately functioning person demonstrates congruence between one's perception of self and self-ideal, that is, one sees oneself as being very similar to the person one wants to be.

In summary, self-ideals are important in maintaining mental health and balance. The self-ideal must neither be too high and demanding nor too vague and shadowy, yet it must be high enough to give continuous support to self-respect.

Self-Esteem

Self-esteem is a person's personal judgment of his or her own worth, based on how well behavior matches up with self-ideal. The frequency with which a person attains goals directly influences feelings of competency (high self-esteem) or inferiority (low self-esteem) (Fig. 19-2). High self-esteem is a feeling based on unconditional acceptance of self, despite mistakes, defeats, and failures, as an innately worthy and important being. It involves accepting complete responsibility for one's own life.

Self-esteem comes from two primary sources: the self and others. It is first a function of being loved and gaining the respect of others. Self-esteem is lowered when love is lost and when one fails to receive approval from others. Conversely, it is raised when love is regained and when one is applauded and praised. The origins of self-esteem can be traced to childhood and are based on acceptance, warmth, involvement, consistency, praise, and respect. The four best ways to promote a child's self-esteem are as follows (Coopersmith, 1967; Mruk, 1995):

- Providing opportunities for success
- Instilling ideals
- Encouraging aspirations
- Helping the child build defenses against attacks to his or her self-perceptions

These should provide the child with a feeling of significance or success in being accepted and approved of by others; a feeling of competence, or an ability to cope effectively with life; and a feeling of power, or control over one's own destiny.

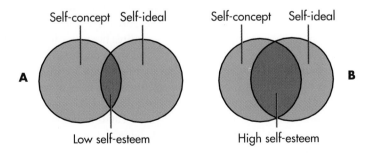

Fig. 19-2 **A,** Person with a low level of self-esteem caused by a large discrepancy between self-concept and self-ideal. **B,** Person with a greater conformity of self-concept and self-ideal and therefore a high level of self-esteem. (From Sundeen SJ et al: *Nurse-client interaction: implementing the nursing process,* ed 6, St Louis, 1998, Mosby.)

Self-esteem increases with age and is most threatened during adolescence, when concepts of self are being changed and many self-decisions are made. The adolescent must choose an occupation and decide whether he or she is good enough to succeed in a given career. Adolescents must also decide whether they are able to participate or are accepted in various social activities.

With adulthood the self-concept stabilizes, and maturity provides a clearer picture of self. The adult tends to be more self-accepting and less idealistic than the adolescent. Adults have learned to cope with many self-deficiencies and to maximize self-strengths. Not all adults attain maturity; some continue to function as adolescents for many of their adult years.

In later life, self-esteem problems again arise because of the new challenges posed by retirement, loss of spouse, and physical disability. The impact of aging on self-esteem is also affected by the status of older people in American society. Being old in a society that values youth often leads to low status and prejudicial attitudes toward the aged. Negative stereotypes of the elderly and the stigmatization that results can decrease self-esteem. Two other potential negative factors are the decreased social interaction of the elderly and their loss of control over their environment, both of which can result in fewer opportunities to validate and confirm one's self-concept.

Research shows a clear relationship between self-reported physical health and self-esteem. The report of a health problem, regardless of its type or severity, is associated with significantly lower self-esteem than is the report of no health problem. In contrast, high self-esteem has been correlated with low anxiety, effective group functioning, and acceptance of others (Bednar et al, 1991). It is a prerequisite to self-actualization; once self-esteem is achieved, the person is free to concentrate on achieving his or her potential.

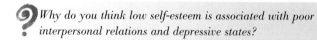
Why do you think low self-esteem is associated with poor interpersonal relations and depressive states?

Role Performance

Roles are sets of socially expected behavior patterns associated with a person's functioning in different social groups. The person assumes various roles that he or she tries to integrate into one functional pattern. Because these roles overlap, an understanding of the person requires the nurse to see him or her in the context of the several roles occupied. On the basis of his or her perception of role adequacy in the most ego-involved roles, the person develops a level of self-esteem. High self-esteem results from roles that meet needs and are congruent with one's self-ideal. Factors that influence a person's adjustment to the role he or she occupies include the following:

- One's knowledge of specific role expectations
- The consistency of the response of significant others to one's role
- The compatibility and complementarity of various roles

- The congruency of cultural norms and one's own expectations for role behavior
- The separation of situations that would create incompatible role behaviors

Gender roles affect performance in other roles. They are particularly significant to family roles but permeate most others as well and are often the cause of role conflict. Another difficult problem faced in growing up is emancipation from one's parents and establishment of an independent life. This primarily occurs during adolescence and early adulthood, when great ambiguity in role definitions occurs. A final crisis is faced during old age, when role behavior must again be changed by aging parents. They rely on their children, yet strive to balance their lives with a sense of independence and a high level of self-esteem.

Role behavior is intimately related to self-concept and identity, and role disturbances often involve conflicts between independent and dependent functioning.

Personal Identity

The word identity is derived from the Latin root **idem**, meaning "the same." It is the organizing principle of the personality. **Identity** is the awareness of being oneself, as derived from self-observation and judgment. It is the synthesis of all self-representations into an organized whole and is not associated with any one accomplishment, object, attribute, or role.

Identity is different from self-concept in that it is a feeling of distinctness from others. It implies consciousness of oneself as an individual with a definite place in the general scheme of things. The person with a sense of identity feels integrated, not diffuse. When a person acts in accordance with his or her self-concept, the sense of identity is reinforced; when he or she acts in ways contrary to the self-concept, he or she experiences anxiety and apprehension. The person with a strong sense of identity sees himself or herself as a unique individual.

Developmental Influences. The concept of ego identity was developed by Erikson (1963) and built within his formulation of the eight stages of human development. For each stage, Erikson describes a psychosocial crisis that must be resolved for further growth and personality development.

In adolescence the crisis of identity versus identity diffusion occurs. At no other phase of life are the promise of finding oneself and the threat of losing oneself so closely aligned. The adolescent's task is one of self-definition as one strives to integrate previous roles into a unique and reasonably consistent sense of self.

Important in achieving identity is the issue of sexuality, the image of oneself as a male or a female and what that implies. Society's ideals of masculinity and femininity are important standards for judging oneself as good, bad, inferior, superior, desirable, or undesirable. These ideals are passed down from generation to generation and become a part of the culture. If males are defined as superior, this idea becomes part of the self-image of both males and females. If passivity and obedience are feminine ideals in a society, most girls will be taught to be unassertive and obedient.

In addition, much of one's identity is expressed in relationships with others. How a person relates to other people is a central personality characteristic. This presents a paradox in that everyone is a part of humanity yet each person is also separate from all others. Achieving identity is a prerequisite for establishing an intimate relationship (Vaillant, 1993). Research has shown that only after a stable sense of identity has been established can one engage in genuinely intimate, mature, and successful relationships.

Healthy Personality

It is possible to describe the healthy personality according to developmental theory and the dynamics of the self. This description may help give perspective to the many aspects of self. A person with a healthy personality would have the characteristics listed in Table 19-1 and be able to perceive both self and the world accurately. This insight would create a feeling of harmony and inner peace.

 How do you compare with the qualities of a healthy personality listed in Table 19-1?

ASSESSMENT
Behaviors

Assessing the various aspects of a patient's self-concept is a challenge to the nurse. Because self-concept is the cornerstone of the personality, it is intimately related to anxiety and depression, problems in relationships, acting out, and self-destructive behavior. All behavior is motivated by a desire to enhance, maintain, or defend the self, so the nurse has much information to evaluate. Behavioral rating scales that the nurse might find useful related to self-concept responses are listed in Box 19-1. The nurse must also go be-

Box **19-1**

Behavioral Rating Scales Related to Self-Concept Responses

- Dissociative Experience Scale
- Dissociative Disorders Interview Schedule
- Menninger Revision of Role Functioning Scale
- Personal Adjustment and Role Skills
- Role Functioning Scale
- Self-Perception Profile for Adults
- Tennessee Self Concept Scale

Table **19-1**

Qualities of the Healthy Personality

Characteristic	Definition	Description
Positive and accurate body image	Body image is the sum of the conscious and unconscious attitudes one has toward one's body, function, appearance, and potential.	A healthy body awareness is based on self-observation and appropriate concern for one's physical well-being.
Realistic self-ideal	Self-ideal is one's perception of how one should behave or the standard by which behavior is appraised.	A person with a realistic self-ideal has attainable life goals that are valuable and worth striving for.
Positive self-concept	Self-concept consists of all the aspects of the person of which one is aware. It includes all self-perceptions that direct and influence behavior.	A positive self-concept implies that the person expects to be successful in life. It includes acceptance of the negative aspects of the self as part of one's personality. Such a person faces life openly and realistically.
High self-esteem	Self-esteem is one's personal judgment of one's own worth, which is obtained by analyzing how well one matches up to one's own standards and how well one's performance compares with others. It evolves through a comparison of the self-ideal and self-concept.	A person with high self-esteem feels worthy of respect and dignity, believes in his or her own self-worth, and approaches life with assertiveness and zest. The person with a healthy personality feels very similar to the person he or she wants to be.
Satisfying role performance	Roles are sets of socially expected behavior patterns associated with functioning in various social groups.	The healthy person can relate to others intimately, receive gratification from social and personal roles, trust others, and enter into mutual and interdependent relationships.
Clear sense of identity	Identity is the integration of inner and outer demands in one's discovery of who one is and what one can become. It is the realization of personal consistency.	The person with a clear sense of identity experiences a unity of or personality and perceives herself himself to be a unique person. This sense of self gives life direction and purpose.

yond objective and observable behaviors to the patient's subjective and internal world. Only by exploring this area can the nurse understand the patient's actions. The nurse can begin the assessment by observing the patient's appearance. Posture, cleanliness, makeup, and clothing provide data. The nurse might discuss the patient's appearance with him or her to determine what values are held related to body image. Observing or inquiring about eating, sleeping, and hygiene patterns gives clues to biological habits and self-care.

These initial observations should lead the nurse to ask: "What does my patient think about himself as a person?" The nurse might ask the patient to describe himself or how he feels about himself. What strengths does he think he has? What areas of weakness? What is his self-ideal? Does he conform to it? Does fulfillment of his self-ideal bring him satisfaction? Does he value his strengths? Does he view his weaknesses as important personality deficits, or are they unimportant to his self-concept? What are his priorities? Does he feel unified and self-directed or diffuse and other-directed?

The nurse can then compare the patient's responses to his behavior, looking for inconsistencies or contradictions. How does he relate to other people? How does he respond to compliments and criticisms? The nurse can also examine his or her own affective response to the patient. Is it one of hopelessness, despair, anger, or anxiety? The nurse's own response to the patient is often a good indication of the quality and depth of the patient's pain.

Associated with Low Self-Esteem. Low self-esteem is a major problem for many people and can be expressed in moderate and severe levels of anxiety. It involves negative self-evaluations and is associated with feelings of being weak, helpless, hopeless, frightened, vulnerable, fragile, incomplete, worthless, and inadequate.

Low self-esteem is a major component of depression, which acts as a form of punishment and anesthesia. Low self-esteem indicates self-rejection and self-hate, which may be a conscious or unconscious process expressed in direct or indirect ways.

Direct expressions of self-hate or low self-esteem may include any of the following areas.

Self-criticism. The patient has negative thinking and believes he or she is doomed to failure. Although the expressed purpose of the criticism may be self-improvement, there is no constructive value to it and the underlying goal is self-demoralization. The patient might describe himself as "stupid," "no good," or a "born loser." He views the normal stressors of life as impossible barriers and becomes preoccupied with self-pity.

Self-diminution. Self-diminution involves minimizing one's ability by avoiding, neglecting, or refusing to recognize one's real assets and strengths.

Guilt and worrying. Guilt and worry are destructive activities by which the person punishes himself or herself. They may be expressed through nightmares, phobias, obsessions, or the reliving of painful memories and indiscretions. They indicate self-rejection.

Physical manifestations. These might include hypertension, psychosomatic illnesses, and the abuse of various substances, such as alcohol, drugs, tobacco, or food.

Postponing decisions. A high level of ambivalence or procrastination produces an increased sense of insecurity.

Denying oneself pleasure. The self-rejecting person feels the need to punish himself and expresses this by denying himself the things he finds desirable or pleasurable. This might be a career opportunity, a material object, or a desired relationship.

Disturbed relationships. The person may be cruel, demeaning, or exploitive with other people. This may be an overt or a passive-dependent pattern of relating, which indirectly exploits others. Another behavior included in this category is withdrawal or social isolation, which arises from feelings of worthlessness.

Withdrawal from reality. When anxiety resulting from self-rejection reaches severe or panic levels, the person may dissociate and experience hallucinations, delusions, and feelings of suspicion, jealousy, or paranoia. Such withdrawal from reality may be a temporary coping mechanism or a long-term pattern indicating a profound problem of identity confusion.

Self-destructiveness. Self-hatred can be expressed through accident proneness or attempting dangerous feats. Extremely low levels of self-esteem can lead to suicide.

Other destructiveness. People who have overwhelming consciences may choose to act out against society. This activity serves to paralyze their own self-hate and displaces or projects it onto victims.

Indirect forms of self-hate. Indirect forms of self-hate complement and supplement the direct forms. They may be chronic patterns and difficult to change in therapy.

Illusions and unrealistic goals. Self-deception is the core element; the person refuses to accept a limited here and now. Illusions increase the possibility of disappointment and further self-hate. Examples of illusions are "If I were married, I would be happy" and "Money brings fulfillment." This indirect form of low self-esteem may make the person sensitive to criticism or overresponsive to flattery. It may also be evident in the defense mechanisms of blaming others for one's failures and becoming hypercritical to create the illusion of superiority.

Exaggerated sense of self. The person may also attempt to compensate by expressing an exaggerated opinion of his ability. He may continually boast, brag of his exploits, or claim extraordinary talents. An extreme compensatory behavior for low self-esteem is grandiose thinking and related delusions. Another example is evident in the perfectionist. Such people strain toward impossible goals and measure their own worth entirely in terms of productivity and accomplishment.

Boredom. This involves the rejection of one's possibilities and capabilities. The person may neglect or reject aspects that have great potential for future growth.

Polarizing view of life. In this case the person has a simplistic view of life in which everything is worst or best, wrong or right. He tends to have a closed belief system that acts as a defense against a threatening world. Ultimately this view of life leads to confusion, disappointment, and alienation from others.

The behaviors associated with low self-esteem are described in the clinical example that follows and are summarized in Box 19-2.

 CLINICAL EXAMPLE

Mrs. G was a 66-year-old woman admitted to the psychiatric hospital with a major depressive episode. She told the admitting nurse that "things have been building up for some time now" and she had been seeing a private psychiatrist for the past 6 months who suggested that she enter the hospital. She had been employed in a community college as a librarian until 18 months earlier, when she was forced to retire. Mrs. G said she had been married for 39 years and had two grown children who were married and lived out of state. Her husband had worked as an accountant but had retired a month before. She said that since her retirement she had felt "useless and lost and closed in" by their apartment. She seldom left the apartment, and had lost contact with many of her friends. She said she worried a great deal about their financial situation, especially now that her husband was also retired. He repeatedly reassured her that they had enough money, but she could not stop worrying about it.

Mrs. G said that she liked her job very much and thought she was good at it. A younger woman took her place at the library, and Mrs. G was very bitter when talking about her. She said that, little by little, this woman took over duties Mrs. G was responsible for and one day even cleaned out Mrs. G's desk and took it as her own. Since her retirement, she said, things had been "going downhill steadily." She said she was not a good housewife and disliked cooking. These tasks had become even more difficult since her husband retired because he was "always underfoot and criticizing" what she did. In the past couple of weeks, she had had

great difficulty sleeping, a decreased appetite, fatigue, and little interest in her appearance. She said it seemed that all she had to do was "wait around to die."

Selected Nursing Diagnoses

- Self-esteem disturbance related to developmental transition, as evidenced by self-criticism and lack of pleasure in life
- Altered role performance related to retirement, as evidenced by feeling useless and failing to complete routine activities
- Social isolation related to low self-worth, as evidenced by lack of contact with friends

---

In this clinical example, Mrs. G's perception of self was closely related to her ability to work. Her retirement created role changes difficult to adapt to. This example points out the close relationship between low self-esteem and role strain. The situation was further compounded by her husband's retirement. Mrs. G's feelings of low self-esteem were evident in her self-criticism, refusal to recognize her own strengths, worrying, physical complaints, and reduced social contacts. The diagnosis of major depressive episode was based on the severity of her feelings of self-depreciation, somatic problems, saddened emotional tone, history of losses, and absence of a manic episode.

Low self-esteem is also a major element of disturbed body image. The following clinical example illustrates the effect of the loss of a body part on a person's self-concept.

 CLINICAL EXAMPLE

Mrs. M was an attractive 32-year-old married woman admitted to the general hospital for a total hysterectomy. Her history was presented in a nursing care conference because she was making many demands and the head nurse noticed that many of the staff were avoiding caring for her. Mrs. M had been married for 2 years and did not have any children. It was observed that Mr. M seldom visited his wife, although she spoke to him over the phone. Mrs. M complained that she was unable to sleep at night and often rang for the nurses with apparently minor requests. She appeared to have established a relationship with one of the evening nurses, who was able to describe some of Mrs. M's concerns.

Mrs. M appeared to have a severe level of anxiety about her hysterectomy. She feared the effect of the surgery on her sexual desires, attractiveness, and ability to have intercourse and respond to her husband. Without her reproductive organs she said she felt "inadequate and no longer like a woman." She said that she and her husband always planned on having children, and she wondered whether her husband might leave her in the future. She also feared that having the hysterectomy would cause her to lose her beauty and youth.

When the nursing staff became aware of Mrs. M's many fears and concerns, they were better able to understand her behavior and plan nursing care. They discussed with her the physiological implications of a hysterectomy and encouraged her to verbalize her feelings. Mr. M was not aware of his wife's concerns, and the nursing staff supported open discussions between them. As the staff were able to identify Mrs. M's concerns, they realized that

---

Box 19-2

Behaviors Associated with Low Self-Esteem

- Criticism of self or others
- Decreased productivity
- Destructiveness
- Disruptions in relatedness
- Exaggerated sense of self-importance
- Feelings of inadequacy
- Guilt
- Irritability or excessive anger
- Negative feelings about one's body
- Perceived role strain
- Pessimistic view of life
- Physical complaints
- Polarizing view of life
- Rejection of personal capabilities
- Self-destructiveness
- Self-diminution
- Social withdrawal
- Substance abuse
- Withdrawal from reality
- Worrying

some of their previous avoidance behavior resulted from their own fears and discomfort. The female nurses had identified with her, and the hysterectomy threatened their own concepts of self, body integrity, and sexual identity.

Selected Nursing Diagnoses

- Body image disturbance related to hysterectomy, as evidenced by expressed fears about her attractiveness and functioning as a woman
- Altered family processes related to lack of ability to bear children, as evidenced by limited communication with husband

---

Associated with Identity Diffusion. Important behaviors that relate to identity diffusion include disruptions in relationships or problems of intimacy. The initial behavior may be withdrawal or distancing. If a person is experiencing an undefined identity, he may wish to ignore or destroy the people who threaten him. The problem is one of gaining intimacy, but it is reflected in isolation, denial, and withdrawal from others. Such patients lack empathy.

A contrasting behavior that may be evident is personality fusing. Erikson has pointed out that true intimacy involves a sense of mutuality, which implies a firm self-delineation of the partners, not a diffused merger of two people. If a person is struggling to cope with a weak or undefined identity, however, he may try to establish his sense of self by fusing or belonging to someone else. This may occur in formal relationships, intense friendships, or brief affairs because each can be seen as a desperate attempt to outline one's own identity. However, personality fusion leads to a further loss of identity. Some of these behaviors are evident in this clinical example.

 CLINICAL EXAMPLE

Mrs. P was seen by a psychiatric nurse in the psychiatric outpatient department of a general hospital. She was a well-dressed 24-year-old woman who had numerous somatic complaints, including decreased appetite, frequent headaches, fatigue, and difficulty falling asleep. She reported that she had no energy or interest in doing anything or being with people. She said she dreaded each day and felt abandoned and alone.

She was married at age 17 to the only boy she ever dated in high school. He was 19 at the time and she "looked up to him tremendously." He established a successful career in the insurance business, and she stayed at home to care for the house. She described herself as centering her whole world around him. Three months earlier, he had told her that he wanted a separation and suggested she begin making a new life for herself. He said he intended to move out of the house at the end of the month, but Mrs. P said she hoped he would not do that when he saw how much she loved and needed him.

Mrs. P also described feelings of being unloved and unlovable. She said she felt empty inside and didn't really know who she was. She complained about her appearance and expressed much fear about living alone, finding a job, and getting along with people, especially men.

Selected Nursing Diagnoses

- Personal identity disturbance related to impending separation, as evidenced by feelings of loneliness and abandonment
- Self-esteem disturbance related to doubts about self and her abilities, as evidenced by expressed fears of living alone, finding a job, and getting along with people

---

Many of Mrs. P's behaviors reflect the problem of identity diffusion. She married at an early age before defining her own sense of self as an autonomous individual. Her only experience in a close relationship was with her husband, and she attempted to establish her own identity by living through his. Within the security of the marriage, she managed to avoid any self-analysis, but the impending separation brought forth her fears and self-doubts. She displayed a low level of self-esteem and an unresolved conflict between dependence and independence.

Personality fusion and problems with identity also have serious implications for the larger family system. Dysfunctional families are often characterized by a fusion of ego mass that may be evident in severe symptomatology by one or more family members. This may be expressed in some form of family violence or abuse (see Chapter 41) or in the scapegoating of one family member, who becomes the "diagnosed" or "symptomatic" psychiatric patient (see Chapter 34).

People with identity diffusion may lack a historical-cultural basis of identity and thus display a peculiar lack of ethnicity. This is evident in their sense of history, cultural norms, group affiliations, lifestyle, and child-rearing practices. A related behavior is the absence of a moral code or any genuine inner value. The behaviors characteristic of identity diffusion are summarized in Box 19-3.

Associated with Depersonalization. A more maladaptive response to problems in identity involving withdrawal from reality occurs when the person experiences panic levels of anxiety. This panic state produces a blocking off of awareness, a collapse in reality testing, and feelings of depersonalization and dissociation (Allen, 1993). Depersonalization is a feeling of unreality in which one is unable to distinguish between inner and outer stimuli. In essence, it is a true alienation from oneself. The person has great difficulty distinguishing self from others, and his or her body has an unreal or strange quality.

Box 19-3

Behaviors Associated with Identity Diffusion

- Absence of moral code
- Contradictory personality traits
- Exploitive interpersonal relationships
- Feelings of emptiness
- Fluctuating feelings about self
- Gender confusion
- High degree of anxiety
- Inability to empathize with others
- Lack of authenticity
- Problems of intimacy

Depersonalization is the subjective experience of the partial or total disruption of one's ego and the disintegration and disorganization of one's self-concept. Because of this, it is the most frightening human experience. It develops as an outcome of uncertainties in human relationships. The person feels unloved and, as a result of his failure to be loved, he fails to love himself.

Depersonalization serves as a defense, but it is destructive because it masks and immobilizes anxiety without diminishing its intensity. It can occur in a variety of clinical illnesses, including depression, schizophrenia, manic states, and organic brain syndromes, and it represents the advanced state of ego breakdown associated with multiple personality disorder and psychotic states.

Many behaviors are associated with depersonalization. Primarily, the patient feels estranged, as though he were hiding something from himself. He experiences a lack of inner continuity and sameness and feels as if life is happening to him rather than his living by his own initiative. The patient may say that the world appears queer, dreamlike, or frightening. He may experience a loss of identity and express confusion regarding his own sexuality. He may describe related feelings of insecurity, inferiority, frustration, fear, hate, shame, and a loss of self-respect and be unable to derive a sense of accomplishment from any activity.

In depersonalization there may be a loss of impulse control and an absence of feeling and emotion that is shown in impersonality and stiffness in social situations. The person may become lifeless and lack spontaneity and animation. He may plod through each day in a state of numbness and may respond to situations ordinarily eliciting emotion without characteristic love, hate, anxiety, or guilt. The person may become increasingly passive, withdrawing from social contacts, failing to assert himself, losing interest in his surroundings, and allowing others to make decisions for him.

Another sign of depersonalization is a disturbance in perception of time, space, and memory (Guralnik et al, 2000). The person may become disoriented and be unable to recognize events as pertaining to yesterday or tomorrow or to plan activities with reference to a schedule. A disturbance of memory may be characterized by aphasia, amnesia, or memory distortion. Thinking and judgment may be impaired and may reflect great confusion and distortion or focus on trivial details. Problems in information processing may be evident in visual hallucinations, and disturbed interpersonal relationships may be reflected in delusions, auditory hallucinations, and incongruent or idiosyncratic communication.

Another behavior associated with depersonalization is a confused or disturbed body image. The person may have a feeling of unreality about parts of the body. He may feel that his limbs are detached or that the size of his body parts is changed, or he is unable to tell where his body leaves off and the rest of the world begins. Some patients describe the feeling that they have stepped outside their bodies and are observing themselves as detached and foreign objects.

Finally, the person may exhibit behaviors related to dissociative identity disorder, formerly known as **multiple personality disorder**. In this case, distinct and separate personalities exist within the same person, each of which dominates the person's attitudes, behaviors, and self-view as though no other personality existed (see A Family Speaks). Because most patients with dissociative identity (multiple personality) disorder usually conceal their condition, there are only limited periods in their lives when they show overt symptoms that can be easily diagnosed. During these times these patients often show subtle dissociative signs in their affects, thoughts, memories, behaviors, object relations, and transferences. The many behaviors associated with depersonalization and dissociation are summarized in Box 19-4. The following clinical example may further clarify these behaviors.

 CLINICAL EXAMPLE

Mr. S was a 40-year-old man with no history of psychiatric hospitalization. Two months before his present admission, he was severely burned while on the job in a steel-making plant. He sustained second- and third-degree burns over his face, hands, chest, and back and was treated in the burn center of a large university hospital. Three days before he was to be discharged from the burn unit, he experienced a psychotic episode. He reported hearing voices telling him to kill himself, and he was unable to recall any events surrounding the accident that produced his burns. He said he felt his arms were withering away and his eyes were falling into his skull. He was unable to change the dressing on his burns even though he had done this before. When he looked at his arms or chest, his face remained impassive and he showed no emotion. He began to talk continuously about returning to work but was unable to identify how long he had been out on sick leave or the amount of time recommended by his physician for recovery.

A Family Speaks

My wife has multiple personality disorder, and it feels like I'm living with several different people. One moment everything is great and the next thing I know she is in a frenzy or a state of rage. There are other problems, too. For example, things keep appearing in our household and no one knows where they came from, or I get calls at work from my wife telling me she is lost and doesn't know how she ended up there. At other times she tells me things and later denies she said them. Sometimes people come up to my wife and talk like they know her, but she says she's never seen them before. And then there are days when she dresses up and acts just like our teenage daughter.

What is it like to live with someone with this illness? Well, it's unreal and very upsetting. Most of all, it's like living in a world of doubt and uncertainty. Who is this woman I married 12 years ago? What is she all about? What is she capable of doing? These are the questions I ask myself each night as I fall asleep. They are the same ones that go unanswered in the early morning hours.

Box **19-4**

Behaviors Associated with Depersonalization

AFFECTIVE

Feelings of loss of identity
Feelings of alienation from self
Feelings of insecurity, inferiority, fear, shame
Feelings of unreality
Heightened sense of isolation
Inability to derive pleasure or a sense of accomplishment
Lack of sense of inner continuity

PERCEPTUAL

Auditory and visual hallucinations
Confusion regarding one's sexuality
Difficulty distinguishing self from others
Disturbed body image
Dreamlike view of the world

COGNITIVE

Confusion
Distorted thinking
Disturbance of memory
Impaired judgment
Presence of separate personalities within the same person
Time disorientation

BEHAVIORAL

Blunted affect
Emotional passivity and nonresponsiveness
Incongruent or idiosyncratic communication
Lack of spontaneity and animation
Loss of impulse control
Loss of initiative and decision-making ability
Social withdrawal

With the onset of these symptoms, he was transferred from the burn unit to the psychiatric unit of the hospital. He remained socially isolated on the unit and refused to participate in ward meetings and group activities. At times he wandered into other patients' rooms and took pieces of their clothing. He was later seen wearing this clothing, and the staff intervened to return it to its owners.

Selected Nursing Diagnoses

- Panic level of anxiety related to severe burn injuries, as evidenced by confusion regarding identity, hearing voices, and reported body distortions
- Altered thought processes related to psychotic state, as evidenced by confusion and disorientation

The various feelings and perceptions associated with depersonalization represent extreme defenses against threats to self that do not alleviate the anxiety and may add to it. The patient views his own behavior as foreign and sees himself as a strong, unknown, and unpredictable being whom he does not recognize. As both a participant and a spectator, he observes himself with great fear because he is unable to control his own impulses. He cannot completely escape the pain of self-awareness. He therefore disowns his behavior, feelings, thoughts, and body and becomes alienated from his true self.

Predisposing Factors

Affecting Self-Esteem. Self-esteem is partly an inheritable trait, and genetic as well as environmental influences are very important (Roy et al, 1995). Specifically, predisposing factors that begin in early childhood can contribute to problems with self-concept. Because the infant initially views himself as an extension of his parents, he is very responsive to both his parents' self-hate and any feelings of hatred toward himself. Parental rejection causes the child to be uncertain of himself and other human relationships. Because of his failure to be loved, the child fails to love himself and is unable to reach out with love to others.

As he grows older, the child may learn to feel inadequate because he is not encouraged to be independent, to think for himself, and to take responsibility for his own needs and actions. Overpossessiveness, overpermissiveness, or overcontrol, exercised by one or both parents, can create a feeling of unimportance and lack of self-esteem in the child. Harsh, demanding parents can set unreasonable standards, often raising them before the child has developed the ability to meet them.

Parents may also subject their children to unreasonable, harsh criticism and inconsistent punishment. These actions can cause early frustration, defeatism, and a destructive sense of inadequacy and inferiority. Another factor in creating such feelings may be the rivalry or unsuccessful imitation of an extremely bright sibling or a prominent parent, often creating a sense of hopelessness and inferiority. In addition, repeated defeats and failures can destroy self-worth. In this instance the failure in itself does not produce a sense of helplessness, but internalization of the failure as proof of personal incompetence does.

Unrealistic self-ideals. With age, other factors emerge that can cause feelings of low self-esteem. The person who lacks a sense of meaning and purpose in life also fails to accept responsibility for his own well-being and to develop his capabilities and potential. He denies himself the freedom of full expression, including the right to make mistakes and fail, and becomes impatient, harsh, and demanding with himself. He sets standards that cannot be met. Self-consciousness and observation turn to self-contempt and self-defeat. This results in a further loss of self-trust.

These self-ideals or goals are often silent assumptions, and the person may not be immediately aware of them. They reflect high expectations and are unrealistic. When the person judges his performance by these unreasonable and inflexible standards, he cannot live up to his ideals and, as a result, experiences guilt and low self-esteem. These inner dictates have been described as the "tyranny of the shoulds," and some of the common ones are identified in Box 19-5.

The person who overemphasizes these rules or ideals often makes a series of deductions such as the following: "Everyone should love me. If he or she doesn't love me, I have failed. I have lost the only thing that really matters. I

Box 19-5

Unrealistic Self-Expectations: the Tyranny of the Shoulds

- I should have the utmost generosity, consideration, dignity, courage, and unselfishness.
- I should be the perfect lover, friend, parent, teacher, student, and spouse. Everyone should love me.
- I should be able to find a quick solution to every problem.
- I should never feel hurt; I should always be happy and serene.
- I should assert myself; I should never hurt anybody else.
- I should always be at peak efficiency. I should not be tired, get sick, or make mistakes.

From Horney K: *Neurosis and human growth*, New York, 1950, WW Norton.

am unlovable. There is no point in going on. I am worthless." This inner punishment results in feelings of depression and despair because no human being can fulfill the demands on self. Slavishly striving for these ideals interferes with other activities, such as living a healthy life and having satisfying relationships with other people. These predisposing factors lay the groundwork for feelings of low self-esteem.

Affecting Role Performance

Gender roles. An important source of strain in contemporary society comes from values, beliefs, and behaviors about gender roles. Research demonstrates that society continues to have clearly defined gender-role stereotypes for men and women. Women are perceived as less competent, less independent, less objective, and less logical than men. Men are perceived as lacking interpersonal sensitivity, warmth, and expressiveness. Moreover, stereotyped masculine traits are more often perceived as desirable than are stereotyped feminine characteristics.

To the extent that these results reflect societal standards of gender-role behavior, both women and men are put in role conflict by the difference in the standards. If a woman adopts behaviors desirable for a man, she risks criticism for her failure to be appropriately feminine; if she adopts behaviors seen as feminine, she is lacking in the values associated with masculinity. Likewise, if a man adopts the behaviors seen as desirable for a woman, his masculinity and sexuality may be questioned and his contributions may be devalued or ignored; if he adopts the behaviors associated with masculinity, he risks not being able to express warmth, tenderness, and responsiveness.

Thus, when a woman steps out of her home, where her gender role has traditionally been defined and confined, and enters the world of work, she may experience heightened role strain. Similarly, the man who arrives home from work in the evening may feel uncertain or in conflict about how he should relate to his school-age son, infant daughter, or working wife.

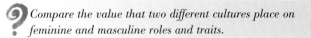

Compare the value that two different cultures place on feminine and masculine roles and traits.

Work roles. Women are still in the minority in most high-status occupations and are clustered near the bottom in terms of professional status and income. In American society, women are socialized to seek an ideal that includes marriage, children, higher education, and satisfying work outside the home. They are increasingly expected to perform in both "feminine" and "masculine" spheres.

This situation has many negative aspects. First, it can be argued that it merely replaces the traditional woman's role with another equally confining one. As the new role is valued, the traditional roles of wife and mother become devalued. Second, although women are expected to assume more "masculine" qualities, there is only a small corresponding trend for men to assume more "feminine" behaviors. Third, the woman who seeks such an expanded role is faced with reconciling the often conflicting goals of work, marriage, homemaking, and parenting.

Despite social and economic changes, there is often little sharing of tasks when men and women are both gainfully employed. Rather, most industrial societies have witnessed a gradual change in the obligations of women, who now perform a dual role: outside employment and continued responsibility for home and children.

The expectation exists that the woman will make the adjustments needed both at home and in her career, including housekeeping and managing; arranging meals, lessons, and appointments; entertaining; caring for the sick; and communicating with the family. There is also the traditional expectation that the wife will be the primary caretaker of the children and will subsume other activities to this end.

Gender and work roles will continue as a source of stress until care of children, home, and career are viewed as equally valuable and important by both sexes and until gender is regarded as irrelevant to the abilities, personalities, and activities of the people involved.

Such a change in attitude should begin with nurses and other mental health clinicians, who indirectly increase role strain by accepting stereotyped views. The cause of mental health might be better served if psychiatric clinicians encourage both men and women to maximize individual potential rather than adjust to existing gender roles.

Affecting Personal Identity.

Constant parental intervention can interfere with adolescent choices. Parental distrust may lead a child to wonder whether his own choices are correct and to feel guilty if he goes against parental ideas. It may also devalue the child's opinions and lead to indecisiveness, impulsiveness, and acting out in an attempt to achieve some identity.

When the parent does not trust the child, the child ultimately loses respect for the parent. It has been found that parents and children do not disagree on significant issues, such as war, peace, race, or religion. Instead, personal and narrow concerns—dating, a party, use of the car, curfews, hairstyles, homework—create the conflict between parents and youth.

Peers may also add to the problem of identity. The adolescent wants to belong, to feel needed and wanted. The peer group, with its rigid standards of behavior, gives him this feeling and provides a bridge between childhood and adulthood. The adolescent loses himself in the fads and the language of the group. However, the group is often a cruel testing ground that can hurt as much as it helps. Taught to be competitive, the young person competes with his friends, putting them down to bring himself up.

Membership in the peer group is bought at a high price; the adolescent must surrender much of his identity to belong. Often there is open destruction of self-esteem and insistence on conformity. In sexual relationships adolescents introduce further uncertainty into their lives, which can interfere with developing a stable self-concept.

 Discuss how belonging to a group affects an adolescent's identity.

Precipitating Stressors

Trauma. Specific problems with self-concept can be brought on by almost any difficult situation to which the person cannot adjust. Specifically, trauma such as physical, sexual, and psychological abuse in childhood has been reported by most patients with dissociative symptoms (Chu et al, 1999), depersonalization disorder (Simeon et al, 1997) and dissociative identity disorder (Kluft, 1999). A small percentage of patients report no abuse but have experienced a trauma they perceive as life threatening to themselves or to someone else, such as a near drowning or witnessing a violent crime. However, it is believed that dissociation usually results from prolonged exposure to sexual or physical abuse rather than from an isolated instance of trauma (see Citing the Evidence).

Role Strain. People who experience stress with expected roles are said to experience role strain. Role strain is the frustration felt when the person is torn in opposite directions or feels inadequate or unsuited to enact certain roles. In the course of a lifetime a person faces numerous role transitions. These transitions may require the incorporation of new knowledge and alterations in behavior. There are three categories of role transitions:

- Developmental
- Situational
- Health-illness

Each of these role transitions can precipitate a threat to one's self-concept.

Developmental transitions. Developmental transitions are normative changes associated with growth. Various developmental stages can precipitate threats to self-identity. Adolescence is perhaps the most critical because it is a time of upheaval, change, anxiety, and insecurity. A serious threat to identity in adulthood is cultural discontinuity. This occurs when a person moves from one cultural setting to another and experiences emotional upheaval. In addition,

---

Citing the Evidence on

Dissociation and Abuse

BACKGROUND: Controversy exists about whether physical abuse and sexual abuse are specifically and causally linked with adult dissociative symptoms. The aim of this study was to examine the relationship between childhood sexual and physical abuse, current psychiatric illness, and measures of dissociation in a nonclinical adult population.

RESULTS: Physical abuse and current psychiatric illness were directly related to a high rate of dissociative symptoms. Sexual abuse was not. The influence of sexual abuse was due to its association with current psychiatric illness and childhood physical abuse.

IMPLICATIONS: About 6% of the general population studied suffered from high levels of dissociative symptoms. All these individuals had higher rates of childhood physical and sexual abuse and current psychiatric illness. However, direct relationships between childhood sexual abuse and dissociative symptoms was not found. The findings from studies such as this suggest that both causal and correlational relationships are complex and that conclusions drawn from only studying clinical populations, rather than general population samples, might lead to false conclusions.

Mulder R et al: Relationship between dissociation, childhood sexual abuse, childhood physical abuse, and mental illness in a general population sample, *Am J Psychiatry* 155(6):806, 1998.

---

problems within the social structure, such as political upheavals, economic depression, and high unemployment, can pose threats to identity. In late maturity and old age, identity problems again arise. Menopause, retirement, and increasing physical disability are problems for which people must work out adaptive responses. Situational transitions involve the addition or subtraction of significant others, occurring through birth or death. An example is the birth of one's first child.

Health-illness transitions. Health-illness transitions involve moving from a well state to an illness state. Some stressors can cause disturbances in body image and related changes in self-concept. One threat is the loss of a major body part, such as an eye, breast, or leg. Disturbances also may result from a surgical procedure in which the relationship of body parts is disturbed. The results of the surgical intervention may be either visible, as with a colostomy or gastrostomy, or invisible, as with a hysterectomy or gallbladder removal. Changes in body size, shape, and appearance can threaten the person's self-perceptions. Threats to body image can result from a pathological process that causes changes in the structure or function of the body, such as arthritis, multiple sclerosis, Parkinson's disease, cancer, pneumonia, and heart disease. The failure of a body part, as in paralysis, is particularly diffi-

Table **19-2**

Factors Influencing Self-Concept Based on Health-Illness Transitions	
Factor	Question
Meaning of the threat for the patient	Does it threaten the patient's ideal of youth or wholeness and decrease self-esteem?
Degree to which the patient's pattern of adaptation is interrupted	Does it jeopardize the patient's security and self-control?
Coping capacities and resources available	What is the response of significant others, and what help is offered?
Nature of the threat, extent of change, and rate at which it occurs	Is the change that of many small adjustments over time or a great and sudden adjustment?

cult to integrate into one's self-perceptions. The physical changes associated with normal growth and development may pose problems, as may some medical or nursing procedures, such as enemas, catheterizations, suctioning, radiation therapy, dilation and curettage, and organ transplantation.

All these stressors can pose a threat to body image, with resultant changes in self-esteem and role perception (Price, 1998). Factors that influence the degree of threat to body image are listed in Table 19-2.

Finally, physiological stressors may also disturb a person's sense of reality, interfere with an accurate perception of the world, and threaten ego boundaries and identity. Such stressors include oxygen deprivation, hyperventilation, biochemical imbalances, severe fatigue, and sensory and emotional isolation. Alcohol, drugs, and other toxic substances may also distort self-concept. Usually these stressors produce only temporary changes.

Appraisal of Stressors

Whether the problem in self-concept is precipitated by psychological, sociological, or physiological stressors, the critical element is the patient's perception of the threat. When assessing behaviors and formulating a nursing diagnosis, the nurse must continue to validate observations and inferences to establish a mutual, therapeutic relationship with the patient.

The incidence of breast cancer is rising in this country. What strategies are women using to promote adaptive self-concept responses?

Coping Resources

It is important that the nurse and patient review possible coping resources. All people, no matter how disturbing their behavior, have some areas of personal strength (Burns, 1991), which might include the following:

- Sports and outdoor activities
- Hobbies and crafts
- Expressive arts
- Health and self-care
- Education or training
- Vocation or position
- Special aptitudes
- Intelligence

- Imagination and creativity
- Interpersonal relationships

When the patient's positive aspects become evident, the nurse should share them with the patient to expand the patient's self-awareness and suggest possible areas for future intervention.

Coping Mechanisms

Short-Term Defenses. An identity crisis may be resolved with either short-term or long-term coping mechanisms. These are used to ward off the anxiety and uncertainty of identity confusion. There are four categories of short-term defenses:

- Activities that provide temporary escape from the identity crisis
- Activities that provide temporary substitute identities
- Activities that temporarily strengthen or heighten a diffuse sense of self
- Activities that represent short-term attempts to make an identity out of meaninglessness and identity diffusion—that try to assert that the meaning of life is meaningless itself

The first category of temporary escape includes activities that seem to provide intense immediate experiences. These experiences so overwhelm the senses that the issue of identity literally does not exist because the person's entire being is occupied with "right now" sensations. Examples include drug experiences, loud rock concerts, fast car and motorcycle riding, some forms of hard physical labor, exercise or sports, and even obsessive television watching.

The category of temporary substitute identity is derived from being a "joiner"; the identity of a club, group, team, movement, or gang may function as a basis for self-definition. The person temporarily adopts the group definition as his own identity in a type of devotion to the larger entity. Temporary substitute identities can also be obtained by playing a certain role within a group, such as clown, bully, or chauffeur, or by buying objects that are marketed with ready-made identities. Thus a certain type of cologne, make of car, or article of dress implies built-in personalities the person can adopt as his own.

The third category of defenses involves confronting or challenging something to feel more intensely alive. This is evident in risk taking for its own sake, which creates a feeling of bravado. Competitive activities, such as sports, academic achievement, and popularity contests, also fit into this category. The idea is that competition and comparison with an outsider more sharply define a sense of self. Another example is bigotry and prejudice. By adopting a bigoted stance toward some outgroup or scapegoat, the person can temporarily strengthen self-esteem or ego integrity.

The final category helps to explain the fads that people indulge in with such fervor and that seem so meaningless to others. The sheer force of commitment to fads is an attempt to transform them into something meaningful.

Long-Term Defenses. Any of these short-term defenses may develop into a long-term one that will be evident in maladaptive behavior. Another type of long-term resolution has been identified as identity foreclosure. This occurs when people adopt the "ready-made" type of identity desired by others without really coming to terms with their own desires, aspirations, or potential. This is a less desirable long-term resolution, as is adopting a deviant or negative identity.

A negative identity is one that is at odds with the values of society. In this case the person tries to define the self in a nonprescribed or antisocial manner. The choice of a negative identity represents an attempt to retain some mastery in a situation in which a positive identity does not seem possible or desirable. The person may be saying, "I would rather be somebody bad than nobody at all." The following clinical example describes the negative identity assumed by an adolescent with a medical diagnosis of conduct disorder—undersocialized, aggressive.

 ## CLINICAL EXAMPLE

Ken was a 17-year-old boy referred to the local community mental health center by his high school nurse. She made the referral after attending a team conference at school about Ken's repeated behavioral problems. He had a history of aggressive and destructive behavior, poor peer relationships, and low academic performance. The school had suspended him on three occasions, and the result of the team conference was to expel him for the remainder of the school year.

Mr. P, a psychiatric nurse at the mental health center, established a contract to work with Ken and his family. He noted that Ken was an obese young man (112.5 kg) who took little interest in his appearance. His dress was sloppy, his complexion unclean, and his hair oily. He sat slumped in the chair in a disinterested and slightly defiant posture.

As Ken talked about himself, he complained of many pressures he experienced in his part-time job at a local hardware store. He thought the work was too difficult and tiring and that he was qualified for better and more prestigious work. When asked for specifics, he could not identify another job in particular. He also expressed a great deal of harassment from his family. His mother and father had been married for 31 years, and he was the only child of the marriage. His mother worked part-time at a bakery, and his father was recently retired from his job as a supervisor at a local utility company, where he was highly regarded.

Ken said that his father "always had things for me to do." He described how his father signed him up for various team sports—baseball, basketball, football—without acknowledging how much Ken hated sports and how uncoordinated he was. His father also stressed good grades and the necessity of college for success in life. Ken described his mother as passive and polite and said he had little respect for her. He said his aggressive outbursts occurred both at home and at school—whenever he was frustrated. People reacted by staying out of his way. He said he never hurt anyone with his temper. He mostly destroyed property and objects.

Ken avoided the subject of peers but, when asked about friends, said he "hung out" with a couple of boys in the neighborhood. They were older than he was. Most had dropped out of high school and were employed in odd jobs. He denied drug use but said he drank heavily, especially on the weekends. He said he had no girlfriends and wasn't interested in complicating his life "with some broad."

Selected Nursing Diagnoses

- Personal identity disturbance related to fear of failure, as evidenced by aggressive and destructive behavior and poor school performance
- Altered family processes related to conflict with parents, as evidenced by avoidance and lack of communication

Ken displays many of the behaviors characteristic of a negative identity. The nurse working with Ken explored his underlying feelings and self-perceptions. Great anger with his father began to surface, and Ken was able to verbalize it. Because he was the only son, he believed he was competing with his father and had to live up to his father's ideals. Ken feared failing in trying to adopt a positive identity and resented the identity his father was trying to impose on him. He thought he had no part in defining it and that it did not represent his real self.

Ego Defense Mechanisms. Patients with alterations in self-concept may use a variety of ego-oriented mechanisms to protect themselves from confronting their own inadequacies. Typical ego defense mechanisms include fantasy, dissociation, isolation, projection, displacement, splitting, turning anger against the self, and acting out. These are described in Chapter 17.

Other, more damaging coping mechanisms can also be used to protect self-esteem. These may include the following:
- Obesity
- Anorexia
- Promiscuity
- Chronic overworking
- Suicide
- Delinquency
- Crime
- Drug use
- Family violence
- Incest

NURSING DIAGNOSIS

Self-concept is a critical aspect of one's overall personality adjustment. Problems with self-concept are associated with feelings of anxiety, hostility, and guilt. These often create a circular, self-propagating process that ultimately results in maladaptive coping responses (Fig. 19-3).

Most people who express dissatisfaction with life, display deviant behavior, or have difficulty functioning in social or work situations have problems related to self-concept.

The primary NANDA nursing diagnoses related to alterations in self-concept are **body image disturbance, self-esteem disturbance, altered role performance**, and **personal identity disturbance**. Nursing diagnoses related to the range of possible maladaptive responses of the patient are identified in the Medical and Nursing Diagnoses box on p. 332.

Examples of complete nursing diagnoses related to self-concept are presented in the Detailed Diagnoses box on p. 333. However, alterations in self-concept affect all aspects of a person's life. Therefore many additional problems may be identified by the nurse.

Related Medical Diagnoses

Maladaptive responses indicating alterations in self-concept can be seen in a variety of people experiencing threats to their physical integrity or self-system. These nursing diagnoses are not limited to the psychiatric setting and do not have a discrete category of medical diagnoses associated with them. Because they pertain to basic personality structure and feelings about oneself, they can emerge with many neurotic and psychotic disorders (see A Patient Speaks on p. 334) and may be related to all the diagnostic categories identified in the *DSM–IV–TR* (American Psychiatric Association, 2000) because all these disorders ultimately reflect on one's view of self.

Several specific medical diagnoses deserve particular attention, however, because their dominant features include alterations in self-concept. They are listed in the Medical and Nursing Diagnoses box on p. 332 and include identity problems and dissociative identity disorder, also known as **multiple personality disorder**.

OUTCOME IDENTIFICATION

The expected outcome when working with a patient with a maladaptive self-concept response is as follows:

The patient will obtain the maximum level of self-actualization to realize his or her potential.

Goals should be as clear and explicit as possible. They should identify realistic steps that the patient can accomplish. In this way the patient's self-confidence will increase, and this will build self-esteem. These goals should emphasize strengths instead of weaknesses. If they are mutually identified, they will motivate the patient and help the patient

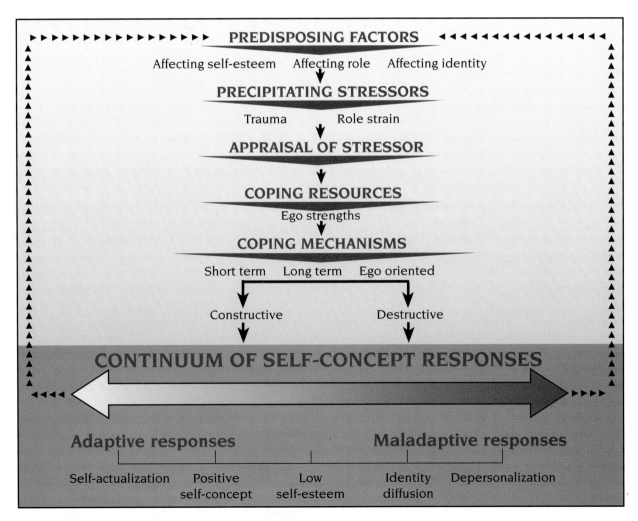

Fig. 19-3 The Stuart Stress Adaptation Model related to self-concept responses.

Medical and Nursing Diagnoses *related to* **Self-Concept Responses**

RELATED MEDICAL DIAGNOSES (*DSM–IV–TR*)*	RELATED NURSING DIAGNOSES (NANDA)†
Identity problem	Adjustment, impaired
Dissociative amnesia	Anxiety
Dissociative fugue	**Body image disturbance‡**
Dissociative identity disorder (multiple personality disorder)	Communication, impaired verbal
Depersonalization disorder	Coping, ineffective individual
	Hopelessness
	Loneliness, risk for
	Personal identity disturbance‡
	Powerlessness
	Role performance, altered‡
	Self-care deficit
	Self-esteem disturbance‡
	Sensory/perceptual alteration
	Sexuality patterns, altered
	Social interaction, impaired
	Social isolation
	Spiritual distress
	Thought processes, altered
	Violence, risk for

*Reprinted with permission from the *Diagnostic and statistical manual of mental disorders*, Fourth Edition, Text Revision. Copyright 2000. American Psychiatric Association.

†From North American Nursing Diagnosis Association: *NANDA nursing diagnoses: definitions and classifications 1999-2000*, Philadelphia, 1999, The Association.

‡Primary nursing diagnosis for alterations in self-concept.

assume increased responsibility for his or her own behavior. Following are examples of goals related to role performance:

Long-term: Mrs. P will resolve role conflict by achieving greater congruency between work and family roles.

Short-term: After 1 week:

- Mrs. P will describe her responsibilities in her work and home roles.
- She will identify aspects of these roles that provide her with satisfaction.
- She will identify areas of role incompatibility.

After 2 weeks:

- She will describe three alternative ways of increasing the complementarity of the roles.
- She will discuss the advantages and disadvantages of each alternative.

After 3 weeks:

- She will take the necessary measures to implement one of the identified alternatives.

PLANNING

The nurse's focus is to help the patient understand himself more fully and accurately so that he can direct his own life in a more satisfying way. This means helping him strive toward a clearer, deeper experience of his feelings, wishes, and beliefs; a greater ability to tap his resources and use them for constructive ends; and a clearer perception of his direction in life, assuming responsibility for himself, his decisions, and his actions.

Self-awareness is crucial in bringing about changes in self-concept, but people usually spend little time in introspec-tion. However, certain conditions or events do stimulate self-awareness. This may occur when stimuli from the body are intensified, as in states of pain, fatigue, or anger, or when stimuli from the environment are decreased, as in sensory deprivation or isolation.

Self-awareness may be triggered when something unexpected or extraordinary takes place, when the person has succeeded or failed, or when the person is confronted with himself by looking in a mirror, listening to his voice on a tape recorder, or reading an old letter. Special occasions, such as birthdays, anniversaries, New Year's Eve, or a death may stimulate introspection. It may also be initiated when others direct their attention to the person through conversation or touch.

Once the person begins to look at and analyze himself, changes in the self become possible. Often they are the result of feelings of failure, unhappiness, anxiety, inadequacy, doubt, or perceived discrepancies between one's concept of self and the demands of the environment or the expectations of others. Usually changes in the self occur only as a result of experiences and occur gradually. Occasionally, however, a change may take place suddenly. A traumatic experience may force a person to see that something drastic must be done. The nurse should take all these factors into consideration when planning nursing care.

Similarly, the family of origin is a source of many people's self-esteem. Adult contact with parents and siblings can correct misconceptions underlying low self-esteem and allow more positive beliefs. Learning to interact with family members with closeness, but without counterproductive forms of fusion and emotionality, can enable a more mature pattern

Detailed Diagnoses *related to* **Self-Concept Responses**

NANDA DIAGNOSIS STEM	EXAMPLES OF COMPLETE DIAGNOSIS
Body image disturbance	Body image disturbance related to fear of becoming obese, as evidenced by refusal to maintain body weight within normal limits
	Body image disturbance related to leukemia chemotherapy, as evidenced by negative feelings about one's body
	Body image disturbance related to cerebrovascular accident, as evidenced by lack of acceptance of body limitations
Self-esteem disturbance	Self-esteem disturbance related to death of spouse, as evidenced by withdrawal from others and feelings of hopelessness
	Self-esteem disturbance related to overly high self-ideals, as evidenced by depressed mood and withdrawal from activities
Role performance, altered	Role performance, altered, related to incompatibility of newly assumed work and family roles, as evidenced by self-criticism and feeling of inadequacy
	Role performance, altered, related to incongruence of cultural and self-role expectations about aging, as evidenced by feelings of frustration and criticism of others
Personal identity disturbance	Personal identity disturbance related to unrealistic parental expectations, as evidenced by running away from home
	Personal identity disturbance related to drug toxicity, as evidenced by confusion and loss of impulse control

DSM–IV–TR DIAGNOSIS	ESSENTIAL FEATURES*
Identity problem	Uncertainty about multiple issues relating to identity such as long-term goals, career choice, friendship patterns, sexual orientation and behavior, moral values, and group loyalties
Dissociative amnesia	The predominant disturbance is episodes of inability to recall important personal information, usually of a traumatic or stressful nature, that is too extensive to be explained by ordinary forgetfulness.
Dissociative fugue	The predominant disturbance is sudden, unexpected travel away from home or one's customary place of work, with inability to recall one's past. Confusion about personal identity or assumption of a new identity.
Dissociative identity disorder (multiple personality disorder)	The presence of two or more distinct identities or personality states (each with its own enduring pattern of perceiving, relating to, and thinking about the environment and self). At least two of these identities or personality states recurrently take control of the person's behavior. Inability to recall important personal information that is too extensive to be explained by ordinary forgetfulness.
Depersonalization disorder	Persistent or recurrent experiences of feeling detached from, and as if one is an outside observer of, one's mental processes or body (for example, feeling as if one is in a dream). During the depersonalization experience, reality testing remains intact. The depersonalization causes clinically significant distress or impairment in functioning.

*Reprinted with permission from the *Diagnostic and statistical manual of mental disorders*, Fourth Edition, Text Revision. Copyright 2000. American Psychiatric Association.

---

to develop. Family relationships would therefore be an appropriate focus for patient education. A Patient Education Plan using family systems is presented on p. 335. Chapter 34 has a more detailed discussion of family systems theory and family interventions.

IMPLEMENTATION

The mutually identified goals can be reached by a problem-solving approach that focuses primarily on the present, removes much of the responsibility from the nurse, and actively engages the patient in working on personal difficulties. This approach increases the patient's self-confidence and self-esteem. It requires that the patient first develop insight into her problems and life situation and take action to effect lasting behavioral changes. The nurse must thus incorporate both the responsive dimensions (insight oriented) and the action dimensions (action oriented) of the therapeutic relationship described in Chapter 2.

The focus of this approach is on the patient's cognitive appraisal of life, which may contain faulty perceptions, beliefs, and convictions. Awareness of feelings and emotions is also important because they too may be subject to misconceptions. Only after examining the patient's cognitive appraisal of the situation and related feelings can one gain insight into the problem and bring about behavioral change (see Cognitive Behavioral Therapy in Chapter 32). There are principles of nursing care for self-concept problems. These principles use a problem-solving approach in a progressive sequence. They focus primarily on the level of the patient. However, they may be implemented with group or family interventions, and the

A Patient Speaks

Thoughts on Mental Illness

It came to me—so clear that I could not deny it, the pain, the hurt, the anger—I am mentally ill. I've tried to pretend that I'd get better putting the hurt away—gutting out the pain hoping it would eventually pass—yes, eventually pass. So I did therapy. I talked about what I had experienced. Perceptual disturbances, they said. I talked about the unrealness, the flatness—like cardboard. Depersonalization, they said. I talked about people making me nervous, about staying to myself. You must think rationally, do self-talk, change your behaviors. Take these drugs, they said because I had heard a voice, or felt something they had not. I had psychotic symptoms—load her up on Mellaril, so what if she gets as fat as a pig—keep increasing the dosage. Too fat? Load her up on Haldol. But I'm not psychotic—oh, but you are schizo-affective; no—let's make that borderline; on second thought, maybe major depression with psychotic features? No, more like depersonalization disorder. Let's check for temporal lobe epilepsy; what the hell—it isn't our money; why are you complaining? And the therapy goes on. I feel worse. The drugs don't work—you're resistant to treatment; take some more drugs—they will help you feel better. So I take the damn drugs—is one antidepressant any different from another? How much of the stuff can you take? It doesn't do any good. How many times do I have

to say that? Why doesn't my doctor listen? Why does she keep writing prescriptions for more of the stuff? Who is taking this stuff—me, or her? I should know if it works.

I do therapy with the silicone people, they who make no mistakes, who are always clinically correct—always clean nice people—but inside I am not clean. I fear that I may be defective, that some loose part may come undone and all will be lost. I'm so scared and I work overtime to find something positive, something good to come out of all this chaos. I don't think he understands when I talk to my therapist. I sometimes feel cheap and shallow because I've bought the time and I know he would not be talking to me if I hadn't. I feel frustrated because I've been trapped in this sickness. How can they feel the humiliation—the stigma. The ones so well—that they can heal? Pain, hurt, and fear are subjectively private, but even for me the loneliness is too much. And so I ask the silicone people, have you ever been afraid? Yes, they say. But they don't feel the fear, and they don't connect with the fear. But I feel it, and I want the silicone folks to feel it, too. I do not want to hurt by myself; I want someone to also feel the hurt. So all you silicone therapists—hear me: to hurt when someone IS there but still is NOT is the worst kind of hurt of all—listen up.

Judy Mays

From South Carolina Self-Help Association Regarding Emotions: *Share the News*, Spring 1993.

---

nurse is expected to include the patient's family, significant others, and community supports whenever possible.

In addition, empirically validated treatments for one of the medical diagnoses related to self-concept responses is summarized in Table 19-3. Recent work in the field suggest that patients with dissociative identity (multiple personality) disorders may respond well to treatment (Ellason & Ross, 1997; Kluft, 1999). Both group therapy (Dallam & Manderino, 1997) and short-term therapy (Applegate, 1997) can result in successful outcomes.

Level 1: Expanded Self-Awareness

To avoid anxiety, most people resist change. In general, change in the self is easier when threat is absent. Threat forces a person to defend himself, perceptions are narrowed, and the person has difficulty forming new perceptions of himself (see Critical Thinking about Contemporary Issues).

To expand the patient's self-awareness and reduce the element of threat, the nurse should adopt an accepting attitude. Acceptance allows the patient the security and freedom to examine all aspects of oneself as a total human being with positive and negative qualities. The basis of a therapeutic relationship is established by listening to the patient with understanding, responding nonjudgmentally, expressing genuine interest, and conveying a sense of caring and sincerity.

Creating a climate of acceptance allows previously denied experiences to be examined. This broadens the patient's concept of self and helps the patient to accept all aspects of one's personality. It also indicates that the patient is a valued person who is responsible for himself and is able to help himself. This is important because the nurse must work with whatever ego strength the patient possesses.

Most patients seen in clinics, the general hospital, and the community setting possess considerable ego strength. However, people who are hospitalized might have limited ego resources. Psychotic patients experiencing depersonalization and identity confusion often present difficult challenges for the nurse (Czuchta & Johnson, 1998). They tend to isolate themselves and withdraw from reality, so little ego strength is available for problem solving. For this type of patient, expanding self-awareness means first confirming the patient's identity. The nurse should attempt to provide supportive measures to decrease the panic level experienced by this patient. Additional interventions related to anxiety and psychotic states are described in Chapters 17 and 22.

The nurse can spend time with the patient in an undemanding way and approach the patient nonaggressively. Initially the nurse may accept the patient's need to remain nonverbal or attempt to clarify and understand the patient's verbal communication even though it may be distorted or lack apparent logic. Attempts should be made to prevent the patient from being isolated by establishing a

PATIENT EDUCATION PLAN *Improving Family Relationships*

CONTENT	INSTRUCTIONAL ACTIVITIES	EVALUATION
Define the concept of self-differentiation within one's family of origin.	Discuss the differences between high and low levels of self-differentiation. Ask the patient to identify level of functioning among family members.	Patient identifies functioning level in family of origin.
Describe the characteristics of emotional fusion, emotional cutoff, and triangulation.	Analyze types and patterns of family relationships. Diagram family patterns.	Patient describes interactional patterns within family. Patient identifies own roles and behavior.
Discuss the role of symptom formation and symptom bearer in a family.	Sensitize the patient to family dynamics and manifestations of stress. Encourage communication with family of origin.	Patient recognizes family contribution to the stress of individual members. Patient contacts family members.
Describe a family genogram and show how it is constructed.	Use a blackboard to map out a family genogram. Assign family genogram as homework.	Patient obtains factual information about family. Patient constructs family genogram.
Analyze need for objectivity and responsibility for changing one's own behavior and not that of others.	Role-play interactions with various family members. Encourage testing out new ways of interacting with family members.	Patient demonstrates a higher level of differentiation in family of origin.

Table **19-3**

Summarizing the Evidence on Treatments that Work for Self-Concept Responses

DISORDER: Dissociative disorders

TREATMENT: ■ Psychodynamic psychotherapy, hypnosis, and amytal narcosynthesis are treatments of choice for these conditions based on case reports

Nathan P, Gorman J: *A guide to treatments that work*, New York, 1998, Oxford University Press.

simple routine for the patient. If the patient displays bizarre behavior, such as inappropriate laughing or mannerisms, the nurse can set limits on the behavior. It is important to orient the patient frequently to reality and reinforce appropriate behavior.

The patient should be helped to increase the activities that provide positive experiences. This may involve the use of occupational therapy, recreational therapy, or activity groups because success at tasks and increased involvement with objects can increase self-esteem. Movement therapy or body ego technique is a goal-directed way to develop identity, body image, and ego structure. It is predominantly a nonverbal therapy because the emphasis is on movement, not on what the person says.

Depersonalization often leads to poor hygiene and an unkempt personal appearance. Nurses who are aware of their own value systems regarding cleanliness and grooming can help patients unable to care for themselves. They can use patience and repetition to establish health routines and can kindly but firmly encourage patients to care for themselves.

? CRITICAL THINKING about **CONTEMPORARY ISSUES**

What Is the Recommended Treatment for Dissociative Identity (Multiple Personality) Disorder?

Reported cases of dissociative identity (multiple personality) disorder have increased dramatically in the last decade, yet there are few data on the preferred treatment of this illness. Most recommendations are made based on the experience of individual clinicians rather than on systematic research. No controlled studies comparing different models of treatment have been published. Work in the field suggests that two or more sessions of psychotherapy a week appear to be the most effective treatment and that the core symptoms of dissociative identity disorder do not respond to psychopharmacology (Kluft, 1999). Antidepressant and antianxiety medications may be useful in treating comorbid conditions.

The length, frequency, and cost of treatment for this illness have major implications for the mental health care system. As a result of managed care and inadequate third-party funding and community resources, it is likely that many of these patients will be unable to obtain adequate treatment despite substantial morbidity and social impairment.

Through verbal and nonverbal messages, nurses can encourage patients to take pride in their appearance and reinforce any progress made.

Another possible nursing intervention is photographic self-image confrontation. This involves taking photographs of patients and then discussing them. This intervention can provide a means for establishing a nurse-patient relationship and mutually exploring some aspects of the self.

Mutuality is often difficult to establish with a patient experiencing depersonalization. Initially the nurse will determine appropriate activities and incorporate the patient into them without asking for a response. Gradually, however, the nurse can expect greater participation and can involve the patient in decision making. Table 19-4 summarizes the nursing interventions appropriate to level 1.

Sometimes the nurse's attitudes or behaviors can block patients from expanding their self-awareness. These behaviors can take the form of criticism, belittlement, condemnation, condescension, indifference, or insincerity. An impersonal attitude can decrease the patient's self-esteem. Excessive demands or direct challenges to self-concept can result in further withdrawal. Nurses should not allow patients to remain alone or inactive, attempt to shame them into improving their habits, or assume total care for them. If they avoid these behaviors and strive for acceptance, they remove themselves as a source of threat and encourage patients to lower their defenses. Patients are then prepared to take the next step in problem solving.

How do you think that the nurse's level of self-esteem affects nursing interventions in patients' self-concept responses?

Level 2: Self-Exploration

At this level of intervention nurses encourage patients to examine feelings, behavior, beliefs, and thoughts, particularly in relation to the current stressor. The cognitive behavioral strategies described in Chapter 32 are very useful at this time. Patients' feelings may be expressed verbally, nonverbally, symbolically, or directly. For example, self-portrait drawing has been found to facilitate awareness and understanding of sense of self for adult survivors of childhood sexual abuse (Glaister, 1996).

Acceptance continues to be important because when nurses accept patients' feelings and thoughts, they are helping them to accept themselves as well. Nurses should facilitate the expression of strong emotions, such as anger, sadness, and guilt. In a sense, patients' emotions or affects serve as clues to inner thoughts and current behavior.

As the patient focuses attention on the meaning that experiences have for him, he is clarifying his perceptions and

Table **19-4**

Nursing Interventions in Alterations in Self-Concept at Level 1		
Principle	Rationale	Nursing Interventions
GOAL: Expand the patient's self-awareness		
Establish an open, trusting relationship.	Reduces the threat that the nurse poses to the patient and helps the patient to broaden and accept all aspects of one's personality.	Offer unconditional acceptance. Listen to the patient. Encourage discussion of thoughts and feelings. Respond nonjudgmentally. Convey to the patient that he is a valued person who is responsible for and able to help himself.
Work with whatever ego strength the patient has.	Some degree of ego strength, such as the capacity for reality testing, self-control, or a degree of ego integration, is needed as a foundation for later nursing care.	Identify the patient's ego strength. Guidelines for the patient with limited ego resources are as follows: 1. Begin by confirming his identity. 2. Provide support measures to reduce his level of anxiety. 3. Approach him in an undemanding way. 4. Accept and attempt to clarify any verbal or nonverbal communication. 5. Prevent him from isolating himself. 6. Establish a simple routine for him. 7. Set limits on inappropriate behavior. 8. Orient him to reality. 9. Reinforce appropriate behavior. 10. Gradually increase activities and tasks that provide positive experiences for him. 11. Help him in personal hygiene and grooming. 12. Encourage the patient to care for himself.
Maximize the patient's participation in the therapeutic relationship.	Mutuality is needed for the patient to assume responsibility for his own behavior and maladaptive coping responses.	Gradually increase the patient's participation in decisions that affect his care. Convey to the patient that he is a responsible person.

concept of himself and his relationship to the people and events around him. The nurse can elicit his perception of strengths and weaknesses and have him describe his self-ideal. He can be made aware of his self-criticisms.

It is important for nurses to accept and deal with their own feelings before becoming involved in the self-exploration of others. Self-awareness limits the potential negative effects of countertransference in the relationship. It also allows nurses to demonstrate authentic behavior that, in turn, can be elicited and reinforced in the patient.

Often patients experience great difficulty in discussing or describing their feelings. This may be because society tends to discourage self-revelation, because some patients are honestly out of touch with their inner self, or because survivors of incest have buried important aspects of the self (Godbey & Hutchison, 1996). In these cases nurses can use themselves therapeutically by sharing feelings, verbalizing how they might feel in the situation, or mirroring their perception of patients' feelings. In this way nurses can help patients explore maladaptive thinking.

The nurse must be careful not to reinforce the patient's self-pity by responding with sympathy. Patients often deny any personal responsibility for their situation and they fail to see how their own behavior precipitates the problem about which they complain. Examples include patients who seek treatment because of things that happened to them (his wife left him, her husband beat her, or his boss fired him, for example) and patients who seek help because of things that have not happened, such as not being happy or not having friends. These patients fail to see that they have a choice in life and that personal growth and satisfaction involve both risk and responsibility.

The nurse can clarify with the patient that he is not helpless or powerless. He is powerless when he sees himself as such and gives up control and responsibility for his behavior. The patient must accept responsibility for logical consequences of the things he chooses to do or not to do. Only if a patient fully understands the implications of his actions and the scope of his choices can he set goals, explore alternatives, and effect change.

In stressing the importance of behavior, the nurse helps the patient see that he chooses to behave in certain ways. If the patient projects his problems onto the environment, the nurse can discuss with him the difficulty in changing other people and explore the possibilities of changing his own self. This means helping the patient realize that when he says, "I can't," he really means "I don't want to." The nurse should not give the impression that she has the power to change a patient's life. That power lies with the patient alone. However, the nurse can help him to maximize his strengths, use available resources, and see that there is more to life than misery and pain.

Self-exploration need not take place solely within the one-to-one relationship. Family sessions and group meetings can help clarify how the patient appears to others. These meetings can supplement the individual sessions with the patient, and similar nursing interventions can be applied within family or group therapy.

Regardless of the setting, the nurse collects information on the patient's thinking about himself, logical or illogical reasoning, and reported or observed reactions. Interventions at this level should see the patient progress from denying or attributing contradictory feelings to the external situation, to recognizing a major conflict within himself (Table 19-5).

Do you believe contemporary society encourages or discourages personal responsibility for behavior? Defend your point of view.

Level 3: Self-Evaluation

This level involves hard work for the patient as he critically examines his own behavior, accepts the consequences for it, and judges whether it is the best possible choice. At this point the problem should be clearly defined and the patient should be helped to understand that his beliefs influence his feelings and behavior. Only by actively and systematically challenging his faulty beliefs and perceptions can he hope for change. Previously identified misperceptions and distortions should be evaluated. Irrational beliefs and unrealistic self-ideals should be identified and analyzed.

The patient's hopelessness should be countered by exploring areas of realistic hope. It is important to point out the mature part of the patient's personality and contrast it to the immature part that causes problems. The behaviors that interfere with effective functioning should be put in perspective so that the patient can see that the maladaptive behavior is only a small part of his or her total personality.

Success and failure must be placed in perspective. Failures occur every moment of every day and are a natural consequence of human activity. As long as people strive to achieve, they will often not reach their goals. The only way to avoid failure is to do absolutely nothing. Failure may be caused by one's own mistakes, a lack of motivation, or circumstances beyond one's control. Whatever the reason, failure is the unavoidable outcome of human effort. The problem arises when people are labeled or label themselves as failures. This is potentially destructive. As an inherent part of life, failure should be seen as either a neutral concept or a positive one for the learning experience it provides.

Unrealistic self-ideals, dependency patterns, and denial are all potential areas that can be analyzed. The patient can be helped to realize that all behavior and coping responses have positive and negative consequences. Contrasts can be drawn between behavior that is destructive, inhibitory, or sabotaging and behavior that is productive, enhancing, or growth producing.

The patient must see that he acts in self-defeating ways because some "payoff" or personal gain is in it for him. The patient is probably well aware of the drawbacks of his maladaptive coping responses. The payoffs, or secondary gains, may be more obscure and well repressed. Following are some common payoffs:

- Procrastination
- Avoiding risks
- Retreating from the present

Table 19-5

Nursing Interventions in Alterations in Self-Concept at Level 2

Principle	Rationale	Nursing Interventions
GOAL: Encourage the patient's self-exploration		
Help the patient to accept his own feelings and thoughts.	When nurses show interest in and accept the patient's feelings and thoughts, they are helping him to do so as well.	Attend to and encourage the patient's expression of his emotions, beliefs, behavior, and thoughts verbally, nonverbally, symbolically, or directly. Use therapeutic communication skills and empathic responses. Note his use of logical and illogical thinking and his reported and observed emotional responses.
Help the patient to clarify his concept of self and his relationship to others through self-disclosure.	Self-disclosure and understanding one's self-perceptions are prerequisites to bringing about future change. This may, in itself, reduce anxiety.	Elicit his perception of self-strengths and weaknesses. Help him to describe his self-ideal. Identify his self-criticisms. Help him to describe how he believes he relates to other people and events.
Be aware and have control of one's own feelings.	Self-awareness allows the nurse to model authentic behavior and limits the potential negative effects of counter-transference in the relationship.	Be open to and accept one's own positive and negative feelings. Practice therapeutic use of self by sharing your own feelings with the patient, verbalizing how another might have felt, or mirroring one's perception of the patient's feelings.
Respond empathically, not sympathetically, emphasizing that the power to change lies with the patient.	Sympathy can reinforce self-pity. The nurse should communicate that the patient's life situation is subject to his own control.	Use empathic responses and monitor oneself for feelings of sympathy or pity. Reaffirm to the patient that he is not powerless in the face of his problems. Convey that the patient is responsible for his own behavior, including his choice of maladaptive or adaptive coping responses. Discuss the scope of his choices, his areas of ego strength, and coping resources that are available. Use the support systems of family and groups to facilitate the patient's self-exploration. Help the patient recognize the nature of his conflict and the maladaptive ways in which he tries to cope with it.

- Evading responsibility for one's actions
- Avoiding working or having to change

Payoffs specific to the patient's problem should be identified by the nurse and patient together. For example, possible secondary gains from being obese include having people feel sorry for you, having an excuse for not dating or being married, being the focus of dieting attention, or being easily recognized and noticed when with other people. Possible secondary gains for an adult remaining dependent on one's parents might include not having to make one's own decisions, having someone else to blame if things go wrong, being protected from risks and venturing out in the world, not establishing lasting intimate relationships, or not having to establish one's own identity, but rather adopting the values and goals of others.

The nurse becomes more active at this level of intervention by confronting, interpreting, persuading, and challenging. The goal is to increase the patient's objectivity in dealing with stressors. For example, the nurse can show the patient that the same person can nurture and gratify as well as anger and frustrate because both negative and positive qualities coexist in the same person. Supportive confrontation may be particularly effective in pointing out inconsistencies in words and actions. The climate of acceptance established by the nurse in level 1 and the empathic communication developed in level 2 provide a basis for confrontation in level 3. This groundwork is necessary to prevent premature confrontation, which can be destructive.

The nurse may use various aspects of role theory during this level, including helping the patient in role clarification by identifying behaviors, clarifying expectations, and specifying goals related to the role. The nurse can also encourage the patient to participate in any activity in which he can observe his own behavior. Role playing may be particularly effective in providing the patient with feedback and increasing his insight. Through it, he may become more objective about the irrationality and self-destructiveness of his self-criticisms.

Table **19-6**

Nursing Interventions in Alterations in Self-Concept at Level 3		
Principle	**Rationale**	**Nursing Interventions**
GOAL: Assist the patient's self-evaluation		
Help the patient to define the problem clearly.	Only after the problem is accurately defined can alternative choices be proposed.	Identify relevant stressors with the patient and his appraisal of them. Clarify that the patient's beliefs influence his feelings and behaviors. Mutually identify faulty beliefs, misperceptions, distortions, illusions, and unrealistic goals. Mutually identify areas of strength. Place the concepts of success and failure in proper perspective. Explore the patient's use of coping resources.
Explore the patient's adaptive and maladaptive coping responses to the problem.	Examine the coping choices the patient has made and evaluate their positive and negative consequences.	Describe to the patient how all coping responses are freely chosen and have both positive and negative consequences. Contrast adaptive and maladaptive responses. Mutually identify the disadvantages of the patient's maladaptive coping responses. Mutually identify the advantages, or payoffs, of the patient's maladaptive coping responses. Discuss how these payoffs have perpetuated the maladaptive response. Use a variety of therapeutic skills (facilitative communication, supportive confrontation, role clarification, and the transference and countertransference reactions occurring in the one-to-one relationship).

Another therapeutic intervention that is particularly useful in promoting the self-esteem and coping mechanisms of the elderly is the use of reminiscence. Reminiscence involves thinking about or relating past experiences, especially those that are personally significant. It has been used to help patients acquire a sense of integrity, enhance self-esteem, and stimulate thinking about oneself. As such, it provides nurses with an opportunity to focus, reflect, and reinforce their patients' uniqueness and enhance their sense of self-worth. Reminiscence is discussed in more detail in Chapter 40.

The nurse-patient relationship is a rich source of information for the patient. Within this relationship the patient is enacting and experiencing many problem areas, and the nurse can use this as a "study in miniature." The nurse can observe how the patient reacts in the one-to-one situation and share reactions with him to give him feedback on how he affects others.

The analysis and use of transference and countertransference reactions constitute the nurse's therapeutic use of self. When a block arises in the relationship or anxiety increases, the nurse should explore its meaning with the patient. The nurse should confront the problem and openly discuss it with him. This can also be done in family or group therapy sessions.

During this level of intervention the patient and nurse critically evaluate the patient's behavior (Table 19-6). Misperceptions, unrealistic goals, and distortions of reality are explored. This provides the patient with sufficient knowledge to progress to the next level of problem solving.

 Think of one of your less desirable habits. What payoff or personal gain does it provide you?

Level 4: Realistic Planning

The nurse and patient are now ready to formulate possible solutions or alternatives. This begins by investigating what solutions were attempted in the past and evaluating their effectiveness.

When the patient holds inconsistent perceptions, he is faced with several choices. He can change his perceptions and beliefs to bring them closer to a reality that cannot be changed. Alternatively, he may seek to change his environment to bring it in line with what he believes. When his behavior is inconsistent with his self-concept, he can change his behavior, change the beliefs underlying his self-concept so that they include his behavior, or change his self-ideal while leaving his self-concept intact.

At this time, all possible solutions should be openly discussed with the patient. Nurses must be careful not to use their influence to persuade the patient to do anything that represents their values rather than the patient's. The nurse should help the patient conceptualize goals. If they are within the patient's reach, his or her efforts can be supported. If the patient has conflicting goals, the nurse helps identify which are more realistic by discussing emotional and practical consequences.

The nurse can work with the patient in various ways. The patient may be encouraged to give up superhuman standards by which he judges his behavior. These standards may set him up for failure. The patient may need to lower his self-ideal and limit his goals. He should be encouraged to renew involvement with life and pursue new experiences for their growth potential.

Role rehearsal, role modeling, and role playing may be used. In role rehearsal the person imagines how a particular situation might take place and how his role might evolve. He mentally enacts his role and tries to anticipate the responses of significant others. Role rehearsal is important in anticipating and planning the course of future action. Role modeling occurs when the patient watches someone else playing a certain role so that he is able to understand and emulate those behaviors. The person he observes may be the nurse, a family member, a group member, or a peer. The nurse can help the patient in his role learning by modeling behavior such as expression of feelings, specific socialization skills, or realistic self-expectations. Proceeding one step further, the nurse and patient may role play certain situations to develop alternative solutions.

Visualization can also be used to enhance self-esteem through goal setting. Through the conscious programming of desired change with positive images, expectations are molded. Strong, positive expectations can then become self-fulfilling. To use visualization the nurse should do the following:

1. Ask the patient to select a positive, specific goal, such as "I will call a friend and suggest we go out together."
2. Help the patient to relax, using a relaxation technique (see Chapter 32).
3. Have the patient repeat the goal phrase several times slowly.
4. Have the patient close his eyes and visualize the goal written on a piece of paper.
5. Have the patient, while relaxed, imagine accomplishing the goal.

The patient should then describe how he feels when the desired goal is reached and how other people respond to him. In this way the patient can gain positive control over his life.

Nursing actions at this level of intervention are summarized in Table 19-7. Ultimately the patient should choose a plan that includes a clear definition of the desired change. Converting a talking decision into an action decision is the final, but most important, step.

Level 5: Commitment to Action

The nurse helps the patient to become committed to his decision and then achieve his goals. The patient's development of self-awareness, self-understanding, and insight is not the ultimate desired outcome of the nursing therapeutic process. Insight alone does not make problems disappear or transform one's world in magical ways. Although a patient may have obtained a high level of insight, he may nevertheless continue to function at a minimum level. Such a patient may be able to discuss with great ease the nature of his problem and the contributing influences, but the problem continues to be unresolved.

Some patients actually use their insights to resist moving forward and avoid the hard work involved in making behavioral changes. The value of having the patient gain insight and increase his self-understanding is that he can gain perspective on why he behaves the way he does and what must be done to break maladaptive patterns.

Table **19-7**

Nursing Interventions in Alterations in Self-Concept at Level 4		
Principle	**Rationale**	**Nursing Interventions**
GOAL: Help the patient formulate a realistic plan of action		
Help the patient identify alternative solutions.	Only when all possible alternatives have been evaluated can change be effected.	Help the patient understand that he can change only himself, not others.
		If the patient holds inconsistent perceptions, help him to see that he can change his beliefs or ideals to bring them closer to reality, and change his environment to make it consistent with his beliefs.
		If his self-concept is not consistent with his behavior, he can change his behavior to conform to his self-concept, change the beliefs underlying his self-concept to include his behavior, or change his self-ideal.
		Mutually review how coping resources may be better used by the patient.
Help the patient develop realistic goals.	Goal setting that includes a clear definition of the expected change is necessary.	Encourage the patient to formulate his own (not the nurse's) goals.
		Mutually discuss the emotional, practical, and reality-based consequences of each goal.
		Help the patient clearly define the concrete change to be made.
		Encourage the patient to pursue new experiences for growth potential.
		Use role rehearsal, role modeling, role playing, and visualization when appropriate.

Providing opportunity for the patient to experience success is essential at this time. To help him commit himself to his goal, the nurse can relate to the patient how she sees him, correcting his own poor self-image. In this mirroring technique the nurse can openly and honestly describe to the patient the healthy parts of his personality and how, by using these parts, he can achieve his goal. The nurse should reinforce his strengths or skills and provide him with opportunities to use them whenever possible.

Sometimes the lack of vocational or social skills is a causative factor for low self-esteem. If so, nursing intervention can be directed toward gaining vocational assistance for the patient. Group and family involvement may be helpful in raising self-esteem. The experience of being accepted by others, the sense of belonging and being important to others, and the opportunity to develop interpersonal competence can all enhance self-esteem.

At this point the patient needs much support and positive reinforcement in effecting and maintaining change. For many patients this means breaking chronic behavior patterns and exposing themselves to real risk. The patient must actively maintain the processes learned to avoid slipping back to the previous behavior. Doing this is difficult and requires that the patient build on the progress made in the other levels. Successful change is a continuing process of modifying not only one's behavior but also one's environment to help ensure that the change to new ways of behaving is permanent. Otherwise a relapse will occur.

The nurse serves as a transition between the pain of the past and the positive gratification of the future. Both nurse and patient must allow sufficient time for change. A significant period may be required for patterns that developed over months or years to be broken and new ones established.

The nurse's role now becomes less active and directive and more confirming of the value, potential, and accomplishments of the patient. A Nursing Treatment Plan Summary for maladaptive self-concept responses is presented below.

NURSING TREATMENT PLAN *Summary* *Maladaptive Self-Concept Responses*

NURSING DIAGNOSIS: Self-esteem disturbance
EXPECTED OUTCOME: The patient will obtain the maximum level of self-actualization to realize his or her potential.

SHORT-TERM GOAL	INTERVENTION	RATIONALE
The patient will establish a therapeutic relationship with the nurse.	Confirm the patient's identity. Provide supportive measures to decrease level of anxiety. Set limits on inappropriate behavior. Work with whatever ego strengths the patient has. Reinforce adaptive behavior.	Mutuality is necessary for the patient to assume responsibility for his or her behavior.
The patient will express feelings, behaviors, and thoughts related to the present stressor.	Help the patient to express and describe feelings and thoughts. Help the patient identify self-strengths and weaknesses, self-ideal, self-criticisms. Respond empathically, emphasizing that the power to change lies within the patient.	Self-disclosure and understanding are necessary to bring about future change. The use of sympathy is not therapeutic because it can reinforce the patient's self-pity. The nurse should communicate that the patient is in control.
The patient will evaluate the positive and negative consequences of his or her self-concept responses.	Identify relevant stressors and the patient's appraisal of them. Clarify faulty beliefs and cognitive distortions. Evaluate advantages and disadvantages of current coping responses.	Only after the problem is defined can alternative choices be examined. It is then necessary to evaluate the positive and negative consequences of current patterns.
The patient will identify one new goal and two adaptive coping responses.	Encourage the patient to formulate a new goal. Help the patient clearly define the change to be made. Use role rehearsal, role modeling, and visualization to practice the new behavior.	Only after alternatives have been explored can change be effected. Goal setting specifies the nature of the change and suggests possible new behavioral strategies.
The patient will implement the new adaptive self-concept responses.	Provide opportunity for the patient to experience success. Reinforce strengths, skills, and adaptive coping responses. Allow the patient sufficient time to change. Promote group and family involvement. Provide the appropriate amount of support and positive reinforcement for the patient to maintain progress and growth.	The ultimate goal in promoting the patient's insight is to have him or her replace the maladaptive coping responses with more adaptive ones.

EVALUATION

Problems with self-concept are prominent in many psychological disorders. To evaluate the success or failure of the nursing care given, each phase of the nursing process should be reviewed and analyzed by the nurse and patient.

The nurse's assessment should include both the objective and the observable behaviors as well as the subjective perceptions of the patient.

- Did the nurse explore the patient's strengths and weaknesses and elicit his self-ideal?
- Was information obtained on his body image, feelings of self-esteem, role satisfaction, and sense of identity?
- Did the nurse compare responses to his behavior, and were any inconsistencies or contradictions identified?
- Was the nurse aware of any personal affective response to the patient, and how did this affect the ability to be therapeutic?

The nurse should have adopted a problem-solving approach that placed responsibility for growth on the patient. The most fundamental nursing action should have been to create a climate of acceptance that confirmed the patient's identity and conveyed a sense of value or worth. In expanding the patient's self-awareness, the following should be evaluated:

- How effective was the nurse in promoting full and pertinent self-disclosure?
- Was the nurse able to show authentic behavior in the relationship and share thoughts and reactions?
- What interventions were used, and which ones were helpful (validation, reflection, confrontation, suggestion, role clarification, role playing)?
- Did the nurse progress on the basis of the patient's readiness and motivation?
- Was the patient able to transfer his new perceptions into possible solutions or alternative behavior?
- Did they both allow sufficient time for changes to occur?

The degree of overall success achieved through nursing care can be determined by eliciting the patient's perception of his own growth and comparing his behavior to the healthy personality described in this chapter. Not everyone will achieve all these characteristics, but success has been achieved if the patient's potential has been maximized.

Summary

1. The continuum of self-concept responses ranges from the most adaptive state of self-actualization to the most maladaptive response of depersonalization. Components of the self include body image, self-ideal, self-esteem, role, and identity.
2. Patient behaviors related to self-concept responses include low self-esteem, identity diffusion, and depersonalization.
3. Predisposing factors affecting self-concept responses are unrealistic self-ideals, sex and work roles, and challenges to personal identity. Precipitating stressors include role strain and developmental, situational, and health-illness transitions.
4. Coping resources focus on the patient's ego strengths, whereas coping mechanisms may be short- or long-term defenses and ego defense mechanisms.
5. Primary nursing diagnoses are body image disturbance, self-esteem disturbance, altered role performance, and personal identity disturbance.
6. Primary *DSM–IV–TR* diagnoses are categorized as dissociative disorders and identity problems.
7. The expected outcome of nursing care is that the patient will obtain the maximum level of self-actualization to realize his or her potential.
8. Interventions include helping the patient expand self-awareness and engage in self-exploration, self-evaluation, realistic planning, and commitment to action.
9. The degree of success achieved through nursing care can be determined by eliciting the patient's perception of his or her own growth and comparing his or her behavior to characteristics of a healthy personality.

Competent Caring   A Clinical Exemplar of a Psychiatric Nurse

MONICA MOLLOY, MSN, RN, CS

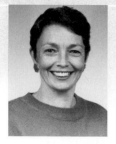

Last week one of my patients died. I have been a nurse for 16 years. I have experienced patients' deaths—many different kinds of deaths, some of them seemingly senseless. I think particularly of young patients with head injuries from motorcycle or automobile accidents. But I understood those deaths. I understood the concept of an accident. What I don't understand is the concept of murder.

In November, a woman was sitting apart from most of the members of a therapy group I lead with a graduate nursing student. I asked her why she didn't join the circle. She replied she was afraid the group didn't want her near them; she thought the odor of her cancer would offend them. When the women in the group responded that they hadn't noticed any odor, she seemed to accept the reassurance offered, but she continued to sit apart. Last week that woman was murdered.

She was a homeless woman, one of the women that embarrass us as a society. She lived in the Family Center of the homeless shelter. I'll call her C. I first met her 2 years ago, when the group began. I remember one group session in particular when she and another shelter guest talked about trust issues in the homeless community. Then she moved away. This past fall she returned to the shelter. In addition to neurofibromatosis, she now had cancer. She looked different; she had lost nearly 40 pounds. She had been discharged from a local hospital to the shelter. Despite her willingness to take a risk and to disclose her fears about the odor she thought she had, she essentially remained alone and apart.

Competent Caring A Clinical Exemplar of a Psychiatric Nurse—cont'd

C's death has given me one more opportunity to examine what it is to practice psychiatric nursing in the community. When nurses practice in inpatient environments, one of our fundamental responsibilities is to ensure patient safety. Sometimes that safety is interpersonal, sometimes it is environmental. Among the homeless population, environmental safety is tenuous at best. One goal for the group intervention in the shelter community is to enable the women to use themselves and each other as resources to create their own safety zone. Somehow that didn't work with C. The day after her death, the graduate nursing student and I spent some time with the women in the Family Center community. We went there to be with the women to provide support. We also went there to

grieve. And perhaps most of all, we went there to try to answer some questions for ourselves, the same questions all clinicians ask when a patient dies: Did we miss some signs? Could we have done something different?

C's death is mentioned in the group weekly now. New guests use her death to reify their fears about being homeless, as a metaphor for their own alienation experience. Through her death C has left a mark on that group and that community. I don't understand the concept of murder any better. I do understand more about the concept of alienation. Acknowledging alienation is a first step to creating a sense of personal safety. It is fundamental to the practice of psychiatric nursing in the community. I learned that from C, and for that I will always be grateful.

MeRLIN Visit **MERLIN: www.mosby.com/MERLIN/Stuart** to find these additional materials and student activities.

- **Worksheets**
- **"Drug of the Month" Updates**
- **"Citing the Evidence" Updates**
- **Critical Thinking Activities and Exercises**
- **Annotated Suggested Readings**
- **Web Links**
- **More!**

Chapter Review Questions

1. **Identify whether the following statements are true (T) or false (F).**

____ **A.** People behave in a manner consistent with what they believe to be true.

____ **B.** There is no evidence that genetics plays a role in the inheritance of self-esteem.

____ **C.** Most people who express dissatisfaction with life, display deviant behavior, or have difficulty functioning in social or work situations have problems related to self-concept.

____ **D.** The optimum outcome desired for a patient with alterations in self-concept is enhanced insight into self-concept and its influence on behavior.

____ **E.** Responding with sympathy is an appropriate nursing intervention to help a patient with self-exploration.

2. **Fill in the blanks.**

A. _____ is a person's perception of how one should behave based on certain personal standards.

B. A person's judgment of his or her own worth obtained by analyzing how well the person's behavior conforms to his or her self-ideal is called

_____ .

C. _____ are sets of socially expected behavior patterns associated with a person's functioning in various social groups.

D. The organizing principle of the personality is called

_____ .

E. _____ is the feeling of unreality in which one is unable to distinguish between inner and outer stimuli.

F. It is believed that _____ is a precipitating stressor for dissociative disorder and multiple personality disorder.

G. Thinking about or relating past experiences, especially those that are personally significant, is called

_____ .

3. **Provide short answers for the following questions.**

A. Describe the four best ways to promote a child's self-esteem.

B. Briefly describe the developmental crisis of adolescence.

C. List six qualities of the healthy personality. Think about someone you admire and evaluate him or her based on each of these qualities.

D. Describe your own body-image, self-ideal, and level of self esteem. What changes would you like to make in each area?

REFERENCES

Allen J: Dissociative processes: theoretical underpinnings of a working model for clinician and patient, *Bull Menninger Clin* 57:287, 1993.

American Psychiatric Association: *Diagnostic and statistical manual of mental disorders,* Fourth Edition, Text Revision. Washington, DC, American Psychiatric Association, 2000.

Applegate M: Multiphasic short-term therapy for dissociative identity disorder, *J Am Psychiatr Nurs Assoc* 3(1):1, 1997.

Bednar R et al: Self-esteem: a concept of renewed clinical relevance, *Hosp Community Psychiatry* 42:123, 1991.

Burns D: Focusing on ego strengths, *Arch Psychiatr Nurs* 5:202, 1991.

Chu J et al: Memories of childhood abuse: dissociation, amnesia and corroboration, *Am J Psychiatry* 156(5):749, 1999.

Coopersmith S: *The antecedents of self-esteem,* San Francisco, 1967, WH Freeman.

Czuchta D, Johnson B: Reconstructing a sense of self in patients with chronic mental illness, *Perspect Psychiatr Care* 34(3):31, 1998.

Dallam S, Manderino M: Peer group supports patients with MPD/DD, *J Psychosoc Nurs* 35(5):22, 1997.

Ellason J, Ross C: Two year follow-up of inpatient with dissociative identity disorder, *Am J Psychiatry* 154(6):832, 1997.

Erikson E: *Childhood and society,* New York, 1963, WW Norton.

Glaister J: Serial self-portrait: a technique to monitor changes in self-concept, *Arch Psychiatr Nurs* 10:311, 1996.

Godbey J, Hutchinson S: Healing from incest: resurrecting the buried self, *Arch Psychiatr Nurs* 10:304, 1996.

Guralnik O et al: Feeling unreal: cognitive processes in depersonalization, *Am J Psychiatry* 157(1):103, 2000.

Horowitz M et al: Self-regard: a new measure, *Am J Psychiatry* 153:382, 1996.

Kluft R: Current issues in dissociative identity disorder, *J Pract Psychiatry Behav Health* 5:3, 1999.

Mruk C: *Self-esteem: research, theory and practice,* New York, 1995, Springer.

Price B: Explorations in body image care: Peplau and practical knowledge, *J Psychiatr Ment Health Nurs* 5:179, 1998.

Putnam F, Lowenstein R: Treatment of multiple personality disorder: a survey of current practices, *Am J Psychiatry* 150:104, 1993.

Roy M et al: The genetic epidemiology of self-esteem, *Br J Psychiatry* 166:813, 1995.

Simeon D et al: Feeling unreal: 30 cases of DSM-III depersonalization disorder, *Am J Psychiatry* 154(8):1107, 1997.

Sullivan HS: *The interpersonal theory of psychiatry,* New York, 1963, WW Norton.

Vaillant G: *The wisdom of the ego,* Cambridge, Mass, 1993, Harvard University Press.

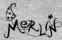

Visit **MERLIN** for *Your Internet Connection*
to websites that are related to the content in this chapter.
www.mosby.com/MERLIN/Stuart

Emotional Responses and Mood Disorders

Gail W. Stuart

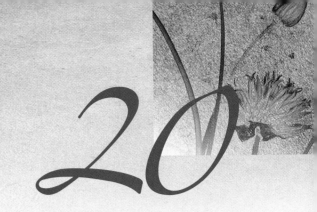

ⶮying awake, calculating the future,
Trying to unweave, unwind, unravel
And piece together the past and the future,
Between midnight and dawn, when the past is all deception,
The future futureless . . .

T.S. Eliot

Variations in mood are a natural part of life. They indicate that a person is perceiving the world and responding to it. Extremes in mood are also linked with extremes in human experience, such as creativity, madness, despair, ecstasy, romanticism, personal charisma, and interpersonal destructiveness.

In this text, mood is a prolonged emotional state that influences the person's whole personality and life functioning. It pertains to prevailing and pervading emotion and is synonymous with the terms **feeling state** and **emotion**. Like other aspects of the personality, emotions or moods serve an adaptive role. The four adaptive functions of emotions are social communication, physiological arousal, subjective awareness, and psychodynamic defense.

CONTINUUM OF EMOTIONAL RESPONSES

Emotions such as fear, joy, anxiety, love, anger, sadness, and surprise are all normal parts of the human condition. The problem arises in trying to evaluate when a person's mood or emotional state is maladaptive, abnormal, or unhealthy. Grief, for example, is a healthy, adaptive, separative process that attempts to overcome the stress of a loss. Grief work, or mourning, is not a pathological process; it is an adaptive response to a real stressor. The absence of grieving in the face of a loss suggests maladaptation.

The continuum of emotional responses is represented in Fig. 20-1. At the adaptive end is emotional responsiveness. This involves the person being affected by and being an active participant in the internal and external worlds. It implies

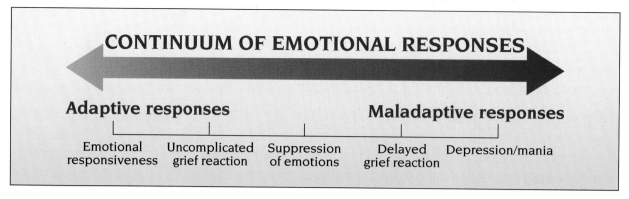

Fig. 20-1   Continuum of emotional responses.

an openness to and awareness of feelings. If used in such a way, feelings provide us with valuable learning experiences. They are barometers that give us feedback about ourselves and our relationships, and they help us function more effectively. Also adaptive in the face of stress is an uncomplicated grief reaction. Such a reaction implies that the person is facing the reality of the loss and is immersed in the work of grieving.

A maladaptive response is the suppression of emotions. This may be a denial of one's feelings or a detachment from them. A transient suppression of feelings may at times be necessary to cope, as in an initial response to a death or tragedy. However, prolonged suppression of emotion, as in delayed grief reaction, will ultimately interfere with effective functioning.

The most maladaptive emotional responses or severe mood disturbances are recognized by their intensity, pervasiveness, persistence, and interference with social and physiological functioning. These characteristics apply to the clinical states of depression and mania, which complete the maladaptive end of the continuum of emotional responses.

Grief Reactions

Grief is the subjective state that follows loss. It is one of the most powerful emotional states and affects all aspects of a person's life. It forces the person to stop normal activities and focus on present feelings and needs. Most often, it is the response to the loss of a loved person through death or separation, but it also occurs following the loss of something tangible or intangible that is highly regarded. It may be a valued object, a cherished possession, an ideal, a job, or status. As a response to the loss of a loved one, grief is a universal reaction. As a person's dependence on others grows, the chance increases of facing loss, separation, and death, which elicit intense feelings of grief. The capacity to form warm, satisfying relationships with others makes a person vulnerable to sadness, despair, and grief when those relationships are terminated.

As a natural reaction to a life experience, grief is universal. It involves stress, pain, and suffering and an impairment of function that can last for days, weeks, or months. Thus the understanding of grief is of great importance because of its effect on both physical and emotional health.

The ability to experience grief is gradually formed in the course of normal development and is closely related to the capacity for developing meaningful relationships. Grief responses may be either uncomplicated and adaptive or morbid and pathological. Uncomplicated grief runs a consistent course that is modified by the abruptness of the loss, the person's preparation for the event, and the significance of the lost object. It is a self-limited process of realization; it makes real the fact of the loss.

A maladaptive response to loss implies that something has prevented it from running its normal course. There are two types of pathological grief reactions: the delayed reaction and the distorted reaction. Depression is one type of distorted grief reaction. Persistent absence of any emotion may signal an undue delay in the work of mourning or a delayed grief reaction. The delay may occur in the beginning of the mourning process or slow the process once it has begun, or both. The delay and rejection of grief may occasionally last for many years. The emotions associated with the loss may be triggered by a deliberate recall of circumstances surrounding the loss or by a spontaneous occurrence in the patient's life. A classic example of this is the anniversary reaction, in which the person experiences incomplete or abnormal mourning at the time of the loss, only to have the grieving response recur at anniversaries of the original loss.

Depression

The person who does not mourn can experience a pathological grief reaction known as depression, or melancholia. It is an abnormal extension or overelaboration of sadness and grief. Depression is the oldest and most common psychiatric illness. It has been described as early as 1500 B.C., and it is as familiar as it is mysterious. The word depression is used in a variety of ways. It can refer to a sign, symptom, syndrome, emotional state, reaction, disease, or clinical entity. In this chapter it is viewed as a clinical illness that is severe, maladaptive, and incapacitating.

Depression may range from mild and moderate states to severe states with or without psychotic features. Psychotic depression is uncommon, however, accounting for less than 10% of all depressions. Major depression can begin at any age, although it usually begins in the mid-twenties and thirties. Symptoms develop over days to weeks. Approximately

(see Critical Thinking about Contemporary Issues)

CRITICAL THINKING about CONTEMPORARY ISSUES

Is There a Difference in the Experience of Depression between Black and White Women in America?

It has been suggested that black women's mental health is affected by their double minority status of being black and female in America. Yet the exact incidence of depression in black women is unclear because of controversy regarding misdiagnosis and lack of clinical research. Although it is known that black women report depression more often than black men, little is known about the sociodemographic indicators of risk and depressive symptoms. The assumption that all women share similar experiences does not allow for differences to emerge regarding the diagnostic process, measurement tools, and successful treatment strategies for various cultural groups.

It is clear that depression is an increasing problem for black women. These women are experiencing role changes and additional stressors. Depressed black women may perceive themselves as being devalued by society and may have fewer support systems to buffer stressful events. Depressive symptoms may develop into clinical depression and further decrease the quality of life for black women. Psychiatric nurses can be instrumental in developing protocols and interventions that respond with cultural sensitivity to the psychological and physiological needs of depressed patients and thus improve their overall quality of life.

Table 20-1

Comorbidity of Depression and Other Psychiatric Illness

	Major Depressive Disorder (%)	Dysthymic Disorder (%)	Depression NOS (%)
Alcohol abuse	10	30	67
Drug abuse	19	30	26
Panic disorder	19	7	21
Obsessive-compulsive disorder	35	15	40

Citing the Evidence on

Depression in Hospitalized Patients

BACKGROUND: This study assessed the relationship among depressed mood, physical functioning, and severity of illness and attempted to determine the relationship between depressed mood and survival time, controlling for severity of illness, baseline functioning, and characteristics of patients.

RESULTS: Greater depressed mood was associated with worse levels of physical functioning and more severity of illness. Depressed mood was also associated with reduced survival time.

IMPLICATIONS: Seriously ill patients should be assessed for the presence of depressed mood even if they have not been given a diagnosis of depression. Further study is needed to determine whether interventions aimed at relieving depressed mood may improve prognosis.

Roach MJ et al: Depressed mood and survival in seriously ill hospitalized adults, *Arch Intern Med* 158:397, 1998.

one out of eight adults may experience major depression in their lifetime, and it affects 11.5 million people each year, 71% of whom are women. Approximately 15% of severely depressed patients commit suicide. Other complications include marital, parental, social, and vocational difficulties (American Psychiatric Association, 2000b).

The lifetime risk for major depression is 7% to 12% for men and 20% to 30% for women. Among women, rates peak between adolescence and early adulthood. This difference holds true across cultures and continents (see Critical Thinking about Contemporary Issues). Other risk factors include a history of depressive illness in first-degree relatives and a history of major depression.

Most untreated episodes of major depression last 6 to 24 months. Although some people have only a single episode of major depression and return to presymptomatic functioning, it is estimated that over 50% of those who have such an episode will eventually have another, and 25% of patients will have chronic, recurrent depression (Solomon et al, 2000).

Depression often occurs along with other psychiatric illnesses (Table 20-1). Up to 43% of patients with major depressive disorders have histories of one or more nonmood psychiatric disorders. These statistics underscore the importance of this health problem and suggest the need for timely diagnosis and treatment. Unfortunately, only one third of all people with depression seek help, are accurately diagnosed, and obtain appropriate treatment.

There is a high incidence of depression among patients hospitalized for medical illnesses. These depressions are largely unrecognized and thus are untreated by health care personnel (see Citing the Evidence). Depression is found in all severities of medical illness, although its intensity and frequency are higher in more severely ill patients. Studies suggest that about one third of medical inpatients report mild or moderate symptoms of depression and up to one fourth may have a depressive illness. Certain medical conditions are often associated with depression, especially cancer, stroke, epilepsy, multiple sclerosis, Parkinson's disease, cardiac disease, and a variety of endocrine disorders. Thus depression is a common accompaniment of many major medical illnesses.

Depressive conditions are also highly prevalent in primary care settings (Ornstein et al, 2000). One out of five patients seeing a primary care practitioner has significant symptoms of depression. Yet only about one in 100 patients cites depression as a reason for the most recent visit, and health care providers fail to diagnose major depression in their patients up to 50% of the time. Finally, it has been estimated that depression costs the American economy $43.7 billion in worker absenteeism, lost productivity, and health care.

> A patient who just underwent cardiac surgery comes for a follow-up visit and tells the physician he is feeling depressed. He is told that depression is a normal response to cardiac illness and he will get over it in time. Do you agree? If not, what nursing actions are indicated?

Mania

In addition to severe depression, manic episodes may occur (Simmons-Alling, 1996). These episodes, like those of depression, can vary in intensity and accompanying level of anxiety from moderate manic states to severe and panic states with psychotic features. Basically, mania is characterized by an elevated, expansive, or irritable mood. Hypomania is a clinical syndrome similar to but not as severe as mania.

In the *DSM–IV–TR* (American Psychiatric Association, 2000a) the major affective disorders are separated into two subgroups—bipolar and depressive disorders—based on whether manic and depressive episodes are involved over time. In this classification, major depression may involve a single episode or a recurrent depressive illness but without manic episodes. When there have been one or more manic episodes, with or without a major depressive episode, the category of bipolar disorder is used (Hilty et al, 1999).

Thus a depressive episode with no manic episodes would be classified as a **depressive disorder.** A depressive episode with previous or current manic episodes would be classified as a bipolar disorder or manic depressive illness because the patient experiences both mania and depression. Although bipolar affective disorders are less common than depressive disorders, it is estimated that 0.6% to 0.88% of the adult population, or approximately 2 million Americans, have bipolar disorder. Risk factors are being female and having a family history of bipolar disorder. The data suggest that people under age 50 years are at higher risk of a first attack, whereas those who already have the disorder face increased risk of a recurrent manic or depressive episode as they grow older. Additional facts about depressive and bipolar disorders are presented in Box 20-1.

ASSESSMENT
Behaviors

Delayed Grief Reaction. Delayed grief reactions may be expressed by excessive hostility and grief, prolonged feelings of emptiness and numbness, an inability to weep or express emotions, low self-esteem, use of present tense instead of past when speaking of the loss, persistent dreams about the loss, retention of clothing of the deceased, an inability to visit the grave of the deceased, and the projection of living memories onto an object held in place of the lost one. The

Box 20-1
Facts about Mood Disorders

MAJOR DEPRESSIVE DISORDER

Major depression is one of the most common clinical problems encountered by primary care practitioners.

Major depression accounts for more bed days (people out of work and in bed) than any other "physical" disorder except cardiovascular disorders, and it is more costly to the economy than chronic respiratory illness, diabetes, arthritis, or hypertension.

Psychotherapy alone helps some depressed patients, especially those with mild to moderate symptoms.

It can be treated successfully by antidepressant medications in 65% of cases.

Success rate of treatment increases to 85% when alternative or adjunctive medications are used or psychotherapy is combined with medications.

BIPOLAR DISORDER

Without modern treatments, patients typically spend one fourth of their adult life in the hospital and fully one half of their life disabled.

Effective medications (lithium and anticonvulsants), often used in combination with psychotherapy, allow 75% to 80% of manic-depressive patients to lead essentially normal lives.

These drugs have saved the U.S. economy more than $40 billion since 1970: $13 billion in direct treatment costs and $27 billion in indirect costs.

following clinical example illustrates some of the behaviors associated with a delayed grief reaction.

 CLINICAL EXAMPLE

Mrs. G was a 38-year-old married woman with no history of depression. She came to the local community mental health center complaining of severe throbbing headaches, difficulty falling asleep, fitful and disturbing dreams when asleep, and poor appetite. She said she felt "disgusted" with herself and "useless" to her family. She was living alone with her husband.

Her family history revealed that she had three children: two boys and a girl. Her eldest son, age 20, was attending college out of state, and her daughter, age 19, was living with a girlfriend in the same city. Her youngest son was killed in an automobile accident 2 years before at age 15. She described him as her "baby" and expressed much guilt for contributing to his death. She scolded herself for allowing him to drive to the seashore for the weekend with friends, and said she now worries a great deal about her other two children. She said she was trying to protect them from the dangers of the world, but they resented her advice and concern. On questioning by the nurse, Mrs. G reported that these feelings of sadness and guilt had emerged in the last month and seemed to be triggered by the graduation of her son's high school class.

Selected Nursing Diagnosis

- Dysfunctional grieving related to son's death, as evidenced by somatic complaints and feelings of sadness and guilt

Table **20-2**

Behaviors Associated with Depression			
Affective	Physiological	Cognitive	Behavioral
Anger	Abdominal pain	Ambivalence	Aggressiveness
Anxiety	Anorexia	Confusion	Agitation
Apathy	Backache	Inability to concentrate	Alcoholism
Bitterness	Chest pain	Indecisiveness	Altered activity level
Dejection	Constipation	Loss of interest and motivation	Drug addiction
Denial of feelings	Dizziness	Pessimism	Intolerance
Despondency	Fatigue	Self-blame	Irritability
Guilt	Headache	Self-depreciation	Lack of spontaneity
Helplessness	Impotence	Self-destructive thoughts	Overdependency
Hopelessness	Indigestion	Uncertainty	Poor personal hygiene
Loneliness	Insomnia		Psychomotor retardation
Low self-esteem	Lassitude		Social isolation
Sadness	Menstrual changes		Tearfulness
Sense of personal worthlessness	Nausea		Underachievement
	Overeating		Withdrawal
	Sexual nonresponsiveness		
	Sleep disturbances		
	Vomiting		
	Weight change		

In this example Mrs. G was experiencing a delayed grief reaction precipitated by the event of her deceased son's would-be graduation. She had failed to progress through mourning at her son's death and was just beginning grief work.

Depression. The behaviors associated with depression vary. Sadness and slowness may predominate, or agitation may occur. The key element of a behavioral assessment is change: Depressed people change their usual patterns and responses. Research indicates that people working through normal mourning respond to their loss with psychological symptoms often indistinguishable from depression, but accepted by them and by their environment as normal. In contrast, patients with depression experience their condition as a change from their usual selves, which often leads them to seek help.

Many behaviors are associated with depression. These can be divided into affective, physiological, cognitive, and behavioral (Table 20-2). The lists describe the spectrum of possible behaviors, and not all patients experience all of them.

The most common and central behavior is that of the depressive mood. This is not necessarily described by the patient as depression but as feeling sad, blue, down in the dumps, unhappy, or unable to enjoy life. Crying often occurs. On the other hand, some depressed people do not cry and describe themselves as "beyond tears." The mood disturbance of the depressed patient resembles that of normal unhappiness multiplied in intensity and pervasiveness. Another mood that often accompanies depression is anxiety: a sense of fear and intense worry. Both depression and anxiety may show diurnal variation, that is, a pattern whereby certain times of the day, such as morning or evening, are consistently worse or better.

Some patients may initially deny their anxious or depressed moods but identify a variety of somatic complaints. These might include gastrointestinal distress, chronic or intermittent pain, irritability, palpitations, dizziness, appetite change, lack of energy, change in sex drive, or sleep disturbances. The person often focuses on these symptoms because they are more socially acceptable than the profound feeling of sadness, inability to concentrate, or loss of pleasure in usual activities. In addition, the physical symptoms may help the person with depression explain why nothing is fun anymore. When patients have a range of somatic symptoms, the nurse should carefully evaluate these complaints but also return to the issues of mood and interest, thus considering the possible diagnosis of depression.

It may also be helpful for the nurse to be familiar with the subgroups of major depressive disorder. The common subgroups and clinical relevance of each are presented in Table 20-3. These subgroups are not all-inclusive and may be varying clinical expressions of the same illness over time, in different age groups, or in relation to specific precipitating stressors. Two of these subgroups merit special attention.

Postpartum onset. Postpartum mood symptoms are divided into three categories based on severity: blues, psychosis, and depression. Postpartum blues are brief episodes lasting 1 to 4 days of labile mood and tearfulness that occur in about 50% to 80% of women within 1 to 5 days of delivery. Treatment consists of reassurance and time to resolve this normal response. **Postpartum psychosis** can be divided into depressed and manic types. The incidence of postpartum psychosis is low, and the symptoms typically begin 2 to 3 days after delivery. The period of risk for postpartum psychosis is within the first month after delivery. The prognosis is good for acute postpartum psychosis. However, many patients subsequently develop a bipolar disorder. The recurrence rate is 33% to 51%. **Postpartum depression** may occur from 2 weeks to 12 months after delivery, but usually occurs within 6 months. The risk of postpartum depression is 10%

Table 20-3

Major Depressive Disorder Subgroups

Subgroup	Essential Features	Diagnostic Implications	Treatment Implications	Prognostic Implications
Psychotic	Hallucinations Delusions	More likely to become bipolar than non-psychotic types May be misdiagnosed as schizophrenia	Antidepressant medication plus a neuroleptic is more effective than are antidepressants alone ECT is very effective	Usually a recurrent illness Subsequent episodes are usually psychotic Psychotic subtypes run in families Mood-incongruent features have a poorer prognosis
Melancholic	Anhedonia Unreactive mood Severe vegetative symptoms	May be misdiagnosed as dementia More likely in older patients	Antidepressant medication is essential ECT is 90% effective	If recurrent, consider maintenance medication
Atypical	Reactive mood Overeating/weight gain Oversleeping Rejection sensitivity Heavy limb sensation Fewer episodes	Common in younger patients May be misdiagnosed as personality disorder	TCAs may be less effective; MAOIs are preferred SSRIs preferred	Unclear
Seasonal	Onset, fall Offset, spring Recurrent	More common in non-equatorial latitudes Pattern occurs in major depressive and bipolar disorders	Medications have questionable efficacy Psychotherapy has questionable efficacy Phototherapy is an option	Recurs
Postpartum psychosis/depression	Acute onset (<30 days) in postpartum period Severe, labile mood symptoms 1/1000 is psychotic form	Often heralds a bipolar disorder	Hospitalize Treat medically Antidepressants, anti-psychotics are effective	50% chance of recurring in the next postpartum period

From Depression Guideline Panel: *Depression in primary care*, vol 1, *Detection and diagnosis, Clinical practice guideline no 5*, Rockville, Md, 1993, US Department of Health and Human Services, Public Health Service, Agency for Health Care Policy and Research, pub no 93-0550.
ECT, Electroconvulsive therapy; *MAOIs*, monoamine oxidase inhibitors; *SSRIs*, selective serotonin reuptake inhibitors, *TCA*, tricyclic antidepressant.

to 15%, but the rate is higher for people with a history of psychiatric disorders (Epperson, 1999).

Seasonal pattern. Seasonal affective disorder (SAD) is depression that comes with shortened daylight in winter and fall and disappears during spring and summer. It is characterized by hypersomnia, lethargy and fatigue, increased anxiety, irritability, increased appetite with carbohydrate craving, and often weight gain. It is believed to be related to abnormal melatonin metabolism (Terman et al, 1998). It has also been noted that two to three times as many people experience the winter recurrence of seasonal mood symptoms as those who actually exhibit behaviors severe enough to merit clinical diagnosis.

> *Conditions of light and darkness have often been noted to affect mood. Evaluate your environment for exposure to light. Compare it with a hospital environment.*

Suicide. Finally, the potential for suicide should always be assessed in severe mood disturbances. Suicide and other self-destructive behaviors are discussed in detail in Chapter 21. The intensity of anger, guilt, and worthlessness may precipi-

tate suicidal thoughts, feelings, or gestures, as illustrated in the following clinical example.

 CLINICAL EXAMPLE

Mr. W was a 60-year-old man who lived alone. His son and daughter were married and lived in the same state. His wife died 2 years before, and since that time his children had often asked him to move in with either of them. He consistently refused to do this, believing that he and his children needed privacy in their lives. Six months before, he was diagnosed as having advanced prostatic cancer with metastasis. After the diagnosis and because of increasing disability, he left his job and began to receive disability compensation. He visited his children and their families about twice a month and kept his regularly scheduled visits with the medical clinic. The nurses and physicians at the clinic noted that he was "despondent and withdrawn" but viewed this as a normal reaction to his diagnosis and family history. No interventions were implemented based on his emotional needs. A week after attending the clinic for a routine follow-up visit, he went to the cemetery where his wife was buried and at her gravestone shot himself in the head. A groundskeeper of the cemetery heard the shot, discovered what had happened, and called an ambulance. Mr. W was

Table **20-4**

Behaviors Associated with Mania			
Affective	**Physiological**	**Cognitive**	**Behavioral**
Elation or euphoria	Dehydration	Ambitiousness	Aggressiveness
Expansiveness	Inadequate nutrition	Denial of realistic danger	Excessive spending
Humorousness	Needs little sleep	Distractibility	Grandiose acts
Inflated self-esteem	Weight loss	Flight of ideas	Hyperactivity
Intolerance of criticism		Grandiosity	Increased motor activity
Lack of shame or guilt		Illusions	Irresponsibility
		Lack of judgment	Irritability or argumentativeness
		Loose associations	Poor personal grooming
			Provocativeness
			Sexual overactivity
			Social activity
			Verbosity

taken to the emergency room of the nearest hospital and, with prompt medical care, survived the suicide attempt.

Selected Nursing Diagnosis

- Risk for self-directed violence related to feelings of depression, as evidenced by gunshot to the head
- Hopelessness related to medical diagnosis of metastatic cancer, as evidenced by withdrawal and despondency

This example dramatically makes three important points. First, medical illness often involves a loss of function, body part, or appearance. Therefore all patients should be assessed for depression. Second, all people experiencing depression and despair have the potential for suicide. Third, nurses can intervene to support the grieving and mourning process, whether it is uncomplicated or pathological. Nursing actions can be preventive, curative, or rehabilitative, based on the nursing assessment and diagnosis.

Mania. The essential feature of mania is a distinct period of intense psychophysiological activation. Some of the behaviors of mania are given in Table 20-4. The predominant mood is elevated or irritable, accompanied by one or more of the following symptoms: hyperactivity, the undertaking of too many activities, lack of judgment in anticipating consequences, pressured speech, flight of ideas, distractibility, inflated self-esteem, and hypersexuality.

If the mood is elevated or euphoric, it is often infectious. Patients report feeling happy, unconcerned, carefree, and devoid of problems. Although such experiences seem enviable, the person has no concern for reality or the feelings of others. The mood is often expansive, and some patients have extraordinary delusions about their power and importance. They characteristically involve themselves in seemingly senseless and risky enterprises.

Alternatively, the mood may be irritable, especially when plans are blocked. Patients can be argumentative and provoked by seemingly harmless remarks. Self-esteem is inflated during a manic episode, and as activity level increases, feelings about the self become increasingly disturbed. Delu-

sional grandiose symptoms are evident, and the patient is willing to undertake any project possible.

In contrast to depressed patients, manic patients are extremely self-confident, with an ego that knows no bounds; they are "on top of the world." Accompanying this magical omnipotence and supreme self-esteem is an equally inordinate lack of guilt and shame. Often they deny realistic danger. The patient's boundless energy, cunning, planning, scheming, and inability to anticipate consequences often lead to irresponsible activities and excessive spending, as well as problems of a sexual, aggressive, or possessive nature. In contrast to depressed patients, manic patients have abundant energy and heightened sexual appetite. Characteristic physical changes are inadequate nutrition, partly because manic patients have no time to eat, and serious weight loss related to their insomnia and overactivity. Extremely manic patients may be dehydrated and require prompt attention.

In addition to mood, speech is often disturbed. As mania intensifies, formal and logical speech is replaced by loud, rapid, and confusing language. As the activated state increases, speech becomes full of plays on words and irrelevancies that can increase to loosened associations and flight of ideas. Some of these behaviors are evident in the next clinical example.

 CLINICAL EXAMPLE

Mr. B was a 30-year-old single man who was admitted to the psychiatric unit of the local community hospital. He had been hospitalized 2 years before for problems related to alcoholism. He was accompanied to the hospital by a friend who lived with him. His friend said that for the past 2 months Mr. B had been "running on 10 cylinders instead of four." He slept and ate little and talked constantly, sometimes so fast that no one could understand what he was trying to say. He had redecorated his bedroom in the apartment twice and had gone into debt buying a new wardrobe. His friend brought him in because his behavior was becoming more erratic and his physical condition was failing.

The nurse who admitted Mr. B asked about his social relationships. He revealed that his girlfriend of 7 years had left him 6 months before for another man. He said that initially he thought she would "see the light," but she had refused to see him since then. Mr. B said this "upset" him a little at the time, but he was sure it was for the best and there were plenty other women waiting for him.

Selected Nursing Diagnosis

- Risk for self-directed violence related to interpersonal rejection, as evidenced by agitated behavior and lack of self-care

Other behaviors found in mania include lability of mood with rapid shifts to brief depression. Such behavior accounts for patients who have loosened associations and alternately laugh and cry. In addition, hallucinations of any type, ideas of reference, and frank delusions may be present with predominant feelings of guilt and thoughts of suicide. Manic episodes are very likely to recur. About 75% of manic patients have more than one episode, and almost all those with manic episodes also have depressive episodes. However, the duration and severity of the manic episodes vary, as do the intervals between relapses and recurrences.

Behavioral rating scales related to mood disorders are listed in Box 20-2. All these clinical examples illustrate the interrelatedness of disturbances of mood with self-esteem and disrupted relationships. Multiple aspects of the patient's life are affected, including physical health. Hypertensive crises, irritable bowel syndromes, coronary occlusions, rheumatoid arthritis, migraine headaches, and various dermatological conditions can occur with severe mood disturbances.

Predisposing Factors

Genetics. There is wide agreement that heredity and environment play an important role in severe mood disturbances. Both bipolar and major depressive disorders run in families, but evidence of heritability is higher for bipolar disorder.

- One parent with bipolar disorder: 25% chance in child
- Two parents with bipolar disorder: 50% to 75% chance in child
- One monozygotic twin with bipolar disorder: 40% to 70% chance in other twin
- One dizygotic twin with bipolar disorder: about 20% chance in other twin
- One parent with depressive disorder: 10% to 13% chance in child

However, studies using only familial aggregations do not necessarily demonstrate the role of genetics because disturbances may be the result of nutritional, infectious, or psychological factors. Some studies using genetic markers such as color blindness suggest that bipolar affective disorder is transmitted by an X-linked dominant gene. Controversy surrounds the mode of genetic transmission in affective disorders, however, because findings from other studies contradict this hypothesis. Most recent research suggests there are different forms of genetic transmission.

Other evidence includes the following:

- A higher frequency of affective disorders in relatives of the patient than in the general population
- A higher frequency of psychiatric problems in relatives of the patient with affective disorder than in the general population
- Onset of the illness at a characteristic age with no evidence of a precipitating event

Thus good evidence exists for the role of genetic factors in mood disorders.

Aggression-Turned-Inward Theory. The aggression-turned-inward theory of Freud views depression as the inward turning of the aggressive instinct, for some reason not directed at the appropriate object and accompanied by feelings of guilt. The process is initiated by the loss of an ambivalently loved object. The person feels angry and loving at the same time and is unable to express anger because it is considered inappropriate or irrational. Also, the person may have developed a pattern throughout life of containing feelings, especially those that are viewed negatively. Angry feelings are then directed inward. Freud believed that if a person went so far as to commit suicide, the act was a strike against the hated and loved object as well as against the self.

Although it is an often quoted theory of depression, little evidence supports it. Furthermore, the redirection of hostility at outside objects has not been consistently correlated with clinical improvement. In some instances it may actually have negative effects on the patient's view of self and problem resolution.

Object Loss Theory. The object loss theory of depression refers to traumatic separation of the person from significant objects of attachment. Two issues are important to this theory: loss during childhood as a predisposing factor for adult depressions and separation in adult life as a precipitating stress. The first issue proposes that a child has ordinarily formed a tie to a mother figure by 6 months of age, and once that tie is ruptured, the child experiences separa-

Box 20-2

Behavioral Rating Scales Related to Mood Disorders

- Apparent Affect Rating Scale (AARS)
- Beck Depression Inventory (BDI)
- Beck Depression Inventory II (BDI-II)
- Carroll Self-Rating Scale
- Center for Epidemiologic Studies Depression Scale (CES-D)
- Dementia Mood Assessment Scale (DMAS)
- Depression Arkansas Scale (D-ARK Scale)
- Depression Outcome Module (DOM)
- Geriatric Depression Scale (GDS)
- Hamilton Depression Scale (Ham-D)
- Inventory for Depressive Symptomatology (IDS)
- Manic-State Scale Montgomery-Asberg Depression Rating Scale (MADRS)
- Profile of Mood States (POMS)
- Raskin Depression Scale
- Young Mania Scale
- Zung Self-Rating Depression Scale (ZSRDS)

tion anxiety, grief, and mourning. Furthermore, this mourning in the early years often affects personality development and predisposes the child to psychiatric illness.

From a research point of view, the connection between early object loss and adult depression is complex. Some cast doubt on the universality of the responses described and suggest that appropriate mothering during the separation period can prevent their occurrence. Other studies indicate that depressed patients seem to experience more parental loss from death, separation, and other causes than do normal and other diagnostic groups. However, that factor alone does not seem to account for all forms of depression. There is even discussion about the beneficial or immunizing effects of having successfully coped with an early loss in the development of resilience.

Another perspective on this theory focuses on the negative impact of maternal depression on infants and children (Field, 1995). This is expressed by the infant as flat affect, lower activity, disengagement, and difficulty in being consoled. Among older children it is seen as sadness, submissive helplessness, and social withdrawal. Older children of depressed parents also have a three to four times higher than average rate of adjustment problems, including a range of emotional disorders. These observations lend a different but related view to the object loss theory. They suggest that emotional unavailability may be more stressful to children than physical separation. They also underscore the need for early and aggressive intervention by nurses for parents suffering from depression (Ferro et al, 2000; Wickramaratne & Weissman, 1998).

Personality Organization Theory. This view of depression focuses on the major psychosocial variable of low self-esteem. The patient's self-concept is an underlying issue, whether expressed as dejection and depression or overcompensated with supreme competence, as displayed in manic and hypomanic episodes. Threats to self-esteem arise from poor role performance, perceived low-level everyday functioning, and the absence of a clear self-identity.

Three forms of personality organization that could lead to depression have been identified (Arieti & Bemporad, 1980). One, based on the "dominant other," occurs because the patient has relied on another for self-esteem. Satisfaction is experienced only through an intermediary. Clinging, passivity, manipulativeness, and avoidance of anger characterize the person with this type of depression. There is a noticeable lack of personal goals and a predominant focus on problems.

Another form of personality disorder results when a person realizes that a desired but unrealistic goal may never be accomplished. This is the "dominant goal" type of depression. This person is usually seclusive, arrogant, and often obsessive. The person sets unrealistic goals and evaluates them with an all-or-nothing standard. An inordinate amount of time is spent in wishful thinking and introverted searches for meaning.

The third type of depression is seen as a constant mode of feeling. These patients inhibit any form of gratification because of strongly held taboos. They experience emptiness, hypochondriasis, pettiness in interpersonal relationships, and a harsh critical attitude toward themselves and others.

This view of depression looks at patients' belief systems in relation to their experiences. Even in the absence of an apparent precipitating stressor, their depression appears to be preceded by a severe blow to their self-esteem. It emphasizes the crucial position of self-concept in adaptation or maladaptation and the importance of patients' appraisal of their life situations.

Cognitive Model. The cognitive model proposes that people experience depression because their thinking is disturbed (Beck et al, 1979). Depression is seen as a cognitive problem dominated by a person's negative evaluation of self, the world, and the future. It suggests that in the course of development certain experiences sensitize people and make them vulnerable to depression. Such people also acquire a tendency to make extreme, absolute judgments.

The depression-prone person, according to this theory, is likely to explain an adverse event as a personal shortcoming. For example, the deserted husband believes "She left me because I'm unlovable," instead of considering the other possible alternatives, such as personality incompatibility, the wife's own problems, or her change of feelings toward him. As he focuses on his personal deficiencies, they expand to the point where they completely dominate his self-concept. He can think of himself only in a negative way and is unable to acknowledge his other abilities, achievements, and attributes. This negative set is reinforced when he interprets ambiguous or neutral experiences as additional proof of his deficiencies. Comparisons with other people further lower his self-esteem, and thus every encounter with others becomes a negative experience. His self-criticisms increase as he views himself as deserving of blame.

Depressed patients become dominated by pessimism. Their predictions tend to be overgeneralized and extreme. Because they see the future as an extension of the present, they expect their failure to continue permanently. Thus pessimism dominates their activities, wishes, and expectations.

Depressed people are capable of logical self-evaluation when not in a depressed mood or when only mildly depressed. When depression does occur, after some precipitating life stressors, the negative cognitive set makes its appearance. As depression develops and increases, the negative thinking increasingly replaces objective thinking.

Although the onset of the depression may appear sudden, it develops over weeks, months, or even years as each experience is interpreted as further evidence of failure. As a result of this tunnel vision, depressed people become hypersensitive to experiences of loss and defeat and oblivious to experiences of success and pleasure. They have difficulty acknowledging anger because they think they are responsible for, and deserving of, insults from others and problems in living. Along with low self-esteem, they experience apathy and indifference. They are drawn to a state of inactivity and withdraw from life. They lack all spontaneous desire and wish only to remain passive. Because they expect failure, they lack the ordinary energy to make an effort.

Suicidal wishes can be viewed as an extreme expression of the desire to escape. Suicidal patients see their life as filled with suffering, with no chance of improvement. Given this negative set, suicide seems a rational solution. It promises to end their misery and relieve their families of a burden, and they begin to believe that everyone would be better off if they were dead. The more they consider the alternative of suicide, the more desirable it may seem, and as their life becomes more hopeless and painful, the desire to end it becomes stronger.

Naturalistic, clinical, and experimental studies have provided substantial support for this cognitive model of depression (see Citing the Evidence). There is also strong evidence of the efficacy of cognitive therapy as a treatment strategy for depressed patients (Gloaguen et al, 1998).

> *Relate the cognitive model of depression to the adage "mind over matter."*

Learned Helplessness-Hopelessness Model. Helplessness is a "belief that no one will do anything to aid you" and hopelessness is a belief that neither "you nor anyone else can do anything." This theory proposes that it is not trauma per se that produces depression, but the belief that one has no control over the important outcomes in life and therefore refrains from adaptive responses (Seligman, 1975). Learned helplessness is both a behavioral state and a personality trait of one who believes that control has been lost over the reinforcers in the environment. These negative expectations lead to hopelessness, passivity, and an inability to assert oneself.

People resistant to depression have high self-efficacy and have experienced mastery in life. Their childhood experiences proved that their actions were effective in producing gratification and removing annoyances. In contrast, those susceptible to depression have low self-efficacy and have had lives devoid of mastery. Their experiences proved that they were helpless to influence their sources of suffering and they did not develop coping responses against failure.

This model has been revised to include the hopelessness theory of depression (Abramson et al, 1989). It suggests that inferred negative consequences and negative characteristics about the self contribute to the formation of hopelessness and, in turn, the symptoms of hopelessness depression. Hopelessness theory thus is very similar to the cognitive model of depression.

Behavioral Model. The behavioral model views people as capable of exercising control over their own behavior (Lewinsohn et al, 1979). They do not merely react to external influences. They select, organize, and transform incoming stimuli. Thus people are not viewed as powerless objects controlled by their environments, but neither are they absolutely free to do whatever they choose. Rather, people and their environment affect each other.

The concept of reinforcement is crucial to this view of depression. Person-environment interactions with positive outcomes provide positive reinforcement. Such interactions strengthen the person's behavior. Little or no rewarding interaction with the environment causes the person to feel sad. Thus the key assumption in this model is that a low rate of positive reinforcement is the antecedent of depressive behaviors.

Two elements of this model are important. One is that the person may fail to provide appropriate responses to initiate positive reinforcement. The other is that the environment may fail to provide reinforcement and thus worsen the patient's condition. This occurs because depressed patients are often deficient in the social skills needed to interact effectively. In turn, other people find the behavior of depressed people distancing, negative, or offensive and often avoid them as much as possible.

Depression is likely to occur if certain positively reinforcing events are absent, particularly those that fall into the following categories:

- Positive sexual experiences
- Rewarding social interaction
- Enjoyable outdoor activities
- Solitude
- Competence experiences

These may be described as "being sexually attractive," "being with friends," "being relaxed," "doing my job well," and "doing things my own way." Depression also occurs in the presence of certain punishing events, particularly those that fall into three categories:

- Marital or interpersonal discord
- Work or school hassles
- Negative reactions from others

The behavioral model of depression emphasizes an active approach to the person and relies heavily on an interactional view of personality. Treatment is aimed at helping the person to increase the quantity and quality of positively reinforcing interactions and to decrease aversive interactions.

Citing the Evidence on

Cognitive Theory

BACKGROUND: This study tested Beck's cognitive theory in depressed inpatients, previously hospitalized and nonhospitalized outpatients, and undiagnosed adults.

RESULTS: Multiple regression indicated that negative views of self, world, and future explained a substantial part of psychosocial functioning in all four groups. In the three depressed groups, views of self and world had a greater impact on psychosocial functioning than did the view of the future.

IMPLICATIONS: Interventions to build self-esteem and enhance self-control may be most effective in improving psychosocial functioning of depressed adults. Because many depressed outpatients seek help from primary care providers, such interventions must be usable by primary care staff as well as mental health specialists.

Zauszniewski J, Rong J: Depressive cognitions and psychosocial functioning: a test of Beck's cognitive theory, *Arch Psychiatr Nurs* 8(6):286, 1999.

How many positive reinforcing events have you experienced this month? How many punishing events? Relate these to your overall mood.

Biological Model. The biological model explores chemical changes in the body during depressed states (see Chapter 6). Whether these chemical changes cause depression or are a result of depression is not yet understood. However, significant abnormalities can be seen in many body systems during a depressive illness. These include electrolyte disturbances, especially of sodium and potassium; neurophysiological alterations; dysfunction and faulty regulation of autonomic nervous system activity; adrenocortical, thyroid, and gonadal changes; and neurochemical alterations in the neurotransmitters, especially in the biogenic amines, which act as central nervous system and peripheral neurotransmitters. The biogenic amines include three catecholamines—dopamine, norepinephrine, and epinephrine—as well as serotonin and acetylcholine. Most researchers agree that no single biochemical model adequately explains the affective disorders.

Endocrine system. The possibility of hormonal causes of depression has been considered for many years. Some symptoms of depression that suggest endocrine changes are decreased appetite, weight loss, insomnia, diminished sex drive, gastrointestinal disorders, and variations of mood. New assay techniques have recently detected alterations of hormone activity concurrent with depression. Mood changes have also been observed with a variety of endocrine disorders, including Cushing's disease, hyperthyroidism, and estrogen therapy. Further support for this theory is evident in the high incidence of depression during the postpartum period, when hormonal levels change.

Current study of neuroendocrine factors in affective disorders emphasizes the disinhibition of the hypothalamic-pituitary-adrenal (HPA) axis and the hypothalamic-pituitary-thyroid (HPT) axis. Two tests based on the neuroendocrine theory and performed clinically may prove to be useful in diagnosing affective illnesses. The first is the corticotropin-releasing factor stimulation test, which evaluates the pituitary's ability to respond to corticotropin-releasing hormone (CRH) and secrete sufficient amounts of adrenal corticotropin hormone (ACTH) to induce normal adrenal activity. The second test is the thyroid-releasing hormone (TRH) infusion test, which differs from CRH infusion by assessing the pituitary's ability to secrete sufficient amounts of thyroid-stimulating hormones (TSH) to produce normal thyroid activity. These tests may be helpful in differentiating unipolar from bipolar depression and mania from schizophrenic psychosis.

Cortisol. Many depressed patients exhibit hypersecretion of cortisol; this has been used in the dexamethasone suppression test (DST) (dexamethasone is an exogenous steroid that suppresses the blood level of cortisol). The DST is based on the observation that, in patients with biological depression, late afternoon cortisol levels are not suppressed after a single dose of dexamethasone. However, many physical illnesses and some medications can interfere with the test results.

Neurotransmission. One of the dominant theories in the neurobiology of mood disorders is the **dysregulation hypothesis,** which proposes that there is a problem in several of the neurotransmitter systems. Some of them have received more attention than others. For example, there is substantial evidence for abnormal regulation of the serotonin (5HT) neurotransmitter system (Fig. 20-2). This dysregulation is in either the amount or the availability of 5HT, in the sensitivity of its receptors in relevant regions of the brain, and in its balance with other neurotransmitters and brain chemicals. Several areas of research support a role for serotonin in depression:

Behavior. 5HT has an important role in brain functions such as aggression, mood, anxiety, psychomotor activity, irritability, appetite, sexual activity, sleep/wakefulness, circadian and seasonal rhythms, neuroendocrine function, body temperature, cognitive function, and pain perception, processes that are abnormal in people with depression.

Biochemistry. Research has shown that there is decreased 5HT availability in patients with depression—too little 5HT, its precursor (tryptophan), or its major metabolite (5HIAA) in the cerebrospinal fluid or blood of people with depression and in the postmortem brains of depressed people who died of other causes and in people who committed suicide.

Neuroimaging. Multiple brain regions, all rich in 5HT pathways, show abnormalities in neuroimaging studies in depressed people. An example is the prefrontal cortex, which shows an abnormal slowing of activity (hypometabolism). It covers the frontal lobes, which have an important role in intellectual and emotional activities. Prefrontal cortex hypometabolism affects the function of many of the brain structures connected with it by way of the 5HT system. It is hypothesized that these interconnections facilitate the varied symptoms of depression (Table 20-5).

Neuroendocrine. 5HT has an important role in the secretion of growth hormone, prolactin, and cortisol, all of which are found to be abnormal in people with depression.

Treatment. Most clinically effective biological antidepressant agents, such as drugs and ECT, have been found to enhance the neurotransmission of 5HT, although the mechanisms of actions differ from each other.

Finally, there are several important implications of viewing depression as a brain-based illness of the prefrontal cortex:

- Cognitive and interpersonal therapies may be viewed as prefrontal rehabilitation because they substitute for, then gradually bring back on line, some of the behaviors and cognitions compromised by prefrontal cortex (PFC) hypoactivity.
- Viewing depression as a disease with identified regional brain dysfunction helps to destigmatize depression and reintegrate mood disorders into modern health care.
- Changes in brain metabolism identified by neuroimaging studies may help with understanding of how psychosocial stressors such as grief (a hyperactivity in the PFC) may evolve into the clinical syndrome of depression (a hypoactivity in the PFC).

Biological rhythms. Mood disorders are also typified by periodic variations in physiological and psychological functions (McEnany, 1996; Giles et al, 1998). Affective illnesses are usually recurrent, with episodes often occurring and remitting spontaneously. Two subtypes of mood disorders are specifically cyclical in nature: rapid cycling bipolar disorder and depressive disorder with seasonal patterns. In the first, cycles may be days, weeks, months, or years. In seasonal affective disorder (SAD), cycles occur annually in the same season each year, as people react to changes in environmental factors such as climate, latitude, or light.

People who are depressed or manic have certain characteristic changes in biological rhythms and related physiology. For instance, body temperature and certain hormones reach their peak earlier than normal; some depressed patients are more sensitive to the absence of sunlight than nondepressed people; and many depressed people experience

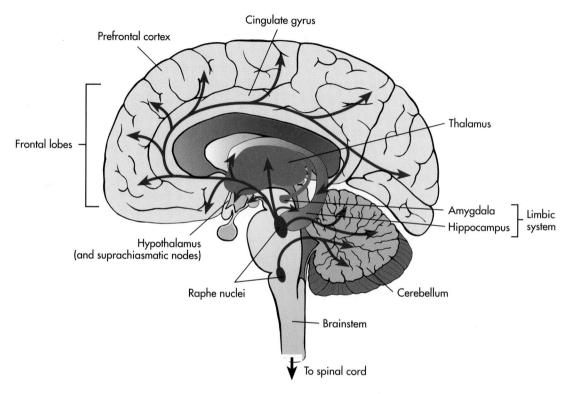

Fig. 20-2   The serotonin neurotransmitter system implicated in depression.

Table 20-5

Prefrontal Cortex and 5HT Interconnections: Implications in Depression	
Interconnected Brain Structures	**Hypothesized Role of These Interconnections in Depression**
Prefrontal cortex	Covering the frontal lobes, it is unique within the CNS for its strong interconnections with all other areas of the brain; it receives information that has already been processed by other sensory areas and then merges this information with other emotional, historical, or relevant information, thus attending to both feelings and intellect.
Limbic system structures	The prefrontal cortex modulates limbic system activities (emotional and instinctive) by way of these three structures:
Hippocampus	Major importance in cognitive function, including memory.
Amygdala	Major importance in modulating feelings such as aggression, anger, love, and shyness.
Cingulate gyrus	Involved in motivation and interest.
Brainstem	Responsible for regulating the general state of arousal and tone of brain function; also the location of structures that manufacture various neurotransmitters, such as serotonin (5HT), norepinephrine (NE), and dopamine (DA).
Raphe nuclei	Located in the brainstem, they manufacture 5HT; they also modulate excessive stimuli, and the organization and coordination of appropriate responses to these stimuli.
Hypothalamus	This interconnection allows for direct prefrontal input into neuroendocrine function via the hypothalamic-pituitary axes.
Suprachiasmatic nucleus	Located in the hypothalamus, it regulates circadian (24-hour) rhythms and circannual rhythms; thus it is also implicated in seasonal affective disorder.

circadian rhythm disturbances such as diurnal variation and early morning awakening. All-night sleep studies of depressed patients show some basic abnormalities. Sleep problems associated with depression have to do with the timing of rapid eye movement (REM) sleep. The strongest finding is that REM sleep begins too early in the night (Fig. 20-3). It also lasts too long—up to twice as long as the first REM period in nondepressed people. This finding may help to explain why patients report feeling tired even after a night's sleep. There is also decreased total sleep time, an increased percentage of dream time, difficulty in falling asleep, and an increased number of spontaneous awakenings. These and other findings in the area of biological rhythmicity may prove to be valuable diagnostic tools for depression.

Research on the biological model has been extensive and of high quality. It has lent support to a biological basis for mood disorders and suggested biological markers of clinical usefulness in diagnosis and treatment. The discovery of neurobiological abnormalities is not surprising and does not preclude psychological causes. Some of the biological bases of depression are shown in Fig. 20-4.

> *A pastor preaches about how depression results from "poor moral character" and "personal weakness." How would you respond?*

Precipitating Stressors

Disturbances of mood are a specific response to stress. Two major types of stress exist. The first is the stress of major life events that is evident to other people. The second type, the minor stress or irritations of daily life, may not be obvious to others. These are the small disappointments, frustrations, criticisms, and arguments that, when accumulated over time and in the absence of compensating positive events, have a major and chronic negative impact. Stressors that may produce disturbances of mood include loss of attachment, major life events, roles, and physiological changes.

Loss of Attachment. Loss in adult life can precipitate depression. The loss may be real or imagined and may include the loss of love, a person, physical functioning, status, or self-esteem. Many losses take on importance because of their symbolic meaning, which makes the reactions to them appear out of proportion to reality. In this sense, even an apparently pleasurable event, such as moving to a new home, may involve the loss of old friends, warm memories, and neighborhood associations. Loss of hope is another significant stressor often overlooked. Because of the actual and symbolic issues involved in loss, the patient's perception is of primary importance.

The intensity of grief becomes meaningful only when the person understands earlier losses and separations. People reacting to a recent loss often behave as they did in previous separations. The intensity of the present reaction therefore becomes more understandable with the realization that the reaction is to earlier losses as well. By definition loss is negative, a deprivation. The ability to sustain, integrate, and recover from loss is a sign of personal maturity and growth.

Uncomplicated grief reactions are the process of normal mourning or simple bereavement. Mourning includes a complex sequence of psychological processes. It is accompanied by anxiety, anger, pain, despair, and hope. The sequence is not a smooth, unvarying course. It is filled with turmoil, regressions, and potential problems (Kissane et al, 1996). Certain factors have been identified that influence the outcome of mourning (Box 20-3).

These factors should be assessed by the nurse for each person experiencing a loss. Two of the factors—the nature of the relationship with the lost person or object and the mourner's perception of the preventability of the loss—have been identified as prime predictors of the intensity and duration of the bereavement. Concurrent crises, the circumstances of the loss, and a pathological relationship with the lost person or object are other factors that contribute to a failure to resolve grief.

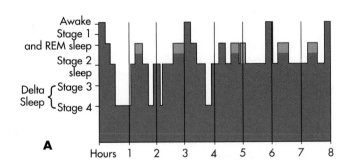

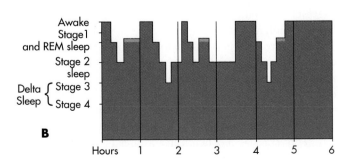

Fig. 20-3 A, Normal sleep architecture. **B,** Depressed sleep architecture. Green areas indicate REM sleep.

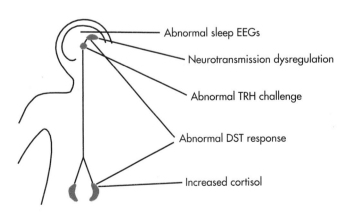

Fig. 20-4 Biological factors related to depression.

Box **20-3**

Factors That Influence the Mourning Process

- Childhood experiences, especially the loss of significant others
- Losses experienced later in life
- History of psychiatric illness, especially depression
- Life crises before the loss
- Nature of the relationship with the lost person or object, including kinship, strength of attachment, security of attachment, dependency bonds, and intensity of ambivalence
- Process of dying (when applicable), including age of deceased, timeliness, previous warnings, preparation for bereavement, expression of feelings, and preventability of the loss
- Social support systems
- Secondary stresses
- Emergent life opportunities

Inhibiting factors. Loss of a loved one is a major stressor for grief reactions. Most people resolve this loss through simple bereavement and do not experience pathological grief or depression. However, various external and internal factors can inhibit mourning. An external factor may be the immersion of the mourner in practical, necessary tasks that accompany the loss but are not directly connected to the emotional fact of the loss. These tasks may include funeral arrangements, unfinished business of the deceased, or a search for immediate employment. All these tasks foster denial of the loss. Denial also may be encouraged by cultural norms that minimize or negate the finality of the loss. The American norm of "courage in the face of adversity" can prevent an open display of grief.

Mourning may also be inhibited when the bereaved lack support from their social network. Nonsupportiveness suppresses grieving when significant others inhibit mourners' expression of sadness, anger, and guilt, block their review of the lost relationship, and attempt to orient them too quickly to the future. Finally, the widespread use of tranquilizers and antidepressant medications may suppress normal grief and encourage pathological reactions.

Internal factors that inhibit mourning are often fostered by a society that encourages the control and hiding of feelings. Crying, for example, may be seen as weakness, especially in men. Grief and anger are particularly repressed in our society, and this repression may create many emotional problems. Another inhibitor is the belief that the quantity and quality of emotion are unique and cannot be communicated.

Finally, some studies have failed to demonstrate a relationship between loss and depression. Other studies support the relationship but suggest that depression may be the cause of alienation and object loss, and not vice versa. Thus the following conclusions may be proposed:

- Loss and separation events are possible precipitating stressors of depression.
- Loss and separation are not present in all depressions.

- Not all people who experience loss and separation develop depressions.
- Loss and separation are not specific to depression but may act as precipitating events for a variety of psychiatric and medical illnesses.
- Loss and separation may result from depression.

Life Events. Research conducted on life events and depression reveals that, on average, depressed patients reported almost three times as many important life events during the 6 months before onset of clinical depressive episode as did normal subjects. The events included loss of self-esteem, interpersonal discord, socially undesirable occurrences, and major disruptions of life patterns. Events perceived as undesirable were most often the precipitants of depression. Analysis of the data showed that exit events (separations and losses) more often than entrance events (additions and introductions) were followed by worsening of psychiatric symptoms, physical health changes, impairment of social role performance, and depressive illnesses. The concept of exit events overlaps with the psychiatric concept of loss.

Certain types of events may also prove to be more important than others. For example, childhood physical and sexual abuse has been found to be associated with high depressive symptoms in women (Giese et al, 1998; Weiss et al, 1999). In addition, the presence of multiple family disadvantages, such as marital or family disruption, parental physical illness, poor physical care of child and home, social dependence, family overcrowding, and poor mothering in early life have been found to be associated with depression in adulthood (Sadowski et al, 1999). Research also suggests that while stressful life events do have a causal relationship with the onset of major depression, some of this effect may be because individuals predisposed to depression select themselves into high-risk environments (Kendler et al, 1999).

Thus any conclusions about life events should be made with caution. All people experience stressful life events, but not all people become depressed. This suggests that specific events can contribute only partially to the development of depression.

Role Strain. In analyzing social role stressors, much of the literature focuses on women. This reflects the predominance of depression among women and the increasing interest in gender socialization processes and women's changing roles. Role strain in marriage emerges as a major stressor related to depression for both men and women. Research also suggests that being married has a protective effect for males but a detrimental effect for females.

Another role-related risk factor for women is exposure to chronic stressors such as those experienced in their classic role as caregivers. These present specific psychosocial and biological challenges, including the following (Beeber, 1996):

- The perinatal period, with its subsequent sleep-disrupting infant care demands, which comes immediately after hormonal, biochemical, and social disruptions associated with pregnancy
- The predominantly female caretaking role for spouses and parents with age- or Alzheimer's-related dementias,

Table **20-6**

Physical Illnesses and Drugs Associated with Depressive and Manic States

	Depression	Mania
Infectious	Influenza	Influenza
	Viral hepatitis	St. Louis encephalitis
	Infectious mononucleosis	Q fever
	General paresis (tertiary syphilis)	General paresis (tertiary syphilis)
	Tuberculosis	
Endocrine	Myxedema	Hyperthyroidism
	Cushing's disease	
	Addison's disease	
	Diabetes mellitus	
Neoplastic	Occult abdominal malignancies (such as carcinoma of head of pancreas)	
	Carcinoid	
	Oat cell carcinoma	
Collagen	Systemic lupus erythematosus	Systemic lupus erythematosus
		Rheumatic chorea
Neurological	Multiple sclerosis	Multiple sclerosis
	Cerebral tumors	Diencephalic and third-ventricular tumors
	Sleep apnea	
	Dementia	
	Parkinson's disease	
	Nondominant temporal lobe lesions	
Cardiovascular	Stroke	
	Coronary artery disease	
Nutritional	Pellagra	
	Pernicious anemia	
Drugs	Steroidal contraceptives	Steroids
	Reserpine	Levodopa
	Alpha-methyldopa	Amphetamines
	Propranolol	Methylphenidate
	Glucocorticoids	Cocaine
	Cycloserine	Monoamine oxidase inhibitors
	Physostigmine	Tricyclic antidepressants
	Alcohol	Thyroid hormones
	Sedative-hypnotics	
	Amphetamine withdrawal	
	Benzodiazepines	
	Neuroleptics	

which can cause the same sleep disruption experienced by mothers of infants

- Achievement-motivated women who take needed time from sleep in order to juggle full-time family and social roles in addition to work and educational commitments
- Shift work that does not follow a forward rotation (days to evenings to nights) with adequate adjustment for each shift change

If these special stressors for women are combined with other rhythm-disrupting processes, such as seasonal light changes, and other risk factors for depression, such as family history and inadequate support systems and primary relationships, a woman has a gender- and role-based risk for depression.

Describe how the early socialization of young girls in contemporary society might affect their cognitive and emotional coping responses. Compare this to the experiences of young boys.

Physiological Changes. Mood may also respond to drugs or a wide variety of physical illnesses (Table 20-6). Drug-induced depressions can follow treatment with antihypertensive drugs, particularly reserpine, and the abuse of addictive substances such as amphetamines, barbiturates, cocaine, and alcohol. Depression may also occur secondary to medical illnesses, such as viral infections, nutritional deficiencies, endocrine disorders, anemias, and central nervous system disorders such as multiple sclerosis, tumors, and cerebrovascular disease (Faller et al, 1999; Wulsin et al, 1999). Most chronic debilitating illnesses, whether physical or psychiatric, are accompanied by depression.

The depressions of the elderly are particularly complex because the differential diagnosis often involves organic brain damage and clinical depression. Diagnostic differentiation is complicated. People with early signs of senile brain changes, vascular disease, or other neurological diseases of aging may be more at risk for depression than the general population (Roberts et al, 1997). In the United States there has been a tendency to overdiagnose arteriosclerosis and senility in people over age 65, without recognizing that depression may manifest itself by a slowing of psychomotor activity. Lowered intellectual function and a loss of interest in sex, hobbies, and activities may be taken as signs of brain disease.

Mania can also be secondary to drugs, particularly steroids, amphetamines, and tricyclic antidepressants. It can be triggered by infections, neoplasms, and metabolic disturbances. The evidence that mania can result from pharmacological, structural, and metabolic disturbances suggests that mania, like depression, is a clinical syndrome with multiple causes. The diversity of causes probably involves more than one pathophysiological pathway and challenges any one model of causation, whether biochemical, psychological, genetic, or structural.

Appraisal of Stressors

Debate continues over the nature of depression, that is, whether depression is a single illness with different signs and symptoms or whether several diseases exist. It is clear, however, that there is an interactive effect among predisposing and precipitating factors that are biological and psychosocial in origin. This underscores the importance of one's appraisal of one's life situation and related stressors. Table 20-7 summarizes these major theories of causation.

Coping Resources

Personal resources include one's socioeconomic status (income, occupation, social position, education), family (nuclear, extended), social support networks, and secondary organizations provided by the broader social environment (see A Family Speaks). The far-ranging effects of poverty, discrimination, inadequate housing, and social isolation cannot be ignored or taken lightly. Thus nursing interventions that foster the person's ability to develop capacities for coping with life's disruptions are very important (Berlanga et al, 1999). The risk factors for depression are listed in Box 20-4.

Coping Mechanisms

Uncomplicated grief reactions can be normal mourning or simple bereavement. Mourning includes all the psychological processes set in motion by the loss. Mourning begins with the introjection of the lost object. In grieving the person's feelings are directed to a mental image of the loved one. Thus the mechanism of introjection serves as a buffering mechanism. Through reality testing the person realizes that the love object no longer exists, and then the emotional investment is withdrawn from it. The ultimate outcome is that reality wins out, but this is accomplished slowly over time. When the mourning work is completed, the ego becomes free to invest in new objects.

A Family Speaks

It's hard for me to imagine how life could be so bad that my beautiful and loving 22-year-old daughter couldn't get out of bed in the morning and cried most of the day. It all started when she quit college and returned home and told us about the biggest mistake she had made in her life. While at school, she accidentally got pregnant and then had an abortion. Since that event, she said she felt worthless, immoral, and extremely guilty.

We talked about it, and I suggested that she get help. She saw two different mental health professionals but dropped out of therapy with each one after only a couple of visits. Then one of my friends recommended a nurse who specialized in working with women with depression. My daughter saw her twice a week initially, then once a week, and finally monthly. My daughter was able to open up to this nurse and together they worked at changing my daughter's negative thoughts, feelings, and behaviors. She kept a diary and began to call friends and socialize.

Today, 8 months later, my daughter has a job and is going to college part-time in the evenings. Sometimes when I look at her, she seems like a different person to me—so much more grown up and mature. I'm sorry for her pain, but I know that now she is a stronger and wiser person for having endured it.

Table **20-7**

Summary of Models of Causation of Severe Mood Disturbances	
Model	**Mechanism**
Genetic	Transmission through hereditary and family history
Aggression turned inward	Turning of angry feelings against oneself
Object loss	Separation from loved one and disruption of attachment bond
Personality organization	Negative self-concept and low self-esteem influence belief system and appraisal of stressors
Cognitive	Hopelessness experienced because of negative cognitive set
Learned helplessness-hopelessness	Belief that responses are ineffectual and that reinforcers in the environment cannot be controlled
Behavioral	Loss of positive reinforcement in life
Biological	Impaired monoaminergic neurotransmission
Life stressors	Response to life stress from four possible sources: loss of attachment, life events, role strain, and physiological changes
Integrative	Interaction of biopsychosocial predisposing and precipitating factors

A delayed grief reaction uses the defense mechanisms of denial and suppression in an attempt to avoid intense distress. Specific defenses used to block mourning are repression, suppression, denial, and dissociation. Denial of the loss in depression results in profound feelings of guilt, anger, and despair that focus on the person's own unworthiness. Manic and hypomanic episodes are more rare than depressive states. Some believe that mania is a mirror image of depression and that, even though the behaviors are dissimilar, the dynamics and coping mechanisms are related. According to this view, manic behavior is a defense against depression because the person attempts to deny feelings of worthlessness and helplessness.

NURSING DIAGNOSIS

The diagnosis of mood disturbances depends on an understanding of many interrelated concepts, including anxiety and self-concept. One task of the nurse in formulating a diagnosis is to determine whether the patient is experiencing primarily a state of anxiety or depression. It is often difficult to distinguish between the two because they may co-exist in one patient and are manifested by similar behaviors. A table distinguishing between anxiety and depression is presented in Chapter 17.

Fig. 20-5 presents the Stuart Stress Adaptation Model with the continuum of emotional responses. The maladaptive responses are a result of anxiety, hostility, self-devaluation, and guilt. This model suggests that nursing care should be centered around increasing self-esteem and encouraging expression of emotions.

The primary NANDA nursing diagnoses related to maladaptive emotional responses are **dysfunctional grieving, hopelessness, powerlessness, spiritual distress,** and **risk for self-directed violence.** Nursing diagnoses related to the

Box 20-4

Risk Factors for Depression

- Prior episodes of depression
- Family history of depression
- Prior suicide attempts
- Female gender
- Age of onset less than 40 years
- Postpartum period
- Medical comorbidity
- Lack of social support
- Stressful life events
- Personal history of sexual abuse
- Current substance abuse

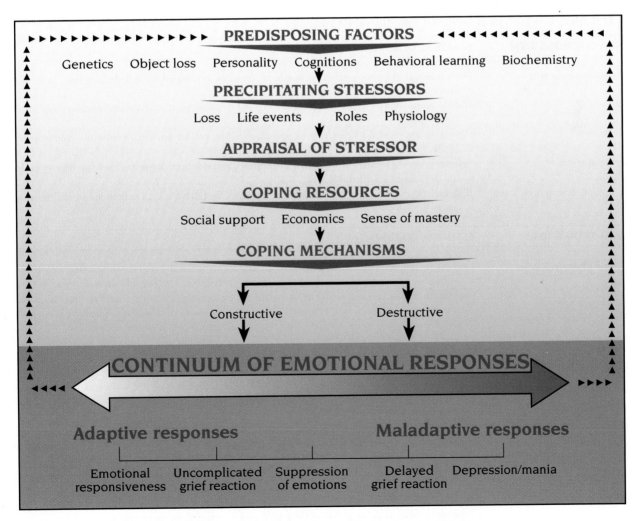

Fig. 20-5   The Stuart Stress Adaptation Model related to emotional responses.

Medical and Nursing Diagnoses *related to* **Emotional Responses**

RELATED MEDICAL DIAGNOSES (*DSM–IV–TR*)*	RELATED NURSING DIAGNOSES (NANDA)†
Bipolar I disorder	Anxiety
Bipolar II disorder	Communication, impaired verbal
Cyclothymic disorder	Coping, ineffective individual
Major depressive disorder	Grieving, anticipatory
Dysthymic disorder	**Grieving, dysfunctional‡**
	Hopelessness‡
	Injury, risk for
	Loneliness, risk for
	Memory, impaired
	Nutrition, altered
	Powerlessness‡
	Self-care deficit
	Self-esteem disturbance
	Sexual dysfunction
	Sleep pattern disturbance
	Social isolation
	Spiritual distress (distress of the human spirit)‡
	Thought processes, altered
	Violence, risk for self-directed‡

*Reprinted with permission from the *Diagnostic and statistical manual of mental disorders*, Fourth Edition, Text Revision. Copyright 2000. American Psychiatric Association.
†From North American Nursing Diagnosis Association: *NANDA nursing diagnoses: definitions and classifications 1999-2000*, Philadelphia, 1999, The Association.
‡Primary nursing diagnosis for disturbances in mood.

 Detailed Diagnoses *related to* **Emotional Responses**

NANDA DIAGNOSIS STEM	EXAMPLES OF COMPLETE DIAGNOSIS
Dysfunctional grieving	Dysfunctional grieving related to death of sister, as evidenced by self-devaluation, sleep disturbance, and dejected mood
Hopelessness	Hopelessness related to loss of job, as evidenced by feelings of despair and development of ulcerative colitis
Powerlessness	Powerlessness related to new role as parent, as evidenced by apathy, uncertainty, and overdependency
Spiritual distress	Spiritual distress related to loss of child in utero, as evidenced by self-blame, somatic complaints, and pessimism about the future
Risk for self-directed violence	Risk for self-directed violence related to rejection by boyfriend, as evidenced by self-destructive acts

DSM-IV–TR DIAGNOSIS	ESSENTIAL FEATURES*
Bipolar I disorder	Current or past experience of a manic episode, lasting at least 1 week, when one's mood was abnormally and persistently elevated, expansive, or irritable. The episode is severe enough to cause extreme impairment in social or occupational functioning. Bipolar disorders may be classified as manic (limited to manic episodes), depressed (a history of manic episodes with a current depressive episode), or mixed (presentation of both manic and depressive episodes).
Bipolar II disorder	Presence or history of one or more major depressive episodes and at least one hypomanic episode. There has never been a manic episode.
Cyclothymic disorder	A history of 2 years of hypomania in which the person experienced numerous periods with abnormally elevated, expansive, or irritable moods. These moods did not meet the criteria for a manic episode, and many periods of depressed mood did not meet the criteria of a major depressive episode.
Major depressive disorder	Presence of at least five symptoms during the same 2-week period, with one being either depressed mood or loss of interest or pleasure. Other symptoms might include weight loss, insomnia, psychomotor agitation or retardation, fatigue, feelings of worthlessness, diminished ability to think, and recurrent thoughts of death. Major depressions may be classified as single episode or recurrent.
Dysthymic disorder	At least 2 years of a usually depressed mood and at least one of the symptoms mentioned for major depression without meeting the criteria for a major depressive episode.

*Reprinted with permission from the *Diagnostic and statistical manual of mental disorders*, Fourth Edition, Text Revision. Copyright 2000. American Psychiatric Association.

range of possible maladaptive responses are identified in the Medical and Nursing Diagnoses box on p. 362. Examples of complete nursing diagnoses are presented in the Detailed Diagnoses box on p. 362.

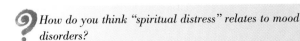 *How do you think "spiritual distress" relates to mood disorders?*

Related Medical Diagnoses

The psychiatric classification of affective disorders has largely reflected the controversies surrounding the nature, cause, and treatment of these disorders. Although these traditional labels are no longer used in the *DSM–IV–TR,* nurses know them because they may continue to have some research and clinical value.

One traditional distinction has been to separate patients into those with **psychotic versus neurotic affective states.** Unfortunately, these terms have acquired multiple meanings and have lost their precision in defining clinical or research practice. Another traditional distinction has been **endogenous versus reactive,** or **exogenous,** types of depression. Endogenous depressions were believed to have resulted from early personality development and intrinsic biological processes, whereas exogenous or reactive types were believed to have occurred in response to external environmental stress, such as recent loss or disappointment. However, research has failed to verify these distinctions. Thus the psychotic-neurotic distinction and the endogenous-reactive dichotomy are better regarded as continuums along which patients may be placed. Most patients are intermediate on the continuum and few are at the extremes. Neither classification is used in the *DSM–IV–TR.*

Another distinction has been made between **primary** and **secondary affective disorders.** Primary affective disorders occur in patients who have been well or whose only previous episodes of psychiatric disease were mania or depression. Secondary affective disorders include feelings of sadness, inadequacy, and hopelessness that occur with another preexisting psychiatric disorder, such as anxiety reactions. They also include symptoms secondary to medical illnesses.

A final distinction is between bipolar and unipolar affective states. It proposes the separation of depressed patients with a history of manic episodes (the bipolar group) from those who have had only recurrent episodes of depression (the unipolar group).

Two major categories of mood or affective disorders are identified in the *DSM–IV–TR:* bipolar disorders and depressive disorders (see the Medical and Nursing Diagnoses box on p. 362. The specific disorders are described in the Detailed Diagnoses box on p. 362. Diagnostic criteria for a major depressive episode and a manic episode are listed in Box 20-5.

OUTCOME IDENTIFICATION

The expected outcome when working with a patient with a maladaptive emotional response is as follows:

The patient will be emotionally responsive and return to a pre-illness level of functioning.

Box 20-5

Diagnostic Criteria for Major Depressive and Manic Episodes

MAJOR DEPRESSIVE EPISODE

At least five of the following (including one of the first two) must be present most of the day, nearly daily, for at least 2 weeks:
Depressed mood
Loss of interest or pleasure
Weight loss or gain
Insomnia or hypersomnia
Psychomotor agitation or retardation
Fatigue or loss of energy
Feelings of worthlessness
Impaired concentration
Thoughts of death or suicide

MANIC EPISODE

At least three of the following must be present to a significant degree for at least 1 week:
Grandiosity
Decreased need for sleep
Pressured speech
Flight of ideas
Distractibility
Psychomotor agitation
Excessive involvement in pleasurable activities without regard for negative consequences

---

Goals of nursing care for patients with severe mood disturbance have the following aims:

- To allow recognition and continuous expression of feelings, including denial, hopelessness, anger, guilt, blame, helplessness, regret, hope, and relief, within a supportive therapeutic atmosphere
- To allow for gradual analysis of stressors while strengthening the patient's self-esteem
- To increase the patient's sense of identity, control, awareness of choices, and responsibility for behavior
- To encourage healthy interpersonal ties with others
- To promote understanding of maladaptive emotions and to acquire adaptive coping responses to stressors

Specific short-term goals should be generated from behaviors of the patient, present areas of difficulty, and relevant stressors. Goal setting should involve a holistic view of the patient and the patient's world. Goals probably will need to be developed regarding the patient's self-concept, physical status, behavioral performance, expression of emotions, and relationships. All these areas can directly relate to the mood disturbance. The patient's participation in setting these goals can be a significant first step in regaining mastery over his or her life.

PLANNING

In planning care the nurse's priorities are the reduction and ultimate removal of the patient's maladaptive emotional responses, restoration of the patient's occupational and psychosocial functioning, improvement in the patient's quality of life, and minimization of the likelihood of relapse and re-

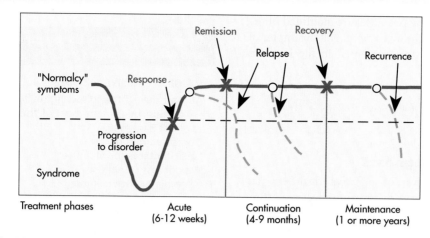

Fig. 20-6 The phases of treatment for mood disorders. (From Kupfer DJ: Long-term treatment of depression, *J Clin Psychiatry* 52[suppl]:28, 1991.)

currence. Treatment consists of three phases: acute, continuation, and maintenance (Fig. 20-6).

Acute Treatment Phase

The goal of acute treatment is to eliminate the symptoms. If patients improve with treatment, they are said to have had a therapeutic response. A successful acute treatment brings patients back to an essentially symptom-free state and to a level of functioning comparable to that before the illness. This phase usually lasts 6 to 12 weeks, and if patients are symptom-free at the end of that time, they are then in remission.

Continuation Treatment Phase

The goal of continuation treatment is to prevent relapse, which is the return of symptoms, and to promote recovery. The risk of relapse is very high in the first 4 to 6 months after remission, and one of the greatest mistakes in the treatment of mood disorders is the failure to continue a successful treatment for a long enough time. This phase usually lasts 4 to 9 months.

Maintenance Treatment Phase

The goal of maintenance treatment is to prevent recurrence, or a new episode of illness. This concept is commonly accepted for bipolar illness, but it is now seen as important for major depressive disorder as well. Studies point out the effectiveness of both pharmacological and cognitive behavioral maintenance therapy in preventing new episodes or lengthening the interval between them. In the maintenance phase, patients may be on medication indefinitely.

Understanding the phases of treatment for mood disorders is critically important. The nurse should discuss them with the patient and family so that they may join in the therapeutic alliance and have clear expectations about the goals and course of treatment.

> *Your patient tells you she stopped taking her medicine after 2 months because she was feeling better. What would you tell her, based on your understanding of the treatment phases of depression?*

IMPLEMENTATION

Maladaptive emotional responses may emerge at unpredicted moments, can vary in intensity from mild to severe, and can be transitory, recurrent, or stable conditions. Episodes of depression and mania can occur in any setting and can arise in conjunction with existing medical problems. Also, the treatment of mood disturbances can take place in various settings: at home, at an outpatient department, or in a hospital. The best treatment setting for the patient depends on the severity of the illness, available support systems, and resources of the treatment center. In timing intervention, remember that help given when maladaptive patterns are developing is likely to be more acceptable and effective than help given after these patterns have been established. Thus early diagnosis and treatment are associated with more positive outcomes.

Empirically validated treatments for major depressive disorder and bipolar disorder are summarized in Table 20-8. Research has also found that the nature of the therapeutic alliance is an important factor with significant impact on treatment outcome in depression (Zuroff et al, 2000).

The nursing interventions described for severe mood disturbances are based on a multicausal, integrative model of affective disorders. Such a model dismisses the notion of one cause or one cure. Rather, it proposes that affective problems have many causes and dimensions that affect all aspects of a person's life. Thus a single approach to nursing care would be inadequate. Nursing interventions must instead reflect the complex nature of the model and address all maladaptive aspects of a person's life. Intervening in as many areas as possible should have the maximum effect in modifying maladaptive responses and alleviating severe mood disturbances. The ultimate aim of these nursing interventions is to teach the patient coping responses and increase the satisfaction gained from interaction with the world.

Environmental Interventions

Environmental interventions are useful when the patient's environment is highly dangerous, impoverished, aversive,

Table **20-8**

Summarizing the Evidence on Treatments That Work for Mood Disorders

DISORDER: Major depressive disorder (MDD)

TREATMENT:
- Tricyclic antidepressants (TCAs), the first antidepressants to be studied extensively, were consistently more efficacious than placebo both in reducing the complex of symptoms of MDD and in managing the disorder over the long term
- Because of their narrow safety margin and significant drug-induced adverse side effects, TCAs have now been largely replaced for the treatment of MDD by selective serotonin reuptake inhibitors (SSRIs), including fluoxetine, setraline, and paroxetine and the new compounds, venlafaxine, bupropion, and nefazodone
- Because of adverse side effects, monoamine oxidase inhibitors (MAOIs) are generally reserved for treatment-refractory MDD patients
- Interventions utilizing behavior therapy, cognitive-behavior therapy, and interpersonal therapy have all yielded substantial reductions in scores on the two major depression rating scales, as well as in the percentage of patients meeting MDD criteria after treatment; all three treatments have also shown significant maintenance of effect after treatment

DISORDER: Bipolar disorder

TREATMENT:
- While pharmacological interventions are treatments of choice, psychosocial treatments, including psychoeducation and cognitive-behavior therapy for medication and adherence, have also shown promise
- Lithium reduced the symptoms of acute mania in bipolar I disorder
- Valproate has shown effectiveness in reducing the symptoms of acute mania in bipolar I disorder
- Carbamazepine has demonstrated effectiveness in treating the symptoms of acute mania
- Lithium has been effective with a substantial percentage of bipolar patients (e.g., 35% to 50%) in preventing or reducing the frequency of recurrent affective episodes; however, side effects have interfered with drug compliance
- Lithium and several antidepressants have also shown moderate effectiveness with acute and chronic bipolar depression

From Nathan P, Gorman J: *A guide to treatments that work*, New York, Oxford University Press.

or lacking in personal resources. In caring for the patient with a severe mood disorder, highest priority should be given to the potential for suicide. Hospitalization is definitely indicated when there is suicidal risk. In the presence of rapidly progressing symptoms and in the absence of support systems, hospitalization is strongly indicated. Nursing care in this case means protecting patients and assuring them that they will not be allowed to harm themselves. Specific interventions for suicidal patients are described in Chapter 21.

Depressed patients must always be assessed for possible suicide. They are at particular risk when they appear to be coming out of their depression because they may then have the energy and opportunity to kill themselves. Acute manic states are also life threatening. These patients show poor judgment, excessive risk taking, and an inability to evaluate realistic danger and the consequences of their actions. In an acute manic episode, immediate measures must be instituted to prevent death.

Another environmental intervention involves changing the physical or social setting by helping the patient to move to a new environment. Sometimes a change in the general pattern of living is indicated, such as a leave of absence from work, a different job, a new peer group, or leaving a family setting. Changes such as these decrease the immediate stress and mobilize additional support.

Nurse-Patient Relationship

Depressed Patients. Depressed patients resist involvement through withdrawal and nonresponsiveness. Because of their negative views, they tend to remain isolated, verbalize little, think that they are unworthy of help, and form dependent attachments.

In working with depressed patients, the nurse's approach should be quiet, warm, and accepting. The nurse should demonstrate honesty, empathy, and compassion. Admittedly, it is not always easy to give warm, personal care to a person who is unresponsive and detached. The nurse may feel angry, resent the patient's helplessness, or fear rejection. Patience and a belief in the potential of each person to grow and change are needed. If this is calmly communicated, both verbally and nonverbally, in time the patient may begin to respond.

Nurses should avoid assuming an overaggressive or lighthearted approach with the depressed person. Comments such as "You have so much to live for," "Cheer up—things are sure to get better," or "You shouldn't feel so depressed" convey little understanding of and respect for the patient's feelings. They will create more distance and block the formation of a relationship. Also, nurses should not sympathize with the patient. Subjective overidentification by nurses can cause them to experience similar feelings of hopelessness and helplessness and can seriously limit therapy.

Rapport is best established with the depressed patient through shared time, even if the patient talks little, and through supportive companionship. The very presence of the nurse indicates belief that the patient is a valuable person. The nurse should adjust to the depressed patient's pace by speaking more slowly and allowing more time to respond. The patient should be addressed by name, talked with, and listened to. By studying the patient's life and interests, the nurse might select topics that lay the foundation for more meaningful discussions.

Manic Patients. In contrast, elated patients may be very talkative and need simple explanations and concise, truthful answers to questions. Although manic patients may appear willing to talk, they resist involvement through manipulation, testing limits, and superficiality. Their hyperactivity, short attention span, flight of ideas, poor judgment, lack of insight, and rapid mood swings all present special problems to the nursing staff.

Manic patients can be very disruptive to a unit and resist engagement in therapy. They may dominate group meetings or therapy sessions by their excessive talking and manipulate staff or patient groups. By identifying a vulnerable area in another person or a group's area of conflict, manic patients are able to exploit others. This provokes defensive and angry responses. Nurses are particularly susceptible to these feelings because they often have the most contact with patients and the responsibility for maintaining the psychiatric unit. When anger is generated, therapeutic care breaks down. Thus the maneuvers of manic patients act as diversionary tactics. By alienating themselves, patients can avoid exploring their own problems.

It is important for nurses to understand how manic patients are able to manipulate others and their reasons for doing so. The treatment plan for these patients should be thorough, well coordinated, and consistently implemented. Constructive limit setting on manic patients' behavior is an essential part of the plan. The entire treatment team must be consistent in their expectations of these patients, and progressive limits must be set as situations arise. Other patients may also be encouraged to carry out the agreed limits. Pressure applied by peers can sometimes be more effective than pressure applied by the staff. Frequent staff meetings are recommended to improve communication, share in understanding the manic patient's behavior, and ensure steady progress.

One goal of nursing care is to increase the patient's self-control, and this should be kept in mind when setting limits. Patients need to see that they can monitor their own behavior and that the staff is there to help them. Also, the nurse should point out that there are many positive aspects to their behavior. The ability to be outgoing, expressive, and energetic is a coping strength that can be maximized.

Physiological Treatments

Physiological treatments include physical care, psychopharmacology, and somatic therapies. They begin with a thorough physical examination and health history to identify

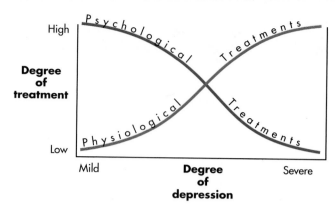

Fig. 20-7   Treatment indications for depression.

health problems and current treatments or medications that may be affecting the patient's mood. The indications for physiological treatment include symptoms that will respond to physiological measures, greater severity of illness, suicidal potential, and need for speed in recovery (Fig. 20-7).

Depressed Patients. In depression, physical well-being may be forgotten or the patient may not be capable of self-care. The more severe the depression, the more important is the physical care. For example, the nurse may need to monitor the diet of a patient who has no appetite and has lost weight. Staying with the patient during meals, arranging for preferred foods, and encouraging frequent small meals may be helpful. Recording intake and output and weighing the patient daily will help evaluate this need.

Sleep disturbances typically occur. It is best to plan activities according to each patient's energy levels; some feel best in the morning and others in the evening. A scheduled rest period may be helpful, but patients should not be encouraged to take frequent naps or remain in bed all day. Patients with depression experience less stage III and IV sleep, and because these stages depend on the period of wakefulness, napping may worsen sleep disturbances. For many patients, eating regularly, staying active during waking hours, and cutting back on caffeine (especially late in the day) may promote more normal sleep patterns.

The patient's appearance may be neglected and all movements slowed. Nurses may have to help with bathing or dressing. They should do this matter-of-factly, explaining that help is being offered because the patient is unable to do it independently right now. Cleanliness and interest in appearance can be noticed and praised. Nurses must allow patients to help themselves whenever possible. Often nurses might rush the patient or do a task themselves to save time, but this does not facilitate the patient's recovery and should be avoided.

Psychopharmacology. Antidepressant medications are often administered to elevate the mood of the depressed patient. They are particularly indicated in severe and recurrent depression. Many antidepressant medications are available on the market (Table 20-9) and new ones can be expected to be released each year. These drugs are equally effective in treating depression and their overall success rate is 60% to

Table **20-9**

Antidepressant Drugs

	Usual Adult Dose (mg/day)	Preparations
SELECTIVE SEROTONIN REUPTAKE INHIBITORS (SSRI)		
Citalopram (Celexa)	20-50	PO
Fluoxetine (Prozac)	20-80	PO
Fluvoxamine (Luvox)	50-300	PO
Paroxetine (Paxil)	20-50	PO
Sertraline (Zoloft)	25-200	PO
OTHER ANTIDEPRESSANT DRUGS		
Amoxapine (Asendin)	200-300	PO
Bupropion (Wellbutrin)	150-450*	PO and SR
Maprotiline (Ludiomil)	50-200*	PO
Mirtazapine (Remeron)	15-45	PO
Trazodone (Desyrel)	50-600	PO
Serotonin Antagonist and Reuptake Blocker (SARI)		
Nefazodone (Serzone)	200-600	PO
Serontonin-Norepinephrine Reuptake Inhibitor (SNRI)		
Venlafaxine (Effexor)	25-375	PO
Selective Presynaptic Noradrenergic Reuptake Inhibitor (SPNRI)		
Reboxetine (Vestra)	4-10	PO
TRICYCLIC DRUGS (TCA)		
Tertiary (parent)		
Amitriptyline (Elavil)	50-300	PO, IM
Clomipramine (Anafranil)	50-250	PO
Doxepin (Adapin, Sinequan)	50-300	PO, L
Imipramine (Tofranil)	50-300	PO, IM
Trimipramine (Surmontil)	50-300	PO
Secondary (metabolite)		
Desipramine (Norpramin)	50-300	PO
Nortriptyline (Pamelor)	50-150	PO, L
Protriptyline (Vivactil)	30-60	PO
MONOAMINE OXIDASE INHIBITORS (MAOI)		
Isocarboxazid (Marplan)	20-60	PO
Phenelzine (Nardil)	45-90	PO
Tranylcypromine (Parnate)	20-60	PO

*Antidepressants with a ceiling dose because of dose-related seizures.
IM, Intramuscular; *L*, oral liquid; *PO*, oral tablet/capsule, *SR*, oral slow-release tablets.

80% (AHCPR, 1999). Fig. 20-8 presents a medication algorithm for treating nonpsychotic major depression.

Despite their success, antidepressant drugs have limitations. Their therapeutic effects usually begin only after 2 to 6 weeks, and they have side effects that can deter some patients from maintenance. Thus patient education is essential. Another major problem with some antidepressant medications is their toxicity. Tricyclics are lethal at high doses, which makes them particularly dangerous for people most in need of them: suicidal patients. In addition, antidepressant medications do not help everyone, and it is difficult to predict who will respond to which drug. Fortunately, those who do not benefit from one drug often do well when switched to another, as seen in the medication algorithm.

What would you say to a patient who tells you that she doesn't want to take medicines for her depression because they are addictive?

Somatic therapies. Electroconvulsive therapy (ECT) is also used with depressed patients, particularly those with recurrent depressions and those resistant to drug therapy. ECT is regarded by many as a specific therapy for patients with severe depressions characterized by somatic delusions and delusional guilt, accompanied by a lack of interest in the world, suicidal ideation, and weight loss.

Sleep deprivation therapy may also be effective in treating depression. Research indicates that depriving some depressed patients of a night's sleep will improve their clinical

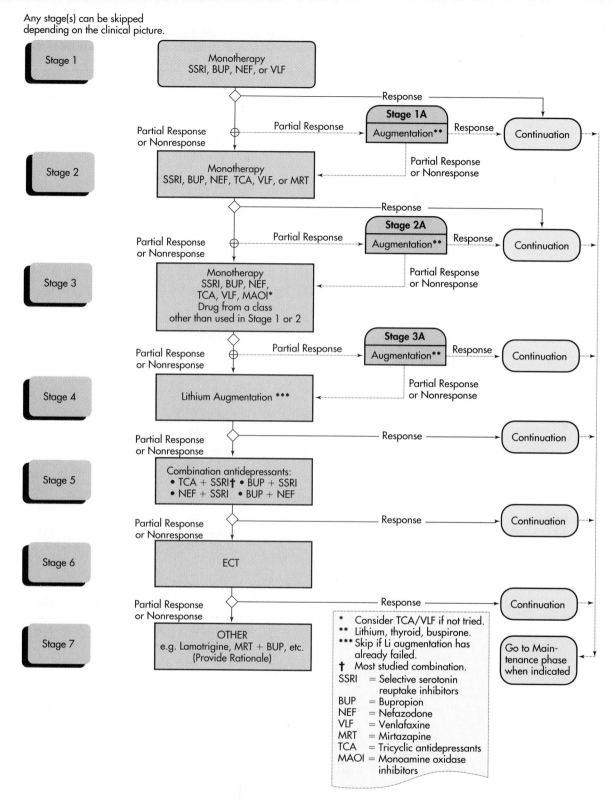

Fig. 20-8 Medication algorithm for treating nonpsychotic major depression. (From Texas Medication Algorithm Project, Depression Module, 1998.)

condition. How sleep deprivation works is not known, and the duration of improvement varies.

Another physiological treatment is that of phototherapy, or light therapy, in which patients are exposed to bright artificial light for a specified amount of time each day. Phototherapy appears to be effective in the short-term treatment of patients with mild to moderate seasonal affective disorder

(SAD). Finally, two new treatments still being researched are transcranial magnetic stimulation (TMS) and vagal nerve stimulation (VNS). These and all of the other somatic therapies are described in detail in Chapter 29.

Manic Patients. Manic patients primarily need protection from themselves. They may be too busy to eat or take care of themselves. Eating problems can be handled in the same

Table **20-10**

Mood-Stabilizing Drugs

Generic (Trade Name)	Usual Adult Dose (mg/day)	Preparations
Lithium (Eskalith, Lithobid, Lithonate)	600-2400	PO, L, SR
Valproic acid (Valproate, Depakote, Divalproex)	750 mg/day +	PO, L
Carbamazepine (Tegretol)	200-1600	PO, Ch
Lamotrigine (Lamictal)	12.5-150+	PO
Gabapentin (Neurontin)	300-1800+	PO
Topiramate (Topamax)	25-200+	PO
Olanzapine (Zyprexa)	10-15	PO

Ch, Chewable tablets; *L*, liquid; *PO*, oral tablet/capsule; *SR*, oral slow-release tablets.

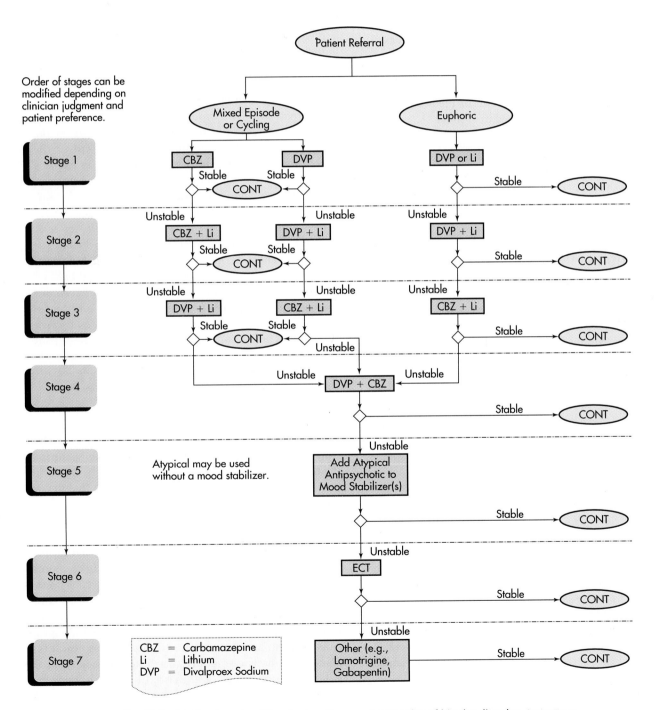

Fig. 20-9 Medication algorithm for treating manic episodes of bipolar disorder. (From Texas Medication Algorithm Project, Bipolar Disorders Module, 1999.)

way as with depressed patients. Manic patients may sleep very little, so rest periods should be encouraged, along with baths, soft music, and whirlpools. These patients may also need help in selecting clothes and maintaining hygiene. Setting limits and using firm actions are effective in physical care.

Psychopharmacology. For many years lithium was considered the drug of choice in the treatment of mania (Friedrich, 1999). Care must be taken regarding the narrow therapeutic index of this drug, which requires frequent blood levels and careful patient monitoring. The anticonvulsants valproate and carbamazepine have added to the treatment alternatives. Most recently, an atypical antipsychotic medication, olanzapine (Zyprexa) was approved for the short-term treatment of acute manic episodes in bipolar disorder (Table 20-10). The overall success rate of these drugs when used to treat bipolar illness is 80%. A medication algorithm for treating manic episodes of bipolar disorder is presented in Fig. 20-9.

Other drugs to treat this illness are being investigated, including substance P blockers that show potential promise in regulating mood. A detailed discussion of medications related to mood disorders is presented in Chapter 28.

> *Your patient with bipolar disorder tells you that she has stopped taking her medication because she misses the highs that she used to feel and the extra energy she used to have. What would your educational approach be to help her comply with treatment?*

Expressing Feelings

Affective interventions are necessary because patients with mood disturbances have difficulty identifying, expressing, and modulating feelings. Feelings that are particularly problematic are hopelessness, sadness, anger, guilt, and anxiety. A range of interventions is available to the nurse in meeting patient needs in this area.

Intervening in emotions requires self-understanding by the nurse. Whether the interventions will be therapeutic depends greatly on the nurse's values regarding the various emotions, the nurse's emotional responsiveness, and the ability to offer genuine respect and nonjudgmental acceptance. Nurses must be able to experience feelings and express them if they expect to help patients.

Depressed Patients. Initially the nurse must express hope for depressed patients. They have a genuine need for repeated reassurance. The nurse can reinforce that depression is a self-limiting disorder and that the future will be better. This can be expressed calmly and simply. The intent is not to cheer the patient but to offer hope that, although recovery is a slow process involving weeks or months, the patient will feel progressively better. The nurse may acknowledge the patient's inability to take comfort from this reassurance. For the depressed, only the depression is real; past or future happiness is an illusion (see A Patient Speaks). By affirming belief in recovery, however, the nurse may make the patient's existence more tolerable.

This initial reassurance is a way of acknowledging the patient's pain and despair while also conveying a sense of hope

A Patient Speaks

In depression this faith in deliverance, in ultimate restoration, is absent. The pain is unrelenting, and what makes the condition intolerable is the foreknowledge that no remedy will come—not in a day, an hour, a month, or a minute. If there is mild relief, one knows that it is only temporary; more pain will follow. It is hopelessness even more than pain that crushes the soul. So the decision making of daily life involves not, as in normal affairs, shifting from one annoying situation to another less annoying—or from discomfort to relative comfort, or from boredom to activity—but moving from pain to pain. One does not abandon, even briefly, one's bed of nails, but is attached to it wherever one goes. And this results in a striking experience—one which I have called, borrowing military terminology, the situation of the walking wounded. For in virtually any other serious sickness, a patient who felt similar devastation would be lying flat in bed, possibly sedated and hooked up to the tubes and wires of life-support systems, but at the very least in a posture of repose and in an isolated setting. His invalidism would be necessary, unquestioned, and honorably attained. However, the sufferer from depression has no such option and therefore finds himself, like a walking casualty of war, thrust into the most intolerable social and family situations. There he must, despite the anguish devouring his brain, present a face approximating the one that is associated with ordinary events and companionship. He must try to utter small talk, and be responsive to questions, and knowingly nod and frown and, God help him, even smile. But it is a fierce trial attempting to speak a few simple words.

From Styron W: *Darkness visible*, New York, 1992, Vintage Books.

in recovery. It is not the premature reassurance of "Don't worry, everything's going to be just fine." It is an openness to the patient's feelings and acknowledgment of them. This is a very important first step. It lets the patient see that the present state is not permanent. For the depressed patient who lacks time perspective, it directs thoughts beyond the present with genuine hope for tomorrow.

Nursing actions in this area should convey that expressing feelings is normal and necessary. Blocking or repressing emotions is partly responsible for the patient's present pain. Nurses can help patients realize that their overwhelming feelings of dejection and worthlessness are defenses that prevent them from dealing with their problems. Encouraging a patient to express unpleasant or painful emotions can reduce their intensity and make the patient feel more alive and masterful. Thus nursing care should be directed toward helping the patient experience feelings and express them. These actions are a prerequisite to interventions in the cognitive, behavioral, or social areas.

Manic Patients. Manic patients may have the opposite problem of patients with depression in that they are often too expressive of their feelings. These patients are often hyperverbal and need help from the nurse in pacing and modulating their expression. The nurse must be careful not to criticize or negate the feelings expressed. Rather, helping patients to speak more slowly and to follow one line of thought are important areas for nursing intervention. Manic patients need feedback on the intensity of their self-expressions, as well as the impact of their behavior on other people. Social skills modeling and reinforcement are nursing care activities that can be incorporated into the daily routine. Setting limits, giving simple directions, and keeping focused are other useful nursing interventions.

When the nurse accepts without criticism the anger, despair, or anxiety expressed by the patient, the patient sees that expressing feelings is not destructive or a sign of weakness. Sometimes, however, patients' expression of anger changes their cognitive set from self-blaming to blaming others. It may allow them to see themselves as more effective because it connotes power, superiority, and mastery. How this anger is expressed is important because aggressive behavior can be destructive and can further isolate them. Many patients experiencing both depressive and manic emotional states have problems with expressing anger and need to learn assertive behavior. This important area of nursing intervention is explored in Chapter 31.

Relaxation techniques may also help both manic and depressed patients deal with their anxiety and tension and obtain more pleasure from life. Reducing anxiety to tolerable levels broadens one's perceptual field and allows the nurse to intervene in the cognitive and behavioral areas. Nursing actions to reduce anxiety are described in Chapters 17 and 32.

To successfully implement any of these nursing actions related to the patient's affective needs, the nurse must use a variety of communication skills (see Chapter 2). Particularly important are empathy skills, reflection of feeling, open-ended feeling-oriented questions, validation, self-disclosure, and confrontation. The patient with a severe mood disturbance will challenge the nurse's therapeutic skills and stringently test the nurse's caring and commitment.

Cognitive Strategies

When intervening in the cognitive area, nurses have three major aims, which require that they begin with the patient's conceptualization of the problem:

- To increase the patient's sense of control over goals and behavior
- To increase the patient's self-esteem
- To help the patient modify dysfunctional thinking patterns

Depressed Patients. Depressed patients often see themselves as victims of their moods and environment. They do not see their behavior and their interpretation of events as possible causes of depression. They assume a passive

---

Citing the Evidence on

Medications versus Cognitive Therapy for Depression

BACKGROUND: The purpose of this study was to compare the acute outcomes of antidepressant medication and cognitive behavior therapy in the severely depressed outpatient subgroups of four major randomized trials.

RESULTS: The overall effect sizes comparing antidepressant medication to cognitive behavior therapy favored cognitive behavior therapy, but tests comparing the two treatments did not show a significant advantage of one treatment over the other.

IMPLICATIONS: Evidence suggests that cognitive behavior therapy has similar efficacy to that of antidepressant medication with severely depressed outpatients in four major comparisons. Depressed patients will benefit from having treatment options that include both pharmacological and psychosocial interventions.

DeRubeis RJ et al: Medications versus cognitive behavior therapy for severely depressed outpatients: meta-analysis of four randomized comparisons, *Am J Psychiatry* 156(7):1007, 1999.

---

stance and wait for someone or something to lift their mood. One task of the nurse, therefore, is to move patients beyond their limiting preoccupation to other aspects of their world that are related to it. To do this, the nurse must progress gradually. The first step is to help patients explore their feelings. This is followed by eliciting their view of the problem. In so doing the nurse accepts the patient's perceptions but need not accept the patient's conclusions. Together they define the problem to give the patient a sense of control, a feeling of hope, and a realization that change may indeed be possible.

Nursing actions may then focus on modifying the patient's thinking (see Citing the Evidence). Depressed patients are dominated by negative thoughts. Often, despite a successful performance, the patient will view it negatively. Cognitive changes may be brought about in a variety of ways, as described in Chapter 32.

Often, negative thinking is an automatic process of which the patient is not even aware. The nurse can therefore help patients identify their negative thoughts and decrease them through thought stopping or substitution. Concurrently, the patient can be encouraged to increase positive thinking by reviewing personal assets, strengths, accomplishments, and opportunities. Next, the patient can be helped to examine the accuracy of perceptions, logic, and conclusions. Misperceptions, distortions, and irrational beliefs become evident. The patient should be helped to move from unrealistic to realistic goals and to decrease the importance of unattainable goals. All these actions enhance the patient's self-understanding and increase self-esteem. More detailed interventions related to alterations in self-concept, which are inherent in disturbances of mood, are explored in Chapter 19.

Also, because the depressed patient tends to be overwhelmed by despair, it is important to limit the amount of negative evaluation in which he or she engages. One way is to involve the patient in productive tasks or activities; another way is to increase the level of socialization. These benefit the patient in two complementary ways: They limit the time spent on brooding and self-criticism and they provide positive reinforcement.

Manic Patients. Manic patients also need to gain control over their thoughts and behaviors. Here, however, the challenge is to bring together a patient's scattered thoughts and ideas to help him or her engage in adaptive, goal-directed behavior. The communication skills of focusing, clarifying, and confrontation are useful in redirecting a patient's self-expressions. Once this is accomplished the nurse can begin to help the patient modify dysfunctional thinking. Manic patients often have problems of grandiosity, overestimation of self, and unrealistic pursuits. As in depression, cognitive interventions can help the patient evaluate these thought problems and identify more realistic and ego-supportive goals.

It is also important for the nurse to realize the meaning, nature, and value the manic patient places on behavior and mood change. For example, research has shown that patients with bipolar disorder receive pronounced short- and long-term positive effects from their illness. These include increases in productivity, creativity, sensitivity to surroundings, social friendliness, and sexual intensity. These effects can provide a great deal of secondary benefit from the illness and can be powerful reinforcers of maladaptive responses, thus making change more difficult. For some patients at some times the perceived positive consequences of the illness may outweigh their perception of the negative consequences.

Behavioral Change

The ability to accomplish tasks and be productive depends on various factors that apply to both depressed and manic patients. First, expectations and goals should be small enough to ensure successful performance, relevant to their needs, and focused on positive activities. Box 20-6 presents a list of rewarding or potentially rewarding activities.

Next, attention should be focused on the task at hand, not what has yet to be done or was done incorrectly in the past. Finally, positive reinforcement should be based on actual performance. If such an approach is used consistently over time, the nurse can expect the patient to demonstrate increasingly productive behavior.

Occupational and recreational tasks are usually easily identified by the nurse. These can be most valuable and are well represented in the positive activities list. Another source of accomplishment is movement and physical exercise. Jogging, walking, swimming, bicycling, and aerobics are popular forms of exercise that may be incorporated in a regular program of activity (Gullette & Blumenthal, 1996). They are beneficial because they improve the patient's physical condition, release emotions and tensions, and can have an antidepressant effect.

Successful behavior is a powerful reinforcer or antidepressant. However, this idea seldom occurs to depressed patients, who use their despondent mood as a rationalization for inactivity. They instead believe that once their mood lifts, they will be productive again. Such an idea is consistent with a negative cognitive set and a sense of helplessness. However, inactivity prevents satisfaction and social recognition. Thus it reinforces a depressive state. Likewise, overactivity or uncompleted activity lowers the self-evaluation of manic patients.

Therefore nursing interventions should focus on activating the patient in a realistic, goal-directed way. Directed activities, strategies, or homework assignments mutually determined by the nurse and patient can reveal alternative coping responses. Many depressed patients benefit from nursing actions that encourage them to redirect their self-preoccupation to interests in the outside world. The timing of these interventions is crucial. Patients should not be

Box 20-6

List of Possible Positive Activities

- Planning something you will enjoy
- Going on an outing (such as a walk, a shopping trip downtown, or a picnic)
- Going out for entertainment
- Going on a trip
- Going to meetings, lectures, or classes
- Attending a social gathering
- Playing a sport or game
- Spending time on a hobby or project
- Entertaining yourself at home (for example, reading, listening to music, or watching television)
- Doing something just for yourself (such as buying something, cooking something, or dressing comfortably)
- Spending time just relaxing (for example, thinking, sitting, napping, or daydreaming)
- Caring for yourself or making yourself attractive
- Persisting at a difficult task
- Completing a routine task or unpleasant task
- Doing a job well
- Cooperating with someone else on a common task
- Doing something special for someone else, being generous, going out of your way
- Seeking out people (for example, calling, stopping by, making a date or appointment, or going to a meeting)
- Initiating conversation (for example, at a store, party, or class)
- Discussing an interesting or amusing topic
- Expressing yourself openly, clearly, or frankly (expressing opinion, criticism, or anger)
- Playing with children or animals
- Complimenting or praising someone
- Physically showing affection or love
- Receiving praise, compliments, or attention

forced into activities initially. Also, they will not benefit from coming into contact with too many people too soon. Rather, the nurse should encourage activities gradually and suggest more involvement on the basis of patients' energy.

For severely depressed hospitalized patients a structured daily program of activities can be beneficial. Because these patients lack motivation and direction, they are slow to initiate actions. The nurse should take into consideration the patient's tolerance to stress and probability of succeeding. The particular task should be neither too difficult nor too time consuming. Success tends to increase expectations of success, and failure tends to increase hopelessness.

Elated patients usually need little encouragement to become involved with others. Because of their short attention span and restless energy, however, they cannot deal with complicated projects. They need tasks that are simple and can be completed quickly. They need room to move about and furnishings that do not overstimulate them.

> *What physiological changes occur as a result of exercise? Relate these to what is currently known about the biology of depression.*

Social Skills

Social factors play a major role in the causation, maintenance, and resolution of affective disorders. Socialization moderates depression by providing an experience incompatible with depressive withdrawal. It also provides increased self-esteem through the social reinforcers of approval, acceptance, recognition, and support.

A major problem is that patients with maladaptive emotional responses are less accomplished in social interaction. In addition, others may avoid them because of their self-absorption, pessimism, or elation. One nursing action to counteract this problem is to help patients improve their social skills. A Patient Education Plan for enhancing social skills is presented below. It applies to patients with either depression or mania.

Involvement with others often is a result of shared activities. The nurse can work with the patient to identify recreational, career, cultural, religious, and personal interests and how to pursue these interests through community groups, organizations, and clubs. Women's groups, single-parent groups, jogging clubs, church groups, and neighborhood associations are all opportunities. Although this may appear to be a simple nursing intervention, it often taxes the nurse's creativity and knowledge of resources.

Family and Group Treatment. In addition to a one-to-one relationship, patients with maladaptive emotional responses can benefit from family and group work. Behaviors associated with depression and mania may be contributed to and supported by other family members. The patient's problems in human relationships are examined in light of family patterns, and all members are expected to take responsibility for their share of the continuing pattern. The theory that friends and partners often reinforce and support the patient's maladaptive behavior has been well documented. Much attention and secondary gain are usually received from others, who respond by being helpful, nurturing, or annoyed. When the patient acts in a more adaptive way, however, attention given is minimal. Therefore one goal of family therapy is to have the family reinforce adaptive behavior and ignore maladaptive mood responses.

Group therapy can also provide multiple benefits. For example, a format for group treatment of patients with depression or mania can have as its overall aim to increase self-worth and self-esteem through identification with the group and awareness of personal strengths. Specifically, group members can do the following:

- Learn more about their own behavior and relationships with others based on feedback from the group
- Increase social support through group relatedness

 PATIENT EDUCATION PLAN   *Enhancing Social Skills*

CONTENT	INSTRUCTIONAL ACTIVITIES	EVALUATION
Describe behaviors interfering with social interaction.	Instruct the patient on corrective behaviors.	Patient identifies problematic and more facilitative behaviors.
Discuss positive social skills that could be used by the patient.	Model effective interpersonal skills for the patient.	Patient describes specific skills that could be acquired.
Analyze the way in which the patient could incorporate these specific skills.	Use role plan and guided practice to allow patient to test these new behaviors.	Patient shows beginning skill in assumed social behaviors.
Encourage patient to test new skills in other situations.	Give the patient homework assignments to do in his or her natural environment.	Patient discusses ability to complete the assigned tasks.
Discuss generalization of new skills to other aspects of the patient's life and functioning.	Give feedback, encouragement, and praise for newly acquired social skills and their generalization.	Patient is able to integrate the new social behaviors in social interactions with others.

- Gain a heightened sense of identity, self-understanding, and control over their own lives
- Realize that other people have problems similar to their own, which helps to reduce their sense of loneliness and isolation, thereby also decreasing feelings of hopelessness, helplessness, and powerlessness
- Learn new ways to cope with stress from others in the group
- More realistically modify their perceptions and expectations of self and others
- Allow for the expression of feelings of hopelessness and frustration within the supportive context of the group

Mental Health Education

A final but important aspect of nursing care related to maladaptive emotional responses is mental health education about the nature, extent, and treatments available for mood disorders. Despite its prevalence, most people with depressive illnesses do not seek treatment because many of them do not know that they have a treatable disease. There is a particular need to target outreach to ethnic and racial minority communities.

Nursing care must also address the specific needs of patients and families for education about mood disorders. A psychoeducational model can be used with families, who are a valuable resource in helping patients deal with their illness (Clarkin et al, 1998; Perry et al, 1999). The overall goal of such a program is to improve patient and family functioning and decrease symptomatology by increasing a sense of self-worth and control for both patients and families. Specific information about the reciprocal impact of depression and family life can be outlined (Box 20-7), along with suggestions and strategies designed to help family members cope more effectively with mood disorders.

In summary, the most important ideas that the nurse should try to communicate through mental health education include the following (Depression Guideline Panel, 1993):

- Mood disorders are a medical illness, not a character defect or weakness.
- Recovery is the rule, not the exception.

Box 20-7

Outline of Topics for Patient-Family Psychoeducational Sessions on Depression

I. Defining depression
   A. Definitions and descriptions of depression and mania
   B. How depression differs from "the blues" we all experience (duration, impact on mood, functioning, self-esteem, responsiveness to the environment)
   C. Possible causes: the Stuart Stress Adaptation Model

II. Depression and the interpersonal environment
   A. What depression looks like: interpersonal difficulties
      1. Oversensitivity and self-preoccupation
      2. Unresponsiveness (to reassurance, support, feedback, sympathy)
      3. Behaviors that appear willful
      4. Apparent lack of caring for others, unrealistic expectations
      5. Apparent increased need to control relationships
      6. Inability to function in normal roles, tasks
   B. Negative interactional sequences
      1. Family attempts to coax, reassure, protect (potential for overinvolvement)
      2. Patient is unresponsive, family escalates attempts to help or withdraws
      3. Patient feels alienated, family becomes withdrawn, angry, or both
      4. Family feels guilty and returns to overprotective stance
      5. Patient feels unworthy, hopeless, infantilized
      6. Families burn out over time but remain caught in guilt/anger dilemma
      7. Alienation or overprotection

III. Treatments
   A. Psychotropic medication
   B. Psychotherapies
   C. Other treatments

IV. Coping with depression
   A. What to avoid
      1. Too rapid reassurance
      2. Taking comments literally
      3. Attempting to be constantly available and positive
      4. Allowing the disorder to dominate family life
   B. Creating a balance (neither overresponsive nor underresponsive)
      1. Recognition of multiple realities
      2. Distinguishing between the patient and the disorder
      3. Decreasing expectations temporarily
      4. Providing realistic support and reinforcement
      5. Avoiding unnecessary criticism (but providing feedback when necessary)
      6. Communicating clearly and simply (proverbially)
      7. Providing activity, structure
   C. Taking care of self and family members other than the patient; skills for self-preservation
      1. Time out (away from patient)
      2. Avoiding martyrdom
      3. Accepting own negative feelings
      4. Minimizing the impact of the disorder
   D. Coping with special problems
      1. Suicide threats and attempts
      2. Medication
      3. Hospitalization
      4. Atypical responses

Modified from Anderson et al: A comparative study of the education vs. process groups for families of patients with affective disorders, *Family Process* 25(2):185, 1986. Reproduced with permission of *Family Process* Inc. via Copyright Clearance Center.

NURSING DIAGNOSIS: Hopelessness
EXPECTED OUTCOME: The patient will be emotionally responsive and return to pre-illness level of functioning.

SHORT-TERM GOAL	INTERVENTION	RATIONALE
The patient's environment will be safe and protective.	Continually evaluate the patient's potential for suicide. Hospitalize the patient when there is a suicidal risk. Help the patient move to a new environment when appropriate (new job, peer group, family setting).	All patients with severe mood disturbances are at risk for suicide; environmental changes can protect the patient, decrease the immediate stress, and mobilize additional resources.

The patient will establish a therapeutic relationship with the nurse.	Use a warm, accepting, empathic approach.
	Be aware of and in control of your own feelings and reactions (anger, frustration, sympathy).
	With the depressed patient:
	  Establish rapport through shared time and supportive companionship.
	  Give the patient time to respond.
	  Personalize care as a way of indicating the patient's value as a human being.
	With the manic patient:
	  Give simple, truthful responses.
	  Be alert to possible manipulation.
	  Set constructive limits on negative behavior.
	  Use a consistent approach by all health-team members.
	  Maintain open communication and sharing of perceptions among team members.
	  Reinforce the patient's self-control and positive aspects of patient behavior.
		Both depressed and manic patients resist becoming involved in a therapeutic alliance; acceptance, persistence, and limit setting are necessary.

The patient will be physiologically stable and able to meet self-care needs.	Help the patient to meet self-care needs, particularly in the areas of nutrition, sleep, and personal hygiene. Encourage the patient's independence whenever possible. Administer prescribed medications and somatic treatments.	Physiological changes occur in disturbances of mood; physical care and somatic therapies are required to overcome problems in this area.
The patient will be able to recognize and express emotions related to daily events.	Respond empathically, with a focus on feelings rather than facts. Acknowledge the patient's pain and convey a sense of hope in recovery. Help the patient experience feelings and express them appropriately. Help the patient in the adaptive expression of anger.	Patients with severe mood disturbances have difficulty identifying, expressing, and modulating feelings.

Continued

NURSING TREATMENT PLAN *Summary* *Maladaptive Emotional Responses—cont'd*

SHORT-TERM GOAL	INTERVENTION	RATIONALE
The patient will evaluate thinking and correct faulty or negative thoughts.	Review the patient's conceptualization of the problem but do not necessarily accept conclusions. Identify the patient's negative thoughts and help to decrease them. Help increase positive thinking. Examine the accuracy of perceptions, logic, and conclusions. Identify misperceptions, distortions, and irrational beliefs. Help the patient move from unrealistic to realistic goals. Decrease the importance of unattainable goals. Limit the amount of negative personal evaluations the patient engages in.	This will help to increase sense of control over goals and behaviors, enhance self-esteem, and modify negative expectations.
The patient will implement two new behavioral coping strategies.	Assign appropriate action-oriented therapeutic tasks. Encourage activities gradually, escalating them as the patient's energy is mobilized. Provide a tangible, structured program when appropriate. Set goals that are realistic, relevant to the patient's needs and interests, and focused on positive activities. Focus on present activities, not past or future activities. Positively reinforce successful performance. Incorporate physical exercise in the patient's care plan.	Successful behavioral performance counteracts feelings of helplessness and hopelessness.
The patient will describe rewarding social interactions.	Assess the patient's social skills, supports, and interests. Review existing and potential social resources. Instruct and model effective social skills. Use role playing and rehearsal of social interactions. Give feedback and positive reinforcement of effective interpersonal skills. Intervene with families to have them reinforce the patient's adaptive emotional responses. Support or engage in family and group therapy when appropriate.	Socialization is an experience incompatible with withdrawal and increases self-esteem through the social reinforcers of approval, acceptance, recognition, and support.

- Mood disorders are treatable illnesses, and an effective treatment can be found for almost all patients.
- The goal of intervention is to not just get better, but to get and stay completely well.
- A Nursing Treatment Plan Summary for patients with maladaptive emotional responses is presented on pp. 375-376.

EVALUATION

The effectiveness of nursing care is determined by changes in the patient's maladaptive emotional responses and the effect they have on functioning. Problems related to self-concept and interpersonal relationships merge and overlap. Because all people experience life stress and related losses, the nurse can ask a fundamental question related to evaluation: "Did I assess the patient for problems in this area?"

Of particular significance are the many special aspects of transference and countertransference that may occur. The patient's heightened attachment and dependency behaviors and lowered defensiveness can lead to intense transference reactions that should be worked through. Themes of loss and fear of loss, control of emotions and lack of control, and ambivalence predominate. Termination of the nurse-patient relationship may be difficult because the patient experiences it as another loss that requires mourning and integration.

Countertransference can be related to the nurse's own bereavements, attitudes about anger, guilt, sadness, and despair, the ability to confront these emotions openly and objectively, and most importantly, conflicts about death and loss. Difficulties with any of these issues can be evident in avoidance behavior, preoccupation with fantasies, blocking of feelings, or shortening of sessions. Nursing care will be more appropriate and effective if the nurse is aware of these issues and sensitive to personal feelings and conflicts regarding loss. Supervision and peer support groups can be of great help in this area.

Summary

1. The continuum of emotional responses ranges from the most adaptive state of emotional responsiveness to the more maladaptive states of delayed grief reaction, depression, and mania.

2. Patient behaviors related to emotional responses include delayed grief reaction, depression, and mania.

3. Predisposing factors affecting emotional responses include genetics, aggression turned inward, object loss, personality organization, cognition, learned helplessness-hopelessness, behavioral learning, and biochemistry. Precipitating stressors include loss of attachment, life events, roles, and physiological changes.

4. Coping resources focus on the patient's social and economic supports and a sense of personal mastery. Coping mechanisms include introjection, denial, and suppression.

5. Primary NANDA nursing diagnoses related to maladaptive emotional responses are dysfunctional grieving, hopelessness, powerlessness, spiritual distress, and risk for self-directed violence.

6. Primary *DSM–IV–TR* diagnoses include bipolar I and II disorders, cyclothymic disorder, major depressive disorder, and dysthymic disorder.

7. The expected outcome of nursing care is that the patient will be emotionally responsive and return to a pre-illness level of functioning.

8. Nursing interventions address environmental issues, nurse-patient relationships, physiological treatments, expressing feelings, cognitive strategies, behavioral change, social skills, and mental health education.

9. The effectiveness of nursing care is determined by changes in the patient's maladaptive emotional responses and the effect they have on functioning. Supervision and peer support groups can be helpful to the nurse working with patients with mood disorders.

Competent Caring A Clinical Exemplar of a Psychiatric Nurse

VIRGINIA A. REUGER, MSN, RN, C

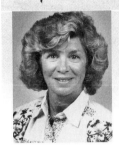

Sure, you read about therapeutic interactions in your nursing textbooks, but every person is not the same, so the only way you learn is by doing, by experiencing. Rarely in school do we have the time to become overly involved with our patients. We are taught on our psychiatric rotation not to let the boundaries between self and others become blurred. Yet the dynamics of a therapeutic relationship are not real until we come face to face with the situation.

It happened to me, subtly, soon after I started working in a private psychiatric hospital. I was working as a staff nurse on the intensive care unit. I was assigned to the next admission. From the intake sheet, I could see it was another depressed, suicidal patient. But when R and her husband walked onto the unit, I was immediately drawn to her with an empathic feeling. She was tiny, frail looking; her face was thin and drawn. Her long, dark hair partially hid her face. She ignored introductions and stared at the floor. My initial challenge was to establish trust to open channels of communication, assess her suicide potential, and provide a secure environment. Her potential for self-harm was quite high. She was put on strict suicidal precautions. Initially, as I worked with R it required observations of her appearance, gestures, and interests, as well as nonverbal communication. I often had to make inferences, and I shared these with her. I felt like she was testing the waters of trust. R would often wrap herself up in her pink blanket and rock back and forth during our interactions. I found myself wondering what she was thinking.

One day during our time together I asked her about how it felt to be depressed. For her, it was the beginning of self-disclosure. She was able to acknowledge her fear and pain and unmet needs. She talked about what it was like growing up in New York City, living in rat-infested row houses. Her father worked at a bakery and sometimes their only food was the bread he brought home. She had two brothers and two sisters. Eventually she told me her uncle and grandfather lived with them, too. As she learned to trust me, she disclosed sexual abuse from her uncle and grandfather. At times

Continued

Competent Caring A Clinical Exemplar of a Psychiatric Nurse—cont'd

the details became so vivid she trembled as she cried. It is hard to express, but there was a sense that we were making contact.

We talked about her present life, her frigidity, her 6-year-old daughter, and the nightmares. She often remarked that her husband and daughter would be better off without her. She believed she could not have a "normal life." R was very bright and talented. She had many hobbies. We started concentrating on these things. I knew her self-esteem was low, and this was the start of some good work. But being her primary nurse and assigned to her one-to-one daily made me realize I was becoming enmeshed in the situation. I went to my nurse manager for supervision. We discussed several options. I questioned whether I was helping her. I think sometimes nurses want to feel like omnipotent rescuers. I was not sure whether I was fostering independence or dependence. It was important to acknowledge my feelings to someone else openly, to discuss them, and then to move on. Even though I felt a bond, I had to help R find strength on her own. We discussed her upcoming discharge date; we talked about prior-ities and decisions she had made. We talked about good choices, bad choices, and no choices. She had suffered many setbacks, but she was making plans.

I remember staying late the day of her discharge to say good-bye. R sent me cards at the hospital, dropped gifts off at the admissions office for me, and once tried to reach me at home. It was difficult to not acknowledge these things; I wanted so much to talk to her. But I knew the boundaries of a therapeutic relationship, and I knew she would be fine. I did talk to her outpatient therapist, and he told me she had completed a course in sign language (during her stay R befriended a deaf elderly woman), and she also was attending clown school, something she had always wanted to do—to make people laugh and feel good.

In psychiatric nursing it is important to remember that the art is to offer what you can without dictating the results while recognizing that you are not the only one to contribute to a person's health and happiness. I learned this important lesson from R.

MERLIN Visit **MERLIN: www.mosby.com/MERLIN/Stuart** to find these additional materials and student activities.

- **Worksheets**
- **"Drug of the Month" Updates**
- **"Citing the Evidence" Updates**
- **Critical Thinking Activities and Exercises**
- **Annotated Suggested Readings**
- **Web Links**
- **More!**

Chapter Review Questions

1. Match each term in Column A with the correct examples in Column B.

Column A	Column B
____ Behaviors related to emotional responses	**A.** Introjection, denial, suppression
____ Coping mechanisms	**B.** Loss, life events, role strain
____ *DSM–IV–TR* diagnoses	**C.** Delayed grief reaction, depression/mania
____ Precipitating stressors	**D.** Bipolar, cyclothymia, depression
____ Predisposing factors	**E.** Genetics, early childhood loss, turning anger inward
____ Seasonal affective disorder	**F.** Depression that comes with shortened daylight

2. Fill in the blanks.

A. The somatic therapy of _____ is often used for patients with severe depression with somatic delusions and delusional guilt, suicidal ideation, and weight loss.

B. There is substantial evidence for abnormal regulation of the _____ neurotransmitter system in depression.

C. Depressed patients with a history of manic episodes are said to have _____ disorder. Depressed patients who have had only episodes of depression are said to have _____ depression.

D. Prior episodes, family history, prior suicide attempts, female gender, and lack of social support are all _____ factors for depression.

E. The brain structure currently the focus of much research for its role in depression is the _____.

F. Two other psychiatric illnesses that often occur with depression are _____ disorders and _____ disorders.

G. When both medications and psychotherapy are used to treat depression and mania, the success rate of treatment is _____ % to _____ %.

H. The goal of the acute phase of treatment for depression is to eliminate symptoms and produce a therapeutic _____ . This phase usually lasts _____ to _____ weeks. If patients are symptom free at the end of that time they are said to be in _____.

I. The goal of the continuation phase of treatment for depression is to promote _____ and prevent _____. This phase usually lasts _____ to _____ months.

J. The goal of the maintenance phase of treatment for depression is to prevent _____. This phase may last _____.

3. **Provide short answers for the following questions.**

A. List the responses on the continuum of emotional responses and give a brief definition of each one.

B. What are the three major aims when intervening in the cognitive area with a depressed patient?

C. You are asked to join a peer support group made up of nurses who work with patients with depression. How can such a group be helpful to you? What can you contribute to the group?

D. Design an intervention program for mothers who are depressed and their young children.

REFERENCES

Abramson L et al: Hopelessness depression: a theory-based subtype of depression, *Psychol Rev* 96:358, 1989.

Agency for Health Care Policy and Research (AHCPR): *Treatment of depression—newer pharmacotherapies, evidence report/technology assessment number 7,* Rockville, MD, 1999, AHCPR.

American Psychiatric Association: *Diagnostic and statistical manual of mental disorders,* Fourth Edition, Text Revision, Washington, DC, American Psychiatric Association, 2000a.

American Psychiatric Association: Practice guideline for the treatment of patients with major depressifve disorder, *Am J Psychiatry* 157(4):489, 2000b.

Arieti S, Bemporad J: The psychological organization of depression, *Am J Psychiatry* 137:1360, 1980.

Beck A et al: *Cognitive therapy of depression,* New York, 1979, The Guilford Press.

Beeber L: Depression in women. In McBride AB, Austin JK, editors: *Psychiatric-mental health nursing: integrating the behavioral and biological sciences,* Philadelphia, 1996, WB Saunders.

Berlanga C et al: Personality and clinical predictors of recurrence of depression, *Psychiatr Serv* 50(3):376, 1999.

Clarkin J et al: Effects of psychoeducational intervention for married patients with bipolar disorder and their spouses, *Psychiatr Serv* 49(4):531, 1998.

Depression Guideline Panel: *Depression in primary care,* vol 2, *Treatment of major depression, Clinical practice guideline,* no 5, Rockville, Md, 1993, U.S. Department of Health and Human Services, Public Health Service, Agency for Health Care Policy and Research, pub no 93-0551.

Epperson C: Postpartum major depression: detection and treatment, *Am Acad Fam Physicians* April 15, 1999.

Faller H et al: Coping, distress, and survival among patients with lung cancer, *Arch Gen Psychiatry* 56:756, 1999.

Ferro T et al: Screening for depression in mothers bringing their offspring for evaluation or treatment of depression, *Am J Psychiatry* 157(3):375, 2000.

Field T: Infants of depressed mothers, *Infant Behav Dev* 18:1, 1995.

Friedrich M: Lithium: proving its mettle for 50 years, *JAMA* 281(24):2271, 1999.

Giese A et al: The impact of a history of childhood abuse on hospital outcome and affective episodes, *Psychiatr Serv* 49(1):77, 1998.

Giles D et al: Controlled comparison of eletrophysiological sleep in families of probands with unipolar depression, *Am J Psychiatry* 155(2):192, 1998.

Gloaguen V et al: A meta-analysis of the effects of cognitive therapy in depressed patients, *J Affective Disorders* 49(1):59, 1998.

Gullette E, Blumenthal J: Exercise therapy for the prevention and treatment of depression, *J Pract Psychiatry Behav Health* 9:263, 1996.

Hilty D et al: A review of bipolar disorder among adults, *Psychiatr Serv* 50(2):201, 1999.

Kendler K et al: Causal relationships between stressful life events and the onset of major depression, *Am J Psychiatry* 156(6):837, 1999.

Kissane D et al: The Melbourne family grief study, I: perceptions of family functioning in bereavement, *Am J Psychiatry* 153(5):650, 1996.

Lewinsohn P et al: Reinforcement and depression. In Depue R, editor: *The psychobiology of the depressive disorders,* New York, 1979, Academic Press.

McEnany G: Part I: Rhythm and blues revisited: biological rhythm disturbances in depression, *J Am Psychiatr Nurs Assoc* 2:15, 1996.

Ornstein S et al: Depression diagnoses and antidepressant use in primary care practice, *J Fam Pract* 49(1):68, 2000.

Perry A et al: Randomized controlled trial of efficacy of teaching patients with bipolar disorder to identify early symptoms of relapse and obtain treatment, *Br Med J* 318:149, 1999.

Roberts R et al: Does growing old increase the risk for depression? *Am J Psychiatry* 154(10):1384, 1997.

Seligman M: *Helplessness: on depression, development and death,* San Francisco, 1975, WH Freeman.

Simmons-Alling S: Bipolar mood disorders: brain, behavior, and nursing. In McBride AB, Austin JK, editors: *Psychiatric-mental health nursing: integrating the behavioral and biological sciences,* Philadelphia, 1996, WB Saunders.

Solomon D et al: Multiple recurrences of major depressive disorder, *Am J Psychiatry* 157(2):229, 2000.

Terman M et al: Seasonal affective disorder and its treatments, *J Pract Psychiatr Behav Health* Sept:287, 1998.

Weiss E et al: Childhood sexual abuse as a risk factor for depression in women: psychosocial and neurobiological correlates, *Am J Psychiatry* 156(6):816, 1999.

Wickramaratne P, Weissman M: Onset of psychopathology in offspring by developmental phase and parental depression, *J Am Acad Child Adolesc Psychiatry* 37(9):933, 1998.

Wulsin L et al: A systematic review of the mortality of depression, *Psychosom Med* 61:6, 1999.

Zuroff D et al: Relation of therapeutic alliance and perfectionism to outcome in brief outpatient treatment of depression, *J Consult Clin Psychol* 68(1):114, 2000.

Self-Protective Responses and Suicidal Behavior

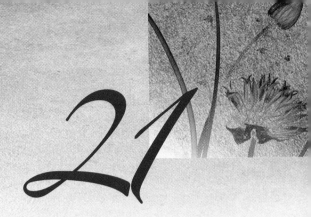

Gail W. Stuart

Out, out brief candle! Life's but a walking shadow, a poor player That struts and frets his hour upon the stage And then is heard no more. It is a tale Told by an idiot, full of sound and fury, Signifying nothing.

WILLIAM SHAKESPEARE, MACBETH, ACT V

Life is full of risk. People must choose the amount of danger to which they are willing to expose themselves. Sometimes these choices are conscious and rational. For instance, the elderly person who decides to stay in the house on an icy day has chosen not to risk falling and possibly fracturing a bone. Other risk-taking behavior is unconscious. Soldiers who volunteer for a suicide mission are probably unaware of their motivation. If asked, they would probably cite patriotism or concern for comrades. Most people go through life accepting some risks as part of their daily routine while carefully avoiding others.

Even though life is risky, most societies have a norm that defines the degree of danger to which people may expose themselves. This norm varies according to age, gender, socioeconomic status, and occupation. In general, the very young, the old, and women are seen as needing to be protected from harm. Some risk takers are admired, particularly athletes, military personnel, those with dangerous occupations, and those who place themselves in danger to help others. At the same time, feelings of admiration may be accompanied by fear and perplexity about the danger-seeking behavior. The varying attitudes toward cigarette smoking are another example of cultural ambivalence. On one hand, smoking is seen as mature behavior, denoting sophistication and social acceptability. On the other, it is seen as socially alienating, unhealthy, and inconsiderate.

CONTINUUM OF SELF-PROTECTIVE RESPONSES

Protection and survival are fundamental needs of all living things. A continuum of self-protecting responses would have self-enhancement as the most adaptive response, whereas indirect self-destructive behavior, self-injury, and suicide would be maladaptive responses. Self-destructive behavior may thus range from subtle to overt.

Direct self-destructive behavior includes any form of suicidal activity, such as suicide threats, attempts, gestures, and completed suicide. The intent of this behavior is death, and the person is aware of the desired outcome. Indirect self-destructive behavior is any activity detrimental to the person's physical well-being that potentially may result in death. However, the person may be unaware of this potential and deny it if confronted. Examples include eating disorders (see Chapter 26) and abuse of alcohol and other drugs (see Chapter 25). Other examples include cigarette smoking, reckless driving, gambling, criminal activity, socially deviant behavior, stress-seeking behavior, participation in high-risk sports, and noncompliance with medical treatment.

Theories of self-destructive behavior overlap with those of self-concept and disturbances in mood. Careful study of Chapters 19 and 20 will help the reader understand the behaviors discussed in this chapter. To think about or attempt destruction of the self, the person must have low self-regard. Low self-esteem leads to depression, which is always present in self-destructive behavior. The range of self-protective responses is shown in Fig. 21-1.

The levels of behavior in the continuum may overlap. For instance, the girl who learns and excels at gymnastics is building her self-esteem and projecting a positive self-concept. However, if she tries movements she is not prepared for and does not take safety measures, her behavior becomes self-injurious or indirectly self-destructive. Similarly, a diabetic man who has never complied completely with his prescribed diet and medication regimen may become discouraged and intentionally take an overdose of insulin. Thus the nurse must be alert to subtle shifts in the mood and behavior of patients when assessing maladaptive self-protective responses.

> *Where do you think patients' requests for assisted-suicide falls in the continuum of self-protective responses?*

Epidemiology of Suicide

About 30,000 people complete the act of suicide each year, making it the eighth leading cause of death in the United States and the third leading killer of young people (NIMH, 1999). Suicides outnumber homicides in the United States by 3 to 2. The rate of suicide among youth has tripled in the past 30 years. The actual number of suicides may be two to three times higher because of the underreporting that occurs. In addition, many single-car accidents and homicides are, in fact, suicides.

Worldwide, at least 1000 suicides occur each day, and 645,680 years of productive life are lost each year in the United States because of deaths by suicide. Of these, 71% occurred among white males, and white females accounted for another 19%. The United States now has one of the highest suicide rates for young men in the world, surpassing Japan and Sweden, countries long identified with high rates of suicide.

Although the base rate of suicide has remained about the same for the past 20 years, the rate has soared for young people ages 15 to 24 and has increased by 25% for the elderly. The highest suicide rate for any group in this country is among people over age 65, especially white men over 85. Although this group constitutes 26% of the total U.S. population, it accounts for about 40% of suicide deaths. White males over the age of 50 represent the greatest number of these deaths (Fig. 21-2).

Teen suicide in the United States is nearly five times as common among boys as among girls. Suicide is also more common among whites than blacks at all ages. The overwhelming majority of completed suicides are committed by males. Well over half of these males shoot themselves, and the use of guns is increasing rapidly. Women attempt suicide twice as often as men, using potentially less lethal means such as medications and wrist slashing. However, one third of women who complete suicide and over half of those 15 to 29 years of age use guns.

Reports of suicide among young children are rare, but suicidal behavior is not. As many as 12,000 children ages 5 to 14 may be hospitalized in this country every year for deliberate self-destructive acts.

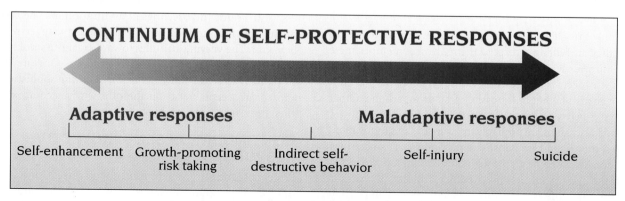

Fig. 21-1 Continuum of self-protective measures.

What factors might contribute to the high rate of suicide among white elderly males?

ASSESSMENT

Behaviors

Noncompliance. It has been estimated that one half of patients do not comply with their health-care treatment plan. People who do not comply with recommended health care activities are generally aware that they have chosen not to care for themselves. They usually have a reason for non-compliance, such as being asymptomatic, not being able to afford the treatment they need, not understanding the treatment, or not having time. Patients may also minimize the seriousness of their problems. Many chronic illnesses are characterized by long periods of stability, during which the person may not be aware of discomfort. This reinforces the noncompliant behavior.

The most prominent behavior associated with noncompliance is refusal to admit the seriousness of the health problem. This denial interferes with acceptance of treatment. Another aspect of noncompliance is that guilt about not following health-care recommendations may also interfere with obtaining regular care. Noncompliant people are also struggling for control. Serious illness is often seen as an attack on the person and a betrayal by the body. Patients need to reassert their control and prove that they are still the master of their fate. Most chronically ill people need to test the limits of their control and the validity of the prescribed self-care regimen. The following clinical example illustrates the problem of noncompliance with a prescribed health-care regimen.

CLINICAL EXAMPLE

Mrs. C was a 61-year-old, white married woman who had been in good health most of her life. She had three grown children who had left home and established their own families. She and her husband were both looking forward to his retirement in 6 months. They planned to buy a recreational vehicle and travel around the United States.

The nurse practitioner did a complete physical examination each time Mrs. C was seen. On her most recent visit, laboratory studies revealed an elevated blood glucose level. Her diagnosis was diabetes mellitus, adult onset. Mrs. C was told that her condition was not serious and could be controlled by diet. She was 20 pounds (9 kg) overweight and was advised that she needed to lose the excess weight. She was instructed about her diet, how to test her urine, and about possible complications of diabetes.

Mrs. C was frightened about her condition but did not mention this because no one else seemed very concerned. At first, she was conscientious about following her diet and testing her urine. She felt very well and was proud when she lost 5 pounds. As time went on, Mrs. C began to wonder whether she was really so sick. She had never felt ill. On her husband's birthday, she fixed a special dinner and baked a cake. She decided she deserved a reward for "being good" and did not follow her diet. She anxiously tested her urine at bedtime and it was negative. Then her son and his family visited for a week. She fixed all their favorite foods and ate with

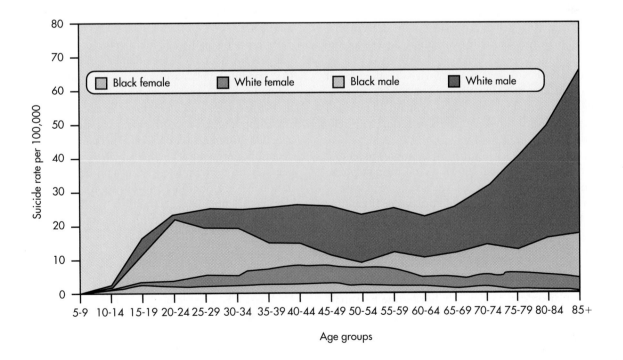

Fig. 21-2 U.S. suicide rates by age, gender, and racial group, 1997. (From National Center for Health Statistics, National Institutes of Mental Health, Washington, DC, 1999.)

them. She still felt fine and decided she did not need to test her urine. When it was time for her next checkup, she postponed calling the nurse practitioner. She was very busy preparing for retirement travel.

Selected Nursing Diagnosis
- Noncompliance related to fear of the diagnosis of diabetes, as evidenced by lack of adherence to medical treatment plan

 Do you think that noncompliance can ever be an adaptive response? Why or why not?

Self-Injury. Society accepts some forms of self-injury as normal. Examples of culturally sanctioned forms include body piercing, cosmetic eyebrow plucking, hair twisting, circumcision, nail biting, and tattoos. Various terms have been used to describe self-injurious behavior: **self-abuse, self-directed aggression, self-harm, self-inflicted injury, and self-mutilation.** Self-injury can be defined as the act of deliberate harm to one's own body. The injury is done to oneself, without the aid of another person, and the injury is severe enough for tissue damage. Common forms of self-injurious behavior include cutting and burning the skin, banging head and limbs, picking at wounds, and chewing fingers (Kehrberg, 1997).

Many nurses mistake self-injury for potential suicide. In fact, these are two separate phenomena. Usually the lethality of self-injury is low, and patients who self-injure typically want relief from the tension they feel rather than to kill themselves. Self-injury is also different from other self-destructive behaviors, such as bingeing, drug abuse, smoking, and high-risk activities. Self-injury is a contained event that occurs in a short time span and with an awareness of the consequences of the act.

Self-injurious behavior may be categorized by the type of patient and clinical context in which the behavior occurs:

- **People with mental retardation.** The mentally retarded may have outward-directed aggression along with self-injurious behavior.
- **Psychotic patients.** Self-injuring acts among psychotic patients tend to be sporadic and often occur in response to command hallucinations or delusions.
- **Prison populations.** Self-injury in prisons is difficult to assess because of poor documentation, drug use, and undiagnosed psychiatric disorders. Many self-injurious events among prisoners may be intentionally manipulative, designed to force transfer to a less restrictive facility.
- **Character disorders, particularly borderline personality disorder.** This group is often young and female with a poor tolerance of anxiety and anger. They also include patients with eating disorders.

Suicidal Behavior. Suicidal behavior is usually divided into the categories of suicide threats, suicide attempts, and completed suicide. In addition, certain suicide attempts may be called **suicide gestures.** The gesture is a suicide attempt directed toward the goal of receiving attention rather than actual destruction of the self. Use of this term is questionable. It implies that it is only an attention-seeking behavior and should not be taken seriously. This is not true. All suicidal behavior is serious, whatever the intent, and deserves the nurse's serious consideration. Therefore, suicide gestures are included in the general category of suicide attempts.

The **suicide threat** may be veiled but usually occurs before overt suicidal activity takes place. The suicidal person may make a statement such as "Will you remember me when I'm gone?" or "Take care of my family for me." In the context of recent stressors and the person's life situation, statements such as these may be ominous. Nonverbal communication often reveals the suicide threat. The person may give away prized possessions, make a will or funeral arrangements, or withdraw from friendships and social activities. Sometimes a person may make a direct verbal suicidal threat, but this occurs less often. The threat is an indication of the ambivalence that is usually present in suicidal behavior. It represents the hope that someone will recognize the danger and rescue the person from self-destructive impulses. It may also be an effort to discover whether anyone cares enough to prevent the person from harming himself or herself.

Suicide attempts include any self-directed actions taken by the person that will lead to death if not stopped. In the assessment of suicidal behavior, much emphasis is placed on the lethality of the method threatened or used. Although all suicide threats and attempts must be taken seriously, vigilant attention is indicated when the person is planning or tries a highly lethal means such as gunshot, hanging, or jumping. Less lethal means include carbon monoxide and drug overdose, which allow time for discovery once the suicidal action has begun.

Assessment of the suicidal person also includes whether the person has made a specific plan and whether the means to carry out the plan are available. The most suicidal person is one who plans a violent death (such as a gunshot to the head), has a specific plan (for example, as soon as his wife goes shopping), and has the means readily available (such as a loaded gun in a desk drawer). This person is exhibiting little ambivalence about a suicide plan. On the other hand, the person who contemplates taking a bottle of aspirin if the situation at work does not improve soon is communicating an element of hope. This person is really asking for help in coping with a poor work situation. The following clinical example illustrates the behavior of a suicidal person.

 CLINICAL EXAMPLE

Mr. Y was a 52-year-old black man employed in the foundry of a large steel mill. He had worked for the company for 20 years. He lived in a rented room in a blue-collar neighborhood near the mill. Most of his neighbors were Appalachian white and southern black families who had moved to the community to work at the mill. There was an undercurrent of racial tension in the neighborhood, but Mr. Y was not involved in conflicts with his neighbors. He had separated from his wife before moving to the community and had no close friends or family. The separation resulted from his violent behavior related to drinking binges.

Mr. Y was seen by the occupational health nurse, Ms. G, when he came to the employee health clinic following a 6-week absence from work. He had been hospitalized for broken ribs and a concussion after he had been beaten and robbed by a gang of adolescents in an alley behind his home. Ms. G was familiar with this patient because he had participated in the company's employee assistance program for alcoholics. When she saw him in the clinic, she immediately noted that he appeared depressed. His face was expressionless, his posture was slumped, and he had lost weight. He appeared disheveled, which was a change from his usual neat appearance. His speech was slow and halting and so soft that he could barely be heard.

He told Ms. G that he had a request to make of her. He knew from past conversations that she was an animal lover. He wanted her to take his pet dog because he did not feel able to care for it adequately, and the neighbors who kept it while he was in the hospital had neglected it. Ms. G was very concerned about Mr. Y and asked him how he was spending his time. He said he kept the television on and he thought a lot. When asked, he said he felt "too shaky" to go outside unless he absolutely had to. He thought the boys who attacked him were still in the neighborhood.

Ms. G asked if he had thought about harming himself. Mr. Y looked startled, then admitted that he saw no other solution to his problem. "It makes sense. I don't have anybody. If you take Rover, I can go." With further questioning, he admitted that he had a loaded revolver at home and planned to use it after he left the clinic. Ms. G realized that Mr. Y needed help immediately and initiated plans for hospitalization.

Selected Nursing Diagnoses

- Risk for self-directed violence related to impoverished social environment, as evidenced by intent to kill self with a gun
- Powerlessness related to recent neighborhood attack, as evidenced by expressed feelings of despair and hopelessness

Completed suicide may take place after warning signs have been missed or ignored. Some people do not give any easily recognizable warning signs. Research done on completed suicide has of necessity been retrospective. However, it can be informative to interview survivors. This procedure is known as the psychological autopsy (Cooper, 1995). It is a retrospective review of the person's behavior before the suicide. Table 21-1 compares the characteristics of suicide completers and suicide attempters (Simpson & Jamison, 1997).

Significant others of suicidal people, including survivors, have many feelings about this behavior. An element of hostility exists in suicidal behavior. Often the message to significant others, stated or implied, is "You should have cared more." At times, when the person survives the attempt, this message may be transmitted in a manipulative way. An example is the adolescent girl who discovers that her boyfriend is dating someone else and takes an overdose of over-the-counter sleeping pills. If she sets the scene so that she will almost inevitably be discovered and makes sure that her boyfriend hears of her behavior, she is behaving in a hostile, manipulative way. A remorseful response by the boyfriend would be reinforcing and increase the likelihood that she will repeat the behavior. It is important to treat these attempts seriously and help the patient develop healthier communication patterns. People who do not really intend to die may do so if they are not discovered in time.

When suicide is successful, the survivors are left with many feelings that they cannot communicate to the involved object, the dead person (see A Family Speaks on p. 386). This may lead to an unresolved grief reaction and depression. Some suicide prevention centers have become involved in postvention. Survivors are helped, either individually or in groups, to express their feelings and work through their grief.

In summary, the suicidal patient may have many different clinical behaviors. Mood disturbances are often present, as are somatic complaints. Hopelessness and helplessness may be more important than depression in explaining suicidal ideation (Lester, 1998). Nurses should take a careful medical and psychiatric history, paying specific attention to the mental status examination described in Chapter 7 and the psychosocial history, and evaluate the patient for recent losses, life stresses, and substance use and abuse (see Critical Thinking about Contemporary Issues on p. 386).

Contrary to common opinion, directly questioning the patient about suicidal thought and plans will not cause the patient to take suicidal action. Rather, most people want to be prevented from carrying out their self-destruction. Most patients are relieved to be asked about these feelings. One of the most important questions to ask of suicidal pa-

Table **21-1**

Characteristics of Suicide Completers and Attempters	
Suicide Completers	**Suicide Attempters**
- Three times as likely to be men - Usually suffer from depression and/or alcohol or substance abuse - Plan the suicide act - Use highly lethal method - Select setting unlikely to be interrupted	- Mainly women under age 40 - Less likely to have depression and other psychiatric conditions - More likely to have personality disorders - Act impulsively - Use method with low lethality - Act in the presence of or notify others

A Family Speaks

My husband died last year. He didn't commit suicide, but he took his own life just as surely as if he had pulled the trigger of a gun. Only his weapon was a cigarette. You see, 2 years ago his doctor discovered a cancer lesion on his lung. At that time my husband was told he needed to lose weight, cut down on his drinking, and most of all, stop smoking. But my husband wasn't a very good patient.

Sometimes I blame myself for not doing more. I nagged for a while, but that only seemed to make our marriage worse. My husband said that what he did with his life was his own choice and that his father had smoked all of his life and lived until he was 84. My husband died at age 62.

One good thing has come out of this tragedy, however. My son has stopped smoking and has vowed he will never touch another cigarette for as long as he lives. That small goodness gives me comfort and some sense of hope.

Box 21-1

Behavioral Rating Scales Related to Suicidal Behavior

- Assessment of Suicidal Potentiality
- Beck Scale for Suicidal Ideation
- Suicide Risk Scale

? CRITICAL THINKING about CONTEMPORARY ISSUES

Are Health-Care Professionals Missing Suicidal Behavior in Their Patients?

It has been reported that 8 out of 10 patients who commit suicide talked about it with someone before completing the act. Often the person they talk with is a health care professional. The problem is that care providers often miss the signs and symptoms of depression and the subtle indicators of self-destructive intentions.

There is evidence, for example, that 60% of people who complete and attempt suicide visit primary care providers within 3 months before their attempt, and 30% within 1 month of their attempt (Pirkis & Burgess, 1998). Among the elderly, more than 80% give clues of their intent. Of the elderly who commit suicide, 75% are known to have visited their personal physician in the month before they took their life (Pearson et al, 1997). In one study, health-care professionals reported a surprisingly small amount of probing for depressive or suicidal symptoms, even when they were mentioned by the patient. Most interesting, patients 55 and older, who were possibly at the highest risk, reported no health professional inquiries about suicidal thinking and perceived the least amount of attention or interest in their mental state (Skoog et al, 1996). It thus appears that much work needs to be done to alert health-care providers to the severity and extent of this problem and to help them to better evaluate patients for potential self-destructive responses.

---

tients is whether they think they can control their behavior and refrain from acting on their impulses. If patients cannot do this, immediate psychiatric hospitalization is indicated.

Finally, the nurse may find it helpful to use an assessment tool to explore self-protective responses such as the one for inpatient settings presented in Fig. 21-3. Box 21-1 lists behavioral rating scales that can be used in any setting with the suicidal patient.

Predisposing Factors

No one theory explains self-destructive responses or guides therapeutic intervention. Behavior theory suggests that self-injury is learned and reinforced in childhood or adolescence. Psychological theory focuses on problems in early stages of ego development, suggesting that early interpersonal trauma and unmanaged anxiety may provoke episodes of self-injury. Interpersonal theory proposes that self-injury may result from interactions that leave the child feeling guilty and worthless. A history of abuse or incest may then precipitate self-destructiveness if negative perceptions have been internalized and acted upon and there is a lack of secure attachments. Other predisposing factors related to self-destructive behavior include the inability to communicate needs and feelings verbally; feelings of guilt, depression, and deperson-

alization; and fluctuating emotions.

Five predisposing factors—psychiatric diagnosis, personality traits and disorders, psychosocial and environmental factors, genetic and familial variables, and biochemical factors—contribute to a biopsychosocial model for understanding self-destructive behavior over the life cycle (Hall et al, 1999; Mann et al, 1999).

Psychiatric Diagnosis. More than 90% of adults who end their lives by suicide have an associated psychiatric illness (Beautrais et al, 1996). There are three broad psychiatric disorders that put people at particular risk for suicide:

- Mood disorders
- Substance abuse
- Schizophrenia

Recent studies suggest that patients with panic disorder also have increased risk of suicide, and adolescents who kill themselves tend to have depression and conduct disorders. In addition, a high percentage of these youth abused alcohol or drugs (Bloch, 1999).

Suicide is the most serious complication of mood disorders, with 15% of those with these illnesses ending their lives by suicide. Suicide is particularly common in depressed elderly men (Conwell et al, 1996). Patients with bipolar disorder and psychotic depression are at greatest risk (Simpson & Jamison, 1999). Alcohol use is associated with 25% to 50% of suicides (Pages et al, 1997). Among patients who are alcohol dependent, suicide often occurs late in the disease and is

INPATIENT SUICIDE/SELF-HARM ASSESSMENT

Complete on admission if indicated by Risk Factor Assessment or any time when suicidal risk is suspected.

Directions: 1.   Answer Question I.
2.   Complete Section II by circling one of the three descriptors for each Key Factor that BEST describes the patient.
3.   Complete Section III.
4.   Add the points for each circled item in Sections I, II, and III to obtain the total score.

I. Is the current admission precipitated by suicide attempt?		Yes 2 No 1	
II. Key Factors	**High Risk** (1:1)	**Moderate Risk** (q15min observation)	**No Precautions**
Contract for safety	Unwilling to contract OR Unable to contract because of impaired reality testing (hallucinations, delusions, dementia, delirium, dissociation) 2	Contracts but is ambivalent or guarded 1	Reliably contracts for safety 0
Suicide plan	Has plan with actual or potential access to planned method 2	Has plan without access to planned method 1	No plan 0
Plan lethality	Highly lethal plan (gun, hanging, jumping, carbon monoxide) 2	Medium lethality of plan (sleeping pills, overdose of aspirin, barbiturates) 1	Low lethality of plan (superficial scratching, head banging, pillow over face, biting, holding breath) 0
Elopement risk	High elopement risk 2	Low elopement risk 1	No elopement risk 0
Suicidal ideation	Constant suicidal thoughts 2	Intermittent or fleeting suicidal thoughts 1	No current suicidal thoughts 0
Attempt history	Past attempts of high lethality 2	Past attempts of low lethality 1	No previous attempts 0
Symptoms (circle those that apply) hopelessness helplessness anhedonia guilt/shame anger/hostility impulsivity impaired problem solving	5-6 symptoms present 2	3-4 symptoms present 1	0-2 symptoms present 0
Current morbid thoughts (reunion fantasies, preoccupation with death, disturbing nightmares)	Constantly 2	Frequently 1	Rarely 0
III. RN's Subjective Appraisal of Patient's Reliability:	Pt. replies not trustworthy; several nonverbal cues		4
	Pt. replies questionably, trustworthy, at least one nonverbal cue		3
	Pt. replies trustworthy		0

Scoring Key: High Risk Precautions   =   10 or more   Total Score   _____
(1:1)

             Moderate Risk Precautions   =   4-9   Assessed by (RN):   _____
(q15min observation)

             Moderate Risk Precautions   =   4-9   Date: _____

             No Precautions   =   0-3   Time: _____

Fig. 21-3   Inpatient suicide/self-harm assessment.

often related to some interpersonal loss or the onset of medical complications.

Schizophrenia, a disease that affects 1% of the population, carries a high incidence of suicide. Among these patients, 40% report suicidal thoughts, 20% to 40% make unsuccessful suicide attempts, and 9% to 13% end their lives by suicide (Meltzer, 1998). The risk is greatest for patients under age 40 who feel hopeless; fear mental disintegration; and had a greater number of depressive episodes, an earlier age of onset of their illness, and an earlier age of first hospitalization (Gupta et al, 1998).

Personality Traits. The three aspects of personality that are most closely associated with increased risk of suicide are hostility, impulsivity, and depression. These traits are important because they cross diagnostic groups. In addition, borderline personality disorder (Brodsky et al, 1997) and antisocial personality disorder are more highly correlated with suicidal behavior (see Chapter 23). The co-existence of antisocial and depressive symptoms appears to be a particularly lethal combination in both adults and young people. The association between hostility and suicide stems from the notion proposed by Freud that the suicidal person turns rage inward against the self. Other studies have found that suicidal people are more socially withdrawn, have lower self-esteem, are less trusting of others, expect bad things to happen to them, feel powerless over their lives, and have a rigid and inflexible way of thinking.

How might the personality traits of hostility, impulsivity, and depression contribute to the development of substance abuse?

Psychosocial Milieu. This domain is concerned with social supports, life events, and chronic medical illnesses. Recent bereavement, separation or divorce, early loss, and decreased social supports are all important factors related to potential suicide. Precipitants of suicidal behavior are often humiliating life events such as interpersonal problems, public embarrassment, loss of a job, or the threat of jail. Evidence also shows that knowing someone who attempted or committed suicide or exposure to suicide through the media may make one more vulnerable to self-destructive behavior. This appears to be a particularly important factor in cluster suicides.

The strength of social supports is also important. There is good evidence that the strength and quality of these supports are important to the etiology of psychiatric problems, compliance with treatment, and response to therapeutic interventions. Finally, diseases with chronic and debilitating courses often precipitate self-destructive behavior. The prevalence of physical illness varies from 25% to 70% of suicides and appears to be an important factor in 11% to 51%. Among the disorders most often associated with suicide are cancer, Huntington's chorea, epilepsy, musculoskeletal disorders, peptic ulcer disease, and HIV/AIDS.

Family History. A family history of suicide is a significant risk factor for self-destructive behavior (Russ et al,

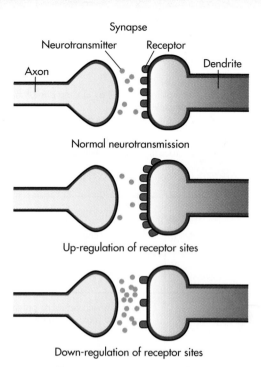

Fig. 21-4 Levels of postsynaptic serotonin (5HT) receptors. There are more receptors when there is too little serotonin (up-regulation) and fewer receptors when there is too much serotonin (down-regulation).

1999). Explanations for this association include identification with and imitation of a family member who has committed suicide, family stress, and transmission of genetic factors. Families of suicide victims have a significantly higher rate of suicide than do families with members who are nonsuicidal but mentally ill. In addition, monozygotic twins have a higher concordance rate for suicide than dizygotic twins.

Biochemical Factors. There is growing evidence of an association between suicide or suicidal tendencies and a low level of the brain neurotransmitter serotonin (5HT). Recent interest in the role of 5HT levels and activity in suicide stems from two main areas of study: an increase in the understanding of abnormal serotonin transmission in the etiology of mental illness, particularly depression and schizophrenia, and a better appreciation that antidepressant drugs enhance the efficacy of serotonin (Mann et al, 1999).

This suggests that 5HT must be in balance for adaptive emotional responses. This balance can be assessed by measuring the amounts of neurotransmitter produced, and the amount of its metabolites (the leftover products of neurotransmitter breakdown, or turnover). Thus, the amount of the metabolite for serotonin, 5HIAA, that can be measured in the blood and spinal fluid is an indication of the amount of serotonin originally available in the brain.

The brain also attempts to regulate or balance neurotransmitter levels in another way. The number of postsynaptic 5HT receptors in the brain is affected by the available levels of 5HT. There are more of these receptors if there is too little 5HT (up-regulation) and fewer of them if there is too much 5HT (down-regulation) (Fig. 21-4). Mood disorders are hypothesized to be the result of an imbalance or deficiency of neurotransmitters, particularly 5HT. Antidepressant drugs generally increase the amount or efficiency of 5HT, thus increasing the amount of metabolites and affecting the numbers of 5HT receptors.

A deficiency in serotonin and its metabolite, 5HIAA, and an increase in one of the 5HT postsynaptic receptors ($5HT_{2A}$) are implicated in suicidal behavior. For example, depressed patients with low serotonin levels have stronger suicidal tendencies than those with normal levels. Among people hospitalized for violent suicide attempts, those with low levels of 5HIAA in their spinal fluid are 10 times more likely to kill themselves within a year. Similarly, schizophrenic patients who have attempted suicide have significantly lower 5-HIAA concentrations than those who do not.

In postmortem studies of the brains of suicide victims, researchers have discovered decreased serotonin activity in the ventrolateral prefrontal cortex. Finally, a combination of impulsive aggressiveness and feelings of hopelessness, associated with serotonin deficiency, is more common in men than in women. This may explain why men kill themselves much more often even though women have a higher rate of depression.

Because of the increased rate of suicide globally and the high suicide risk in psychiatric patients, it would be beneficial to be able to identify high-risk people for suicide prevention and treatment. Thus, in addition to demographic, psychosocial, personality, and behavioral indicators for suicide risk, a simple blood test that could provide an additional method for identifying those at greatest risk for suicide would be a significant advantage for the mental health field. Although there is currently no biological test that shows a differentiation between people who commit suicide and those who do not, there is a great deal of interest in finding such a biological marker for suicide. Neuroimaging techniques, such as PET scans, also offer an opportunity to visualize serotonin function in vivo in more direct ways than has been previously available. This technology and emerging genetic research may provide the possibility of timely therapeutic intervention in patients at high risk for suicide.

 Do you believe suicide is a fundamental human right and should be allowed by society? Why or why not?

Precipitating Stressors

Self-destructive behavior may result from any stress the person feels as overwhelming (see Citing the Evidence). Stressors are somewhat individualized, as is the person's ability to tolerate stress. All self-destructive behaviors may be seen as attempts to escape from uncomfortable or intolerable life situations. Anxiety is therefore central to self-destructive behavior.

The anxiety associated with a deliberate attempt at self-destruction is overwhelming. It is difficult to imagine if it has not been experienced. Most people cringe from contemplating their own deaths, much less initiating self-destruction. Self-death is experienced differently from the death of

---

Citing the Evidence on

Suicide and Stress

BACKGROUND: Among the victims of floods, earthquakes and hurricanes, there is an increased prevalence of post-traumatic stress disorder (PTSD) and depression, which are risk factors for suicidal thinking. This study was conducted to determine whether natural disasters affect suicide rates.

RESULTS: Suicide rates increased in the four years after floods; in the two years after hurricanes; and in the first year after earthquakes. The increases for suicide rates were found for both sexes and for all age groups. The suicide rates did not change significantly after tornadoes or severe storms.

IMPLICATIONS: Mental health support is needed after severe disasters. It should be available for varying periods of time and take into account the needs of the different age groups. Prevention could include providing social support and facilitating aid to victims. In addition, disaster prone areas could be targeted for programs that reduce the conditions that predispose people to commit suicide.

Krug E et al: Suicide after natural disasters, *New Engl J Med* 338(6): 373, 1998.

---

another because self-death literally cannot be experienced. In a sense, those who destroy themselves actually destroy everything else but themselves.

In contrast, people engaged in gradual self-destructive behavior tend to deny their eventual deaths, usually believing that they can assume control at any time. This fantasy of control, although it relieves anxiety, also helps to perpetuate the behavior. When the sense of self-worth is extremely low, self-destructive behavior reaches its peak. At this point, suicidal behavior is likely. Suicide implies a loss of the ability to value the self at all.

Appraisal of Stressors

Suicide prediction is not possible to any meaningful degree (Hughes, 1995; Kessler et al, 1999). What is possible and essential is for the nurse to assess each patient for the suicidal risk factors listed in Box 21-2. In addition, risk factors for suicide in special populations are presented in Box 21-3.

Coping Resources

Patients with chronic, painful, or life-threatening illnesses may engage in self-destructive behavior. Often these people consciously choose to kill themselves. Quality of life becomes an issue that overrides quantity of life. An ethical dilemma may arise for nurses who become aware of the patient's choice to engage in this behavior. There are no easy answers to the question of how to resolve this conflict

Box **21-2**

Risk Factors in the Assessment of the Self-Destructive Patient

ASSESSING CIRCUMSTANCES OF AN ATTEMPT

Precipitating humiliating life event
Preparatory actions: acquiring a method, putting affairs in order, suicide talk, giving away prized possessions, suicide note
Use of violent method or more lethal drugs/poisons
Understanding of lethality of chosen method
Precautions taken against discovery

PRESENTING SYMPTOMS

Hopelessness
Helplessness
Self-reproach, feelings of failure and unworthiness
Depressed mood
Impaired problem solving
Agitation and restlessness
Persistent insomnia
Weight loss
Slowed speech, fatigue, social withdrawal
Suicidal thoughts and plans

PSYCHIATRIC ILLNESS

Previous suicide attempt
Mood disorders
Alcoholism or other substance abuse

Borderline or antisocial personality disorder
Schizophrenia
Panic disorder
Conduct disorders and depression in adolescents
Early dementia and confusional states in the elderly
Combinations of these illnesses

PSYCHOSOCIAL HISTORY

Recently separated, divorced, or bereaved
Lives alone
Unemployed, recent job change or loss
Multiple life stresses (move, early loss, breakup of important relationship, school problems, threat of disciplinary crisis)
Chronic medical illness
Excessive drinking or substance abuse

PERSONALITY FACTORS

Impulsivity, aggressivity, hostility
Cognitive rigidity and negativity
Low self-esteem

FAMILY HISTORY

Family history of suicidal behavior
Family history of mood disorder, alcoholism, or both

Box **21-3**

Risk Factors for Suicide in Special Populations

IN HOSPITALIZED DEPRESSED PATIENTS

- High levels of anxiety
- First week of admission
- First month after discharge

IN OLDER PATIENTS

- Death of a loved one

IN ALCOHOLICS

- Loss of a close relationship within 6 weeks
- Concurrent use of other drugs
- Late in the course of illness

IN DEPRESSED ADOLESCENTS

- Comorbid substance abuse
- Prior suicide attempt
- Family history of major depression
- Previous antidepressant treatment
- History of legal problems
- Handgun available in the house

(Rosenbluth et al, 1995). Nurses must do so according to their own belief system.

Self-destructive behavior may be related to many social and cultural factors. The structure of society has a great influence on the individual. Society may either help or sustain individuals or lead them to self-destruction (see A Patient Speaks). Social isolation may lead to loneliness and increase the person's vulnerability to suicide. People who are actively involved with others in their communities are more able to tolerate stress. Those who do not participate in social activities are more likely to turn to self-destructive behavior. Religious involvement is particularly supportive to many people during difficult times.

> *Did you know that the U.S. suicide rate of 30,000 people per year is higher than the homicide rate, which was 17,000 in 1998? That means once every 17 minutes an American commits suicide. Do you think this fact requires a reallocation of social resources? If so, in what way?*

Coping Mechanisms

A patient may use a variety of coping mechanisms to deal with self-destructive feelings, including denial, rationalization, and regression. In addition, the patient might display magical thinking. These coping mechanisms may stand between the person and self-destruction. They defend the person from strong emotional responses to life events that are a serious threat to the ego. If they are removed, underlying depression will become overt and may lead to suicidal behavior.

Suicidal behavior indicates the imminent failure of the coping mechanisms. A suicidal threat may be a last-ditch effort to get enough help to be able to cope. Completed suicide represents the total failure of adaptive coping mechanisms.

A Patient Speaks

The following are notes left by patients who committed suicide.

- *Please forgive me and please forget me. I'll always love you. All I have was yours. No one ever did more for me than you; oh please pray for me, please.*

- *To Whom It May Concern,*
  I, Mary Smith, being of sound mind, do this day make my last will as follows: I bequeath my rings, diamond and black opal to my daughter-in-law, Doris Jones, and any other of my personal belongings she might wish. What money I have in my savings account and my checking account goes to my dear father, as he won't have me to help him. To my husband, Ed Smith, I leave my furniture and car.

- *I hate you and all of your family and I hope you never have peace of mind. I hope I haunt this house as long as you live here and I wish you all the bad luck in the world.*

- *Dear Daddy:*
  Please don't grieve for me or feel that you did something wrong, you didn't. I'll leave this life loving you and remembering the world's greatest father. I'm sorry to cause you more heartache, but the reason I can't live anymore is because I'm afraid. Afraid of facing my life alone without love. No one ever knew how alone I am. No one ever stood by me when I needed help. No one brushed away the tears. I cried for "help" and no one heard. I love you Daddy, Jeannie.

NURSING DIAGNOSIS

When considering the nursing diagnosis of self-destructive behavior, the nurse must incorporate information about the seriousness and immediacy of the patient's harmful activity. The nurse must consider the information obtained in the assessment to identify accurately the patient's need for nursing intervention (Fig. 21-5). Validation of the nursing diagnosis with the patient is essential. However, denial is a prominent defense with most self-destructive disorders. The patient may not be able to agree with a statement that confronts this behavior. The primary concern is to communicate, through the diagnosis, the level of protection the patient needs. In the case of self-destructive behavior, caution is recommended in determining the level of risk. It is better to overestimate the patient's level of risk than to allow serious injury to occur.

Primary NANDA nursing diagnoses related to maladaptive self-protective responses are **risk for self-mutilation, noncompliance,** and **risk for self-directed violence.** Because of the nature of the disorders associated with self-destructive behavior, other nursing diagnoses are often applied in the care of these patients. Nursing diagnoses related to the range of possible maladaptive responses are listed in the Medical

and Nursing Diagnoses box on p. 392. Examples of complete nursing diagnoses related to self-protective responses are presented in the Detailed Diagnoses box on p. 393.

Related Medical Diagnoses

Suicidal behavior is not identified as a separate diagnostic category in *DSM–IV–TR* (American Psychiatric Association, 2000). Several medical diagnostic classifications of the *DSM–IV–TR* include actual or potential self-destructive behavior among their defining criteria. The medical diagnoses in which this behavior is listed as possible include bipolar disorder, major depression, noncompliance with treatment, schizophrenia, and substance use disorders. Their essential features are described in the Detailed Diagnoses box on p. 393.

OUTCOME IDENTIFICATION

The expected outcome when working with a patient with maladaptive self-protection responses is as follows:
The patient will not physically harm oneself.

Careful setting of priorities is necessary with the self-destructive patient. Highest priority should be given to preservation of life. The nurse must identify goals related to immediately life-threatening behavior. For example, the actively suicidal person must first be prevented from acting on impulses.

In dealing with self-destructive behavior, the nurse and the patient may appear to have incompatible goals. Suicidal patients may resist attempts to protect them and may actively try to evade their observers. However, most of these patients have some ambivalence. The nurse, in setting positive, life-preserving goals, is appealing to the healthy part of the person's self that wants to survive and be better able to cope with life. The very act of seeking help is an expression of this healthy aspect of the personality. The positive attitude of the nurse in setting constructive goals conveys a sense of hope to a patient who may be feeling hopeless. Communicating hope is often the most therapeutic element in any nursing intervention with a suicidal patient.

PLANNING

The nursing care plan for the person with self-destructive behavior must focus first on protecting the patient from harm. In addition, the plan must address the factors that contributed to the patient's dangerous behavior. Later, the nurse can attend to the development of insight into the suicidal behavior and substitution of healthy coping mechanisms.

Suicidal patients can be treated in a variety of settings. The decision about which setting is most appropriate for a given patient is based on the assessment of risk. The algorithm presented in Fig. 21-6 on p. 394 begins with the issue of the nature of the suicidal ideation. People who seem very intent, have a specific plan for action, and cannot contract for safety should be admitted to an inpatient setting where they can be monitored closely. Another important factor in determining the treatment setting is the patient's judgment. Anything that impairs a patient's judgment and rational de-

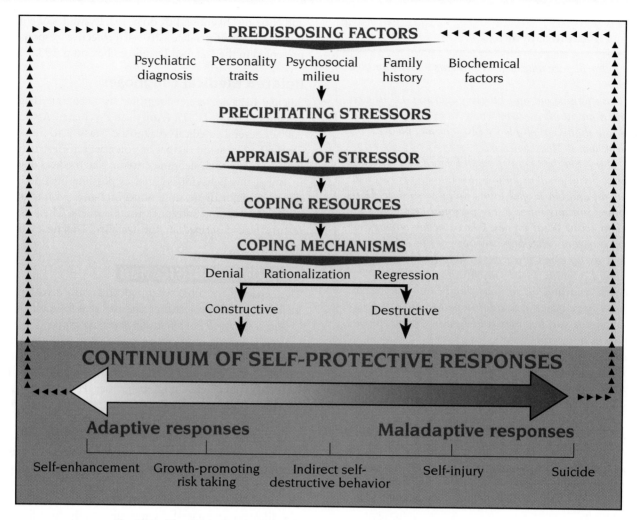

Fig. 21-5 The Stuart Stress Adaptation Model related to self-protective responses.

Medical and Nursing Diagnoses *related to* Self-Protective Responses

RELATED MEDICAL DIAGNOSES (*DSM–IV–TR*)*	RELATED NURSING DIAGNOSES (NANDA)†
Bipolar disorder	Adjustment, impaired
Major depressive disorder	Anxiety
Noncompliance with treatment	Body image disturbance
Schizophrenia	Coping, individual, ineffective
Substance use disorders	Denial, ineffective
	Noncompliance‡
	Self-esteem disturbance
	Self-mutilation, risk for‡
	Spiritual distress
	Violence, risk for self-directed‡

*Reprinted with permission from the *Diagnostic and statistical manual of mental disorders*, Fourth Edition, Text Revision. Copyright 2000. American Psychiatric Association.
†From North American Nursing Diagnosis Association: *NANDA nursing diagnoses: definitions and classifications 1999-2000*, Philadelphia, 1999, The Association.
‡Primary nursing diagnosis for self-destructive behavior.

cision-making capacity greatly increases the risk of a suicide attempt and is a good indication for inpatient treatment. Another issue is the availability of a responsible family member or close friend willing to stay with the patient through the immediate crisis until the suicidal ideation abates. Sometimes this may require several family members taking shifts and watching the patient around the clock. In the final analysis, however, the safety of the patient is the top priority.

Detailed Diagnoses *related to* Self-Protective Responses

NANDA DIAGNOSIS STEM	EXAMPLES OF COMPLETE DIAGNOSIS
Risk for self-mutilation	Risk for self-mutilation related to feelings of tension and worthlessness, as evidenced by cutting of arms and legs
	Risk for self-mutilation related to command hallucinations, as evidenced by dissection of calf
Noncompliance	Noncompliance with taking antihypertensive medication related to asymptomatic behavior, as evidenced by unchanged elevation of blood pressure
	Noncompliance with 1800-calorie-per-day diabetic diet related to denial of illness, as evidenced by gain of 10 pounds since last clinic visit
Risk for self-directed violence	Risk for self-directed violence related to loss of spouse, as evidenced by purchase of a gun and discussions of death
	Risk for self-directed violence related to phencyclidine (PCP) abuse, as evidenced by extreme psychotic disorganization and lack of body boundaries

DSM–IV–TR DIAGNOSIS	ESSENTIAL FEATURES*
Bipolar disorder	Presence of a manic episode and no past depressive episodes (see Chapter 19 for details)
Major depressive disorder	The presence of at least five symptoms nearly every day during the same 2-week period, with one being either depressed mood or loss of interest or pleasure (see Chapter 19 for details)
Noncompliance with treatment	Noncompliance with an important aspect of the treatment for a mental disorder or a general medical condition
Schizophrenia	Presence of two or more of the following symptoms for a 1-month period: delusions, hallucinations, disorganized speech, disorganized behavior, negative symptoms (see Chapter 22 for details)
Substance use disorders	Presence of substance dependence or substance abuse (see Chapter 25 for details)

*Reprinted with permission from the *Diagnostic and statistical manual of mental disorders*, Fourth Edition, Text Revision. Copyright 2000. American Psychiatric Association.

IMPLEMENTATION

Common elements exist in nursing intervention with all patients who exhibit self-destructive behavior. First, nurses must consider their own responses to people who are trying to harm themselves. It can be difficult for a person who is happy and involved in life to imagine the depth of despair that leads to suicidal impulses or the lack of caring for the self that results in physically, psychologically, and socially damaging behavior, even if not immediately lethal. On the other hand, nurses who are depressed and dissatisfied with their own life may be threatened by interacting with patients who are more upset because they may fear similar consequences for themselves. These nurses may also overidentify with the patient, which limits their ability to help. A therapeutic approach is empathic and nonjudgmental, with subjective responses limited by awareness of one's own attitudes.

All possible efforts must be made to protect patients and to motivate them to choose life. Nurses should align themselves with the patients' wish to live and then help them to be responsible for their own behavior. However, nurses must also understand that some patients will choose death despite their best efforts to intervene. Nurses must therefore develop a realistic understanding of the patient's responsibility for his or her own life and accept the possibility of losing a suicidal patient even with the best nursing care.

 A friend tells you that suicidal patients are intent on dying and will ultimately succeed despite all intervention. How would you respond?

Protection

The highest priority nursing activity with self-destructive patients is to protect them from inflicting further harm on themselves and, if suicidal, from killing themselves. Lawsuits related to suicides began to increase in the 1980s and are now one of the most common reasons for litigation against nurses and hospitals (Wysoker, 1999). The message of protection is conveyed to patients verbally and nonverbally.

Verbally, patients are informed of the nurse's intention not to allow harm to come to them. The nurse might say, "I understand that you are feeling impulses to harm yourself. I will be here with you to help you control those impulses. I will do whatever is necessary to protect you. I'd like to talk with you about how you are feeling whenever you are able to share that with me."

The nonverbal communication should reinforce and agree with the verbal. Obviously, dangerous objects such as belts, sharp implements, glass, and matches should be taken from the suicidal patient. It is impossible to make an environment perfectly safe. Even walls and floors can cause injury if patients throw themselves against them.

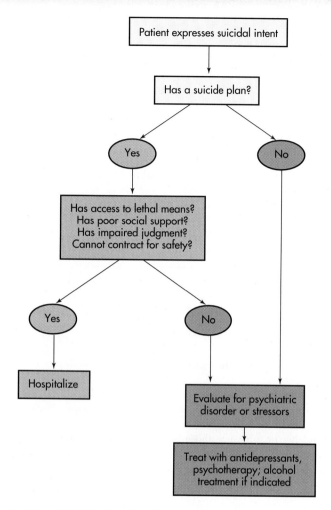

Fig. 21-6 Clinical algorithm for planning treatment for the suicidal patient.

Citing the Evidence on

Safety

BACKGROUND: Constant observation is a staff-intensive, costly intervention that entails continuous supervision of suicidal inpatients until they no longer express suicidal intent or behavior. This qualitative study explored patients' experiences of constant observation to determine whether they derived any therapeutic benefits beyond the intended protective benefit.

RESULTS: Thirteen of the 20 participants expressed positive feelings toward observers, particularly when they perceived them as friendly and willing to help. Therapeutic benefits other than protection were related to observers who were optimistic, who acknowledged the patient as a human being, who provided distraction with activities and conversation, and who gave emotional support. Nontherapeutic aspects were observers' lack of empathy, lack of acknowledgment, and failure to provide information about constant observation, as well as a lack of privacy and a feeling of confinement.

IMPLICATIONS: Constant observation can be enhanced if observers engage patients in actively supportive interventions. However observers' perceived attitudes and behaviors can also cause patients distress, which reaffirms the need for careful supervision of observers.

Cardell R, Pituala C: Suicidal inpatients' perceptions of therapeutic and nontherapeutic aspects of constant observation, *Psych Services* 50(8): 1066, 1999.

However, the removal of dangerous objects gives a message of concern.

One-to-one observation of the suicidal patient also communicates caring. This observation should be carried out sensitively, with the nurse neither hovering over nor remaining aloof from the patient (see Citing the Evidence on Safety). The patient's nonverbal cues can guide the one-to-one interaction. It is important to remain alert until the mental health team and the patient agree that the self-destructive crisis is over.

Suicidal patients may appear to be feeling much better immediately before making an attempt. This is due to the feeling of relief experienced when the decision has been made and the plans finalized. Nurses have been fooled by this behavior pattern, relaxing their vigilance, only to have patients kill themselves when they are allowed to be alone for a moment.

Contracting for Safety

An important aspect of protecting the patient involves coming to an agreement about the nature of the therapeutic relationship (see Citing the Evidence on No-Suicide Contracts). This can involve the use of contracts in which the patient agrees not to inflict self-harm for a specified period of time

(Egan et al, 1997; Goin, 1998). The patient further agrees to contact the clinician if he or she is tempted to act on self-destructive impulses. The patient also agrees to give away any possibly lethal articles such as guns or pills. Hospitalization is indicated if the patient is not willing to agree to these terms. Outpatients and clinicians need names and telephone numbers to cover any emergencies. Finally, supportive others should be involved in the contracting process. Families and friends are important allies in caring for a suicidal patient.

After a trustworthy contract has been made, the nurse can take some additional steps to ensure the patient's safety. First, the patient should be supervised at all times. The patient should never be left alone. Second, the nurse can monitor any medications the patient receives. For example, some antidepressants are fatal in overdose. This suggests that the patient should have only a few days' supply if treated as an outpatient. The nurse should note that tricyclic antidepressants are associated with a higher rate of death in the event of overdose than the newer SSRI antidepressants. The nurse should also be prepared to inform patients and families that, contrary to what is discussed in the media, fluoxetine (Prozac) decreases rather than increases the risk of suicide (Leon et al, 1999). In con-

Citing the Evidence on

No-Suicide Contracts

BACKGROUND: Many people hospitalized on psychiatric units are at high risk of suicide. Among the strategies recommended for suicide prevention is the negotiation of a no-suicide or no-harm contract. In spite of the conventional acceptance of these interventions, there is little research done in this area.

RESULTS: No-suicide contracts were used by 79% of the hospitals. Contracts were generally negotiated after suicidal ideation was expressed, after self-harm, or after a patient was admitted who had made a suicidal attempt. In all but one hospital, nurses negotiated contracts with patients. Contracts were usually verbal or handwritten rather than preprinted.

IMPLICATIONS: No-suicide contracting is a common nursing practice in psychiatric inpatient settings. Contracts are not indiscriminately used but are negotiated when high suicide risk is assessed.

Drew B: No-suicide contracts to prevent suicidal behavior in inpatient psychiatric settings, *J Am Psych Nurses Assoc* 5(1): 23, 1999.

trast, the benzodiazepines may disinhibit a patient, resulting in less control over self-destructive impulses (see Chapter 28).

Your depressed patient has been prescribed a tricyclic antidepressant because it is less expensive than the newer antidepressants. However, she lives in a rural area and cannot have the prescription filled every few days. You are worried about potential overdose. What alternatives can you identify?

Increasing Self-Esteem

Self-destructive people have low self-esteem. The nurse may intervene by treating the patient as someone deserving attention and concern. Positive attributes of the patient should be recognized with genuine praise. An attempt to make up reasons to praise the patient is usually recognized as artificial and lowers the patient's self-esteem. The message is that the patient is so bad that one has to search for positive characteristics. When getting to know the patient, the nurse should be alert to strengths that can be built on to provide the patient with positive experiences. It is also important to reinforce reasons for living and promote the patient's realistic expectations. Chapter 19 describes interventions the nurse can use to enhance a patient's self-esteem.

Regulating Emotions and Behaviors

Nursing care should also be directed toward helping patients become aware of their feelings, label them, and express them appropriately. Anger is often a difficult feeling for these patients. The angry patient must be helped to deal constructively with anger through anger management skills. These are described in Chapter 31. Anxiety can also be overwhelming. Chapter 17 discusses anxiety-reducing interventions.

It may be helpful to assist patients with self-destructive responses to explore the predisposing and precipitating factors influencing their behavior. Once the acute crisis is over, the nurse can help the patient understand high-risk times and triggers, the feelings that are stimulated, dysfunctional thinking patterns, and resultant maladaptive coping responses (Reilly, 1998). Plans can then be made to test out new coping mechanisms. For instance, during times of stress, the patient can do the following:

- Increase involvement with others
- Initiate a physical activity
- Engage in relaxation and tension-reducing activities
- Process feelings by talking with someone or writing in a journal

These and other examples of cognitive behavioral strategies are described in Chapter 32

Mobilizing Social Support

Self-destructive behavior often reflects a lack of internal and external resources. Mobilization of social support systems is an important aspect of nursing intervention. Significant others probably have many feelings about the patient's self-destructive behavior. They need an opportunity to express their feelings and make realistic plans for the future. Family members must be made aware of control issues and helped to encourage self-control by the patient. Both the patient and the family may need help to see that caring can be expressed by fostering self-care, as well as by providing care.

Families of suicidal patients may be frightened of future suicidal activity. They need to be aware of behavioral clues to suicide and of community resources that can help with crises. Suicidal behavior often recurs. False reassurance should be avoided. A better approach is to foster improved communication and an ability to cope in the family. The nurse may help people sort out their feelings and may want to refer significant others for individual intervention or family therapy.

If a patient commits suicide, it is important to intervene with the survivors, who may themselves be at risk for suicidal behavior (Constantino & Bricker, 1996). They need someone who can listen to them and let them know that their feelings are not abnormal. They need to be able to discuss their beliefs about why the death occurred and helped to find some meaning in the experience. Family members should be encouraged to support one another. Survivors are often stigmatized and may need assistance in dealing with this.

Community resources may also be important for the long-term care of the self-destructive person. Self-help groups may provide the recovering patient with needed peer support. Family therapy may help in the reintegration of a family group that has been disrupted by the patient's recent experiences. Public health nurses, clergy, and other community-based helping people can provide the patient and family with day-to-day support. The nurse may be active in explaining resources to the patient and initiating referrals to other agencies.

Patient Education

Patient education is an important nursing intervention. Education must be timed carefully. Patient readiness is essential if behavior change is to result. Patients who are noncompliant with prescribed health-care regimens may not understand the nature of their problem. The nurse should assess the patient's knowledge and initiate appropriate teaching. A Patient Education Plan for a patient who is noncompliant with medical treatment is presented below. Many patients are willing to participate in self-care if it makes sense to them. Teaching ways to monitor health status may also be helpful. For example, if hypertensive patients learn to check their blood pressure, they can learn to associate their health care activities with their physiological response.

Patients following medication regimens, such as psychotropic medication for the previously suicidal patient, should know the prescribed dosage, frequency, and side effects. Information about how to handle any future crises should be provided to the patient. If the nurse has explained the possible reason for the patient's behavior, this may be reinforced at termination of the relationship to help the patient integrate the experience into his or her self-concept. Helping a patient to work through self-destructive behavior can be an extremely rewarding aspect of psychiatric nursing.

Suicide Prevention

In 1999 the Surgeon General released a *Call to Action to Prevent Suicide,* which introduced a blueprint for reducing suicide in the United States. As both evidence-based and highly prioritized by leading experts, the 15 key recommendations from the report are listed in Box 21-4. The 15 key recommendations are intended to serve as a framework for immediate action and are categorized as Awareness, Intervention, and Methodology, or AIM.

Nurses, in particular, need to be aware of several specific strategies that may help to prevent suicide. These are listed in Box 21-5. Educational measures and suicide curricula in schools are other helpful interventions. These programs try to break down taboos about suicide and describe the symptoms of depression to students, teachers, and parents (Shaffer & Craft, 1999). The development of prevention clinics in communities may also be helpful. Such clinics might offer expert clinical assessment and treatment combined with strong community links, increased social supports, family education, and hotlines staffed with mental health professionals. Another effective suicide prevention strategy is telephone services to the elderly that provide home assistance, need assessment, and emotional support (DeLeo et al, 1995). In addition, education of the public and health-care providers is needed to increase knowledge about the early warning signs of self-destructive behavior and implement effective treatment strategies. A Nursing Treatment Plan Summary for patients with maladaptive self-protective responses is presented on p. 398.

EVALUATION

Evaluation of the nursing care of the self-destructive patient requires careful daily monitoring of the patient's behavior. Patient involvement in evaluation of his or her progress can provide reinforcement and an incentive to work toward a

 PATIENT EDUCATION PLAN   *Compliance Counseling*

CONTENT	INSTRUCTIONAL ACTIVITIES	EVALUATION
Assess patient's knowledge of self-care activities.	Ask patient to describe usual diet, exercise, and medication patterns. Validate whether described behaviors match self-care instruction received in the past.	Patient describes usual behavior. Patient repeats directions.
Identify areas in which patient behavior differs from healthy self-care practices.	Describe healthy self-care behavior to patient, provide written patient education materials, encourage patient to describe reasons for not performing recommended self-care.	Patient discusses compliance problems.
Discuss alternative approaches to self-care.	Help patient to identify alternative self-care behaviors that would be more acceptable. Enable patient to talk about feelings related to illness and treatment regimen.	Patient decides on different approach and shares feelings related to illness.
Agree on a reward for compliant behavior.	Ask patient what reward he or she would choose for taking good care of him- or herself.	Patient identifies reward.
Reinforcement.	Praise patient for making a commitment to a healthier lifestyle.	Patient recognizes renewed commitment to self-care.

Box 21-4

Recommendations from the Surgeon General's Call to Action to Prevent Suicide, 1999

AWARENESS: Broaden the public's awareness of suicide and its risk factors.

- Promote public awareness that suicide is a public health problem and, as such, many suicides are preventable.
- Use information technology to make facts about suicide and suicide prevention widely and appropriately available to the general public and health-care providers.
- Expand awareness of and enhance access to resources for suicide prevention programs in communities.
- Develop and implement strategies to reduce the stigma associated with mental illness, substance abuse, and suicide and with seeking help for such problems.

INTERVENTION: Enhance services and programs, both population-based and clinical care.

- Extend collaboration with and between public and private sectors to complete a National Strategy for Suicide Prevention.
- Improve ability of primary care providers to recognize and treat depression, substance abuse, and other major mental illnesses associated with suicide risk.
- Increase the referral to specialty care when appropriate.
- Eliminate barriers in public and private insurance programs for provision of quality mental health treatments and create incentives to treat patients with coexisting mental and substance abuse disorders.
- Institute training for all health, mental health, and human service professionals (such as clergy, teachers, correctional workers, and social workers) concerning suicide risk assessment and recognition, treatment, management, and aftercare interventions.
- Develop and implement effective training programs for family members of those at risk and for natural community helpers on how to recognize, respond to, and refer people showing signs of suicide risk. Natural community helpers are people such as educators, coaches, hairdressers, and faith leaders, among others.

- Develop and implement safe and effective programs in educational settings for youth that address adolescent distress and crisis intervention and incorporate peer support for seeking help.
- Enhance community care resources by increasing the use of schools and workplaces as access points for mental and physical health services and providing comprehensive support programs for persons who survive the suicide of someone close to them.
- Promote a public/private collaboration with the media to ensure that entertainment and news coverage represent balanced and informed portrayals of suicide and its prevention, mental illness, and mental health care.

METHODOLOGY: Advance the science of suicide prevention.

- Enhance research to understand risk and protective factors, their interaction, and their effects on suicide and suicidal behaviors. Additionally, increase research on effective suicide prevention programs, clinical treatments for suicidal individuals, and culture-specific interventions.
- Develop additional scientific strategies for evaluating suicide prevention interventions and ensure that evaluation components are included in all suicide prevention programs.
- Establish mechanisms for federal, regional, and state interagency public health collaboration toward improving monitoring systems for suicide and suicidal behaviors and develop and promote standard terminology in these systems.
- Encourage the development and evaluation of new prevention technologies to reduce easy access to lethal means of suicide.

---

goal. Modifications of the care plan are often necessary as patients reveal more of themselves and their needs to the nurse.

Unfortunately, self-destructive behavior tends to recur. Nurses sometimes become discouraged and angry with patients who return again and again with the same behavior (Loughrey et al, 1997). When this occurs, nurses may be caught in the trap of feeling responsible for patient behavior. Nurses who have given the best nursing care possible have done as much as they can for the patient. It is impossible to change the total life situation for the patient. The nurse can only help to identify alternative behaviors and provide encouragement for change. If the patient returns, the nursing process must begin again with an attitude of hope that this time the patient will learn and grow more and be better able to live a satisfying life.

A final issue related to suicidal behavior is the impact of a completed suicide on the clinical staff. Psychiatric nurses will inevitably experience a patient suicide. When a patient commits suicide, staff response can split the interdiscipli-

Box 21-5

Suicide Prevention Strategies

- Gun control and decreased availability of lethal weapons
- Limitations on the sale and availability of alcohol and drugs
- Increased public and professional awareness about depression and suicide
- Less attention and reinforcement of suicidal behavior in the media
- Establishment of community-based crisis intervention clinics
- Campaigns to decrease the stigma associated with psychiatric care
- Increased insurance benefits for psychiatric and substance abuse disorders

NURSING TREATMENT PLAN *Summary*   *Maladaptive Self-Protective Responses*

NURSING DIAGNOSIS: Potential for self-directed violence
EXPECTED OUTCOME: The patient will not physically harm himself or herself.

SHORT-TERM GOAL	INTERVENTION	RATIONALE
The patient will not engage in self-injury activities.	Observe closely. Remove harmful objects. Provide a safeenvironment. Provide for basic physiological needs. Contract for safety if appropriate. Monitor medications.	Highest priority is given to life-saving patient care activities. The patient's behavior must be supervised until self-control is adequate for safety.
The patient will identify positive aspects of oneself.	Identify patient's strengths. Encourage the patient to participate in activities that he or she likes and does well. Encourage good hygiene and grooming. Foster healthy interpersonal relationships.	Self-destructive behavior reflects underlying depression related to low self-esteem and anger directed inward.
The patient will implement two adaptive self-protective responses.	Facilitate the awareness, labeling, and expression of feelings. Help the patient to recognize unhealthy coping mechanisms. Identify alternative means of coping. Reward healthy coping behaviors.	Maladaptive coping mechanisms must be replaced with healthy ones to manage stress and anxiety.
The patient will identify two social support resources that can be helpful.	Help significant others to communicate constructively with the patient. Promote healthy family relationships. Identify relevant community resources. Initiate referrals to community resources.	Social isolation leads to low self-esteem and depression, perpetuating self-destructive behavior.
The patient will be able to describe the treatment plan and its rationale.	Involve patient and significant others in care planning. Explain characteristics of identified health-care needs, nursing care needs, medical diagnosis, and recommended treatment and medications. Elicit response to nursing care plan. Modify plan based on patient feedback.	Understanding of and participation in health-care planning enhance compliance.

nary treatment team. Thus interventions must be aimed not only at helping the individual clinician heal, but also at preserving the integrity of the treatment team. The following activities can help this process (Bultema, 1994):

- Have an immediate review of the event by the treatment team to acknowledge feelings, and plan care for the other patients.
- Hold a patient community meeting to help patients accept the reality of the loss.
- Call an additional meeting of the treatment team 2 to 3 days after the suicide to further process the suicide.
- Conduct an in-house memorial service to facilitate grieving.
- Participate in a continuous quality improvement critical incident review to help staff understand the suicide and objectively review the treatment.
- Identify opportunities for continuous process improvement.

- Acknowledge anniversary reactions.
- If a variety of these activities are provided for the healing of other patients and the treatment team, recovery can occur and growth result.

Summary

1. The continuum of self-protective responses ranges from the most adaptive state of self-enhancement to the maladaptive responses of indirect self-destructive behavior, self-injury, and suicide.
2. Self-destructive behaviors may range from subtle to overt and include noncompliance with medical treatment plan, self-injury, and suicidal behavior.
3. Predisposing factors affecting self-protective responses include psychiatric diagnosis, personality traits, psychosocial milieu, family history, and biochemical factors. Precipitating stressors may be any stress the person perceives as overwhelming.

4. Coping resources focus on social support systems, and coping mechanisms may include denial, rationalization, and regression.
5. Primary nursing diagnoses are high risk for self-mutilation, noncompliance, and risk for self-directed violence.
6. Suicide is not identified as a separate diagnostic category in the *DSM–IV–TR*. Medical diagnostic classifications of the *DSM–IV–TR* that include actual or potential self-destructive behavior are bipolar disorder, major depression, schizophrenia, and substance use disorder.

7. The expected outcome of nursing care is that the patient will not physically harm himself or herself.
8. Nursing interventions include protecting the patient, contracting for safety, increasing self-esteem, regulating emotions and behaviors, mobilizing social support, educating the patient, and preventing suicide.
9. Evaluating nursing care requires daily monitoring of the patient's behavior. The nurse must not become discouraged if self-destructive behavior recurs, but approach the patient with the hope that this time the patient will grow and be better able to live a satisfying life.

Competent Caring A Clinical Exemplar of a Psychiatric Nurse

PHILIP MACAIONE, BS, RN

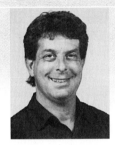

After 18 years of acute care nursing practice with a specialty in ICU, ER, and trauma nursing, I sought a new challenge and began psychiatric nursing practice. Having had the opportunity to associate professionally with hundreds of patients over the years who were experiencing critical and life-threatening situations, I felt well equipped to deal with psychiatric emergencies, until that seemingly routine day shift on an inpatient adult unit.

Ms. W had been committed to our unit as a dual-diagnosis patient. She was referred from our county emergency room. She had been found near-stuporous, wandering the city streets, and was thought to be homeless. She was addicted to heroin, cocaine, and alcohol. She also suffered from multiple personality disorder, anxiety disorder, major depression, and schizotypical disorder. She was 6'2" and weighed more than 300 pounds. Her hospital course over the previous week was highlighted by her continued acting-out behaviors. These included disrupting the milieu; verbal, physical, and sexual threats to others; seeking the medication of other patients; noncompliance with her treatment plan; and defiance of unit rules and policies. Needless to say, she was a nursing challenge and required a firm, consistent approach by the staff and a constant vigil over her behavior. One morning her behavior deteriorated to the point where staff intervened by placing her in scrubs and escorting her to the seclusion room to maintain her safety and that of the other patients. I explained to her that during this time-out I would help her to begin processing her behavior and identify more effective coping strategies. I gave her a PRN medication for her agitation and anxiety and suggested that she begin writing her thoughts and feelings down in her journal. After about a half hour, she verbally contracted for safety, seemed aware of her actions, and was resting quietly on her mattress. She also said that she was "feeling much better now" and thanked me for my help. I decided to put her on

15-minute checks but leave her in open-door seclusion until we agreed that she was ready to return to the milieu. I remember thinking, "Wow, I did a good job with this patient, and she is really making progress."

After years of nursing practice I notice that I have developed a sixth sense when I feel that something is just not right. On the surface Ms. W seemed to be in control, but my sixth sense drew me back to the seclusion room only minutes after I had left her. As I walked into the room I did a double take and thought to myself, "This can't be happening." Unfortunately, it was. Ms. W had managed, in the moments that had elapsed since I had left her side, to tear up her journal into small pieces, place the scraps between her legs, and ignite them with a cigarette lighter we later discovered she had hidden in her vagina. She was madly waving the fire between her legs to produce more flames. Her scrub pants and mattress were now on fire. At this point I just reacted. I ran to her, pulled away the mattress, patted down the flames on her pants, and yelled for help. The smoke alarm had gone off, and within seconds other staff arrived. I instructed them to remove the patient to the corridor and give her first aid. This was no easy task given the patient's size and level of agitation. I then activated the fire procedure, grabbed the fire extinguisher, and returned to the seclusion room. By now the smoke was thick, but I pulled the pin of the fire extinguisher, aimed, and released the foam. Within seconds, the fire was extinguished. The fire department had now arrived and moved in to deal with the smoldering mattress. Ms. W suffered no injuries and was discharged to a boarding house about 1 week later.

I learned a great deal from this incident and think I am a better nurse because of it. The staff response and teamwork in reacting to this crisis were extraordinary. I also think that the many years of critical decision-making opportunities afforded me throughout my nursing practice made me well equipped to handle this seemingly routine shift on our unit. Most of all, I have a greater appreciation and respect for the sixth sense of nurses, which may be the mark of truly competent nursing care.

Visit MERLIN: www.mosby.com/MERLIN/Stuart to find these additional materials and student activities.

- **Worksheets**
- **"Drug of the Month" Updates**
- **"Citing the Evidence" Updates**
- **Critical Thinking Activities and Exercises**
- **Annotated Suggested Readings**
- **Web Links**
- **More!**

Chapter Review Questions

1. Identify whether the following statements are true (T) or false (F).

_____ A. Suicide rates are highest for adolescent males.

_____ B. The most prominent behavior associated with noncompliance is refusal to admit the seriousness of the health problem.

_____ C. A suicide gesture is an attention-seeking behavior and should not be reinforced by focusing on it.

_____ D. Physical diseases with chronic and debilitating courses often precipitate self-destructive behavior.

_____ E. There is currently no biological test that is an accurate predictor of suicide.

_____ F. The newer SSRI antidepressant medications have a higher rate of death by overdose than the older tricyclics.

_____ G. Most people who commit suicide have sought medical help before their suicide attempt.

_____ H. Asking a person if he or she is planning to kill oneself will give the person the idea and lead to a suicide attempts.

2. Fill in the blanks.

A. The retrospective review of a person's behavior in the time preceding the suicide is called the

_____.

B. The psychiatric disorders that put people at particular risk for suicide are _____,

_____, and

_____.

C. Mood disorders are hypothesized to be the result of an imbalance or deficiency of neurotransmitters, particularly _____.

D. _____ is often the most therapeutic element in any nursing intervention with a suicidal patient.

E. The three personality traits most closely associated with increased risk of suicide are _____,

_____, and

_____.

F. When a patient agrees not to inflict self-harm for a specified period of time it is called

_____.

G. The _____ issued a *Call to Action to Prevent Suicide* in 1999.

3. Provide short answers for the following questions.

A. It has been observed that patients often act less depressed and seem to be in better spirits immediately before attempting suicide. Explain the reason for this behavior.

B. Identify the five factors to assess in the self-destructive patient.

C. Describe how you would determine the best treatment setting for a patient expressing suicidal thoughts.

D. There is currently much discussion about the wisdom and the ethics of assisted suicide. Discuss your position on this subject, first as a consumer of health care and then as a nurse.

REFERENCES

American Psychiatric Association: *Diagnostic and statistical manual of mental disorders,* Fourth Edition, Text Revision. Washington, DC, American Psychiatric Association, 2000.

Beautrais A et al: Prevalence and comorbidity of mental disorders in persons making serious suicide attempts: a case-control study, *Am J Psychiatry* 153:1009, 1996.

Bloch D: Adolescent suicide as a public health trust, *J Child Adol Psych Nurs* 13(1):26, 1999.

Brodsky B et al: Characteristics of borderline personality disorder associated with suicidal behavior *Am J Psychiatry,* 154(12):1715, 1997.

Bultema J: Healing process for the multidisciplinary team: recovering post-inpatient suicide *J Psychosoc Nurs* 32:19, 1994.

Constantino R, Bricker P: Nursing postvention for spousal survivors of suicide *Issues Ment Health Nurs* 17:131, 1996.

Conwell Y et al: Relationships of age and axis I diagnoses in victims of completed suicide: a psychological autopsy study *Am J Psychiatry* 153:1001, 1996.

Cooper C: Psychiatric stress debriefing, *J Psychosoc Nurs* 33:21, 1995.

DeLeo D et al: Lower rates associated with a tele-help/tele-check service for the elderly at home *Am J Psychiatry* 152:632, 1995.

Egan M et al: The "no-suicide contract" helpful or harmful? *J Psychosoc Nurs,* 35(3):31, 1997.

Goin M: Treating the suicidal patient: the no-suicide contract—who benefits? *J Prac Psych Behav Health* 4:243, 1998.

Gupta S et al: Factors associated with suicide attempts among patients with schizophrenia, *Psych Services* 49(10): 1353, 1998.

Hall R et al: Suicide risk assessment: a review of risk factors for suicide in 100 patients who made severe suicide attempts, *Psychosomatics* 40(1):18, 1999.

Hughes D: Can the clinician predict suicide? *Psychiatr Serv* 46:449, 1995.

Kehrberg C: Self-mutilating behavior, *J Child Adoles Psych Nurs* 10(3): 35, 1997.

Kessler R et al: Prevalence of and risk factors for lifetime suicide attempts in the national comorbidity survey, *Arch Gen Psych* 56:617, 1999.

Leon A et al: Prospective study of fluoxetine treatment and suicidal behavior in affectively ill subjects, *Am J Psych* 156(2):195, 1999.

Lester D: Helplessness, hopelessness and haplessness and suicidality, *Psychol Report* 82:946, 1998.

Loughrey L et al: Patient self-mutilation: when nursing becomes a nightmare, *J Psychosoc Nurs* 35(4):30, 1997.

Mann J et al: The neurobiology suicide risk: a review for the clinician, *J Clin Psych* 60(suppl 2):7, 1999.

Mann J et al: Toward a clinical model of suicidal behavior in psychiatric patients, *Am J Psych,* 156(2):181, 1999.

Meltzer H: Suicide in schizophrenia: risk factors and clozapine treatment, *J Clin Psych* 59(suppl 3):15, 1998.

NIMH: Suicide Fact Sheet, December 1999.

Pages K et al: Determinants of suicidal ideation: the role of substance use disorders, *J Clin Psych* 58(11):510, 1997.

Pearson J et al : Late-life suicide and depression in the primary care setting. In Schneider L, editor. *Developments in geriatric psychiatry. New directions for mental health services,* 76:13, San Francisco, 1997, Jossey-Bass.

Pirkis J, Burgess P: Suicide and recency of health care contacts, *Br J Psych* 173:462, 1998.

Reilly C: Cognitive therapy for the suicidal patient: a case study, *Perspect Psych Care* 34(4): 26, 1998.

Rosenbluth M et al: Suicide: the interaction of clinical and ethical issues, *Psychiatr Serv* 46:919, 1995.

Russ M et al: Assessment of suicide risk 24 hours after psychiatric hospital admission, *Psychiatr Serv* 50(11):1491, 1999.

Shaffer D, Craft L: Methods of adolescent suicide prevention, *J Clin Psych* 60(suppl 2):70, 1999.

Simpson S, Jamison K: Suicide and mood disorders, *Primary Psych* 59, May 1997.

Simpson S, Jamison K: The risk of suicide in patients with bipolar disorders, *J Clin Psych* 60(suppl 2):53, 1999.

Skoog I et al: Suicidal feelings in a population sample of nondemented 85-year-olds, *Am J Psychiatry* 153:1015, 1996.

Surgeon General's call to action to prevent suicide, Washington, DC, 1999, US Public Health Service.

Wysoker A: Suicide: risk management strategies, *J Am Psych Nurses Assoc* 5(5):164, 1999.

Visit **MERLIN** for *Your Internet Connection*
to websites that are related to the content in this chapter.
www.mosby.com/MERLIN/Stuart

22 Neurobiological Responses and Schizophrenia and Psychotic Disorders

Mary D. Moller

Millene F. Murphy

LEARNING OBJECTIVES

After studying this chapter the student should be able to:

- Describe the continuum of adaptive and maladaptive neurobiological responses
- Discuss the prevalence of schizophrenia and other psychotic disorders
- Identify behaviors associated with maladaptive neurobiological responses
- Analyze predisposing factors, precipitating stressors, and appraisal of stressors related to maladaptive neurobiological responses
- Describe coping resources and coping mechanisms related to maladaptive neurobiological responses
- Formulate nursing diagnoses related to maladaptive neurobiological responses
- Examine the relationship between nursing diagnoses and medical diagnoses related to maladaptive neurobiological responses
- Identify expected outcomes and short-term nursing goals related to maladaptive neurobiological responses
- Develop a family education plan to promote adaptive neurobiological responses
- Analyze nursing interventions related to maladaptive neurobiological responses
- Evaluate nursing care related to maladaptive neurobiological responses

TOPICAL OUTLINE

How do I get away from you–voices? How do I leave you behind me forever? You who echo my feelings haunt my thoughts and ravage my nights . . . How do I get away from you? I sing at the top of my voice and still I hear you. I talk loud and listen to people and still I hear you. Is there a me without you? No, the answer comes loud and clear, there is no me without you. As long as I have feelings you will be my echo. As long as I have thoughts you will be the ghost. As long as there is night you will be in the darkness.

SHARON LeCLAIRE

Psychiatric nurses are often challenged when providing nursing care to patients with schizophrenia and other psychotic disorders. These are complex neurobiological brain diseases involving a number of syndromes. The behaviors associated with these disruptions in brain function are difficult to understand and are usually severe and long lasting. Patients who experience psychosis are often frightened by their experiences, have difficulty forming close relationships, are severely disabled, and tend to be alienated from society. Competent nurses should strive to make contact with patients who are psychotic and help them toward rehabilitation and wellness. A Patient Speaks box describes one person's experience with psychosis.

Read the patient's description of psychosis a second time. Focus on identifying the feelings that might be associated with these experiences.

CONTINUUM OF NEUROBIOLOGICAL RESPONSES

The range of neurobiological responses includes a continuum from adaptive responses such as logical thought and accurate perceptions to maladaptive responses, such as thought distortions and hallucinations (Fig. 22-1). The symptoms of

A Patient Speaks

Psychosis is real. Its main feature is a loss of consciousness of the self in such a way that I can no longer discern my relationship to the reality that my body is in. This would not be destructive, except that I have done it inadvertently; I have done it without consciousness and have not provided for my body. My body, then, goes on without me. It wanders aimlessly and does not know to keep warm in the cold. It does not know how to avoid attack by violence. It does not know to protect itself from fire and deep water and the traffic that races down the highway.

My brain comes up with fantastical ideas about who I might be, since I am not there to tell it. Perhaps I am the Queen of Hearts, or a messenger from another planet, or even Jesus Christ himself. And why not? My brain distorts the reality of the senses: Is this burner hot or cold? Is this coat wet or dry? Is this chair a chair, or what exactly is this anyway, and for that matter, what in the world are you?

Maybe bugs are jumping out of my mind and onto that wall over there. Maybe there's a current coming up from the earth and into my feet and trying to pull me in. My brain can think of every kind of combination and defini-

tion, every kind of idea that it can put together, for it has a nearly infinite number of choices. It has all it has ever experienced, all the sounds, all the sights, all the sensations, all the dreams, all the fantasies, all the nightmares.

My brain chooses its manifestation according to what emotions were available to it when I was in charge. Only I am not there to add my discernment, my wisdom, and my awareness according to what I have learned. My brain goes haywire then. It has no person to guide it, no captain, no helm, and no rudder. It has no fingers at the keyboard. It wanders through its inner space like the steel ball that is thrown into nothing and bounces at random from arbitrarily placed spots in the pinball machine.

What is this I, then, that is gone, and where did it go? It is consciousness. It is awareness. It is the presence of the I in me. It is ego. It is my separation. It is the part in me that tells me the difference between me and the world. It is the I-ness of me that holds me upright like a spine and says, "You will not fall into this tree, or this song, or this ocean of water or air, and it will not fall into you. The I that is gone is the intelligence that says I am me, and you are you."

From Corday R: *Psychosis, the inner experience,* Boulder, Colo, 1991, Common Loon Productions.

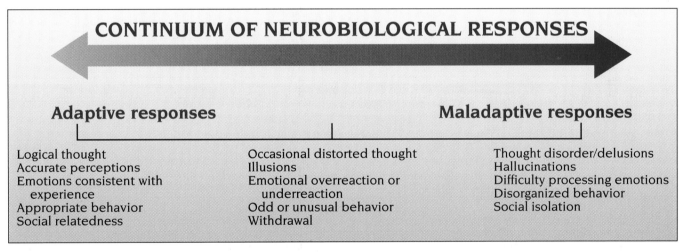

Fig. 22-1   Continuum of neurobiological responses.

psychosis are at the maladaptive end of this continuum. Schizophrenia is a serious and persistent neurobiological brain disease. It is a clinical syndrome of profoundly disruptive psychopathology that results in responses that severely impair the lives of individuals, their families and communities. Table 22-1 presents information on the impact of schizophrenia on the individual and society.

ASSESSMENT

Schizophrenia is one of a group of related disorders that are heterogeneous in pathophysiology, predisposing factors, pre-

cipitating stressors, and related behaviors. Other psychotic disorders include schizophreniform disorder, schizoaffective disorder, delusional disorder, brief psychotic disorder, shared psychotic disorder (folie a deux), psychotic disorder due to a general medical condition, and substance-induced psychotic disorder (American Psychiatric Association, 2000). In addition, psychosis is sometimes present in other disorders such as depression with psychotic features and manic episodes of bipolar disorder.

Although descriptions of the symptoms of what is called schizophrenia today are found throughout recorded history,

Table **22-1**

Impact of Schizophrenia on the Individual and Society

- About one in every 100 people suffers from schizophrenia, or 2.5 million Americans, regardless of race, ethnic group, or gender.
- In three out of four cases it begins between the ages of 17 and 25 years.
- 95% of people with schizophrenia have it for their lifetime.
- The annual cost of family caregiving and crime- and welfare-related expenditures as a result of schizophrenia is $33 billion in the United States.
- More than 75% of taxpayer dollars spent on treatment of mental illness are used for people with schizophrenia.
- People with schizophrenia occupy 25% of all inpatient hospital beds.
- An estimated one third to one half of homeless people in the United States have schizophrenia.
- Schizophrenia is ranked fourth worldwide in terms of burden of illness. The top three are unipolar depression, alcohol use, and bipolar disorder.
- Schizophrenia is a chronic illness, five times more common than multiple sclerosis, six times more common than insulin-dependent diabetes, 60 times more common than muscular dystrophy, and 80 times more common than Huntington's disease.
- Of patients with schizophrenia, 25% do not respond adequately to traditional antipsychotic medication.
- 20% to 50% of patients with schizophrenia attempt suicide; 10% succeed.

the term schizophrenia was not introduced until 1911 by the Swiss psychiatrist Eugene Bleuler. He believed that the "schizophrenias" were multidimensional and organic in nature and that these illnesses were strongly influenced and could be shaped by psychological factors. The word **schizophrenia** is a combination of two Greek words, **schizein**, "to split," and **phren**, "mind." Bleuler's reference was not to a "split personality," which refers to separate identities, but to his belief that a split occurred between the cognitive and emotional aspects of the personality.

The symptoms of schizophrenia have been organized in various ways over time, depending on the evolving understanding of brain function in this disorder, as well as the increasing efficacy of antipsychotic drugs. A prominent system for categorizing the symptoms of schizophrenia lists them as "positive" (additional behaviors) and "negative" (deficit of behaviors) symptoms (Table 22-2). Another useful categorization defines five core symptom clusters, presented in Fig. 22-2. With minimum overlap, this model incorporates the positive and negative symptoms described above plus other aspects of schizophrenia, including cognitive symptoms, mood symptoms, and some of the social and occupational dysfunction common in schizophrenia.

Assessment of this devastating and costly illness involves an understanding of the way in which the brain processes information from the senses and the behavioral responses to these processes. These behaviors are organized into the following categories: cognition, perception, emotion, behavior and movement, and socialization. Be-

Table **22-2**

Positive and Negative Symptoms of Schizophrenia

POSITIVE SYMPTOMS

An excess or distortion of normal function, usually responsive to traditional antipsychotic drugs

Psychotic Disorders of Thinking

Delusions (paranoid, somatic, grandiose, religious, nihilistic, or persecutory themes, and thought broadcasting, insertion, or control); hallucinations (auditory, visual, tactile, gustatory, olfactory)

Disorganization of Speech and Behavior

Positive formal thought disorder (incoherence, word salad, derailment, illogicality, loose associations, tangentiality, circumstantiality, pressured speech, distractible speech, or poverty of speech); bizarre behavior (catatonia, movement disorders, deterioration of social behavior)

NEGATIVE SYMPTOMS

A diminution or loss of normal function, usually unresponsive to traditional antipsychotics and more responsive to atypical antipsychotics.

Problems of Emotion

Affective flattening: limited range and intensity of emotional expression
Anhedonia/asociality: inability to experience pleasure or maintain social contacts

Impaired Decision-Making

Alogia: restricted thought and speech
Avolition/apathy: lack of initiation of goal-directed behavior
Attentional impairment: inability to mentally focus

havioral rating scales related to psychotic disorders are listed in Box 22-1.

Behaviors

Cognition. Cognition is the act or process of knowing. It involves awareness and judgment that enable the brain to process information in a way that ensures accuracy, storage, and retrieval. People with schizophrenia are often unable to produce complex logical thoughts and express coherent sentences because neurotransmission in the brain's information processing system is malfunctioning. Information processing involves the organization of sensory input by brain processes into behavioral responses (Fig. 22-3). Sensory input is screened according to the focus of the person's attention and ability to remember, learn, discriminate, interpret, and organize information.

Describe how your cognitive processing differs from that of a person of the opposite sex, an older generation, another race, and another socioeconomic class. What are the results of these differences?

The information processing of people with schizophrenia may be altered by brain deficits. However, interferences with cognitive function often keep people with schizophrenia from realizing that their ideas and behavior are different from others. This is particularly evident in their self-perception of worth and abilities. They tend to dramatically

Box 22-1

Behavioral Rating Scales Related to Psychotic Disorders

- Behavioral Observation Schedule
- Brief Psychiatric Rating Scale (BPRS)
- Life Skills Profile: Schizophrenia (LSP)
- Positive and Negative Syndrome Scale (PANSS)
- Scale for Assessment of Negative Symptoms (SANS)
- Scale for Assessment of Positive Symptoms (SAPS)
- Schizophrenia Outcomes Module (SOM)
- University of Washington Paranoia Scale

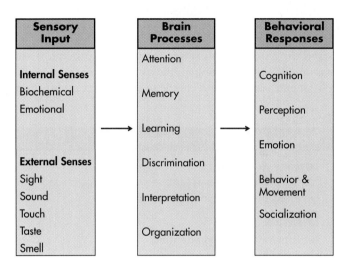

Fig. 22-3 Brain information processing model.

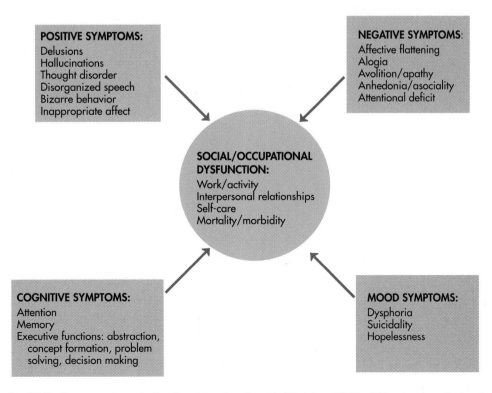

Fig. 22-2 Core symptom clusters in schizophrenia. (Modified from Eli Lilly: *Schizophrenia and related disorders: a comprehensive review and bibliography slide kit,* Indianapolis, 1996, Lilly Neuroscience.)

overestimate or underestimate their own capability. The increased brain dysfunction during an acute episode makes it difficult for the patient to realize his or her need for help.

Symptoms related to problems in information processing associated with schizophrenia are often called cognitive deficits. They include problems in cognitive functioning in all aspects of memory, attention, form and organization of speech, decision-making, and thought content (Box 22-2).

Memory is the retention or storage of knowledge about the world. Memory is a biological function carried out in several parts of the brain. Additional information about memory and its assessment can be found in Chapters 6, 7, and 24. Memory problems associated with schizophrenia can include forgetfulness, disinterest, problems learning, and lack of compliance. It is important for the nurse to understand the frustration these symptoms cause patients. They commonly seek validation for the correctness of task accomplishment, ask whether it is time to attend a group function

Box 22-2

Problems in Cognitive Functioning

MEMORY
Difficulty retrieving and using stored memory
Impaired short-term/long-term memory

ATTENTION
Difficulty maintaining attention
Poor concentration
Distractibility
Inability to use selective attention

FORM AND ORGANIZATION OF SPEECH (FORMAL THOUGHT DISORDER)
Loose associations
Tangentiality
Incoherence/word salad/neologism
Illogicality
Circumstantiality
Pressured/distractible speech
Poverty of speech

DECISION MAKING
Failure to abstract
Indecisiveness
Lack of insight
Impaired concept formation
Impaired judgment
Illogical or concrete thinking
Lack of planning and problem-solving skills
Difficulty initiating tasks

THOUGHT CONTENT
Delusions
Paranoid
Grandiose
Religious
Somatic
Nihilistic
Thought broadcasting
Thought insertion
Thought control

or an appointment, and seek permission to make a telephone call just to verify whether they remember phone numbers. Staff may place restrictions on these patients if they fail to differentiate symptoms from manipulative behaviors. When people with schizophrenia repeatedly ask the same question, such as what time it is or how to get somewhere, it is important for the nurse to provide the requested information in a kind and matter-of-fact manner that does not cause embarrassment or decrease the person's self-worth and that continues to reinforce the alliance with the patient.

Attention is the ability to focus on one activity in a sustained, concentrated manner. Disrupted attention is an impairment in the ability to pay attention, observe, and concentrate on external reality. Disturbances in attention are common in schizophrenia and include difficulty completing tasks, difficulty concentrating on work, and easy distractibility. Distractibility refers to a patient's attention being drawn easily to irrelevant external stimuli such as noises, books out of order on a bookshelf, or people passing by. In addition, the patient who is experiencing auditory hallucinations often is distracted by them and thus has problems with attention.

These impairments are not constant and may fluctuate, depending on the brain activity required. This generates much frustration for the patient, who often complains about his inability to complete tasks because "my mind wanders." The nurse should be prepared to redirect the patient back to the task at hand. The nurse will also need to repeat directions often and in short, simple phrases.

The parents of a young man who has schizophrenia tell you that they are frustrated by their son's unwillingness to return to work. Based on your understanding of the cognitive disorders related to schizophrenia, how would you respond?

Form and organization of speech are at the core of communication. Malfunctions in information processing produce disturbances in relaying thoughts that interfere with coherent communication. Problems with form and organization of speech (formal thought disorders) may include loose associations, word salad, tangentiality, illogicality, circumstantiality, pressured speech, poverty of speech, distractible speech, and clanging. These behaviors are described in Chapter 7. Box 22-3 presents nurse-patient dialogues that reflect problems in the form and organization of speech related to psychotic disorders. Recognizing that speech is a reflection of cognitive processing helps the nurse appreciate the considerable difficulties a person with schizophrenia has in communicating clearly. The nurse will need to focus attention and use active listening to understand the patient. The nurse who is attempting to identify and clarify what a patient wants should not be afraid of offending the patient by seeking to understand. It is essential to remember that the patient is trying to answer, no matter how difficult or bizarre the answer is. The nurses' responsibility is to identify one or two key verbal or nonverbal responses and seek validation. This is usually achieved through simple trial and error.

Decision making means arriving at a solution or making a choice. Components of decision making include insight, judgment, logic, decisiveness, planning, ability to carry out decisions, and abstract thought. Lack of insight is probably one of the greatest problems in schizophrenia because patients generally do not believe that they are ill or different in any way. Unfortunately, many clinicians confuse lack of insight with denial and treat people who have schizophrenia as if their symptoms were willful and within conscious control. Faulty logic is often identified through the speech of people with schizophrenia who display the behaviors of thought disorder. When there are cognitive deficits in decision-making, the patient makes decisions based on incorrect inferences, yet cannot understand that the judgment was faulty.

Some people with schizophrenia are simply unable to reach a decision. For them, life is difficult at best. They wrestle with even simple decisions such as which coffee cup to use. Plans based on faulty decision-making do not serve the intended purpose. This symptom creates much of the frustration related to schizophrenia. Following through on decisions is also a problem for people who have schizophrenia. Often this is mistaken for lack of motivation. Motivation involves having a desire, not having the ability to follow through. People with schizophrenia typically have difficulty initiating tasks of any kind because of problems related to decision making.

Concrete rather than abstract thinking is characteristic of schizophrenia, particularly during acute episodes. As a result, patients often have difficulty with multiple-step commands. In other words, if the nurse presents a patient with the daily schedule and, at the same time, gives directions about the time and place of group and occupational therapies, all of the information will not be processed as the brain perceives an overload. Thus the patient will probably miss one or more of the directions.

Another example of concrete thinking is difficulty with time management. People with schizophrenia describe this behavior as "trying to tell time with clocks that have no minute or second hands." This is why patients often are late or miss events and appointments altogether. This may create fear in patients who have to be alone for long periods of time

---

Box 22-3

Form and Content of Speech Related to Psychotic Disorders

LOOSE ASSOCIATIONS

Nurse: "Do you have enough money to buy that candy bar?"

Patient: "I have a real yen for chocolate. The Japanese have all the yen and have taken all our money and marked it. You know, you have to be careful of the Marxists because they are friends with the Swiss and they have all the cheese and all the watches and that means they have taken all the time. The worst thing about Swiss cheese is all the holes. People have to be careful about falling into holes."

Nurse: "It sounds like you are worried about your money."

Patient: "Yes, I have it all here in my wallet and you can't have it and the bank can't have it either."

INCOHERENCE

Nurse: "What does your family like to do at Christmas?"

Patient: "I believe they took Christmas from the Russians to get all the cars into the ocean and make jello. You could go and get the Christmas but you could not do it because the keylars have the fan."

TANGENTIALITY

Nurse: "I'm interested in learning more about your landscape paintings."

Patient: "My interest in art goes back to my parents who lived on a farm in Indiana. They had lots of haystacks, kind of like they do in Ohio, but you know, the hay is different colors in different states so that gave me the ability to paint so many different colors of yellow. Some people do not really like bright yellow hay, but I do. If I make the hay really bright yellow, then I make the barns a dull red, because barns really should not be painted with bright red paint. Bright red should be saved for fire engines and fire hydrants and stop signs."

ILLOGICAL SPEECH

Nurse: "Do you think your medicine is helping you think more clearly?"

Patient: "I used to think my medicine helped me think. But I realized that it was me who took the medicine, so it wasn't the medicine that helped me think. Medicine cannot think, don't you realize that? Maybe you should take some medicine to help you think better. But if you do, I would have to give it to you because it is the fact I took it myself that my thinking is better, so, no, I do not think the medicine is helping me think better."

DISTRACTIBLE SPEECH

Nurse: "I would like to talk with you about your understanding of schizophrenia."

Patient: "I know it's got something to do with my brain. What perfume are you wearing? It must be from France. Is that where that picture was taken? Your hair is different than when that picture was taken. Was that about 4 years ago?"

CLANG ASSOCIATIONS

Patient: "I got a new shirt but the buttons became loose. Do you suppose Lucifer's buttons become lucent or are they lucid like Lucy's lucky ducky?"

"I want to sing ping pong that song wong kong long today hey way."

POVERTY OF CONTENT OF SPEECH

Nurse: "Do you want to go to the grocery store?"

Patient: "Yeah, uh huh, well what would I do with the, uh, the stuff that is over there on top of it? Do they, uh, have the, the, you know, the thing to do it with the wheels on the floor. I, uh, guess they should let me."

or are required to be places at specific times. Some patients have developed clever ways to determine time, such as getting watches with built-in alarms and monitoring certain television programs.

Difficulty managing money is another result of concrete thinking. People with schizophrenia often lose their ability to understand the concept of dollars and cents and are exploited by other people. A patient may agree to buy items without having enough money just because he sees some money in his wallet. He may not remember to pay for items he gets in a store or leave a restaurant without paying for the meal. Unfortunately, many patients get into legal trouble because of this cognitive problem.

Literal interpretation of words and symbols is one of the most problematic behaviors related to concrete thinking. People with schizophrenia have difficulty abstracting the English language. Patients' descriptions of literal interpretation are presented in the following clinical examples.

"I was standing in the medication line and the nurse asked me to take my pills. So I took the medicine cup and held it in my hand. The nurse asked me again to take my pills and I did not know what to do. She began to lose her patience as I stood there holding the medicine cup. She then told me to put the pills in my mouth and to swallow them with the water she handed me. I could follow each of the instructions and eventually 'took my pills.'"

An example of literal interpretation of symbols is described by this patient: "It took me at least 15 minutes to walk down the street because I stopped every time the light changed from green to red. I did not understand that the traffic signal was only for cars."

Sometimes this problem advances to the point where the patient interprets a metaphor literally, as seen in this example: "I remembered the expression 'step on a crack and break your mother's back.'" One day I was walking down the street and stepped on a crack in the sidewalk. That same day my mother had fallen off a step stool after getting a can of soup from the kitchen cupboard and fractured two vertebrae in her back. For 9 months I believed that I had caused this accident to happen." This is also called magical thinking.

Nursing implications regarding patient teaching for the person experiencing concrete thinking are profound. Consider this example: During the admission of a new patient, a nurse instructed the patient to collect a sterile urine specimen. The patient exhibited terror and strongly resisted. When the nurse gently asked him why he was so frightened, he replied, "I do not want to become sterile."

The role of the nurse is to help with decision making in a nonpunitive, supportive manner, recognizing that these symptoms represent neurological disabilities over which the patient has little control. The nurse functions in a rehabilitative role and needs to provide information as clearly and concretely as possible. The language used should involve simple words in short phrases that are easy to understand. The nurse also needs to seek validation regarding how instructions were heard to clarify confusion and misunderstanding.

It is important to involve the patient in planning nursing care. Describe how you would accomplish this if the patient has cognitive problems that interfere with decision-making ability.

Thought content is the final domain for assessment of cognitive functioning and includes evaluation for the presence of delusions in persons with schizophrenia. A delusion is a personal belief based on an incorrect inference of external reality. One of the mind's primary functions is to produce thoughts. Thoughts provide a sense of identity. Thoughts are produced as a result of intricate processes that involve screening and filtering internal and external stimuli and the use of multiple feedback loops in the brain. Recognizing the complexity of this process helps the nurse appreciate the unyielding way in which a person defends personal beliefs.

Recalling the cognitive deficits already described helps the nurse understand why people with schizophrenia sometimes have different beliefs from others. It is also important to realize that a delusion does not always last. It is common for a belief to be fixed for only a few weeks or few months, particularly in the less severe forms of schizophrenia. The inability of the brain to process data accurately can result in paranoid, grandiose, religious, nihilistic, and somatic delusions. The delusions can be complicated further by thought withdrawal, thought insertion, thought control, or thought broadcasting. Types of delusions are described in Chapter 7.

Delusions represent an elaborate interplay between brain physiology, current environmental stimuli, and the person's frame of reference regarding the world. Delusions have several characteristics that must be identified before effective interventions can be planned. Delusions can become intertwined with hallucinations. They may be a single thought or pervade the person's entire cognitive process. They can represent a complete thought or only a portion of an idea. Delusions may be systematized, which means they are restricted to a specific area of belief such as family or religion, or nonsystematized, meaning they extend into many areas of a person's life, so new people and new information are incorporated into the delusion. Many patients have reported the relief they experienced as their symptoms remitted and they realized the belief was really a delusion, just a symptom, not the actual truth.

Perception. Perception is identification and initial interpretation of a stimulus based on information received through sight, sound, taste, touch, and smell. Given the complex interplay of brain functions among brain stem, diencephalon, and cortex for each of the five senses, it is important to recognize that perceptual problems are often the first symptoms in many brain illnesses. Hallucinations and delusions are perceptual distortions that occur in maladaptive neurobiological responses. Although hallucinations are most commonly associated with schizophrenia, only about 70% of people with this illness experience them. They can also occur in a manic or depressive illness, as well as in delirium. It is essential to stress that hallucinations and delusions can occur in any illness that disrupts brain function. Hallucinations arise from any of the five senses. They are described in Table 22-3.

A young woman is hospitalized in a forensic psychiatric unit because she attempted to kill her preschool children. She says her dead mother's voice told her to do this because the devil would get them unless they were in heaven with her. Is this a delusion, a hallucination, or both? Would knowing the woman's sociocultural background influence your response? Why or why not?

Another category of perceptual behaviors involves sensory integration and includes pain recognition, stereognosis, graphesthesia, right/left recognition, and recognition and perception of faces. Symptoms related to these perceptions are common in schizophrenia yet often are assessed inaccurately within a behavioral instead of a perceptual context. Sensory integration disruptions often lead to deliberate acts of self-harm, as described in this clinical example.

CLINICAL EXAMPLE

During an initial physical assessment a nurse noted many superficial scars on the left arm of a young woman who had just completed an 8-week education program on symptom management in schizophrenia. The nurse said, "Tell me about those scars," to which the patient replied: "Before I knew it was okay to talk about my symptoms I often lost sensation in my left arm and hand and thought my arm was poisoned or dead. I tried to determine if I was alive or not. I could see myself walking and see and feel my right arm, so I thought I was probably alive but I did not know for sure, so I used to take a knife and poke tiny holes in my skin. I could not feel the knife yet I saw blood. It was when I saw the blood that I knew I was still alive."

Selected Nursing Diagnoses

- Altered sensory perception, tactile, related to disrupted sensory integration, as evidenced by explanation of scars on right arm

- Risk for self-mutilation related to perceptual disturbance, as evidenced by scars from past episodes of cutting left arm

The concept of pain and **pain recognition** has been well studied. Knowing that the parietal lobe is the major site of pain recognition helps the nurse to see this as a neurobiologically based symptom. Visceral pain recognition involves integration of stimuli from the spinal cord through the brainstem, diencephalon, and cortex using intricate feedback circuits. People with schizophrenia generally have poor visceral pain recognition and need to have an in-depth assessment of physical complaints, as described by the patient in the next clinical example.

CLINICAL EXAMPLE

"I told my case manager that I had a stomachache, some diarrhea, and vomiting and felt like I had the flu. I had a fever, so she took me to the doctor, who said I probably had the flu and should just go home and rest. After a few days I got real sick and had to be taken to the emergency room, where they discovered my appendix had ruptured, and I had to have a very long and complicated surgery."

It is not uncommon for people with schizophrenia to think they just have a bad cold and have it diagnosed as pneumonia. Unfortunately, the physical needs of psychiatric patients can often be neglected or disregarded.

Sensory integration perceptions are included in standard neurological examinations under the category *soft signs*, meaning that they represent a neurological deficit in an undetermined location but are consistent with brain injury to the frontal or parietal lobes. These terms refer to the ability to identify objects by touch. **Stereognosis** is the ability to recognize an object only by touch, such as reaching into a paper bag filled with objects and identifying a key. **Astereognosis** is the inability to do this. **Graphesthesia** is the recognition of

Table **22-3**

Sense	Characteristics
Sensory Modalities Involved in Hallucinations	
Auditory	Hearing noises or sounds, most commonly in the form of voices. Sounds that range from a simple noise or voice, to a voice talking about the patient, to complete conversations between two or more people about the person who is hallucinating. Audible thoughts in which the patient hears voices that are speaking what the patient is thinking and commands that tell the patient to do something, sometimes harmful or dangerous.
Visual	Visual stimuli in the form of flashes of light, geometric figures, cartoon figures, or elaborate and complex scenes or visions. Visions can be pleasant or terrifying, as in seeing monsters.
Olfactory	Putrid, foul, and rancid smells such as blood, urine, or feces; occasionally the odors can be pleasant. Olfactory hallucinations are typically associated with stroke, tumor, seizures, and the dementias.
Gustatory	Putrid, foul, and rancid tastes such as blood, urine, or feces.
Tactile	Experiencing pain or discomfort with no apparent stimuli. Feeling electrical sensations coming from the ground, inanimate objects, or other people.
Cenesthetic	Feeling body functions such as blood pulsing through veins and arteries, food digesting, or urine forming.
Kinesthetic	Sensation of movement while standing motionless.

letters "drawn" on the skin, such as recognizing the letters C-A-T "drawn" on one's back. **Agraphesthesia** is the inability to do this. Table 22-4 lists several neurological soft signs common in schizophrenia that should be assessed carefully during a baseline evaluation of each patient. Problems in these functions contribute to difficulty with fine motor actions of the hand, and the patient may appear clumsy. Problems with right/left discrimination also contribute to lack of coordination and ability to carry out directions involving concepts of right and left.

Misidentification and perception of faces can contribute to fear, aggressiveness, withdrawal from interactions, and hostility. This symptom involves self-recognition as well and often is present when patients refuse to look in a mirror or avoids eye contact.

Environmental factors can stimulate hallucinations. In general, objects that are reflective, such as television screens, photo frames, and fluorescent lights can contribute to visual hallucinations. Auditory hallucinations can be caused by excessive noise and by sensory deprivation. The nurse should be acutely aware of environmental stimuli and the patient's response or lack of response. Patients may withdraw from sensory stimuli in an attempt to decrease sensory responses.

When perceptions are altered, concurrent symptoms in cognitive functions are common. Studies have shown that 90% of people who experience hallucinations also have delusions, whereas only 35% who experience delusions also have hallucinations. Approximately 20% of patients have mixed sensory hallucinations, usually auditory and visual.

Emotion. In psychiatry, emotions are described in terms of mood and affect. Mood is defined as an extensive and sustained feeling tone that can be experienced for a few hours or for years and can noticeably affect the persons' world view. (Chapter 20 includes a complete description of mood and mood disorders.) Affect refers to behaviors such as hand and body movements, facial expression, and pitch of voice that can be observed when a person is expressing and experiencing feelings and emotions. Terms related to affect include **broad, restricted, blunted, flat,** and **inappropriate.** What is considered normal varies greatly among cultures. **Broad** and **restricted** are usually considered within the range of normal, whereas **blunted, flat,** and **inappropriate** represent symptoms of an underlying problem. Disorders of affect refer to expression of emotion, not the experience of emotion. Patients describe affective symptoms in the following examples:

- "I remember trying to smile for 3 years, but my face did not work."
- "My face was as stiff as your fingers would be if you tied them to popsicle sticks for 3 months and then tried to use them to thread a needle."

Patients describe tremendous frustration with these affective symptoms because others assume that they do not experience any emotion. These descriptions demonstrate why patients are commonly misjudged as appearing bored, disinterested, and unmotivated.

Emotion refers to moods and affects that are connected to specific ideas. Emotions are generated from an interplay of neural activity between the hypothalamus, limbic structures (amygdala and hippocampus), and higher cortex centers such as the association cortices. The hypothalamus, in addition to its hormonal functions, is the emotional coordinating center. Emotions can be hyperexpressed or hypoexpressed. People with schizophrenia commonly have symptoms of hypoexpression. Some patients perceive that they no longer have any feelings. Problems of emotion usually seen in schizophrenia include alexithymia, apathy, anhedonia, and a decreased ability to feel intimacy and closeness:

- **Alexithymia:** difficulty naming and describing emotions
- **Apathy:** lack of feelings, emotions, interests, or concern
- **Anhedonia:** inability or decreased ability to experience pleasure, joy, intimacy, and closeness

In addition to problems with emotions and affect, people with schizophrenia can also have mood disorders. A major depression may develop in up to 60% of people with schizophrenia. Ten percent to 13% of people with schizophrenia complete suicide (Harkavy-Friedman & Nelson, 1997). A diagnosis of schizoaffective disorder is given to the patient who meets the diagnostic criteria for schizophrenia as well as bipolar disorder or major depression.

Understanding the effect of brain malfunctions on the emotions and affect of the person with schizophrenia is important for promoting constructive communication and problem solving. One should also recognize that people with brain illnesses often have an uncanny ability to sense the emotions of others, yet they may have difficulty identifying their own emotions. This creates special problems in caring

Table **22-4**

Neurological Soft Signs: Prefrontal Cortical Dysfunction in Schizophrenia

- Astereognosis: inability to recognize objects by the sense of touch (such as differentiating a nickel from a dime)
- Agraphesthesia: inability to recognize numbers or letters traced on the skin
- Dysdiadochokinesia: impairment of the ability to perform smooth, alternating movements (such as turning the hand face up and face down rapidly)
- Mild muscle twitches, choreiform and ticlike movements, grimacing
- Impaired fine motor skills and abnormal motor tone
- Increased rate of eye blinking
- Abnormal smooth pursuit eye movements (SPEM): difficulty following movement of objects
- Neurological hard signs: loss of function, weakness, diminished reflexes, paralysis caused by a CVA, tumor, traumatic injury, etc

for the patient and requires the nurse to be aware of and in control of her own emotional reactions.

Caregivers often confuse feelings that are a direct result of brain malfunction and those that are an indirect product of social difficulties resulting from illness. Examples of feelings that are a direct result of brain malfunction include paranoid hostility and emotional flattening. An example of feelings that are an indirect product of social difficulties caused by illness is frustration over not being able to achieve one's potential. When patients and caregivers have difficulty identifying feelings and emotions, barriers to good communication usually result.

Behavior and Movement. Definition of "normal" behavior and movement is based on culture, age appropriateness, and social acceptability. Maladaptive neurobiological responses cause behaviors and movements that are odd, unsightly, confusing, difficult to manage, dysfunctional, and puzzling to others. With exploration, many behaviors can be explained and movements can be understood. Some make sense in the context of information provided by the patient or of the patient's neurobiological illness.

> *Describe unusual behaviors or movements that you have observed in patients with maladaptive neurobiological responses. Were you able to discover the reason for the behaviors or movements? Can you think of possible explanations for wearing several layers of clothing in very hot weather? Refusing to bathe? Hugging oneself and rocking?*

Maladaptive behaviors in schizophrenia include deteriorated appearance, lack of persistence at work or school, avolition, repetitive or stereotyped behavior, aggression and agitation, and negativism. Deterioration in appearance includes disheveled and dirty clothes, sloppy and unkempt appearance, poor or absent personal grooming, and lack of personal hygiene. This is often the first set of symptoms to occur and is a signal to the family that something is happening to their loved one. Accompanying deterioration in appearance is lack of persistence at work or school. As problems in brain function begin to appear, the cognitive skills seem to "short circuit" and the person can no longer perform routine tasks. As deterioration continues the person begins to experience avolition, which means lack of energy and drive. This is a result of the brain changes (which may be occurring rapidly) and frustration with the inability to accomplish tasks that required little effort in the past. Unfortunately, at this point most people with schizophrenia are mislabeled as lazy, disinterested, and unmotivated.

As deterioration continues, patients often engage in repetitive or stereotyped behaviors. These appear similar to obsessive-compulsive behavior but are related to a private meaning rather than to thoughts. Examples include having to eat foods in a certain way, wearing only certain clothes, walking four steps forward and one step back, or being able to drink only half a glass of water at a time.

Aggression, agitation, and the potential for violence unfortunately are often used to describe the typical person with schizophrenia. The person with schizophrenia generally is the victim rather than the aggressor. However, people experiencing psychoses are sometimes violent, especially when their illness is out of control. Agitation is common for anyone who is living with a chronic illness for which there is no cure. It is important to identify and document situations that seem to be triggers for agitated behavior (see Chapter 31). People who have schizophrenia tend to become agitated when experiencing performance anxiety, particularly related to carrying out tasks that previously posed no difficulty. Abnormal behaviors and movements in schizophrenia are summarized in Box 22-4.

Maladaptive movements associated with schizophrenia include catatonia, abnormal eye movements, grimacing, apraxia/echopraxia, abnormal gait, mannerisms, and extrapyramidal side effects of psychotropic medications (see Chapter 28). Catatonia is a stuporous state in which the patient may require complete physical nursing care, similar to that for a comatose patient, sometimes interspersed with unpredictable outbursts of aggressive behavior or strange posturing. Grimacing refers to abnormal facial movements that are beyond the patient's control and are not caused by psychotropic medications. Abnormal eye movements include difficulty following a moving target, absence or avoidance of eye contact, decreased or rapid eye blinking, and frequent staring. These are common ocular motor symptoms found in 40% to 80% of people with schizophrenia. Apraxia is difficulty carrying out a purposeful, organized task that is somewhat complex, such as dressing. Echopraxia is defined as purposeless imitation of movements made by other people. This symptom may not always be purposeless but can illustrate a delusion, as described by the patient in the following clinical example.

CLINICAL EXAMPLE

"I thought the nurse was my mirror and I had to do what the mirror showed me, so I copied everything she did. As long as I could see her I could feel connected to myself and my surroundings, but

---

Box 22-4

Abnormal Behaviors and Movements in Schizophrenia

BEHAVIORS

Appearance
Aggression/agitation/violence
Repetitive or stereotyped behavior
Avolition
Impersistence at work or school

MOVEMENTS

Catatonia, waxy flexibility, posturing
Extrapyramidal side effects of psychotropic medications
Abnormal eye movements
Grimacing
Apraxia/echopraxia
Abnormal gait
Mannerisms

she did not understand how important it was for me to be around her and watch what she did. Of course I could not explain what was happening to me at the time because I was psychotic, so she put me in seclusion and restraints."

Selected Nursing Diagnosis
- Altered thought processes related to maladaptive information processing, as evidenced by belief that the nurse was a mirror

Staggering, intentional stepping, and walking with the toes touching the ground first are abnormal gaits common in people with schizophrenia. Mannerisms involve gestures that seem contrived and are not appropriate to the situation, such as stopping in the middle of a sentence to whirl two fingers around.

Socialization. Socialization is the ability to form cooperative and interdependent relationships with others. This was placed last among the five major brain functions because problems with the others must be understood to appreciate the relational consequences of maladaptive neurobiological responses. Social problems are often the major source of concern to families and health-care providers because these tangible effects of illness are often more prominent than the symptoms related to cognition and perception.

Social problems may result from the illness directly or indirectly. Direct effects occur when symptoms prevent the person from socializing within accepted sociocultural norms or when motivation deteriorates. Regardless, the result is social withdrawal and isolation from life's activities. Behaviors directly causing these problems include inability to communicate coherently, loss of drive and interest, deterioration of social skills, poor personal hygiene, and paranoia.

Indirect effects on socialization are secondary consequences of the illness. An example is low self-esteem related to poor academic and social achievement. Significant social discomfort and further social isolation may result. Specific problems in the development of relationships include social inappropriateness, disinterest in recreational activities, inappropriate sexual behavior, and stigma-related withdrawal by friends, families, and peers.

Social inappropriateness relates directly to cognitive deficits and results in behaviors such as suddenly beginning loud, evangelistic prayer in public, toileting in public, standing in the middle of a street trying to direct traffic, dressing bizarrely, and engaging in intimate conversation with total strangers. Social inappropriateness often involves bizarre sexual behavior such as public masturbation, running nude in the street, or making inappropriate sexual advances. Sometimes bizarre sexual behavior is related to gender identity confusion. It is not uncommon, particularly with temporal lobe involvement, for people with schizophrenia to be unable to recognize their genitalia as their own. This often is the reason for sudden undressing and what appears to be public masturbation, when it actually may be a patient's futile attempt at reality testing.

Stigma also presents major obstacles to developing relationships and adversely affects quality of life. Stigma, which literally means mark of shame, is a major cause of the social isolation of people with schizophrenia. Stigma often spreads to the whole family, who may be having their own schizophrenia-related social problems stemming from embarrassment about having the illness in the family (see Chapters 15 and 16). They may avoid talking about it, or if they do want to talk they may not know how. Stigma and rejection may discourage them from talking. Family members may feel like social outcasts for having this illness in the family. One family member explained, "For the rest of my life I will be dealing not only with the heartbreak of my brother's illness, but with negative response, stigma, and ignorance in my hometown that will affect me deeply. I know, because the last 10 years of it already has been sheer hell."

Describe your own attitudes and behaviors and those of your peers toward people who have maladaptive neurobiological responses and their families.

Predisposing Factors

Biological. Behaviors related to maladaptive neurobiological responses have been described in writing and art since biblical times. Causes proposed for these strange behaviors ranged from demon possession, bad blood, and witchcraft to the full moon. Fortunately, modern science is now identifying many clues to the biological causes of these disorders (see Chapter 6).

Schizophrenia is a heterogeneous neurodevelopmental brain disorder. It is not known what accounts for the disruptions in brain function causing the many symptoms of schizophrenia. Nonetheless, there are interesting research results that hypothesize an integrative model of schizophrenia as a disorder of brain neural circuits.

Genetics. The specific genetic defects that cause schizophrenia have not yet been identified, but there has been progress towards identifying a potential location on chromosome 6, with additional genetic contributions associated with chromosomes 4, 8, 15, and 22 (Buchanan & Carpenter, 2000). Family, twin, and adoptive studies have long shown increased risk for the disease in people with a first-degree relative (parent, sibling, offspring) with schizophrenia. Whereas there is a 1% lifetime risk of developing schizophrenia in the general population, the monozygotic (identical) twin of a person with schizophrenia has a 50% risk for the disorder, and a dizygotic (fraternal) twin has a 15% risk for the disorder. Children with a biological parent with schizophrenia have a 15% risk for it, and if both parents have schizophrenia the risk goes up to 35%. Children with a biological parent with schizophrenia who were adopted at birth by a family with no incidence of the disorder have the same risk as if they had been raised by their biological parents. Thus there is compelling evidence for both a genetic predisposition for the disorder and additional environmental or random factors, as evidenced by the fact that identical twins share 100% of genes, but only 50% of the risk for schizophrenia.

Neurobiology. Multiple studies show anatomical, functional, and neurochemical abnormalities in the living and postmortem brains of people with schizophrenia. Research suggests that the prefrontal cortex and the limbic cortex may never fully develop in the brains of persons with schizophrenia. The two most consistent neurobiological research findings in schizophrenia are imaging studies showing decreased brain volume and abnormal function, and neurochemical studies showing alterations of numerous neurotransmitter systems. Particular focus has been on the frontal cortex, implicated in the negative symptoms of schizophrenia; the limbic system (in the temporal lobes), implicated in the positive symptoms of schizophrenia; and the neurotransmitter systems connecting these regions, particularly dopamine and serotonin, and more recently, glutamate. Therefore, psychotic behaviors may be related to lesions in the frontal, temporal, and limbic regions of the brain and dysregulation of neurotransmitter systems connecting these regions. Another recent theory (Andreasen, 1999) describes a misconnection syndrome between the cortex and the cerebellum, mediated by the thalamus (this circuitry normally coordinates both motor and mental activity), as a theoretical framework for strategies to explore etiology, pathophysiology, intervention, and prevention of schizophrenia.

Imaging studies. Computed tomography (CT) and Magnetic resonance imaging (MRI) studies of brain structure show decreased brain volume in people with schizophrenia. There are larger lateral and third ventricles; atrophy in the frontal lobe, cerebellum, and limbic structures (particularly the hippocampus and amygdala); and increased size of sulci (fissures) on the surface of the brain. These findings all suggest loss (atrophy) or underdevelopment of brain tissue. There is a trend for enlarged ventricles to be associated with two indicators of poor prognosis: early age of onset and poor premorbid functioning (functioning before the first diagnosis).

PET scans usually demonstrate decreased cerebral blood flow to the frontal lobes during specific cognitive tasks in people with schizophrenia. This frontal hypometabolism is thought to account for some problems with attention, planning, and decision-making. The thalamus (which lies in the center of the brain, near the temporal lobes and hippocampus, and regulates sensory input, serving as a filter or relay station between the cerebral cortex and the rest of the brain) was also found in several studies to be smaller than average and to have reduced activity in some schizophrenic patients. This may explain some of the problems in sensory filtering and information processing in many people with schizophrenia. The basal ganglia, part of the extrapyramidal system, are responsible for various aspects of movement, such as the inhibition of unwanted movement and the promotion of motor learning and planning, and may also play a role in cognitive function with their rich connectivity to the frontal lobes. The basal ganglia are overactive in people with schizophrenia, perhaps accounting for movement and speech abnormalities.

Neurotransmitter studies. During the past several decades, research in the area of neurotransmission has led to the dysregulation hypothesis of schizophrenia: a persistent impairment in one or more neurotransmitter or neuromodulator homeostatic regulatory mechanisms causing unstable or erratic neurotransmission. This theory proposes that there are overactive dopamine pathways in the mesolimbic area while prefrontal mesocortical dopaminergic pathways are hypoactive and that there is an imbalance between dopamine and serotonin neurotransmitter systems (and probably others as well).

Dopamine has been implicated the longest in neurotransmitter studies of schizophrenia. This is because it has long been known that mind-altering drugs such as amphetamines and cocaine increase brain levels of dopamine and produce psychosis and because early on it was understood that the conventional antipsychotic drugs exerted their therapeutic effects by blocking dopamine receptors. Dopamine is important in responses to stress, and has many connections to the limbic system. The prefrontal cortex has few dopamine receptors of its own, but it may regulate dopamine in other circuits in the brain. Also, dopamine is present in high levels in the brain during late adolescence, when schizophrenia usually first appears. Dopamine is found in three parts of the brain:

- Substantia nigra motor center, affecting movement and coordination
- Midbrain, involving emotion and memory
- Hypothalamic-pituitary connection, involving emotional responses and stress-coping patterns

Dopamine has four major pathways in the brain (Fig. 22-4):

- Mesocortical: innervates the frontal lobes. Function: insight, judgment, social consciousness, inhibition, and highest level of cognitive activities (reasoning, motivation, planning, decision-making). Negative symptoms: affective flattening or blunting, poverty of speech or speech content, blocking, poor grooming, lack of motivation, anhedonia, social withdrawal, cognitive defects, and attention deficits
- Mesolimbic: innervates the limbic system. Function: associated with memory, smell, automatic visceral effects, and emotional behavior. Positive symptoms: hallucinations, delusions, disorganized speech, and bizarre behavior
- Tuberoinfundibular: originates in the hypothalamus and projects to the pituitary. Function: endocrine function, hunger, thirst, metabolism, temperature control, digestion, sexual arousal, and circadian rhythms (implicated in some of the endocrine abnormalities seen in schizophrenia and some of the side effects of antipsychotic drugs)
- Nigrostriatal: originates in the substantia nigra and terminates in the caudate nucleus–putamen complex (neostriatum). Function: innervates the motor and extrapyramidal systems (implicated in some of the movement side effects of antipsychotic drugs)

Serotonin, in addition to mediating many brain functions, has also been implicated in schizophrenia. It has a modulating effect on dopamine, and some atypical antipsychotic drugs (clozapine, risperidone, olanzapine, and quetiapine) are combination serotonin/dopamine blocking agents, accounting for their improved efficacy over the typi-

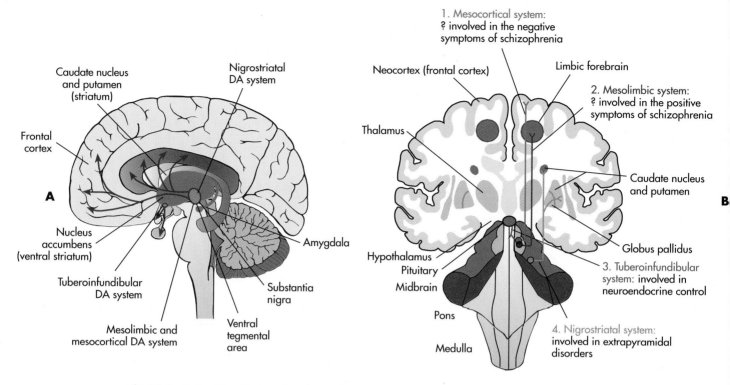

Fig. 22-4 A, A midsagittal section shows the approximate anatomical routes of the four dopamine tracts. **B,** A coronal section shows the sites of origin and the targets of all four tracts. (Modified from Kandel E, Schwartz J, Jessell T: *Principles of neural science,* ed 3, New York, 1991, Elsevier.)

cal antipsychotics in the treatment of the negative symptoms of schizophrenia.

Glutamate is the major excitatory neurotransmitter in the brain. Research on the effect of PCP (phencyclidine), a drug that seems to mimic the symptoms of schizophrenia in normal volunteers, has led to a better understanding of how glutamate interacts with dopamine. The function of glutamates' major receptor complex, NMDA (N-methyl-D-aspartate), is interrupted by PCP. This important brain communication system is abnormal in the prefrontal cortex and thalamus in post mortem studies of schizophrenics. Experimental psychotropic agents that activate the NMDA receptor complex and its coagonist site for glycine are proposed as potential future treatments for schizophrenia.

Neurodevelopment. It is now clear that the multiple structural, functional, and chemical brain deviations seen in schizophrenia are usually present long before the symptoms appear, probably from the earliest years of life, and perhaps before birth. It is not clear yet whether these changes are caused by genetic programming defects or environmental injury, or both, creating a vulnerability that remains dormant until later developmental events occur. Several brain structures are abnormal in patients with schizophrenia as compared with controls that interfere with working memory (prefrontal cortex and hippocampus), and these brains were found to have increased cortical folding (a sign of early developmental abnormality in the infant brain). Also, the volume of grey matter in the fusiform gyrus, a structure that participates in facial recognition and naming, a cognitive function commonly disturbed in psy-

chosis, was 13% less in patients with schizophrenia compared with controls (Lindsay, 2000).

Research has shown that some preschizophrenic children show subtle abnormalities involving attention, coordination, and emotional responses long before they exhibit overt symptoms of schizophrenia (Duzyurek & Wiener, 1999). In some monozygotic twin pairs, the schizophrenic twin was noted to become permanently different from the unaffected identical twin by the age of 5 years, although symptoms of schizophrenia did not appear until young adulthood. These early childhood differences included excessive shyness, hyperactivity, bed-wetting, aggressiveness, poor concentration and coordination, tantrums, hand-washing compulsions, reversion to baby talk, and delays in learning to walk and speak (Torry et al, 1994). Identification of these prodromal symptoms in children at risk for adult schizophrenia can result in early intervention strategies, perhaps avoiding or delaying the onset of illness or minimizing its effects.

It has not been agreed that the intrauterine environment or early infant events are linked to the development of schizophrenia. Some research has found a greater frequency of prenatal and perinatal complications among schizophrenics, such as preeclampsia or trauma or oxygen deprivation at the time of delivery, extreme prematurity, or maternal problems such as poor nutrition, stress, tobacco, alcohol, street drugs, caffeine, viral infection, and pharmacological agents. This research suggests that some disruption in fetal neural development may change the way the brain matures throughout childhood and adolescence, affecting the myelination, migration, and interconnections of young neurons as they mature in utero and in the first few decades after birth and thus may contribute to brain abnormalities common in schizophrenia (Dalman et al, 1999).

Viral theories. There is mixed evidence that prenatal exposure to the influenza virus, particularly during the second trimester, may be one of the factors in the etiology of schizophrenia in some people but not in others. This theory is supported by research findings that more people with schizophrenia are born in the winter or early spring and in urban settings. These findings suggest a potential season and place of birth impact on the risk for schizophrenia. Viral infections are more common in crowded places and in winter and early spring, and may occur in utero or in early childhood in some vulnerable people (Battle et al, 1999).

Psychological. In the past, in the absence of identified biological causes for schizophrenia, psychological, sociological, and environmental influences became the focus of psychodynamic and other theories and beliefs about the illness. For most of the twentieth century schizophrenia was thought to be an illness caused partly by the family and partly by some individual character flaw. The mother was believed to be anxious, overprotective, or cold and unfeeling; the father was distant or overbearing. Marital conflict and families that stayed together for the sake of the children were blamed. There were theories describing a "schizophrenogenic" mother and theories that described how communicating in double messages could "double bind" a person into developing schizophrenia.

Schizophrenia was also proposed by some to be a failure to accomplish an early stage of psychosocial development. For example, an infant's inability to form a trusting relationship could lead to a lifetime of intrapsychic conflict. Schizophrenia was seen as the most severe example of inability to cope with stress. Disturbances in identity, inability to attach to a love object, and inability to control basic drives also served as key theories.

It is important for psychiatric nurses and the health-care community in general to realize that with the psychobiological discoveries of recent years, these psychodynamic theories have no scientific evidence to support them. In addition, they can have a very negative impact on patient and family alliances with mental health-care professionals, can perpetuate stigma associated with these illnesses, and may contribute to a delay of appropriate interventions that could impact negatively on treatment outcome.

The "schizophrenogenic" mother was described as one who gave her child conflicting and confusing messages about their relationship, resulting in schizophrenia. How would this unsupported theory affect the mothers of people with schizophrenia, their relationships with their ill children, and their relationships with care providers?

Sociocultural and Environmental. Some theorists proposed that poverty, society, and cultural disharmony could cause schizophrenia or that people chose to become schizophrenic to cope with the insanity of the modern world. Others proposed that schizophrenia was caused by living in the city or living in isolation in the country. Although accumulated stress related to sociocultural and environmental factors is likely to be a contributing factor to the onset of schizophrenia and to relapses, neurobiological findings point to other causes for the primary development of psychotic disorders.

Precipitating Stressors

Biological. Interference in a brain feedback loop that regulates the amount of information that can be processed at a given time has been identified as one possible biological stressor. Normal information processing occurs in a predetermined series of neural activities. Visual and auditory stimuli are initially screened and filtered by the thalamus and sent for processing by the frontal lobe. If too much information is sent at once, or if the information is faulty, the frontal lobe sends an overload message to the basal ganglia. The basal ganglia in turn send a message to the thalamus to slow down transmissions to the frontal lobe. The decreased function of the frontal lobe impairs the ability of this feedback loop to perform. There is less ability to regulate the basal ganglia, and ultimately, the message to slow down transmissions to the frontal lobe never occurs. The result is information-processing overload and the neurobiological responses described in the beginning of this chapter.

Another possible biological stressor is the abnormal gating mechanisms that may occur in schizophrenia. Gating is an electrical process involving electrolytes. It refers to inhibitory and excitatory nerve action potentials and the feedback occurring within the nervous system related to completed nerve transmissions. Decreased gating is demonstrated by a person's inability to selectively attend to stimuli (Perry et al, 1999). For example, at a baseball game the person with schizophrenia would be unable to differentiate the noise from the crowd, the organ, the team, or the public address system. Normally, when people hear a loud noise they become startled; however, when the noise is repeated, there is a decreased startle response. For example, if you hear a neighbor setting off firecrackers on the Fourth of July, you become startled. When you hear a second explosion, you are generally less startled. The person with schizophrenia is just as startled the second time, and maybe even more than the first. This inability to gate a noise stimulus causes people to become frightened in crowds or wherever there is increased noise.

Symptom triggers. Precursors and stimuli or combinations of them often precede a new episode of the illness. The word **trigger** is used to describe these stressors. Common triggers of neurobiological responses related to health, environment, attitudes, and behaviors are listed in Table 22-5. Patients with schizophrenia can learn to recognize triggers that they are particularly reactive to, and they can be taught to avoid them if possible, and to contact their mental health-care provider for help if they cannot.

Appraisal of Stressors

Stress Diathesis. There is no scientific research indicating that stress causes schizophrenia, but it is increasingly clear that it is a disorder that not only causes stress, but is also

Table 22-5

Neurobiological Response Symptom Triggers

HEALTH

Poor nutrition
Lack of sleep
Out-of-balance circadian rhythms
Fatigue
Infection
Central nervous system drugs
Lack of exercise
Barriers to accessing health care

ENVIRONMENT

Hostile/critical environment
Housing difficulties (unsatisfactory housing)
Pressure to perform (loss of independent living)
Changes in life events, daily patterns of activity
Interpersonal difficulties, disruptions in interpersonal
  relationships
Social isolation
Lack of social support
Job pressures (poor occupational skills)
Stigmatization
Poverty
Lack of transportation (resources)
Inability to get/keep a job

ATTITUDES/BEHAVIORS

"Poor me" (low self-concept)
"Hopeless" (lack of self-confidence)
"I'm a failure" (loss of motivation to use skills)
"Lack of control" (demoralization)
Feeling overpowered by symptoms
"No one likes me" (unable to meet spiritual needs)
Looks/acts different from others who are of the same
  age, culture
Poor social skills
Aggressive behavior
Violent behavior
Poor medication management
Poor symptom management

strongly influenced by stress. Studies of relapse and symptom exacerbation provide evidence that stress, one's appraisal of the stressor, and problems with coping with the stress may predict the return of symptoms (Perese, 1997). The stress diathesis model described in a classic work by Liberman and colleagues (1984) states that schizophrenic symptoms develop based on the relationship between the amount of stress that a person experiences and an internal stress tolerance threshold. This is an important model because it integrates biological, psychological, and sociocultural factors. In this way it is similar to the Stuart Stress Adaptation Model, which is used as the organizing conceptual framework of this text (Fig. 22-5). Wuerker (2000) provides an adaptation of a model from which to understand the integration of stress in this neurobiological brain disease (Fig. 22-6).

Coping Resources

Coping skills tend to be learned from parents. Children and young adults with schizophrenia need to be actively taught these skills because they have difficulty internalizing them from observation. Family resources such as parental understanding of the illness, finances, availability of time and energy, and ability to provide ongoing support influence the course of illness.

It is important to remember that the mix of disabilities and resources of a particular patient is related to the type and location of the brain dysfunction. Thus it is essential to assess mental status carefully to identify the person's strengths. For instance, some people with maladaptive neurobiological responses are highly intelligent but unable to express themselves well. Others may be artistically talented but not skilled at verbal communication. Exploring these areas of strength helps the nurse in planning individualized nursing interventions.

Coping Mechanisms

Patients attempt to protect themselves from the frightening experiences caused by their illnesses. Regression is related to information-processing problems and expenditure of large amounts of energy in efforts to manage anxiety, leaving little for activities of daily living. Projection is an effort to explain confusing perceptions by assigning responsibility to someone or something. Withdrawal is related to problems establishing trust and preoccupation with internal experiences. Families often express denial when they first learn of their relative's diagnosis. This is the same as the denial that occurs whenever one receives information that causes fear and anxiety. It allows the person to gather internal and external resources and adapt to the stressor gradually.

NURSING DIAGNOSIS

In formulating the nursing diagnosis the nurse should review the complete nursing assessment as illustrated in the Stuart Stress Adaptation Model (Fig. 22-5). Nursing diagnoses take into account the functional level, stressors, and support systems of the patient and should be prioritized according to the patient's stage of illness (crisis, acute, maintenance, or health promotion). Nursing diagnoses associated with maladaptive neurobiological responses are presented in the Medical and Nursing Diagnoses box on p. 418. Primary NANDA nursing diagnoses include **impaired verbal communication, sensory/perceptual alterations, impaired social interaction, social isolation,** and **altered thought processes.** Examples of complete nursing diagnoses are presented in the Detailed Diagnoses box on p. 419.

Related Medical Diagnoses

The medical diagnoses associated with maladaptive neurobiological responses include the schizophrenias, schizophreniform disorder, schizoaffective disorder, delusional disorder, brief psychotic disorder, and shared psychotic disorder. These diagnoses and related essential features are presented in the Detailed Diagnoses box on p. 419.

OUTCOME IDENTIFICATION

The expected outcome of patient care is as follows:

The patient will live, learn, and work at a maximum possible level of success, as defined by the individual.

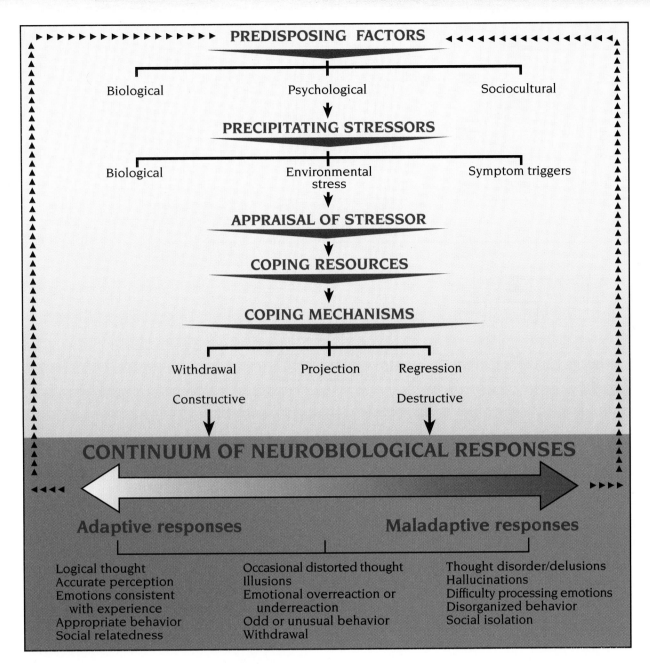

Fig. 22-5   The Stuart Stress Adaptation Model related to neurobiological responses.

Prevention of relapse and early intervention are key components of a successful outcome. Relapse is the return of symptoms severe enough to interfere with activities of daily living. It can be prevented only by thorough, ongoing symptom monitoring (Herz, 1999). Planning therapeutic interventions depends on goals related to diagnosis and level of wellness.

Short-term goals identify the steps that will lead the patient to successfully accomplish the expected outcome. Examples include the following:

- The patient will initiate conversation with at least one person daily.
- The patient will participate in medication education group.
- The patient will identify medications and describe the prescribed dose, expected effects, possible side effects, and actions to take if questions arise.

- The patient will engage in a wellness lifestyle.
- The patient will describe preferred living situation following hospital discharge.
- The patient will practice community living skills such as food preparation, housekeeping, care of clothing, money management, and use of public transportation.

PLANNING

When a person is in the crisis or acute stage of illness, care is often given in a hospital. The overall goal is to help the patient to reach stability while establishing a foundation for habilitation. Because of the complex psychosocial needs of patients with maladaptive neurobiological responses, planning for discharge begins with admission. All patient resources must be studied. The family resources are particularly important because families are the providers of care for

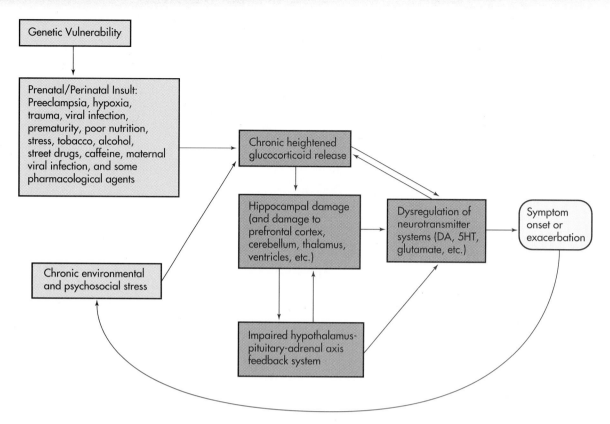

Fig. 22-6 Neural stress – diathesis model of schizophrenia. (Modified from Wuerker A: *Issues Ment Health Nurs* 21:123, 2000.)

 Medical and Nursing Diagnoses *related to* **Maladaptive Neurobiological Responses**

RELATED MEDICAL DIAGNOSES (*DSM–IV–TR*)*	RELATED NURSING DIAGNOSES, NANDA†
Schizophrenia	Adjustment, impaired
Paranoid type	Activity intolerance
Disorganized type	Anxiety
Catatonic type	**Communication, impaired verbal‡**
Undifferentiated type	Confusion
Residual type	Coping, family: potential for growth
Schizophreniform disorder	Coping, ineffective family: compromised
Schizoaffective disorder	Coping, ineffective individual
Delusional disorder	Decisional conflict
Brief psychotic disorder	Denial, ineffective
Shared psychotic disorder	Management of therapeutic regimen, individual or family: effective or ineffective
	Personal identity disturbance
	Role performance, altered
	Self-care deficit (bathing/hygiene, dressing/grooming)
	Self-esteem disturbance
	Sensory/Perceptual alterations (specify)‡
	Social interaction, impaired‡
	Social isolation‡
	Thought processes, altered‡
	Caregiver role strain, risk for

*Reprinted with permission from the *Diagnostic and statistical manual of mental disorders*, Fourth Edition, Text Revision. Copyright 2000. American Psychiatric Association.
†From North American Nursing Diagnosis Association: *NANDA nursing diagnoses: definitions and classifications 1999-2000*, Philadelphia, 1999, The Association.
‡Primary nursing diagnosis for maladaptive neurobiological responses.

Detailed Diagnoses *related to* **Maladaptive Neurobiological Responses**

NANDA DIAGNOSIS STEM	EXAMPLES OF COMPLETE DIAGNOSIS
Impaired verbal communication	Impaired verbal communication related to formal thought disorder, as evidenced by loose associations.
Sensory/perceptual alteration (specify)	Sensory/perceptual alteration (auditory) related to physiological brain dysfunction, as evidenced by verbal reports of "hearing voices that say bad things about me."
Social isolation	Social isolation related to inadequate social skills, as evidenced by inappropriate sexual advances toward members of both sexes.
Altered thought processes	Altered thought processes as related to physiological brain dysfunction, as evidenced by stated belief that staff members are really actors who were hired by parents to watch him.

DSM–IV–TR DIAGNOSIS	ESSENTIAL FEATURES*
Schizophrenia	At least two of the following, each present for a significant portion of time during a 1-month period: Delusions Hallucinations Disorganized speech Grossly disorganized or catatonic behavior Negative symptoms For a significant portion of the time since the onset of the disturbance, one or more major areas of functioning such as work, interpersonal relations, or self-care is markedly below the level achieved before the onset. Continuous signs of the disturbance persist for at least 6 months.
Paranoid type	Preoccupation with one or more delusions or frequent auditory hallucinations.
Disorganized type	All of the following are prominent: disorganized speech, disorganized behavior, flat or inappropriate affect; does not meet the criteria for catatonic type.
Catatonic type	At least two of the following dominate the clinical picture: motor immobility as evidenced by catalepsy or stupor; excessive motor activity; extreme negativism or mutism; peculiarities of voluntary movement, as evidenced by posturing, stereotyped movements, prominent mannerisms, or prominent grimacing; echolalia or echopraxia.
Undifferentiated type	Symptoms meeting the first general criteria for schizophrenia are present, but criteria for other types are not met.
Residual type	Criteria for schizophrenia are not met, nor are those for any other subtype. There is continuing evidence of the disturbance, indicated by negative symptoms or attenuated presence of two or more symptoms included in the general criteria.
Schizophreniform disorder	Meets criteria for schizophrenia and an episode lasts at least 1 month but less than 6 months. Specify with or without good prognostic features based on at least two of the following: onset of prominent psychotic symptoms within 4 weeks of first noticeable change in behavior or functioning, confusion or perplexity at the height of the psychosis, good premorbid social and occupational functioning, and absence of blunted or flat affect.
Schizoaffective disorder	An interrupted period of illness including a major depressive episode or manic episode concurrent with symptoms of schizophrenia. During the same period of illness, there have been delusions or hallucinations for at least 2 weeks in the absence of prominent mood symptoms. Symptoms of a mood episode are present during a substantial part of the illness.
Delusional disorder	Nonbizarre delusions (situations that could occur, such as being followed, poisoned, or having a disease) lasting at least a month. Has never met criteria for schizophrenia. Apart from the impact of the delusion, functioning and behavior are not markedly affected.
Brief psychotic disorder	Presence of at least one of the following: delusions, hallucinations, disorganized speech, or grossly disorganized or catatonic behavior. (Behaviors are not culturally sanctioned.) Duration between 1 day and 1 month, with eventual return to premorbid functioning. The presence (brief reactive) or absence of marked stressors should be noted, as should onset within 4 weeks postpartum.
Shared psychotic disorder (folie a deux)	A delusion develops in a patient in the context of a close relationship with someone who already has a delusion. The delusions of the people involved are similar in content.

*Reprinted with permission from the *Diagnostic and statistical manual of mental disorders*, Fourth Edition, Text Revision. Copyright 2000. American Psychiatric Association.

at least 65% of patients with schizophrenia (Hatfield, 1997). Federal law requires that patients and, with patients' permission, family members be present at treatment planning meetings. This facilitates a smooth transition from the hospital to home. Recognizing the burden of caring for loved ones with schizophrenia, families must decide what resources they are able to use to assist the patient (Lukens et al, 1999). These resources may include time, energy, knowledge, and money. The discharge plan must be based on the reality of available resources.

Care of the patient in the maintenance phase occurs at home or in another community setting. The focus of this phase is to assist with habilitation. The process of habilitation begins with learning to identify symptom triggers and

Citing the Evidence on

Patterns of Usual Care

BACKGROUND: This survey of 719 persons with schizophrenia examined the current patterns of usual care they received to the Schizophrenia Patient Outcomes Research Team (PORT) Treatment Recommendations.

RESULTS: The rates at which patients' treatment conformed to the recommendations were modest at best, generally below 50%. Specifically:

Only 29% of patients received the appropriate dose of antipsychotic medication over the long-term

Fewer than half of people who also suffered symptoms of depression received antidepressant medication

Only half of those suffering serious side effects of medication received appropriate and effective treatment to counteract those problems

African Americans were almost twice as likely to be overmedicated with antipsychotic medications and suffer higher rates of side effects

Fewer than one in 10 families received even minimal education and support

Fewer than one in 4 patients who could have benefited from employment received any such support

As few as 2% of patients received assertive community treatment (ACT), which is highly effective in preventing relapse (see Chapter 36).

IMPLICATIONS: The findings indicate that current usual treatment practices related to schizophrenia fall substantially short of what is recommended based on the best evidence on treatment efficacy. This disparity points to the need for greater efforts to ensure that treatment research results are translated into practice in order to improve the quality of care provided to patients.

Lehman A et al: Patterns of usual care for schizophrenia: initial results from the schizophrenia Patient Outcomes Research Team (PORT) client survey, *Schizophr Bull* 24(1): 11, 1998.

early symptoms. Successful habilitation also involves the identification of symptom management techniques that reduce the potential for relapse and maintain stability. Additional information about the rehabilitation of people with maladaptive neurobiological responses is included in Chapter 15. Finally, it is important for nurses to be aware that while there are effective treatments for schizophrenia, for the most part, people facing this serious brain disease are not receiving them (see Citing the Evidence). Thus the nurse has a significant responsibility to patients, families and communities to educate, advocate and promote effective treatment strategies for neurobiological illnesses.

When stability has been attained, the health promotion phase begins. The goal is to collaboratively develop and implement symptom management techniques that prevent relapse. When patients and families recognize that relapse prevention is possible, they become empowered and can enjoy a quality of life that places the patient rather than the illness in control.

IMPLEMENTATION

Intervention modalities encompass the full range of psychosocial and psychobiological treatments and must include the patient, family, and caretaker if possible (American Psychiatric Asociation, 1997; Lehman et al, 1998). The modality chosen should be based on predisposing factors, precipitating stressors, coping resources, coping mechanisms, and the patient's responses.

The core problems related to cognition, perception, emotion, behavior and movement, and socialization create significant difficulties for people with schizophrenia. These problems affect the implementation of the nursing treatment plan. Table 22-6 outlines areas of difficulty and related nursing interventions in working with a patient who is psychotic. These issues must be addressed in order to maximize the patient's recovery and enhance compliance with the treatment plan. Empirically validated treatments related to schizophrenia are summarized in Table 22-7.

Interventions in the Crisis and Acute Phases

Unstable neurobiological responses require constant observation and monitoring of health, behavior, and attitudes. Research has shown that aggressive early intervention improves both prognosis and quality of life (Jarboe et al, 1998; Ho et al, 1998). Nursing interventions in this phase should focus on restoring adaptive neurobiological responses while providing for the safety and well-being of the patient.

Patient Safety. Patient safety is a critical issue during the crisis and acute phases, particularly in light of the fact that 10% of patients with schizophrenia commit suicide (see Citing the Evidence on Suicide, p. 422). Environmental safety factors should be attended to, including the availability of sharp and dangerous objects, as well as the placement of furniture, art objects, and pictures (see Chapter 21). It is important to maintain constant vigilance with the patient and carefully explain all actions involving the patient. Patients may accidentally harm themselves because of impaired judgment or responding to hallucinations or delu-

Table **22-6**

Behavioral Strategies for People with Psychosis

Core Problems	Nursing Interventions
Anxiety	Teach patient the symptoms related to anxiety. Help patient to identify what triggers anxiety. Help patient use symptom management techniques to cope with anxiety. Assess whether anxiety is a relapse trigger and, if so, make a plan to reduce anxiety while still in the moderate stage.
Depression	Teach patient the symptoms related to depression. Help patient use symptom management techniques to cope with depression. Assess whether depression is a relapse trigger and, if so, make a plan to reduce depression while still in a mild stage because there is a high correlation between depression and being able to perform activities of daily living.
Inability to learn from experience	Review both positive and negative experiences. Identify what was successful in helping the patient achieve the desired goal and what was not successful.
Problems with cause-and-effect reasoning	Analyze each experience to see what went well and what did not. Help patient sequence events leading to the outcome in each experience. Rehearsal may be helpful in enacting an event before it occurs.
Difficulty assessing passage of time	Teach patient how to use clocks to tell time. Teach patient to use environmental cues such as the sun going down or a certain radio program to orient oneself to time of day. Help patient create and maintain a calendar of scheduled activities.
Concrete thinking	Realize that the patient sees every problem as having one solution. Teach patient to look at other possible solutions to problems. Realize that the patient often thinks there is only one way to do a task. Create alternative ways to approach situations.
Difficulty telling background from foreground information	Teach patient to distinguish between important and unimportant information. Teach patient to focus on only the important information. Help patient learn to avoid or minimize confusion caused by excess stimulation from noise and large crowds.
Slowed information processing	Give patients time to process and respond to information. Minimize anxiety because this increases information processing difficulties. Demonstrate genuine interest in trying to understand what the patient is saying. Be clear and simple when communicating with patient.
Difficulty screening information to share	Teach patient to identify people who are safe to talk to about one's illness. Teach patient to go to these people when the symptoms are creating problems. Let patient know that you understand the illness and are a safe person to talk with.
Communication difficulties	Use active listening to understand the patient. Clarify what the patient is trying to tell you. Listen for the theme. Seek validation from patient on what is communicated. Help patient with vocabulary as needed. Use the literal meaning of words. Have patient repeat back what was heard. Help patient understand the words and phrases used.
Problems expressing needs	Help patient to identify and prioritize needs. Help patient to express needs in ways that others will understand. Role play conversations and practice negotiating with others.
Low self-concept	Help patient identify and maximize his or her strengths and positive characteristics. Use role play to handle common situations patients face. Give positive feedback when patient handles a situation well. Analyze a problem to determine how it could have been better handled.
Forced isolation due to stigma	Maximize patient's understanding of his or her illness. Teach patient to minimize stigmatizing behaviors when possible. Identify comments that are difficult to handle. Teach ways to handle stigma and rude comments. Develop concrete humorous comebacks. Role play various situations with the nurse being the patient.
Difficulty with perception and interpretation of sensory stimuli	Review problematic situations with the patient. List and assess the thought processes in interpreting events. Help patient reality test and reframe problematic interpretations. Reinforce positive and productive processes.
Poor attention span and difficulty completing tasks	Help patient break tasks into small sequential steps. Help the patient keep focused on a single task, a step at a time. Do not emphasize completing the task. Give directions to patient one step at a time.
Inappropriate social behaviors	Identify the patient's thought processes that lead to the behavior. Ask patient about the behavior. Help correct inaccurate perceptions. Help patient identify undesirable outcomes of the behavior. Teach appropriate social skills.
Difficulty with decision making	Help patient to determine desired outcomes. Help patient to prioritize goals and categorize them into short and long term. Help patient establish a time line for attainment of each goal. Help establish small, concrete steps to achieve desired goals. Ensure that these small steps are achievable by the patient and are culturally and value congruent.

Table **22-7**

Summarizing the Evidence on Treatments that Work for Neurobiological Responses
DISORDER Schizophrenia
TREATMENT: ■ Conventional antipsychotic medications (e.g., chlorpromazine, fluphenazine, haloperidol, loxapine, perphenazine, trifluoperazine, thiothixene, and thioridazine) markedly reduced the positive symptoms of schizophrenia and significantly decreased the risk of symptomatic relapse and rehospitalization. However, serious neurological side effects made these drugs difficult to tolerate for many patients with schizophrenia.
■ More recently, a group of "atypical" antipsychotic drugs (e.g., clozapine, risperidone, and olanzapine) have demonstrated comparable—or better—efficacy with schizophrenic symptoms with significantly less risk of adverse neurological events. These drugs may be especially effective in treating the negative symptoms of schizophrenia.
■ Behavior therapy and social learning/token economy programs helped structure, support, and reinforce prosocial behaviors in treatment refractory persons with schizophrenia. Structured, educational family interventions helped maintain gains achieved with medication and customary case management. Social skills training enabled persons with schizophrenia to acquire instrumental and affiliative skills to improve functioning in their communities.

From: Nathan P, Gorman J: *A guide to treatments that work*, New York, 1998, Oxford University Press.

Citing the Evidence on

Suicide

BACKGROUND: This study explored the association between psychosocial variables and symptoms among patients with schizophrenia who have attempted suicide and those who have not attempted suicide.

RESULTS: There was a 29.2% rate of one or more suicide attempts among the study subjects with schizophrenia. Compared with patients who had not attempted suicide, patients who had made an attempt had a greater number of lifetime depressive episodes, an earlier age of onset of their illness, and an earlier age of first hospitalization.

IMPLICATIONS: These results may be important risk factors for suicidal behavior among patients with schizophrenia and other psychotic disorders. Depressive symptoms, especially in patients with early age of onset, should be recognized early and treated. The results also suggest that psychosocial variables may be less valuable predictors of suicide than clinical variables.

Gupta S, Black D: Factors associated with suicide attempts among patients with schizophrenia, *Psychiatr Serv* 49:1353, 1998.

sions. For example, a patient with a badly abscessed tooth refused to go to the dentist. He was afraid the dentist would plant a radio in his tooth that would broadcast his thoughts to those who were trying to harm him. The concern of the health-care providers was that the infection was interfering with the patient's health and making the psychosis worse. Unfortunately, patients often have difficulty distinguishing between people who are trying to help them and those they believe seek to harm them.

Staff can create safety issues for patients when they fail to respond to patient needs in a caring and appropriate manner. Patients should not feel threatened, belittled, anxious, ignored, rejected, boxed in, or controlled by staff. Helping the patient to reduce anxiety and feel safe and accepted decreases the incidence of harmful behaviors toward self and others.

Managing Delusions. Patients cope with delusions in several ways. Some adapt by learning to live with them. Others deny the presence of these troublesome symptoms. Still others seek to understand the symptom and become empowered to manage delusions when they occur. The art of communicating with people who have delusions requires the development of trust. Patients with cognitive disorders have difficulty processing language; therefore, the beginning of trust is more readily accomplished through nonverbal communication. Patients with delusions perceive the environment as much more stimulating than others do. It is essential for the nurse to approach the patient with calmness, empathy, and gentle eye contact. Patients report they can literally "feel the vibrations" of others and can "sense if the nurse is with me or against me." Once trust is established, the use of clear, direct, and simple statements becomes significant in communicating with people who have delusions.

Describe nonverbal nursing approaches that would foster the development of trust between a nurse and a delusional patient.

These patients are keenly sensitive to rejection. When they sense anxiety and avoidance in the nurse they often feel annoyed, inadequate, and hopeless. Sensing rejection by health-care professionals can also lead to anger on the part of the patient.

If patients perceive that the nurse is going along with the delusion, they become confused, particularly if they sense that the nurse is trying to get their cooperation. The nurse should not attempt a logical explanation of the delusion be-

Box 22-5

Strategies for Working with Patients with Delusions

PLACE THE DELUSION IN A TIME FRAME AND IDENTIFY TRIGGERS

Identify all of the components of the delusion by placing it in time and sequence.

Identify triggers that may be related to stress or anxiety.

If delusions are linked to anxiety, teach anxiety management skills.

Develop a symptom management program.

ASSESS THE INTENSITY, FREQUENCY, AND DURATION OF THE DELUSION

Fleeting delusions can be worked out in a short time frame.

Fixed delusions, endured over time, may have to be temporarily avoided to prevent them from becoming stumbling blocks in the relationship.

Listen quietly until there is no need to discuss the delusion.

IDENTIFY EMOTIONAL COMPONENTS OF THE DELUSION.

Respond to the underlying feelings rather than the illogical nature of the delusions.

Encourage discussion of fears, anxiety, and anger without assuming that the delusion is right or wrong.

OBSERVE FOR EVIDENCE OF CONCRETE THINKING

Determine whether the patient takes you literally.

Determine whether you and the patient are using language in the same way.

OBSERVE SPEECH FOR SYMPTOMS OF A THOUGHT DISORDER

Determine whether the patient exhibits a thought disorder (is talking in circles, going off on tangents, easily changing subjects, and unable to respond to your attempts to redirect).

It may not be the appropriate time to point out discrepancy between fact and delusion.

OBSERVE FOR THE ABILITY TO ACCURATELY USE CAUSE-AND-EFFECT REASONING

Determine whether the patient can make logical predictions based on past experiences.

Determine whether the patient can conceptualize time.

Determine whether the patient can access and use meaningfully his or her recent and long-term memory.

DISTINGUISH BETWEEN THE DESCRIPTION OF THE EXPERIENCE AND THE FACTS OF THE SITUATION

Identify false beliefs about real situations.

Promote the patient's ability to reality test.

Determine whether the patient is hallucinating, as this will strengthen the delusion.

CAREFULLY QUESTION THE FACTS AS THEY ARE PRESENTED AND THEIR MEANING

Sometimes talking with the patient about the delusion will help him or her see that it is not true.

If you take this step before the previous steps are completed it may reinforce the delusion.

DISCUSS CONSEQUENCES OF THE DELUSION WHEN THE PERSON IS READY

When the intensity of the delusion lessens, discuss the delusion when the patient is ready.

Discuss the consequences of the delusion.

Allow the patient to take responsibility for his or her behavior, daily activities, and decision making.

Encourage the patient's personal responsibility for and participation in wellness and recovery.

PROMOTE DISTRACTION AS A WAY TO STOP FOCUSING ON THE DELUSION

Promote activities that require attention to physical skills and will help the patient use time constructively.

Recognize and reinforce healthy and positive aspects of the personality.

---

cause it will not be possible to identify one. Only the patient understands the logic behind the delusion and is not able to express it until after the delusion has reached conscious awareness. On gaining insight into the illness and symptoms, the patient can differentiate experiences with delusions from those that are reality based. In the meantime, the nurse should not underestimate the power of a delusion and the patient's inability to differentiate the delusion from reality.

It is normal for the nurse to feel confused by a delusion. The nurse must carefully assess the content of the delusion without appearing to probe. It is also important to assess the context and environmental triggers for the delusional experience. The nurse must avoid becoming incorporated into the delusion. However, this is difficult if the nurse has achieved a trusting relationship with the patient because people who are significant to the patient in reality may also become part of the delusional world.

Box 22-5 identifies strategies helpful in working with the patient who is delusional, and Box 22-6 identifies barriers to intervening. The intervention plan should be followed consistently by the entire treatment team. If the nurse resorts to "trying anything" to gain compliance, care will be inconsistent and will create an even more chaotic environment for the patient, who already has great difficulty identifying reality.

Managing Hallucinations. Approximately 70% of hallucinations are auditory, 20% are visual, and the remaining 10% are gustatory, tactile, olfactory, kinesthetic, or cenesthetic. Therapeutic nursing interventions for hallucinations involve understanding the characteristics of the hallucination and identifying the related anxiety level. Table 22-8 describes intensity levels, characteristics, and observable behaviors commonly associated with hallucinations.

The goal of intervention with patients who are hallucinating is to help them to increase awareness of these symptoms so that they can distinguish between the world of psychosis and the world of reality experienced by others without schizophrenia. The first step toward achieving this goal is facilitative communication. Unfortunately, patients experiencing these symptoms are often laughed at, belittled, and ignored when these symptoms emerge.

Box **22-6**

Barriers to Successful Intervention for Delusions

BECOMING ANXIOUS AND AVOIDING THE PERSON

Anxiety leads to annoyance, anger, a sense of hopelessness and failure, feelings of inadequacy, and potential laughing at or discounting the patient.

REINFORCING THE DELUSION

Do not go along with the delusion, especially to get the co-operation of the patient.

ATTEMPTING TO PROVE THE PERSON IS WRONG

Do not attempt a logical explanation.

SETTING UNREALISTIC GOALS

Do not underestimate the power of a delusion and the patient's need for it.

BECOMING INCORPORATED INTO THE DELUSIONAL SYSTEM

This will cause great confusion for the patient and make it impossible to establish boundaries of the therapeutic relationship.

FAILING TO CLARIFY CONFUSION SURROUNDING THE DELUSION

If the complexity and many intricacies of the delusion are not clearly understood, the delusion will become more elaborate.

BEING INCONSISTENT IN INTERVENTION

The intervention plan must be firmly adhered to; if you resort to "trying anything," approaches will become inconsistent and the patient less able to identify reality.

SEEING THE DELUSION FIRST AND THE PERSON SECOND

Avoid saying "the person who thinks he's being poisoned."

Table **22-8**

Levels of Intensity of Hallucinations

Level	Characteristics	Observable Patient Behaviors
Stage I: Comforting Moderate level of anxiety Hallucination is generally pleasant.	The hallucinator experiences intense emotions such as anxiety, loneliness, guilt, and fear and tries to focus on comforting thoughts to relieve anxiety. The person recognizes that thoughts and sensory experiences are within conscious control if the anxiety is managed. **Nonpsychotic**	Grinning or laughter that seems inappropriate. Moving lips without making any sounds. Rapid eye movements. Slowed verbal responses as if preoccupied. Silent and preoccupied.
Stage II: Condemning Severe level of anxiety Hallucination generally becomes repulsive.	Sensory experience is repulsive and frightening. The hallucinator begins to feel a loss of control and may attempt to distance self from the perceived source. Person may feel embarrassed by the sensory experience and withdraw from others. **Mild psychotic**	Increased autonomic nervous system signs of anxiety such as increased heart rate, respiration, and blood pressure. Attention span begins to narrow. Preoccupied with sensory experience and may lose ability to differentiate hallucination from reality.
Stage III: Controlling Severe level of anxiety Sensory experiences become omnipotent.	Hallucinator gives up trying to combat the experience and gives in to it. Content of hallucination may become appealing. Person may experience loneliness if sensory experience ends. **Psychotic**	Directions given by the hallucination will be followed rather than objected to. Difficulty relating to others. Attention span of only a few seconds or minutes. Physical symptoms of severe anxiety such as perspiring, tremors, inability to follow directions.
Stage IV: Conquering Panic level of anxiety Generally becomes elaborate and interwoven with delusions.	Sensory experiences may become threatening if person does not follow commands. Hallucinations may last for hours or days if there is no therapeutic intervention. **Severe psychotic**	Terror-stricken behaviors such as panic. Strong potential for suicide or homicide. Physical activity that reflects content of hallucination such as violence, agitation, withdrawal, or catatonia. Unable to respond to complex directions. Unable to respond to more than one person.

Learning about a person's hallucinations helps avoid the roadblocks to communication these symptoms can create when unrecognized. Left unattended, hallucinations will continue and may escalate. Nurses may become so involved in planning what to say that they forget about the importance of listening. Listening and observing are the keys to successful intervention with the person who is hallucinating.

Hallucinations are very real to the person having them, just as dreams during sleep are very real. The hallucinating person may have no way to determine whether these perceptions are real. It usually does not even occur to the person to verify the experience. An analogy might be hearing an ordinary weather report on the radio and not thinking to question whether the voice is from a real person. Inability to perceive reality accurately can make life difficult. Therefore, hallucinations can be considered problems needing a solution. This is best accomplished when the person can talk freely about the hallucinations. Nurses also need to be able to talk about hallucinations because they are useful indicators of the current level of symptoms in ongoing monitoring of a psychotic illness. To facilitate monitoring, the patient needs to be comfortable telling the nurse about symptoms.

Patients often learn not to discuss their unusual experiences with anyone because they have received negative responses from people who think their ideas are strange. The experience of hallucinations can be especially troublesome for the patient who does not have anyone to talk to about them. Being able to talk about one's hallucinations is a greatly reassuring and self-validating experience. This discussion can take place only in an atmosphere of genuine interest and concern.

For those who have never experienced a hallucination, it can be difficult to understand that the person has no control over it. People with true psychosis have no direct voluntary control over the brain malfunction that causes hallucinations. This means that they cannot just will them away. Ignoring hallucinations may increase the confusion of the already chaotic brain filled with delusional ideas and disjointed thoughts. If the person is left alone to sort out reality without the input of trusted health-care providers, the symptoms may overwhelm available coping resources. Interactive discussion of hallucinations is a vital element in the development of reality-testing skills. Communicating right at the time of the hallucination is particularly helpful. Honesty, genuineness, and openness are the foundation for effective communication during hallucinations.

Modulation of sensory stimulation to an optimal level is another useful technique for helping the patient minimize the perceptual confusion. Some patients do well with minimal environmental stimulation, whereas others find that noise and distraction help to drown out the hallucinations. It is essential to find out how the patient has previously managed hallucinations.

Command hallucinations are a special type of hallucination that are potentially dangerous. They may lead a person to perform harmful acts such as cutting off a body part or striking out at someone at the instruction of voices. Fear caused by these often frightening hallucinations can also lead to dangerous behaviors such as jumping out a window. Because of the potential seriousness of this symptom, intervention is crucial.

Intervening during the acute phase of hallucinations requires patience and the ability to spend time with the patient. Box 22-7 outlines strategies useful in working with patients who experience hallucinations. Four basic principles are helpful during this phase: maintain eye contact, speak simply in a slightly louder voice than usual, call the patient by name, and use touch. The patient needs sensory validation to override the abnormal sensory processes that are occurring in the brain. Unfortunately, traditional interventions focus on isolating the patient. Isolating a person during this time of intense sensory confusion often reinforces the psychosis. As with delusions, consistency is the essential ingredient to a successful intervention plan.

Psychopharmacology. Psychopharmacology as a treatment for maladaptive neurobiological responses is described in Chapter 28. Drugs that are more site and symptom specific and provide a better response with fewer side effects will ultimately improve patient adherence and patient outcome. Typical (traditional) antipsychotics have provided some measure of symptom relief for the majority of patients for the past 50 years, but these drugs have problematic side effects and are not effective for all symptoms of schizophrenia. Clozapine is the first of the newer atypical antipsychotic drugs. Because of the potential for it to cause agranulocytosis, its use is usually limited to the treatment of those patients who are treatment resistant to several trials of antipsychotic drugs. It is estimated that clozapine is effective for approximately 30% of the 20% not responding to the traditional antipsychotics (Littrell & Littrell, 1997). Risperidone, olanzapine, and quetiapine, examples of other atypical antipsychotic drugs, do not have the life-threatening side effects associated with clozapine, and are more efficacious with fewer side effects than the typical antipsychotics. Thus they are considered by most experts to be cost-effective first line treatments for schizophrenia (see Citing the Evidence on Atypical Antipsychotics, p. 426). Table 22-9 summarizes the medications most often prescribed for maladaptive neurobiological responses. Figure 22-7 provides a medication algorithm for the treatment of schizophrenia.

Cognitive-Behavioral Therapy. Cognitive-behavioral therapy (CBT), originally developed and evaluated with affective disorders, has been used successfully to treat persistent hallucinations and delusions as an adjunct to medication (Tarrier et al, 1998). This treatment has also been shown to be effective in those schizophrenic patients who were resistant to medication. CBT is a method of changing patients' thought processes, behavior, and emotion. Giving CBT in addition to routine care can reduce hallucinations and delusions, common positive psychotic symptoms in patients with chronic schizophrenia (see Citing the Evidence on Cognitive Behavioral Therapy, p. 428).

Interventions in the Maintenance Phase

Nursing interventions that focus on teaching self-management of symptoms and identifying symptoms indicative of

Box 22-7

Strategies for Working with Patients with Hallucinations

ESTABLISH A TRUSTING, INTERPERSONAL RELATIONSHIP

If the nurse is anxious or frightened, the patient will be anxious or frightened.

Be patient, show acceptance, and use active listening skills.

ASSESS FOR SYMPTOMS OF HALLUCINATIONS INCLUDING DURATION, INTENSITY, AND FREQUENCY

Observe for behavioral clues that indicate the presence of hallucinations.

Observe for clues that identify the level of intensity and duration of the hallucination.

Help the patient to record the number of hallucinations that are experienced each day.

FOCUS ON THE SYMPTOM AND ASK THE PATIENT TO DESCRIBE WHAT IS HAPPENING

Empower the patient by helping him or her to understand the symptoms experienced or demonstrated.

Help the patient gain control of the hallucinations, seek helpful distractions, and minimize intensity.

IDENTIFY WHETHER DRUGS OR ALCOHOL HAVE BEEN USED

Determine whether the person is using alcohol or drugs (over-the-counter, prescription, or street drugs).

Determine whether these may be responsible for or exacerbate the hallucinations.

IF ASKED, POINT OUT SIMPLY THAT YOU ARE NOT EXPERIENCING THE SAME STIMULI

Respond by letting the patient know what is actually happening in the environment.

Do not argue with the patient about differences in perceptions.

When a hallucination occurs, do not leave the person alone.

SUGGEST AND REINFORCE THE USE OF INTERPERSONAL RELATIONSHIPS AS A SYMPTOM MANAGEMENT TECHNIQUE

Encourage the patient to talk to someone trusted who will give supportive and corrective feedback.

Help the patient in mobilizing social supports.

HELP THE PATIENT DESCRIBE AND COMPARE CURRENT AND PAST HALLUCINATIONS

Determine whether there is a pattern to the patient's hallucinations.

Encourage the patient to remember when hallucinations first began.

Pay attention to the content of the hallucination; it may provide clues for predicting behavior.

Be especially alert for command hallucinations that may compel the patient to act in certain way.

Encourage the patient to describe past and present thoughts, feelings, and actions as they relate to hallucinations.

HELP THE PATIENT IDENTIFY NEEDS THAT MAY BE REFLECTED IN THE CONTENT OF THE HALLUCINATION

Identify needs that may trigger hallucinations.

Focus on the patient's unmet needs and discuss the relationship between them and the presence of hallucinations.

DETERMINE THE IMPACT OF THE PATIENT'S SYMPTOMS ON ACTIVITIES OF DAILY LIVING

Provide feedback regarding the patient's general coping responses and activities of daily living.

Help the patient recognize symptoms, symptom triggers, and symptom management strategies.

Citing the Evidence on

Atypical Antipsychotics

BACKGROUND: This study tested the efficacy of novel (atypical) antipsychotics in the treatment of cognitive impairment in early phase schizophrenia.

RESULTS: The results showed a significantly better benefit from treatment with olanzapine relative to risperidone, but no significant difference shown between risperidone and haloperidol.

IMPLICATIONS: These data suggest that olanzapine has some superior cognitive benefits relative to risperidone and haloperidol, although a larger study is needed to confirm and generalize these observations.

Purdon S et al: Neuropsychological changes in early phase schizophrenia during 12 months of treatment with olanzapine, risperidone, or haloperidol, *Arch Gen Psychiatry* 57:249, 2000.

relapse are most useful in the maintenance phase. Patient teaching should involve caregivers whenever possible (see A Family Speaks on p. 429) (Dixon et al, 1999). A Family Education Plan for understanding the world of psychosis is presented on p. 430. Behavioral interventions that teach patients skills for coping with psychotic symptoms include cognitive reframing regarding the cause of symptoms, gaining control over symptoms, and behavioral coping strategies. Patients and families should also be taught the following classic stages of relapse (Docherty et al, 1978).

Stages of Relapse. The first two of these five stages of relapse do not involve symptoms that indicate psychosis. This is relevant because this is the crucial time to intervene. In the first two stages the patient can seek and use feedback constructively.

Stage one is **overextension.** In this stage the patient complains of feeling overwhelmed. Symptoms of anxiety are intensified and great energy is used to overcome them. Patients describe feeling overloaded, being unable to concentrate on or complete tasks, and tend to forget words in the middle of

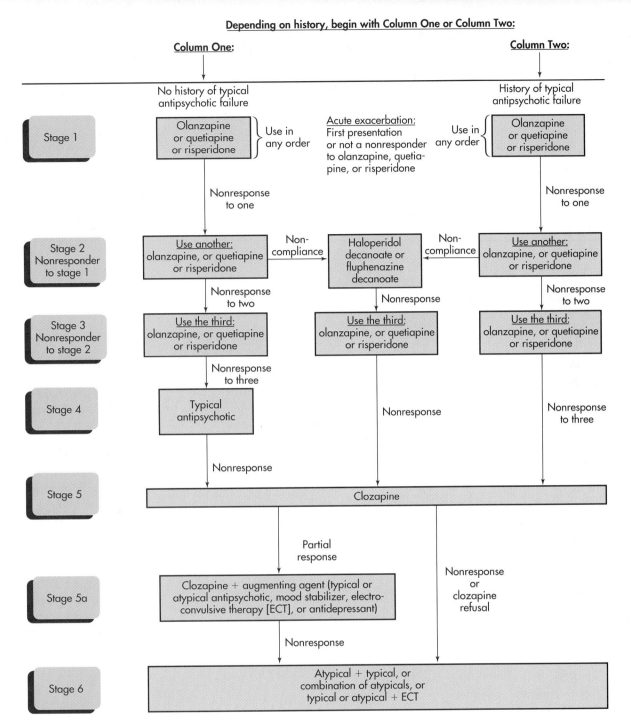

Fig. 22-7 Algorithm for the pharmacological treatment of schizophrenia. (From Chiles J et al: The Texas Medication Algorithm Project: development and implementation of the Schizophrenia Algorithm, *Psych Serv* 50(1):69, 1992.)

sentences. Other symptoms of overextension include increasing mental efforts to perform usual activities, decreasing performance efficiency, and easy distractibility.

Stage two is **restricted consciousness**. The previous symptoms of anxiety are joined by symptoms of depression. The depression is more intense than usual daily mood variations. There are added dimensions of appearing bored, apathetic, obsessional, and phobic. Somatization may occur. The pa-

tient seems to withdraw from everyday events and limits external stimulation as a way to protect against the upcoming loss of control.

The first appearance of psychotic features occurs in stage three, **disinhibition**. Symptoms may resemble those of hypomania and usually include the emergence of hallucinations and delusions that the patient no longer is able to control. Previously successful defense mechanisms tend to break down.

Table **22-9**

Antipsychotic Drugs		
Generic Name (Trade Name)	Drug Dosage Equivalence (mg)	Usual Maintenance Dosage Range (mg/day)
TYPICAL DRUGS		
Chlorpromazine (Thorazine)	100	300-1400
Thioridazine (Mellaril)	100	300-600*
Mesoridazine (Serentil)	50	100-500
Perphenazine (Trilafon)	10	8-64
Trifluoperazine (Stelazine)	5	10-80
Fluphenazine (Prolixin)	2	5-40
Thiothixene (Navane)	4-5	10-60
Haloperidol (Haldol)	2	5-50
Loxapine (Loxitane)	15	50-250
Molindone (Moban)	10-15	25-250
ATYPICAL DRUGS		
Clozapine (Clozaril)	100	300-600
Risperidone (Risperdal)	—	4-6
Olanzapine (Zyprexa)	10	5-20
Quetiapine (Seroquel)	150	150-750

*Upper limit to avoid retinopathy.

Citing the Evidence on

Cognitive Behavioral Therapy

BACKGROUND: This study examined the efficacy of CBT in people with treatment resistant schizophrenia by utilizing research methods that would withstand scientific scrutiny. Prior studies showed methodological limitations.

RESULTS: CBT was compared with a nonspecific befriending control intervention for 9 months. Results showed similar improvement in positive and negative symptoms and in depression in both groups. At the 9 month follow-up evaluation, the CBT patients continued to improve while the control group did not. These results were not attributable to changes in medication.

IMPLICATIONS: CBT is effective in treating negative as well as positive symptoms in schizophrenia resistant to standard antipsychotic drugs, with its efficacy sustained over 9 months of follow-up.

Sensky T et al: A randomized controlled trial of Cognitive-Behavioral Therapy for persistent symptoms in schizophrenia resistant to medication, *Arch Gen Psychiatry* 57:165, 2000.

In stage four, **psychotic disorganization**, clearly psychotic symptoms occur. Hallucinations and delusions intensify and the patient ultimately loses control. This stage is characterized by three distinct phases:

- The patient no longer recognizes familiar environments or people and may accuse family members of being impostors. Extreme agitation is possible. This phase is called **destructuring of the external world**.

- The patient loses personal identity and may refer to the self in the third person. This subphase is called **destructuring of the self**.
- Total fragmentation is the total loss of the ability to differentiate reality from psychosis and may be called **loudly psychotic**. The patient experiences complete loss of control. Hospitalization is usually required at this point, and family members may have to enlist law enforcement officers to take the patient to the hospital. When this happens it is extremely devastating and embarrassing to both the patient and the family.

Stage five, **psychotic resolution**, usually occurs in the hospital. The patient is generally medicated and still experiencing psychosis, but the symptoms are "quiet." The person may appear to follow instructions in a robotic manner and often looks dazed. Unfortunately, many patients are discharged in this stage because they are compliant or they no longer have insurance benefits.

Identify how you would approach a patient and family regarding the need for a change in the treatment plan at each stage of the relapse process. Why is it important to identify relapse as soon as possible?

An example of how well patients can recognize their symptoms compared with staff and families is described in the following clinical example.

CLINICAL EXAMPLE

During a class on relapse and symptom management, a patient was asked what symptoms caused a return to the hospital. The patient responded, "It was my red dots." When asked to explain, he said, "I see red dots all the time, but when they change in a way that I

A Family Speaks

When our daughter, Sue, was in college, she began to change quite suddenly. She had been almost a perfect child. She got good grades all the way through high school, and we never worried that she would get into trouble. In fact, we used to feel sorry for our friends who suspected that their children were experimenting with drugs and sex, hanging out with wild friends, and failing at school.

What a shock it was when we visited Sue and she had completely changed. Her room was a mess. She was wearing sloppy clothes and obviously needed a bath. When we asked what was wrong, she denied there was a problem and then became angry and refused to say anything more to us at all. When we got home, we called a counselor at the college, who told us that Sue was about to flunk out. She had not been attending classes, and other students had been reporting that she was "living in her own world."

We returned to the college to take our daughter home. We immediately took her to a psychiatrist who said that she was schizophrenic and referred her to a hospital. We were frightened, confused, and depressed. We had little understanding of schizophrenia, except that it is a terrible disease that people never recover from and they usually end up in a hospital forever. We also felt guilty that we had perhaps failed Sue in some way. What a relief it was to talk with her primary nurse. She immediately scheduled us for a family education group that met at the hospital. Every time that she was working when we visited, she made sure to spend time so that we could ask questions, and we had a million of them. Most important, she told us about the Alliance for the Mentally Ill. It was so reassuring to meet and talk with other family members who knew what we were going through. We know now that our daughter may never achieve the potential that we thought she once had, but she can lead a productive life. We continue to learn with her about how that will happen for her.

can no longer tell the difference between my red dots, brake lights of the car in front of me, or stop lights, I know it's time to go back to the hospital for a medication check." A staff member said, "So that's why you are always staring at the exit sign, because it's red?" The patient nodded, and the staff member continued with, "So why didn't you tell us?" The patient simply said, "You didn't ask."

This example clearly demonstrates the need not only to teach patients about symptoms indicative of relapse, but also to ask what they already know about their own symptoms.

Managing Relapse. The key to managing relapse is awareness of the onset of behaviors indicating relapse. About 70% of patients and 90% of families are able to notice symptoms of illness recurrence. It has been evident for the past sev-

eral decades that almost all patients know when symptoms are intensifying (Donlon & Blacker, 1975). These and other studies also identify a prodromal phase before relapse. A prodromal phase is the time between the onset of symptoms and the need for treatment. With the majority of patients and families indicating a prodromal period longer than 1 week, it is essential that nurses collaborate with the patient, family, and residential staff regarding the onset of relapse. Box 22-8 presents a guide for patients on how to best handle a potential relapse. Identifying and managing symptoms help to decrease the number and severity of relapses. Teaching this to patients and families is a cost-effective intervention that can provide control over one's life and decrease the number or length of hospitalizations. A growing number of studies have demonstrated a significant reduction in relapse rates as a result of psychoeducational interventions (Lukens et al, 1999).

Tools such as the Moller-Murphy symptom management assessment tool (MM-SMAT) (Murphy & Moller, 1993) can help the patient to self-report symptoms, difficulties in activities of daily living, problems with medications, and ways of managing symptoms. Once patients can validate their experiences they are empowered to manage symptoms rather than have the symptoms rule their lives.

 In what ways is self-assessment of symptoms an empowering experience for patients? How might it positively affect the nurse-patient relationship?

When assessing symptom stability of any chronic illness, it is important to evaluate whether daily symptoms are better, about the same, or worse than usual. Some patients with schizophrenia have psychotic symptoms daily yet are able to maintain adaptive responses and carry out activities of daily living. Relapse for these patients is usually indicated by an increase in symptom intensity.

The nurse conducting discharge teaching or working in an outpatient or residential setting must stress the lengthy recuperation process, with special emphasis on the sedative qualities of the medication used to prevent relapse. When families and residential supervisors who do not understand the length of time needed for recuperation complain that the patient just wants to sit around, smoke, and watch television, the nurse is encouraged to provide information. This clinical example illustrates this behavior.

CLINICAL EXAMPLE

A 26-year-old man with a medical diagnosis of schizophrenia who experienced a lengthy relapse was discharged from the acute care setting and admitted to a residential group home affiliated with a local mental health center. He was later asked to leave both community-based treatment programs because he was not able to actively engage in the required therapies. He was discharged to the care of his parents, who were to motivate him to take his medications and engage him in some type of therapy eventually leading to a job. The parents were active in the Alliance for the Mentally Ill. After months of frustration the parents attended a program on relapse and learned about the lengthy rehabilitation period required.

FAMILY EDUCATION PLAN   *Understanding Psychosis*

CONTENT	INSTRUCTIONAL ACTIVITIES	EVALUATION
Describe psychosis.	Introduce participants and leaders. State purpose of group. Define terminology associated with psychosis.	The participant will describe the characteristics of psychosis.
Identify the causes of psychotic disorders.	Present theories of psychotic disorders. Use audiovisual aids to explain brain anatomy, brain biochemistry, and major neurotransmitters.	The participant will discuss the relationship between brain anatomy, brain biochemistry, and major neurotransmitters and the development of psychosis.
Define schizophrenia according to symptoms and diagnostic criteria.	Lead a discussion of the diagnostic criteria for schizophrenia. Show a film on schizophrenia.	The participant will describe the symptoms and diagnostic criteria for schizophrenia.
Describe the relationship between anxiety and psychotic disorders.	Present types and stages of anxiety. Discuss steps in reducing and resolving anxiety.	The participant will identify and describe the stages of anxiety and ways to reduce or resolve it.
Analyze the impact of living with hallucinations.	Describe the characteristics of hallucinations. Demonstrate ways to communicate with someone who is hallucinating.	The participant will demonstrate effective ways to communicate with a person who has hallucinations.
Analyze the impact of living with delusions.	Describe types of delusions. Demonstrate ways to communicate with someone who has delusions. Discuss interventions for delusions.	The participant will demonstrate effective ways to communicate with a person who has delusions.
Discuss the use of psychotropic medications.	Provide and explain handouts describing the characteristics of psychotropic medications that are prescribed for schizophrenia.	The participant will identify and describe the characteristics of medications prescribed for self/family member.
Describe the characteristics of relapse and the role of compliance with the therapeutic regimen.	Help the participants to describe their own experiences with relapse. Discuss symptom management techniques and the importance of complying with the therapeutic regimen.	The participant will describe behaviors that indicate an impending relapse and discuss the importance of symptom management and compliance with the therapeutic regimen.
Analyze behaviors that promote wellness.	Discuss the components of wellness. Relate wellness to the elements of symptom management.	The participant will analyze the effect of maintaining wellness on the occurrence of symptoms.
Discuss ways to cope adaptively with psychosis.	Lead a group discussion focused on coping behaviors and the daily problems of living with psychosis. Propose ways to create a low-stress environment.	The participant will describe ways to modify lifestyle to create a low-stress environment.

Box **22-8**

A Patient Guide for Handling Potential Relapse

- Go to a safe environment with someone who can help you if help is needed. This person should be able to monitor behavior that indicates the relapse is getting worse.
- Reduce the stress and demands on you. This includes reducing stimuli. Some people find a quiet room where they can be alone, perhaps with soft music. Relaxation techniques or distraction techniques may work for you. A quiet place where you can talk with one person you trust is often helpful.

- Take medications if this is part of your program. Work with your prescriber to determine whether medications may be useful to reduce relapse. Medications are most helpful when used with a safe, quiet environment and stress reduction.
- Talk to a trusted person about what the voices are saying to you or about the thoughts you are having. The person needs to know ahead of time that you will call them if you need help.
- Avoid negative people who say such things as, "You are thinking crazy" or "Stop that negative talk."

They were encouraged to make sure their son ate well and kept up daily hygienic practices, to stop trying to force him to go out, and to support his basic needs based on the wellness model. After 6 months he said one day that he wanted to play a sport at which he had previously excelled. He was encouraged to practice and entered competition. After that positive experience he was able to reenter life within the limits of his neurobiological responses.

Selected Nursing Diagnoses

- Social isolation related to low energy during recovery, as evidenced by resistance to involvement in activities
- Caregiver role strain related to parents' unrealistic expectations for rapid recovery, as evidenced by positive response to education about relapse and recovery

Anxiety and depression are often overlooked as major contributors to poor health-related practices of people with schizophrenia. Common observable behaviors related to anxiety include pacing, restlessness, irritability, quickness to anger, or withdrawal. The high incidence of suicide in people with schizophrenia mandates the importance of assessing lethality, potential dangerousness toward self, and risk of leaving treatment against medical advice. Because of impaired information processing, patients should also be assessed for potential dangerousness to others.

Finally, a variety of symptom management techniques have been found useful by patients. Box 22-9 categorizes these techniques. Patients who have found other symptom management techniques should be encouraged to use them as long as the technique is not harmful to self or others. The following six steps can serve as a guide to the teaching of effective symptom management techniques:

1. Identify problem symptoms.
2. Identify current symptom management techniques.
3. Identify specific support systems.
4. Discuss additional symptom management techniques.
5. Eliminate nonproductive symptom management.
6. Develop new symptom management plan.

Relapse and Medications. The most common causes of relapse relate in some way to medications. Unfortunately, one of the first things nurses often do in assessing relapse is to blame the patient for not taking medications. The nurse should realize that relapse is likely to occur whether the patient is taking medications or not, particularly if the patient has poor health practices. However, there will be a distinct difference in the onset, quality, and length of relapse based on compliance with the treatment regimen.

Caffeine and nicotine can affect the action of psychotropic medications (see Critical Thinking about Contemporary Issues on p. 432). Predicting the success of any medication is impossible if the patient consumes alcohol or other drugs. Research on a variety of ethnic groups has also determined that enzyme variations among population groups cause medications to act and metabolize differently in people of different backgrounds.

Box 22-9

Symptom Management Categories and Techniques

CATEGORY I: DISTRACTION

Talking with friends
Listening to music or dancing
Prayer/meditation
Watching television
Working
Writing
Going for a walk or a ride

CATEGORY II: FIGHTING BACK

Positive self-talk
Positive thinking
Yelling at the voices
Not paying attention to the thoughts
Avoiding situations that increase symptoms

CATEGORY III: HELP SEEKING

Going to a mental health treatment center
Talking with a health-care professional
Seeking the support of a family member

CATEGORY IV: ATTEMPTS TO FEEL BETTER

Eating
Taking a bath or shower
Hugging a pillow or stuffed animal
Taking medication
Relaxation exercises

CATEGORY V: ISOLATION

Going to bed
Staying home

Studies consistently show that without medication, people with schizophrenia relapse at a rate of 60% to 70% within the first years of diagnosis. For those who are faithful to the medication regimen, the relapse rate is approximately 40%, but drops to 15.7% with a combination of medications, group education, and support (Olfson et al, 2000). This statistic has tremendous implications for the role of patient education.

Patients who are compliant yet still experience relapse tend to have a rapid onset of mood-related symptoms and recover quickly with minimal or no change in their antipsychotic medications. These patients usually volunteer for treatment and are generally able to trace the onset of their relapse to an identifiable stressor. Nonadherent patients tend to have a gradual onset of relapse with prominent psychotic features and generally enter treatment through an involuntary hospital commitment. They usually require a longer hospitalization and a change in medication. Typically they cannot trace the onset of the relapse to any specific trigger.

Even with support, education, and adherence to the treatment regimen relapse still occurs. This emphasizes the need for ongoing symptom monitoring and identification of factors leading to nonadherence. Cooperative medication man-

CRITICAL THINKING about CONTEMPORARY ISSUES

Should Inpatient and Residential Mental Health-Care Facilities Be Caffeine and Nicotine Free?

Many patients are faithful to their treatment regimens, but because of a daily intake of over 250 mg of caffeine, experience a decrease in effectiveness of most antipsychotic and antianxiety drugs as well as lithium. In addition, a nicotine intake of more than 10 to 20 cigarettes daily dramatically decreases the effectiveness of antipsychotic drugs (Hughes et al, 1998; Lyon, 1999). Because of the effects of nicotine and caffeine on maladaptive neurobiological responses and the effectiveness of medications, many inpatient psychiatric units have eliminated use of these substances. Smoking has also been banned because of the direct and indirect impact on health.

This is a major change in psychiatric settings. Until recently, coffee and cigarettes were an important part of the inpatient culture. Cigarettes, in particular, were used as rewards in token economy behavioral management plans. Patients often measured the course of the day from one cigarette break to the next. Given this history of reinforcement of these habits, some believe that it is cruel to deprive chronically hospitalized people of one of their few pleasures. Others believe that these restrictions are not in keeping with the philosophy of individual choice and the value that adults should make their own health-related decisions.

Limits on smoking and caffeine are based on the obligation of a health-care program to promote healthful behavior. Careful attention should be paid to patient education and programs that help with withdrawal. An issue that needs more attention is the impact on a newly admitted person of sudden withdrawal from these highly addictive substances. Nurses need to assess preadmission use of caffeine and nicotine carefully. The impact of withdrawal must be considered when evaluating response to medications. In addition, the nurse should be aware of the possibility of withdrawal symptoms, help the patient understand them, and design alternatives to sudden withdrawal from these substances if the patient is addicted to them.

Box 22-10

Nursing Interventions to Prevent Relapse

- Identify symptoms that signal relapse.
- Identify symptom triggers.
- Select symptom management techniques.
- Identify coping strategies for symptom triggers.
- Identify support system for future relapse.
- Document action plan in writing and file with key support people.
- Facilitate integration into family and community.

---

surprising because all patients had attended both group and individual medication instruction classes during the hospitalization. Considering the cognitive symptoms of an acute episode of schizophrenia, the results are less surprising and implications for ongoing post discharge medication instruction become clear.

Interventions in the Health Promotion Phase

Teaching in the health promotion phase focuses on prevention of relapse and symptom management through engaging in a healthy lifestyle (Holmberg & Kane, 1999). Patient teaching methods that involve simple, clear, and concrete instructions including repetition and return demonstrations are the most helpful. One of the keys to preventing relapse includes identifying symptom triggers and strategies for managing them. Box 22-10 summarizes nursing interventions to prevent relapse.

Relatives often do not know how to react to more autonomous functioning and need as much teaching and support as the patient. Psychotherapy may also be helpful in the rehabilitative phase of recovery as patients deal with the neurobiological deficits that often become apparent to them only then. The focus of the psychotherapy is usually supportive and nonconfrontational.

Many families make comments such as, "When we learned our son's diagnosis was schizophrenia, it was like he had died." Thus it is understandable that schizophrenia remains a closely held secret in many households. These attitudes often prevent families from effectively coping with schizophrenia.

The situation may be complicated by incorrect advice from health professionals who tell or imply to families that they caused or perpetuated the illness. Parental guilt stemming from self-blame further blocks communication within the family. Parents often do not know how to talk with their ill child and perhaps even fear him or her. Clearly this situation does not help parents face the many problems they encounter in their additional roles of case manager, residential supervisor, and legal guardian.

Parents must also act as negotiators between the assigned case manager, guardian, and an adult child. No one knows a person better than the family, but it can be emotionally painful and draining to be a loving, nurturing, advocating

---

agement can be fostered if the patient is included as an equal partner in treatment (Ruscher et al, 1997). This only occurs when the patient is taught about the effects and side effects of the medication and staff and family are sensitive to feedback from the patient about how the medication makes him or her feel.

Even with education, medication nonadherence still occurs. In a classic study of 253 psychiatric inpatients interviewed on the day of discharge from a short hospital stay, more than half did not know the name and dosage of the psychiatric medications prescribed for them or why they were supposed to take them; 38% of the patients knew the names of all their psychiatric medications, but only 53% knew when to take them (Clary et al, 1992). These results are

NURSING TREATMENT PLAN *Summary* *Maladaptive Neurobiological Responses*

NURSING DIAGNOSIS: Altered thought processes
EXPECTED OUTCOME: The patient will live, learn, and work at a maximum possible level of success, as defined by the individual.

SHORT-TERM GOAL	INTERVENTION	RATIONALE
The patient will participate in brief, regularly scheduled meetings with the nurse	Initiate a nurse-patient relationship contract mutually agreed on by nurse and patient. Schedule brief (5- to 10-minute), frequent contacts with the patient. Consistently approach the patient at the scheduled time. Extend length of sessions gradually based on patient's agreement.	The establishment of a trusting relationship is fundamental to developing open communication. A patient with altered thought processes cannot tolerate extended, intrusive interactions and functions best in a structured environment.
The patient will describe delusions and other altered thought processes.	Demonstrate attitude of caring and concern. Validate the meaning of communications with the patient. Help the patient to identify the difference between reality and internal thought processes.	Patients are very sensitive to others' responses to their symptoms. A respectful, interested approach will enable the patient to discuss unusual and frightening thoughts. Identification of reality by a trusted person is helpful.
The patient will identify and describe the effect of brain disease on thought processes.	Provide information about causes of psychoses. Discuss the relationship between the patient's behaviors and brain function. Involve significant others in educational sessions.	Understanding of the physiological basis for altered thought processes helps the patient to recognize symptoms and feel in control of the illness. Significant others can provide support and experience less stigma if they are informed about the illness.
The patient will identify signs of impending relapse and describe actions to take to prevent relapse.	Help patient and significant others to identify behaviors related to altered thought processes that indicate threatened relapse. Identify community resources and mutually plan actions directed toward prevention of relapse.	Relapse can be predicted if the patient and family are alert to warning signs. Early intervention allows the patient to control the course of the illness. Family members can help the patient to identify symptoms and provide support for seeking assistance.
The patient will describe symptom management techniques that are helpful in living with altered thought processes.	Describe symptom management techniques that other patients have used. Ask the patient to describe techniques used to manage symptoms. Encourage the patient to take control of the illness by using symptom management techniques. Discuss the advantages of engaging in a wellness lifestyle.	Many patients with psychoses continue to have delusions after the acute phase of the illness has passed. Patients can function better if they learn ways to manage the symptom. Symptom self management promotes personal empowerment. Elimination of substances that interfere with healthy CNS function improves cognition and perception.
The patient will engage in a trusting relationship with the nurse.	Initiate a nurse-patient relationship contract mutually agreed on by nurse and patient. Establish mutual goals related to social interaction. Establish trust by consistently meeting the elements of the plan and engaging in open and honest communication.	Patients who have maladaptive neurobiological responses often have difficulty trusting others. Difficulty with information processing causes problems interpreting the communication of others.

Continued

NURSING TREATMENT PLAN *Summary* *Maladaptive Neurobiological Responses—cont'd*

SHORT-TERM GOAL	INTERVENTION	RATIONALE
The patient will discuss personal goals related to social interaction.	Encourage the patient to describe current relationship patterns. Discuss past relationship experiences. Identify problems associated with social interaction. Explore goals.	The patient may be unaware of the characteristics of mutually satisfying interpersonal relationships. Honest feedback from the nurse can help the patient to identify the reasons for past problems. Knowledge of the patient's relationship goals leads to the development of realistic behavioral change.
The patient will identify behaviors that interfere with social relationships.	Share observations about the patient's behavior in social situations.	Identification of problematic behavior helps the patient and nurse target changes.
The patient will practice alternative social behaviors with the nurse.	Discuss possible behavioral changes that will facilitate the establishment of social relationships. Role play alternative behaviors. Provide feedback.	Practice will help the patient to gain comfort with new behaviors. Feedback provides reinforcement for successful behavioral change.
The patient will select one person and practice social interaction skills.	Discuss experience of practicing new behavior with another person. Discuss ways of maintaining a relationship.	The patient will need ongoing feedback and support related to maintaining behavioral change.

parent in one situation, a treatment-enforcing case manager in another, and residential supervisor to an outside case manager in yet another. Simultaneous patient/family teaching about symptom management and medication compliance is useful at this stage. Patient and family education may also dispel myths and provide suggestions for improving communication with the treatment team.

Research shows that structured rehabilitation programs provide significant improvement in function and coping skills (see Chapter 15). There are four programs with structured curricula and participant manuals that have as their main goal either to rehabilitate the patient or to help the family cope more effectively with chronic mental illness.

The **Three Rs Psychiatric Rehabilitation Program** is for patients with chronic mental illness and their families (Moller & Murphy, 1997a; 1997b; 1998). The three Rs are relapse, recovery, and rehabilitation. The aim of the program is to teach patients to use a wellness model to manage their illness and integrate back into the community. Developed by advanced practice psychiatric rehabilitation nurses, this program has shown a significant decrease in hospitalization of its participants.

Liberman's Skill Training Program has as its aim the rehabilitation of patients by teaching life skills (Liberman, 1994). The patient is taken through a structured set of modules that teach coping strategies in order to effect life changes.

McFarlane's Family Education Program is aimed at teaching families about schizophrenia and helping them to cope with the illness (McFarlane, 1992). This is the only program that is exclusively for families and uses professionals specifically trained to conduct the program.

Family to Family is a self-help program developed by NAMI (National Alliance for the Mentally Ill) for families of people with chronic mental illness. It is a scripted program that uses family members trained to facilitate the program. It is further described in Chapter 16.

A Nursing Treatment Plan Summary for the patient with maladaptive neurobiological responses is presented on pp. 434-435.

EVALUATION

Evaluation of the nursing care provided to patients who have maladaptive neurobiological responses is based on input from the patient and family. Because these are serious, long-term illnesses, care is often episodic. Relapse should not be interpreted as a failure of the nursing intervention but should be considered in the context of the patient's life situation.

To evaluate the nursing intervention, the following questions may be asked:

- Is the patient able to describe the behaviors that characterize the onset of a relapse?
- Is the patient able to identify and describe the medications prescribed, reason for taking them, frequency of taking them, and possible side effects?
- Does the patient participate in relationships with other people at a comfortable level?
- Is the patient's family aware of the characteristics of the illness and able to participate in a supportive relationship with the patient?
- Are the patient and family informed about available community resources such as rehabilitation programs, mental health-care providers, educational programs, and support groups, and do they use them?

Summary

1. Maladaptive neurobiological responses are related to disruptions in brain functioning and affect cognition, perception, emotion, behavior, and socialization. Adaptive neurobiological responses include logical thought, accurate perceptions, emotions consistent with experiences, behavior consistent with cultural norms, and relatedness. Maladaptive neurobiological responses include thought disorder (delusions), misperceptions (hallucinations), inability to experience emotions, bizarre behavior, and social isolation.

2. The behaviors associated with maladaptive neurobiological responses include cognitive, perceptual, emotional, behavioral, and relational responses.

3. Predisposing factors for maladaptive neurobiological responses are described from biological, psychological, and sociocultural perspectives. Precipitating stressors include biological characteristics, environmental stress, and symptom triggers.

4. Coping resources are individualized and depend on the nature and extent of the neurobiological disruption. Family resources are very important. Coping mechanisms may include regression, projection, and withdrawal and represent the person's attempt to control the illness.

5. Primary NANDA nursing diagnoses are impaired verbal communication, sensory/perceptual alterations, impaired social interaction, social isolation, and altered thought processes.

6. Primary *DSM–IV–TR* diagnoses are schizophrenia, schizophreniform disorder, schizoaffective disorder, delusional disorder, brief psychotic disorder, and shared psychotic disorder.

7. The expected outcome of nursing care is that the patient will live, learn, and work at a maximum possible level of success as defined by the individual.

8. The nursing care plan must be based on an understanding of the patient's disabilities, strengths, and preferences. Patient and family education about symptom management and relapse prevention is a critical element of the plan.

9. Primary nursing interventions for patients with maladaptive neurobiological responses include intervention in delusions, intervention with hallucinations, medication management, and patient and family education about symptom management and relapse.

10. Evaluation is based on the patient's satisfaction with the level of functioning and on the ability to communicate improvement or impending relapse.

Competent Caring   A Clinical Exemplar of a Psychiatric Nurse

MELODY SEWELL, MSN, RN

I had the unique opportunity to broaden my skills as a psychiatric nurse by working with J, a psychotic patient. I learned invaluable lessons in patience and acceptance as I watched the thought processes of this young man unfold. He also taught me important lessons in caring as we built our therapeutic relationship.

J was a well-groomed, handsome 26-year-old white man with a 9-year history of paranoid schizophrenia. He displayed an intense facial expression. He was admitted to our 22-bed adult psychiatric unit for a second time within the year. Although he had a high level of functioning, he neglected to acknowledge his limits. This was evidenced by his working more than 60 hours per week in landscaping for the previous 6 months. The patient had been followed up on an outpatient basis monthly since his discharge last year. The psychiatrist working with him noted increasing symptoms of paranoia exacerbated by job-related stress.

J was admitted to the unit with a marked weight loss, guarded affect, and minimal interaction. Reiterating that "I need to get back to my job—the bills must be paid," he expressed the importance of maintaining his independence from his parents and retaining his employment and apartment. He was on the unit 1 week. A pending discharge date was set for 2 days hence despite his minimal disclosure and apparent lack of progress. I was concerned he would return to the same environmental demands and deteriorate further if our treatment was not effective. This might also increase his risk for rehospitalization, which would further threaten his self-esteem and feelings of independence. When I arrived at work, another patient reported to me that J was tearful, expressing feelings of helplessness and worthlessness. From my perspective he clearly was not ready for discharge without prompt constructive intervention. I realized that this would be difficult, however, because he withdrew from almost all interaction.

I approached J, providing a quiet, comfortable area free from distractions and allowing for privacy. When I expressed my observation of his red and swollen eyes, he immediately responded, "I wear contacts." I provided an atmosphere of trust, building on my rapport with him that dated back to his previous hospitalization and continued to offer myself in a nonjudgmental manner, encouraging him to explore issues that were perpetuating internal conflicts. This time my intervention worked. His once-guarded affect softened as tears filled his eyes. He spoke of job-related stressors, his need to maintain independence from his parents, and his desire to provide for himself without government financial assistance. He elaborated on his feelings of failure as a son. When further explored, issues of his father's difficulty accepting the limitations associated with the mental illness of his only son became apparent. J explored this and realized that he had to accept responsibility for his own actions and provide boundaries for himself to maintain his sense of independence. To do so, he could no longer overextend himself and be able to maintain good functioning.

When encouraged to continue talking, he expressed concerns about his sexuality. He greatly desired companionship

Competent Caring A Clinical Exemplar of a Psychiatric Nurse—cont'd

but realized the chronicity of his illness. Painfully exploring the insight of his diminished ability to provide financially for a family, he cried. I empathized with his pain but also confirmed that he was a sexual being with options. At the end of our discussion, we established concrete steps to implement on discharge. One of these included finding a job with fewer physical and time demands. He also expressed his gratitude to me, since he could now see that his symptoms had prevented any constructive interactions or positive outcomes previously.

Throughout the discussion with J, I maintained an atmosphere of mutual interaction. He vacillated between tearfulness and guarded behavior, expressing that our interaction was uncomfortable for him at times. I also observed occasional twitching of his thumbs, which I assessed for possible extrapyramidal

symptoms. J was discharged with plans to implement the changes we had discussed. He expressed hope, admitting that he had previously thought of leaving the hospital and "traveling around the country to get away from everything and just see where I might end up." Now, with some pertinent education coupled with concrete steps to guide him, he was leaving the hospital with a sense of direction and hopeful intentions for his life. Through a comprehensive care approach and expressed respect for my patient, J and I were able to set attainable goals for his discharge, allowing him to leave the hospital with a sense of control and hope. I think about him often, especially on my hectic and sometimes discouraging days in psychiatric nursing, and quietly smile, knowing the difference one nurse can make.

MERLIN Visit MERLIN: **www.mosby.com/MERLIN/Stuart** to find these additional materials and student activities.

- **Worksheets**
- **"Drug of the Month" Updates**
- **"Citing the Evidence" Updates**
- **Critical Thinking Activities and Exercises**
- **Annotated Suggested Readings**
- **Web Links**
- **More!**

Chapter Review Questions

1. Match each term in Column A with the correct definition in Column B.

Column A

____ Attention
____ Perception
____ Hallucinations
____ Mood
____ Cognition
____ Anhedonia
____ Affect
____ Decision making

Column B

A. The act or process of knowing
B. The retention and storage of knowledge learned
C. The ability to focus on one activity in a sustained, concentrated manner
D. Identification and initial interpretation of a stimulus based on information from the senses
E. Perceptual distortions
F. Neurological deficits consistent with frontal or parietal lobe damage
G. An extensive and sustained feeling tone affecting the person's world view
H. Inability to experience pleasure, joy, intimacy, and closeness

____ Memory
____ Soft signs

I. Behaviors and expressions that show during experiences of feelings
J. Insight, judgment, logic, decisiveness, planning, and abstract thought

2. Fill in the blanks.

A. The five areas affected by maladaptive neurobiological responses related to disruptions in brain functioning are _____, _____, _____, _____, and _____.

B. Difficulty carrying out a purposeful, organized, complex task is called _____.

C. One of the current dominant biological theories of schizophrenia that proposes abnormal neurotransmission is the _____.

D. _____ are precursors and stimuli that often precede a new episode of schizophrenia and can serve as warnings to the patient and mental healthcare provider.

E. The five stages of relapse in schizophrenia are

_____ , _____ ,

_____ , _____ ,

and _____ .

3. **Identify whether the following statements are true (T) or false (F).**

____ A. Studies show multiple abnormalities in the brains and behaviors of many people with schizophrenia before they become symptomatic.

____ B. The majority of hallucinations experienced by people with schizophrenia are visual.

____ C. Atypical antipsychotic drugs should be used only when the patient does not respond to typical (conventional) treatments.

____ D. Teaching during the health promotion phase focuses on relapse prevention and symptom management.

____ E. The self-help program developed by the National Alliance for the Mentally Ill is called the Three Rs.

4. **Provide short answers for the following questions.**

A. Review the positive and negative symptoms of schizophrenia. How would their presence or absence affect the treatment plan you design for your patient?

B. One of your patients with schizophrenia and her husband tell you they would like to have children. They ask you to explain the risk factors for having children with the disorder. How would you respond?

C. Spend some time in a crowded place and make a detailed list of the things you notice about people that make them stand out or blend into the crowd. How can you use this knowledge to help your socially isolated patients?

References

American Psychiatric Association: *Diagnostic and statistical manual of mental disorders,* Fourth Edition, Text Revision. Washington, DC, American Psychiatric Association.

American Psychiatric Association: Practice guideline for the treatment of patients with schizophrenia, *Am J Psychiatry* 154(Suppl) 1997.

Andreason N: A unitary model of schizophrenia, *Arch Gen Psychiatry* 56:781, 1999.

Battle Y et al: Seasonality and infectious diseases in schizophrenia: the birth hypothesis revisited, *J Psychiatr Res* 33:501, 1999.

Buchanan R, Carpenter W: Schizophrenia: introduction and overview. In Saddock B, Saddock V, editors: *Comprehensive textbook of psychiatry,* Philadelphia, 2000, Williams & Wilkins.

Clary C et al: Psychiatric inpatients' knowledge of medication at hospital discharge, *Hosp Community Psychiatry* 43:140, 1992.

Dalman C et al: Obstetric complications and the risk of schizophrenia, *Arch Gen Psychiatry* 56:234, 1999.

Dixon L et al: Services to families of adults with schizophrenia: from treatment recommendations to dissemination, *Psychiatr Serv* 50:233, 1999.

Docherty J et al: Stages of onset of schizophrenic psychosis, *Am J Psychiatry* 135:420, 1978.

Donlon P, Blacker K: Clinical recognition of early schizophrenic decompensation, *Dis Nervous System* 35:223, 1975.

Duzyurek S, Wiener J: Early recognition in schizophrenia: the prodromal stages, *J Pract Psych Behav Health* 7:187, 1999.

Harkavy-Friedman J, Nelson E: Management of the suicidal patient with schizophrenia, *Psychiatr Clin North Am* 20:625, 1997.

Hatfield A: Families of adults with severe mental illness: new directions in research, *Am J Orthopsychiatry* 67:254, 1997.

Herz M: Early intervention in different phases of schizophrenia. *J Pract Psych Behav Health* 5:197, 1999.

Ho B et al: Two year outcomes in first-episode schizophrenia: predictive value of symptoms for quality of life, *Am J Psychiatry* 155:1196, 1998.

Holmberg S, Kane C: Health and self-care practices of persons with schizophrenia, *Psychiatr Serv* 50:827, 1999.

Hughes J et al: Caffeine and schizophrenia, *Psychiatr Serv* 49:1415, 1998.

Jarboe K et al: Diagnosis, neurobiology and treatment of first episode schizophrenia, *J Am Psych Nurses Assoc* 4:S2, 1998.

Lehman A et al: Translating research into practice: the schizophrenia Patient Outcomes Research Team (PORT) treatment recommendations, *Schizophr Bull* 24(1): 1, 1998.

Liberman R et al: The nature and problem of schizophrenia. In Bellack AS, editor: *Schizophrenia: treatment, management, and rehabilitation,* New York, 1984, Grune & Stratton.

Liberman R et al: Biobehavioral treatment and rehabilitation of schizophrenia, *Behav Ther* 25:89, 1994.

Lindsay H: Neurodevelopment of schizophrenia revealed, *Clin Psychiatr News* 3:34, 2000.

Littrell K, Littrell S: Choosing an antipsychotic in the treatment of schizophrenia: conversions to olanzapine, *J Am Psychiatr Nurses Assoc* 3:S18, 1997.

Lukens E et al: Family psychoeducation in schizophrenia: emerging themes and challenges. *J Pract Psych Behav Health* 5:314, 1999.

Lyon E: A review of the effects of nicotine on schizophrenia and antipsychotic medications, *Psychiatr Serv* 50:1346, 1999.

McFarlane W: From research to clinical practice: dissemination of New York State's family psychoeducation project, *Hosp Community Psychiatry* 44:265, 1992.

Moller M, Murphy M: *Recovering from psychosis: a wellness approach,* Nine Mile Falls, Wash, 1998, Psychiatric Rehabilitation Nurses.

Moller M, Murphy M: The three R's rehabilitation program: a prevention approach for the management of relapse symptoms associated with psychiatric diagnoses, *J Psychiatr Rehab* 20, 3, 42-48, 1997a.

Moller M, Murphy M: Reintegration and schizophrenia: the three R's approach, *Continuum* 4:17, 1997b.

Murphy M, Moller M: Relapse management in neurobiological disorders: the Moller-Murphy Symptom Management Assessment Tool, *Arch Psychiatr Nurs* 7: 226, 1993.

Olfson M et al: Predicting medication noncompliance after hospital discharge among patients with schizophrenia, *Psychiatr Serv* 51:216, 2000.

Perese E: Unmet needs of persons with chronic mental illness: relationship to their adaptation to community living, *Issues Ment Health Nurs* 18:19, 1997.

Perry W et al: Sensorimotor gating and thought disturbance measured in close temporal proximity in schizophrenic patients, *Arch Gen Psychiatry* 56:277, 1999.

Ruscher S et al: Psychiatric patients attitudes about medication and factors affecting noncompliance, *Psychiatr Serv* 48:82, 1997.

Tarrier N et al: Randomized controlled trial of intensive cognitive behavior therapy for patients with chronic schizophrenia, *Br Med J* 317:303, 1998.

Torrey E et al: Prenatal origin of schizophrenia in a subgroup of discordant monozygotic twins, *Schizophr Bull* 20:423, 1994.

Wuerker A: The family and schizophrenia, *Issues Ment Health Nurs* 21:127, 2000.

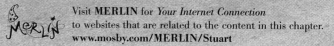
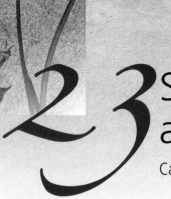

23 Social Responses and Personality Disorders

Carol K. Perlin

The emptiness caused by dissatisfaction with mere achievement and the helplessness that results when the channels of relation break down have brought forth a loneliness of soul such as never existed before.

         Karl Jaspers, *Existenzphilosophie*

In order to find satisfaction in life, people must be able to establish positive and healthy interpersonal relationships. Such people experience closeness with others while keeping their separate identities. This closeness is called **intimacy** and is characterized by sensitivity to the other person's needs. Other classic characteristics of healthy relatedness include open communication of feelings, acceptance of the other person as valued and separate, and empathic understanding (Rogers, 1961). To become intimately involved with another person, an individual must be willing to risk revealing private thoughts and feelings. This can be frightening, especially if one has had past difficulty sharing feelings with other people. Fear of exposing private feelings makes some people reluctant to become involved in intimate relationships. People who have extreme difficulty in relating intimately to others may have behaviors that are characteristic of a personality disorder.

"Personality" is a set of deeply ingrained, enduring patterns of thinking, feeling, and behaving. A personality disorder is a set of patterns or traits that hinder a person's ability to maintain meaningful relationships, feel fulfilled, and enjoy life. It is an enduring pattern of inner experience and behavior that deviates markedly from the expectations of the individual's culture, is pervasive and inflexible, has onset in adolescence or early adulthood, is stable over time, and leads to distress or impairment (APA, 2000; Grilo et al, 1998). These disorders are attitudes toward self, others, and the world expressed in everything a person thinks, feels, and does. They often decrease in severity of expression as a person ages (mainly as a result of corrective life experiences). Personality disorders are continuous rather than episodic, and they are pervasive across a wide range of circumstances in the individual's life, although the appearance and severity of a particular symptom can vary at times (Kay & Tasman, 2000).

    The concept of personality "disorder" implies that one knows what a normal personality is even though it is very difficult to define. It is doubtful that research and therapeutic efforts to date have significantly increased clinical insights into personality or succeeded in modifying it. It is clear, however, that while a healthy individual is able to adjust and adapt to the demands or expectations of different people and different situations, individuals with personality disorders have a persistent impairment in their interpersonal relationships and other aspects of functioning (Pringle, 1998).

It can be difficult to separate the differences between "personality" and mood, anxiety, responses to stress, demands of social roles, or situational reactions. Although the border between normal and abnormal personality can be elusive, the distinction involves significant maladaptation. A limitation of the current diagnostic system is that the criteria for the different personality disorders overlap. Two thirds of patients with one personality disorder meet criteria for another personality disorder (Grinspoon, 2000). This can confuse efforts to determine etiologies, make a diagnosis, select specific treatments, and measure outcomes. Research and debates among experts to clarify the current system are in process. Regardless, since patients with these problems are among the most challenging in the health-care system, the nurse should be able to identify the different personality disorders in their patients and intervene appropriately.

There are three features of personality disorders (Millon & Davis, 1995):

1. The individual has acquired few strategies for relating, and their approach to relationships and to the environment is inflexible and maladaptive.
2. There is a tendency for the individual's needs, perceptions, and behavior to foster vicious cycles that continue unhelpful patterns and provoke negative reactions from others.
3. The individual's adaptation is characterized by tenuous stability, fragility, and lack of resilience when faced with stressful situations.

Prevalence estimates of personality disorders in the general population range from 10% to 18%, and at least some of these disorders are associated with a high mortality rate as a result of suicide (Brodsky et al, 1997). Suicide victims with personality disorders almost always also have a depressive illness, substance abuse disorder, or both (Isometsa et al, 1996).

The fixed, enduring quality of specific personality disorder symptoms is an essential element to the diagnosis. Even with treatment, it is not possible to completely change someone's personality. However, it is possible to help people with personality disorders improve the quality of their life. Research shows that specific treatment modalities may lead to significant improvement in the symptoms, distress, and general functioning of patients with personality disorders (Hampton, 1997; Miller et al, 1998).

> *Based on your experiences, compare the relationships you have had with family, with friends, and with patients in a nurse-patient relationship. How they are alike and different?*

CONTINUUM OF SOCIAL RESPONSES

Every person has the potential to be involved in many levels of relationships, from intimacy to casual contact. Intimate and interdependent relationships provide security and instill the self-confidence necessary to cope with the demands of daily life. A lack of intimacy with family members and friends leaves only superficial encounters, taking away many of life's most meaningful experiences.

Adaptive and Maladaptive Responses

Within a relationship the participants usually develop a continuum of dependent and independent behavior. Ideally, these behaviors are balanced, which is described as interdependence. The interdependent person can decide when to rely on others and when it is appropriate to be independent. An interdependent person can let another be dependent or independent without needing to control that person's behavior. All people are responsible for controlling their own behavior while receiving support and help from significant others as needed. Adaptive social responses therefore include the ability to tolerate solitude and the expression of autonomy, mutuality, and interdependence.

Interpersonal relationship behaviors may be represented on a continuum that ranges from healthy interdependent interactions to those involving no real contact with other people (Fig. 23-1). At the midpoint of the continuum, a person experiences loneliness, withdrawal, and dependence. The maladaptive end of the continuum reflects the dominance of manipulation, impulsivity, and narcissism. People with these responses often have a history of problematic relationships in the family, on the job, and in the social arena.

Development Through the Life Cycle

Researchers do not agree on much beyond the fact that personality is shaped by biology and social learning, and that whether it develops a healthy or pathological form depends on the nature, timing, and interaction of these influences. As more is learned about child development and the structure and function of the brain, it is becoming clear that the seed of personality is "temperament"—hereditary biological dispositions, evident almost from birth, that affect mood and activity level, attention span, and responsiveness to stimulation (Grinspoon, 2000).

Infancy. From birth until 3 months the infant does not perceive physical separation between self and mother. Although physical differentiation occurs at about 3 months, psychological differentiation does not begin until 18 months. This period between 3 and 18 months is the symbiotic stage of development. The infant is completely dependent on others. Trust develops as needs are met consistently and predictably. The infant experiences the environment as unconditionally loving, nurturing, and accepting. Feelings of positive self-worth result from the infant's complete dependence on an environment that is good and loving. This creates a capacity for empathic understanding in future relationships.

Preschool Years. The period between 18 months and 3 years of age is the separation-individuation stage. Separation includes all the experiences, events, and developmental achievements that promote self-differentiation and a sense of being separate and unique. Individuation is the evolution of the child's internal psychological structure and growing sense of separateness, wholeness, and capability. The toddler ventures away from the mother to explore the environment. During this phase, a sense of object constancy develops. This means that the child knows that a valued person or object continues to exist when it cannot be directly perceived. Games such as peek-a-boo teach object constancy. At the beginning of the separation-individuation process, the child seeks the parents' reassurance, support, and encouragement. If the response to autonomous behavior is positive and reinforcing, there is a foundation for building a solid sense of self and future relationships characterized by interdependence, commitment, and a capacity for interpersonal growth.

Childhood. The internal development of morality and empathic feelings occurs between the ages of 6 and 10 years. During this period a supportive environment that encourages the budding sense of self fosters development of a positive, adaptive self-concept. Conflict occurs as adults set limits on behavior, often frustrating the child's efforts toward independence. However, loving, consistent limit-setting communicates caring and helps the child develop interdependence. The older child adopts the parents' guidelines for behavior and a value system begins to appear. In school the child begins to learn cooperation, competition, and compromise. Peer relationships and approval of adults from outside the family, such as teachers, scout leaders, and friends' parents become important.

Preadolescence and Adolescence. By preadolescence the person becomes involved in an intimate relationship with a friend of the same sex, a best friend. This relationship involves sharing. It offers another chance to clarify values and recognize differences in people. This is usually a very dependent relationship. There are often active efforts to exclude others. However, as adolescence develops, the dependence on a close friend of the same sex usually yields to a dependent heterosexual relationship. While young people are involved in these dependent relationships with peers, they are asserting independence from their parents. Friends support each other in this struggle, which often includes re-

bellious behavior. Parents can help the adolescent grow by providing consistent limits and a caring tolerance of rebellious outbursts. Another step toward mature interdependence is taken as the person learns to balance parental demands and peer group pressures.

Young Adulthood. Adolescence ends when the person is self-sufficient and maintains interdependent relationships with parents and peers. Decision making is independent, taking the advice and opinions of others into account. The person may marry and begin a new family. Occupational plans are made and a career begun. The mature person demonstrates self-awareness by balancing dependent and independent behavior. Others are allowed to be dependent or independent as appropriate. Being sensitive to and accepting the feelings and needs of oneself and others is critical to this level of mature functioning. Interpersonal relationships are characterized by mutuality.

Middle Adulthood. Parenting and adult friendships test the person's ability to foster independence in others. Children gradually separate from parents, and friends may move away or drift apart. The mature person must be self-reliant and find new supports. Pleasure can be found in the development of an interdependent relationship with children as they grow. Decreased dependent demands by children creates freedom that can be used for new activities.

Late Adulthood. Change continues during late adulthood. Losses occur, such as the physical changes of aging, the death of parents, loss of occupation through retirement, and later the deaths of friends and one's spouse. The need for relatedness must still be satisfied. The mature person grieves over these losses and recognizes that the support of others can help resolve the grief. However, new possibilities arise, even with a loss. Old friends and relatives cannot be replaced, but new relationships can develop. Grandchildren may become important to the grandparent, who may delight in spending time with them. The aging person may also find a sense of relatedness to the culture as a whole. Life has deeper meaning in relation to one's perception of personal accomplishments and contributions to the welfare of society. The mature older person can accept whatever increase in dependence is necessary but also retain as much independence as possible. Even loss of physical health does not nec-

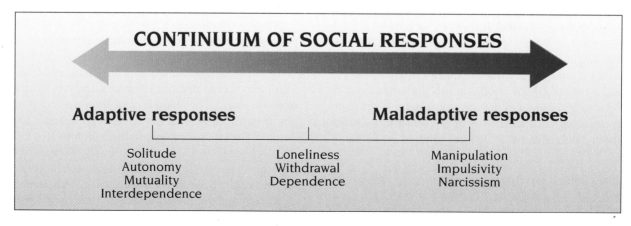

Fig. 23-1 Continuum of social responses.

essarily force the person to give up all independence. The ability to maintain mature relatedness throughout life enhances one's self-esteem (Masterson, 1985).

ASSESSMENT
Behaviors

The behaviors observed in people with personality disorders are characterized by chronic, maladaptive social responses. The *DSM–IV–TR* (APA, 2000) has grouped the personality disorders into three clusters based on descriptive similarities:

- Cluster A includes personality disorders of an odd or eccentric nature (paranoid, schizoid, and schizotypical personality disorders).
- Cluster B are of an erratic, dramatic, or emotional nature (antisocial, borderline, histrionic, and narcissistic personality disorders).

- Cluster C includes disorders of an anxious or fearful nature (avoidant, dependent, and obsessive-compulsive personality disorders).

There are two additional personality disorder diagnoses that are under consideration in the *DSM–IV–TR* (passive-aggressive and depressive). A specific classification of interpersonal and behavioral characteristics associated with each of the personality disorders is presented in Box 23-1. The patient usually reports or exhibits more than one of these traits in the course of the nursing assessment.

People with Cluster B personality disorders have unique character features that can make the provision of nursing care complicated and difficult (Greene & Ugarriza, 1995). Borderline personality disorder, in particular, has one of the highest suicide rates (3% to 9.5%) of all the personality disorders (Brown & Dodson, 1999). Impulsive aggression is the hallmark of borderline personality disorder, and it plays

---

Box 23-1

Classification and Features of *DSM–IV–TR* Personality Disorders

DISORDERS	FEATURES
Cluster A: Odd, Eccentric, General Tendency Toward Social and Emotional Withdrawal	
Paranoid	Distrust: persistent suspiciousness, secretive, withholding, hypervigilant, jealous, envious; suspects without sufficient basis that others are exploiting, harming, or deceiving them.
Schizoid	Social detachment: self-absorbed; restricted emotionality; cold and indifferent; neither desires or enjoys close relationships; anhedonic, indifferent to others; less disturbed than schizotypical.
Schizotypical	Interpersonal deficits; cognitive distortions; eccentricities; paranoid; difficulty feeling understood and accepted; odd beliefs, magical thinking, unusual perceptual experiences; social isolation.
Cluster B: Overemotional, Dramatic, Erratic, Impulsive	
Antisocial	Disregard for rights of others; lies; manipulates; exploitative; seductive; repeatedly performs acts that are grounds for arrest.
Borderline	Instability; impulsivity; hypersensitivity; self-destructive behavior; profound mood shifts; unstable and intense interpersonal relationships.
Histrionic	Excessive emotionality; attention seeking; superficial and stormy relationships; lively; uncomfortable when not the center of attention.
Narcissistic	Arrogance; need for admiration; lack of empathy; seductive; socially exploitative; manipulative; grandiose sense of self-importance.
Cluster C: Anxious, Fearful	
Avoidant	Social inhibition; withdraw from social and occupational situations that involve significant interpersonal contact; longs for relationships; inadequacy; hypersensitivity to negative criticism, rejection, or shame.
Dependent	Submissive behavior; low self-esteem; dependency in relationships; extreme self-consciousness; urgently and indiscriminately seeks another relationship when close relationship ends; inadequate; helpless.
Obsessive-Compulsive	Unable to express affection; overly cold and rigid; crippling preoccupation with trivial detail, orderliness, perfectionism, and control (i.e., attends to rules, lists, organization, schedules, to the extent that the major point of the activity is lost); superior attitude.
Suggested Personality Diagnoses in *DSM–IV–TR* Needing Further Study	
Passive-Aggressive	**Negativistic Attitudes:** Sullen and argumentative, resents others, resists fulfilling routine obligations, complains of being unappreciated
Depressive	**Depressive Cognitions:** Gloomy, brooding, pessimistic, guilt-prone, highly critical of self and others, cheerless

Reprinted with permission from the *Diagnostic and statistical manual of mental disorders*, Fourth Edition, Text Revision. Copyright 2000. American Psychiatric Association; Kay J, Tasman A: *Psychiatry: behavioral science and clinical essentials*, Philadelphia, 2000, WB Saunders.

a pivotal role in the borderline person's self-mutilation, unstable relationships, violence, and completed suicides. Moreover, the results of one study found that patients with borderline personality disorder and antisocial personality characteristics are more likely to have attempted suicide than those without such comorbidity (Brodsky et al, 1997). Another study found that a diagnosis of borderline personality disorder as well as the total number of Cluster B personality traits in depressed inpatients, and not the severity of the depression, correlated with the number and lethality of previous suicide attempts (Corbitt et al, 1996). For these reasons, the nursing assessment and implementation of care for people with borderline, antisocial, and narcissistic personality disorders are emphasized in this chapter. Common maladaptive responses of people with Cluster B personality disorders include manipulation and narcissism and the impulsivity that often overlaps both.

Manipulation. People who use manipulative behaviors present a particularly difficult nursing problem. They tend to treat others as objects, and their behavior is easily misunderstood, as illustrated in the following clinical example:

 CLINICAL EXAMPLE

Mr. Y was a 20-year-old single man who was committed to an inpatient psychiatric unit by a judge for a psychiatric evaluation. He had been charged with the sale of illicit drugs, statutory rape of his 15-year-old pregnant girlfriend, and contributing to the delinquency of a minor. He had been arrested on the grounds of a junior high school, where he was selling PCP and barbiturates to a group of young teenagers.

In jail Mr. Y had been observed to be "crazy" by the guards. He paced his cell, chanted, and threw his food on the floor. Because of this behavior, the judge agreed to order a psychiatric evaluation. On arrival at the psychiatric unit Mr. Y continued to behave in the same manner. However, his behavior did not seem typical of psychosis. There was no evidence of hallucinations or disorders of thought or affect. When unaware that he was observed, Mr. Y seemed relaxed and was noted at one time to be talking with another patient. By the day after admission he seemed to be free of his symptoms. At this point the staff began to describe him as a "nice guy." He complimented female staff members and behaved toward them in a pleasantly seductive manner. He was respectful to the physicians and agreed to abide by all the rules. He was helpful with other patients. In group meetings he admitted that he had behaved badly in the past and described how he had been led astray by his friends. He said he became involved in drugs because he wanted to be "one of the gang" and he needed money so he "had to" start selling drugs. By the end of his first week in the hospital he had received the sympathy of all the other patients and the staff.

Nine days after admission, after visiting hours, it was noted that Mr. Y and two other patients looked lethargic. Their speech was slurred and their gaits ataxic. The nursing staff immediately collected urine and blood specimens for toxicological analysis. The unit was searched for hidden drugs, but none were found. The results of the toxicology screening tests were positive for barbiturates. Suspicion was immediately focused on Mr. Y because the

other patients involved were young adolescents with no history of drug abuse. When confronted, Mr. Y seemed amazed that he could be suspected and pointed out his past behavior as a model patient. He admitted that he had behaved strangely and wondered whether someone had "slipped" him some drugs. He was convincing but was warned that if he was involved in any way with drugs, he would be sent directly back to jail.

Mr. Y convinced his family of his good intentions, and they agreed to allow him to move into their house. On the basis of these indications of positive behavioral change, Mr. Y received a recommendation for probation, which was carried out by the judge.

Three months after discharge from the hospital, Mr. Y and a friend were arrested for operating a PCP manufacturing laboratory in a friend's garage.

Selected Nursing Diagnoses

- Impaired social interaction related to need for control, as evidenced by illegal behavior and treating people like objects.
- Defensive coping related to inability to identify relationship problems, as evidenced by manipulation of others.

These patients usually have little motivation to change because manipulative behavior often has rewards for them, facilitating the accomplishment of a desired goal. The manipulator is goal-oriented or self-oriented, not other-oriented. However, the person is skilled at giving the impression of involvement with others. In this clinical example, Mr. Y was able to gain the confidence of the staff in order to have support in court. This is typical of a person with an antisocial personality disorder.

Antisocial personality disorder is a complex disorder that is particularly difficult to diagnose and treat. To meet *DSM–IV–TR* criteria, an individual must be at least 18 years of age but must demonstrate a pattern of breaking rules since the age of 15 years (APA, 2000). The diagnosis is applied when an individual consistently ignores social rules; is manipulative; exploitative; dishonest; lacks remorse for actions; and is frequently involved in criminal activity. Although this diagnosis occurs in only 3% of men and 1% of women, these individuals are responsible for a large proportion of crime, violence, and social distress (Kaylor, 1999).

The manipulative person is unaware of a lack of relatedness and assumes that all interpersonal relationships are formed to take advantage of others. This person cannot imagine an intimate, sharing relationship. The manipulator believes in maintaining control at all times to avoid being controlled. Patients with borderline personality disorder are often manipulative. This results in their inability to participate in mature interpersonal relationships, as illustrated in the next clinical example.

 CLINICAL EXAMPLE

Ms. S is a 23-year-old woman who was admitted to a general hospital psychiatric unit. She had lacerated her wrists superficially three times during the week before admission. Each time she cut herself, she had telephoned her therapist, a psychiatric clinical nurse specialist. Because her therapist was about to leave for vacation and she was concerned about the safety of Ms. S, the nurse decided to hospitalize her.

On admission Ms. S appeared mildly depressed. She gave the impression of a guilty child who had been punished. She denied any current self-destructive thoughts. During the physical assessment, the nurse noted that there were many scars on the patient's body. When asked about these, she claimed she was abused as a child. Her therapist's records described the scars as the result of much self-mutilation since the age of 16 years. This had been her main reason for seeking therapy. There was also a history of sexual promiscuity.

Ms. S described herself as a failure, stating that she had "the best parents in the world, but they did not get the daughter they deserve." She said she was a drifter who had never been able to settle on a career, a lifestyle, or any consistent friends. She didn't know who or what she was. When asked how she felt, she responded, "Most of the time, I don't feel anything, just empty." She had no signs of psychosis.

Ms. S was placed on constant observation to prevent further cutting. All sharp objects were removed from the room. At first she was very cooperative and superficially friendly to other patients. Because of her smooth adjustment, constant observation was discontinued after 3 days. She was also given a schedule of activities and informed that she was responsible for following it.

The next day, an X-Acto knife was missing from the activities therapy room. Ms. S was found in the bathroom, bleeding from several small cuts on her ankles. This sequence was repeated several times. Each time the constant observation was discontinued, she found a sharp object and cut herself.

She was also very labile emotionally. She had unpredictable outbursts of anger, similar to temper tantrums. However, these outbursts passed as quickly as they came, never lasting more than a few minutes. She also began to categorize the staff as "good guys and bad guys." When she was with staff members she liked, she was pleasant, complimenting them on their kind and understanding attitudes toward her. With staff she disliked, she was sullen and uncooperative, comparing them unfavorably to the others. Eventually the staff began to bicker about her care, some believing she was spoiled and others that she was neglected.

Ms. S remained in the hospital during her therapist's absence. When the therapist returned, Ms. S refused to see her. The frequency of angry outbursts increased dramatically. However, following frequent visits from her therapist, Ms. S began to request discharge. Behavioral criteria for discharge were set, including no self-mutilation and no temper tantrums. She met the criteria and was discharged back to outpatient treatment.

Selected Nursing Diagnoses

- Risk for self-mutilation related to anxiety about her therapist's vacation, as evidenced by lacerating her wrists
- Self-esteem disturbance related to unclear goals and expectations, as evidenced by describing herself as a failure
- Impaired social interaction related to inability to tolerate close relationships, as evidenced by splitting staff into " good guys" and "bad guys"

The diagnosis of **borderline personality disorder** occurs in 2% to 3% of the general population and is the most prevalent personality disorder in clinical settings (Nehls, 1998). The diagnosis is three times more often in women than in men, and theories that may explain this include the following (Brown & Dodson, 1999):

1. Women may be more biologically vulnerable than men.
2. Sociocultural expectations of perceived roles and attitudes may contribute to this problem in women.
3. Similar symptoms may generate a diagnosis of narcissistic personality disorder in men.

Research shows that women with borderline personality disorder feel that the label is difficult to live with, their self-destructive behavior is seen as manipulative, and they have limited access to care (see Citing the Evidence).

Developmental theory (Masterson, 1985) proposes that the borderline person fails to achieve object constancy during the separation-individuation stage of psychosocial development. Because of this, the person relates to another as a series of disconnected parts rather than as a whole. The borderline person cannot recall the image of someone who is absent. He or she is not able to mourn the loss of another person. When someone fails to meet the borderline person's needs, the relationship is likely to end.

People who fail to complete separation from the mother (or primary caretaker) and develop autonomy in childhood often repeat this developmental crisis at adolescence. Behaviors characteristic of this phase include the following:

- Clinging
- Depression accompanied by rage and defended by acting out or neurotic behavior
- Detachment and withdrawal

Many of these behaviors can be seen in the preceding clinical example. Because of their inability to become involved in reciprocal interpersonal relationships and the related manipulativeness, these patients are frustrating for nursing staff

Citing the Evidence on

Women with Borderline Personality Disorder

BACKGROUND: This qualitative study described the experience of 30 women living with the diagnosis of borderline personality disorder.

RESULTS: Three themes were identified: living with a label, living with self destructive behavior perceived as manipulation, and living with limited access to care.

IMPLICATIONS: Mental health care for persons with borderline personality disorder could be improved by confronting prejudice, understanding self-harm, and safeguarding opportunities for dialogue.

Nehls N: Borderline personality disorder: the voice of patients, *Res Nurs Health* 22:285, 1999.

to interact with and treat. It must be remembered that their behavior is not consciously planned but is a defense against a fear of loneliness.

Narcissism. The term narcissism comes from the Greek myth of Narcissus, who fell in love with his own reflection in the waters of a spring and died. The flower that bears his name sprang up at the site of his death. Many successful people are narcissistic. Acting, modeling, professional sports, and politics are usually attractive occupations to people with this personality trait. In these contexts self-centeredness is usually expected. However, problems occur when the person does not gain the status they think they deserve or loses status, or tries to have interpersonal relationships. The frustration caused by lack or loss of recognition may be expressed as anger, depression, substance abuse, or other maladaptive behaviors.

People with narcissistic personality disorders have fragile self-esteem, driving them to search constantly for praise, appreciation, and admiration. The clinical example that follows demonstrates narcissistic entitlement, which describes an egocentric attitude, envy, and rage when others are seen as critical or not supportive.

 ## CLINICAL EXAMPLE

Ms. T, the psychiatric clinical nurse specialist, was called to the emergency room to see a new patient, Mr. F. He was accompanied by his wife. The nurse knew from the intake form that Mr. F was a 44-year-old man with no psychiatric history. His chief complaint was that he had gone into a "blind rage" when he had an argument with his wife earlier in the evening and he had punched her in the arm. He was frightened by his loss of control and said that he felt like a failure. Both Mr. and Mrs. F denied any history of violence, although Mr. F said that his first marriage ended "because of my anger."

Mr. F appeared quite anxious; he was tapping his foot and wringing his hands, and he avoided eye contact with Ms. T. After a short time, however, he became more verbal, and he willingly explained what had led to the "blow up." He had been self-employed for the past 10 years and had been "highly successful," expanding his company nationally. He told Ms. T that his father was a "multimillionaire" and that he had been on his way to exceeding his father's wealth. It seemed important to impress Ms. T by dropping the names of well-known people, whom he described as his friends.

Mrs. F angrily interrupted him, saying "that's important to you—who you know and how it looks." Mrs. F then explained that business began slipping 2 years ago. Despite several profitable years, he had never invested or saved money. When sales fell, instead of cutting expenses and downsizing the company, he continued to live lavishly, making extravagant purchases. It was this situation that led to their argument. When Mrs. F accused her husband of taking them to the brink of financial collapse, he went into a rage and punched her. Mrs. F began sobbing, and Mr. F seemed not to notice. He said he felt like his life was falling apart and that he must be the failure his father always said he was. He angrily referred to his "rich brother," who, in his father's eyes, was the perfect son. He became tearful, and Mrs. F then turned to her husband, attempting to provide support and reassurance.

Selected Nursing Diagnoses

- Impaired social interaction related to the need for approval by others, as evidenced by attempts to impress others and inability to respond to wife's distress
- Risk for violence directed at others related to impulsivity as evidenced by acts engaged in during "blind rage"
- Altered family processes related to inconsistency between goals of husband and wife, as evidenced by wife's reaction to patient's description of his problem
- Defensive coping related to fear of failure as evidenced by bragging and name-dropping
- Chronic low self-esteem related to perceived lack of caring and approval from father, as evidenced by stated need to exceed his father's success and description of himself as "a failure" in his father's eyes

Mr. F's impulsiveness was demonstrated by his extravagance, inability to establish and follow a life plan, failure to learn by experience, poor judgment, and unreliability. The behaviors related to maladaptive social responses are summarized in Table 23-1. Patients often exhibit combinations of these behaviors. The nurse should be able to identify the complex behaviors associated with high levels of stress and anxiety. In some cases, a usual mode of behavior, such as manipulation, may be exaggerated or combined with a change in behavior. For instance, manipulative people may withdraw when confronted about their manipulations and may be rejected by those they have been trying to manipulate. In other instances, the behavior resulting from stress may be different from the person's usual style of relatedness. A person who is usually outgoing may withdraw when under great stress. It is helpful to include a description of the patient's usual relationships in the nursing assessment. This provides a baseline of behavior for that person against which the nurse measures the patient's progress.

Table **23-1**

Behaviors Related to Maladaptive Social Responses	
Behavior	**Characteristics**
Manipulation	Others are treated as objects
	Relationships center around control issues
	Person is self-oriented or goal-oriented, not other-oriented
Narcissism	Fragile self-esteem
	Constant seeking of praise and admiration
	Egocentric attitude
	Envy
	Rage when others are not supportive
Impulsivity	Inability to plan
	Inability to learn from experience
	Poor judgment
	Unreliability

Predisposing Factors

Current research supports the multifactorial origins of personality disorders, including a variety of predisposing neurobiological, early developmental, and sociocultural factors. The nurse should explore all relevant areas during the nursing assessment.

Biological Factors. Many researchers believe that for severe mental illness, such as borderline personality disorder or antisocial personality disorder, there must be an inherited biological vulnerability or a genetic susceptibility, which sets the stage for environmental influences (Brown & Dodson, 1999). Recent studies suggest a genetic link for antisocial personality disorder and a biological hypothesis that impulsive and violent behavior may be caused by brain dysfunction, a low threshold of excitability of the limbic system, low levels of serotonin, or toxic chemical substances. One recent study found that people with antisocial personality disorder have a subtle structural brain dysfunction that may underlie their low arousal, poor fear conditioning, lack of conscience, and decision-making deficits (see Citing the Evidence). Personality disorders have been linked to alcohol and drug abuse. Findings reveal that first-degree relatives of people with personality disorders have a higher than normal rate of being substance abusers, thus they are considered to have a probable genetic link. Borderline personality disorder and antisocial personality disorder in particular are associated with a wide variety of substance use disorders, and the combination results in severe global impairment (Skodol et al, 1999).

Researchers are looking for the biological basis of very early infant and childhood characteristics. For instance, about 20% of children are inhibited from an early age, and can be upset easily by age 4 ½ months. There is evidence that these children show a high heart rate, even in the womb, and their amygdala (the brain region that governs learned fear and emotion) may be more excitable than average. In contrast, antisocial personality is apparently correlated with abnormal brain processing of emotionally charged words, an unusually low heart rate, and slow responses to experimental rewards and punishments from an early age (Grinspoon, 2000). Further research is needed to clarify the role of inheritance and brain structure and function in the development of personality disorders.

Developmental Factors. Early studies of the childhood experiences of patients with personality disorders focused on the etiological role of early separations and disturbed parental involvement. More current research has focused specifically on the developmental consequences of childhood abuse and its role in the etiology of Cluster B personality disorders, particularly borderline personality disorder.

Research has shown that patients with borderline personality disorder compared with patients with other personality disorders were significantly more likely to report having been emotionally and physically abused by a caretaker and sexually abused by a noncaretaker. However, the results suggest that sexual abuse by itself is neither necessary nor sufficient for the etiology of borderline personality disorder, therefore there are other predisposing factors involved (Zanarini et al, 1997). Moreover, approximately 25% of patients with borderline personality disorder are also given a diagnosis of posttraumatic stress disorder, a condition that results from an overwhelming psychological assault (Brown & Dodson, 1999). Similarly, childhood histories of people with antisocial personality disorder often reveal abuse, neglect, and the absence of an early emotional attachment. It is theorized by some that lack of parental caring is internalized, and the individual becomes incapable of bonding with others. People with antisocial personality disorder never develop a sense of trust or a capacity for guilt or remorse (Kaylor, 1999).

In a longitudinal study of childhood behaviors that preceded a diagnosis of personality disorders in adolescence, four childhood conditions were found: conduct problems, depressive symptoms, anxiety or fear, and immaturity. Thus antecedents of adolescent personality disorder can be identified 10 years earlier through an accurate assessment of emotional and behavioral problems (Bernstein et al, 1996).

Theories of family impact on personality are controversial. Some research supports the fact that, apart from genetic similarity, children raised in the same family do not resemble one another more closely than strangers. Thus influences outside the family (i.e., peer groups) are greater than parental influences during childrearing. Other theorists support the notion that many people with maladaptive social responses are enmeshed in a family system that blocks further development and makes change difficult and hazardous. Families of borderline and narcissistic people often operate with the unspoken ground rule that independence and separation from the family imply rejection of family val-

---

Citing the Evidence on

Brain Deficit in Antisocial Personality Disorder

BACKGROUND: Major damage from trauma to gray and white brain matter in the prefrontal cortex results in pseudopsychiatric personality in patients with neurological disorders. Do people with antisocial personality disorder who do not have discernible brain trauma, have subtle prefrontal deficits?

RESULTS: The patients with antisocial personality disorder were found to have 11% reduction in prefrontal gray matter volume in the absence of brain trauma, and reduced autonomic activity during stress.

IMPLICATIONS: These findings suggest a structural brain deficit in antisocial personality disorder that may cause the low arousal, low fear, lack of conscience, and decision-making deficits that characterize this disorder.

Raine A et al: Reduced prefrontal gray matter volume and reduced autonomic activity in antisocial personality disorder, *Arch Gen Psychiatry* 57:119, 2000.

ues. The parents often reenact their own developmental conflicts through their children, and role reversals (for example, parent as child) are common. Features of these families include various degrees of restrictiveness from the extrafamilial world, absence of clear-cut lines of authority, confusion of parental executive and nurturing roles, blurred generational boundaries, generations of family patterns in which people are labeled as good and bad, and the generational transmission of irrational forms of thinking and relating (see Chapter 34).

The nurse should assess the nature of family interactions and gather information related to early child behaviors, child abuse and alcohol abuse as part of a comprehensive data collection (Kaylor, 1999).

Sociocultural Factors. Sociocultural factors can also influence the person's ability to establish and maintain relatedness. Many forces in American culture make people feel isolated and lonely. Friendships are often short term because of the mobility involved in many occupations. Family relationships are more distant as adult children move away and see their parents only occasionally. Friends are often closer than siblings.

Involuntary social isolation also affects the disabled and chronically ill of any age. People with chronic or terminal illnesses or disfiguring disorders are often stigmatized and avoided by others. This is also true for people with long-term psychiatric problems. Although an effort has been made to decrease chronic institutionalization, many people continue to resist integrating disabled people into their community. This involuntary isolation may result in a variety of maladaptive social responses as the person tries to cope with loneliness.

Immigration continues to be an active cultural force in the United States and many other parts of the world. As people move into entirely different cultures, they may feel alienated and frightened about customs they do not understand. Sometimes immigrants form separate communities to preserve their traditions. These close-knit communities help to meet relationship needs but create barriers to broader community participation and integration. Unfortunately, they also focus attention on the group, often attracting discriminatory behavior.

Closeness is the ideal in American culture. At the same time, people are given the message that they need to be careful in deciding whom to trust. This can cause confusion and a feeling of insecurity. Rising crime rates cause fear and reluctance to risk closeness or contact with strangers. Some urban residents, particularly the elderly, become lonely prisoners in their own homes.

Precipitating Stressors

Maladaptive social responses are the result of experiences that negatively influence the person's emotional growth. In most instances a series of life events predisposes a person to have relationship problems. Many people cope with their interpersonal problems and say they are reasonably satisfied with their relationships. However, additional stress can cause

a somewhat satisfying interpersonal life to become disrupted. Response to stressors is highly individual, and the nurse should remember that the person experiences an increase in anxiety as a result of the stressor, and this is often at the root of behavioral disruption.

Sociocultural Stressors. Stressors leading to relationship difficulties may be sociocultural in nature. For instance, there can be instability in the family. Divorces are common. Mobility has broken up the extended family, depriving people of all ages of an important support system. Less contact occurs between the generations. Tradition, which provides a powerful link with the past and a sense of identity, is less observable when the family is fragmented. Interest in ethnicity and "roots" may reflect the efforts of isolated people to associate themselves with a specific identity. The many stresses on the family have made it more difficult for family members to accomplish the developmental tasks related to intimacy.

Nurses who work in general hospitals often encounter patients with maladaptive social responses. Even a reasonably well-adjusted person may have difficulty maintaining a satisfying level of intimacy while hospitalized. The patient's feeling of isolation is enhanced by the impersonal hospital environment. Sometimes patients need to be isolated because of infection, or in the psychiatric setting, to control behavior. They are then susceptible to the effects of sensory deprivation. Creative nursing care is needed to minimize this problem. For instance, a patient who is in isolation for infection control could be given a schedule of times when staff will be present. This should include time to talk. Family members should be encouraged to visit, telephone, and share current activities. On the other hand, sensory overload may be a problem for patients in critical care units. This can also lead to loneliness and separation from others.

Psychological Stressors. Many psychological theories have been proposed to explain problems in establishing and maintaining satisfying relationships. It is known that high anxiety levels result in impaired ability to relate to others. A combination of prolonged or intense anxiety with limited coping ability is believed to cause severe relationship problems.

It has been suggested that the person with borderline personality disorder is likely to experience an incapacitating level of anxiety in response to life events that represent increased autonomy and separation (such as high school or college graduation, going away to camp, marriage, birth of a child, employment, job promotion). The person who has narcissistic personality disorder tends to experience high anxiety, causing relationship difficulties, when the significant other no longer adequately nourishes the person's fragile self-esteem. These relationships often move through predictable stages:

1. Idealization and overvaluation
2. Disappointment when unrealistic needs for maintaining self-esteem are not met
3. Rationalization and devaluation
4. Rejection of the other person based on "narcissistic injury"

Typically, these people go through life repeating this pattern on the job, in marriages, and in friendships.

Appraisal of Stressors

The mature person who can participate in healthy relationships is still vulnerable to the effects of psychological stress. A person's appraisal of the stressor is critically important in this regard. A series of losses or a single significant loss may lead to problems in establishing future intimate relationships. The pain of a loss can be so great that the person avoids future involvements rather than risk more pain. This response is more likely if the person had difficulty with developmental tasks pertinent to relatedness. Losses of significant others may cause difficulty with future relationships, but other types of losses may do the same. For example, the loss of a job decreases a person's self-esteem. This can also result in future withdrawal and emotional problems unless the person has a well-established support system.

Coping Resources

When a person is having problems with relationships, it is important for the nurse to assess the person's coping resources. For many people, when one relationship is troublesome or lost, others are available to offer support and reassurance. Those who have broad networks of family and friends have many resources to draw on. Sometimes they need encouragement to reach out for help.

Some people do not have readily available human supports but have other ways of managing interpersonal problems. Pets can be an important way of expressing relatedness. Isolated elderly people often focus their need to give and receive affection on a dog or cat. Sometimes a person who is troubled about a relationship will use creative ways to express feelings. Use of expressive media such as art, music, or writing allows the person to explore and resolve an upsetting experience. Others are helped by reading, exercise, looking at art, dancing, or listening to music.

> *Identify a novel, a popular song, or a work of art that would have meaning for a person who is trying to cope with an interpersonal loss. How do such things help you?*

Coping Mechanisms

Behaviors associated with maladaptive social responses are attempts to cope with anxiety related to threatened or actual loneliness. However, they are not healthy and sometimes have the unintended effect of driving people away. Thus the person is always caught in the approach-avoidance conflict of the need-fear dilemma, searching for some degree of human contact on one hand and pushing people away on the other.

Manipulative people view other people as objects. Their defenses protect them from potential psychological pain related to the loss of a significant other. People with antisocial personality disorder often use the defenses of projection

and splitting. **Projection** places responsibility for antisocial behavior outside oneself. For instance, a patient may rationalize using drugs by saying, "Everybody I know uses cocaine. Why shouldn't I?" **Splitting** is characteristic of people with borderline and narcissistic personality disorders as well. It is the inability to integrate the good and bad aspects of oneself and objects. An object is anything outside of the self, animate or inanimate, to which the person has an attachment. An object could be a parent, a friend, or a teddy bear. The process of splitting by a borderline patient in an inpatient setting results in different staff members seeing the borderline patient in very different ways (Quaytman & Scharfstein. 1997).

Projective identification is a complex defense mechanism. When the borderline patient projects parts of himself or herself onto others, these people are often not consciously aware of this. However, they may begin to behave like the projected parts (Brown & Dodson, 1999). For example, a patient projects onto a nurse cruel, punishing parts of himself. The projection reverberates with something in the nurse that had been submerged, and the nurse will tend to react to the patient in a cruel, punishing manner. Likewise, staff who have received idealized projected parts of the patient will tend to respond in an overly involved, protective, indulgent manner. An example of projective identification is demonstrated by Ms. T in the following clinical example.

 CLINICAL EXAMPLE

A nurse, Ms. M, was describing her relationship with a borderline patient, Ms. T, who had been on the unit for approximately 2 weeks. She explained that Ms. T had become negativistic and increasingly demanding to the point that her demands had no bounds. For the past week Ms. T had been calling Ms. M "Nurse Ratched." If that was not difficult enough, Ms. T was also telling new patients on the unit about what a tyrant Ms. M was. Further inquiry made it clear that soon after Ms. T had cast Ms. M into "Nurse Ratched," she started to react to the patient far more rigidly than was typical for her. Indeed, most of her interactions with Ms. T were now focused on policy adherence and strict limit setting. Without knowing it, Ms. M was on her way to repeating a script straight out of the movie *One Flew Over the Cuckoo's Nest*.

Selected Nursing Diagnosis

- Self-esteem disturbance related to use of the defense mechanism of splitting, as evidenced by need to belittle the nurse

Finally, the defense mechanisms of splitting and projective identification help explain why different staff members often see the same patient in very different ways, as illustrated in Fig. 23-2.

> *Compare the processes of empathic understanding and projective identification. Give some examples of each from your experience.*

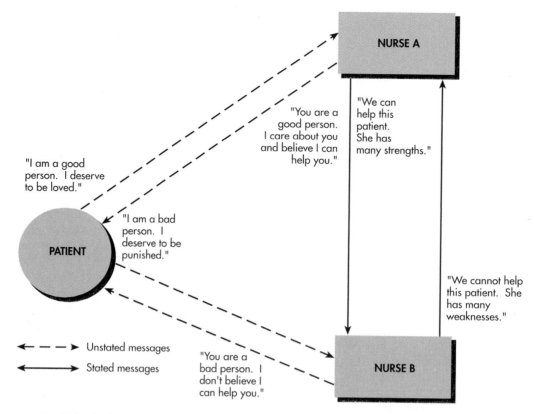

Fig. 23-2 Projective identification and splitting affects patient-to-nurse and nurse-to-nurse communication.

NURSING DIAGNOSIS

When diagnosing maladaptive social responses, the nurse should consider the extent and nature of maladaptive behaviors, coping mechanisms, and the predisposing factors and precipitating stressors leading to the behaviors. The nurse may formulate a nursing diagnosis by using the Stuart Stress Adaptation Model (Fig. 23-3) as a guide. Nursing diagnoses associated with maladaptive social responses and related medical diagnoses are presented in the Medical and Nursing Diagnoses box on p. 449. Primary NANDA diagnoses include **personal identity disturbance, self-esteem disturbance, risk for self-mutilation, impaired social interaction,** and **risk for violence.** Examples of complete nursing diagnoses are presented in the Detailed Diagnoses box on p. 450.

Related Medical Diagnoses

Medical diagnoses related to maladaptive social responses are categorized as personality disorders. Personality is composed of temperament, which is inherited, and character, which is learned (Bates et al, 1995).

In general, distinguishing characteristics of personality disorders include the fact that they tend to be:

- Chronic and long-standing
- Not based on a sound personality structure
- Difficult to change

Personality disorders are described in the Detailed Diagnoses box.

Describe one of your own personality traits that is due to temperament and one that is due to character. How have each affected your life?

OUTCOME IDENTIFICATION

The expected outcome for nursing care of the patient with maladaptive social responses is the following:

The patient will obtain maximum interpersonal satisfaction by establishing and maintaining self-enhancing relationships with others.

Short-term goals are more specific to the patient's problems. They may progress from simpler to more complex changes in behavior. It can be difficult to set mutual nursing care goals with a patient who has problems with relatedness. This is partly because mutuality must be based on a strong nurse-patient relationship. It is difficult to develop a strong relationship with a patient who fears intimacy. In addition, setting a goal implies a commitment to change. Many patients who have maladaptive social responses are reluctant to commit themselves to change. Because most of these behavioral problems also serve as coping mechanisms, there is additional resistance to change.

For these reasons, even though it is desirable to have the patient's full participation, it may be necessary for the nurse to set initial goals. To overcome a problem with relatedness, the person must be involved with others. At first, the other person may be the nurse, but eventually others will take the nurse's place.

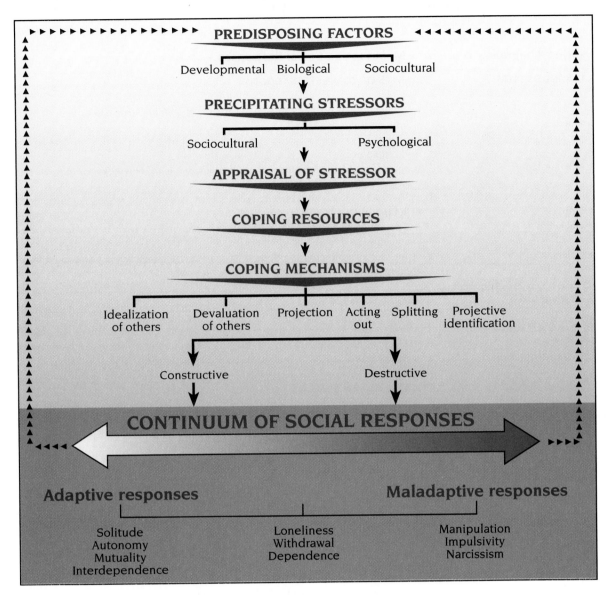

Fig. 23-3 The Stuart Stress Adaptation Model related to social responses.

Medical and Nursing Diagnoses *related to* Maladaptive Social Responses

RELATED MEDICAL DIAGNOSES (*DSM–IV–TR*)*	RELATED NURSING DIAGNOSES (NANDA)†
Paranoid personality disorder	Adjustment, impaired
Schizoid personality disorder	Anxiety
Schizotypical personality disorder	Coping, ineffective family
Antisocial personality disorder	Coping, ineffective individual
Borderline personality disorder	Family processes, altered
Histrionic personality disorder	Management of therapeutic regimen, individual or family: effective or ineffective
Narcissistic personality disorder	**Personal identity disturbance‡**
Avoidant personality disorder	Role performance, altered
Dependent personality disorder	**Self-esteem disturbance‡**
Obsessive-compulsive personality disorder	**Self-mutilation, risk for‡**
	Social interaction, impaired‡
	Social isolation
	Thought processes, altered
	Violence, risk for‡
	Self-directed
	Directed at others

*Reprinted with permission from the *Diagnostic and statistical manual of mental disorders*, Fourth Edition, Text Revision. Copyright 2000. American Psychiatric Association.
†From North American Nursing Diagnosis Association: *NANDA nursing diagnoses: definitions and classifications 1999-2000*, Philadelphia, 1999, The Association.
‡Primary nursing diagnosis for maladaptive social responses.

Detailed Diagnoses *related to* **Maladaptive Social Responses**

NANDA DIAGNOSIS STEM	EXAMPLES OF COMPLETE DIAGNOSIS
Personal identity disturbance	Personal identity disturbance related to early developmental arrest, as evidenced by difficulty defining self boundaries
Self-esteem disturbance	Self-esteem disturbance related to physical abuse during childhood, as evidenced by verbalized unhappiness with personal accomplishments
Risk for self-mutilation	Risk for self-mutilation related to fear of rejection, as evidenced by cutting self after visits from parents
Impaired social interaction	Impaired social interaction related to rejection of sociocultural values, as evidenced by stated belief that rules do not pertain to self
Risk for violence: self-directed	Risk for self-directed violence related to need to punish self, as evidenced by repeated burning of hands and feet when criticized
Risk for violence: directed at others	Risk for violence directed at others related to use of projection as evidenced by blaming, argumentativeness, and recent purchase of a handgun

DSM–IV–TR Diagnosis	ESSENTIAL FEATURES*
Paranoid personality disorder	A pervasive distrust and suspiciousness of others such that their motives are interpreted as malevolent, beginning in early adulthood and present in a variety of contexts
Schizoid personality disorder	A pervasive pattern of detachment from social relationships and a restricted range of expression of emotions in interpersonal settings, beginning in early adulthood and present in a variety of contexts
Schizotypical personality disorder	A pervasive pattern of social and interpersonal deficits marked by acute discomfort with and reduced capacity for close relationships and by cognitive and perceptual distortions and eccentricities of behavior, beginning in early adulthood and present in a variety of contexts
Antisocial personality disorder	A pervasive pattern of disregard for and violation of the rights of others occurring since age 15 years
Borderline personality disorder	A pervasive pattern of instability of interpersonal relationships, self-image, and affects, and marked impulsivity beginning by early adulthood and present in a variety of contexts
Histrionic personality disorder	A pervasive pattern of excessive emotionality and attention-seeking, beginning by early adulthood and present in a variety of contexts
Narcissistic personality disorder	A pervasive pattern of grandiosity (in fantasy or behavior), need for admiration, and lack of empathy beginning by early adulthood and present in a variety of contexts
Avoidant personality disorder	A pervasive pattern of social inhibition, feelings of inadequacy, and hypersensitivity to negative evaluation, beginning by early adulthood and present in a variety of contexts
Dependent personality disorder	A pervasive and excessive need to be taken care of that leads to submissive and clinging behavior and fears of separation, beginning by early adulthood and present in a variety of contexts
Obsessive-compulsive personality disorder	A pervasive pattern of preoccupation with orderliness, perfectionism, and mental and interpersonal control, at the expense of flexibility, openness, and efficiency, beginning by early adulthood and present in a variety of contexts

*Reprinted with permission from the *Diagnostic and statistical manual of mental disorders*, Fourth Edition, Text Revision. Copyright 2000. American Psychiatric Association.

Short-term goals with these patients may focus on reducing acting-out behaviors and modifying specific communication patterns. Examples include the following:

- The patient will use verbal communication as an alternative to acting out.
- The patient will verbally identify angry feelings when they occur during a one-to-one interaction.

These goals should be developed with the patient's active participation.

Learning to relate more directly and openly causes anxiety. Therefore, the patient's ability to tolerate anxiety must be considered when setting goals. Increasing the anxiety level before the patient has increased coping ability and environ-

mental supports may reinforce use of maladaptive coping behaviors.

PLANNING

The nursing treatment plan provides a guide for intervention and promotes consistency among the nursing staff members who provide care to the patient. This is particularly important when working with patients with maladaptive social responses (Doenges et al, 1995). Planning also includes attending to the patient's educational needs. A Patient Education Plan for modifying impulsive behavior is presented on p. 451. It is an important and challenging part of the nurse's responsibility to help patients and their families

PATIENT EDUCATION PLAN   *Modifying Impulsive Behavior*

CONTENT	INSTRUCTIONAL ACTIVITIES	EVALUATION
Describe characteristics and consequences of impulsive behavior.	Select a situation in which impulsive behavior occurred. Ask the patient to describe what happened. Provide the patient with paper and a pen. Instruct the patient to keep a diary of impulsive actions, including a description of events before and after the incident.	The patient will identify and describe an impulsive incident. The patient will maintain a diary of impulsive behaviors. The patient will explore the causes and consequences of impulsive behavior.
Describe behaviors characteristic of interpersonal anxiety and relate anxiety to impulsive behavior.	Discuss the diary with the patient. Help the patient to identify interpersonal anxiety related to impulsive behavior.	The patient will connect feelings of interpersonal anxiety with impulsive behavior.
Explain stress-reduction techniques.	Describe the stress response (see Chapters 18). Demonstrate relaxation exercises (see Chapter 34). Help the patient to return the demonstration.	The patient will perform relaxation exercises when signs of anxiety appear.
Identify alternative responses to anxiety-producing situations.	Using situations from the diary and knowledge of relaxation exercises, help the patient to list possible alternative responses.	The patient will identify at least two alternative responses to each anxiety-producing situation. Practice using alternative responses to anxiety-producing situations.
Role-play each of the identified alternative behaviors.	Discuss the feelings associated with impulsive behavior and the alternatives.	The patient will describe the relationship between behavior and feelings. The patient will select and perform anxiety-reducing behaviors.

to understand the nature and treatment of any of the disorders that cause maladaptive social responses.

IMPLEMENTATION

Patients with personality disorders come to treatment for help with depression, anxiety, alcoholism, or difficulties in work or personal relationships, not to have their personalities changed. In fact, they often regard any attempt to change their personality as unnecessary and intrusive. The focus of therapy therefore is to help patients change the thinking and the behavior that result from personality traits or limit the consequences, and treat their symptoms of depression or other disorders (Perry et al, 1999; Grinspoon, 2000). Empirically validated treatments for some of the medical diagnoses related to personality disorders are summarized in Table 23-2. The various therapies include corrective learning experiences in which the patient's relationship with the therapist serves as a model.

Establishing a Therapeutic Relationship

No matter what type of maladaptive social response the patient is experiencing, nursing care is based on accessibility. The nurse must be physically present with the patient regularly so that there is an opportunity for interaction. There must also be psychological accessibility. This means that the nurse shows interest in the patient. The nurse tries to understand the patient by clarifying meanings and validating perceptions. The

nurse is also empathic. If the nurse-patient relationship is a healthy one, the patient can learn how to find satisfaction in other human relationships (see A Patient Speaks on p. 452).

Family Involvement

Because intimate relationships are always affected by maladaptive social responses, significant others must be involved in the plan of care (see A Family Speaks on p. 453). This is especially important for manipulative patients, who often shift attention away from themselves by creating conflict between the family and the staff. For instance, the patient may complain to family members about poor nursing care. At the same time the patient may tell the staff about mistreatment by the family. Staff and family are then in conflict. Attention is distracted from the patient, who avoids the discomfort of self-examination. When the staff finally realizes what is happening, the result is usually anger at the patient. Nurses should be aware of this tendency and avoid a punitive response. When manipulative patients are hospitalized, this behavior occurs many times. The patient returns home, still relating to others as objects. Family involvement is also important to promote and maintain positive change for the patient and family.

 How would you help family members to participate in the treatment of a person with a personality disorder?

Table **23-2**

Summarizing the Evidence for Personality Disorders
DISORDER: Borderline personality disorder
TREATMENT: ■ Dialectical behavioral therapy (DBT) produced lower attrition, fewer and less severe episodes of parasuicidal behavior, and fewer days of hospitalization compared with a control condition ■ Noradrenergic agents tended to improve mood but not irritability or dyscontrol, whereas serotonergic agents may act to decrease impulsivity; there are inconsistent data for the utility of antipsychotic and anticonvulsive agents
DISORDER: Mixed personality disorder (excluding Cluster A disorders)
TREATMENT: ■ An average of 40 weeks of brief dynamic therapy yielded substantial symptomatic improvement at both the end of treatment and after 1.5 years ■ Medications may be useful for several of these disorders, although many methodological problems remain to be worked out
DISORDER: Schizotypal personality disorder (and other Cluster A disorders)
TREATMENT: ■ Dopamine antagonists may be useful in reducing some of the symptoms of these disorders

From Nathan P, Gorman J: *A guide to treatments that work*, New York, 1998, Oxford University Press.

A Patient Speaks

When I was hospitalized, the nurses were my link with the outside world. They were with me more than anyone else. They were also my link to the treatment that was prescribed by my psychiatrist. The doctor left PRN orders because he thought I was a mature woman who could decide when I needed medication. I often felt a loss of dignity when the nurse questioned my need for the PRN medication. Because the medicine decreased my anxiety, I think I was the best judge of when I needed it. Because the doctor made me responsible for requesting the medication, it was not the nurse's job to question my need for it unless I asked for more than was prescribed. Even if someone is in the hospital, they need to be treated with dignity and respect. They are sick, not children and not stupid. Nothing hurts more than being treated like a second-class citizen by people who are in a more powerful position. It is much easier to work with a nurse who is kind and supportive.

Milieu Therapy

Because it is difficult and takes a long time to change maladaptive social responses, most patients are treated in the community rather than an inpatient setting. However, hospitalization is sometimes needed. For instance, the person with a borderline personality disorder may be self-destructive, or the antisocial person may require a structured environment with limit setting. Day treatment or partial hospitalization programs can have advantages for the treatment of patients with borderline personality disorder by offering them an acceptable level of intensiveness and containment, resulting in less regressive dependency and acting-out behavior (Miller, 1995).

The milieu, as found in hospitals, residential treatment, or outpatient programs, can effectively provide patients with an opportunity to gain insight into their behavior. Aside from staff limit setting, patients with maladaptive social responses learn from other patients about how much acting out will be tolerated. The patient responds well to a therapeutic milieu in which mature, responsible behavior is expected. Milieu work with these patients is most effective if it focuses on the following:

- Realistic expectations
- The process of decision making
- The process of interactional behaviors in the here and now

Nursing roles in milieu therapy include the following:

- Provide a structured environment
- Serve as an emotional sounding board
- Clarify and diagnose conflicts

Consistent clinical supervision is also very important because transference (intense emotional attachment of rejection derived from feelings about earlier personal relationships) and countertransference (the therapist's strong reaction to the patient, such as excessive sympathy, impatience, anger, contempt, fantasies of rescue, moralistic disdain, impulses to accept compliments from or identify with or hurt the patient) are usually an issue when caring for these patients (Dychoff, 1996) (see Chapter 2). Positive countertransference by some staff members, and negative by others, leads to splitting and staff conflict. Whenever these behavioral patterns emerge while there is a manipulative patient on the psychiatric unit, the staff must examine their level of involvement with the patient (Hartman, 1995).

The principles of milieu treatment for patients with Cluster B personality disorders include the following:

- Establish control with no option to escape involvement
- Provide an experienced, consistent staff
- Implement a strict hierarchical structure with rules that are firm and consistently enforced

A Family Speaks

It seems like my brother was always a problem. When we were growing up, he got us both into trouble all the time. Finally I learned to ignore his schemes and stay away from him. As he got older, the situation got worse. Our parents kicked him out of the house, but he would come back and promise to change and they would let him back in. Then it would start all over again. He began to get into trouble with the law. First there was vandalism for spray-painting graffiti on a building; then he was with a gang of kids who stole a car. He said he was just along for the ride, but I didn't really believe him.

The rest of the family was pretty embarrassed about his behavior. I thought about telling people I was adopted so they wouldn't think I was like him. I didn't do that because I knew it would hurt my parents and they had enough trouble already. I'll never forget the night when the phone rang at 4:00 AM and it was my brother saying he was in jail. He had been caught with drugs in a stolen car and had also resisted arrest. My parents refused to bail him out and he didn't have any money. The next day he called again to say that he was at the local psychiatric hospital. He had threatened to kill himself in jail, so they sent him to the hospital to see whether he was really mentally ill. My parents were really upset about this development. I think it was actually a good thing because the doctors and nurses at the hospital explained to us that he has a personality disorder. It did help to know that there might be a reason for his behavior, although he hasn't really changed much. I think my parents are beginning to accept this, but I know it's really hard for them.

- Provide support while the patient learns to experience painful feelings

Limit Setting and Structure

The way the nurse approaches limit setting can make the difference between a productive hospital experience and one that is nonproductive or counterproductive. Angry, punitive limit setting confirms the patient's expectations. Suppressive and rigid limits create obstacles to self-exploration and therapeutic change. This approach also confirms the patient's belief of having little or no control over life situations. It is essential that the nurse not view limits as a way of controlling the patient. For example, a patient with antisocial personality structure engages in physically aggressive acting-out behavior. One way of dealing with this might be to emphasize the need for medications and to tighten up restrictions. The treatment team might also issue an ultimatum, such as "One more similar episode, and we're going to have to transfer you to another hospital." A more positive way of approaching the situation could be: "You seem to want to put the treatment team in the position of having to reassess continuation of

your stay in this hospital. Has there been some change about wanting to help yourself?" The difference in the latter approach is emphasis on the idea that the patient has responsibility for life situations; the control and the decisions are the patient's. It also communicates an attitude of respect, which could boost the patient's self-esteem. The more the nurse is able to align with the nonregressed aspects of the patient's ego, the better are the chances for improved functioning.

Manipulative patients should also be held responsible for their behavior. They are skilled at placing responsibility on others. Staff members should communicate with each other so that consistent messages are given. These patients recognize any inconsistency and use it to focus attention on others. They usually resist rules. Staff and family members should collaborate in enforcing clear limits. Manipulative patients sometimes lie. It is important to confront the patient who consciously lies.

Guidelines for treating borderline patients include several principles (Masterson, 1985). There is a need for availability of staff attention combined with structured discipline. There must be an expectation that the patient will meet standards of healthy behavior. Failure to meet the standard is identified, and acting out is confronted. Loss of control may be dealt with by room restriction, with the patient instructed to think about the episode so that it may be discussed in therapy. The length of the restriction should be based on the seriousness of the behavior. These approaches may lead to depression. The depressed feelings should be directed into formal psychotherapy sessions, but the staff can act as role models for appropriate behavior. A school program, occupational therapy, and the milieu may be used to teach age-appropriate social and achievement skills. Reality orientation may also be necessary.

Protection from Self-Harm

The deliberate self-destructive or self-mutilating behavior of the borderline patient is very difficult to treat (see Chapter 21). Often the nursing staff must observe the patient constantly to prevent serious physical harm. At the same time, these patients have intense dependency needs related to an unresolved separation-individuation developmental phase. This makes it extremely difficult to wean them from constant staff attention, and contact must be decreased very gradually. Observation may need to be increased again if the patient seems out of control. Patient involvement in planning for decreased observation may be helpful. The patient must be reassured that less contact does not equal no contact. Consistent, scheduled time with a staff member is recommended. Primary nursing is particularly effective with a patient who needs to work through these separation issues (see Critical Thinking about Contemporary Issues).

You believe that a manipulative adolescent patient is exploiting another patient by "borrowing" money, clothing, and snacks. When confronted, the first patient claims that the items were gifts, "because we're friends." Do you think that limit setting is needed? If so, how would you set appropriate limits?

CRITICAL THINKING about CONTEMPORARY ISSUES

Should Constant Close Observation Be the Primary Nursing Approach for Borderline Patients with Impulsive Self-harming Behavior?

Patients with borderline personality disorder are most often hospitalized because of impulsive attempts at self-mutilation or suicide. The nursing intervention of constant close observation is usually initiated to protect the patient from impulsive behavior. This intervention activates the patient's conflicts about close relationships. Splitting may become evident as the patient establishes preferences for the staff assigned to observation. The patient is challenged to outwit the staff and find opportunities to act out. When efforts are made to decrease the level of observation, the patient's attachment conflicts become evident. There is often an effort to maintain the undivided attention of staff by renewed self-harming behavior.

Much attention in the media recently has been directed toward an exploration of the use of restrictive environments, such as restraint and seclusion, in psychiatric settings. There has been a focus on alternative interventions that are less restrictive or intrusive, staff training regarding the use of these interventions, and careful documentation. It is important to assist the patient to understand the purpose of these interventions, enlist the patient's help whenever possible, and encourage the patient to participate in the necessary steps to change to a less restrictive modality as soon as he is ready. The nurse should encourage the patient's help in defining and describing the harmful behavior.

Identification of cues and triggers allows the patient to request assistance, thereby becoming an active participant in the therapeutic process. Nurses are less judgmental about the patient if they understand the source of the behaviors and if they are in touch with the patient's feelings. The challenges to nurses are to maintain the patient's safety, facilitate the patient's participation in care, select the least restrictive intervention, facilitate behavioral change, and help the patient assume responsibility for his behaviors.

Focusing on Strengths

Patients with maladaptive social responses often are effective leaders within the patient group. A useful nursing approach is to encourage them to identify and use their strengths. They may be given responsibilities within the patient care unit and can be helpful to other patients. They are often intelligent and can participate actively in planning their own care. However, they are extremely resistant to recognizing or dealing with feelings and need consistent encouragement to verbalize these emotions.

Nurses become frustrated with these patients because they seem to be so aware of what is happening and in control of most situations, yet so unaware of others' needs. Nurses should remember that these patients have little tolerance for intimacy. Their maneuvering of others is a way to keep them at a safe distance. These patients are often charming, and it is easy to become involved with them. However, as soon as other people make demands or show signs of emotional closeness, the patients dilute the relationship by withdrawing, frustrating others, or distracting attention from themselves.

Journal writing is a nursing intervention that can be helpful to patients who have difficulty with close relationships. Keeping a diary of their thoughts and feelings helps them identify the various aspects of their interpersonal experiences and review them over time. It gives them an opportunity to see continuity of people and relationships. Interpersonal strengths can be identified and reinforced. The nurse can also note behavioral strengths that the patient has not yet identified and help the patient in recognizing these as well.

Behavioral Strategies

Various behavioral strategies can help decrease antisocial behavior (see Chapter 32). The patient is usually impatient with delays in gratification. Material rather than emotional rewards are preferred. Thus reinforcers used in a behavior modification program should be concrete and readily available. For example, points may be accumulated to qualify for privileges, such as a trip to the canteen. Other reinforcers might be a visit or a favorite food. Ignoring undesirable behavior is the least reinforcing but is not always possible. If behavior is disruptive and there must be a response, it should be matter of fact and one not desired by the patient. For instance, removal from contact with others for a specific period of time may discourage undesirable behavior, whereas a lecture that attracts attention may be a reinforcer.

Behavioral contracting can be helpful with borderline patients as a tool to structure treatment. Although useful for many patients, they may not be helpful for involuntarily admitted patients who are exhibiting self-destructive behaviors (O'Brien, 1998).

A specific kind of cognitive-behavioral therapy called dialectical behavior therapy (DBT) is an empirically validated treatment approach designed initially for suicidal women with borderline personality disorder (Linehan, 1993; Simpson et al, 1998). DBT uses behavioral and cognitive techniques that include psychological education, problem-solving, training in social skills, exercises in monitoring moods, modeling by the therapist, homework assignments, and meditation. It is based on the assumption that temperament and an unresponsive environment have made them unable to trust their own emotional responses or soothe themselves. It has shown a high rate of effectiveness in decreasing hospital stays, suicide attempt frequency, visits to emergency rooms, and therapy attrition (Hampton, 1997; Miller et al, 1998).

Medications. The use of drugs have a limited role in the treatment of personality disorders (see Table 23-2). They are used primarily to relieve symptoms (anxiety, mood swings, impulsive aggression, psychotic delusion, hallucinations), thus facilitating other treatments. The patient must be stable enough to take the medications as prescribed. Personal attention and reassurance by the nurse and the rest of the health-care team are important (Grinspoon, 2000).

A Nursing Treatment Plan Summary for the patient with maladaptive social responses is presented on the opposite page.

NURSING TREATMENT PLAN *Summary* *Maladaptive Social Responses*

NURSING DIAGNOSIS: Impaired social interaction
EXPECTED OUTCOME: The patient will obtain maximum interpersonal satisfaction by establishing and maintaining self-enhancing relationships with others.

SHORT-TERM GOAL	INTERVENTION	RATIONALE
The patient will participate in a therapeutic nurse-patient relationship.	Initiate a nurse-patient relationship contract mutually agreed on by patient and nurse. Develop mutual behavioral goals. Maintain consistent behavior by all nursing staff. Communicate honest responses to the patient's behavior. Provide honest, immediate feedback about behavioral change. Maintain confidentiality. Demonstrate accessibility.	An atmosphere of trust facilitates open expression of thoughts and feelings. A trusting relationship enables the patient to risk sharing feelings. Honest responses reinforce openness. Staff consistency creates a predictable environment that creates trust.
The patient will describe interpersonal strengths and weaknesses.	Provide opportunities to demonstrate strengths, such as helping other patients, assuming leadership roles. Help to analyze experiences that are perceived as failures. Communicate acceptance of the patient as a person while not accepting maladaptive social behavior.	Patients with maladaptive social responses are unable to identify accurately their interpersonal strengths and weaknesses, leading to fear of closeness and fear of failure. It is important to help the patient to separate behavioral incidents from total self-worth and recognize that one can be liked even if imperfect.
The patient will establish or reestablish one interpersonal relationship that is mutually satisfying and adaptive.	Provide consistent feedback about adaptive and maladaptive social behavior. Encourage patient to describe successful and unsuccessful relationship experiences orally or in a written journal. Help patient in initiating or resuming a relationship with one other person. Review aspects of this relationship with the patient. Reinforce the patient's adaptive social responses. Evaluate with the patient alternatives to maladaptive social responses.	Describing and evaluating one's behavior requires taking responsibility for the behavior and its consequences. Patients need to go beyond understanding or insight to engaging in actual behavioral change. It is important for the nurse to help the patient evaluate whether one's responses are adaptive or maladaptive. Alternatives can then be identified to further the patient's goal achievement.

NURSING DIAGNOSIS: Risk for self-mutilation
EXPECTED OUTCOME: The patient will select constructive rather than self-destructive ways of coping with interpersonal anxiety.

SHORT-TERM GOAL	INTERVENTION	RATIONALE
The patient will not engage in self-mutilation.	Develop a contract with the patient to notify staff when anxiety is increasing. Provide close 1:1 observation of the patient when necessary to maintain safety. Remove all potentially dangerous objects from the patient and the environment. Provide prescribed medications.	When the patient is unable to cope with anxiety, safety is the nurse's highest priority. A contract helps the patient assume responsibility and explore healthier coping responses.
The patient will describe self-mutilating episodes.	Help the patient review these events. Identify cues and triggers that precede self-mutilating behavior. Help the patient explore feelings related to these episodes.	Self-mutilation is often a way of relieving extreme anxiety. Structured interpersonal support can help the patient review these events.

Visit **MERLIN** for *Your Internet Connection* to websites that are related to the content in this chapter. www.mosby.com/MERLIN/Stuart

24 Cognitive Responses and Organic Mental Disorders

Michele T. Laraia

Sandra J. Sundeen

Cogito, ergo sum. I think, therefore I am.

DESCARTES

The ability to think and reason and to behave accordingly is a distinguishing feature of human beings. This ability created civilization and allowed the progression from the Stone Age to the Space Age and beyond. Information is growing at such a rapid rate that there is an overwhelming demand for each person to assimilate new information daily. Society has moved from the time when power meant physical strength, to the use of money to acquire power, to an era in which power lies in having the latest information.

Intellectual functioning is highly valued in Western society. Most people fear the possibility of losing their cognitive abilities (reasoning, memory, judgment, orientation, perception, and attention). These functions allow a person to make sense of experience and interact productively with the environment. Maladaptive cognitive responses leave the affected person in a state of confusion—unable to understand and learn from experience and unable to relate current to past events or to interact reasonably with the people in his or her life. Maladaptive cognitive responses change the way in which individuals think of themselves and the world in which they find themselves, as well as how the world thinks of and relates to them in return.

CONTINUUM OF COGNITIVE RESPONSES

Learning may be defined as any relatively permanent change in behavior that results from experience. Learning involves biological changes in the brain that are affected by external environments (the experience of the world in which humans are raised) and internal environments (genetic characteristics, developmental events, neurotransmission). All organisms can modify their behavior by instinctive, reflexive, and maturational responses to the environment, but human behavior is particularly affected by the ability to learn from experience, to remember what is learned, and to modify behavior in response.

Memory is defined as the storage and retrieval of past experience and, like learning, is a neurochemical process mediated by the brain. Memory is a key cognitive ability; to exercise judgment, make decisions, or even be oriented to time and place, a person must remember past experiences. Therefore memory loss is a particularly frightening symptom.

There are several types of memory, each with specific biological correlates and clinical implications; these different types of memory work together in most learning situations. Fig. 24-1 depicts different types of learning and memory and their behavioral and biological correlates.

In some people with brain dysfunction, cognitive responses either do not develop fully or deteriorate once they have developed. In general, maladaptive cognitive responses that occur during childhood are called developmental disabilities or mental retardation. The reader is referred to a textbook of pediatric nursing for a discussion of these disorders. This chapter considers maladaptive cognitive responses in the adult. Although maladaptive cognitive responses may occur at any age, they are most common in the elderly. It is recommended that this chapter be read in conjunction with Chapter 40, because the content of these two chapters is complementary.

Maladaptive cognitive responses include an inability to make decisions, impaired memory and judgment, disorientation, misperceptions, decreased attention span, and difficulties with logical reasoning. They may occur episodically or be present continuously. Depending on the stressor, the condition may be reversible or characterized by a progressive deterioration in functioning. Fig. 24-2 illustrates the continuum of cognitive responses.

> *The knowledge of how to get to school or work is a mixture of learned habits, attention, procedures, and remembered facts. Explain this using the biological and behavioral model of learning and memory to the caregiver of a patient with Alzheimer's disease.*

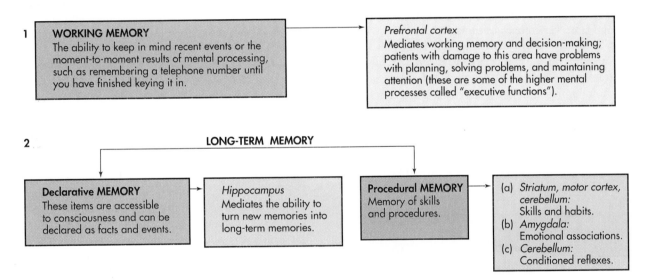

Fig. 24-1 Behavioral and biological correlates of learning and memory. (Modified from Nolte J: *The human brain: an introduction to its functional anatomy,* ed 4, St Louis, 2000, Mosby).

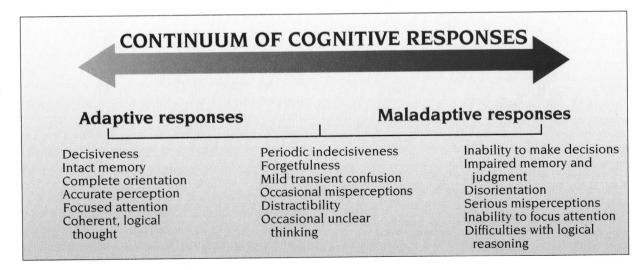

Fig. 24-2 Continuum of cognitive responses.

ASSESSMENT
Behaviors

Maladaptive cognitive responses are most apparent in people who have a psychiatric diagnosis of delirium, dementia, and amnestic and other cognitive disorders as described in the *DSM–IV–TR* (American Psychiatric Association, 2000). Such responses are classified as cognitive because they feature as a cardinal symptom an impairment in important functions such as memory, language, or attention. Discussions in this chapter focus primarily on delirium and dementia because these are the psychiatric diagnostic categories that nurses encounter most often. Assessment relies heavily on both biological findings (see Chapter 6) and on the results of the mental status examination (see Chapter 7). Box 24-1 lists behavioral rating scales related to the measurement of maladaptive cognitive responses.

Cognitive activity is dependent on intelligence, education, experience, and culture. These variables among patients can affect test scores, but not all scales or raters take them into account. The nurse should consider that some measures may have these shortcomings when assessing patients with varied abilities and from varied backgrounds.

Associated with Delirium. Delirium is the behavioral response to widespread disturbances in cerebral metabolism; it usually represents a sudden decline from a previous level of functioning and is usually considered a medical emergency. It is a syndrome with many possible causes, all of which result in **disturbances in consciousness** (reduced clarity or awareness of the environment), attention (impaired ability to direct and maintain mental focus, resulting in problems with processing stimuli into information), cogni-tion (recent memory impairment, disorientation to time and person, or language disturbance), and perception (misinterpretations, illusion, or hallucinations). The patient thus experiences a diminished awareness of the environment involving sensory misperceptions and disordered thought. Disordered thought processes include disturbed attention, memory, thinking, and orientation. There are also disturbances of psychomotor activity and the sleep-wake cycle.

These disturbances develop rapidly (hours to days) and tend to fluctuate over the course of the day, with occasional periods of mental clarity. The disturbances usually worsen at night. The clinical example that follows illustrates the behavior typical of a patient who is delirious.

 CLINICAL EXAMPLE

Ms. S was brought to the emergency department of a general hospital by her parents. This 22-year-old single woman was described as having been in good health until 2 days before admission, when she complained of malaise and a sore throat and stayed home from work. She worked as a typist in a small office and had a stable employment record. According to her parents, she had an active social life, and there were no significant conflicts at home.

On admission, Ms. S was extremely restless and had a frightened facial expression. Her speech was garbled and incoherent. When approached by an unfamiliar person, she would become agitated, try to climb out of bed, and strike out aimlessly. Occasionally she would slip into a restless sleep. Her temperature on admission was 104° F (40° C) rectally, her pulse was 108 beats per minute, and her respirations were 28 per minute. Her skin was hot, dry, and flushed. According to her mother, Ms. S had only a few sips of water in the last 24 hours and had not urinated at all, but she had experienced several episodes of profuse diaphoresis.

Ms. S's ability to cooperate with a mental status examination was limited. She would respond to her own name by turning her head. When her mother asked her where she was, she said "home," but she could not say where her home was. She would give only the month when asked for the date and said it was January (the actual date was February 19). She also refused to give the day of the week. A neurological examination was negative for signs of increased intracranial pressure or for localized signs of CNS disease.

The tentative medical diagnosis was delirium secondary to fever of unknown origin. Symptomatic treatment of the fever, including intravenous fluids, an aspirin suppository, and a cool water mattress, was begun immediately while further diagnostic studies were performed. Nurses caring for Ms. S noticed that she continued to be restless and disoriented and that her speech was still incoherent. They also noticed that she was picking at the bed clothing. Suddenly she became extremely agitated and tried to get out of bed while crying out, "Bugs, get away, get bugs away!" She was brushing and slapping at herself and the bed. As her mother and the nurse talked with her and held her, she gradually became calmer but periodically continued to slap at "the bugs" and needed reassurance and reorientation.

Additional laboratory results became available later in the day. A lumbar puncture was normal, as was magnetic resonance imaging (MRI) of the head. Results of a toxicological screening of the blood

Box 24-1

Behavioral Rating Scales Related to Cognitive Responses

CONTENT AREA: ORGANIC MENTAL DISORDERS
- Alzheimer's Disease Assessment Scale (ADAS)
- Behavior Pathology in Alzheimer's Disease
- Blessed Dementia Scale
- Brief Cognitive Rating Scale
- Clinical Dementia Rating Scale
- Cognitive Abilities Screening Instrument (CASI)
- Cohen-Mansfield Agitation Inventory
- Confusion Assessment Method
- Cornell Scale for Depression in Dementia
- Delirium Index
- Delirium Rating Scale
- Delirium Symptom Interview
- Disruptive Behavior Scale
- Face-Hand Test
- Haycox Dementia Behavioral Scale
- Memory and Behavior Problems Checklist
- Mini-Mental State Examination (MMSE)
- Multidimensional Observation Scale for Elderly Subjects
- NEECHAM Confusion Scale
- Neurobehavioral Rating Scale for Dementia (NRS)
- Overt Agitation Severity Scale
- Short Portable Mental Status Questionnaire (SPMSQ)

were also negative. However, the electroencephalogram revealed diffuse slowing. In addition, the elevated white blood count and electrolyte imbalance were consistent with severe dehydration. Cultures of Ms. S's throat and blood were both positive for beta-hemolytic streptococci, and intravenous antibiotic therapy was begun at once while other supportive measures were continued.

Ms. S's mental state improved as the infection gradually came under control and the fever decreased. Her cognitive functioning was completely normal when she was discharged from the hospital a week later, with the exception of amnesia for the time during which she was delirious.

Selected Nursing Diagnoses

- Hyperthermia related to infection, as evidenced by elevated temperature; hot, dry, flushed skin; and diaphoresis
- Fluid volume deficit related to decreased fluid intake, as evidenced by anuria for 24 hours and hot, dry, flushed skin
- Risk for injury related to fear and disorientation, as evidenced by agitated behavior
- Impaired verbal communication related to altered brain chemistry, as evidenced by garbled and incoherent speech
- Sensory-perceptual alterations (visual) related to altered brain chemistry, as evidenced by the hallucination of bugs
- Altered thought process related to altered brain chemistry, as evidenced by disorientation

Ms. S demonstrates many behaviors often seen in patients with delirium. These behaviors have a sudden onset and are related to alterations in neurochemical and electrical responses in the brain as a result of the stressor that causes the maladaptive response. Disorientation is generally present and is sometimes present in all three spheres of time, place, and person. Thought processes are usually disorganized. Judgment is poor, and little decision-making ability exists. Stimuli may be misinterpreted, resulting in illusions or distortions of reality. An example of such an illusion is the perception that a polka-dot drape is actually covered with cockroaches. Delirious patients may hallucinate. These hallucinations are usually visual and often take the form of animals, reptiles, or insects. They are real to the person and are very frightening. Assaultive or destructive behavior may be the patient's attempt to strike back at a hallucinated image. At times, patients with delirium also exhibit a labile affect, changing abruptly from laughter to tearfulness and vice versa for no apparent reason. There may also be a loss of usual social behavior, resulting in acts such as undressing, playing with food, and grabbing at others. Delirious patients tend to act on impulse.

Other behaviors may be specifically related to the cause of the behavioral syndrome. For example, Ms. S's brain syndrome and the fever and dehydration she experienced were a result of her systemic streptococcal infection. It is very important that observations of behavior be described carefully, because this helps to identify the stressor. Treatment is usually conservative until a specific stressor has been isolated. Although most patients recover, it is possible for the person to develop long-term disabilities or to die as a result of the severity of the stressor. Delirium is commonly found in hospitalized patients, particularly in intensive care units, geriatric psychiatry units, emergency departments, alcohol treatment units, and oncology units. If adequate intervention does not take place, delirium may become dementia.

Associated with Dementia. Dementia is a maladaptive cognitive response that features a loss of intellectual abilities and interferes with the patient's usual social or occupational activities. The loss of intellectual ability includes an impairment of memory, judgment, and abstract thought. The patient with dementia does not have the clouding of awareness or the rapid onset that is seen with delirium. The onset of dementia is usually gradual. It may result in progressive deterioration, or the condition may become stable. Personality changes often occur and may appear either as an alteration or as an accentuation of the person's usual character traits. In some cases the process of dementia can be reversed, and the person's intellectual functioning improves if the underlying stressors are identified and treated. In many cases, however, dementia involves a continual and irreversible decline in mental function and behavior. **Senility** or **senile** are nonspecific terms with negative connotations, and therefore the use of these terms is discouraged.

Dementia may occur at any age but most often affects the elderly. This condition results from structural and neurochemical changes in the brain as a result of trauma, infection, cerebrovascular disruptions, substance use, or an unknown cause. Alzheimer's disease (AD) is the most common type of dementia and accounts for approximately 65% of cases of dementia. It is estimated that 4.8 million people in the United States have AD at an annual cost of $80 billion. The prevalence of AD doubles every 5 years between 65 and 85 years of age. The onset of symptoms occurs after 40 years of age in 96% of cases and between 45 and 65 years of age in 80% of cases. Early-onset AD is associated with a more rapid course and genetic predisposition compared with later-onset AD. AD is the fourth leading cause of death after 75 years of age. Fig. 24-3 graphically presents the increase in AD in the United States. The following clinical example demonstrates the behaviors associated with dementia.

CLINICAL EXAMPLE

Mr. B is a 73-year-old widower who has resided in a retirement home for 3 years. He chose to move to the retirement home after his wife's death even though his son encouraged him to live with him and his family. Mr. B stated that he did not want to burden his family and would be happier with others of his same age. He did well for the first 18 months. He was an active participant in social groups both in the home and in his church, which he continued to attend regularly. He also visited his son once a week and enjoyed seeing his grandchildren and puttering around his son's house.

Approximately 18 months ago Mr. B began to seem forgetful. He would ask the same question several times and on occasion prepared for church on a Friday or Saturday. He also became irritable and accused his son of not caring about him and of abandoning him in "that place." Mr. B spent many hours taking papers from his desk and studying them. When asked what he was doing,

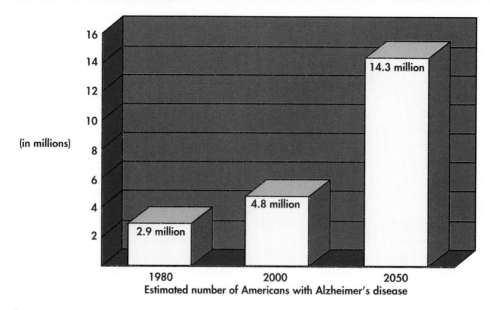

(in millions)

2.9 million

4.8 million

14.3 million

1980   2000   2050

Estimated number of Americans with Alzheimer's disease

Fig. 24-3 Alzheimer's disease in the United States. (From Evans D et al: Estimated prevalence of Alzheimer's disease in the United States, *The Millbank Quarterly,* 1990).

he would say, "Attending to my business." He began to withdraw from activities and make flimsy excuses to avoid playing his favorite card game, gin rummy. When persuaded to play, he usually quit in frustration because he could not remember which cards had been played. Mr. B was quite anxious at times. He seemed well oriented periodically and expressed great concern about the changes he was experiencing, wondering if he was "going crazy."

Because of the concern of the retirement home staff, Mr. B was scheduled for a complete physical examination by his family physician and for a psychiatric evaluation by the geriatric psychiatric nurse consultant who came to the retirement home each week. The physical examination revealed Mr. B to be in generally good health for a man his age. He had a mild hearing loss and slight prostatic hypertrophy. Hypertension had been diagnosed 10 years before this examination but was well controlled by diuretics. A neurological examination revealed normal reflexes, normal muscle strength, a slight intention tremor, normal responses to sensation, normal cranial nerves, and no disturbance of gait. An electroencephalogram was normal, as were the results of laboratory studies of blood and urine. Computed tomography studies of the brain revealed some atrophy of the cerebral cortex.

The mental status examination confirmed the deficits in cognitive functioning observed by the nursing home staff and Mr. B's son. He was oriented to person and place but stated the date as April 6, 1958 (the real date was January 21, 2001). He also thought the day of the week was Friday, and it was actually Tuesday. He correctly identified the season of the year as winter. Mr. B was able to give correctly his birth date, the date of his son's birth, and the year he began to work at his first job. He spoke at length and with great detail about his exploits as a young man. His vocabulary was excellent, as was his fund of general information. However, he could not repeat the names of three objects after 5 minutes and could not remember what he had eaten for lunch or the last name of the man who shared his room. He became distressed while trying to answer these questions. He was unable to remember the names of the two most recent presidents but could recite the names of the eight presidents preceding them.

Mr. B's judgment was somewhat impaired. When asked what he would do if he found a stamped, addressed, sealed envelope, he said he would "read it, then mail it." His ability for abstract thinking was slightly concretized, as was demonstrated by his difficulty in interpreting proverbs. His attention span and ability to concentrate were normal. His eye-hand coordination was disrupted, as demonstrated by his difficulty in copying simple figures. A hand tremor was evident both when he was drawing and when he was signing his name.

Mr. B's affect was appropriate to the content of the discussion both in quality and in quantity. He appeared depressed when talking about his memory loss but cheerful and proud when describing his grandchildren. No abrupt mood swings were noted. His flow of speech was of a normal rate and volume. The content of his speech was logical and coherent but became somewhat disjointed when he tried to remember and describe recent events.

As a result of the data gathered in the physical and mental status examinations, Mr. B was diagnosed as having dementia not otherwise specified. Over the next several months his condition continued to deteriorate gradually. He became increasingly forgetful and began to confabulate and fabricate stories. He was less conforming to social norms and needed to be reminded about hygiene and appropriate dress. He also became seductive with female residents and staff, making suggestive remarks and occasionally fondling someone. Visits to his son's home became impossible as his behavior deteriorated. His memory of the identity of family members was sometimes confused. He would misidentify his daughter-in-law as his wife and his grandson as his son. His conversation increasingly consisted of rambling reminiscences about his life in his youth. His son and health-care providers began to discuss plans to move him to the Assisted Living Program associated with his retirement home. Because he was surrounded by caring people, Mr. B continued to live with dignity and respect despite his progressively limited ability to communicate and to take care of himself.

Selected Nursing Diagnoses

- Impaired verbal communication related to cognitive impairment, as evidenced by recent memory loss and confabulation

Table **24-1**

Association of Areas of Brain Pathology to Behavioral Changes in Dementia		
Anatomical Structure	**Function**	**Dysfunction**
Occipital lobe	Visual processing	Blindness, loss of depth perception, color agnosia (lack of recognition), persistent after-images
Frontal lobe	Organization of words into fluent speech	Difficulty using "little words" (e.g., in, on, he, she, or); changes in personality, judgment, and behavior
Parietal lobe	Association area for integrating sensory input	Alexia (inability to read), agraphia (inability to write), neglect syndrome, inability to perceive pain, agnosia, apraxia, aphasia, visual-spatial disturbances, loss of executive functions, psychosis
Temporal lobe	Recognition and comprehension of sensory input, hearing, memory consolidation, association of memory, thought, perception, and emotion	Agnosia, apraxia, aphasia, visual-spatial disturbances, loss of executive functions, disorientation in space and time, psychosis, memory loss, misinterpretation of emotional events, misinterpretation of relationships
Limbic system	Emotions, storage of short-term memory, mood	Memory dysfunction, no affective dimension to memory, apathy, unstable affect, personality changes, poor learning ability, memory loss

Modified from Garand L et al: The biological basis of behavioral symptoms in dementia, *Issues Ment Health Nurs* 21:91, 2000.

- Impaired social interaction related to altered thought processes, as evidenced by a loss of conformity to social norms
- Self-care deficit (bathing/hygiene) related to cognitive impairment, as evidenced by a failure to perform personal hygiene activities without reminders
- Self-care deficit (dressing/grooming) related to cognitive impairment, as evidenced by a need for assistance in selecting appropriate clothing
- Altered thought processes related to cognitive impairment, as evidenced by disorientation and memory loss

The behaviors associated with dementia reflect the brain tissue alterations that are taking place (Table 24-1). Behavioral change occurs slowly in the early and late stages of AD and rapidly in the middle stage. Cognitive changes are related to the actions of stressors that interfere with the functioning of the cerebral cortex and the hippocampus. Other areas of the brain are also affected, which is one reason for performing a complete medical and neurological examination. Another reason is that although the condition may be irreversible, progression may be stopped or slowed by identifying the stressor and treating the underlying dysfunction. For example, the treatment of hypertension may prevent a further occurrence of small brain hemorrhages, which are a possible cause of dementia.

Depression in the elderly is often misinterpreted as dementia and therefore is not treated appropriately. **Pseudodementia** is a cognitive impairment secondary to a functional psychiatric disorder such as depression (lapses in memory and judgment, poor concentration, and seemingly diminished intellectual capacity); this condition is reversible with appropriate treatment of the depression (Draper, 1999). Aggression in patients with dementia is strongly linked to the presence of depressive symptoms; appropriate treatment of the depression may be a means of preventing and managing the physically aggressive behavior (Lyketsos et al, 1999). Be-

Elderly adults with depression are often misdiagnosed as having dementia, and the diagnosis of delirium is often missed. What nursing observations help to determine whether a patient's mental disorder is primarily affective or cognitive, and how would this affect treatment?

haviors related to delirium, dementia, and depression are compared in Table 24-2.

A common behavior related to dementia is disorientation. Time orientation is usually affected first, then place and, finally, person. This behavior can be distressing to the patient, who may be aware of this difficulty and embarrassed or frightened by it. This is particularly true if the person's mental acuity is fluctuating. In these instances the person is aware, during periods of lucidity, of the confusion and disorientation experienced at other times.

Memory loss is another prominent characteristic of dementia. There are five abstract concepts of memory: sensory memory (visual or auditory), primary memory (immediate or short-term), secondary memory (storage of information that one intends to retain), tertiary memory (long-term), and working memory (operates with primary memory and includes the simultaneous storage and processing of information over a short time). These abstract concepts of memory do not correlate with brain structures but can be predictably demonstrated with functional testing and are evaluated during a mental status examination. In the last clinical example, Mr. B had trouble remembering the three objects he heard 5 minutes before and what he had eaten for lunch, but he gave accurate dates for significant events earlier in his life. Most aging people dwell on the past, but people with recent memory loss have difficulty shifting to the present and at advanced stages may seem to live in the past. This is exemplified by Mr. B's misidentification of his grandson and his daughter-in-law.

Another behavior related to memory loss is confabulation. Confabulation is a confused person's tendency to make

Table **24-2**

	Delirium	**Depression**	**Dementia**
Onset	Rapid (hours to days)	Rapid (weeks to months)	Gradual (years)
Course	Wide fluctuations; may continue for weeks if cause is not found	May be self-limited or may become chronic without treatment	Chronic; slow but continuous decline
Level of consciousness	Fluctuates from hyperalert to difficult to arouse	Normal	Normal
Orientation	Patient is disoriented, confused	Patient may seem disoriented	Patient is disoriented, confused
Affect	Fluctuating	Sad, depressed, worried, guilty	Labile; apathetic in later stages
Attention	Always impaired	Difficulty concentrating; patient may check and recheck all actions	May be intact; patient may focus on one thing for long periods
Sleep	Always disturbed	Disturbed; excess sleeping or insomnia, especially early-morning waking	Usually normal
Behavior	Agitated, restless	Patient may be fatigued, apathetic; may occasionally be agitated	Patient may be agitated or apathetic; may wander
Speech	Sparse or rapid; patient may be incoherent	Flat, sparse, may have outbursts; understandable	Sparse or rapid; repetitive; patient may be incoherent
Memory	Impaired, especially for recent events	Varies day to day; slow recall; often short-term deficit	Impaired, especially for recent events
Cognition	Disordered reasoning	May seem impaired	Disordered reasoning and calculation
Thought content	Incoherent, confused, delusional, stereotyped	Negative, hypochondriac, thoughts of death, paranoid	Disorganized, rich in content, delusional, paranoid
Perception	Misinterpretations, illusions, hallucinations	Distorted; patient may have auditory hallucinations; negative interpretation of people and events	No change
Judgment	Poor	Poor	Poor; socially inappropriate behavior
Insight	May be present in lucid moments	May be impaired	Absent
Performance on mental status examinations	Poor but variable; improves during lucid moments and with recovery	Memory impaired; calculation, drawing, following directions usually not impaired; frequent "I don't know" answers	Consistently poor; progressively worsens; patient attempts to answer all questions

From Holt J: How to help confused patients, *Am J Nurs* 93:32, 1993.

up a response to a question when he or she cannot remember the answer. For instance, when Mr. B was asked whether he knew one of the female residents of the home, he replied, "Of course I know her. I used to play gin with her husband." Actually, the woman's husband had been dead for many years and Mr. B had never met him. This behavior should not be viewed as lying or as an attempt to deceive but rather as a way of trying to save face in an embarrassing situation. Mr. B is aware that he should know the answer to the question and gives an answer that seems reasonable, not entirely disbelieving it himself. It is not unlike the situation in which a person meets an acquaintance and cannot recall the other's name or where they met. The person acts as if these facts are remembered, hoping that the other will offer clues about his or her identity. Denial of memory loss may also be related to the effect of dementia on the cognitive abilities needed for awareness of the problem.

As AD progresses, patients often develop aphasia, apraxia, agnosia, and amnesia:

- Aphasia is difficulty finding the right word.

- Apraxia is an inability to perform familiar skilled activities.
- Agnosia is a difficulty in recognizing well-known objects, including people.
- Amnesia is significant memory impairment in the absence of clouded consciousness or other cognitive symptoms.

These behaviors are related to the effect of the illness on the temporal-parietal-occipital association cortex.

Vocabulary and general information may be less affected by dementia until its late stages and depends on when the information was learned. Facts learned early in life may be recalled well, whereas those learned recently may be quickly forgotten, as demonstrated by Mr. B's performance in listing the last 10 presidents.

Patients with dementia may have labile affective behavior, particularly if the limbic system has been affected by the disease process. There may also be some deterioration in social skills. Impulsive sexual advances may occur, which reflects decreased inhibition and impaired judgment as well as dete-

Table **24-3**

| **Disturbing Behaviors Characteristic of Dementia** | | |
Behavior	Description	Examples
Aggressive psychomotor behavior	An increase in gross motor movement that has the effect of harming or repelling another	Hitting, kicking, pushing, scratching, assaultiveness
Nonaggressive psychomotor behavior	An increase in gross motor movement that does not have an apparent negative effect on others but draws attention because of its repetitive nature	Restlessness, pacing, wandering
Verbally aggressive behavior	Vocalizations that have the effect of repelling others	Demanding, disruptive, manipulative behaviors; screaming; complaining; negativism
Passive behavior	A diminution of behavior, that is, a decrease in gross motor movement accompanied by apathy and a lack of interaction with the environment	Decreased activity, loss of interest, apathy, withdrawal
Functionally impaired behavior	Loss of ability to perform self-care, the expression of which may be aversive and burdensome	Vegetative behaviors, incontinence, poor personal hygiene

Modified from Kolanowski AM: Disturbing behaviors in demented elders: a concept synthesis, *Arch Psychiatr Nurs* 9:188, 1995.

rioration in the limbic system. Often this behavior is an attempt to establish interpersonal contact and is a way of asking for caring from others. It is also a way of reinforcing an important part of the person's identity—a part that becomes less secure as mental functioning declines. An alteration in sexual functioning associated with AD causes great concern for patients and their partners. Loss of erection ability is a common problem among men with AD, and it is uncertain whether this is physiological or psychological in origin. However, both the patient and the sexual partner can benefit from continued sexual intimacy.

Restlessness and agitation are other behaviors that occur with dementia. Extreme agitation may occur at night; this is sometimes called the sundowning syndrome. Sundowning syndrome probably results from tiredness at the end of the day combined with fewer orienting stimuli, such as planned activities, meals, and contact with people.

> *Based on your understanding of sundowning syndrome, describe nursing interventions that would decrease the severity of this problem in patients with dementia at home, in the hospital, or in the nursing home.*

Disorientation can result in fear and agitation. Behavior that becomes extremely agitated is called a **catastrophic reaction. It is a medical emergency.** The following precipitating factors related to catastrophic reactions have been identified (Swanson et al, 1993):

- A change in cognitive status that results in difficulty organizing and interpreting information; sensory or cognitive overload or misinterpretation of sensory stimuli may be contributing factors.
- Side effects of medications.
- Psychosocial factors that results in increased demands to remember, such as fatigue, changes in routines or caregivers, and disorienting stimuli.
- Environmental factors, including environmental changes, noise, and decreased light.

The term **confusion** is often used when referring to a person with cognitive impairment. Although widely accepted as nursing and medical jargon, this term has not been specifically defined. It is better to use specific terms when describing a patient's behavior. Five types of disturbing behaviors characteristic of dementia are summarized in Table 24-3.

Some people with maladaptive cognitive responses function at a level that is lower than would be expected on the basis of objective measurements of their impairment. This type of functional deficit is called **excess disability** (Beck et al, 1991). This problem adds to the frustration of the patient and to the burden placed on caregivers. Caregivers may contribute to the development of excess disability by performing activities for the patient rather than coaching and assisting when needed. Functional abilities are lost more rapidly as the patient becomes more passive in his or her self-care routines.

Patients with a cognitive impairment are often referred to a clinical psychologist for testing. This referral should be made for a specific purpose because the testing is time consuming, expensive, and tiring for the patient. Reasons for psychological testing include measuring the extent of the disability, identifying the stressors causing the disruption, understanding the dynamics of the problem, developing guidelines for therapeutic intervention, and obtaining a prognosis for recovery.

Predisposing Factors

Maladaptive cognitive responses are usually caused by a biological disruption in the functioning of the central nervous system (CNS). The CNS requires a continuous supply of nutrients, including oxygen, in order to function. Any interference with the provision of supplies to the brain or with the removal of waste products will cause functional disruptions in cognition.

Aging. In the United States, the number of people over 65 years of age is projected to reach almost 80 million by 2045; in 1990 there were just over 30 million in this age-group. Aging itself predisposes the person to maladaptive cognitive responses. It is now accepted that a loss of mental abilities is not automatically associated with aging. Although a cumulative degeneration of brain tissue *is* associated with aging, it is not extensive enough to be particularly noticeable in most people. As people age normally, their cognitive functions slow down but remain intact. If other stressors are added, the person may experience difficulty. Exposure to a toxic chemical or heavy metal, disease, or injury may result in maladaptive cognitive responses, which disrupts normal cognitive responses at any age. Advanced age, however, is one of the risk factors for dementia associated with AD.

Neurobiological. AD is the most prevalent cause of maladaptive cognitive responses. Intensive research has focused on identifying its causes, characteristics, and treatment. Investigators have found that characteristic alterations occur in brain tissue:

- Neuritic plaques, which consist of beta-amyloid (a starchlike protein), and remains of dying nerve cells. Plaques also contain altered glial cells.
- Neurofibrillary tangles, which are twisted clumps of protein fibers. Tangles contain a substance called tau protein, which seems to interfere with internal transport in neurons.

These phenomena are found in the cortex (cognition, judgment), the amygdala (emotion), and the hippocampus (consolidation of short-term memory). This is consistent with the emotional changes and short-term memory loss characteristic of AD (see Citing the Evidence). In addition, there is atrophy of the associational areas of the cortex.

Citing the Evidence on

Amygdalar Changes in Alzheimer's Disease

BACKGROUND: Everyday experience suggests that highly emotional events are the most memorable. Experimental work with animals and humans has demonstrated that the amygdala plays a crucial role in emotional memory (memory of events arousing strong emotions). This study measured damage to the amygdala and impaired memory of real-life emotional events in 36 patients with probable AD by asking them to recall specific events of a recent earthquake.

RESULTS: Emotional memory was correlated with amygdalar volume as measured by magnetic resonance imaging and regardless of generalized brain atrophy, cognitive impairments, or size of hippocampus.

IMPLICATIONS: The impairment of emotional event memory in patients with AD is related to the intensity of amygdalar damage. This result provides evidence of the involvement of the amygdala in emotional memory in humans.

More E et al: Amygdalar volume and emotional memory in Alzheimer's disease, *Am J Psychiatry* 156:216, 1999.

Alterations have also been noted in the neurotransmitter systems; in particular, there is a significant deficiency of acetylcholine. Table 24-4 lists the relationships between neurotransmitters and behavior in dementia. See Chapter 6 for additional information about the biology of AD.

Vascular dementia is much less common than dementia of the Alzheimer's type. Vascular dementia was previously called multiinfarct dementia because of the underlying cause—disruptions in the cerebral blood supply. Patients with hypertensive vascular disease may experience this type of dementia as a result of the sudden closure of the lumen of arterioles related to pressure changes. Atherosclerosis may lead to the formation of thrombi or emboli. In either case, the outcome is infarction of the brain tissue in the area supplied by the affected blood vessels. The resulting cognitive problems are related to the area of the brain involved. Another brain disorder that results in dementia is associated with the dementia complex of HIV/AIDS, which is discussed in Chapter 42.

Genetic. Genetic predisposition may also be a cause of maladaptive cognitive responses. An example of a hereditary degenerative brain disease is Huntington's chorea, which is inherited as an autosomal dominant trait. Progress has been made in identifying the genetic markers that indicate a potential for developing AD; the risk for development of AD is greater for relatives of people with the illness than it is for those with no family history (Li et al, 1995). The risk is greatest for relatives of people who developed AD before age 55. It also occurs more often in people with Down syndrome, another genetic brain disorder that affects normal growth and development and cognitive abilities.

Underlying Psychiatric and Medical Disorders. A degree of cognitive impairment may be found along with other maladaptive psychiatric responses. For instance, people with delusions may seem disoriented because they misidentify their location. People who have affective disorders may have short attention spans. Depression may also result in memory disorders, although it is often difficult to determine whether the problem is related to memory loss or to a lack of motivation. Patients with mental disorders resulting from a general medical condition can also exhibit symptoms of cognitive impairment. Such medical conditions include thyroid disease, adrenal dysfunction, hypoglycemia, brain lesions, and degenerative disorders. The predisposing factors related to maladaptive cognitive responses as a result of psychiatric and medical disorders are related to the underlying primary problem.

Precipitating Stressors

Associated with Delirium. Any major dysregulation in the balance of body functions can disrupt cognitive functioning. The underlying conditions most commonly associated with delirium can be categorized into five major groups: CNS disorders, metabolic disorders, cardiopulmonary disorders, systemic illnesses, and sensory deprivation or stimulation (Table 24-5). The psychiatric nurse should be alert for possible causes of delirium when evaluating each patient with maladaptive cognitive responses and

Table **24-4**

Relationship Between Neurotransmitter and Behavior in Dementia

Neurotransmitter System/ Neurotransmitter	Anatomical Origin	Function	Dysfunction and Behavior
Cholinergic system/ acetylcholine (Ach)	Synthesized by an enzyme, choline acetyltransferase, in the nucleus basalis of Meynert in the basal forebrain	Promotes hippocampal and cerebral cortex function; necessary for selective attention, learning, memory, and the sleep-wake cycle	Diminished levels of Ach lead to amnesia, agitation, and psychotic symptoms Possible direct relationship to severity of disease Imbalance in the DA system
Noradrenergic system/norepinephrine (NE)	The locus ceruleus in the rostral pons of the brainstem	Modulates mood and stress response; produces psychotic symptoms	Increased NE: hypervigilance, decreased appetite, insomnia, anxiety, agitation, psychosis Decreased NE: depressed mood Imbalance in the 5HT system
Serotonergic system/serotonin (5HT)	The raphe nuclei in the brainstem	Regulates body temperature, cardiovascular system, respiratory system, sleep/alertness, mood, aggression, sensory perception, sexual behavior, and feeding behavior	Decreased 5HT: anxiety, agitation, psychomotor activity, insomnia, psychosis, depressed mood, possibly suicidal behavior Imbalance in the NE system
Dopaminergic system/dopamine (DA)	The substantia nigra in the brainstem, with projections directly communicating with the frontal lobe, limbic system, and motor areas	Regulates emotional responses (limbic system), executive functions (frontal lobes), and complex movements (motor striatum)	Decreased DA: difficulty initiating movement, rigidity, postural abnormalities, parkinsonian tremor (akinesia or bradykinesia), blunted affect, apathy Imbalance in the Ach system

Modified from Garand L et al: The biological basis of behavioral symptoms in dementia, *Issues Ment Health Nurs* 21:91, 2000.

Table **24-5**

Underlying Conditions Commonly Associated with Delirium

Type	Disorder
Central nervous system disorder	Head trauma, seizures, post-ictal state, vascular disease (e.g., hypertensive encephalopathy), degenerative disease, tumor, brain abscess, meningitis, encephalitis
Metabolic disorder	Renal failure, hepatic failure, anemia, hypoxia, hypoglycemia, vitamin deficiency (thiamine, folate, B_{12}, nicotinic acid), endocrinopathy, fluid or electrolyte imbalance, acid-base imbalance, low albumin, malnutrition
Cardiopulmonary disorder	Myocardial infarction, congestive heart failure, cardiac arrhythmia, shock, respiratory failure, severe hypertension
Systemic illness	Substance intoxication or withdrawal (e.g., alcohol, antidepressants, antipsychotics, anesthetics, benzodiazepines, opiates, anticholinergics, nonsteroidal antiinflammatory drugs [NSAIDs], corticosteroids), toxins (insecticides, carbon monoxide, fuel, paint), infections (urinary tract, pneumonia, HIV, septicemia), neoplasm (primary and metastatic tumors), severe trauma (burns, surgery, and fractures, especially hip), sensory deprivation, temperature dysregulation, postoperative state
Sensory deprivation or stimulation	Sensory deprivation (underload), sensory stimulation (overload)

Modified from American Psychiatric Association: Practice guideline for the treatment of patients with delirium, *Am J Psychiatry* 156(5 suppl):1, 1999.

when assessing a change of cognitive status from a previous level of functioning for each patient.

Central nervous system disorder. Any major assault on the brain is likely to disrupt cognitive functioning. Severe head trauma and other brain diseases and infections such as meningitis and encephalitis cause changes in the normal function of the brain. When these disorders occur in areas of the brain responsible for cognitive function, the patient exhibits symptoms that are indicative of maladaptive cognitive responses.

Metabolic disorder. Metabolic disorders often affect mental functioning, especially when they are severe or of long duration. Endocrine malfunctioning, whether it involves underproduction or overproduction of hormones, can adversely affect cognition. For example, thyroid hormone greatly influences mental alertness. People with hypothyroidism are sluggish and dysfunctional in their thinking. Those with severe hypothyroidism (myxedema) may develop psychotic behavior characterized by delusional thinking. Other endocrine disorders that may cause cognitive disruptions include hypoglycemia, hypopituitarism, and adrenal disease.

Hypoxia can result in cognitive dysfunction because the brain is not getting its normal oxygen supplies. Hypoxia resulting from anemia may be insidious in onset. Possible stressors include aspirin ingestion that results in occult bleeding; other occult blood loss; or deficiencies of iron, folic acid, or vitamin B_{12}. Other causes of hypoxia can include dehydration, hyperthermia, hypothermia, or increased intracranial pressure resulting from a tumor, subdural hematoma, or normal pressure hydrocephalus.

Nutrition in general can affect cognitive functioning. Malnutrition increases a person's risk of organic brain disease and is often a problem in the elderly, who may lack the physical or financial resources needed for an adequate diet. Young people with anorexia nervosa or bulimia nervosa are also at risk for cognitive impairment. Vitamin B–complex deficiency, particularly thiamine, is believed to cause the Wernicke-Korsakoff syndrome found in some chronic alcoholics. A prominent feature of this syndrome is a severe deficit in cognitive functioning.

> *Based on a review of neurophysiology, compare the effects of hypoxia, hypothyroidism, and hypoglycemia on cerebral functioning.*

Cardiopulmonary disorder. Heart disease that compromises the flow of blood to the brain or to the lungs to exchange carbon dioxide for oxygen is likely to cause maladaptive cognitive responses. Respiratory illnesses such as chronic obstructive lung disease, acute respiratory infection, and cardiac conditions such as congestive heart failure, atherosclerosis, hypotension, and hypertension are common problems and may be underlying causes of changes in cognitive function.

Systemic illness. Substances such as alcohol and drugs, even many drugs commonly used in the treatment of psychiatric disorders, can cause changes in sensorium during ingestion. Some substances may cause these changes during withdrawal. Prescription and over-the-counter drugs can be potential toxic stressors. A thorough assessment of drug use is critical with all patients. It is especially critical with elderly patients because of their increased sensitivity to drugs associated with normal aging and because confusion can lead to difficulty in following the directions for taking drugs. Interactions between drugs or between drugs and other substances, particularly alcohol, may also lead to disruptions in cognitive functioning.

Toxic and infectious agents may also result in the behavior typical of maladaptive cognitive responses. Toxins may originate within the patient or in the external environment. An example of an internally generated toxin is the elevated blood level of urea found in a patient with renal failure. Environmental toxins include various poisonous substances, such as toxic wastes and animal venoms. Infections in any body system may also impair the CNS if body temperature is extremely elevated. People who are infected with HIV often develop an organic brain syndrome called AIDS dementia complex.

Sensory deprivation or stimulation. Sensory deprivation or sensory overload can result in cognitive dysfunction. People who are placed in environments with minimal stimuli seem to develop internally produced stimuli in the form of hallucinations. In contrast, the constant light and activity in intensive care units (ICUs) can lead to confusion, delusions, and hallucinations; this is sometimes called ICU psychosis. It is difficult to determine the extent to which the cognitive impairment results from the sensory experience as opposed to other concurrent stressors, such as the introduction of multiple drugs into the system, the result of massive assaults on physical integrity, and changes in the normal sleep cycle imposed upon ICU patients.

> *Sensory overload or sensory deprivation may lead to maladaptive cognitive responses. In what way is this information significant in planning the nursing care of a patient who is confined to a seclusion room on a psychiatric unit?*

Associated with Dementia. The underlying conditions most commonly associated with dementia are the subject of much research and conjecture. The most common underlying conditions associated with dementia across the life span are listed in Table 24-6. In addition to age, family history of AD, and Down syndrome, apolipoprotein E (APOE), a serum lipoprotein involved in the transport of cholesterol, is implicated in the formation of neuritic plaques, which in turn cause the neuronal and synaptic loss seen in AD. Different studies have shown varying levels of association between the different APOE genotypes and either a risk for AD (APOE e4) or protection from AD (APOE e2 or e3) (Desai & Grossberg, 1999). Factors that may precede AD are depression, mild cognitive impairment, hippocampal atrophy, and delayed paragraph recall on neurocognitive testing. Table 24-7 lists the risk factors and proposed protective factors for AD.

Appraisal of Stressors

Unfortunately, the specific stressor related to cognitive impairment often cannot be identified. Understanding the biochemical process of the brain and the response of the brain and nervous tissue to stressors is the subject of intense research. As knowledge advances, specific biological components may be identified as part of the etiology of all psychiatric disorders. For example, severe deficiency in the neurotransmitter acetylcholine has been observed in patients with AD. It is not known whether this is a cause or effect of the illness, but psychopharmacologic treatment approaches include drugs designed to preserve this neurotransmitter in the brain.

In general, when assessing maladaptive cognitive responses, physiological causes are ruled out first, and then psychosocial stressors are considered. Even when physiological factors are present, psychosocial stress may further compromise the person's thought process; therefore appraisal of this stressor is critically important. Each patient should receive a complete assessment so that nursing care can be planned in a competent and thorough manner.

Coping Resources

Individual and interpersonal resources are important to the person who is attempting to cope with maladaptive cognitive responses. A person who has a varied repertoire of skills may be able to substitute for functional losses. For instance, it has been noted that people with AD who have attained higher levels of education and who have remained active and involved in their lives deteriorate less rapidly than those who have less education and have remained sedentary and socially isolated.

Interpersonal resources are extremely important to the person with a cognitive impairment. Family members and friends often have a calming influence on the agitated person. They can provide the nurse with information about the person's usual lifestyle and ensure that the environment contains familiar objects. Caregivers also need coping resources, which can often be found by attending self-help groups such as the Alzheimer's Disease and Related Disorders Association. The importance of family involvement is illustrated in A Family Speaks.

Coping Mechanisms

How a person copes with maladaptive cognitive responses is greatly influenced by past experience. A person who has

A Family Speaks

My mother, Margaret, is 78 years old and has been in a nursing home for the past 3 years. She is diagnosed with dementia. There are days when she does not recognize me and there are some days when she does, but her mood may not be very pleasant. Many days she just sits in her chair and responds to nothing. Often she cannot feed herself or express her needs. I visit her nearly every day.

The nurses in the home are my only link to my mother. The doctor visits weekly but rarely communicates with me unless there is an emergency. The nurses give me information about my mother's condition and listen to me when I have concerns about her. In the beginning the nurses were indifferent to me, and I worried that they were the same with my mother. I brought pictures of the family to the nursing home and shared them with the nurses. These pictures allowed the nurses to see a person instead of a patient. They began to see that her life had been very different, and this helped them to treat her with more respect and dignity. Now I really depend on the nurses to let me know how my mother is doing from day to day.

Table 24-6

Underlying Conditions Commonly Associated with Dementia Across the Life Span	
Elderly	**Degenerative brain disorders:** Alzheimer's disease, frontotemporal dementia, and dementia with Lewy bodies, Parkinson's disease, Huntington's disease, Pick's disease, and late-onset extrapyramidal symptoms **Cerebrovascular dementia:** multiinfact dementia, Binswanger's disease, cerebral hemorrhage **Toxic-metabolic disturbances:** iatrogenic drug-induced dementia, alcoholism, poisons, inhalants, heavy metals, cardiopulmonary disease, B_{12} deficiency, hypothyroidism **Central nervous system infections:** chronic meningitis, neurosyphilis, Creutzfeldt-Jacob disease, AIDS, kuru, subacute sclerosing panencephalitis **Miscellaneous:** traumatic brain injury, brain tumors, hydrocephalus, depression, thyroid disease
Adolescents	Huntington's disease (juvenile type), Wilson's disease (hepatolenticular degeneration), subacute sclerosing panencephalitis, AIDS, substance abuse (especially inhalants), head trauma
Children	Head trauma (including child abuse), subacute sclerosing panencephalitis, AIDS

Modified from Kay J, Tasman A: Dementia, delirium, and cognitive disorders. In Kay J, Lieberman JA, Tasman A: *Psychiatry: behavioral science and clinical essentials*, Philadelphia, 2000, WB Saunders.

Table 24-7

Risks and Proposed Protective Factors for Alzheimer's Disease			
RISK FACTORS			**PROTECTIVE FACTORS**
Definitive	Probable	Possible	Proposed
Age Family history APOE e4 Down's syndrome	Female gender Low level of education	Head injury with loss of consciousness Vascular brain lesions Aluminum Insulin-dependent diabetes mellitus Solvent exposure Electromagnetic exposure Elevated thyrotropin Hypertension Myocardial infarction	Estrogen APOE e2 and e3 Higher education Antiinflammatory medications Vitamin E Smoking Lifestyle issues: social, physical, and intellectual activity

Modified from American Psychiatric Association: Practice guideline for the treatment of patients with delirium, *Am J Psychiatry* 156(5 suppl):1, 1999.

developed many effective coping mechanisms is better able to handle the onset of a cognitive problem than one who has not.

Because the basic behavioral disruption in delirium is altered awareness (which reflects the severe biological disturbance in the brain), psychological coping mechanisms are not generally used. Therefore the nurse must protect the patient from harm and provide a substitute for the patient's coping mechanisms by constantly reorienting him or her and reinforcing reality during the treatment process.

The patient's response to the onset of dementia often mirrors his or her basic personality. For instance, a person who has usually reacted to stress with anger toward other people and the environment will probably react similarly when limitations in intellectual abilities occur. A person who is more apt to direct anger inward and become depressed will be more likely to respond with depressive behaviors. A person who has relied on a mechanism such as intellectualization will be more threatened by the loss of intellectual ability than a person who has used a mechanism such as reaction formation.

One characteristic of early dementia is the mechanism of denial. Those with dementia attempt to pursue their usual daily routine and make light of memory lapses. They may be able to use some environmental resources to help them cope. For instance, a businessman who is experiencing difficulty with recent memory might ask his secretary to remind him of all his appointments and to provide him with the names of the people with whom he is meeting and the meeting's purpose. As the impairment progresses, the person may become very resistant to any limitations on independence. For example, the family of a woman with AD might become very concerned about her ability to continue to drive a car safely. She probably would be very reluctant to give up her driver's license and would deny having any problem.

Regression is often used to cope with advanced dementia and may be caused in part by a deterioration in mental function. It probably also results from the behavioral manifestations of dementia, which cause the patient to become more dependent on others for the fulfillment of basic needs such as nutrition and hygiene. Encouraging patients to perform self-care also supports their use of healthier coping mechanisms.

As cognitive ability decreases, efforts to cope become more obvious. For instance, a family member may complain that a relative has "always been irritable but is now belligerent when he doesn't get his way." In other cases the person's behavior may be perceived as a personality change. Behaviors that are probably attempts to cope with a loss of cognitive ability include suspiciousness, hostility, joking, depression, seductiveness, and withdrawal. Because it is threatening to admit that a close relative has dementia, family members may focus on the coping mechanism instead of on the real problem, thus participating in the denial of the underlying cognitive impairment.

NURSING DIAGNOSIS

The nursing diagnosis of the patient with cognitive impairment should consider both the possible underlying stressors and the patient behaviors. Fig. 24-4 summarizes the Stuart Stress Adaptation Model related to maladaptive cognitive responses.

Most cognitive impairment disorders are physiological in origin. Therefore the nurse should consider both the patient's physical needs and the psychosocial behavioral problems. For example, a delirious patient may be reacting to an infection or a drug overdose. The identified problem and all its effects should be reflected in a complete nursing diagnosis. Many people with dementia are also elderly; they experience many effects of the aging process in addition to impaired cognitive functioning. A thorough nursing diagnosis reflects all of these influences on the patient's behavior. In addition, the nature of a cognitive impairment may inhibit the patient's ability to participate in the care-planning process. The nurse should rely on observational skills and on the input of significant others to arrive at an accurate, relevant diagnosis. If the nursing diagnosis cannot be validated with the patient, a family member familiar with his or her behavioral patterns should be involved. The primary NANDA nursing diagnosis related to maladaptive cognitive response is **altered thought processes**. The range of common NANDA nursing diagnoses and the *DSM–IV–TR* psychiatric diagnoses are included in the Medical and Nursing Diagnoses box on p. 474. The primary NANDA diagnoses and examples of complete nursing diagnoses are presented in the Detailed Diagnoses box on p. 475.

OUTCOME IDENTIFICATION

The expected outcome related to the patient who has maladaptive cognitive responses is the following:

The patient will achieve optimum cognitive functioning.

Goals may be directed toward an improved ability to process information (if this is realistic) or toward optimum use of the abilities the patient retains (if the impairment is irreversible). For example, a goal for a patient who is disoriented because of drug withdrawal might be to verbalize the complete date within 3 days.

In contrast, a goal for a patient who is disoriented because of chronic alcoholism and who is not in withdrawal might be to find his or her own bed every night without assistance after 1 month.

The second patient may never be able to remember the exact date, but he or she may not need that information if he or she will be functioning in a protected setting. The first patient, however, will need that information. In addition, the nurse can use the assessment of the patient's orientation to time to assess the current status of mental functioning.

Goals should be realistic to avoid discouragement. If the second patient is required to learn the date, frequent confrontation with deteriorated cognitive skills might result and lead to frustration, higher anxiety, and possibly less effective coping.

If an identified stressor is causing the patient's behavioral disruption, goals that focus on that stressor should also be developed. For instance, if a person is delirious because of a fever, a goal might state that the patient's temperature will be maintained below 100° F (37.8° C).

When the cause of the elevated temperature is identified, appropriate goals are written to address that problem. For example, dehydration may be a stressor that contributes to an elevated temperature. A related nursing goal would be

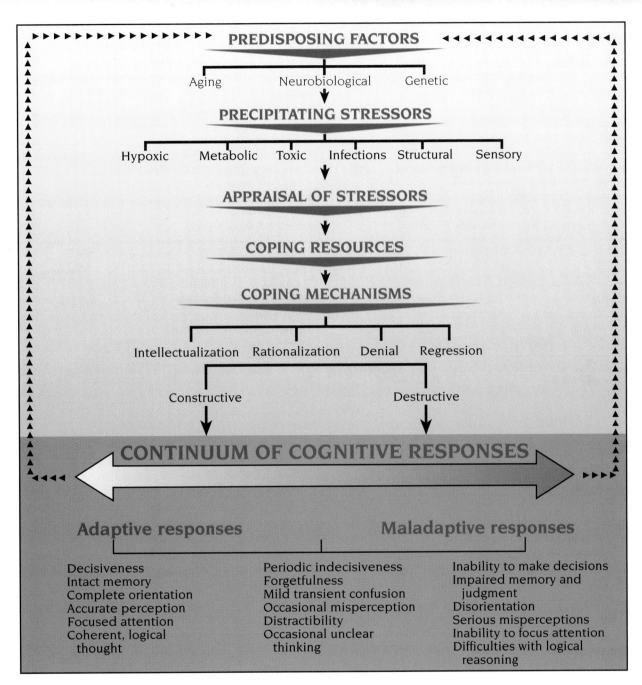

Fig. 24-4 The Stuart Stress Adaptation Model related to cognitive responses.

that the patient's fluid intake is at least 3000 ml in each 24-hour period. As the various elements of the patient's behavior are explored and documented, nursing goals must be updated and modified, new goals must be added, and accomplished goals must be deleted.

PLANNING

The nursing care plan for a patient with maladaptive cognitive responses must address all of his or her biopsychosocial needs. In most cases, the patient either has or is at risk for physiological problems in addition to the psychosocial disruption. Life-threatening problems always receive the highest priority for nursing intervention. Protection of safety is almost always a concern with these patients.

Mental health education related to patients with impaired cognition is often directed toward the family, who are often the caregivers for these patients (see Citing the Evidence on p. 476). The nurse can help caregivers cope with this difficult and demanding responsibility by providing them with information about problematic behaviors and problem solving. A Family Education Plan for the families of cognitively impaired people is presented on p. 476. Another strategy to facilitate family involvement in caring for individuals with dementia is to develop a formal protocol. This approach details a negotiated partnership with staff caregivers and family and includes education about caregiving, negotiation of a partnership agreement, and evaluation and renegotiation of the partnership as needed (Kelley et al, 2000).

Medical and Nursing Diagnoses *related to* **Maladaptive Cognitive Responses**

RELATED MEDICAL DIAGNOSES *(DSM–IV–TR)**	RELATED NURSING DIAGNOSES (NANDA)†
Delirium due to a general medical condition	Anxiety
Substance-induced delirium	Communication, impaired verbal
Delirium due to multiple etiologies	Coping, ineffective family: compromised
Dementia of the Alzheimer's type	Coping, ineffective individual
Vascular dementia	Health maintenance, altered
Dementia due to other general medical conditions	Home maintenance management, impaired
Substance-induced persisting dementia	Injury, risk for
Dementia due to multiple etiologies	Mobility, impaired physical
Amnestic disorder due to a general medical condition	Role performance, altered
Substance-induced persisting amnestic disorder	Self-care deficit (specify)
	Bathing/hygiene, feeding, dressing/grooming, toileting
	Sensory-perceptual alterations (specify)
	Visual, auditory, kinesthetic, gustatory, tactile, olfactory
	Sleep pattern disturbance
	Social interaction, impaired
	Social isolation
	Thought processes, altered‡
	Trauma, risk for

*Reprinted with permission from the *Diagnostic and statistical manual of mental disorders*, Fourth Edition, Text Revision. Copyright 2000. American Psychiatric Association.

†From North American Nursing Diagnosis Association: *NANDA nursing diagnoses: definitions and classifications 1999-2000*, Philadelphia, 1999, The Association.

‡Primary nursing diagnosis for maladaptive cognitive responses.

IMPLEMENTATION

Intervening in Delirium

Physiological Needs. Highest priority is given to nursing interventions that will maintain life. If the patient is too disoriented or agitated to attend to his or her basic physiological needs, nursing care should be planned to meet these needs. Nutrition and fluid balance may be maintained by intravenous therapy. If the patient is very agitated or restless, restraint may be necessary to keep the intravenous line open. However, restraints can increase agitation and anxiety and thus should be used only when absolutely necessary. A disoriented patient should never be restrained and left alone.

Sleep deprivation may be another problem. Intervention is important because a lack of sleep can add to an already existing cognitive dysfunction. Because sedative medications may complicate attempts to identify the original stressor, the physician or advanced practice nurse medication prescriber may be reluctant to prescribe a sedative. Nursing measures such as a back rub, a glass of warm milk, and gentle but persistent orientation so that patients are continually reminded of their surroundings are low-tech interventions that decrease the incidence of delirium in elderly patients (Inouye, 1999). The presence of a family member is also reassuring to the patient. Disoriented patients need to be in a lighted room. Shadows may be misinterpreted and add to the patient's fear. Environmental objects also help the patient orient to place and person.

Do you think it is safer and more effective to use physical (mechanical) restraints than to use chemical restraints (medication) with an agitated, delirious patient?

Hallucinations. Disoriented patients may need to be protected from hurting themselves or others, particularly when they are having hallucinations. Visual hallucinations of delirium are often very frightening. Patients may try to run away or even jump out a window. Patients' rooms must be safe, with security screens and a minimum of extra furniture or other objects that might cause harm. These patients often require one-on-one nursing observation and repetitive verbal reorientation.

It is tempting to help a frightened patient eliminate the hallucinated object. For instance, the patient might request help in brushing the bugs off the sheets. Agreeing to do this is not usually therapeutic. By participating in this activity, the nurse is nonverbally communicating to the patient that the hallucinated objects are real. This can make the patient even more frightened. In reality the hallucinations will continue until the underlying stressor is eliminated. A more appropriate response is to orient the patient continually to the reality of being sick and hospitalized. In addition, the patient can be assured that the nursing and medical staff are there to help and to keep the patient safe. Family members should also be helped to respond in a supportive way.

Communication. Patients with maladaptive cognitive responses need clear messages and instructions. Choices should be kept to a minimum. Independent decision making can be introduced into the plan of nursing care as the patient improves. Decisions related to orientation may be especially difficult for the patient. Responding appropriately to the question "What time would you like to take your bath?" requires knowledge of the present time and some idea of the usual routine.

Detailed Diagnoses *related to* **Maladaptive Cognitive Responses**

NANDA DIAGNOSIS STEM	EXAMPLES OF COMPLETE DIAGNOSIS
Altered thought processes	Altered thought processes related to severe dehydration, as evidenced by hypervigilance, distractibility, visual hallucinations, and disorientation to time, place, and person
	Altered thought processes related to barbiturate ingestion, as evidenced by altered sleep patterns, delusions, disorientation to time and place, and decreased ability to grasp ideas
	Altered thought processes related to brain disorder, as evidenced by inaccurate interpretation of environment, deficit in recent memory, impaired ability to reason, and confabulation

DSM–IV–TR DIAGNOSIS	ESSENTIAL FEATURES*
Delirium (general criteria) (to be applied to all other categories of delirium)	Disturbed consciousness accompanied by a cognitive change that cannot be accounted for by dementia
	Impaired ability to focus, sustain, or shift attention
	Cognitive changes that include impaired recent memory, disorientation to time or place, language disturbance, or perceptual disturbance
	Develops over a short time; tends to fluctuate during the course of a day
Delirium due to a general medical condition	Evidence that the cognitive disturbance is the direct result of a general medical condition
Substance-induced delirium	Evidence of substance intoxication or withdrawal, medication side effects, or toxin exposure judged to be related to the delirium
Delirium due to multiple etiologies	Evidence of multiple causes for the delirium
Dementia (general criteria) (to be applied to all other	Development of multiple cognitive deficits, including memory impairment and at least one of the following: aphasia, apraxia, agnosia, or disturbed executive functioning (ability to think abstractly categories of dementia) and plan, initiate, sequence, monitor, and stop complex behavior)
	Must cause severe impairment in social or occupational functioning
Dementia of the Alzheimer's type	Gradual onset with continuing cognitive decline; all other causes of dementia must be ruled out
Vascular dementia	Focal neurological signs and symptoms or laboratory evidence of cerebrovascular disease that are judged to be related to the dementia
Dementia due to other general medical conditions	Evidence that the general medical condition (such as HIV, traumatic brain injury, Parkinson's disease, Huntington's disease, Pick's disease, Creutzfeldt-Jakob disease, normal-pressure hydrocephalus, hypothyroidism, brain tumor, vitamin B_{12} deficiency) is etiologically related to the dementia
Substance-induced persisting dementia	Deficits do not occur exclusively during delirium and persist beyond the usual duration of substance intoxication or withdrawal
	Evidence that the deficits are related to persisting effects of substance use (e.g., drug of abuse, medication)
Dementia due to multiple etiologies	Evidence that the dementia has more than one etiology
Amnestic disorder (general criteria)	Development of memory disorder, as evidenced by impaired ability to learn new information or to recall previously learned information
	Disturbance causes significant impairment in social or occupational functioning and represents a significant decline from a previous level of functioning
	Does not occur exclusively during the course of delirium or dementia
Amnestic disorder due to a general medical condition	Evidence that the disturbance is directly related to a general medical condition (including physical trauma)
Substance-induced persisting amnestic disorder	Evidence that the memory disturbance is etiologically related to the persisting effects of substance use (e.g., drug of abuse, medication)

*Reprinted with permission from the *Diagnostic and statistical manual of mental disorders*, Fourth Edition, Text Revision. Copyright 2000. American Psychiatric Association.

Simple, direct statements are reassuring and are most likely to result in an appropriate response. Orienting phrases such as "here at the hospital" or "now that it's June" can be woven into a conversation. Patients who have difficulty dressing or feeding themselves need matter-of-fact, specific directions. Confused patients need to be fed or dressed in a manner that allows them to maintain their dignity. Families can often help with this. Helping the patient can lessen the family's anxiety, and the patient may be reassured by the family's physical closeness and concern.

Citing the Evidence on

Caregiving

BACKGROUND: Caregivers of persons with dementia have stressful and complex lives. This study sought to describe the experience of control as perceived by family caregivers of relatives with dementia in order to determine how caregivers manage caregiving at home, how they evaluate their resources, and how their perception of "control" affects their coping.

RESULTS: The experience of control was directly related to how caregivers coped with their caregiving situations. Dimensions of control were either maintaining control (positive identification of resources, anticipating the future, and asking for help) or lacking control (negative identification of resources, failure to anticipate the future); these were related to caregivers beliefs about caregiving. How caregivers experienced control seemed directly related to how they perceived they coped in the caregiving situation.

IMPLICATIONS: The results of this study can help nurses intervene more effectively with family caregivers by recognizing how caregivers manage or cope in the caregiving situation and determining whether they need assistance to continue to provide care. The proposed model is a starting point for further research on control and coping, and it also provides direction for practice.

Szabo V, Stang V: Experiencing control in caregiving, *Image J Nurs Sch* 31:71, 1999.

Patient Education. While recovering, patients may be concerned about what happened to them. The health-care team needs to discuss this issue and arrive at a conclusion about the disruption in functioning that occurred. This should then be explained to patients and their families. The nurse should assess the patient's understanding of the nature of the problem, the stressors that were involved, any ongoing therapy that is required, and preventive measures that will decrease the probability of a recurrence. Teaching may need to be repeated several times before the patient can cope with personal feelings and understand the information. Written materials can be helpful to patients who are having residual problems processing information. The teaching should include at least one responsible family member so that the information will be reinforced when the patient goes home.

A community health nursing referral may be helpful if the patient is discharged from the hospital with a residual deficit in cognitive functioning. The community health nurse can then continue to implement the nursing care plan and validate the patient's compliance with the treatment plan.

Intervening in Dementia

Nursing care of the patient with dementia is similar in some respects to that of the patient with delirium. In dementia, the stressors involved usually do not present an immediate threat to life; thus highest priority is given to nursing care that will help the patient to maintain an optimum level of functioning. This will differ for each patient. An attitude of hopelessness often evolves in those who work with chronically ill people. This can lead to stereotyping and a decreased ability to see and appreciate the uniqueness of each person. It is challenging to search for this uniqueness and rewarding to find it. Individualized nursing care is probably most

 FAMILY EDUCATION PLAN *Helping a Family with a Cognitively Impaired Member*

CONTENT	INSTRUCTIONAL ACTIVITIES	EVALUATION
Explain possible causes of maladaptive cognitive responses.	Describe predisposing factors and precipitating stressors that may lead to impaired cognition; provide printed reference materials.	The family identifies possible causes of the patient's disorder.
Define and describe orientation to time, place, and person.	Define the three spheres of orientation; role play interpersonal responses to disorientation.	The family identifies disorientation and provides reorientation.
Relate level of cognitive functioning to ability to communicate.	Describe the impact of maladaptive cognitive responses on communication; demonstrate effective communication techniques; videotape and discuss return demonstration.	The family adjusts communication approaches to the patient's ability to interact.
Describe effect of maladaptive cognitive responses on self-care behaviors.	Describe the usual progression of the gain or loss of self-care ability related to the nature of the disorder; encourage the family to help in providing care to patient; provide written instructional materials.	The family helps with activities of daily living as required by the patient's level of biopsychosocial functioning.
Refer to community resources.	Provide a list of community resources; arrange to meet with staff members of selected community programs; visit meetings of selected programs and self-help groups.	The family describes various programs that provide services relevant to the patient's and family's needs and contacts appropriate programs or self-help groups when needed.

important for those who will be institutionalized for a long time. Empirically validated treatments for dementia are summarized in Table 24-8.

Nursing approaches should address the patient's need for social interaction. Interventions that may be helpful include discussion groups with structured agendas, exercise groups to promote physical activity, reality orientation groups, sensory stimulation, and parties that are appropriate to the time of year or that recognize important events such as birthdays. Arranging for visits from community volunteer groups provides stimulation as well as an opportunity to socialize. Referral to other members of the treatment team, especially the occupational, recreational, art, music, and dance therapists, may be indicated.

Pharmacological Approaches. The goal of AD research is to identify agents that prevent the occurrence, defer the onset, slow the progression, or improve the symptoms of disease (Cummings & Jeste, 1999). Pharmacological approaches to the treatment of dementia are related to theories about the cause of the disorder. Cholinesterase inhibitors improve cognitive symptoms or temporarily reduce the rate of cognitive decline (Cummings, 2000). Tacrine (Cognex) was the first of several cholinesterase inhibitors to receive approval as a specific treatment for the cognitive symptoms of this disorder. In dosages up to 160 mg/day, it has been found to delay the progression of AD for a time in most patients. It maximizes the function of cholinergic neurons by inhibiting the enzyme acetylcholinesterase; such inhibition prevents the metabolism of acetylcholine, the neurotransmitter that is associated with memory and learning and is found to be lower than normal in AD. Donepezil (Aricept) is also an acetylcholinesterase inhibitor for the treatment of mild to moderate AD. Like tacrine, donepezil allows a greater concentration of acetylcholine in the brain, thereby improving cholinergic function.

Much current research is focused on identifying pharmacological agents that can protect neurons from the progressive death caused by AD. Brain functions involving glutamate, calcium, and free radicals are being targeted in this research. Other brain research related to cognitive disorders involves investigating the role of phospholipid metabolism and the usefulness of antiinflammatory drugs, nerve growth factor, and estrogen (Kumar et al, 1996). Some authorities recommend the use of small amounts of antipsychotic medications, such as phenothiazines and butyrophenones, to help patients rest; barbiturate sedatives may cause paradoxical agitation in patients with organic brain syndromes. The use of the atypical antipsychotic drugs, such as risperidone (Risperdal), has been shown to decrease the agitation in patients with dementia (Masand, 2000).

Medications must be used with care when treating persons with dementia. Elderly people are very sensitive to medications and combinations of medications. Drugs with anticholinergic effects and benzodiazepines (which interfere with learning) should be avoided. Table 24-9 lists the categories of pharmacological treatment options for symptoms of AD.

Orientation. Disorientation is a common problem of people with cognitive impairment. Nursing interventions should help the patient function in the environment. In an institution it is helpful to mark patient rooms with large, clearly printed signs indicating the occupant's name. This also reminds forgetful people of others' names. Everyone needs a personal space. A favorite rocking chair, a handmade afghan, or a family picture gives the patient a sense of identity and helps to identify a personal area of the institution. Personal possessions can also be orienting devices. A light in the room at night helps the patient remain oriented and decreases nighttime agitation. Clocks with large faces help with orientation to time. A digital clock is not recommended because the confused person may not identify it as a clock. Calendars with large writing and a separate page for each day also help with time orientation. Newspapers provide other orienting stimuli and help to stimulate interest in current events. An institutional newspaper provides a creative outlet

---

Table **24-8**

Empirically Validated Treatments in Dementia

The efficacy of dihydroergotoxine mesylate (Hydergine), one of two drugs currently approved by the FDA for alleviation of the cognitive deterioration of dementia, remains in question.

Acetylcholinesterase inhibitors (tacrine and donepezil) are the other FDA-approved drugs for this disorder; they have shown modest clinically significant benefits.

From Nathan P, Gorman J: *A guide to treatments that work,* New York, 1998, Oxford University Press.

Table **24-9**

Pharmacologic Treatment Options in Alzheimer's Disease

Category	Target Symptoms
Cholinesterase inhibitors	Apathy, psychosis (delusions, hallucinations), agitation, anxiety, nighttime behavior; positive effects have been shown on cognition, activities of daily living, and global functioning
Antipsychotics	Psychosis (delusions, hallucinations), hostility, aggression, agitation, violent behavior
Antidepressants	Depressive symptoms, anxiety disorders
β-Blockers	Agitation
Benzodiazepines	Anxiety, agitation
Estrogen	Agitation
Anticonvulsants	Agitation, aggression, mood swings
Serotonergic agents	Psychosis, agitation

Modified from Academic highlights: new insights into genetics and pathophysiology of Alzheimer's disease: what are the clinical and therapeutic implications? *J Clin Psychiatry* 61(4):307, 2000.

that focuses on patient strengths and helps patients maintain an awareness of their environment.

In general, reality orientation is helpful to patients with cognitive impairments. Systematic reality orientation includes attention to the dimensions of time, place, and person. This approach often takes place in a group and is most effective if the group meets daily, if possible, and at a consistent time. A pattern of group activity should be established. For instance, the group might begin with each person introducing himself or herself, after which everyone is informed of the date and time. A review of the schedule for the day is often helpful. A brief time is allowed for questions. In general, this type of group should last only 15 to 20 minutes. If the members become fatigued, their cognitive ability will deteriorate.

Communication. Recent memory loss is another common problem. Patients may be frustrated when constantly confronted with evidence of failing memory. Conversational focus can be directed toward topics that the patient initiates. Most patients feel more comfortable talking about remote memories and may derive pleasure from discussing past experiences. Misperceptions of the present can be dealt with gently and diplomatically. For example, if an elderly woman who has been widowed for 10 years says that she expects her husband to come home soon, the nurse might reply, "You must have loved your husband very much. Sometimes it seems to you that he's still here." Explicitly or implicitly agreeing that her husband will "come home" fosters false hope, perhaps leading to a disappointment. Abrupt confrontation with the reality of her husband's death is cruel and will increase her anxiety. Considerations about reality orientation are discussed in Critical Thinking about Contemporary Issues.

The nurse should introduce herself at each interaction with the patient. There should be an attitude of unconditional positive regard. Empathy, warmth, and caring are important, and verbal communication should be clear, concise, and unhurried. A pleasant, calm, supportive tone of voice should be used, with the voice modulated in relationship to the patient's ability to hear. Shouting may be interpreted as anger by a person who hears well. The use of pronouns should be avoided. Questions that require "yes" and "no" answers are best. Behavior should be requested one step at a time; if repetition is required, it should be stated in exactly the same way as the first time. Nonverbal communication skills are also important, and verbal and nonverbal communication must be congruent. Nonverbal techniques, especially touch, are sometimes reassuring to the patient. The nurse should try to understand who the patient was in the past. This can be accomplished by encouraging reminiscence and talking with family members. Pictures or music may help the patient to remember past experiences. The patient's daily schedule should be predictable and unhurried. Distraction or diversion along with decreased stimulation should be used if a patient appears to become agitated. An appropriate use of humor and flexibility by the nurse helps the patient to function in the environment.

Reinforcement of Coping Mechanisms. Previously helpful coping mechanisms are often used by patients

CRITICAL THINKING about CONTEMPORARY ISSUES

Is Reality Orientation Always the Best Nursing Intervention for Patients Who Are Experiencing Progressive Memory Loss?

Reality orientation is often recommended as a nursing intervention for patients who are disoriented. The rationale is that patients are reassured by being in touch with where they are in time and place. For the same reason, clocks and calendars are placed where patients can see them. Reality orientation is appropriate for patients who can process the information given to them. However, in the case of progressive memory loss related to dementia, the question arises regarding whether repeated efforts at reality orientation serve patients' needs.

For example, consider a situation in which a patient was distressed at attempts by the nursing staff to convince him that he was in a hospital. When a nurse participated in his life situation as he was experiencing it and responded as if she were in his workplace with him, he was much happier. The nurse's rationale for this intervention was that she was helping him to reminisce, which is an important developmental task for the elderly. Nurses must maintain a delicate balance between providing the patient with needed information about the environment and denying the patient's inability to process that information in a meaningful way. This means that nurses must question the automatic use of reality orientation as the best intervention for every disoriented patient.

with maladaptive cognitive responses. Sometimes these attempts to cope may be hard to understand unless placed in the appropriate context. An older man who pats and pinches nurses and makes lewd remarks may have had past success dealing with his anxiety by behaving seductively. An elderly woman who hoards food in her room may equate food with security. An aging person who has been suspicious of others in the past may become more suspicious over time. These behaviors have a protective nature and therefore should not be actively confronted. The nurse should instead try to discover the source of the patient's anxiety and attempt to alleviate it, thus allowing the person to behave less defensively.

Wandering. Wandering is a behavior that causes great concern to caregivers. In fact, it often leads to institutionalization or to the use of restraints. Nurses should observe patients carefully in order to understand such behavior, identify the situations that contribute to it, and plan appropriate interventions. In some cases medications may cause agitation and restlessness. Some patients are extremely sensitive to stress and tension in the environment, and their wandering may be an attempt to get away. Similarly, if patients are aware that an activity they dislike is about to occur (e.g., bathing or medication administration), they may try to

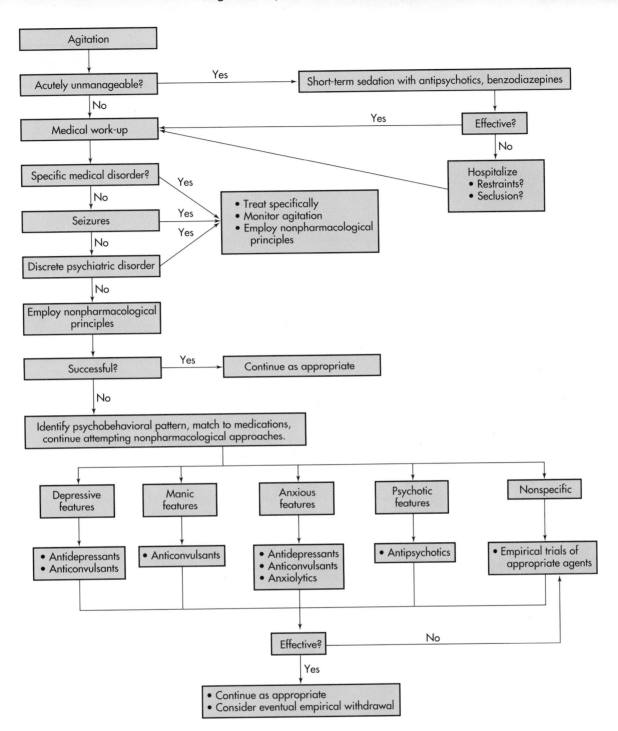

Fig. 24-5 Clinical algorithm for the treatment of agitation in dementia. (Modified from Tariot P: Clinical algorithm for the treatment of agitation in dementia, *J Clin Psychiatry* 60[suppl 8]:11, 1999.

avoid it. If wandering meets a patient's needs for attention, efforts to control the behavior may actually reinforce it.

The nurse should decrease stress in the patient's environment, especially at night, when many people have decreased stress tolerance. Eliminating distracting background noise or shadows may help. Safe areas should be provided where patients can move about freely. If possible, this should include an outside area with adequate staff supervision to ensure safety. Environmental design can be used to camouflage doorways or

to incorporate distractions. Any method of increasing orientation can also decrease the need to wander. However, it is important to base nursing interventions on observations and an analysis of the motivation for the patient's behavior.

Decreasing Agitation. Patients may also become agitated when pushed to do something unfamiliar or unclear. Expectations should be explained simply and completely. If the patient can make choices, they should be offered. An individual daily schedule of activities can help the person pre-

Table **24-10**

Practical Recommendations for Caregivers of Agitated and Aggressive Patients with Dementia

DECREASE ESCALATION

Decrease environmental stimuli and modify the environment.
Approach in a calm manner.
Use distraction: food, drink, music.
Maintain eye contact and a comfortable posture with arms/hands relaxed.
Use more than one sensory modality to send a calm message.
Match verbal and nonverbal signals.
Identify the affect observed in the patient; verbalize this for him or her.
Do not add more demands at this time.
Slow down pace and simplify your actions.
Maintain physical comfort.
Identify what is fueling the fire (e.g., triggers and reactions).
Maintain safety.

COMMUNICATE EFFECTIVELY

Capture the patient's attention; stay in view.
Use simple, direct statements.
Limit choices.
Use gestures to assist with verbal directions.
Use one-step commands.
Speak clearly and slowly; allow time for response.
Lower tone if voice needs to be raised.
Communicate your desire to help.

REVIEW THE BASICS

Behavior is symptomatic of the illness; separate the behavior from the person.
A damaged mind gets stuck in one activity and has trouble shifting gears; what worked an hour ago may not work now.
The caregiver is the only security in a shrinking world.
Persons with dementia lose the ability to plan.
Know the person and structure his or her environment accordingly.
Having a daily pattern of repetitive behaviors at predictable times and by familiar persons helps those with memory
  impairment to help themselves.
A loving voice, attentiveness, touch, and consistency are enormously important.
Remember, a caregiver is not always an angel; there are times when frustration and anger are expressed; no one is
  perfect.
The caregiver's needs must also be recognized and respected.
Maintain the patient's religious/spiritual identity.
Humor can help.

From Tariot P: Treatment of agitation in dementia, *J Clin Psychiatry* 60(suppl 8):11, 1999.

pare for and plan his or her day. If a patient refuses to participate in an activity, continued insistence usually leads to increased agitation and sometimes to a loss of behavioral control, resulting in a catastrophic response. The best approach may be to wait a few minutes and then return to see if the patient will agree to the request. Meanwhile the approach to the patient can be examined to see if the nurse might have contributed to the problem. Perhaps the patient thought the nurse was too controlling and a power struggle developed, or perhaps the nurse initiated the request abruptly and did not allow the patient a time for transition. Fig. 24-5 is a clinical algorithm that can assist the nurse in caring for the patient with dementia and agitation (Tariot, 1999).

Family and Community Interventions. Many people with dementia live in the community with their families. It is important to support the caregivers, because the patient usually derives great benefit from being with them. When hospitalization occurs, careful discharge planning is needed to help the family prepare to receive the patient back home. Table 24-10 provides practical recommendations that may be helpful to caregivers.

Families of patients with AD may need support in identifying and coping with feelings such as denial, anger, and guilt—feelings much like those experienced by individuals who are grieving over a dying loved one. They may need assistance in providing 24-hour care for the patient. Home care agencies may provide nursing and homemaking services to enable patients to remain in their own homes. If family members are not available during the day, adult daycare centers are available in some communities. These programs provide help with activities of daily living, recreation, health supervision, rehabilitation, exercise, and nutrition. Families also receive support and assistance, particularly during the first few weeks of attendance, when the patient may be resistant because he or she is having difficulty adapting to a new experience. A Nursing Treatment Plan Sum-

NURSING TREATMENT PLAN *Summary* *Maladaptive Cognitive Responses*

NURSING DIAGNOSIS: Altered thought processes
EXPECTED OUTCOME: The patient will achieve optimum cognitive functioning.

SHORT-TERM GOAL	INTERVENTION	RATIONALE
The patient will meet basic biological needs.	Maintain adequate nutrition, monitor fluid intake and output, and monitor vital signs. Provide opportunities for rest and stimulation. Help with ambulation if necessary. Help with hygiene activities as needed.	Basic biological integrity is necessary for survival. Interventions related to survival are given high priority for nursing intervention.
The patient will be safe from injury.	Assess sensory and perceptual functioning. Provide access to items such as eyeglasses, hearing aids, canes, and walkers. Observe and remove safety hazards (e.g., obstacles, slippery floors, open flames, and inadequate lighting). Supervise medications if necessary. Protect from injury during periods of agitation with one-to-one nursing care; use restraints only if absolutely necessary.	Maladaptive cognitive responses usually involve sensory and perceptual disorders that can endanger the patient's safety.
The patient will experience an optimum level of self-esteem.	Provide reality orientation. Establish a trusting relationship. Encourage independence. Identify interests and skills; provide opportunities to use them. Give honest praise for accomplishments. Use therapeutic communication techniques to help patient communicate thoughts and feelings.	Cognitive impairment is a threat to self-esteem. A positive nurse-patient relationship can help the patient to express fears and feel secure in the environment. The recognition of accomplishments also raises self-esteem.
The patient will maintain positive interpersonal relationships.	Initiate contact with significant others. Encourage patient to interact with others; involve in group activities. Teach family and patient about the nature of the problem and the recommended health-care plan. Allow significant others to help with patient care if they wish. Meet with significant others regularly and provide them with an opportunity to talk. Involve patient and family in discharge planning.	Caring relationships with others promote a positive self-concept. Communication from significant others can often be understood more easily than communication from strangers. Family and friends can provide help in knowing the patient's habits and preferences. Involvement of significant others in caregiving often helps them cope with the stress of the patient's health problem.

mary for patients who have maladaptive cognitive responses is presented on the opposite page.

EVALUATION

Expectations of the patient who has cognitive difficulty must be realistic but not pessimistic. One evaluation criterion is the appropriateness of the nursing goal to the patient. The nurse should assess whether the expectation is too high or too low. Levels of expectation can be increased until the patient is clearly unable to function and then lowered to the realistic level.

The evaluation of the nursing care of the patient who has maladaptive cognitive responses is based on achievement of

the identified nursing care goals. If these goals are not achieved, the nurse should ask the following questions:

- Was the assessment complete enough to correctly identify the problem?
- Were the goals individualized for the patient?
- Was enough time allowed for goal achievement?
- Did I have the skills needed to carry out the identified interventions?
- Were there environmental factors that affected goal achievement?
- Did additional stressors affect the patient's ability to cope?
- Was the goal achievable for this patient?

- What alternative approaches could be tried?

Colleagues are helpful in evaluating the nursing care plan. They may suggest alternative interventions or provide feedback about transference-countertransference issues. For instance, nurses who work with aging patients with dementia may respond to concerns about their own aging or that of their parents and have difficulty seeing patients as unique persons. Hallucinating patients often arouse anxiety in nurses, who may then respond with their own defense mechanisms. Regular supervision can help nurses to develop enhanced self-awareness and to determine when a particularly anxiety-provoking situation has bothered them and why.

Summary

1. The continuum of cognitive responses is related to behavioral and biological models of learning and memory.
2. Behaviors related to cognitive responses vary depending on whether the maladaptive response is acute and likely to resolve (as in delirium) or progressive and chronic (as in dementia). Behaviors are related to disturbances in thought, memory, reasoning, judgment, orientation, perception, and attention.
3. Predisposing factors related to dementia are aging, neurobiological functioning, genetic factors, and underlying psychiatric and medical conditions. Precipitating stressors related to delirium are categorized as CNS disorders, metabolic disorders, cardiopulmonary disorders, systemic illness, and sensory deprivation or stimulation. Precipitating stressors related to dementia are categorized as degenerative brain disorders, cerebrovascular causes, toxic-metabolic disturbances, CNS infections, and miscellaneous causes.
4. Coping resources are based on individual and interpersonal supports. Coping mechanisms include intellectualization, rationalization, denial, and regression.
5. The primary NANDA nursing diagnosis is altered thought processes.
6. The primary *DSM–IV–TR* diagnoses addressed in this chapter are categorized as delirium and dementia.
7. The expected outcome of nursing care is that the patient will achieve the optimum level of cognitive functioning.
8. Interventions related to delirium include caring for physiological needs, responding to hallucinations, therapeutic communication, and patient education. Interventions related to dementia include pharmacological approaches, orientation, therapeutic communication, reinforcement of coping mechanisms, responding to wandering, decreasing agitation, and family and community approaches.
9. Evaluation of nursing care is based on goal accomplishment and involves feedback from the patient, significant others, peers, and supervisors.

Competent Caring   A Clinical Exemplar of a Psychiatric Nurse

ALISON MEEKS, RN, MS

I worked on a unit that was set up to care for patients with behavioral problems as a result of their dementia. I vividly remember one call we received about a patient who was described as violent, explosive, confused, and in need of total care in activities of daily living. When the patient arrived on the unit I discovered that Ms. S weighed 90 pounds, had long beautiful hair up in a bun, and was ambulatory. She thought she was going to a hotel, so we took her bags and served her lunch while we interviewed her husband, who was her primary caregiver.

His was a very sad story. Tearfully he reported that his wife no longer loved him, that she was very malicious, and that she became physically violent at least once a day. He wanted to go on vacation while she was in the hospital, which some of the staff felt was probably the reason for this admission. However, he has been caring for his wife for 5 years with little or no help from the community or family members, and it was clear that he needed a break. It would be hard, however, because this would be the first time they had been apart from each other in their 58 years of marriage.

Ms. S had a mini-mental state examination score of 12 and had great difficulty visually interpreting her environment. For example, she thought a comb was a knife and the garbage can, her purse. She was also very sensitive to her environment. If the unit was loud and a lot of people were walking around, she became more active and often had the potential for getting hurt or hurting someone else. During periods of activity on the unit, such as a shift change, we escorted Ms. S to her room, where she would fold clothes or go through one of four pocketbooks we put together for her. We needed four pocketbooks because she would misplace one and we would not be able to find it. This symptom presented great problems at home for the caregiver because anything left out would be moved and often never found. Our solution was to set up several baskets of safe items for Ms. S to rummage through.

Ms. S became physically violent three times during her 10-day hospitalization. Each incident occurred when staff members entered her room and she accused them of breaking into her home. We started to knock on her door before entering and would have something for her such as a pocketbook, a book, or her stockings in our hands. That seemed to solve that problem. Another intervention that worked for Ms. S was music. She always liked ballet and now thought she was a retired dancer. We never challenged this and listened to her wonderful stories about dance and other dancers.

Ms. S did not recognize her husband when he came back from vacation. He was hurt and said we had done nothing to help her. We worked extensively with her husband by having him come and observe our interventions with Ms. S. Our goal was to help him realize the level of her impairment. He soon realized that her actions were not malicious. We diagnosed a

Competent Caring A Clinical Exemplar of a Psychiatric Nurse

urinary tract infection during her admission, which we treated, and we prescribed 0.5 mg of haloperidol each morning, which helped to decrease her explosive episodes. We also enlisted the help of family members, friends, and a home health provider to care for Ms. S. I made one home visit after discharge and gave suggestions on how to make the home safe for Ms. S.

Four weeks after discharge Mr. S mailed the nurses a letter thanking us for giving him his life back. He explained that he felt he should have been better able to care for his wife on his own before her hospitalization and that he had even contemplated suicide because of the overwhelming burden of caring for his wife. It seemed to us that in this case, we touched the lives of two rather than one.

 Visit **MERLIN: www.mosby.com/MERLIN/Stuart** to find these additional materials and student activities.

- **Worksheets**
- **"Drug of the Month" Updates**
- **"Citing the Evidence" Updates**
- **Critical Thinking Activities and Exercises**
- **Annotated Suggested Readings**
- **Web Links**
- **More!**

Chapter Review Questions

1. Match each term in Column A with the correct definition in Column B.

Column A

____ Delirium

____ Denial

____ Dementia

____ Agnosia

____ Pseudodementia

____ Sundowning syndrome

____ Amygdala

____ Aphasia

____ Apraxia

____ Excess disability

Column B

A. Responsible for emotion and emotional memory

B. Difficulty recognizing well-known objects

C. Disturbed consciousness and cognitions developing over a short time

D. May ignore memory loss, interfering with treatment planning

E. Depressed, missed in the elderly, not treated appropriately

F. Gradual onset with continuing cognitive decline

G. Difficulty finding the right word

H. Extreme agitation, occurring at night

I. Cognitive responses functioning at a lower level than one would expect

J. Inability to perform familiar skilled activities

2. Fill in the blanks.

A. The brain lesions that are characteristic of Alzheimer's disease are _____ and _____.

B. Cholinesterase inhibitors are pharmacological interventions for _____.

C. The term _____ refers to extreme agitation related to dementia.

D. _____ is usually sudden and a medical emergency.

3. Provide short answers for the following questions.

A. Describe the behavioral and biological differences between working memory and long-term memory.

B. List three coping strategies that you would suggest to the caregiver of a person who has a moderate level of cognitive impairment due to dementia.

C. Describe a discharge plan for a person who has been hospitalized for the treatment of delirium related to combining prescription medicine and alcohol.

REFERENCES

American Psychiatric Association: *Diagnostic and statistical manual of mental disorders,* Fourth Edition, Text Revision. Washington, DC, American Psychiatric Association, 2000.

Beck C et al: Dressing for success: promoting independence among cognitively impaired elderly, *J Psychosoc Nurs Ment Health Serv* 29:30, 1991.

Cummings J: Cholinesterase inhibitors: a new class of psychotropic compounds, *Am J Psychiatry* 157:4, 2000.

Cummings J, Jeste D: Alzheimer's disease and its management in the year 2010, *Psychiatr Serv* 50(9):1173, 1999.

Desai A, Grossberg G: Risk factors and protective factors for Alzheimer's disease, *Clin Geriatr* 7(11):43, 1999.

Draper B: The diagnosis and treatment of depression in dementia, *Psychiatr Serv* 50(9):1151, 1999.

Inouye S: A multicomponent intervention to prevent delirium in hospitalized older patients, *N Engl J Med* 340:669, 1999.

Kelley L et al: Family involvement in care for individuals with dementia protocol, *J Gerontol Nurs* 2:13, 2000.

Kumar V et al: Advances in pharmacotherapy for decline of memory and cognition in patients with Alzheimer's disease, *Psychiatr Serv* 47:249, 1996.

Li G et al: Age at onset and familial risk in Alzheimer's disease, *Am J Psychiatry* 152:424, 1995.

Lyketsos C et al: Physical aggression in dementia patients and its relationship to depression, *Am J Psychiatry* 156:1, 1999.

Masand P: Atypical antipsychotics for elderly patients with neurodegenerative disorders and medical conditions, *Psychiatr Ann* 30(3):202, 2000.

Swanson EA et al: Catastrophic reactions and other behaviors of Alzheimer's residents: special unit compared with traditional units, *Arch Psychiatr Nurs* 7:292, 1993.

Tariot P: Treatment of agitation in dementia, *J Clin Psychiatry* 60(suppl 8):11, 1999.

Visit **MERLIN** for *Your Internet Connection*
to websites that are related to the content in this chapter.
www.mosby.com/MERLIN/Stuart

Chemically Mediated Responses and Substance-Related Disorders

Linda V. Jefferson

Sleepmonger, deathmonger, with capsules in my palms each night, eight at a time from sweet pharmaceutical bottles I make arrangements for a pint-sized journey. I'm the queen of this condition. I'm an expert on making the trip and now they say I'm an addict. Now they ask why. Why!

                ANNE SEXTON, *THE ADDICT*

Psychoactive substances have been used by people in almost all cultures since prehistoric times. These substances have been seen as enhancers of individual and social functioning. People continue to use them for relief of negative emotional states, such as depression, fear, and anxiety; relief from fatigue or boredom; and as a break from daily routines through altered states of consciousness. Alcohol and drugs also continue to be used in various religious ceremonies. Ethical and legal considerations aside, moderate use for any of these purposes would probably not result in major social or individual harm. However, all cultures have recognized the negative effects of alcohol and drug use. Excessive use of these substances has contributed to profound individual and social problems.

Any drug that can produce pleasurable changes in mental or emotional states has potential for abuse. Drugs that cause the most marked and immediate desirable effects have the greatest abuse potential. Alcohol and cocaine are very popular because they produce effects on the brain within minutes. Drugs of abuse include legal drugs, such as alcohol and prescription drugs; illegal drugs, such as heroin, cocaine, and marijuana; and household products, such as inhalants.

CONTINUUM OF CHEMICALLY MEDIATED RESPONSES
Definition of Terms

A person may achieve a state of relaxation, euphoria, stimulation, or altered awareness in several ways. The range of these chemically mediated coping responses is illustrated in Fig. 25-1. Although there is a continuum from occasional drug use to frequent drug use to abuse and dependence, not everyone who uses drugs becomes an abuser, nor does every abuser become dependent. The definitions of the terms **use,** **abuse,** and **dependence** have changed through the years and vary greatly in the addiction literature. The nurse must realize that what one person or health-care professional means by addiction is not necessarily meant by another. Reading and discussion should start with agreement about the meanings of terms.

Substance abuse, as described in the *Diagnostic and Statistical Manual of Mental Disorders,* fourth edition (*DSM–IV–TR*) (American Psychiatric Association, 2000), refers to continued use despite related problems. The term substance dependence, related to either drugs or alcohol, indicates a severe condition, usually considered a disease. There may be physical problems as well as serious disruptions in the person's work, family, and social life. The psychosocial behaviors related to substance dependence are often called addiction. For most purposes, the terms **dependence** and **addiction** are used interchangeably. Dual diagnosis is the co-existence of substance abuse and psychiatric disorders within the same person.

Withdrawal symptoms and tolerance are signs that the person is physically dependent on the drug. Withdrawal symptoms result from a biological need that develops when the body becomes adapted to having the drug in the system. Characteristic symptoms occur when the level of the substance in the system decreases. Tolerance means that with continued use, more of the substance is needed to produce the same effect.

Physical dependence can occur independently from the symptoms of substance dependence. For example, a patient who receives narcotics for chronic pain may develop both tolerance and withdrawal, yet not have any of the other problems related to substance dependence, such as preoccupation with getting the drug, loss of control, or use despite problems. This person would be described as physically dependent on the narcotic but would not be called a drug addict.

Many people progress from use to abuse at some time in their lives. However, only about 1 in 10 people progress from use to abuse to dependence. Once use has begun, the risk of becoming dependent is influenced by many biological, psychological, and sociocultural factors.

Attitudes Toward Substance Abuse

Substance abuse is viewed differently, depending on the substance used, the person using it, and the setting in which it is used. Nurses should be aware of these social and cultural attitudes and recognize their impact on individual users and people close to them. For instance, a businessman who starts arguments after a few drinks with his associates would not usually be considered an alcohol abuser. If the same person was caught nipping from a bottle in his desk, he would probably be considered to have a drinking problem. Tobacco abuse is still widely accepted in the United States, despite convincing evidence of medical problems related to smoking and the effects of secondary smoke inhalation and the release of a number of practice guidelines for the treatment of patients with nicotine dependence (Box 25-1). On the other hand, a person who smokes opium would be considered deviant, even if the behavior took place in private.

> *Can you describe other examples of sociocultural mixed messages about the use of tobacco, caffeine, alcohol, and marijuana? How would you as a health professional go about changing these attitudes?*

Changing laws related to consumption, sale, and serving of alcohol and drugs may reflect changing attitudes toward their use. Driving while intoxicated (DWI) laws are becoming tougher. When groups of friends go out, it is common for one to be the designated driver and not drink. Places where alcoholic beverages are served can be held liable if a customer overindulges and then causes an accident. Manda-

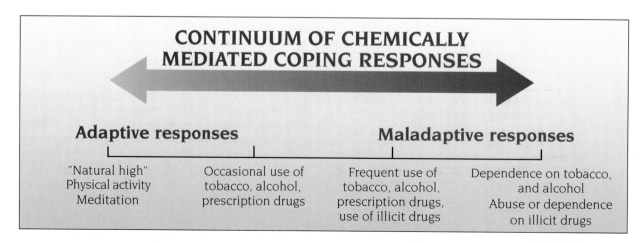

Fig. 25-1 Continuum of chemically mediated coping responses.

tory sentencing for certain drug offenses is intended to show an unaccepting attitude toward drug abuse.

Many nurses have negative attitudes toward alcoholics and other drug abusers. Some have had negative experiences with family members or friends who have had substance-related problems. This may influence the nurse's ability to assess and care for these patients. Nurses often see substance abusers at their worst, during a medical or psychiatric crisis. They see these patients returning repeatedly for alcohol or drug-related health problems. Nurses rarely have contact with alcoholics and drug addicts who have recovered from their addiction because they are ill less often. When they do seek health care, these patients may try to hide their substance abuse history. The best way for nurses to change negative attitudes is to attend open meetings of self-help groups, where they will meet recovering alcoholics and addicts who have overcome tremendous odds to remain sober and lead healthy, productive lives.

Prevalence

The United States has one of the highest levels of substance abuse in the world. Substance abuse is involved in numerous chronic illnesses, hospitalizations, emergency room visits, and deaths. Data from the 1998 National Household Survey on Drug Abuse revealed that about 81% of people in the United States age 12 and older have used alcohol sometime in their lives. About 6% reported heavy alcohol use in the past month. In contrast, 36% had used illicit drugs (NIDA, 1999). Cigarette use was at 28%, a drop from 39% in 1985.

Overall, use of alcohol and illicit drugs appears to increase into the mid-20s, level off, and then decrease with age. Both the lifetime prevalence and the intensity of alcohol use were greater among males. In addition, whites reported higher levels of alcohol use than blacks or Hispanics. Those with more education were more likely to use alcohol, but heavy use was more common among the less educated and unemployed. Most people with alcohol use disorders do not seek treatment. Research estimates that from 75% to 93% of adults in the United States who need alcohol treatment do not actually receive it. The most frequently cited reasons for not seeking alcohol treatment are displayed in Fig. 25-2.

Adolescence is the most common period for the first experience with drugs. Although teenagers who use psychoactive substances tend to progress from nicotine to alcohol to marijuana (also known as the "gateway" drugs) and then to drugs that are perceived to be more dangerous, drug use patterns seem to be most related to availability. About 31% of youth report current alcohol use, 15% report binge drinking, and 17% describe their alcohol use as "heavy." The percentage of high school seniors who had ever used an illicit drug peaked at 65% in the United States in 1981, then steadily decreased to 41% by 1992. However, by 1997 the rate had again risen to 54%. Information about substance abuse by adolescents is provided in Chapter 39.

Multiple Substance Use. Simultaneous or sequential use of more than one substance is very common. People do this to enhance, lessen, or otherwise change the nature of their intoxication or to relieve withdrawal symptoms. Use of alcohol with cocaine or use of alcohol with heroin ("speedballing") is especially common. Heroin users often combine alcohol, marijuana, and benzodiazepines with heroin. Multiple drug use is particularly dangerous if synergistic drugs, such as barbiturates and alcohol, are used. It also complicates substance abuse assessment and intervention because the patient may be demonstrating effects of or withdrawal from several drugs at the same time.

Dual Diagnosis. In the addicted population, there is no greater prevalence of psychiatric illness than in the general population. However, up to 51% of individuals with a serious mental illness are also dependent on or addicted to alcohol or illicit drugs (Kessler et al, 1996). For example, people with schizophrenia are more than four times as likely to have a substance use disorder during their lifetimes, and those with bipolar disorder are more than five times as likely to have such a diagnosis than people in the general population. This poses unique challenges for clini-

Box 25-1

Nicotine as a Substance of Abuse

After a long and steady increase in smoking among American teens that began in the early 1990s, smoking rates among high school students have started to decrease (SAMHSA, 1999b). In 1997, smoking decreased among 8th and 10th graders, whereas smoking among 12th graders continued to rise. However, in 1998, all three grade levels showed some decrease in smoking. Although 28% of the U.S. population smokes, the vast majority of new smokers are younger than 18.

The federal government has been trying to reduce smoking among children and adolescents. In 1996, President Clinton signed an executive order that subjected tobacco to regulation by the Food and Drug Administration (FDA). The FDA then issued a regulation that included provisions to reduce youth access to tobacco products, require more explicit labeling or packaging and advertising, and to limit tobacco product advertising and promotion that appeals to children. However, the tobacco companies, the advertising industry, and the convenience store owners filed lawsuits against the FDA, challenging the agency's authority over tobacco products. In 2000, the Supreme Court supported the lawsuit, ruling that Congress had never granted FDA the authority to regulate tobacco products. It is now up to Congress to act to grant this authority to the FDA.

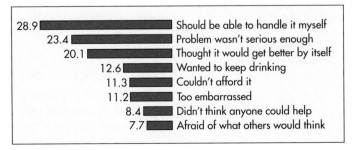

28.9	Should be able to handle it myself
23.4	Problem wasn't serious enough
20.1	Thought it would get better by itself
12.6	Wanted to keep drinking
11.3	Couldn't afford it
11.2	Too embarrassed
8.4	Didn't think anyone could help
7.7	Afraid of what others would think

Fig. 25-2 Reasons why people (%) do not seek alcohol treatment. (From Grant B: NLAES identifies treatment beliefs as barriers to access, 1999.)

cians, because these patients are often treatment-resistant with high relapse rates.

Despite their prevalence, substance disorders are frequently underdetected and underdiagnosed in acute-care psychiatric settings. Failure to detect substance abuse disorder results in misdiagnosis of the psychiatric disorder, suboptimal pharmacological treatment, neglect of appropriate interventions for substance abuse, and inappropriate treatment planning and referral. This underdetection can be caused by a combination of factors, including clinicians' lack of awareness of the high rates of substance disorders in psychiatric populations; the inadequacy of standardized assessment tools in this population; patients' denial, minimization, and failure to acknowledge their substance-related problems; and patients' cognitive, psychotic, and other impairments related to their psychiatric illness (Miele et al, 1996).

Substance-Related Disorders in Nurses. Despite claims that health-care professionals have a higher rate of substance abuse than the general public, there are data to support this. The following rates of substance use in the past year among nurses have been reported: 16% binge drinking, 14% cigarette smoking, 7% prescription-type drug use, 4% marijuana/cocaine use (Trinkoff, 1998).

State board of nursing disciplinary records provide additional information. According to the National Council of State Boards of Nursing, 53% of all disciplinary actions taken against registered nurses in 1995 were drug related, down from 94.4% in 1987 and 68% in 1991. These figures could reflect a decrease in the problem, a decrease in reporting of the problem, or earlier and more effective treatment. Unfortunately, it is still a common practice to deal with a nurse who has a drug problem by ignoring the problem, firing the nurse, or asking for the nurse's resignation rather than reporting it to the state licensing board. Therefore, these data may only reflect a small segment of the problem.

Alcohol is the drug of choice for nurses, as in the general population. Also, as in the general population, the nurse's choice of substance is influenced by availability and exposure. Of all health-care professionals, physicians and nurses use parenteral narcotics the most in their practices. Therefore, they are more likely to choose these drugs for their own use. Among narcotics, the drug of choice for nurses is meperidine (Demerol). Anesthesiologists and nurse anesthetists who abuse substances tend to favor fentanyl, a potent, short-acting narcotic. In general, health-care professionals tend to abuse prescription drugs rather than "street" drugs, whether they acquire them by prescription or diversion.

ASSESSMENT

Although accurate assessment of a patient's patterns of drug and alcohol use is important, it is sometimes very difficult to accomplish. Alcohol and drug addicts may use many defense mechanisms when discussing their chemical use. They tend to deny how much they use and its relationship to problems in their lives. They often rationalize their substance use. Patients should not be criticized for these unconscious mechanisms. They are often not aware of the extent or effects of their use. It is also true that some patients purposely distort the truth about drug use to avoid feared consequences. The nurse must be aware of these behaviors and take them into account. On the other hand, the nurse should be aware that only about 1 in 10 people who drink develop substance dependence at some point in their lives. Thus, one should not jump to the conclusion that a person is in denial if he or she relates no alcohol-related problems.

Screening for Substance Abuse

One must first be asking the right questions. People who drink, take drugs, or do both tend to be around others who drink and use drugs as they do. They do not have a good idea of what "normal" use patterns are. Therefore, even people who deny drug and drinking problems are apt to answer certain questions truthfully. These questions are included in screening tools, which are the first level of assessment for alcohol and drug dependence.

Simple screening tools are available that are useful in identifying people who may be addicted to alcohol or drugs. Box 25-2 lists behavioral rating scales related to substance use. Because screening tools are only suggestive, findings from them should be followed by a full diagnostic assessment.

CAGE. The simplest tool that can be used in any health setting to screen for alcoholism is the CAGE questionnaire. CAGE is an acronym for the four questions it contains (Box 25-3). Answering "yes" to two or more questions indicates

---

Box 25-2

Behavioral Rating Scales Related to Substance Use Disorders

CONTENT AREA: SUBSTANCE USE DISORDERS
- Addiction Severity Index (ASI)
- Alcohol Dependence Scale (ADS)
- Alcohol/Substance Abuse Questionnaire (ASAQ)
- Alcohol Use Disorders Identification Test (AUDIT)
- Alcohol Use Inventory (AUI)
- Alcohol Use Scale (AUS)
- Brief Drug Abuse Screening Test (B-DAST)
- CAGE Questionnaire
- Chemical Use, Abuse and Dependence Scale (CUAD)
- Children of Alcoholics Screening Test (CAST)
- Clinical Institute Narcotic Assessment (CINA)
- Clinical Institute Withdrawal Assessment-Alcohol, Revised (CIWA-AR)
- Drug Use Scale (DUS)
- Drug Abuse Screening Test (DAST)
- Drug Use Screening Inventory (revised) (DUSI)
- Family Alcohol and Drug Survey (FADS)
- Follow up Drinker Profile
- Inventory of Drinking Situations (IDS)
- Michigan Alcoholism Screening Tool (MAST)
- Rapid Alcohol Problems Index (RAPS)
- Rutgers Alcohol Problem Index (RAPI)
- Substance Abuse Outcome Module (SAOM)
- Substance Abuse Subtle Screening Inventory (SASSI)
- Substance Abuse Treatment Schedule (SATS)
- Treatment Services Review (TSR)

probable alcoholism. Further assessment would be needed to make a diagnosis. The CAGE questionnaire is recommended as an initial screening tool because its questions and scoring can be remembered easily and included in any interview.

? Given that CAGE is such a simple screening tool, why do you think it is not used more often in routine nursing assessments?

B-DAST. The Brief Drug Abuse Screening Test (B-DAST) is the quickest drug abuse screening tool (Box 25-4). Each item has a one-point value. Scores of 6 or more suggest significant drug-abuse problems. Patients who score above established cutoff scores are considered to be addicted.

Breathalyzer. The simplest biological measure to obtain is blood alcohol content (BAC) by use of a Breathalyzer. Alcohol in any amount has an effect on the central nervous system (CNS). The behaviors that can be expected from a nontolerant person at different concentrations of alcohol in the blood are shown in Table 25-1. Remember that a person who has developed tolerance to alcohol would not demonstrate these behaviors and could have a high BAC without showing any signs of impairment. A level greater than 0.10% without associated behavioral symptoms indicates the pres-

---

Box 25-3

The CAGE Questionnaire

- Have you ever felt you ought to **C**ut down on your drinking?
- Have people **A**nnoyed you by criticizing your drinking?
- Have you ever felt bad or **G**uilty about your drinking?
- Have you ever had a drink first thing in the morning to steady your nerves or get rid of a hangover (**E**ye-opener)?

Scoring: Two "yes" answers indicate probable alcoholism

From Ewing JA: *JAMA* 252:1905, 1984.

Table **25-1**

Comparison of Blood Alcohol Concentrations with Behavioral Manifestations of Intoxication

Blood Alcohol Level	Behaviors
0.05 to 0.15 g/dl	Euphoria, labile mood, cognitive disturbances (decreased concentration, impaired judgment, loss of sexual inhibitions)
0.15 to 0.25 g/dl	Slurred speech, staggering gait, diplopia, drowsiness, labile mood with outbursts
0.3 g/dl	Stupor, aggressive behavior, incoherent speech, labored breathing, vomiting
0.4 g/dl	Coma
0.5 g/dl	Severe respiratory depression, death

Box 25-4

Brief Drug Abuse Screening Test (B-DAST)

Instructions: The following questions concern information about your involvement and abuse of drugs. Drug abuse refers to (1) the use of prescribed or over-the-counter drugs in excess of the directions and (2) any nonmedical use of drugs. Carefully read each statement and decide whether your answer is yes or no. Then circle the appropriate response.

YES NO	1.	Have you used drugs other than those required for medical reasons?
YES NO	2.	Have you abused prescription drugs?
YES NO	3.	Do you abuse more than one drug at a time?
YES NO	4.	Can you get through the week without using drugs (other than those required for medical reasons)?
YES NO	5.	Are you always able to stop using drugs when you want to?
YES NO	6.	Have you had "blackouts" or "flashbacks" as a result of drug use?
YES NO	7.	Do you ever feel bad about your drug abuse?
YES NO	8.	Does your spouse (or parents) ever complain about your involvement with drugs?
YES NO	9.	Has drug abuse ever created problems between you and your spouse?
YES NO	10.	Have you ever lost friends because of your use of drugs?
YES NO	11.	Have you ever neglected your family or missed work because of your use of drugs?
YES NO	12.	Have you ever been in trouble at work because of drug abuse?
YES NO	13.	Have you ever lost a job because of drug abuse?
YES NO	14.	Have you gotten into fights when under the influence of drugs?
YES NO	15.	Have you engaged in illegal activities in order to obtain drugs?
YES NO	16.	Have you ever been arrested for possession of illegal drugs?
YES NO	17.	Have you ever experienced withdrawal symptoms as a result of heavy drug intake?
YES NO	18.	Have you had medical problems as a result of your drug use (e.g., memory loss, hepatitis, convulsions, bleeding, etc.)?
YES NO	19.	Have you ever gone to anyone for help for a drug problem?
YES NO	20.	Have you ever been involved in a treatment program specifically related to drug use?

From Skinner HA: *Addict Behav* 7:363, 1982.
(Items 4 and 5 are scored in the "no," or false, direction.)

ence of tolerance. The higher the level without symptoms, the more severe the tolerance. High tolerance is a sign of physical dependence.

Blood and Urine Screening. Blood and urine are the body fluids most often tested for drug content, although saliva, hair, breath, and sweat analysis methods have been developed and are being refined. Identification and measurement of drug levels in the blood are useful for treating drug overdoses or complications in emergency room and other medical settings. Otherwise, urine drug screening is the method of choice because it is noninvasive. Urine drug screening is sometimes used to test prospective employees and athletes for evidence of drug use. Drug treatment personnel also use it to determine whether patients have used drugs while in treatment. Urine drug screening is often used in court to validate a person's drug use related to criminal activity.

The person being tested may try to alter the sample to hide drug use. The most common ways to do this are diluting the specimen with water from the toilet or substituting a "clean" specimen donated by a friend for the "dirty" specimen. To help prevent these practices, the specimen is often collected on random days under direct observation of a same-sex staff member. Another way is to have the person leave jackets, sweaters, purses, and so forth outside the stall, place drops of dye in the toilet water to alter its color, and test the specimen for temperature. Fresh, undiluted urine should feel warm through the cup and should be approximately 37° C.

The length of time that drugs can be found in blood and urine varies according to dosage and the metabolic properties of the drug. All traces of the drug may disappear within 24 hours or may still be detectable 30 days later.

 Random urine testing for drugs is required for members of some occupations, including some nurses. This practice has been challenged as an invasion of privacy and an intrusion on professional integrity. What is your opinion about random urine testing for nurses?

Behaviors of Abuse and Dependence

There are many consequences of using alcohol and drugs. Some are very serious and have led to great social concern. Lifestyles associated with drug abuse carry risks. Accidents are frequent, and violence is common. Self-neglect is the norm, contributing to physical and mental disease. The drugs and associated lifestyle also can lead to complications during pregnancy and the risk of fetal abnormalities and fetal drug dependence.

Intravenous drug users and their sexual partners are at high risk for infection with bloodborne pathogens, particularly hepatitis B (HBV) and the human immunodeficiency virus (HIV), which causes the acquired immunodeficiency syndrome (AIDS). It is common for addicts to share needles when they are using drugs in a group. Because the needles are not cleaned, blood is transferred from one person to the others. This is an ideal situation for the transmission of HIV or HBV.

CNS Depressants. This term is used for any drug that depresses excitable tissues at all levels of the brain. These drugs are also called sedative-hypnotics. Their primary effects are to reduce anxiety (the calming, antianxiety, or sedative effect), induce sleep (the hypnotic effect), or both. Included in this class are alcohol, barbiturates, and benzodiazepines. The signs and symptoms of the use of, overdose by, and withdrawal from CNS depressants are listed in Table 25-2. It should be noted that cross-tolerance develops among all drugs in this category. This means that as tolerance develops to one drug, it develops to all other drugs in this category as well. For example, a chronic alcoholic will need very high doses of benzodiazepines to control signs of withdrawal.

Alcohol. Although alcohol is a sedative, it creates an initial feeling of euphoria. This is probably related to decreased inhibitions. Symptoms of sedation of different CNS structures increase as the amount drunk increases.

Approximately 15% of drinkers progress to alcoholism. A person's drinking may begin like everyone else's, or a person may be able to drink more alcohol than others before feeling intoxicated. In either case, the person likes the feeling and continues to drink whenever possible. Gradually, drinking occurs more often and in larger quantities. As this happens, drinking begins to cause problems in the person's life, which are quickly explained away. The problems increase, the drinking increases, physical and psychological dependence develops, and the person begins to drink to avoid withdrawal symptoms. Or, the person drinks in binges. Not everyone progresses in the same way or displays all of these characteristics, and the time period over which the progression occurs varies widely. The following clinical example illustrates many of the behaviors described. Mr. H has the medical diagnoses of alcohol dependence and alcohol withdrawal delirium.

CLINICAL EXAMPLE

Mr. H was admitted to the detoxification center of a large metropolitan hospital in acute alcohol withdrawal. He was delirious and having visual hallucinations of bugs in his bed. He was extremely frightened, thrashing around in bed, and mumbling incoherently. Because he had a long and well-documented history of alcohol abuse, family members were contacted and confirmed that he had recently stopped drinking after a 2-week binge.

The patient had been a successful lawyer with a large practice. He specialized in corporate law and conducted much business over lunch or dinner. He also kept a well-stocked bar in his office to offer clients a drink. Without his really being aware of it, Mr. H's drinking gradually increased. After a few years he was drinking almost nonstop from lunchtime to bedtime. He then began to have a Bloody Mary with breakfast "just to get myself going."

His wife reported that he had become irritable, particularly if she questioned his drinking. On two occasions he had hit her during their arguments. She was seriously considering divorce. He had also become alienated from his children, who appeared frightened of him. Infrequently he would feel guilty about his neglect of his family and plan a special outing. Most of the time, though, he was too drunk to carry out his plans. The family had also become less involved in activities with friends. Mrs. H and the children felt embarrassed about his behavior and did not invite anyone to their home. On two occasions, Mr. H had tried to stop drinking. The first time he went to a private hospital, where he was detoxified. He abstained from drinking for about 1 month after discharge.

He then lost an important case and decided to have "just one drink" to carry him through the crisis. Soon his drinking was again out of control. His second hospitalization was at a general hospital with an active alcoholism rehabilitation program. He was introduced to Alcoholics Anonymous (AA) and started taking disulfiram (Antabuse). This program worked until he decided that he could manage without medication. A couple of weeks later his co-workers persuaded him to "help celebrate" at an office party. This was the start of a binge that ended when he had an automobile accident on the way home from a bar. A passenger in the other car was killed, and Mr. H was charged with vehicular homicide and driving under the influence of alcohol. He stopped drinking abruptly, which resulted in his current hospital admission 3 days later.

Selected Nursing Diagnoses

- Sensory-perceptual alteration (visual), related to neurobiological changes induced by acute alcohol withdrawal, as evidenced by hallucinations of bugs in the bed
- Ineffective individual coping related to repeated drinking, as evidenced by work and family problems and denial of drinking problems
- Risk for injury related to drinking and driving, as evidenced by recent automobile accident
- Risk for violence directed at others related to lack of control of behavior when drunk, as evidenced by past pattern of violent behavior

Barbiturates. Barbiturates include barbital, amobarbital (Amytal), phenobarbital, pentobarbital (Nembutal), secobarbital (Seconal), and butabarbital. These drugs were once widely prescribed for their sedative and hypnotic effects. However, many problems were associated with their use, and they have been the major cause of overdose death from accidental poisonings and suicide. They produce excessive drowsiness, even at therapeutic doses. Also, tolerance to them develops rapidly. Like alcohol, barbiturates are depressants that cause an initial response of euphoria. Thus they are popular street drugs. Barbiturate use leads to both physical and psychological dependence. The combination of alcohol and barbiturates produces a synergistic effect, meaning that either drug potentiates the effects of the other. For this reason, combinations of these drugs are particularly dangerous and can lead to accidental overdose and death. Despite these drawbacks, barbiturates are very useful for the treatment of epilepsy and general depressant withdrawal syndromes.

Benzodiazepines. In the 1960s benzodiazepines replaced barbiturates as the preferred treatment for anxiety and related disorders. This was based on the following three beliefs about these drugs:

- They would relieve anxiety without drowsiness.

- They had a wide therapeutic index (the difference between the therapeutic dose and the lethal dose).
- They were nonaddicting.

It is now known that benzodiazepines do cause drowsiness, although less than barbiturates. They are also addictive, causing both physical and psychological dependence. In addition, they lead to the same withdrawal symptoms as alcohol. Because benzodiazepines are longer acting, the symptoms are less intense and continue over a longer period. They are safer in terms of overdoses. Despite their drawbacks, they are still widely prescribed in the United States. The clinical uses of benzodiazepines are described in Chapter 28.

Stimulants. The stimulants have the ability to stimulate the CNS at many levels. The most common of these are the amphetamines and cocaine. People use these drugs for the feelings of euphoria, relief from fatigue, added energy, and alertness that they provide. The signs and symptoms of use, overdose, and withdrawal are basically the same for all drugs in this class (see Table 25-2).

Amphetamines. The amphetamine drugs include amphetamine, methamphetamine, dextroamphetamine, and benzphetamine. Amphetamines are thought to act by crowding norepinephrine and dopamine out of storage vesicles and into the synapse. The increase of these catecholamines at the receptors causes increased stimulation. It was once believed that amphetamines did not cause physical dependence, but clear patterns of tolerance and withdrawal have been described. Tolerance develops to the euphoria and the pleasant effects of these drugs but not to the wakefulness effects. Prolonged or excessive use of amphetamines can lead to psychosis, which is almost identical to paranoid schizophrenia.

In the 1950s and 1960s, amphetamines were widely prescribed for weight loss and relief of fatigue and depression. Their effectiveness for both conditions was only temporary and often led to dependency. In 1970 the FDA restricted the legal use of amphetamines to three types of conditions: narcolepsy, hyperkinetic behavior in children, and short-term weight reduction programs. Today it is clear that the abuse potential of amphetamines outweighs the benefit of their medical use for almost any reason. Safer treatments for these conditions have been found and are generally preferred.

Cocaine. Cocaine may be a drug of recent popularity, but it has been around for thousands of years. Cocaine is usually inhaled as a powder, injected intravenously, or smoked.

The form of cocaine that is smoked is produced by a process called freebasing. The "crack" form of freebase cocaine is produced by "cooking" street-grade cocaine in a baking soda solution. Its name is derived from the cracking sound it makes when it is smoked.

The euphoria caused by cocaine is short acting, starting with a 10- to 20-second rush and followed by 15 to 20 minutes of less intense euphoria. A person who is high on cocaine feels euphoric, energetic, self-confident, and sociable. Although cocaine was not initially thought to produce physical dependence, a pattern of withdrawal symptoms very similar to that seen in amphetamine users has been observed, beginning with intense craving and drug-seeking be-

Text continued on p. 496

Table **25-2**

Characteristics of Substances of Abuse

Substance	Route (most common first)	Common Street Names	Dependence: Physical/ Psychological	Use Signs and Symptoms of Class
DEPRESSANTS				
Alcohol	Ingestion	Booze, brew, juice, spirits	Yes/Yes	Depression of major brain functions such as mood, cognition, attention, concentration, insight, judgment, memory, affect, and emotional rapport in interpersonal relationships. Extent of depression is dose dependent and ranges from lethargy through anesthesia and death. Psychomotor impairment, increased reaction time, interruption of hand-eye coordination, motor ataxia, nystagmus. Decreased REM sleep leading to more dreams and sometimes nightmares.
Barbiturates	Ingestion, injection	Barbs, beans, black beauties, blue angels, candy, downers, goof balls, G.B., nebbies, reds, sleepers, yellow jackets, yellows	Yes/Yes	
Benzodiazepines	Ingestion, injection	Downers	Yes/Yes	
STIMULANTS				
Amphetamines	Ingestion, injection	A, AMT, bam, bennies, crystal, diet pills, dolls, eye-openers, lid poppers, pep pills, purple hearts, speed, uppers, wake-ups	Yes/Yes	Sudden rush of euphoria, abrupt awakening, increased energy, talkativeness, elation. Agitation, hyperactivity, irritability, grandiosity, pressured speech. Diaphoresis, anorexia, weight loss, insomnia. Increased temperature, blood pressure, and pulse. Tachycardia, ectopic heartbeats, chest pain. Urinary retention, constipation, dry mouth. *High dose:* Slurred, rapid, incoherent speech. Stereotypic movements, ataxic gait, teeth grinding, illogical thought processes, headache, nausea, vomiting. *Toxic psychosis:* Paranoid delusions in clear sensorium; auditory, visual, or tactile hallucinations. Very labile mood. Unprovoked violence.
Cocaine	Inhalation, smoking, injection, topical	Bernice, bernies, big C, blow, C, charlie, coke, dust, girl, heaven, jay, lady, nose candy, nose powder, snow, sugar, white lady. Crack = conan, freebase, rock, toke, white cloud, white tornado	Yes/Yes	

Overdose Signs and Symptoms of Class	Withdrawal Signs and Symptoms of Class	Special Considerations/Consequences of Use of Class
Unconsciousness, coma, respiratory depression, death.	*General depressant withdrawal syndrome:* Tremors, agitation, anxiety, diaphoresis, increased pulse and blood pressure, sleep disturbance, hallucinosis, seizures, delusions, delirium tremens (DTs) *High-dose sedative-hypnotic withdrawal:* For short-acting sedative hypnotics (including alcohol), symptoms begin between several hours to 1 day after the last dose and peak after 24 - 36 hours. For long-acting sedative hypnotics, symptoms peak after 5 - 8 days. *Low-dose sedative-hypnotic withdrawal:* Usually transient "symptom rebound" effects (anxiety, insomnia) for 1 - 2 weeks. May have more severe symptoms: perceptual hyperacusis, psychosis, cerebellar dysfunction, seizures. *Postacute (protracted) withdrawal:* Irritability, anxiety, insomnia, mood instability may occur for months.	Chronic alcohol use leads to serious disruptions in most organ systems: malnutrition and dehydration; vitamin deficiency leading to Wernicke's encephalopathy and alcoholic amnestic syndrome; impaired liver function, including hepatitis and cirrhosis; esophagitis, gastritis, pancreatitis; osteoporosis; anemia; peripheral neuropathy; impaired pulmonary function; cardiomyopathy; myopathy; disrupted immune system; and brain damage. High susceptibility to other dependencies. Dependence on barbiturates and benzodiazepines may develop insidiously; users may underreport the actual amount taken because of guilt about multiple prescriptions and abuse.
Seizures. Cardiac arrhythmias, coronary artery spasms, myocardial infarctions, marked increase in blood pressure and temperature that can lead to cardiovascular shock and death.	*Acute withdrawal (after periods of frequent high-dose use):* Intense and unpleasant feelings of depression and fatigue, and sometimes suicidal ideation. *Otherwise:* Milder symptoms of depression, anxiety, anhedonia, sleep disturbance, increased appetite, and psychomotor retardation, which decrease steadily over several weeks. Sometimes a user stops stimulants purposely to decrease tolerance, decreasing the amount needed to get high.	Certain amphetamines prescribed for attention deficit hyperactivity disorder in children because of a paradoxical depressant action. Sometimes these medications are stolen and abused. May be used alternately with depressants. Cocaine use may lead to multiple physical problems: destruction of the nasal septum related to snorting, coronary artery vasoconstriction, seizures, cerebrovascular accidents; transient ischemic episodes, sudden death related to respiratory arrest, and myocardial infarction. Intravenous use of stimulants may lead to the serious physical consequences described under Opiates.

Continued

Table 25-2

Characteristics of Substances of Abuse—cont'd

Substance	Route (most common first)	Common Street Names	Dependence: Physical/ Psychological	Use Signs and Symptoms of Class
OPIATES				
Heroin	Injection, ingestion, inhalation	H, horse, harry, boy, scag, shit, smack, stuff, white junk, white stuff	Yes/Yes	Euphoria, relaxation, relief from pain, "nodding out" (apathy, detachment from reality, impaired judgment, and drowsiness); constricted pupils, nausea, constipation, slurred speech, respiratory depression.
Morphine	Injection		Yes/Yes	
Meperidine	Injection, ingestion		Yes/Yes	
Codeine	Ingestion, injection		Yes/Yes	
Opium	Smoking, ingestion		Yes/Yes	
Methadone	Ingestion		Yes/Yes	
MARIJUANA				
	Smoking, ingestion	Acapulco gold, aunt mary, broccoli, dope, grass, grunt, hay, hemp, herb, J, joint, joy stick, killer weed, maryjane, pot, ragweed, reefer, smoke, weed	No/Yes	Altered state of awareness, relaxation, mild euphoria, reduced inhibition, red eyes, dry mouth, increased appetite, increased pulse, decreased reflexes, panic reaction.
HALLUCINOGENS				
	Ingestion, smoking	Acid, big D, blotter, blue heaven, cap, D, deeda, flash, L, mellow yellows, microdots, paper acid, sugar, ticket, yello		Distorted perceptions and hallucinations in the presence of a clear sensorium. Distortions of time and space, illusions, depersonalization, mystical experiences, heightened sense of awareness. Extreme mood lability. Tremor, dizziness, piloerection, paresthesias, synesthesia, nausea, and vomiting. Increased temperature, pulse, blood pressure, and salivation. Panic reaction, "bad trip."
LSD			No/No	
DMT			No/No	
Mescaline			No/No	
MDMA		Ecstacy	No/No	
PHENCYCLIDINE (PCP)				
	Smoking, ingestion	Angel dust, DOA, dust, elephant, hog, peace pill, supergrass, tic tac	No/No	Intensely psychotic experience characterized by bizarre perceptions, confusion, disorientation, euphoria, hallucinations, paranoia, grandiosity, agitation. Anesthesia. Apparent enhancement of strength and endurance. Rage reactions. May be agitated and hyperactive with tendency toward violence or catatonic and withdrawn or vacillate between the two conditions. Red, dry skin; dilated pupils, nystagmus, ataxia, hypertension, rigidity, and seizures.

Overdose Signs and Symptoms of Class	Withdrawal Signs and Symptoms of Class	Special Considerations/Consequences of Use of Class
Unconsciousness, coma, respiratory depression, circulatory depression, respiratory arrest, cardiac arrest, death. Anoxia can lead to brain abscess.	*Initially:* Drug craving lacrimation, rhinorrhea, yawning, diaphoresis. *In 12-72 hr:* Sleep disturbance, mydriasis, anorexia, piloerection, irritability, tremor, weakness, nausea, vomiting, diarrhea, chills, fever, muscle spasms, flushing, spontaneous ejaculation, abdominal pain, hypertension, increased rate and depth of respirations. *Protracted withdrawal:* Hypersensitivity to sensory stimuli, paresthesias, perceptual distortions, muscle pains, twitching tremors, headache, and sleep disturbances; tension, irritability, lack of energy, impaired concentration, derealization, and depersonalization. May last for several months.	Intravenous use leads to risk for infection with bloodborne pathogens, such as HIV or hepatitis B. Other infections (skin abscesses, phlebitis, cellulitis, and septic emboli causing pneumonia, pulmonary abscess, or subacute bacterial endocarditis) may occur as a result of lack of asepsis or contaminated substances. Chronic use leads to lack of concern about physical well-being, resulting in malnutrition and dehydration. Criminal behavior may occur to acquire money for drugs.
Toxic psychosis	No acute symptoms, but irritability and difficulty sleeping may last for a couple days.	Pulmonary problems. Interference with reproductive hormones. May cause fetal abnormalities.
Rare with LSD: convulsions, hyperthermia, death	None	Flashbacks may last for several months. Permanent psychosis may occur.
Seizures, coma, and death.	None	If flashbacks occur, they are mild and usually not disturbing.

Continued

Table **25-2**

Characteristics of Substances of Abuse—cont'd

Substance	Route (most common first)	Common Street Names	Dependence: Physical/ Psychological	Use Signs and Symptoms of Class
INHALANTS				
Gasoline Glue Aerosol sprays Paint thinner	Inhalation	Spray, rush, bolt, huffing, bagging, sniffing	Yes/Yes	*Psychological:* Belligerence, assaultiveness, apathy, impaired judgment. *Physical:* Dizziness, nystagmus, incoordination, slurred speech, unsteady gait, depressed reflexes, tremor, blurred vision, euphoria, anorexia.
Nicotine	Smoking, chewing, buccal	Cigarettes, cigars, bidis, kreteks, pipe tobacco, snuff, chewing tobacco	Yes/Yes	Feelings of pleasure, increased alertness, enhanced mental performance, increased heart rate, increased blood pressure, restricts blood flow to heart muscle.

havior. The relapse rate for patients who try to discontinue cocaine use is very high. Cocaine use has been known to result in sudden death.

Biochemically, cocaine blocks the reuptake of norepinephrine and dopamine. Because more neurotransmitter is present at the synapse, the receptors are continuously activated. It is believed that this causes the euphoria. At the same time, presynaptic supplies of dopamine and norepinephrine are depleted. This causes the "crash" that happens when the effect of the drug wears off.

Cocaine use has been glamorized by the publicity given to it by movie stars, sports figures, and other well-known people. This makes it particularly inviting to adolescents who regard famous people as role models.

Addiction to barbiturates ("downers") and stimulants ("uppers"), particularly the amphetamines, often occurs simultaneously. Sometimes a patient who has been using downers develops a need for uppers to provide enough energy to function. The next clinical example illustrates this pattern. Ms. W's pattern is not uncommon. Aside from street use, many people slip into drug abuse without being aware of the consequences of their behavior.

 CLINICAL EXAMPLE

Ms. W was a 34-year-old woman who was moderately overweight. She had tried various diets on her own with little success. A friend told her about a "diet doctor" who had a reputation for helping his patients lose weight with minimum deprivation. Ms. W decided to see the physician and was accepted for treatment. She was given a diuretic and appetite depressant medication. The latter contained amphetamines. She began to lose weight as soon as she started the prescribed regimen and was delighted. She also liked the additional burst of energy she felt every time she took her medication. She completed projects that she had been planning to work on for months. However, her family began to complain because she was irritable and very restless. In addition, she developed insomnia and roamed about the house at night.

On the urging of her husband, she went to her family physician. She felt guilty about seeing another physician for her weight problem, so did not tell her regular physician about this. With the history of insomnia, irritability, and recent weight loss, her physician thought she might be depressed. He ordered an antidepressant medication and a barbiturate sedative. Ms. W soon found that she was able to sleep well with her sedative. However, she felt slightly hung over in the morning and still wanted to lose more weight, so she continued with her diet pills as well. For a while she was able to function well. Gradually, however, she found that she needed two sedatives, and then she also began to use extra stimulants. Her husband questioned her drug use. Ms. W had read about drug abuse and with her husband's help identified that she had a problem. She decided to see her family physician again and this time told him the whole story. He then advised a brief hospitalization so that she could be withdrawn from both drugs under medical supervision. Ms. W was very embarrassed by her addiction. While in the hospital, she needed a great deal of nursing support to integrate this experience.

Selected Nursing Diagnoses

- Ineffective individual coping related to dependence on stimulants and depressants, as evidenced by inability to function without the drugs and the development of tolerance

Overdose Signs and Symptoms of Class	Withdrawal Signs and Symptoms of Class	Special Considerations/Consequences of Use of Class
Lethargy, stupor/coma, respiratory arrest, cardiac arrhythmia.	Symptoms similar to alcohol withdrawal.	Death from inhalants can occur in different ways: • Sudden death is caused by cardiac arrhythmia—sometimes this happens the first time the child uses inhalants. • Suicide may be a result of impaired judgment. Injury: Under the influence of inhalants, youth feel invulnerable. Burns and frostbite can also be caused by these chemicals. Permanent cognitive impairment may require an individual to reside in a structured setting.
N/A	Anger, anxiety, depressed mood, difficulty concentrating—all of which subside within 3-4 weeks; increased appetite and craving for nicotine, which may persist for months.	Smoking by pregnant women contributes to low birth weight, increased incidence of stillborn, and premature babies.

- Altered role performance related to drug dependence, as evidenced by family concern over her behavior
- Altered nutrition, more than body requirements, related to repeated dieting failures, as evidenced by seeking out a doctor who would help her lose weight with minimal deprivation

Opiates. The opiates include opium, heroin, meperidine, morphine, codeine, and methadone. Meperidine, morphine, and codeine are commonly used analgesics. Methadone is used to treat addiction to other opiates. It can be used either to aid withdrawal or to provide maintenance at a stable dose. It is useful because it does not interfere with the ability to function productively, as other narcotics do. Patients taking a maintenance dose of methadone may work and live normally, although still addicted to narcotics.

Opiate use is less widespread than depressant or stimulant use but is still a serious social problem. Although some people use opiates for years with few problems, people with opiate addiction often deteriorate mentally and physically until they are unable to function productively. Illegal behavior, such as stealing or prostitution to acquire money for drugs, may result from addiction. Obtaining and using drugs becomes an all-consuming passion.

One characteristic of narcotic addiction is the development of tolerance, which also increases the expense of the habit. Physiological effects of narcotics are included in Table 25-2.

The most important psychological response to opiate use is euphoria, or feeling high. This powerful, pleasurable response causes the person to use the drug repeatedly, leading to addiction. Other psychological effects of narcotics include apathy, detachment from reality, and impaired judgment. The phrase "nodding out" describes this group of behaviors combined with drowsiness. The next clinical example demonstrates the behaviors associated with opiate abuse.

 CLINICAL EXAMPLE

Mr. C was a 35-year-old man who had been jailed for auto theft. He was believed to be a member of a large ring of automobile thieves in a major metropolitan area. His arrest record included several episodes of armed robbery and breaking and entering. A few hours after he had been jailed, Mr. C complained of abdominal cramps and appeared very anxious. His nose and eyes were running, there were beads of perspiration on his brow, and he was rocking back and forth on his bunk. The guard called Ms. V, the correctional health nurse.

Ms. V observed Mr. C and performed a brief physical assessment. She noted that his pupils were dilated, his blood pressure was elevated, and he had gooseflesh. In addition, there were multiple needle tracks on his arms. She asked him directly about drug use, and he admitted that he had been addicted to heroin. He stated that his addiction began in 1967 while he was stationed with the army in Vietnam. When he returned to the United States, he remained in the army for 18 months and was able to stop using drugs altogether. He planned to get a job and attend school after leaving the service. He related that he was disturbed by the attitude of people toward Vietnam veterans. While he was still in the service, he was able to use peer support to cope with his feelings. However, after his discharge, he was reluctant to talk about his military experience. Others seemed disinterested, embarrassed, or hostile when he talked about it.

Mr. C had difficulty finding a civilian job. He was an artillery specialist in the army and found that it was difficult to apply this experience. He began to have nightmares and flashbacks of his combat experiences. Because of the anxiety associated with this, he returned to drugs. Without a job, he used illegal means to finance his habit and therefore repeatedly went to jail.

Ms. V discussed Mr. C's problem with the physician in the prison health department. They decided to assess Mr. C's eligibility for a methadone drug treatment program and to request consultation from a counselor at the local veterans counseling center.

Selected Nursing Diagnoses

- Ineffective individual coping related to inability to obey the law, as evidenced by repeated arrests
- Altered role performance related to difficulty adjusting to civilian life, as evidenced by inability to find a job or seek out peer support
- Social isolation related to unresolved stressful military experiences, as evidenced by reliance on drugs rather than people
- Risk for violence directed at others, related to compelling need for drugs, as evidenced by history of armed robbery

---

Withdrawal from narcotics is extremely uncomfortable but is not usually life threatening. Overdosage of narcotics, on the other hand, is very dangerous. It can rapidly lead to coma, respiratory depression, and death. Accidental overdoses among narcotic addicts sometimes occur, particularly because the user is uncertain of the drug's strength. Drugs are usually cut with inert (and sometimes toxic) substances before they are sold, resulting in the availability of varied strengths on the streets.

Natural opiates. In 1975 natural substances that acted very much like morphine were isolated in the brain. It was later learned that these biochemicals, known as endorphins or enkephalins, were neurotransmitters that bond with opiate receptors in the brain and pituitary gland. Release of these "natural opiates" results in a feeling of euphoria. This understanding has led to a theory of drug cravings: When large amounts of artificial opiates are taken over a long period, the brain responds by cutting off production of endorphins in an attempt to restore homeostasis. As the artificial opiates leave the system, there are no natural opiates to take their place. This deprivation is experienced as craving. Details of these mechanisms continue to be studied.

Marijuana. Marijuana is sometimes classified as a hallucinogenic drug, but it rarely causes hallucinations. It causes sedation, but is not primarily a CNS depressant. The active ingredient in marijuana is tetrahydrocannabinol (THC). The marijuana cigarette can be smoked as it is or through a water-pipe, or "bong," to cool the hot vapors. Marijuana generally produces an altered state of awareness accompanied by a feeling of relaxation and mild euphoria. Effects depend on the potency of the drug, as well as the setting and the experience of the user. Strength can vary widely from 1% to 30%.

Prolonged use may lead to apathy, lack of energy, loss of desire to work or be productive, diminished concentration,

poor personal hygiene, and preoccupation with marijuana. This cluster of symptoms is known as the **amotivational syndrome.** Although study findings are controversial, there seems to be general support for the existence of such a syndrome. Use of very large doses can lead to a toxic psychosis that clears as the substance is eliminated from the body. Marijuana may also precipitate psychosis when used by schizophrenics, whose symptoms are otherwise controlled with antipsychotic drugs. It does not appear to lead to psychosis in nonschizophrenic people.

The main physiological effects of marijuana are mild (see Table 25-2). Tolerance develops in heavy users, but there is no withdrawal pattern. Marijuana has been reported to have medicinal benefits in alleviating glaucoma as well as the nausea and vomiting associated with chemotherapy used in cancer treatment. However, its effectiveness for these purposes is controversial. It appears at best to have no greater efficacy than drugs already on the market. Thus its use for medicinal purposes has been limited legally in the United States.

> *Supporters of legalization of marijuana say that the penalties are too severe for the behavior and that marijuana is no more harmful than legal substances such as alcohol and nicotine. What is your position on the legalization of marijuana?*

Hallucinogens. Drugs that create experiences very similar to those typical of a psychotic state have been called **hallucinogens,** although they generally produce perceptual distortions, not true hallucinations. They have also been called psychedelic or mind-revealing drugs. LSD, peyote, mescaline, and psilocybin are commonly used hallucinogens, with LSD being the most commonly used.

LSD is generally swallowed. It is colorless and tasteless and is often added to a drink or food, such as a sugar cube. It may be given to a person without that person knowing. Pleasurable effects of hallucinogen use include intensification of sensory experiences. Colors are described as more brilliant, and sounds, smells, and tastes are heightened. Sometimes users of these drugs report synesthesia, or a crossover of sensory experiences during which music may be seen or colors may be heard. Space and time are distorted.

The hallucinogens do not appear to cause physical dependence, but tolerance develops if they are used regularly. Hallucinogens also lead to self-destructive behavior because they cause impaired judgment. Vulnerable people who take these drugs may experience "bad trips," sometimes resulting in psychotic episodes. They may experience paranoid, grandiose, or somatic delusions, usually accompanied by vivid hallucinations. The hallucinatory experience may be pleasant or frightening. Patients who are psychotic are not in contact with reality and often misinterpret environmental events. They may be unable to attend to any of their biological needs and may inadvertently hurt themselves or others in response to hallucinations or while trying to escape from the frightening experience. Because there is no physical dependence, withdrawal symptoms do not occur. Usually there is a gradual decrease in psychotic behavior, although the patient may have flashbacks for several months. These brief recurrences of the hallucinogenic experience can be frightening. Patients often express the fear that they are crazy and will never be free of the after effects of the drug.

> *A college classmate who is not a nursing major tells you that she overheard her 12-year-old brother talking with a friend about "doing microdots." You suspect that he was talking about LSD. What would you advise her to do?*

PCP. As a street drug, PCP (phencyclidine) may be ingested, but it is often smoked in a mixture with another substance, such as marijuana. Severity of symptoms are dose dependent. At low doses (less than 5 mg) the user experiences a euphoric, floating feeling, along with heightened emotionality and incoordination. Distorted perceptions such as objects floating or growing in size, inability to judge distance, or feelings of being outside one's body are common. At higher doses, PCP use may precipitate an intensely psychotic experience characterized by extreme agitation. Patients may become violent toward themselves or others. Because the drug is an anesthetic, PCP-intoxicated people feel little or no pain and may pound their heads into a wall or strike out violently, causing serious injury to themselves or others. Physical manifestations of PCP intoxication are noted in Table 25-2.

PCP may cause or exacerbate a previously controlled psychosis. The unpredictability of the reaction to PCP makes it an extremely dangerous drug.

Inhalants. There are approximately 1400 products that can be inhaled. The most common inhalants include butane (lighter fluid), gas, air fresheners, rubber cement, correction fluid, and nitrous oxide (whippets). It is estimated that approximately 21% of eighth graders in the United States have used inhalants at least once in their lives. Children and adolescents choose inhalants as a means of obtaining a high because of the quality of the high, the rapid onset of the effect, the low cost, and the ease of availability.

The nurse must be alert to the physical indicators of inhalant abuse when completing an assessment. These signs include residue from paint, glue, or substances noted on the clothes, hands, or face, especially around the nose. Youth may also have symptoms of a cold, such as a runny nose, or pimples or sores around the mouth. These are caused by the abrasive effect of the chemicals on the skin. Finally, it is essential that nurses take a leadership role in educating children and adults about the nature of inhalant abuse.

> *You are working as a nurse in a local high school in which a 15-year-old student recently died while inhaling butane. The principal approaches you requesting that students not be told that inhalants were involved in the death because it might "give other students ideas." How would you respond?*

Nicotine. Nicotine is the active substance found in cigarettes, cigars, pipe tobacco, snuff, bidis (small brown cigarettes with up to 7 times the nicotine of regular cigarettes),

and kreteks (clove cigarettes that anesthetize the throat thus promoting deeper inhalation). It is both a stimulant and a depressant. Because smoke is a lung irritant, a person must learn how to inhale and must adjust to the body's natural rejection of this substance. Once inhaled, the nicotine in tobacco is readily absorbed into the blood stream and has an almost immediate effect on the reward systems in the brain.

Caffeine. Caffeine is the active ingredient in coffee, tea, and many carbonated beverages. It is also found in substances such as chocolate. Major effects of use are increased alertness and increased blood pressure. Overuse can cause jitteriness. Although caffeine increases alertness, it does not affect the dopaminergic brain structures related to reward, motivation, and addiction, as do the drugs of abuse and nicotine. Therefore, it is not addictive. However, heavy use of caffeine can lead to withdrawal symptoms, a sign of physical dependence. These symptoms include headache, sleepiness, fatigue, problems in attention and concentration, and decreased vigor. They are generally transient and mild, with relatively little interference in a person's daily life. However, the presence of theses withdrawal symptoms may be the main factor for the continued use of the substance (Nehlig, 1999).

Co-Dependence. When the term **co-dependency** was first coined in 1979, it referred to people who had become dysfunctional as a result of living in a committed relationship with an alcoholic. It was said that the alcoholic was addicted to the bottle, and the co-dependent was addicted to the alcoholic. The major focus was initially on the spouse of the alcoholic.

The concept is really not a new one. Al-Anon was created in the 1930s specifically to help family members of alcoholics cope with their own problems that stem from living with an alcoholic. However, the co-dependency movement stresses the lasting effects of growing up in an alcoholic home. Adult children of alcoholics (ACOA) are believed to share certain characteristics as adults because they all struggled to survive the chaos of growing up with an alcoholic parent. The major aspects of the condition are:

- Overinvolvement with a dysfunctional person
- Obsessive attempts to control the dysfunctional person's behavior
- A strong need for approval from others
- Constantly making personal sacrifices to help the dysfunctional person be "cured" of the problem behavior

As the movement has grown, however, the definition has broadened to include almost anyone who has had anything to do with a dysfunctional person, either while growing up or as an adult. Anyone who can identify with the laundry list of symptoms associated with co-dependency (most notably low self-esteem, need to please others, and over-responsibility for others) can identify with the term.

The positive aspect of this movement is that it may allow many people who are unhappy with themselves to reframe their life situation and improve their functioning in very significant ways, with or without formal counseling. In fact, many people who otherwise would never have recognized their own dysfunction identify with the characteristics of co-dependency and are motivated to seek specific counseling and self-help groups.

ACOA and co-dependency self-help groups, based on the 12-step recovery program of AA, have sprung up all over the country. Dozens of self-help books have been published by people who self-identify with the concept and who offer recommendations about how to recover from it. Clinicians have also developed specific recovery programs for co-dependents. The negative side of the movement is that some people use the label to blame problems on current or past relationships without taking responsibility for their own part in the process.

Despite the popularity of this movement, there is no evidence to support the existence of a clinical syndrome distinct for ACOA. A number of studies have shown that adults raised in alcoholic homes share many characteristics with adults raised in nonalcoholic but otherwise seriously dysfunctional homes. Furthermore, symptoms of adults raised in dysfunctional alcoholic or nonalcoholic homes vary from none to very severe. Thus, the environment, family system, and individual all must be assessed when working with ACOA (Brown & Schmid, 1999).

Whether a clearly identifiable and unique syndrome exists or not, it is easy to understand how children who grow up in alcoholic homes can develop low self-esteem. As an adult this is often expressed in a preoccupation with the lives, feelings, and problems of others. Although co-dependents want their loved ones to stop drinking or using drugs, their behavior may have the opposite effect and enable the person to continue drug or alcohol use.

The nurse may observe some of these behaviors in family members of substance-dependent patients, in the patients themselves, or in nurses and other professionals. Simple questions to family members about efforts they have made to try to control the addict's use may uncover the pattern. Questions to patients about relationships with others may indicate that growing up in an alcoholic home may have contributed to their own substance abuse problem. Listening to colleagues talk about their family and friends may reveal similar patterns in their relationships. Nurses tend to find great satisfaction in caring for others. When this behavior is the person's only source of self-esteem, it is done at the expense of personal health and welfare. It takes on a compulsive quality that is evidence of co-dependence.

Dual Diagnosis

A patient may have a substance use disorder, a psychiatric disorder, or both concurrently. The types of relationships between substance use and psychiatric disorders are listed in Box 25-5. One can precede and cause the other, such as when the alcoholic becomes severely depressed or when the depressed person uses alcohol to treat the depression. It is often impossible to distinguish the two disorders, especially early in the assessment process. To complicate matters further, substance abuse may cause psychiatric symptoms such as hallucinations or paranoia, even though the person has no separate psychiatric diagnosis. Therefore, assessment of peo-

ple with potential co-existing conditions is best done in the following three stages (Drake et al, 1996b):

1. Detection
2. Diagnostic assessment
3. Specialized assessment

Because substance use problems are so common among psychiatric patients, mental health clinicians should routinely assess all patients for these problems.

Detection of substance abuse in patients with psychiatric illness is most effective when multiple instruments or types of assessment are used. A combination of interview, screening tools, information from collateral sources, and laboratory tests including urine drug screens should be used. **Diagnostic assessment** is done according to *DSM–IV–TR* criteria. However, the nurse should be aware that psychiatric patients may be especially vulnerable to small amounts of substances. For example, even small amounts of cocaine may precipitate a psychotic episode in a patient with schizophrenia. **Specialized assessment** can follow the more general diagnostic assessment to obtain more detailed information necessary for treatment planning. The special problems posed by patients who are dually diagnosed can be seen in the following clinical example.

 CLINICAL EXAMPLE

Robbie is a 25-year-old, single, white male who began using alcohol and drugs at age 16, around the time he dropped out of school. He continued to live with his mother and spent most of his time in his room, although there were long periods of time when

---

Box 25-5

Relationships between Substance Use and Psychiatric Disorders

- Substance use may be causing the psychopathology (a substance-induced mental disorder). This is the most common situation. Some of the more common substance-induced disorders are alcohol-induced depressive disorders, cocaine-induced psychotic disorders, and stimulant-induced anxiety disorders.
- Substance use may be secondary to the psychopathology in various ways:
- Patients may use substances to self-medicate the symptoms of their mental disorder (for example, alcohol may be used to try to alleviate the symptoms of an anxiety disorder, such as social phobia).
- Patients may use substances to enhance symptoms of the mental disorder (as in the use of stimulants by manic patients).
- Patients may use substances in an attempt to counter side effects of medications that they are taking for a mental disorder (for example, a patient with schizophrenia may use cocaine in an attempt to counter neuroleptic side effects).
- The mental disorder and the substance-use problems may be coincidental and not related to each other.

From Miele G, Trautman K, Hasin D: Assessing comorbid mental and substance-use disorders: a guide for clinical practice, *J Pract Psychiatry Behav Health* 2:272, 1996.

she did not know where he was. His mother reported that he increasingly isolated himself and acted so strangely that others did not feel comfortable around him.

Over the next couple of years, Robbie's behavior became increasingly bizarre until one day his mother observed him pacing, talking to himself, saying strange and threatening things aloud, and pounding his fists together. She obtained an emergency petition, and the police took him to the emergency room for an evaluation. He was diagnosed with schizophrenia, stabilized with medication, and returned to his mother's home with an appointment for outpatient follow-up. However, he did not return to the clinic, stopped taking his medication, and was rehospitalized 1 month later. This time, he was prescribed fluphenazine (Prolixin) and promised to return to the clinic as scheduled in 2 weeks. He seemed to do well for a few days until he resumed drinking and smoking marijuana. He disappeared for several weeks, then was found by his mother wandering the city streets, dirty, unkempt, reeking of alcohol, and talking to himself again. During the subsequent rehospitalization, he admitted also using cocaine and heroin occasionally. He was referred to AA and assigned to a social worker, who helped him to obtain social services.

Soon he was getting a disability check every month, which exacerbated his problems. Every month he cashed his check as soon as he got it and went on a binge of drug and alcohol use until his money was gone, usually in about 1 week. Unable to afford such heavy use for the remainder of the month, Robbie approached people on the streets and demanded money. Eventually, he was picked up by the police for aggressive panhandling. By the time he was 24, Robbie was well-known by the police and emergency rooms in town. He'd been hospitalized at least a dozen times and arrested for numerous petty crimes. His mother, doctor, and social worker were totally exasperated by his failure to comply. When the new Dual Diagnosis Clinic opened in the Mental Health Center, Robbie was one of the first referrals.

Predisposing Factors

Several models or etiological factors have been proposed for substance abuse. Belief in a particular model influences the assessment and intervention. Awareness of the differences between these models helps the nurse understand why patients, as well as other professionals, hold many different views about substance abuse treatment. Much research has been conducted concerning the factors that predispose a person to becoming chemically dependent. These factors may be biological, psychological, or sociocultural.

Biological. A key biological factor is the tendency of substance abuse to run in families. Most genetic research has focused on alcoholism, but there is a growing body of knowledge on the genetics of other drugs of abuse as well. There is much evidence from adoption, twin, and animal studies that heredity is significant in the development of alcoholism. Some research has identified subtypes of alcoholism that differ in inheritability. One type of alcoholism is associated with an early onset, inability to abstain, and an antisocial personality. This type appears to be limited to

males and is primarily genetic in origin. Another type tends to be associated with onset after age 25, inability to stop drinking once started, and a passive-dependent personality. This type seems to be influenced much more by the environment. However, there is controversy in the field as to whether such subtypes actually exist and with regard to the precise nature of their characteristics.

The discovery in 1990 that the A1 allele of the DRD2 gene appeared to be associated with alcoholism gave rise to much genetic research over the next decade. There is also some evidence that the DRD2 gene is associated with other substance abuse disorders as well (Anthenelli & Schuckit, 1998; Nobel, 1998). It is theorized that these genetic abnormalities block feelings of well-being. This results in a tendency toward anxiety, anger, low self-esteem, and other negative feelings as well as a craving for a substance that will take the bad feelings away. People with such a disorder need alcohol or some other psychoactive drug just to feel "normal." These genetic findings are only one of many predisposing factors in the etiology of substance abuse. It is important to understand that a larger role appears to be played by environmental factors and still unidentified genes.

> *If genetic factors are clearly identified as major influences on the development of alcoholism in some people, what ethical issues are likely to be debated?*

Biological differences in the response to alcohol may also influence susceptibility. For example, many Asian people experience a physiological response to alcohol including flushing, tachycardia, and an intense feeling of discomfort. This appears to be related to the tendency for Asians to have a genetically inactive form of the enzyme aldehyde dehydrogenase. This leads to a buildup of the toxic substance acetaldehyde, an alcohol metabolite, which causes the symptoms. This response may help explain why Asian-Americans have the lowest level of alcohol consumption and alcohol-related problems of the major racial and ethnic groups in the United States.

Psychological. Many psychological theories have attempted to explain the factors that predispose people to developing substance abuse. Psychoanalytic theories see alcoholics as fixated at the oral stage of development, thus seeking need satisfaction through oral behaviors such as drinking. Behavior or learning theories view addictive behaviors as overlearned, maladaptive habits that can be examined and changed in the same way as other habits. Cognitive theories suggest that addiction is based on a distorted way of thinking about substance use. Family system theory emphasizes the pattern of relationships between family members through the generations as an explanation for substance abuse. Belief in any particular theory influences assessment and treatment.

Clinicians have observed a link between substance abuse and several psychological traits such as depression, anxiety, antisocial personality, and dependent personality. There is little evidence that these psychological problems existed before or caused substance abuse. It is just as likely that they resulted from drug and alcohol use and dependence.

Many studies have tried to find common personality traits among people addicted to alcohol or drugs. No addictive personality has been identified. Studies show a wide variety of personality types among alcoholics. Observed personality patterns result from the effects of the alcohol or drug on previously normal psychological functions, combined with ineffective responses to these effects.

Another theory of substance abuse focuses on the human tendency to seek pleasure and avoid pain or stress. Drugs create pleasure and reduce physical or psychological pain. Because pain returns when the effect of the drug wears off, the person is powerfully attracted to repeated drug use. It has been suggested that some people are more sensitive to the euphoric effects of drugs and are more likely to repeat their use. This repeated drug use leads to more problems and initiates the downhill spiral of substance use.

Some substance abusers have psychological problems related to childhood experiences. Many have histories of childhood physical or sexual abuse. Most have low self-esteem and difficulty expressing emotions. These problems may have influenced the initial use of drugs and progression into dependence.

Sociocultural. Several sociocultural factors influence a person's choice whether to use drugs, which drugs to use, and how much to use. Attitudes, values, norms, and sanctions differ according to nationality, religion, gender, family background, and social environment. Assessment of these factors is necessary to understand the whole person. Combinations of factors may make a person more susceptible to drug abuse and interfere with recovery.

Nationality and ethnicity influence alcohol use patterns. For example, it has been found that northern Europeans have higher alcoholism rates than southern Europeans. Values may influence the way in which addiction is viewed. Some believe that addiction results from moral weakness or lack of willpower. Unfortunately, a moralistic approach may cause the person to feel guilty, often resulting in drinking to alleviate the guilt.

Formal religious belief can also affect drinking behavior. Members of religions that discourage the use of alcohol have much lower rates of alcohol use and alcoholism than members of those that accept or encourage its use. Of the major religious groups in the United States, Roman Catholics have the highest rate of alcoholism and Jews the lowest. During assessment, however, the nurse should not assume certain use or nonuse patterns related to ethnic or religious factors.

Gender differences also have been noted in the prevalence of substance abuse. Research is needed to determine the influence of biological as opposed to sociocultural reasons for this. However, powerful gender-related cultural factors help shape substance-using behaviors. There is much less acceptance of female alcoholism, which is often hidden. Women tend to deny having a drinking problem even longer than men do. In the United States more women than men abuse prescription drugs, such as diazepam. This is more socially acceptable and sometimes even encouraged. In contrast, use of antianxiety drugs is viewed as weak and unmasculine, whereas the ability to drink large amounts of alcohol is considered manly.

Finally, sociocultural factors influence drug use, abuse, and treatment. Multiple social crises can contribute to the risk for drug abuse in poor neighborhoods. Affordable and decent housing and shelter are difficult to find. Job opportunities are limited, and many jobs are low paying. Social programs often inadvertently foster development of single-parent families. The dropout rate in inner-city schools is high, and advanced education is difficult to obtain. Living in neighborhoods dominated by these problems, along with poor health-care access, crime, and violence, creates vulnerability to the escape some people find in drugs and alcohol. However, it is important to recognize that the majority of people living in these circumstances are not addicted to drugs, which supports the belief that many factors influence the development of drug use patterns.

 What sociocultural factors have you observed that encourage the use of drugs and alcohol?

Precipitating Stressors

Withdrawal. If a person becomes physically dependent on a substance, substance abuse may continue simply to avoid withdrawal symptoms. The person may no longer get much effect from the substance other than its ability to prevent withdrawal. Symptoms of withdrawal from specific drugs of abuse are listed in Table 25-2. There is debate as to whether drug cravings also should be considered part of the withdrawal syndrome. However they are categorized, it is clear that the emergence of withdrawal symptoms and cravings together serve as powerful precipitating stressors for continued drug use.

General depressant drug withdrawal. Withdrawal from all depressant drugs (including alcohol) is similar and sometimes is referred to as the **general depressant withdrawal syndrome.** The main difference in the time course of symptoms depends on the half life of the particular drug. The main difference in the severity of symptoms depends on the drug dose and length of use. For example, substances with short half-lives, such as alcohol and the short-acting benzodiazepines and barbiturates, lead to earlier appearance of withdrawal symptoms and a shorter withdrawal syndrome. The shorter-acting drugs are considered to be more addictive because the effect is quicker. However, these drugs also leave the system more quickly, increasing the chance of withdrawal.

Prescribed depressants/sedative-hypnotics withdrawal. The use of depressants at higher-than-therapeutic doses for more than 1 month can produce physical dependence and can result in "high dose withdrawal syndrome." Symptoms may peak within 24 hours for the short-acting drugs but take as long as 8 days for long-acting ones. Patients who have taken regular, therapeutic doses of sedative-hypnotics for at least 4 months (or less with higher doses) may experience a "low dose withdrawal syndrome" when the dosage is decreased or discontinued. These effects may be due to an intensified return of the symptoms for which the drug was prescribed in the first place, a phenomenon called **symptom rebound**. Although many patients have no or mild symptoms after cessation of therapeutic doses, a few may experience a more severe syndrome.

Alcohol withdrawal. When a large amount of alcohol is ingested, unpleasant symptoms usually occur. If overindulgence is short-lived, symptoms are caused by the direct effect of alcohol on body cells. This results in headache and stomach and intestinal distress—the typical hangover. However, if heavy drinking occurs over a long time, a decrease in blood alcohol level may cause symptoms of withdrawal. Alcohol sedates the CNS. When alcohol is withdrawn, the symptoms resemble a rebound reaction in the CNS. Fig. 25-3 presents information on the alcohol withdrawal syndrome (Mayo-Smith et al, 1998).

Neurobiology. Most abused drugs interact with specific nerve cell receptors, either imitating or blocking the actions of normally working neurotransmitters in the brain. Heroin and other opiates, for example, activate opioid receptors that normally respond to the brain's natural opioid-like neurotransmitters (such as endorphin, enkephalin, and dynorphin). Alcohol both activates some receptors (for the neurotransmitter GABA) and blocks others (for the neurotransmitter glutamate). In contrast, cocaine and other stimulants block the reuptake of various neurotransmitters, including dopamine, serotonin, and norepinephrine, with the effect of prolonging the action of these brain chemicals on target cells.

Other aspects of neurobiology account for the reinforcing and addicting aspects of drugs of abuse. The mesolimbic dopamine system is a pathway in the brain that originates from dopamine-producing cells in the brainstem and targets higher regions of the brain (see Chapter 6). This brain pathway regulates natural drives such as the desire for food, drink, and sex. Taking drugs of abuse repeatedly produces long-lasting changes in these areas of the brain, leading to the negative feelings during withdrawal and strong drug cravings. They also produce cognitive changes, making the risk of relapse over many years and even a lifetime quite high.

Most drugs also inhibit the cAMP (cyclic adenosine monophosphate) pathway, which is an intracellular messenger system. cAMP is one of the chemicals within target cells that can either be activated or inhibited when a neurotransmitter locks into a receptor. Most drugs of abuse inhibit the cAMP response, and this is thought to contribute to the reinforcing actions of the drugs. As the person continues to use drugs, the brain cells try to compensate for the lack of cAMP by making more cAMP and other molecules involved with its action. This is what leads to drug tolerance. Due to changes in gene expression, the brain cells continue to overproduce cAMP, which leads to withdrawal symptoms, such as dysphoria and lack of motivation. These unpleasant feelings are countered by taking more drug, thus leading to drug dependence. With chronic drug exposure, certain other nerve cells become more excitable, making the drug user more sensitive to the drugs or to conditioned cues associated with drug exposure, or even to stress. This sensitization is thought to be a powerful factor in drug relapse and thus a powerful precipitating stressor for the continued use of drugs (Nestler & Aghajanian, 1997).

Appraisal of Stressors

The reasons a person initiates use of substances vary widely. Curiosity, desire to be grown up, desire to rebel against authority, peer pressure, desire to ease the pains of living, desire to feel good—all of these are stressors and may apply. If

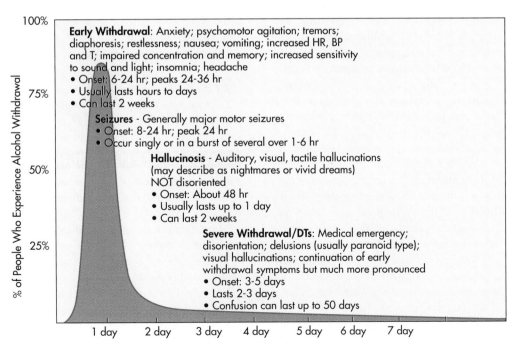

Fig. 25-3 Alcohol withdrawal syndrome.

use of the substance brings about the desired effects, then use is likely to continue. As the amount and frequency of substance use increase, so do the perceived stressors, which lead to more use. If substance use becomes associated with relief from emotional and social pain in the person's mind, then these stressors will lead to more substance use. Perceiving the substance as the answer to these problems, the person fails to develop healthier coping mechanisms. Gradually it takes more and more of the substance to get the same effect.

Coping Resources

Comprehensive assessment of a patient with a substance abuse problem must include assessment of the personal, social, and material assets available to the person. Assessment of motivation and social supports is particularly important. What is the patient's motivation to change the substance use pattern? It could be that the patient is sick and tired of being sick and tired, or may have been ordered to complete a treatment program after receiving a DWI charge. What social supports does the patient have? Family, friends, and coworkers may be available for support, or the patient may be homeless and have no family or friends. What is the status of the patient's health? The health status may be perfect, or the patient may have hepatitis, AIDS, or other complications of abuse. What social skills does the patient have? Some patients are very adept in social interactions, and some are withdrawn, quiet, and isolated. Patients may or may not have developed problem-solving skills in other areas of their lives. They may or may not have other social, material, and economic assets to support recovery. They may or may not have intellectual skills and personality traits that contribute to positive change.

Coping Mechanisms

Although the patient may have used substances in response to certain stressors, the substance use may have escalated to the point in which it has become an additional stressor. Patients who use problem-focused coping mechanisms will take responsibility for the substance-use problem and either find ways to change or seek help in doing so. These are constructive coping mechanisms. Patients may also use destructive coping mechanisms, such as when they change the meaning of the substance-abuse problem so that it becomes a nonproblem, saying that there is no problem ("It's just the thing to do") or devaluing a desired object ("I didn't want that job anyway"). Patients may also try to decrease emotional stress by minimization of the extent of use ("I only had a couple of beers") or the consequences of use ("We don't fight about it too much"), denial ("I don't have a problem. I can quit anytime I want"), and rationalization ("If you had the problems I have, you'd drink, too"). It is impossible in the initial assessment to sort out the facts from the distortions caused by these coping mechanisms. This is one reason why assessment is an ongoing process. Information from collateral sources and continued observation of behavior over time are essential.

NURSING DIAGNOSIS

After completion of the nursing assessment, the nurse synthesizes the data regarding the patient's drinking or drug use behavior. Using the Stuart Stress Adaptation Model (Fig. 25-4) and the NANDA classification system, appropriate nursing diagnoses are identified.

Addiction problems are very complex. They affect nearly every aspect of the patient's functioning. The nurse should be sure that the nursing diagnoses selected reflect the whole person. At least 27 nursing diagnoses are common in addiction nursing practice, which can be grouped into four categories: biological, cognitive, psychosocial, and spiritual (American Nurses' Association & National Nurses' Society of Addictions, 1988). Nursing diagnoses related to chemically mediated responses and medical diagnoses for substance-related disorders are listed in the Medical and Nursing Diagnoses box on p. 506. The primary NANDA diagnoses include **sensory-perceptual alteration, altered thought processes, ineffective individual coping,** and **altered family processes.** Examples of complete nursing diagnoses are presented in the Detailed Diagnoses box on p. 507.

Related Medical Diagnoses

Disorders that are related to substance abuse are included in *DSM–IV–TR* in two ways. First, diagnoses that are primarily related to alcohol or drug use are categorized as substance-related disorders. The essential features of these are presented in the Detailed Diagnoses box. A patient with a substance-related disorder who is also diagnosed with another Axis I psychiatric disorder is considered to be dually diagnosed.

Second, if substance-induced intoxication or withdrawal is associated with another type of mental disorder, the diagnosis is located in the substance-induced category. For example, if a person is depressed related to alcohol withdrawal, the medical diagnosis would be substance-induced (withdrawal) mood disorder. The categories that include substance-induced diagnoses are delirium, dementia, amnestic, psychotic, mood, anxiety, sex, and sleep.

> *How would you respond to a patient who prefers street drugs over prescribed medication because of the side effects of the medication?*

OUTCOME IDENTIFICATION

The expected outcome related to withdrawal is as follows:
The patient will overcome addiction safely and with minimum discomfort.

Short-term goals related to this phase of recovery may include the following:

- The patient will withdraw from dependence on the abused substance.
- The patient will be oriented to time, place, person, and situation.
- The patient will report symptoms of withdrawal.
- The patient will correctly interpret environmental stimuli.

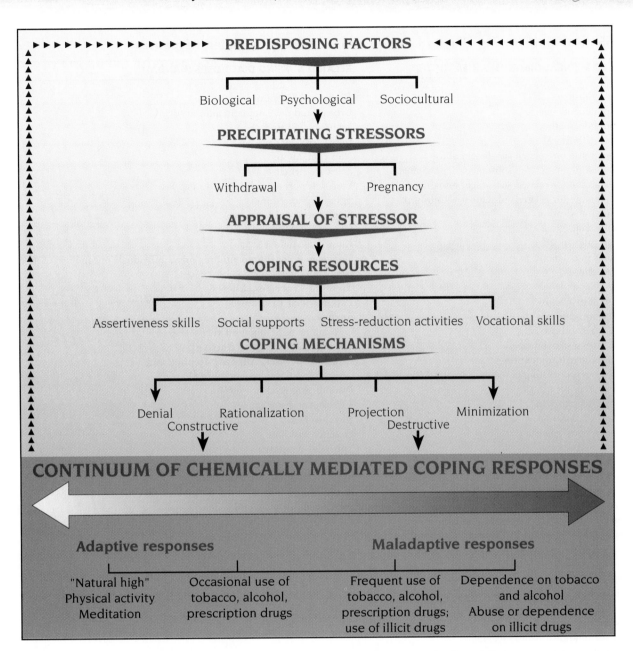

Fig. 25-4 The Stuart Stress Adaptation Model related to substance abuse.

- The patient will recognize and talk about hallucinations or delusions.

For people dependent on drugs or alcohol, the expected outcome is that:

The patient will abstain from all mood-altering chemicals.

Studies have shown that most people who are dependent on a drug or alcohol cannot safely return to any level of use of any addictive drug. If they do, eventually the vast majority return to their old addictive patterns. However, patients often become very anxious at the thought of never again using the substance to which they are addicted. Therefore it may be helpful to focus on short-term goals. Short-term goals related to abstinence may include the following:

- The patient will agree to remain drug and alcohol free for 1 week, with the agreement to be renewed weekly.

- The patient will make a daily commitment to abstain.
- The patient will attend at least two support group meetings weekly.
- The patient will contact a supportive person if he or she experiences an urge to use an addictive substance.

Development of some kind of support system is an essential expected outcome for drug-dependent patients. Once abstinence and support system goals are established, attention can turn to learning about dependence and recovery and developing alternative coping skills. Goals related to the person's job, relationships, or education should be deferred until later, unless any are a roadblock to recovery. For instance, a person is usually encouraged to focus on self and not on a relationship. However, if the person's spouse is an alcoholic and violence in the home is

Medical and Nursing Diagnoses *related to* Chemically Mediated Responses

RELATED MEDICAL DIAGNOSES (*DSM–IV–TR*)*	RELATED NURSING DIAGNOSES (NANDA)†
Alcohol abuse	**Biological Responses**
Alcohol dependence	Growth and development, altered
Alcohol intoxication	Infection, risk for
Alcohol withdrawal	Injury, risk for
Amphetamine (or related substance) abuse	Nutrition, altered
Amphetamine (or related substance) dependence	Self-care deficit
Amphetamine (or related substance) intoxication	**Sensory/perceptual Alterations‡**
Amphetamine (or related substance) withdrawal	Sexual dysfunction
Caffeine intoxication	Sleep pattern disturbance
Cannabis abuse	**Cognitive Responses**
Cannabis dependence	Knowledge deficit
Cannabis intoxication	Management of therapeutic regimen, individuals or families: ineffective
Cocaine abuse	Noncompliance
Cocaine dependence	**Thought Processes, Altered**
Cocaine intoxication	**Psychosocial Responses**
Cocaine withdrawal	Anxiety
Hallucinogen abuse	Communication, impaired verbal
Hallucinogen dependence	**Coping, Individual Ineffective‡**
Hallucinogen intoxication	**Family Processes, Altered: Alcoholism‡**
Hallucinogen persisting perception disorder (flashbacks)	Growth and development, altered
Inhalant abuse	Parenting, altered
Inhalant dependence	Self-esteem disturbance
Inhalant intoxication	Social isolation
Nicotine dependence	Violence, risk for
Nicotine withdrawal	**Spiritual Responses**
Opioid abuse	Grieving, dysfunctional
Opioid dependence	Hopelessness (also psychological)
Opioid intoxication	Powerlessness
Opioid withdrawal	Spiritual distress
Phencyclidine (or related substance) abuse	
Phencyclidine (or related substance) dependence	
Phencyclidine (or related substance) intoxication	
Sedative, hypnotic, or anxiolytic abuse	
Sedative, hypnotic, or anxiolytic dependence	
Sedative, hypnotic, or anxiolytic intoxication	
Sedative, hypnotic, or anxiolytic withdrawal	
Polysubstance dependence	
Other (or unknown) substance abuse	
Other (or unknown) substance dependence	
Other (or unknown) substance intoxication	
Other (or unknown) substance withdrawal	

*Reprinted with permission from the *Diagnostic and statistical manual of mental disorders*, Fourth Edition, Text Revision. Copyright 2000. American Psychiatric Association.
†From North American Nursing Diagnosis Association: *NANDA nursing diagnoses: definitions and classifications 1999-2000*, Philadelphia, 1999, The Association.
‡Primary nursing diagnosis for chemically mediated response.

common, then the priority shifts to finding a safe place to live.

Goals should be worded so that it is clear that the patient is responsible for behavior. Addicted patients often want others to do the work for them. Nurses sometimes comply because they want to be helpful. However, such behavior does not help in the long run. Writing the goals and a specific plan of action into a contract and providing the patient with a copy of the contract will reinforce the patient's re-

sponsibility. The contract should be signed by both the nurse and the patient.

PLANNING

Long-range goals of treatment for patients with substance use disorders include the following (American Psychiatric Association, 1995):

- Abstinence or reduction in the use and effects of substances

Detailed Diagnoses *related to* Chemically Mediated Responses

NANDA DIAGNOSIS STEM	EXAMPLES OF COMPLETE DIAGNOSIS
Sensory-perceptual alteration	Sensory-perceptual alteration related to hallucinogen ingestion, as evidenced by visual hallucination of snakes in the bed
Altered thought processes	Altered thought processes related to alcohol withdrawal, as evidenced by disorientation to time, person, and place
Ineffective individual coping	Ineffective individual coping related to cocaine abuse of 6 months' duration, as evidenced by loss of job and lack of personal goals
Altered family processes: alcoholism	Altered family processes related to alcoholism, as evidenced by marital conflict and avoidance of the family and home by the children

DSM–IV–TR DIAGNOSIS	ESSENTIAL FEATURES*
Substance dependence	Maladaptive pattern of substance use characterized by any three of the following within 12 months: tolerance; withdrawal; using more of the substance or using for longer than planned; persistent desire or unsuccessful efforts to cut down or control use; much time spent in efforts to obtain, use, or recover from use; interference with social, occupational, or recreational activities; continued use despite knowledge of use-related recurrent physical or psychological problems
Substance abuse	Maladaptive pattern of substance use characterized by one or more of the following within 12 months: recurrent use resulting in failure to meet role obligations, recurrent use in physically hazardous situations, recurrent use–related legal problems, continued use despite persistent or recurrent use–related social or interpersonal problems, has never met the criteria for dependence for this class of substance

*Reprinted with permission from the *Diagnostic and statistical manual of mental disorders*, Fourth Edition, Text Revision. Copyright 2000. American Psychiatric Association. The essential features of intoxication and withdrawal vary according to the substance and are listed in Table 25-2.

- Reduction in the frequency and severity of relapse
- Improvement in psychological and social functioning

Priority must be given to the most immediate needs. For patients who are experiencing drug withdrawal, the highest priority is given to stabilization of the patient's physiological status until the crisis of withdrawal has subsided. Once safety needs are met, abstinence and support system issues must be addressed. Plans related to these needs must be made in collaboration with the patient with consideration of the overall assessment and the patient's current life situation and desires. Family members and supportive friends should be included in the planning process; this will help them to understand the problems that the patient may encounter as recovery continues.

The nurse must be aware that it is rare for an addicted person suddenly to stop substance use forever. Most addicts try at least once and usually several times to use the substance in a controlled way. It is important for addicts to know that they should return to treatment after these relapses. They can learn from what they did and try to prevent further relapses. These issues should be addressed openly in the planning process.

IMPLEMENTATION

The nurse encounters patients with substance abuse problems in all health-care settings. The types of interventions recommended depend largely on the setting in which the nurse works. When encountering these patients outside addiction treatment programs, the nurse may be able to refer the person to treatment. If a patient has a history of seizures or serious withdrawal symptoms or is at risk for developing symptoms because of a heavy, chronic use pattern, the first referral should be to a detoxification program. Otherwise, referral should be to the program that appears to match the patient's level of severity. Studies to determine which kinds of treatment programs are best for which kinds of patients have found similar efficacy rates for various alcohol treatment strategies (Project MATCH Research Group, 1997). More specific research involving matching patients to different services within a treatment program may be more promising. Substance abusers often come into contact with the health-care system because of a physiological crisis. It may be related to overdose, withdrawal, allergy, or toxicity. There may be physical deterioration caused by the damaging effects of drugs, including conditions such as malnutrition; dehydration; and various infections, including HIV. When an acute physical condition is present, it takes priority over the other health needs of the patient. It is particularly important to attend to the condition that the patient has identified as the problem. The nurse is then seen as potentially helpful and will have more credibility when other aspects of the addiction are addressed.

Intervening in Withdrawal

Interventions depend on the current and potential withdrawal symptoms that the patient may experience. Substances with potentially life-threatening courses of withdrawal include alcohol, benzodiazepines, and barbiturates. Withdrawal from the general depressants and opiates is generally treated by substitution with a longer-acting drug in the same class, which is then gradually tapered. Withdrawal from opiates and stimulants can be extremely uncomfortable but is generally not dangerous, although a patient may become suicidal during the acute phase of cocaine withdrawal. Symptom-specific medications may be used to treat symptoms of stimulant withdrawal. Phenobarbital may be prescribed for inhalant withdrawal symptoms. There is no identified acute withdrawal pattern associated with marijuana, hallucinogens, or PCP.

Withdrawal symptoms may occur despite efforts to prevent them. Substance abusers do not always give accurate drug use histories, although it is extremely important to obtain as specific an assessment as possible. If the amount of substance used has been understated or if multiple abuse is undetected, withdrawal symptoms may occur unexpectedly. The possibility of seizures should always be anticipated. Emergency equipment should be at hand. Drug abuse should always be considered possible when unexpected seizures occur. If drug abuse is suspected, the physician should be informed so that blood and urine specimens can be collected for laboratory analysis and an appropriate treatment plan initiated.

The process of helping an addict safely through withdrawal is called detoxification. Actually, the liver detoxifies the substance. Medications and nursing actions only help to relieve the symptoms.

Detoxification is best accomplished in a setting in which there can be close monitoring of the patient. This can be an inpatient medical or psychiatric unit or a crisis stabilization unit. Outpatient detoxification may also be possible.

It is best to maintain a quiet, calm environment for patients experiencing the general depressant withdrawal syndrome. This helps the patient relax and decreases nervous system irritability. Reassurance in a calm, quiet tone of voice is also helpful. To help maintain the patient's orientation, the nurse should place a clock within sight and give frequent, low-key reminders about who he or she is, where the patient is, the nurse's name, and the day of the week. If possible, another patient who is further along in detoxification may be assigned as a buddy so that the patient is not left alone. A family member may also help.

The patient in withdrawal should be treated symptomatically. Fluids should be encouraged only if the person is dehydrated. Eating should be encouraged, and vitamins are usually ordered. Acetaminophen (Tylenol) or attapulgite (Kaopectate), if ordered, may be given for discomfort or diarrhea. A small amount of milk may be offered frequently to help manage epigastric distress. Seizure precautions should be taken. A cool washcloth can be offered for use on the forehead if the patient is feeling warm or diaphoretic. Position changes, assistance with ambulation, and changing damp clothing are also indicated. Evidence suggests that offering this type of intense, supportive care can reduce withdrawal symptoms rapidly and often dramatically without medications. If the patient is receiving large doses of benzodiazepines, the nurse should monitor for signs of toxicity, such as ataxia (difficulty walking) and nystagmus (involuntary rhythmic movement of the eyeball). The patient always should be treated with respect and dignity.

Management of Alcohol Withdrawal. The principles of alcohol detoxification, according to evidence based practice guidelines are as follows (Mayo-Smith et al, 1997):

- The long-acting benzodiazepines are the drugs of choice in treating alcohol withdrawal because they effectively reduce signs and symptoms of withdrawal, prevent seizures, and have a better margin of safety than many other drugs. The dosing regimens recommended in the practice guidelines are listed in Table 25-3.
- A symptom-triggered dosing regimen is preferred over fixed-schedule dosing because it is effective, requires significantly less medication, and appears to prevent seizures as well as fixed schemes.
- The use of a clinically valid and reliable withdrawal assessment tool such as the CIWA–AR (Clinical Institute Withdrawal Assessment–Alcohol, Revised) is recommended as the basis for medication determinations. This reduces overmedication due to patient overreporting of symptoms or fixed regimens and undermedication due to staff reluctance to treat.
- A fixed schedule, with prn dosing, may be indicated if used on a unit where the staff have no training in the use of a withdrawal assessment tool.

Table **25-3**

Management of Alcohol Withdrawal

Monitor patient q 4-8 hr with the CIWA–AR until score has been less than 8 to 10 for 24 hr. Use additional assessments as needed.

Symptom-Triggered Regimen	Fixed-Schedule Regimen

Administer one of the following every hour when CIWA–AR scores > 8 – 10:
  Chlordiazepoxide, 50-100 mg
  Diazepam, 10-20 mg
  Lorazepam, 2-4 mg
Repeat CIWA–AR 1 hr after every dose to assess need for further medication
	Chlordiazepoxide, 50 mg q 6 h for 4 doses; then 25 mg q 6 h for 8 doses
	Diazepam, 10 mg every 6 hr for 4 doses, then 5 mg q 6 h for 8 doses
	Lorazepam, 2 mg q 6 h for 4 doses then 1 mg q 6 h for 8 doses
	Provide additional medication as needed when symptoms not controlled (i.e., CIWA–AR >8-10) with above measures
	Other benzodiazepines may be used at equivalent doses.

- Although neither magnesium nor thiamine reduces seizures, administration of thiamine is recommended to prevent Wernicke's disease and Wernicke-Korsakoff syndrome.

Symptoms of alcohol withdrawal do not always progress from mild to severe in a predictable manner. A grand mal seizure may be the first sign of acute withdrawal. However, initial assessment and ongoing monitoring with the CIWA–AR may be effective in preventing the onset of more severe symptoms. A score of 9 or less on the CIWA–AR indicates mild withdrawal, 10 to 18 indicates moderate withdrawal, and a score greater than 18, severe withdrawal. The CIWA–AR should be used with caution in patients with co-occurring medical or psychiatric illnesses and in those with concurrent withdrawal from other drugs because it rates signs and symptoms that may be caused by the other conditions and not by the alcohol withdrawal. The CIWA–AR should be repeated every 1 to 2 hours. Increasing scores signify the need for additional medication according to a predetermined scale, whereas decreasing scores indicate a therapeutic response to the treatment regimen. Scores less than 10 do not generally require use of medication.

There is some evidence that symptom-triggered medication shortens the length of treatment and requires significantly less medication. There is also evidence that the use of the CIWA–AR as a basis for medication need results in significantly less medication being given with no reduction in efficacy (Substance Abuse and Mental Health Services Administration [SAMHSA], 1995a).

Management of Benzodiazepines, Barbiturates, and Other Sedative-Hypnotics Withdrawal.

These drugs are generally prescribed for therapeutic purposes, sometimes for long periods of time. When this occurs, development of physical dependence on the drug is sometimes unavoidable. As long as the drug is taken as prescribed, such a physical dependence is not considered substance abuse and the term **detoxification** should be replaced by the term **therapeutic discontinuation**. Heroin and stimulant users sometimes use these drugs as part of their drug abuse pattern. When individuals use the drug other than prescribed, obtain the drug by illegitimate means, or when the drug use interferes with their lives, then such use can lead to dependence, which requires detoxification. Whether used therapeutically or abused, abrupt cessation from these drugs can lead to severe withdrawal and even death. Therefore, careful medical management is required.

High-dose withdrawal may be treated by a gradual reduction of the drug used, or phenobarbital may be substituted during the detoxification process. The dosing regimen starts with the patient's average daily dose (as self-reported) of all sedative-hypnotic drugs, including alcohol. This dose is then converted to phenobarbital equivalents and the daily amount divided into three doses. Before each dose, the nurse checks for signs of phenobarbital toxicity (sustained nystagmus, slurred speech, or ataxia). Since nystagmus is the most reliable sign, if present, the dose is withheld. If all three signs are present, the next two doses of phenobarbital are withheld, and the daily dosage of phenobarbital for the following day is reduced by half.

If the patient is in acute withdrawal and is at risk for withdrawal seizures, the first dose of phenobarbital is administered intramuscularly (IM). If nystagmus and other signs of intoxication develop 1 to 2 hours after IM dosing, then the patient is in no immediate danger from barbiturate withdrawal. In this case, patients continue to receive the initial dosing schedule for 2 days. Then, if the patient displays neither signs of withdrawal nor toxicity nor has an unsteady gait, doses are decreased by 30 mg per day. If toxicity develops, the daily dose is decreased by 50% and the 30 mg per day withdrawal is continued from the reduced dose. If the patient has objective signs of withdrawal, the daily dose is increased by 50% and the patient is restabilized before continuing withdrawal.

Low-dose withdrawal is dependent on the patient's symptoms. Seizures are uncommon unless the patient has an underlying seizure disorder, in which case anticonvulsants should be administered and other medications that lower the seizure threshold should be avoided. If symptoms are severe, 200 mg of phenobarbital is given per day initially, then slowly tapered over several months.

Management of Opiate Withdrawal.

All opiates produce similar withdrawal signs and symptoms, but the time of onset and the duration vary. Treatment is aimed at alleviating the acute symptoms. This may be done by substitution of the long-acting opiate methadone or by management of the withdrawal symptoms with medications such as clonidine.

- Methadone substitution involves initial administration of methadone—an opiate agonist—to stabilize symptoms of heroin withdrawal, usually 10 to 40 mg in the first 24 hours. Once the patient is stabilized, the dose can be slowly tapered to 0. Tapering by 5 mg/day is common, but slower tapering may be more comfortable for the patient. The detoxification of patients from longer-acting opioids, such as methadone, requires an even longer period of time.

- Clonidine is available in oral, sublingual, or transdermal patch preparations. The protocol for clonidine administration usually involves 0.1 to 0.3 mg in three divided doses on the first day (perhaps higher doses for inpatients who can be closely monitored). The dose is then adjusted until withdrawal symptoms are reduced. The blood pressure should initially be checked every 45 minutes, since some patients are extremely sensitive to clonidine and experience profound hypotension, even at low doses. If the blood pressure drops below 90/60 mm Hg, the next dose should be withheld and subsequent doses adjusted according to patient response. Although clonidine effectively relieves several symptoms of opiate withdrawal, it is not helpful for muscle aches, insomnia, or drug craving, which then require additional medication.

Just as the CIWA–AR is useful in rating alcohol withdrawal, the CINA (Clinical Institute Narcotic Assessment) rating scale may be helpful in the assessment and monitoring of opiate withdrawal.

Management of Nicotine Withdrawal. Nicotine gum and the nicotine patch both provide mechanisms for nicotine to be delivered into the body without the carcinogens and carbon monoxide present in cigarettes. Nicotine in these forms serves to replace the nicotine in cigarettes, thus relieving withdrawal symptoms and allowing for tapering of the dose to 0 over time. The optimum length of treatment before tapering is 4 to 6 weeks. Dosing is most effective at 2 to 4 mg per hour for the gum, which comes in 2 and 4 mg sticks. Patches are available in 21 to 22 mg/24-hour patch and 15 mg/16-hour patch (for use while awake). Other available, but less popular, forms of nicotine are nasal sprays and inhalers.

The use of clonidine to relieve withdrawal symptoms does not have as high a level of scientific support as does nicotine replacement, but it is appropriate for those who prefer to discontinue nicotine in all forms. Bupropion can also be prescribed for smokers who prefer a non-nicotine treatment or who might experience depression upon cessation. It has been shown to be as effective as nicotine replacement and produces no significant side effects (American Psychiatric Association, 1996).

Management of Caffeine Withdrawal. Although not classified as a drug of abuse, caffeine has a well-defined physical withdrawal syndrome. Symptoms are relieved with caffeine. There is no published regimen of caffeine administration for the purpose of relieving withdrawal.

Intervening in Toxic Psychosis. Users of lysergic acid diethylamide (LSD), PCP, and stimulants often come to the emergency room in acute toxic psychosis. Their behavior may be quite similar to that of the patient with schizophrenia. However, there may be no history of abnormal behavior. Careful assessment of an acute psychotic reaction, particularly in an adolescent or young adult, should include exploration of drug use. It may be necessary to interview friends of the patient to obtain this information. An attempt should be made to identify the specific drug used, although LSD and PCP may be taken without the knowledge of the person involved.

There is an important difference in the nursing approach to users of PCP and amphetamine as opposed to those who have an adverse reaction to LSD. Unless the psychiatric symptomatology is severe, LSD users experiencing a "bad trip" often respond to reassurance and may be "talked down." Patients should be oriented frequently and discouraged from closing their eyes because this may make the symptoms worse.

However, victims of PCP-induced psychosis do not respond well to attempts at interaction. Agitated PCP and amphetamine users are more likely to strike out in response to their misperceptions and panic. They are potentially more harmful to themselves and others. This aggression may be totally unprovoked. In addition, because PCP is also an anesthetic, these patients feel little or no pain. For this reason, they seem to have enormous strength. They do not feel pain when they exceed the limits of their muscular capability and may continue pushing, pulling, or hitting until they seriously injure themselves or others.

Other elements of treatment are basically the same for acutely agitated LSD and PCP users. Both require a safe environment that has minimum stimulation. Staff should not perform any procedures without a thorough explanation, should not touch the patient without permission, and should avoid rapid movements in the patient's presence. Adequate staff should be present to control impulsive behavior. Vital signs should be monitored, and other physiological needs should be met. Although restraints may exacerbate muscle damage and agitation, they may be necessary, especially if a seclusion room is not available. Benzodiazepines are the treatment of choice, followed by high-potency antipsychotic medications if benzodiazepines are ineffective. Gastric lavage may be necessary for persistent symptoms or if an overdose has been taken, although this is not recommended for PCP users because it increases agitation.

Intervening to Maintain Abstinence

Once the individual is through the initial withdrawal phase, interventions to maintain abstinence can begin. The first months after cessation of substance use represent the highest risk for relapse and offer the greatest opportunity for pharmacological interventions that can help patients decrease cravings and maintain abstinence. However the drugs currently available are of limited usefulness, mainly because patients stop taking them. The effects are generally temporary unless the drugs are used as part of a broader program of psychosocial treatment.

Antabuse. A long-term biological approach to substance abuse is the prescription of disulfiram (Antabuse) for alcoholics. This drug interrupts the metabolism of alcohol, causing a buildup of a toxic substance in the body if the person uses alcohol in any form. The physiological response may include a severe headache, nausea and vomiting, flushing, hypotension, tachycardia, dyspnea, diaphoresis, chest pain, palpitations, dizziness, and confusion. Rarely, it can lead to respiratory and cardiac collapse, unconsciousness, convulsions, and death.

Antabuse should never be given without the patient's stated willingness to comply. It is also important that the patient agree to take Antabuse only after careful instruction about the potential consequences of drinking while taking the drug. This instruction should include a written list of alcohol-containing preparations to be avoided, including cough medicines, rubbing compounds, vinegar, aftershave lotions, and some mouthwashes.

Drinking must be avoided for 14 days after Antabuse has been discontinued. This medication cannot prevent someone who is determined to drink from drinking. This person can simply wait until the Antabuse has been excreted. However, it helps to prevent impulsive drinking because the person has to wait to be able to drink safely. This treatment should be used in conjunction with other supportive therapies, not by itself.

Describe the information that should be provided to a patient who is to be treated with Antabuse. What issues related to informed consent should be considered in the use of this drug?

Naltrexone. Naltrexone was approved by the FDA in 1994 for the treatment of alcohol dependence. Naltrexone, an opiate antagonist, has demonstrated effectiveness in helping the alcoholic to maintain abstinence. It diminishes craving during the early stages of abstinence and works best when accompanied by psychosocial interventions (see Citing the Evidence). It is believed to act in the following way: Alcohol intake increases the number of endorphins (naturally occurring opioids) in the brain. Naltrexone, in doses of approximately 50 mg/day, appears to block the effects of these endorphins, thus reducing the reinforcing effects of alcohol (SAMHSA, 1998). Limitations of this medication include discontinuation from side effects (primarily nausea) and dose-dependent hepatotoxic effects, which are particularly concerning considering the damaging effects of alcohol on the liver.

Nalmefene. Nalmefene is a newer opioid antagonist that is structurally similar to naltrexone but with a number of pharmacological advances for the treatment of alcohol dependence. These include no dose-dependent association with toxic effects to the liver, greater oral bioavailability, longer duration of antagonist action, and more complete binding with opioid receptor subtypes that are thought to

reinforce drinking. It has been found to be effective in preventing relapse to heavy drinking and has few side effects (Mason et al, 1999).

Opiate Agonists. Long-term opiate addicts who meet federal criteria for opiate dependence may be eligible for maintenance with methadone or LAAM. LAAM is a longer-acting opiate agonist. Patients in maintenance programs take stable doses of one of these substitute drugs for years—even for the rest of their lives. They must report to the clinic daily (for methadone) or every other day (for LAAM). Since LAAM has not been approved for take-home dosing, if LAAM patients cannot get through the weekend free of withdrawal symptoms, they may be given a Sunday take-home dose of methadone (SAMHSA, 1995b). This treatment approach is controversial because these substitution drugs are narcotics. However, addiction to methadone does not cause impaired functioning; thus the person can be productive while addicted. Those in favor of methadone maintenance point out the benefits of avoiding the debilitating effects of heroin addiction and the lifestyle associated with obtaining illegal drugs on the streets.

Methadone maintenance is essentially substituting a legal narcotic for an illegal one. Do you believe that this is a responsible practice? State the reasons for your position.

Acamprosate. Acamprosate is a new drug that shows promise in the maintenance of abstinence from alcohol. Acamprosate (calcium acetylhomotaurinate) is a synthetic compound, similar in chemical structure to gamma-aminobutyric acid (GABA). It appears to work by lowering the activity of receptors for the excitatory neurotransmitter glutamate. Chronic alcohol abuse increases the number of these receptors, and their resultant latent excitability may account for the high rate of relapse in the first few months after withdrawal (Wilde & Wagstaff, 1997). Side effects, which are generally mild, include occasional diarrhea and headache. Large scale studies in Europe show that it reduces drinking frequency and appears to be effective without having an abuse potential of its own (Garbutt et al, 1999).

Cocaine Vaccine in Development. One of the most exciting breakthroughs in the field is the development of a cocaine vaccine that is designed to be part of a comprehensive approach to treating cocaine addiction. A therapeutic vaccine that induces anticocaine antibodies and prevents the drug from crossing the blood/brain barrier is being used in experimental animal trials with some success. It may prove to be a powerful tool to inhibit the reinforcing activity of the drug.

Pregnancy. Because most of the drugs that are abused cross the placental barrier, women should be counseled about the possible effects of substance use during pregnancy. Congenital abnormalities have occurred in infants of mothers who have taken drugs. A fetal alcohol syndrome has been identified, which involves a pattern of physical growth and mental deficiencies. In addition, during pregnancy use of drugs that cause physical dependence can result in the birth of an addicted baby who must be withdrawn from the drug. The safest pregnancy is one in which the mother is totally

---

Citing the Evidence on

Pharmacological and Psychosocial Therapies

BACKGROUND: In a few studies with limited sample sizes, naltrexone has been shown to be effective when combined with psychosocial therapies for the treatment of alcohol dependence. The goal of this study was to obtain additional information regarding its efficacy with a well-defined psychosocial therapy. One hundred thirty-one recently abstinent alcohol-dependent outpatients were treated with 12 weekly sessions of manual-guided cognitive behavioral therapy and either 50mg/day of naltrexone or placebo in a double-blind randomized clinical trial.

RESULTS: Naltrexone treated patients drank less, took longer to relapse, and had more time between relapses. They also showed more resistance to and control over alcohol-related thoughts and urges. Over the study period, 62% of the naltrexone group did not relapse into heavy drinking, compared with 40% of the placebo group.

IMPLICATIONS: Motivated individuals with moderate alcohol dependence can be treated with greater effectiveness when naltrexone is used in conjunction with weekly outpatient cognitive behavioral therapy. The therapeutic effects of cognitive behavioral therapy and naltrexone may be synergistic.

Anton R et al: Naltrexone and cognitive behavioral therapy for the treatment of outpatient alcoholics: results of a placebo-controlled trial, *Am J of Psych* 156(11):1758, 1999.

drug and alcohol free with one exception: For pregnant women addicted to heroin, methadone maintenance is safer for the fetus than acute opiate detoxification.

> **?** *Some policymakers have proposed that pregnant women who abuse substances should be jailed, placed under house arrest, or committed to a mental hospital until the baby is born. Do you agree with this? Support your position. Do you have the same opinion related to all abused substances, including alcohol and nicotine?*

Psychological Interventions

Before initiating nursing intervention with a substance-abusing patient, the nurse must develop self-awareness of feelings and attitudes about the problem (see A Patient Speaks). It is recommended that a value clarification approach be used, as described in Chapter 2. Most people have had personal contact with substance abuse by family, friends, or colleagues. This problem creates many negative feelings. It is important that the nurse be able to differentiate feelings associated with past situations from those aroused by contacts with patients and their families. A supervisor, teacher, or senior clinical nurse can be of assistance when a nurse is having difficulty sorting out these feelings.

Traditional addiction treatment is based on the concepts of addiction as a disease, total abstinence from all substances, immersion in 12-step recovery programs, direct confrontation of denial and other defense mechanisms (generally in group sessions), and a lifelong recovery process. Groups are usually led by recovering alcoholic/addict counselors. Ambivalence, resistance, and denial are viewed as characteristics of the disease of addiction. Confrontation is viewed as necessary to break through these defenses. Through the years, a practice of using very harsh and confrontational counseling techniques has evolved. Although some people respond well to these approaches, others do

---

A Patient Speaks

I have abused drugs and alcohol for many years. One thing that has been important is for nurses to spend time with me so I can learn to trust them. It helps when they make sure I schedule treatment appointments and keep them. Substance abuse education is very important, and it has to be repeated over and over.

I've been through detoxification many times. Some of the nurses in those programs have coddled me. This makes it easy for me to dance around issues of sobriety. I've had the best success with the nurse who will hang in there with me and not let me make excuses, get in my face, and cut me no slack. The nurses who have high expectations leave me enough room to help myself, but not enough to be dishonest. There needs to be a balance of empathy and toughness. It's not easy, but that's the role for the nurse to establish.

---

not. Despite their popularity, clinical outcome studies do not support such confrontational strategies, and some of the traditional programs have adopted gentler approaches.

In the past, traditional addiction treatment was offered in specialized programs, whereas psychiatric patients with substance abuse problems were treated in psychiatric and mental health programs. Many psychiatric professionals viewed alcoholism and other drug addictions as secondary to psychiatric disorders. They believed that the substance abuse would cease when the person's primary psychiatric disorder was resolved. Psychiatric patients often were given tranquilizers to treat what was believed to be their underlying pathology. However, instead of abstaining from their substance of choice, many of these patients became addicted to the tranquilizers as well. Psychiatric treatment models operated from a different philosophical base, which was effective in dealing with psychiatric problems but less effective in dealing with addiction. Differences in treatment philosophies and backgrounds of providers contributed to a developing rift between psychiatric clinicians and addiction counselors. Dually diagnosed patients were often caught in the middle of this rift.

Over the years, however, approaches have been developed for the treatment of addictions that incorporates knowledge of both addictions and mental health strategies. Addiction counselors now include family counseling and cognitive behavioral techniques into their treatment strategies. So too, psychiatric clinicians better understand addiction as a separate disorder. Dual diagnosis programs have been developed, and mental health approaches have been adapted for the primary treatment of addiction.

Although these newer approaches vary, they generally involve creation of an alliance between the therapist and the patient, inclusion of the patient in the setting of treatment goals (even if the patient's goal is not total abstinence), avoidance of confrontation, brevity of treatment, and use of professional therapists. More than just a series of techniques, they offer a new type of relationship between clinician and patient. Even more important, they have demonstrated efficacy in the treatment of patients with substance abuse disorders. Some of these newer approaches are now described.

Motivational Approaches. Motivational counseling is a relatively new approach to helping patients with substance abuse problems. It is based on the concept that motivation for change is not static but dynamic, and that the clinician can influence change by developing a therapeutic relationship that respects and builds on the patient's autonomy and by making the patient a partner in the change process (SAMHSA, 1999a). Although many different techniques can be used, the most important element of treatment is the attitude of the clinician. Five basic principles are used with this approach:

- **Express empathy through reflective listening**. This communicates respect for and acceptance of patients and their feelings. It also establishes a safe and open environment that helps in examining issues and exploring personal reasons for change.

- **Develop discrepancy between patients' goals or values and their current behavior.** Focus patients' attention on how current behavior differs from behavior described as ideal or desired.
- **Avoid argument and direct confrontation.** Trying to convince a patient that a problem exists or that change is needed could precipitate even more resistance. Arguments can rapidly degenerate into a power struggle and do not enhance motivation for beneficial change.
- **Roll with resistance.** Resistance is a signal that the patient views the situation differently. There are four types of resistance: arguing, interrupting, denying, or ignoring. The clinician's job is to ask questions in a way that helps the patient to understand and work through resistance.
- **Support self-efficacy.** This requires the clinician to recognize the patient's strengths and bring these to the forefront whenever possible. It involves supporting hope, optimism, and the feasibility of accomplishing change.

Critical components of effective motivational interventions include the FRAMES approach and Decisional Balance exercises. FRAMES is an acronym for the basic elements of motivational counseling and is described in the following:

- **F**eedback regarding personal risk or impairment is given to the patient after assessment of substance use patterns and related problems.
- **R**esponsibility for change is placed explicitly on the patient, with respect for the patient's right to make his or her own choices.
- **A**dvice about changing substance use is clearly given to the patient, nonjudgmentally, by the clinician.
- **M**enus of self-directed change options and treatment alternatives are offered.
- **E**mpathic counseling—showing warmth, respect, and understanding—is emphasized.
- **S**elf-efficacy—or optimistic empowerment is engendered in the patient to encourage change.

Decisional Balance exercises are specific ways that the clinician can assist the patient to explore the pros and cons of old and new behaviors for the purpose of tipping the scales toward a decision for positive change. The items are identified by the patient with gentle assistance from the clinician and written in blocks, as in Fig. 25-5. The four blocks add a new twist to the traditional two-column "pros and cons" list. One advantage of the four-block grid is recognition of the fact that there are positive elements about the old behavior that must be faced. For example, if drinking helps the patient to relax, part of recovery may include finding other ways to relax without alcohol. Even more important than the number of items in each block is the weight of each item. For example, the negative impact on the family may more than outweigh the social pleasures of drinking. The clinician then summarizes the list of concerns and presents them to the patient in a way that expresses empathy, develops discrepancy, and weights the balance toward change. The objective is to meet the patients where they are and walk with them through the process.

All of these motivational approaches are designed to help improve patient participation in the treatment process. They are based on the **stages of change** model, which identifies five stages of change (Fig. 25-6): precontemplation, contemplation, preparation, action, and maintenance (Prochaska & DiCelemente, 1986). Goals and approaches differ for each stage. For instance, if a patient is in the precontemplation stage of change, the decisional-balance would be an appropriate tool to help patients recognize they have a problem. Presenting these patients a menu of treatment options, however, would not be helpful since they would not be ready to accept help for a problem they do not yet acknowledge having. However, options would be appropriate during the preparation stage.

Cognitive-Behavioral Strategies. Cognitive-behavioral approaches are aimed at improving self-control and social skills in order to reduce drinking. Self-control strategies

DECISIONAL BALANCE GRID	
Old Behavior	**New Behavior**
Pros/Benefits Like the taste of alcohol Helps me to relax Source of fun and socialization Makes me forget my problems	Pros/Benefits Better relationship with spouse No more DWIs Save money Feel better about myself More time for other activities and 　people in my life
Cons/Costs Costs a lot of money Led to DWI—costly, embarrassing, and 　inconvenient Spouse gets upset Poor role model for children Feel bad about myself If I lose my driver's license, I could lose 　my job	Cons/Costs Will miss my drinking friends Don't know how to have fun without it It will be harder to face my problems I'll feel left out, "different" I'll be more up-tight, less relaxed

Fig. 25-5 Decision Balance Grid.

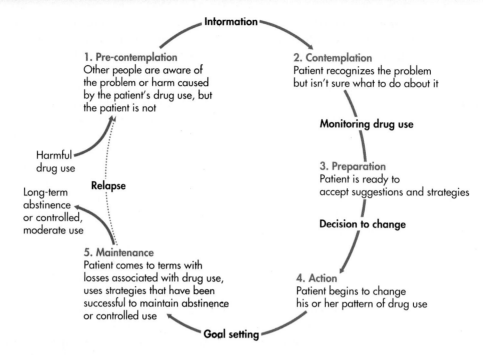

Fig. 25-6   A model of change in substance use disorders.   (Modified from Prochaska J, DiClemente C: Towards a comprehensive model of change. In Miller W, Heather N, editors: *Treating addictive behaviors: process of change.* New York, 1986, Plenum).

include goal-setting, self-monitoring, functional analysis of drinking antecedents, and learning alternative coping skills. Social-skills training focuses on learning skills for forming and maintaining interpersonal relationships, assertiveness, and drink refusal. Contingency management is another behavioral approach that has been successfully applied in many substance abuse treatment programs. In this strategy, rewards (often in the form of vouchers that can be exchanged for desired items) are given for adaptive behavior (such as compliance with treatment or clean urine). Behavioral contracting is also a useful approach. It involves creating a written agreement with the patient that specifies targeted patient behavior and consequences.

In general, cognitive-behavioral strategies adapt well to briefer interventions that have been necessitated by managed care programs. They appear to be as effective as longer-term therapies. Cognitive-behavioral treatment strategies are discussed in more detail in Chapter 32.

> *Discuss the significance of the substance abuser's level of self-esteem to the recovery process. Describe nursing interventions designed to enhance self-esteem.*

Working with Co-Dependency.   Whether or not co-dependency exists as an independent phenomenon is not important in treatment planning. However, it is important not to discount the patient's identification with the co-dependency movement or the syndrome. Having a label for problems makes them more legitimate and easier to accept for some people. The co-dependency label has popular appeal. It is nonstigmatizing because the cause does not lie within the self, but with another person. The nurse should

accept the patient's view of the problem as a legitimate starting point for a therapeutic alliance. Then the patient can be helped to understand how behavior that once allowed survival in a dysfunctional family no longer serves this purpose. The nurse can help the patient to move gradually away from anger and fear and toward responsibility for self-fulfillment.

Interventions center around the patient's primary identified problems and may include assertiveness training, challenging cognitive distortions, teaching self-affirmations, and relaxation training. Because physical and sexual abuse are common in alcoholic families, specific assessment and intervention strategies must be implemented to identify and help patients with these types of problems. Referral to specialized programs may be useful. Additional information about appropriate interventions for survivors of abuse and violence is in Chapter 41. ACOA self-help groups may be useful. The nurse should suggest that the patient try several self-help groups before deciding to be actively involved in any one group. The nurse should also monitor how the patient responds to participation in these groups. Some groups are more positive and forward-focused than others.

Alcoholism is known to run in families. People who grew up in an alcoholic home often develop alcohol problems themselves or may marry alcoholics. It is clear that both biological and environmental factors contribute to generational transmission of this disorder. Thus it is common for a patient to be alcoholic and have an alcoholic parent. Intervention is most effective if it addresses intergenerational patterns.

Intervening in Relapse.   Behavior change is always difficult, but change related to addiction is even more difficult because of the chemical imbalance in the brain induced by the substance. It is rare, therefore, for a person to make a sudden and drastic behavioral change and maintain it with no return to the old behaviors. Since there are very few medications to counteract the effects on the brain, the patient must be assisted to make behavioral and lifestyle changes in spite of extremely powerful chemical forces in the brain luring him or her to return to the substance that would temporarily restore the chemical brain balance.

Most people who try to stop using an addictive substance are not successful on the first attempt. The nurse who is a smoker can generally identify with this phenomenon. The nurse who has never used an addictive substance but may have tried dieting can understand through this experience the difficulty of making behavioral changes that have strong physiological forces pulling in the opposite direction. Such personal identifications can help the nurse to empathize with the patient and reduce negative judgments, which are essential to being a credible counselor.

In a sense, it would be better to abandon the notion of relapse altogether since it represents dichotomous thinking that does not fit well with the complexities of human behavior (such as a person is either abstinent or relapsed, sober or drinking). Behavior change is actually a process that occurs over time. Nurses can help those who are trying to change by helping them learn from whatever works and does not work in their behavior change efforts. This seems to have a more positive focus than a focus on failures or "relapses."

Relapse prevention strategies have been widely used in substance abuse recovery programs and have been shown to be effective in assisting patients to staying clean and sober (Irvin et al, 1999).

In these strategies, relapse is seen as a process, not an event. Rather than being viewed as an indicator of treatment failure, it is dealt with as an error from which to learn—a temporary setback on the road to recovery. Recovery is not an all-or-nothing proposition. Rather "success" is measured by improvements—such as increasing lengths of time being clean between relapses and shorter time periods of relapse.

It is important for the nurse to accept the patient without judging and to assist the patient in learning from the relapse. The nurse should help the patient identify external and internal triggers that may precipitate cravings and thus lead to drug use. External triggers include the people, places, and things that have been associated with previous drug use. The nurse helps the patient figure out ways to avoid these triggers. Situations that include one or all of these triggers are called high-risk situations. Since these cannot always be avoided, the nurse should assist the patient to manage them successfully. For example, if alcohol will be served at a family wedding and it is important to the patient to attend, the nurse can encourage the patient to attend the wedding with a relative who will support one's decision to remain abstinent. Major lifestyle changes—such as making new friends, moving to a different neighborhood—may need to be made in order to avoid these triggers. The nurse should also help the patient to identify internal triggers, which are the thoughts and feelings contributing to past drug use, such as loneliness, boredom, or anger. The nurse can then help the patient develop healthy coping skills to deal with these negative emotional states without using substances (Marlatt, 1996).

The nurse will generally need to help patients restructure their time. So much time may have been spent in obtaining and using drugs that patients may have no idea what to do with their new free time. Lastly, the nurse should teach patients how to identify and deal with cravings. At the time they occur, it sometimes seems that the only way to satisfy cravings is to use the substance of choice. However, the nurse can reassure patients that the cravings will pass if they get involved in some other nondrug-related activity. Patients should also be taught that there are many decision points on the road to relapse—one being before using, others being after the first use, etc. This can help patients avoid the **abstinence violation effect**, in which patients feels so guilty about violating a period of abstinence, that they figure they may as well keep using and "start again tomorrow. . . Monday. . . next week. . . after this run," etc. The goal is for the patient to want to avoid the use altogether, but if it happens, to minimize the amount and the time involved.

Social Interventions

Family Counseling. Reliable support from caring people is crucial to the recovery of substance abusers. However, the family is often frustrated with the patient's behavior and finds it difficult to be supportive. The family seldom understands the nature of addiction and generally does all the wrong things in its attempt to help the substance abuser. The family often tries to protect the patient from consequences. Many times, family members cover up by making excuses to employers and other family members for the person's erratic behavior. They also tend to blame themselves for the behavior and go to great lengths to avoid confrontation with the user. All of these behaviors are called enabling behaviors. By shielding the person from the consequences of drug use, the family enables the person's continued use of the drug.

Addiction is a family problem (see A Family Speaks). Everyone in the family suffers, not just the alcoholic or drug addict. Some problems that families experience include guilt, shame, resentment, insecurity, delinquency, financial troubles, isolation, fear, and violence. Families think their problems would be solved if their loved one simply stopped using drugs or alcohol. However, they can get help even if the user refuses. They should also realize that without help, many of the negative patterns of behavior developed over years of dysfunctional family life will continue after sobriety.

The nurse should encourage family members to seek counseling from a professional experienced in addiction treatment. Referral to Al-Anon, a support group for friends and family of alcoholics, or NarAnon, for friends and family of narcotic addicts, is also helpful. These groups are based on the same 12 steps as AA and NA except that they are powerless over their alcoholic/addict instead of the substance itself. These families must learn to pay attention to their own needs. They should stop covering up for the addict. They need to be direct in their communication. They also need to know that they are not alone. These issues are evident in the following clinical example.

CLINICAL EXAMPLE

Mr. B was a 45-year-old man who was admitted to the medical unit of a general hospital with a diagnosis of gastritis. He complained of abdominal pain, nausea, and vomiting. He had a slightly elevated temperature of 37.5° C (100° F). When the admitting nurse who was completing the nursing assessment asked Mr. B about alcohol use, he said he had "a couple of beers" after work every day. He also reported that his wife had left him the day before admission. He said he was not sure why she left, but he was sure she would be back. Mrs. B did come to the hospital to visit her husband. His primary nurse met with them together and asked Mrs. B why she left. She said she was tired of putting Mr. B to bed every night after he passed out from drinking and did not want to continue to call his employer saying he was sick when he was really hung over. She had threatened to leave before, but Mr. B had always begged her to stay and she had relented. She had married him because she felt sorry for him. He had been living alone and was not taking good care of himself. She revealed that her first husband was also an alcoholic and her father had been one as well. She would agree to try again to make the marriage a success if he would agree to stop drinking and seek counseling. Mr. B said to the nurse, "I'll be good and do what she says. You tell her I'll be good."

Selected Nursing Diagnoses

- Ineffective individual coping related to reluctance to be responsible for his behavior, as evidenced by denial of why his wife left
- Altered family processes related to alcoholism, as evidenced by cycles of drinking, threats to leave, and promises to change

Mr. B used alcohol to avoid responsibility for his actions and his life. He used his wife in a similar way. When Mrs. B confronted him with her expectations, he responded in a childlike way and tried to place the nurse in the parental role.

Mrs. B appears to be drawn to dependent men. She is probably a very maternal person who likes to take care of others. This increases the possibility that she will assume the role of enabler. The enabler perpetuates the substance abuse problem by not confronting the substance abuser and by helping to cover up the problem. When Mrs. B called Mr. B's employer to say he was sick, she was being an enabler. When significant others play an enabling role, family counseling or family support groups help the family accept and support the changing behavior of the patient.

Group Therapy. Group psychotherapy is the usual method of treatment in traditional substance abuse treatment programs. Chapter 33 provides detailed information about therapeutic groups.

History sharing and feedback are important elements in traditional program groups. Patients share their substance abuse histories and talk about their daily efforts to stop drinking or taking drugs. The therapist and group members listen closely and give feedback to patients about their recovery efforts. Feedback is the honest reaction of group members to what the speaker says. It is based on the content of what the person says and on previous experiences with the speaker. Although feedback from one person, especially the therapist, may be discounted, it is difficult for the addict to ignore feedback from several group members, especially if they have experienced the same type of behavior at some point. The style of giving feedback varies from person to person. It may be gentle and facilitative or direct and confrontational. The best feedback is that which is focused and shows respect for the person.

In traditional programs, another major group focus is participation in 12-step self-help programs. Patients may be required to attend a certain number of AA or NA meetings each week in order to remain in the group. Patients share their reactions to the meetings that they have attended and are encouraged to obtain a sponsor, do service work (such as set up the chairs or make coffee for meetings), and actively

A Family Speaks

When I met Jim in 1983, I knew he dabbled in drugs but I still married him. I had no idea how his growing drug abuse problem would affect my life over the next decade. In 1986, Jim entered treatment for his heroin addiction for the first time. I was impressed with the nurses in that program. They were compassionate, understanding, and knowledgeable about addiction. They taught Jim the first steps in the recovery process and supported him through the difficult changes that he had to make to maintain a drug-free lifestyle.

One nurse was particularly helpful to me as a family member of a newly recovering addict. She stood out because she consistently showed genuine concern for Jim and me. She always asked about Jim by name. She talked like he was an individual, not just one of the patients in the program. This allowed me to open up to her. I was finally able to ask if some of the things he was going through were normal, and I was very relieved to find out that they were! In contrast, another nurse on the staff talked down to all the patients. Neither the patients nor the family members felt they could talk to her.

Despite all the help he received, Jim relapsed after a few months of being clean. I was disappointed, but I had learned about relapse and I refused to give up on him. After 5 more years, Jim entered a methadone maintenance program. By then our marriage was falling apart. A nurse in the program had special training in working with families. We saw her together. With her help, Jim was able to recognize that he, not I, was responsible for his addiction. He became more responsible for himself. I learned about how I had enabled his addiction and how I would have to change for our drug-free marriage to succeed. It seemed like each of us could hear what the nurse said better than we could hear each other. Now, 4 years later, Jim is still taking methadone, and we are still together. I want nurses to know that little kindnesses as well as bigger interventions can make a positive difference in the lives of drug addicts and their families.

work the steps of the program. Successes and difficulties with maintaining abstinence during the past week are shared and discussed. Less traditional groups may encourage trials or active involvement with 12-step programs but not require it. Expectations for work done outside of the group are more individualized. In all groups, homework may be assigned that emphasizes an important recovery topic.

> *A group member says he has read that studies have found that some alcoholics can learn to drink in a controlled way. How would you respond?*

Self-help groups. The most common type of self-help group for substance abusers is the 12-step group. AA is the model for 12-step support groups. It is composed entirely of alcoholics who have a desire to stop drinking. They believe that mutual support can give the alcoholic strength to abstain. AA aims for total abstinence. The member must admit to alcoholism openly and publicly by introducing himself or herself at meetings, saying, "My name is (John) and I am an alcoholic." At speaker meetings, one or more members share their life histories with the group. This shows that members are more alike than different, removing a common resistance to involvement. AA members also commit themselves to helping each other. Some AA members serve as sponsors, a role that involves availability and accessibility to another member whenever a member feels the need to drink. The sponsor also teaches the person how to work the 12 steps of the program. This reciprocal relationship gives the new member caring support and the sponsor improved self-esteem. AA also involves a strong spiritual orientation that is experienced as supportive by some alcoholics. The 12 steps of AA are listed in Box 25-6. It is easy to see the therapeutic benefit of these steps. For example, admitting the problem, making amends for past behavior, and reaching out to others who need help are sound therapeutic processes.

Some aspects of 12-step programs do not appeal to everyone. One of these is the powerlessness that must be acknowledged. Many people believe that the power to change lies within oneself. Some people are upset by the need to turn over one's will to a higher power. Members are told that this higher power can be the AA group, the sponsor, or anything else they want. Although the higher power does not have to be God in the religious sense, the meetings generally have a religious overtone and usually end with the Lord's Prayer. Some members have formed AA groups especially for agnostics.

Other self-help groups have emerged. One of these is Women for Sobriety (WFS) (Kirkpatrick, 1999). This program shows women how to change their way of life through a change of thinking. The program serves women's needs by teaching them to overcome depression, guilt, and low self-esteem. WFS helps women overcome their drinking problems with the support of other group members who have the same problems and needs. The difference from AA is evident in the first statement of the WFS acceptance program: "I have a drinking problem that once had me." All of the 13 statements of WFS are worded positively.

Another very popular self-help program is the Rational Recovery (RR) movement, which is based on Albert Ellis' Rational Emotive Therapy (see Chapter 3). This program asserts that alcohol dependence is not biologically determined nor beyond our control. Rather, it is seen as a way of thinking. Irrational thoughts keep the alcoholic drinking. Rational thoughts can get and keep the alcoholic sober. RR philosophy is one of personal power; there is no reference to a higher power. RR groups have professional advisors who provide occasional rational input and observe members for problems that indicate a need for a higher level of care. Group meetings operate by discussion, also known as crosstalking. This is in contrast to AA, which strongly discourages interrupting or responding to others. Group members read rational literature, learn to think rationally, and become rational counselors to themselves and others (Trimpey, 1996).

It should be noted that total abstinence is the goal of each of these programs. Patients who choose to try controlled drinking will get no support for this goal from these programs. Controlled drinking for a person who has experienced the loss of control characteristic of addiction has mixed support in the research literature (see Critical Thinking About Contemporary Issues).

Box 25-6

The 12 Steps of Alcoholics Anonymous

1. We admitted we were powerless over alcohol—that our lives had become unmanageable.
2. Came to believe that a Power greater than ourselves could restore us to sanity.
3. Made a decision to turn our will and our lives over to the care of God as we understood Him.
4. Made a searching and fearless moral inventory of ourselves.
5. Admitted to God, to ourselves, and to another human being the exact nature of our wrongs.
6. Were entirely ready to have God remove all these defects of character.
7. Humbly asked Him to remove our shortcomings.
8. Made a list of all persons we had harmed and became willing to make amends to them all.
9. Made direct amends to such people whenever possible except when to do so would injure them or others.
10. Continued to take personal inventory and when we were wrong promptly admitted it.
11. Sought through prayer and meditation to improve our conscious contact with God as we understood Him, praying only for knowledge of His will for us and the power to carry that out.
12. Having a spiritual awakening as the result of these steps, we tried to carry this message to alcoholics and to practice these principles in all our affairs.

The Twelve Steps are reprinted with permission of Alcoholics Anonymous World Services, Inc. Permission to reprint this material does not mean that AA has reviewed or approved of the contents of this publication. AA is a program of recovery from alcoholism only; use of the 12 Steps in connection with programs and activities that are patterned after AA, but address other problems, does not imply otherwise.

CRITICAL THINKING about CONTEMPORARY ISSUES

Is Abstinence Necessary?

For several decades, experts have been debating about whether alcoholics can return to moderate drinking. According to AA and many mental health professionals, abstinence is necessary because alcoholics will inevitably lose control once they start to drink. Advocates of controlled drinking believe that most alcoholics are not powerless over the drug and that they can change their drinking behavior without giving up alcohol entirely. One way to approach the issue is to distinguish degrees of severity. Perhaps dependent alcoholics need to quit cold, but controlled drinking may be possible in milder cases. Aiming for abstinence can also be a way to achieve moderation, just as a lower speed limit causes people to drive more slowly even if they still break the law.

Community Treatment Programs. A variety of community programs are available for drug abusers. Medical detoxification is most often done in hospitals, either on medical, psychiatric, or special substance abuse units. Criteria for admission to these programs may be strict due to managed care restrictions. Length of stay is generally very short—just long enough to stabilize the person medically. Attempts to secure the patient's agreement to participate in aftercare programs is a major part of the intervention. Sometimes, detoxification can be done safely on an outpatient basis. For patients not requiring intense medical monitoring, but still in need of strict environmental controls, there are still many residential, free-standing rehabilitation programs that provide services for weeks to months. Some patients receive court orders to enter into these treatment programs after drug-related arrests, with the costs being covered by the state.

The next level of care after inpatient and residential care is day or evening partial hospitalization. In these programs, the patient spends most of the day in treatment and returns home at night, or spends the day at work and several evenings a week in treatment. Methadone maintenance programs offer methadone maintenance or withdrawal for opiate addicts. Patients must attend daily to obtain their methadone. Methadone programs must have special licensure to operate and follow federal guidelines.

Regular outpatient programs that are attended once or twice per week are even less intensive. Most programs provide a mix of group, individual, and family therapy; vocational counseling; drug and health education; and involvement with 12-step self-help programs. 12-step programs such as AA may be an adjunct to or substitute for professionally run programs.

Employee Assistance Programs. Another potential resource for the substance-abusing patient is the employee assistance program that may be part of an employee health service. Many businesses have found that it is profitable for them to help substance-abusing employees. These programs gener-

ally offer counseling and health education. Employees with a substance abuse problem are usually required to participate in the program to retain their job. Nurses are often key staff members in employee assistance programs. The health-care system has been rather slow in developing these programs for health-care providers. Because there are nurses and physicians who also have problems with drugs and alcohol, there is a need for programs that can focus on their problems.

A Nursing Treatment Plan Summary for patients who abuse substances is presented on the opposite page.

Working with Dually Diagnosed Patients

The dually diagnosed patient needs treatment for both disorders. The problem is that the substance abuse and mental health fields have developed approaches that appear to conflict with each other. For instance, many substance abuse counselors rely on direct confrontation of behavior. Such an approach could be detrimental to a person with severe mental illness. Substance abuse counselors also tend to have a limited understanding of the medications used for psychiatric disorders. In fact, the chronically mentally ill are often excluded from substance abuse programs. Mental health clinicians, on the other hand, often do not understand substance abuse and may overlook symptoms of continued use. They tend to think that the substance abuse will stop when the person's psychiatric illness is under control. Patients can suffer from these differences, either missing out on some important treatments or getting caught in the middle of two different approaches with two different clinicians (called parallel treatment). To avoid this, treatment is sometimes offered in sequence (first psychiatric treatment, then substance abuse treatment or vice versa).

The best possible treatment is an integrated one, with both services offered by program staff qualified in both areas and excellent coordination of other community services (Mueser et al, 1998). The chronically mentally ill can benefit more from these programs, which generally are less confrontational and more supportive than traditional substance abuse programs. They have professional staff to prescribe and follow medication effectiveness. They often practice assertive case management, in which case workers seek out patients when they fail to show for treatment and help patients to meet multiple psychosocial needs, including basic living arrangements. Such specialized treatment programs offer special treatment groups for the mentally ill, chemically addicted (MICA) patient (also called mentally ill, substance abusing, or MISA) and refer patients to community self-help groups developed for such people, called double trouble groups. Nurses who understand both conditions are in an ideal position to work with dually diagnosed patients.

Appropriate treatment is linked to correct assessment of co-existing conditions. If the causative disorder can be isolated, it should be the focus of initial treatment unless the secondary disorder has become life-threatening, as when the alcoholic develops a suicidal depression. However, it should not be assumed that resolution of primary psychiatric problems will automatically resolve associated substance abuse problems. If substances are used chronically, substance abuse

NURSING DIAGNOSIS: Ineffective individual coping
EXPECTED OUTCOME: The patient will abstain from using all mood-altering chemicals.

SHORT-TERM GOALS	INTERVENTION	RATIONALE
The patient will substitute healthy coping responses for substance-abusing behavior.	Help the patient to identify the substance-abusing behavior and its consequences. Help the patient to identify the substance abuse problem. Involve the patient in describing situations that lead to substance-abusing behavior. Consistently offer support and the expectation that the patient has the strength to overcome the problem.	Motivation for change is related to recognition of a problem that is upsetting to the patient. Identification of predisposing factors and precipitating stressors must precede planning for more adaptive behavioral responses.
The patient will assume responsibility for behavior.	Encourage the patient to participate in a treatment program. Develop with the patient a written contract for behavioral change that is signed by the patient and nurse. Help the patient to identify and adopt healthier coping responses.	Denial and rationalization are dysfunctional coping mechanisms that can interfere with recovery. Personal commitment will enhance the likelihood of successful abstinence.
The patient will identify and use social support systems.	Identify and assess social support systems that are available to the patient. Provide support to significant others. Educate the patient and significant others about the substance abuse problem and available resources. Refer the patient to appropriate resources and provide support until the patient is involved in the program.	Substance abusers are often dependent and socially isolated people who use drugs to gain confidence in social situations. Substance-abusing behavior alienates significant others, thus increasing the person's isolation. It is difficult to manipulate people who have participated in the same behaviors. Social support systems must be readily available over time and acceptable to the patient.

NURSING DIAGNOSIS: Sensory-perceptual alteration
EXPECTED OUTCOME: The patient will overcome addiction safely and with a minimum of discomfort.

SHORT-TERM GOALS	INTERVENTION	RATIONALE
The patient will withdraw from dependence on the abused substance.	Supportive physical care: vital signs, nutrition, hydration, seizure precautions. Administer medication according to detoxification schedule.	Detoxification of the physically dependent person can be dangerous and is always uncomfortable. The patient's physical safety must receive high priority for nursing intervention
The patient will be oriented to time, place, person, and situation.	Assess orientation frequently, orient the patient if needed, and place a clock and calendar where they can be seen by the patient.	Cognitive function is usually affected by addiction; disorientation is frightening.
The patient will report symptoms of withdrawal.	Observe carefully for withdrawal symptoms and report suspected withdrawal immediately.	Withdrawal symptoms provide powerful motivation for continued substance abuse; judgment may be impaired by substance use.
The patient will correctly interpret environmental stimuli.	Explain all nursing interventions, assign consistent staff, keep soft light on in room, avoid loud noises, and encourage trusted family and friends to stay with the patient.	Sensory and perceptual alterations related to use of drugs or alcohol are frightening; consistency reduces the need to interpret stimuli.
The patient will recognize and talk about hallucinations or delusions.	Observe for response to internal stimuli, encourage patient to describe hallucinations or delusions, and explain the relationship of these experiences to withdrawal from addictive substances.	Helping the patient to identify delusional or hallucinatory experiences and relate them to withdrawal is reassuring.

can develop into a primary disorder, taking on a life of its own. In these cases, the initial emphasis of treatment must be on the most serious problem at the time. Although the relative importance of symptoms may vary with time and influence the focus of treatment, both disorders must be treated.

Comprehensive treatment for co-occurring disorders usually requires a combination of pharmacological treatment, psychosocial treatment, and supportive services. Successful psychosocial programs for patients with psychiatric and substance abuse disorders provide behavioral skill-building interventions as the primary ingredient of active treatment, which has been shown to be more effective than case management or 12-step intervention (Jerrell, 1996). In addition, the following five therapeutic tasks or steps that can serve as guidelines for structuring treatment of dual-diagnosis patients have been identified (Carey, 1996):

- Establish a therapeutic alliance with the patient.
- Help the patient evaluate the costs and benefits of continued substance use.
- Individualize goals for change with the patient that include harm reduction as an alternative to total abstinence.
- Help the patient build an environment and lifestyle supportive of abstinence.
- Acknowledge that recovery is a long process, and help the patient cope with crises by anticipating triggers of relapse and coping with setbacks as they occur.

Because both mental illness and substance abuse are chronic, relapsing conditions, the course of treatment can be expected to take considerable time. Stages of treatment have been identified and are used as the basis for treatment planning in many dual diagnosis treatment programs today. Interventions appropriate to each stage have been identified and are listed along with goals in Table 25-4 (Drake et al, 1996a). Counselors and interdisciplinary teams are also useful, as can be seen in the following clinical example.

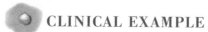

CLINICAL EXAMPLE

Bobby was a 17-year-old who was admitted to the hospital acutely psychotic with a history of recent use of PCP. The emergency room nurse noted scarring of the veins in Bobby's arm and surmised that he also used heroin. Blood and urine testing confirmed this suspicion. Bobby recovered from his psychotic episode in 24 hours but was extremely uncomfortable due to opiate withdrawal. The decision was made to use titrated doses of methadone to help with the withdrawal. Mr. L, a young nurse, established a close relationship with Bobby during this time. Bobby requested the nurse's help in planning for his future, but doubted that he had the strength to stay away from drugs. He was advised to take a day at a time. Mr. L took Bobby on a visit to a drug treatment program, and he agreed to try membership in one of the groups at this center. Bobby did well in the group and was very helpful to new members, describing his experiences and encouraging them to "take 1 day at a time." Bobby expressed an interest in finishing school and said he would like to become a drug counselor. The staff of the drug treatment program agreed that Bobby seemed to have an aptitude for that role and encouraged him to pursue his goal.

Selected Nursing Diagnoses

- Altered thought processes related to PCP use, as evidenced by uncontrolled behavior in the emergency room
- Situational low self-esteem related to pessimism about ability to stop using drugs, as evidenced by expressed self-doubt

Mr. L used his relationship with Bobby to communicate his belief that he could successfully give up drugs. This message has a core of positive regard for Bobby's potential strength. The staff of the drug treatment program added to this seed of self-esteem by encouraging Bobby to help others in the program and then to aim higher at becoming a counselor himself. This taught Bobby that there were re-

Table **25-4**

Treatment Stages, Goals, and Interventions for Dually Diagnosed Patients	
Stage of Treatment	**Suggested Goals and Interventions**
Engagement	**Goal:** Development of working relationship between patient and nurse. **Interventions:** Intervene in crises, help with practical living problems, establish rapport with family members, demonstrate caring and support, listen actively.
Persuasion	**Goal:** Patient acceptance of having a substance abuse problem and the need for active change strategies. **Interventions:** Help to analyze pros and cons of substance use, educate patient and family, arrange peer group discussions, expose patient to double trouble self-help groups, adjust medication, persuade patient to comply with medication regimen (motivational interviewing skills is particularly helpful during this stage).
Active treatment	**Goal:** Abstinence from substance use and compliance with medication. **Interventions:** Help to change thinking patterns, friends, habits, behaviors, and living situations as necessary to support goals; teach social skills; encourage to develop positive social supports through double trouble self-help groups; enlist family support of changes; monitor urine and breath for substances; offer medication.
Relapse prevention	**Goal:** Absence or minimization of return to substance abuse. **Interventions:** Reinforce abstinence, compliance, and behavioral changes; identify risk factors and help to practice preventive strategies; encourage continued involvement in double trouble groups; continue laboratory monitoring.

wards in life other than those attached to drug use. Gradually, he learned to value the interpersonal rewards more than the drug rewards while making positive use of his past difficulties.

Intervening with Impaired Colleagues

It is usually difficult for nurses to respond to a colleague who is showing signs of a substance abuse problem. This is true of supervisors as well as peers. For the safety of the nurse, as well as the nurse's patients, it is necessary to identify the problem and take action. In addition, many states have laws that require health-care professionals to report colleagues who show signs of working while impaired. In these states, reporting is both an ethical and a legal obligation.

It is not usually easy to be sure that a nurse's practice is impaired by drug or alcohol use. However, particular patterns of behavior and signs are characteristic of this problem (Box 25-7). The concerned colleague should report incidents of this nature to the supervisor. It is also important that these incidents be documented in writing, with the time, date, place, description of the incident, and the names of others who were present. This documentation will make it easier to intervene.

If the pattern of behavior indicates that impairment exists, an intervention should be planned. An advisor should be selected who has expertise in the area of impaired nursing practice. This advisor could be someone from the state nurse rehabilitation committee, if there is one. A team of people who have meaningful relationships with the nurse should be asked to prepare written statements demonstrating their observations of probable impaired practice. The team should consist of co-workers, the supervisor or other nurse administrator, and perhaps a family member. The team rehearses the statements in a meeting without the nurse present to work out any details and to ensure a non-moralistic tone. They also anticipate various reactions the nurse may have and decide how to respond to these. Treatment options are discussed and plans made to escort the nurse directly from the meeting to a treatment facility.

After this preparation, a meeting is called in which the team members read their statements to the nurse, who is informed of the disciplinary action recommended by the team, which usually requires that the nurse enter treatment or resign from nursing and potentially lose the license to practice. The nurse is escorted to either an inpatient treatment program or an outpatient appointment. Because the suicide risk for nurses who have just gone through an intervention is great, the nurse should not be left alone after the intervention.

During treatment the supervisor should maintain contact with the treatment program to see how the nurse is progressing. It is strongly advised that a return-to-work contract be written that clearly describes the nurse's responsibilities upon return. If the state has a nurse rehabilitation or peer assistance program, it can assume some responsibility for monitoring the nurse's progress and in developing treatment and return-to-work contracts (Finke et al, 1996). This type of intervention makes it possible for the chemically dependent nurse to get the treatment needed, yet remain employed, a situation in which everyone benefits.

Box **25-7**

Signs of Impaired Nursing Practice

JOB PERFORMANCE CHANGES
Controlled Drug Handling/Records (potential drug diversion)

- Drug counts incorrect
- Excessive errors
- Excessive wastage, often not countersigned
- Medicine signed out to patient who has not been in pain
- Two strengths of drug signed out to same patient, same time
- Packaging appears to be tampered with
- Patient complaints of ineffective pain control
- Volunteers to give controlled drugs
- Comes in early or stays late
- Disappears into the bathroom after handling controlled drugs
- Unexplained absences from the unit

General Performance

- Medication errors
- Poor judgment
- Euphoric recall for involvement in unpleasant situations, or confrontations on the job
- Illogical or sloppy charting
- Absenteeism, especially in conjunction with days off
- Requesting leave time just before the assigned shift
- Tardiness with elaborate excuses

- Job shrinkage (does the minimum work required to get by)
- Missed deadlines

BEHAVIOR/PERSONALITY CHANGES

- Sudden changes in mood
- Periods of irritability
- Forgetfulness
- Wears long sleeves, even in hot weather
- Socially isolates from co-workers
- Inappropriate behavior
- Has chronic pain condition
- History of pain treatment with controlled substances

SIGNS OF USE

- Alcohol on the breath
- Constant use of perfumes, mouthwash, and breath mints
- Flushed face, reddened eyes, unsteady gait, slurred speech
- Hyperactivity, accelerated speech
- Increasing family problems that interfere with work

SIGNS OF WITHDRAWAL

- Tremors, restlessness, diaphoresis, pupil changes
- Watery eyes, runny nose, stomach aches, joint pains, gooseflesh

> *An enabler is a person who supports someone in maintaining an addiction. Describe behaviors that would enable a colleague to continue drug or alcohol use that impairs performance of nursing roles. What alternative behaviors would be more helpful?*

Preventive Interventions

Primary prevention programs aimed at preventing drug use among children are in place in many elementary schools in this country (see Citing the Evidence). School nurses can be involved in education efforts in the schools. Nurses can also support legislation designed to reduce the incidence of use and abuse. Nurses can serve as public speakers in the community on drug abuse issues.

Secondary prevention efforts are aimed at people with mild to moderate drinking problems. For every person with a severe drinking problem, there are several more people with mild to moderate drinking problems. Several brief therapies have evolved to address their special needs. These range from simple advice to stop drinking to more elaborate programs involving early identification, presentation of assessment findings, education (see the Patient Education Plan below), advice regarding the need to reduce drinking with an emphasis on personal responsibility, self-help manuals, and periodic follow-up. People with mild to moderate drinking problems are increasingly being referred to treatment programs through the courts after DWI charges.

Tertiary prevention involves decreasing the complications of addiction. Medical and psychiatric treatment settings still serve a major role here, as do more current case management, community outreach, and dual diagnosis programs.

EVALUATION

The evaluation of substance abuse treatment is based on accomplishment of the expected outcomes and short-term goals. The nurse and patient together should evaluate progress toward these goals on a regular basis. If progress is not being made, together they should re-evaluate both the goal and the progress to see where the problem lies and what needs to be done about it.

Relapse does not automatically mean failure. Progress toward a lifelong goal of abstinence from substances of abuse can be measured in many ways. For example, a significant increase in the periods of time that a chronic alcoholic patient stays sober between binges or relapses can be viewed as

Citing the Evidence on

Preventing Drug Abuse

BACKGROUND: The use of illegal substances in childhood and adolescence occurs at an alarming rate. In response to this problem, there has been a growth of schoolwide intervention programs designed to curb, if not eliminate, substance use in this population. Project DARE (Drug Abuse Resistance Education) is one of the most widely used of these programs. This study examined the impact of Project DARE 10 years after its administration.

RESULTS: Few differences were found between those young people who had received DARE or a standard drug-education curriculum in terms of actual drug use, drug attitudes, or self-esteem. In no case did the DARE group have a more successful outcome than the comparison group.

IMPLICATIONS: The widespread popularity of DARE is interesting, given the lack of evidence for its efficacy. Research suggests that DARE, which is more expensive and longer running than conventional drug education programs, should be reconsidered by schools wishing to implement a drug education program.

Lynn D et al: Project DARE: no effects at 10-year follow-up, *J Consult Clin Psychol* 67(4):590, 1999.

 PATIENT EDUCATION PLAN *Promoting Adaptive Chemically Mediated Responses*

CONTENT	INSTRUCTIONAL ACTIVITIES	EVALUATION
Elicit perceptions of substance use.	Lead group discussion regarding knowledge about chemical use and experience with it; correct misperceptions.	The patient will describe accurate information about substance use.
Demonstrate negative effects of substance abuse.	Show films of physical and psychological effects of substance abuse; provide written materials.	The patient will identify and describe physical and psychological effects of substance abuse.
Interaction with peer who has abused chemicals.	Small group discussion with peer group member who has abused substances and quit because of negative experiences.	The patient will compare advantages and disadvantages of using mind-altering substances.
Obtain agreement to abstain from use of mind-altering substances.	Discuss future plans for refusing abused chemicals if offered.	The patient will verbally agree to abstain from using mind-altering substances.

improvement. A decrease in the amount of time that the alcoholic patient remains in relapse before returning to sobriety can likewise indicate improvement. The patient who returns to treatment after relapse should be commended for previous successes and for the decision to keep trying. Then the nurse and patient together can analyze what worked and what did not work in the patient's attempts to maintain sobriety. This information should be used to modify the patient's relapse prevention plan.

It is also recommended that several measures of success toward abstinence goals be used, not just patient self-report. Objective measures such as breath analysis and urinalysis should be used as well as information from collateral sources such as spouses and employers (with a signed release of information). Success toward goals in other areas of living such as obtaining or keeping a job, improvements in health, and improvements in family relationships are interrelated with abstinence goals and important in the total recovery process.

Summary

1. Adaptive chemically mediated responses include "natural highs," which may be related to physical activity or meditation. Maladaptive responses include dependence on tobacco and alcohol and abuse of or dependence on illicit drugs.

2. After reaching its highest peak in 1979, drug use decreased for several years until 1991. Since then, drug use among high school seniors increased every year until it leveled off in 1997 and 1998, and even decreased in some cases. Among the general population age 12 and older, drug use levels have remained fairly constant since 1992. Multiple-substance abuse and dual diagnosis continue to be major problems.

3. Patient behaviors related to chemically mediated responses are related to dependence, intoxication, or overdose and vary according to the abused substances. Abused substances may include CNS depressants (alcohol, barbiturates, benzodiazepines), marijuana, stimulants, opiates, hallucinogens, PCP, inhalants, and nicotine.

4. Predisposing factors that lead to maladaptive chemically mediated responses are described from the biological, psychological, and sociocultural perspectives. Precipitating stressors include withdrawal from addiction.

5. Coping resources include motivation, social supports, health, social skills, material and economic assets, and intellectual and personality traits. Maladaptive coping mechanisms include denial, rationalization, and minimization.

6. Primary NANDA nursing diagnoses related to maladaptive chemically mediated responses are sensory-perceptual alteration, altered thought processes, ineffective individual coping, and altered family processes related to alcoholism.

7. Primary *DSM–IV–TR* diagnoses are dependence, abuse, intoxication, or withdrawal related to a particular substance.

8. The expected outcome of nursing care is that the patient will abstain from using all mood-altering chemicals.

9. Planning is based on providing first for safe withdrawal, followed by developing ways to maintain abstinence. Support systems, including family, friends, and self-help groups, should be involved whenever possible.

10. Interventions include biological, psychological, and social interventions; working with dually diagnosed patients; intervening with impaired colleagues; and preventive interventions.

11. Evaluation criteria for nursing care related to chemically mediated responses include goal achievement, increases in amount of sober time, negative breath and urinalysis tests, and improved psychosocial dimensions.

Competent Caring A Clinical Exemplar of a Psychiatric Nurse

S.W Jernigan, BS, RN, C

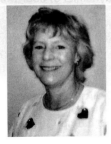

One Sunday morning I was doing a dressing change on a patient in for her third admission. This patient's right knee had been injured during a "bust" for possession of narcotics. Though the dressing change was a simple one, she seemed talkative and jumped at the chance to complete the procedure in the treatment room. She talked at length about her Baltimore neighborhood where she had lived all her life, her deep roots in the community, and her mother's recent death.

At the time I had perhaps the easiest job in the world—saying "mmmhh," and "uh-uh," to an interesting person who wanted to talk. But it wasn't long before she got to the subject of her repeated failures to stay off drugs. Then she began to speak more slowly and with intense feeling, obviously looking for answers—of which I had few. The old standards, she'd already heard, "Keep trying," "Don't give up," "Go to NA," and her facial expressions confirmed this. A silence ensued. Quietly she said, "This is going to kill me. What can I do?" Another silence. Finally I said to her, "I have heard from some who said the only way they could 'stay clean' was to move; to get totally away from the old neighborhood, leave all the old friends, and start a new life. It is a radical, shocking change, but for some people it is the only way." Her shoulders straightened. She nodded.

She was discharged several days later, and hasn't "reappeared"—maybe because she moved to another state.... maybe because of being "clean"—or so we heard. In retrospect, I think this patient didn't just have something to say—there was something she wanted to hear, and on some level she knew what she needed to hear. Patients in difficulty often have a sort of homing instinct about what they need in order to be well—it might be attention; it might be solitude; it might be, as in this case, permission to take the next step.

The gender differences in the prevalence of eating disorders may result from biological, sociocultural, and psychodynamic factors, as well as the fact that men may be more reluctant to seek treatment. Although there are differences in the prevalence of eating disorders in men and women, men and women have more similarities than differences in terms of the illness, rates of comorbid psychiatric disorders, and satisfaction with body image.

Bulimia and anorexia may be present in the same patient. As many as 50% of individuals with anorexia develop bulimic symptoms, and some people with bulimia develop anorexia. Bulimia usually occurs in people of normal weight, but it may also occur in obese people and thin people (Fig. 26-2).

Binge Eating Disorder. Individuals with binge eating disorder consume large amounts of calories but do not attempt to prevent weight gain. This disorder has a prevalence of approximately 2% to 4% of the population. It has been estimated that 19% to 40% of obese people who seek treatment for weight control have binge eating disorder; this suggests that assessing for eating disorders should be an important part of weight management programs (Brewerton et al, 1998; Grilo, 1998). The differences among people who are obese but do not binge, those who are obese and do binge, and nonobese patients with bulimia who both binge and purge are summarized in Table 26-1.

ASSESSMENT

Patients with maladaptive eating regulation responses need to receive a comprehensive nursing assessment that includes complete biological, psychological, and sociocultural evaluations. A full physical examination should be performed, with particular attention given to vital signs, weight for height and age, skin, the cardiovascular system, and evidence of laxative or diuretic abuse and vomiting. A dental examination may be indicated, and it is useful to assess growth, sexual development, and general indicators of physical development. A psychiatric history, substance use history, and family assessment are also needed.

Specific attention should focus on the assessment of eating regulation responses. Several questionnaires and rating scales have been developed to screen for the presence of eating disorders (Box 26-1). However, one study found that asking only the following two questions may be as effective as more extensive questionnaires in identifying women with eating disorders (Freund et al, 1993):

- Are you satisfied with your eating patterns?
- Do you ever eat in secret?

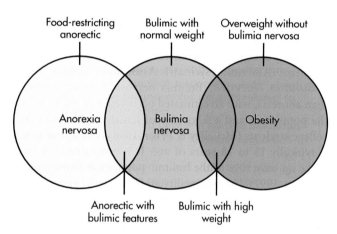

Fig. 26-2 The overlapping relationship between eating disorders and obesity. (Modified from Santmeyer K: Interventions for clients with anorexia nervosa and bulimia nervosa. In Ignatavicius D et al, editors: *Medical-surgical nursing across the health care continuum*, ed 3, Philadelphia, 1999, WB Saunders.)

Box 26-1

Behavioral Rating Scales Related to Eating Disorders

- Body Attitudes Test
- Diagnostic Survey for Eating Disorders (DSED)
- Eating Habits Checklist
- Eating Behaviors Diary
- Eating Disorders Inventory 2 (EDI-2)

Table 26-1

	Obese Nonbingers	Obese Bingers	Nonobese Bulimic Patients
Differences in Obese Nonbingers, Obese Bingers, and Nonobese Bulimic Patients			
Body image distortion	Low or none	Moderate to low	High level
Amount of binging	Once per month or less	High amount but less than bulimic patients of normal weight	Very high level
Mood disturbance	Same as general population	One third chronic	One third to one half chronic and 75% to 80% lifetime
Purging	Rare	Infrequent (tend to use laxatives)	High level
Degree of control regarding binging	High	Medium to low	Low
Interest in food	Preoccupied at times	Obsessed	Obsessed
Problems with self-esteem	Same as general population	Low self-esteem	Low self-esteem
Substance abuse	Same as general population	Moderate to high	High

These two questions can be easily incorporated into the nursing assessment of all patients. If a patient is being evaluated for an eating disorder, additional information should be obtained, including the following (Erickson & Yager, 1998):

- Actual and desired weight
- Onset and pattern of menstruation
- Food avoidances, restrictions, dieting and fasting patterns
- Frequency and extent of binge eating and purging
- Unusual beliefs about nutrition
- Use of laxatives, diuretics, diet pills, and so on
- Chewing and spitting food
- Weight and shape preoccupations
- Body image disturbances
- Food preferences and peculiarities
- Compulsive exercise patterns

It is also helpful to ask the patient how the illness developed and its impact on school, work, and social relationships so that a holistic view of the patient's world can be obtained.

Behaviors

Binge Eating. Binge eating involves the rapid consumption of large quantities of food in a discrete period of time, although there is no agreement on exactly how many calories constitutes a binge. Patients with anorexia who binge may describe a binge of several hundred calories. Patients with bulimia who are not also anorectic may ingest several thousand calories at a sitting. An emphasis on the patient's perception of loss of control and perceived excessive caloric intake is more important to the nursing assessment than the total number of calories consumed during a binge. Therefore it is important that the nurse carefully assess exactly what each patient means by a binge.

People usually binge secretively, and there is often considerable shame associated with their binging behavior. A person with bulimia typically is of average weight or is slightly overweight and has a history of unsuccessful dieting. The severity of the binging can vary greatly, ranging from several times a week, to more than 10 times a day, to only occasional binges related to stressful situations.

Fasting or Restricting. People with anorexia often do not consume more than 500 to 700 calories daily and may ingest as few as 200 calories daily, yet they see their intake as adequate for their energy needs. They may follow an unbalanced vegetarian diet, eliminating all meat, poultry, fish, and dairy products without substituting nonanimal sources of protein and other important nutrients. They may be obsessive-compulsive about their eating habits and food choices, such as eating the same foods, eating foods in a predetermined order, or eating at the same time every day. They may have bizarre food preferences, avoid foods that are considered fattening, and fast for days at a time.

Despite these restrictions, many people with anorexia are preoccupied or obsessed with food and may do much of the family cooking or be employed in a food-related occupation. The following clinical example describes the fasting behavior seen in people with anorexia.

 CLINICAL EXAMPLE

Barbara is a 15-year-old white female who has been restricting her food intake for 6 months because she feels too fat. Her weight at the beginning of her food restriction was 128 pounds. This weight was appropriate for her age, her height (5 feet, 5 inches), and her small body frame. Her current weight is 102 pounds, which is approximately 80% of what she should weigh. The patient denies having any eating problems and believes that her family is overreacting to her weight loss. She is willing to come for treatment only because her family wants her to do so.

Barbara was age 13 at menarche and had regular periods until they stopped 2 months ago. She says she never tried or planned to lose weight but admits to becoming a vegetarian 6 months ago. Despite her low weight, Barbara thinks she needs to lose another 10 pounds because she thinks her thighs are too large. She is an avid ballet dancer and practices dancing 2 to 3 hours a day. Her family describes her as the perfect daughter.

Selected Nursing Diagnoses

- Altered nutrition: less than body requirements related to restricted food intake, as evidenced by weight loss
- Body image disturbance related to eating disorder, as evidenced by continued desire to lose weight
- Ineffective denial related to eating problems, as evidenced by a lack of acceptance of realistic weight parameters

Purging. A variety of purging behaviors may be used by people with maladaptive eating regulation responses to prevent weight gain. These behaviors include excessive exercise, over-the-counter and prescription diuretics, diet pills, laxatives, and steroids. Laxatives are commonly abused by people with eating disorders, yet they are one of the most inefficient ways to lose calories.

Laxative abuse often begins gradually but can increase to 60 per week in some people. Less well-known substances used to counteract weight gain include insulin, cocaine, heroin, thyroid replacements, nicotine, hallucinogens, analgesics, benzodiazepines, antidepressants, ipecac, and sorbitol. Many patients engage in more than one purging behavior.

For these patients, exercising often becomes a grueling, time-consuming affair. Running or participating in high-impact aerobics for 2 to 3 hours each day is typical of the compulsive exerciser. Many patients with an eating disorder exercise so much that they sustain major skeletal injuries, but this still does not deter them from continuing this maladaptive behavior. Such behavior is seen in the following clinical example.

 CLINICAL EXAMPLE

Bill is a single, 30-year-old man with a 7-year history of anorexia nervosa and bulimia nervosa. Bill exercises compulsively at least 3 hours daily; from age 23 until age 29 he exercised 6 to 7 hours daily. Examples of current and previous exercise rituals include running 25 miles followed by a 2- to 3-mile swim and bicycling 25 miles before allowing himself to eat a meal. His athletic abilities have been rewarded with numerous trophies. He is receiving fewer trophies lately because of damage to his knees from overuse.

In addition to exercising compulsively, Bill also vomits after binging and has periods of fasting that last 2 to 3 days. When he does eat a regular meal, he eats only certain foods and eats them in a certain order. Bill also writes obsessively and is methodical about the order of his personal hygiene. He is depressed about the fact that his life revolves around his eating, hygiene, and exercise rituals, and he is eager to receive treatment.

Selected Nursing Diagnoses

- Altered nutrition: less than body requirements related to anxiety about body size, as evidenced by binging and fasting
- Body image disturbance related to fears of gaining weight, as evidenced by excessive exercise and food restrictions
- Risk for injury related to excessive exercise, as evidenced by knee injuries

---

Binging, fasting, and purging are sometimes described as addictive behaviors. Compare these behaviors to smoking, gambling, and substance abuse.

Medical Complications. Every person with a maladaptive eating regulation response usually has some type of associated physical problem. The various complications associated with eating disorders are listed in Box 26-2.

An assessment of the patient's physical status can reveal the seriousness of the eating problem. For example, patients 20% below or 40% above their ideal body weight demonstrate more physical abnormalities than those who are closer to their ideal weight. Patients who are 30% below or 100% above their ideal body weight will have clinical and laboratory findings that are often life threatening. People who vomit and use laxatives or diuretics, regardless of their weight, usually have significant and sometimes life-threatening clinical findings and laboratory abnormalities.

In anorexia nervosa, metabolic and endocrine abnormalities result from the reaction of the body to the malnutrition associated with starvation. All body systems are affected. Most commonly seen are amenorrhea, osteoporosis, and hypometabolic symptoms such as cold intolerance and bradycardia. Starvation may cause hypotension, constipation, and acid-base and fluid-electrolyte disturbances, including pedal edema.

In bulimia nervosa, potassium depletion and hypokalemia are often seen as a result of vomiting and laxative or diuretic abuse. Symptoms of potassium depletion include muscle weakness, cardiac arrhythmias, conduction abnormalities, hypotension, and other problems associated with electrolyte imbalance. Gastric, esophageal, and bowel abnormalities are common complaints in patients with bulimia. Those who vomit are subject to erosion of the dental enamel and enlargement of the parotid glands.

Serious health problems caused by excess weight or prior health problems exacerbated by increased weight are com-

---

Box 26-2

Medical Complications of Eating Disorders

CENTRAL NERVOUS SYSTEM
Cortical atrophy
Decreased rapid eye movement and shortwave sleep
Fatigue
Seizures
Thermoregulatory abnormalities
Weakness

RENAL
Hematuria
Proteinuria
Renal calculi

HEMATOLOGICAL
Anemia
Leukopenia
Thrombocytopenia

GASTROINTESTINAL
Dental caries and erosion
Diarrhea (laxative abuse)
Esophagitis, esophageal tears
Gastric dilation
Hypercholesterolemia
Pancreatitis
Parotid swelling

METABOLIC
Acidosis
Dehydration
Hypocalcemia
Hypochloremic alkalosis
Hypokalemia
Hypomagnesemia
Hypophosphatemia
Osteoporosis

ENDOCRINE
Amenorrhea
Decreased luteinizing hormone and follicle-stimulating hormone
Decreased triiodothyronine, increased reverse triiodothyronine, rT3, normal thyroxin and thyroid-stimulating hormone
Irregular menses
Regression of secondary sex characteristics

CARDIOVASCULAR
Bradycardia
Dysrhythmia, sudden death
Postural hypotension
Ventricular enlargement

mon for individuals with binge eating disorder and concurrent morbid obesity. Many have hypertension, cardiac problems, sleep apnea, difficulties with mobility, and diabetes mellitus. Some of the medical consequences of eating disorders are seen in the following clinical example.

 CLINICAL EXAMPLE

Audrey is a 25-year-old black woman with a 4-year history of restrictive intake and a 3-year history of binge eating and laxative abuse. Audrey has been concerned about her weight since high school, when she was a star basketball player, a competitive swimmer, and a participant in track, volleyball, and tennis. She bypassed her senior year in high school. She began to diet at age 20, and her severe restriction of food at age 21 led to a 20-pound weight loss and amenorrhea. At age 22 she began to binge and use laxatives. Since that time she has binged two to three times each week and uses an average of 30 to 60 laxatives each week.

Audrey is constantly preoccupied with food and her weight and has periods of mood lability, sadness, lack of energy, social isolation, anxiety, irritability, and difficulty concentrating. Audrey also reports chronic constipation; bloating; edema of the hands, feet, legs, and face; and lightheadedness. She recently consulted a gastroenterologist for her severe constipation and was advised that her large intestine is grossly oversized. Audrey became very frightened by the report and immediately called a local eating disorder program for help.

Selected Nursing Diagnoses

- Altered nutrition: less than body requirements related to fear of gaining weight, as evidenced by binging
- Body image disturbance related to anxiety about body size, as evidenced by excessive use of laxatives
- Constipation related to maladaptive eating patterns, as evidenced by pain, bloating, and enlarged intestine

Psychiatric Complications. Many patients seeking treatment for eating disorders show evidence of other psychiatric disorders. Comorbid major depression or dysthymia has been reported in 50% to 75% of people with anorexia and bulimia, and obsessive-compulsive disorder may be found in as many as 25% of patients with anorexia. Among patients with bulimia, there are increased rates of anxiety disorders, posttraumatic stress disorder, substance abuse, and mood disorders. People with antisocial personality disorders are six to seven times more likely to have bulimia than the general population. Finally, binge eating disorder has been found to be associated with higher rates of major depression, panic disorder, bulimia nervosa, borderline personality disorder, and avoidant personality disorder (American Psychiatric Association, 2000a).

Predisposing Factors

Researchers have identified biological, psychological, and sociocultural factors that may predispose a person to the development of an eating disorder. These factors are involved in the regulation and control of food intake and reflect a combination of genetic, neurochemical, developmental, characterological, social, cultural, and familial factors (Fig. 26-3).

Biological. Both anorexia nervosa and bulimia nervosa are familial (Strober et al, 2000). There is a higher risk for eating disorders in first-degree female relatives of people with eating disorders than in the general population. The concordance rates for eating disorders are 52% in monozygotic twins and 11% in dizygotic twins. There is also a higher risk for other eating disorders, depression, and substance abuse in first-degree relatives of people with eating disorders (Wade et al, 2000). The development of an eating disorder in a vulnerable person may be caused by complex relationships among personality traits, environmental and familial factors, and genetic predisposition (Lilenfeld et al, 1998).

Biological models of the etiology of eating disorders focus on the appetite regulation center in the hypothalamus, which controls specific neurochemical mechanisms for feeding and satiety. It has been hypothesized that the neurotransmitters, neuromodulators, and hormones that control feeding and satiety are dysregulated in patients with eating disorders.

Studies in animals and humans indicate that reduced serotonin is associated with reduced satiety, increased food intake, and dysphoric mood. When dietary tryptophan (the amino acid necessary for the brain to manufacture serotonin) is reduced, women with bulimia show a marked increase in eating behavior and show mood changes such as irritability, lability, and fatigue; this suggests a disturbance of serotonin activity in this disorder (Brewerton, 1995; Weltzin et al, 1995; Jimerson et al, 1997). It has also been reported that 3-methoxy-4-hydroxyphenylglycol (MHPG), the major

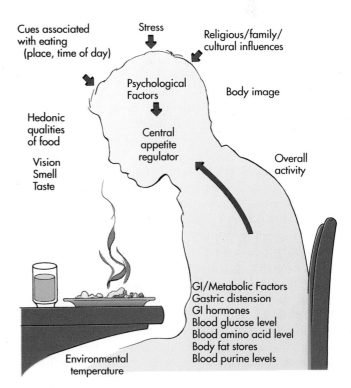

Fig. 26-3 Major peripheral inputs influencing appetite.

metabolite of norepinephrine, is reduced in eating disorders, which suggests a role for this neurotransmitter.

Other hypotheses propose that eating disorders may be a type of mood disorder or may be a type of disorder caused by decreased endogenous opioid activity. This last theory is based on the clinical observation that carbohydrates, particularly sugar, play a role in binge eating and obesity; many binge eaters prefer to eat sweets during a binge. Beta-endorphin has an appetite-stimulating mechanism; if sugar stimulates beta-endorphin production, it can eventually lead to increased eating. Positron emission tomography (PET) scans are also being conducted on patients with anorexia, and abnormal findings on computed tomography (CT) scans of the brain have been reported in more than half of these patients. All of these models are still in the developmental stage, and ongoing research promises to shed more light on the biological factors that may predispose a person to maladaptive eating regulation responses.

> *Analyze the hypothesized role of serotonin in the development of both eating disorders and depressive disorders, as well as the implications this has for the use of selective serotonin reuptake inhibitors as a medication strategy for both disorders.*

Psychological. Most patients with eating disorders exhibit psychological symptoms such as rigidity, ritualism, and meticulousness. When studied years after treatment, women who had long-term weight recovery continued to show an obsessive need for perfectionism, exactness, and symmetry, as well as greater risk avoidance, restraint, and impulse control (Pollice et al, 1997; Srinivasagam et al, 1995). Early separation and individuation conflicts, a pervasive sense of ineffectiveness and helplessness, difficulty interpreting feelings and tolerating intense emotional states, and a fear of biological or psychological maturity may predispose a person to an eating disorder. Women who binge also report great fluctuations of self-esteem, negative affect, shame, and guilt (Sanftner & Crowther, 1998; Greeno et al, 2000).

Environmental. A variety of environmental factors may predispose a person to developing an eating disorder. Early histories of patients with eating disorders are often complicated by medical and surgical illnesses, separations, and family deaths. Women with bulimia also describe growing up in a detached family environment and experiencing more behavioral disturbances such as drug abuse, suicide attempts, truancy, and other emotional problems. Sexual abuse has been reported in 20% to 50% of patients with bulimia and anorexia—a rate higher than in the general population (Wonderlich et al, 1997).

Parents who overemphasize athletics, reward slimness, or express disapproval of overweight people are placing their children at risk for developing eating disorders (Chally, 1998; Brink et al, 1999). Parents who continually skip meals, eat when distressed, and otherwise model poor nutritional habits are not teaching children about the appropriate value of food as nourishment. An important preventive nursing intervention involves educating the parents of young children regarding healthy eating behaviors (see the Family Education Plan for preventing childhood eating problems on the opposite page).

Sociocultural. In the past 50 years there has been a steady increase in the incidence of diagnosed eating disorders, subclinical eating problems, and body image disturbances. Eating disorders are thought to be rare in cultures where plumpness is accepted or valued. Shifting cultural norms for young women have forced them to face multiple, ambiguous, and often contradictory role expectations. Thinness is highly valued, culturally rewarded, and associated with achievement. The contemporary American ideal woman is lean, strong, graceful, and feminine (Barber, 1998). One advantage to this profile is its emphasis on fitness and health. A disadvantage is the demand this norm places on women to focus on and control their bodies, often as a means for achieving desired goals. This leads to intense social pressure on women for self-discipline, rigorous exercise, dieting, and often obsessive concern about weight and body image (Taylor et al, 1998). The result is that at least 50% of American women are on a diet at any given time, with Americans spending more than $5 billion on dieting products.

Children, adolescents, and young adults living in communities or going to schools where emphasis is placed on weight and size are often prone to developing eating disorders (see Citing the Evidence). Activities or occupations that emphasize beauty or fitness also promote a preoccupation with weight and eating behaviors. Ballet dancers, models, actors, athletes, fashion retailers, cooks, and flight attendants have demands placed on them concerning body weight and size. Although

---

Citing the Evidence on

Eating Disorders in Adolescent Girls

BACKGROUND: This longitudinal study examined the stability of the body weight and shape self-schema in middle adolescent girls during their transition from junior high to high school, as well as the relationship between these self-cognitions and emotional distress and disordered eating behaviors.

RESULTS: Girls in the fat/out-of-shape group had lower self-esteem, appearance, and athletic competence scores and higher dieting and depression scores than the slim/athletic group. In addition, the girls' self-schema was a stronger predictor of outcomes than weight.

IMPLICATIONS: Body weight/shape self-schema plays an important role in adolescent girls' emotional health. The development of interventions that influence the content of the body weight and shape self-schema holds the potential for improving emotional well-being and physical health in adolescent girls.

Stein K, Hedger K: Body weight and shape self-cognitions, emotional distress, and disordered eating in middle adolescent girls, *Arch Psychiatr Nurs* 11(5):264, 1997.

FAMILY EDUCATION PLAN   *Preventing Childhood Eating Problems*

CONTENT	INSTRUCTIONAL ACTIVITIES	EVALUATION
Describe self-demand feeding and its importance in healthy eating behaviors.	Explore parents' current feeding practices and understanding of healthy eating. Provide information to enhance knowledge of healthy eating behaviors.	Parents will identify healthy eating behaviors and self-demand feeding and begin to explore how their relationship with food influences their children's eating.
Describe the physiological and psychological signs of hunger and satiety, as well as the meaning and difference of both types of signs.	Explore parents' own signs of hunger and satiety, and have parents describe children's signs.	Parents will keep a hunger diary to record physical and psychological signs of hunger and satiety for themselves and their children.
Describe the danger of psychological hunger.	Explain the use of a hunger diary, which is a daily journal regarding signs of hunger.	Parents will be able to distinguish between psychological and physical hunger.
Explore myths about feeding, such as "cleaning the plate" and "eating because other children are starving."	Describe the importance of allowing children to determine their feeding needs and the relationship of healthy eating to the children's ability to differentiate between physical and psychological signs of hunger and satiety. Give a homework assignment for each parent to interview three other adults about their current eating practices and memories of eating.	Parents will complete homework assignment, discuss interview experiences, and describe how perpetuating myths about feeding can harm their children.
Implement self-demand feeding at particular developmental stages of children.	Review the eating stages children experience and the potential problems they may have at each stage.	Parents will discuss the developmental stages of their children and plan to implement self-demand feeding.
Discuss parental experiences related to implementing self-demand feeding.	Review parents' expectations and experiences with implementing self-demand feeding.	Parents will relate any problem with implementing self-demand feeding. Nurse will evaluate family for further education and plan for follow-up if necessary.

these occupations and activities in themselves do not cause eating disorders, they do attract people who may measure their self-esteem, self-worth, and attractiveness by their body parameters rather than by their accomplishments and personal satisfaction. Psychosocial predisposing factors for the development of eating disorders are summarized in Box 26-3.

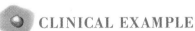 *Watch television for an evening and count the number of men and women who are overweight. Explain any socio-cultural bias you observe.*

Precipitating Stressors

Having one or more predisposing factors puts a person at risk for an eating disorder. People who are predisposed are especially vulnerable to environmental pressures and stress. Lacking an integrated self-concept and realistic body image, they rely on external feedback such as the reactions of others to their appearance and actions. They are unable to perceive or interpret stimuli from within the body, have difficulty describing their feelings and self-concepts, and lack an internal center of initiative and regulation. Thus they must rely on external cues

to regulate themselves. Food becomes one of these cues and is used as an external replacement for a deficient internal regulator and an inadequate integration of the body and mind.

Appraisal of Stressors

The person with an eating disorder is very susceptible to the impact of life stressors, such as the loss of a significant other, interpersonal rejection, and failure. Some researchers have suggested that people predisposed to eating disorders exercise not as a way to lose weight but as an attempt to experience the reality of their bodies. Controlling their eating or vomiting is another attempt to avoid the anguish of emptiness, boredom, or tension. Although binge eating may momentarily release this tension, it sets in motion a cycle of binging and purging that, once begun, is very difficult to stop. The importance of a person's appraisal of stressors related to eating disorders is seen in the following clinical example.

CLINICAL EXAMPLE

Lydia is a 15-year-old female with a 6-year history of binging, a 9-month history of purging, and a 2-year history of restricting food intake. She is the only child of parents who separated when she was 3 and divorced when she was 6. Her father has a history of frequent mood swings and has been diagnosed with and treated for bipolar disorder. He has always been overly concerned not only about his bodily appearance but also about the appearance of his family. When Lydia was 9, her father moved to a city 500 miles away, and 2 years later he remarried. Lydia's mother remarried several months later, but her marriage lasted less than a year. Her new husband had concealed an alcohol problem, and Lydia and her mother were verbally abused by this man on many occasions.

After her second divorce, Lydia's mother socialized very little and became overprotective of Lydia. She has often criticized Lydia's father for his extramarital behavior during their marriage. She supported him through college and dental school and was angry about her lowered standard of living since their divorce.

Lydia's parents continue to have a stormy relationship, and she feels caught between them at times. She avoids conflict by siding with her custodial parent (her mother) and by avoiding any discussion about her mother with her father. Lydia tries to be the perfect daughter and strives not to displease either parent. She has become very overprotective of her mother and secretly despises her father. She feels that a number of people have hurt her mother and that she and her mother must protect each other. She is afraid to grow up because her mother will be left alone. She states, "I'm the center of my mom's universe. If she's alone, her world will crumble.... I'm happiest when I'm worrying about my mom." Lydia does not think she has any eating problems and is very resistant to treatment. Her parents feel otherwise.

Selected Nursing Diagnoses

- Altered nutrition: less than body requirements related to unrealistic self-image, as evidenced by binging, purging, and restricting food
- Ineffective denial related to family conflict, as evidenced by overprotection of mother and ambivalence toward father

Coping Resources

One of the most important parts of the assessment of patients with maladaptive eating regulation responses is their motivation to change their behavior. This may be determined by asking patients to rate their desire for treatment on a scale of 1 to 10, with 10 representing high motivation and 1 representing low motivation for change. Patients may also be asked to identify the advantages and disadvantages of giving up the behavior; this information can be used to evaluate a patient's insight, to identify coping resources, and to stimulate therapeutic issues for future discussion. Four specific areas have been found to be crucial in engaging patients who are reluctant to treat their eating disorder: provision of psychoeducational material, an examination of the advantages and disadvantages of symptoms, the use of focused strategies, and an exploration of personal values (Vitousek et al, 1998).

Box 26-3

Psychosocial Predisposing Factors for the Development of Eating Disorders

PERSONAL FACTORS
Weight
Puberty/maturation
Restrained eating/dieting
Body image dissatisfaction
Problems regulating affect
Depression
Perfectionism
Low self-esteem
Stress
Low resiliency/confidence
Poor coping skills
Alcohol and substance use
Sexual/physical abuse
Dating

FAMILY FACTORS
Parental attitudes
Family functioning
Socioeconomic status

PEERS
Attitudes about weight
Behaviors
Teasing

CULTURE
Media influences

ACTIVITIES
Gymnastics
Professional dance
Modeling

From Taylor C, Altman T: Priorities in prevention research for eating disorders, *Psychopharmacol Bull* 33(3):413, 1997.

The nurse might also ask patients how their binging, fasting, and purging serve as a form of coping. Asking patients what precedes these episodes and how they feel afterward are important elements of the nurse's assessment. The patient should also be asked how stress and tension have been handled adaptively in the past and what supports in the environment can help in the treatment process (see Citing the Evidence). Such supports may include family members, friends, work, and leisure activities.

Coping Mechanisms

People with anorexia nervosa are happiest when fasting, losing weight, or achieving their weight goals. Their use of denial is severely maladaptive, and they are unlikely to seek help on their own. Concerned family members, primary practitioners, nurses, or school counselors are usually the ones who identify a problem and attempt to obtain help. People with anorexia are usually angry or impatient with the concern shown by others. Interestingly, as the family be-

Citing the Evidence on

Coping in Eating Disorders

BACKGROUND: Recent research has supported the role of stress in the development and maintenance of eating disorders. However, coping and crisis support have received little systematic attention. This study used semistructured interviews to measure coping and crisis support in response to severe events in women with anorexia, bulimia, or no eating disorder.

RESULTS: Women with eating disorders were more likely to use cognitive avoidance or cognitive rumination and were less likely to downplay their problems. In addition, women with bulimia were more likely to blame themselves and were less likely to receive crisis support. Overall, women with eating disorders were less likely to be masterful and more likely to be helpless in response to crises than women without eating disorders.

IMPLICATIONS: Women with eating disorders are less effective in their coping than women without eating disorders. Results suggest that the cognitive aspects of coping, rather than merely problem solving techniques, should be the main focus of treatment for eating disorders. However, these two aspects are likely to overlap.

Troop et al: Stress, coping and crisis support in eating disorders, *Int J Eat Disord* 24:157, 1998.

---

comes more distraught about the loss of weight or signs of malnutrition, the insistence of normalcy by the person with anorexia increases.

For people with anorexia, the issue is not about weight—it is about controlling life and fears. Those who fear maturity, independence, failure, sexuality, or parental demands believe they have found a solution to the problem by controlling their food intake and their bodies. With the increasing concerns of the family, people with anorexia are now able to control the focus of significant others as well. For them, this seems to be the perfect solution.

The defense mechanisms used by people with bulimia include avoidance, denial, isolation of affect, and intellectualization. Regardless of their weight, people with bulimia are usually very upset about their binging and purging behavior. They realize that their behavior is a sign that they are not in control or coping adaptively, but they do not know why. They are more likely to acknowledge that they have a problem than are patients with anorexia. However, they may regard the symptoms as preferable to the prospect of weight gain, and it may be years before they accept treatment.

People with binge eating disorder share the bulimic patient's distress about binging, but it is unclear how motivated they are to seek treatment. Obese binge eaters are more likely to seek assistance on their own or to be willing to be referred by their primary practitioner.

NURSING DIAGNOSIS

In formulating the nursing diagnosis, the nurse should review all aspects of the assessment phase as identified in the Stuart Stress Adaptation Model (Fig. 26-4). Nursing diagnoses related to eating disorders encompass biological, psychological, and sociocultural concerns; because of the complexity of these disorders, many NANDA nursing diagnoses may be appropriate. The primary NANDA diagnoses for working with patients with maladaptive eating regulation responses include **anxiety, body image disturbance, fluid volume deficit, risk for self-mutilation, altered nutrition, powerlessness,** and **self-esteem disturbance.** The Medical and Nursing Diagnoses Box on p. 537 presents nursing diagnoses and medical diagnoses associated with the range of possible maladaptive eating regulation responses. Primary NANDA nursing diagnoses and examples of complete nursing diagnoses are presented in the Detailed Diagnoses Box on p. 537.

Patients with moderate to extreme nutritional deficiencies exhibit symptoms of malnutrition that may be mistakenly related to other causes. Irritability, apathy, depression, obsessiveness, difficulty with concentration, anxiety, decreased interest in sex, and negativism are psychological symptoms that usually reverse with adequate nutrition. The nurse may see a very different outward presentation in a patient who is no longer malnourished. Family members may offer important insights into the patient's premorbid functioning and be able to give a clearer picture of the patient's personality before the eating disorder developed.

Related Medical Diagnoses

The medical diagnoses associated with maladaptive eating regulation responses include anorexia nervosa, bulimia nervosa, and binge eating disorder (American Psychiatric Association, 2000b). These medical diagnoses and their essential features are described in the Medical and Nursing Diagnoses Box. The key features distinguishing anorexia nervosa from bulimia nervosa are listed in Box 26-4.

OUTCOME IDENTIFICATION

The expected outcome for the patient with maladaptive eating regulation responses is the following:

The patient will restore healthy eating patterns and normalize physiological parameters related to body weight and nutrition.

For patients with anorexia nervosa or bulimia nervosa, this means eating 100% of all meals without binging, purging, or engaging in other compensatory behavior. Obese patients with binge eating disorder should be encouraged to leave something (no more than 5% and no less than 2%) on their plate at the end of the meal.

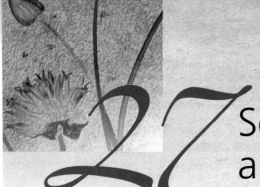

Visit **MERLIN** for *Your Internet Connection* to websites that are related to the content in this chapter.
www.mosby.com/MERLIN/Stuart

27 Sexual Responses and Sexual Disorders

Susan G. Poorman

I locked myself away from you Too long, Tossing aside my feelings For you. Looking for a way out, an excuse Not to touch you; Because I want to, Inciting a riot within me. To reach out for you Is difficult, But less difficult Than turning away.

LESLIE BERTEL

Sexuality broadly refers to all aspects of being sexual and is one dimension of the personality. It includes more than the act of intercourse and is an integral part of life. It is evident in the person's appearance and in beliefs, behaviors, and relationships with others. Four aspects of sexuality are as follows:

- **Genetic identity,** which is a person's chromosomal gender
- **Gender identity,** which is a person's perception of his or her own maleness or femaleness
- **Gender role,** which is the cultural role attributes of one's gender, such as expectations regarding behavior, cognitions, occupations, values, and emotional responses
- **Sexual orientation,** which is the gender to which one is romantically attracted

Accepting a broad concept of sexuality allows nurses to explore ways in which people are sexual beings and understand more fully their feelings, beliefs, and actions. Nurses are often called on to intervene in the sexual concerns of patients when providing holistic patient care. Therefore it is important to develop skills and competence in addressing sexual issues by increasing awareness through education.

As nurses become educated in the basic principles of sexuality, they will better understand sexual needs and problems. If nurses are comfortable with sexual issues, they will convey this to the patient, who will feel more comfortable in discussing these issues. Patients are often experiencing pain and change as a result of threats to health or even as a part of normal growth and development. Thus it is important that the nurse-patient relationship allow for honest discussions about sexuality.

In answering the question, What do nurses need to know about sexuality?, several factors emerge. First, nurses need to know themselves and be aware of their feelings and values regarding sexuality. If nurses are not aware of their feelings,

Citing the Evidence on

Coping in Eating Disorders

BACKGROUND: Recent research has supported the role of stress in the development and maintenance of eating disorders. However, coping and crisis support have received little systematic attention. This study used semistructured interviews to measure coping and crisis support in response to severe events in women with anorexia, bulimia, or no eating disorder.

RESULTS: Women with eating disorders were more likely to use cognitive avoidance or cognitive rumination and were less likely to downplay their problems. In addition, women with bulimia were more likely to blame themselves and were less likely to receive crisis support. Overall, women with eating disorders were less likely to be masterful and more likely to be helpless in response to crises than women without eating disorders.

IMPLICATIONS: Women with eating disorders are less effective in their coping than women without eating disorders. Results suggest that the cognitive aspects of coping, rather than merely problem solving techniques, should be the main focus of treatment for eating disorders. However, these two aspects are likely to overlap.

Troop et al: Stress, coping and crisis support in eating disorders, *Int J Eat Disord* 24:157, 1998.

comes more distraught about the loss of weight or signs of malnutrition, the insistence of normalcy by the person with anorexia increases.

For people with anorexia, the issue is not about weight—it is about controlling life and fears. Those who fear maturity, independence, failure, sexuality, or parental demands believe they have found a solution to the problem by controlling their food intake and their bodies. With the increasing concerns of the family, people with anorexia are now able to control the focus of significant others as well. For them, this seems to be the perfect solution.

The defense mechanisms used by people with bulimia include avoidance, denial, isolation of affect, and intellectualization. Regardless of their weight, people with bulimia are usually very upset about their binging and purging behavior. They realize that their behavior is a sign that they are not in control or coping adaptively, but they do not know why. They are more likely to acknowledge that they have a problem than are patients with anorexia. However, they may regard the symptoms as preferable to the prospect of weight gain, and it may be years before they accept treatment.

People with binge eating disorder share the bulimic patient's distress about binging, but it is unclear how motivated they are to seek treatment. Obese binge eaters are more likely to seek assistance on their own or to be willing to be referred by their primary practitioner.

NURSING DIAGNOSIS

In formulating the nursing diagnosis, the nurse should review all aspects of the assessment phase as identified in the Stuart Stress Adaptation Model (Fig. 26-4). Nursing diagnoses related to eating disorders encompass biological, psychological, and sociocultural concerns; because of the complexity of these disorders, many NANDA nursing diagnoses may be appropriate. The primary NANDA diagnoses for working with patients with maladaptive eating regulation responses include **anxiety, body image disturbance, fluid volume deficit, risk for self-mutilation, altered nutrition, powerlessness,** and **self-esteem disturbance.** The Medical and Nursing Diagnoses Box on p. 537 presents nursing diagnoses and medical diagnoses associated with the range of possible maladaptive eating regulation responses. Primary NANDA nursing diagnoses and examples of complete nursing diagnoses are presented in the Detailed Diagnoses Box on p. 537.

Patients with moderate to extreme nutritional deficiencies exhibit symptoms of malnutrition that may be mistakenly related to other causes. Irritability, apathy, depression, obsessiveness, difficulty with concentration, anxiety, decreased interest in sex, and negativism are psychological symptoms that usually reverse with adequate nutrition. The nurse may see a very different outward presentation in a patient who is no longer malnourished. Family members may offer important insights into the patient's premorbid functioning and be able to give a clearer picture of the patient's personality before the eating disorder developed.

Related Medical Diagnoses

The medical diagnoses associated with maladaptive eating regulation responses include anorexia nervosa, bulimia nervosa, and binge eating disorder (American Psychiatric Association, 2000b). These medical diagnoses and their essential features are described in the Medical and Nursing Diagnoses Box. The key features distinguishing anorexia nervosa from bulimia nervosa are listed in Box 26-4.

OUTCOME IDENTIFICATION

The expected outcome for the patient with maladaptive eating regulation responses is the following:

The patient will restore healthy eating patterns and normalize physiological parameters related to body weight and nutrition.

For patients with anorexia nervosa or bulimia nervosa, this means eating 100% of all meals without binging, purging, or engaging in other compensatory behavior. Obese patients with binge eating disorder should be encouraged to leave something (no more than 5% and no less than 2%) on their plate at the end of the meal.

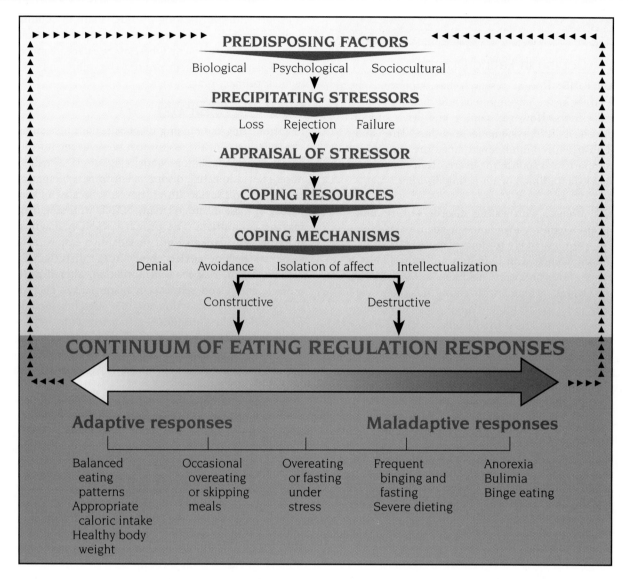

Fig. 26-4 The Stuart Stress Adaptation Model related to eating regulation responses.

Short-term goals may further specify the steps the patient needs to take to demonstrate adaptive eating regulation responses. These steps might include the following:

- The patient will identify cognitive distortions about food, weight, and body shape.
- The patient will develop a week's menu of nutritionally balanced meals.
- The patient will accurately describe body dimensions.
- The patient will exercise in moderate amounts only when nutritionally and medically stable.
- The patient will demonstrate positive family interactions and successful movement toward the achievement of separation and individuation issues.

PLANNING
Choice of Treatment Setting

Nursing care varies to some degree based on the treatment setting of the patient with maladaptive eating regulation responses (White & Litovitz, 1998). A number of factors affect the choice of treatment setting, including the patient's physical and psychological condition, financial resources, availability of treatment specialists, and patient preference (see Citing the Evidence on Treatment Settings for Anorexia Nervosa, p. 538). Clinical criteria for inpatient treatment of eating disorders are listed in Box 26-5.

Outpatient treatment is often the best because it allows the patient the greatest opportunity for self-control and autonomy. It requires a high level of patient motivation, the active support and involvement of family members, and ongoing physiological monitoring. Contingencies for outpatient treatment should be mutually agreed on expectations of behavioral change, including weight gain and decreased binging or purging, as well as the acceptance of inpatient or more intense day treatment programs if the patient is not making progress.

Outpatient settings, including day treatment or partial hospitalization programs, are the current standard treatment settings. This is because of the unavailability of reimbursement for inpatient programs except under dangerous or severe conditions, such as suicidal intent. An advantage to inpatient

Medical and Nursing Diagnoses *related to* **Eating Regulation Responses**

RELATED MEDICAL DIAGNOSES *(DSM–IV–TR)**	RELATED NURSING DIAGNOSES (NANDA)†
Anorexia nervosa	**Anxiety‡**
Binge eating disorder	**Body image disturbance‡**
Bulimia nervosa	Coping, ineffective individual
	Decisional conflict
	Denial, ineffective
	Family processes, altered
	Fatigue
	Fluid volume deficit‡
	Growth and development, altered
	Hopelessness
	Injury, risk for
	Nutrition, altered‡
	Personal identity disturbance
	Powerlessness‡
	Role performance, altered
	Self-esteem disturbance‡
	Self-mutilation, risk for‡
	Sexual dysfunction
	Social interaction, impaired
	Thought processes, altered

*Reprinted with permission from the *Diagnostic and statistical manual of mental disorders*, Fourth Edition, Text Revision. Copyright 2000, American Psychiatric Association.
†From North American Nursing Diagnosis Association: *NANDA nursing diagnoses: definitions and classifications 1999-2000*, Philadelphia, 1999, The Association.
‡Primary nursing diagnosis for eating problems.

 Detailed Diagnoses *related to* **Eating Regulation Responses**

NANDA DIAGNOSIS STEM	EXAMPLES OF COMPLETE DIAGNOSIS
Anxiety	Anxiety related to fear of weight gain, as evidenced by rituals associated with food preparation and eating
Body image disturbance	Body image disturbance related to fear of weight gain, as evidenced by verbalization of being "fat" while actually being 30% below ideal body weight
Fluid volume deficit	Fluid volume deficit related to purging activities, as evidenced by weakness, poor skin turgor, hypokalemia, and hypotension
Risk for self-mutilation	Risk for self-mutilation related to feelings of inadequacy, as evidenced by injuries caused by excessive exercise and self-induced vomiting
Nutrition, altered	Altered nutrition related to excessive intake of calories, as evidenced by being 40% above ideal body weight, sleep apnea, and difficulty with mobility
Powerlessness	Powerlessness related to perceived lack of control over eating behaviors, as evidenced by inability to stop binge eating and the avoidance of food-related settings
Self-esteem disturbance	Self-esteem disturbance related to feelings of low self-worth, as evidenced by verbalization of sole standard of success being related to physical attractiveness

DSM–IV–TR DIAGNOSIS	ESSENTIAL FEATURES*
Anorexia nervosa	An intense fear of gaining weight, even when underweight. There is a disturbance in the way the body is experienced and a refusal to maintain body weight above a minimal normal weight for age and height; this leads to a body weight 15% below expected. In females there is also the absence of at least three consecutive menstrual cycles. Two subtypes of anorexia nervosa are (1) restricting type, and (2) binge-eating/purging type.
Bulimia nervosa	Recurrent episodes of binge eating with a feeling of lack of control over the eating behavior and a persistent overconcern with body shape and weight. The person also regularly engages in self-induced vomiting; the misuse of laxatives, diuretics, enemas, or other medications; fasting; or excessive exercise.
Binge eating disorder	Recurrent episodes of binging that are a cause of distress, with a feeling of lack of control over the eating behavior but without behaviors used to prevent weight gain.

*Reprinted with permission from the *Diagnostic and statistical manual of mental disorders*, Fourth Edition, Text Revision. Copyright 2000, American Psychiatric Association.

Box 26-4

Key Features of Anorexia Nervosa and Bulimia Nervosa

ANOREXIA NERVOSA (WITHOUT BINGING OR PURGING)

Rare vomiting or diuretic/laxative abuse
More severe weight loss
Slightly younger
More introverted
Hunger denied
Eating behavior may be considered normal and a source of esteem
Sexually inactive
Obsessional and perfectionistic features predominate
Death from starvation (or suicide, in chronically ill)
Amenorrhea
Fewer behavioral problems (these increase with level of severity)

BULIMIA NERVOSA

Frequent vomiting or diuretic/laxative abuse
Less weight loss
Slightly older
More extroverted
Hunger experienced
Eating behavior considered foreign and source of distress
More sexually active
Avoidant, dependent, or borderline features as well as obsessional features
Death from hypokalemia or suicide
Menses irregular or absent
Drug and alcohol abuse, self-mutilation, and other behavioral problems

Citing the Evidence on

Treatment Settings for Anorexia Nervosa

BACKGROUND: Clinicians are under increasing pressure to transfer inpatients with anorexia nervosa to less intensive treatment early in their hospital course. This study identified the prognostic factors clinicians can use in determining the earliest time to transfer an inpatient with anorexia to a day hospital program.

RESULTS: A greater risk of day hospital program treatment failure and inpatient readmission was associated with patients who had been ill for more than 6 years, had amenorrhea for more than 2.5 years, and had a body mass index 75% less than normal at the time of inpatient admission.

IMPLICATIONS: Inpatients with anorexia who have the poor prognostic indicators found in this study are in need of continued inpatient care to avoid immediate relapse and a higher cost and longer duration of treatment.

Howard W et al: Predictors of success or failure of transition to day hospital treatment for inpatients with anorexia nervosa, *Am J Psych* 156(11):1697, 1999.

Box 26-5

Clinical Criteria for Hospitalization of Patients with an Eating Disorder

MEDICAL

Need for extensive diagnostic evaluation
Weight loss greater than 25% of body weight over 3 months
Heart rate less than 40 beats/min or greater than 110 beats/min
Temperature less than 97.0° F
Systolic blood pressure >70 mm Hg or marked orthostatic hypotension <20 mm Hg/minute standing
Serum potassium less than 2.5 mEq/L despite oral potassium replacement
Severe dehydration or vomiting of blood
Concurrent somatic illnesses (e.g., infection)

PSYCHIATRIC

Risk of suicide or self-mutilation
Severe depression
Substance abuse
Psychosis
Family crisis
Failure to comply with treatment contract or poor motivation
Inadequate response to outpatient treatment

treatment, however, is the availability of 24-hour nursing care to ensure patient safety, support needed behavioral change, and monitor physiological responses. Patients with eating disorders can present a unique challenge to staff, and care requires a high level of interdisciplinary collaboration, coordination, and consistency. Empirically validated treatments for bulimia nervosa are summarized in Table 26-2.

Nurse-Patient Contract

Nurse-patient contracts can be formulated for patients with eating disorders who are seen in either inpatient or outpatient settings. The terms of the contract may vary, but the goal is the same: to engage the patient in a therapeutic alliance and to obtain commitment to the treatment process.

Before a patient is admitted to an eating disorder treatment program, the patient's cooperation should be obtained with a nurse-patient contract. By signing such a contract, patients will understand the treatment they will be receiving and will be able to make informed decisions about their commitment to the treatment process and their ability to honor the contract.

Table **26-2**

Summarizing the Evidence on Eating Disorders

DISORDER:	Bulimia Nervosa (BN)
TREATMENT:	■ Several different classes of antidepressant drugs produced significant, short-term reductions in binge eating and purging. ■ Cognitive-behavioral therapy (CBT) was most effective in eliminating the core features of BN; roughly half the patients receiving CBT reduced binge eating and purging; long-term maintenance of improvement was good.

From Nathan P, Gorman J: *A guide to treatments that work*, New York, Oxford University Press.

How would you respond to a patient who wants to receive treatment for an eating disorder but does not want to sign the nurse-patient contract because it is "too restrictive"?

? CRITICAL THINKING about CONTEMPORARY ISSUES

Should Tube Feeding Be a Part of an Eating Disorders Treatment Program?

The positive and negative consequences of nasogastric tube feeding or even total parenteral nutrition for patients with an eating disorder have been debated among clinicians and researchers. Current guidelines recommend that refeeding interventions be used only rarely and in life-threatening situations (American Psychiatric Association, 2000a). Specifically, there is recognition of the danger of rapid refeeding, which includes severe fluid retention and cardiac failure, and of forced nasogastric or parenteral feeding. Therefore these procedures should not be used routinely. However, some severely malnourished patients with anorexia may accept nasogastric feeding more willingly than eating, especially in the early stages of renourishment.

If forced feeding is being considered, careful thought should be given to the patient's clinical condition, the patient's and family's opinion, and the legal and ethical dimensions of the patient's treatment. Each of these areas merits a full discussion by the interdisciplinary health-care team, and treatment decisions should include specific timelines, outcomes, and alternatives.

IMPLEMENTATION

Nutritional Stabilization

Stabilizing the patient's nutritional status is a high priority for nursing intervention. Healthy target weights and expected rates of controlled weight gain or loss should be set. In life-threatening circumstances, patients who are malnourished may need refeeding interventions (see Critical Thinking about Contemporary Issues), but these cases are exceptional. Specific nursing interventions to promote weight stabilization and restore healthy eating patterns can be facilitated by program protocols that identify treatment goals, program components, and patient and staff responsibilities. Some of these items might include the following:

- The time, frequency, and procedure for weighing the patient and whether the patient may see the weight
- The time when meals will be served and how many meals are to be eaten each day
- How the staff is to interact with the patient during mealtimes to maximize their therapeutic value
- The amount of time the patient will be allowed to spend eating each meal, and the consequences if the meal is not completed
- Whether diet foods, condiments, or food substitutions are allowed
- The amount of water the patient may drink each day
- The frequency of obtaining the patient's vital signs, intake and output, and required laboratory work
- Conditions regarding bathroom privileges
- Indications for close observation by staff

Once patients are able to master their meals, they can move toward more independence with eating and food se-

lection. Selecting their own menus with assistance is next. The patient can then progress to shopping for and cooking food with supervision. By discharge the patient should have gained a high level of comfort with food and its preparation.

For outpatients with anorexia nervosa, stabilizing nutrition and promoting weight gain usually require a motivated patient and cooperative family. Obtaining the patient's agreement to stop trying to lose weight is the first obstacle the nurse must overcome; patients are often very resistant to such an idea. Getting a patient with anorexia to gain weight is an even more difficult task. Nurse-patient contracts can be effective tools with these patients because their need for control of food is so great. For example, the nurse and patient may set a realistic goal of gaining 1 pound per week. If the patient fails to gain 4 pounds in a month, the contract would stipulate that the patient would agree to enter a hospital, day treatment program, or some other more intensive type of care.

Counseling about healthy eating patterns and behaviors is an essential aspect of nursing care for all patients, regardless of whether they need to gain, lose, or maintain weight. The nurse should also clarify with patients the effect of poor nutrition on the body. Collaboration with a dietitian may be helpful in teaching patients about proper eating habits and in planning menus with patients. Nurses should teach, clarify, and reinforce knowledge about proper nutrition and the importance of planning healthy meals. Patients should be encouraged to make shopping lists, and the nurse may even accompany the patient to the grocery store. Nutritional assessment, education, and ongoing support are essential nursing care activities.

The patient who is struggling with major issues regarding food will not be ready for intensive psychological interventions. As the patient feels less need to be in control of food and eating, issues underlying the eating disorder may start to surface. This can be a difficult time for the patient, who may actually begin to feel worse than when treatment began. Patients in a hospital or a partial hospitalization program always have someone available to talk with, but this is not always true for the outpatient. Thus the outpatient may need more frequent sessions with the nurse or more phone contacts between sessions. When sufficient progress has been made toward nutritional rehabilitation, the patient will be better prepared both cognitively and emotionally to begin the next phase of treatment.

Exercise

As the patient's eating increases, the need to increase exercise or engage in a new purging or compensatory behavior also increases. Patients on an inpatient or partial hospitalization unit can be closely monitored to prevent such compensatory activity. It is often appropriate to begin a gradual exercise program as the patient stabilizes and responds to treatment. For some patients who exercise compulsively, this can be the most difficult period of treatment. The nurse should initially allow patients limited amounts of exercise, with gradual increases over time. The focus of the exercise program should be on physical fitness rather than on working off calories. Consultation with a recreational therapist or exercise physiologist may be helpful to maximize the therapeutic value of the exercise regimen.

Cognitive Behavioral Interventions

Cognitive-behavioral therapy has been found to be the single most effective treatment for patients with eating disorders (Fairburn et al, 1999; Whittal et al, 1999; Wilson et al, 1999). It is important for the nurse to work with patients around their cognitive distortions and faulty thinking about body shape, weight, and food. Box 26-6 presents a list of cognitive distortions common among patients with eating disorders, as well as an example of each. Cognitive behavioral therapy is discussed in detail in Chapter 32.

Helping the patient to become aware of his or her cognitive distortions is the first step in changing them. The patient should be asked to monitor and record eating, binging, and purging behavior and his or her thoughts and feelings regarding weight, shape, and food. The goal of these exercises is for the patient to better understand the following:

- The cues that trigger problematic eating responses
- The thoughts, feelings, and assumptions associated with the specific cues
- The connection between these thoughts, feelings, assumptions and eating regulation responses
- The consequences resulting from the eating responses

Cues. Cues that trigger maladaptive eating behavior can be social, situational, physiological, and psychological. Examples of social cues are loneliness, interpersonal conflict, social awkwardness, and holiday celebrations. Examples of situational cues include diet advertisements and walking by a store that sells food for binging. Hunger and fatigue are the two most common physiological cues. Memory and mental images are two examples of psychological cues.

Specific cues such as these can trigger cognitive distortions and lead to maladaptive eating regulation responses (Jansen, 1998). For example, when stepping on the scale a patient may see that she has gained a pound. She then may use dichotomous thinking: "Since I've gained 1 pound, I will probably gain 20 pounds in the next week. I'd better take a package of laxatives so that I can lose the pound by tomorrow."

- Stepping on the scale is the cue.
- Believing she will gain 20 pounds is the related irrational thought.
- Taking the laxatives is the maladaptive eating regulation response connected to the cognitive distortion.
- Beginning another purge cycle is the consequence resulting from the maladaptive response.

Cues can be used as a strategy for change. Rearranging cues, avoiding a cue, and changing the response to a cue are ways of altering maladaptive responses. After continued learning about eating, binging, and purging behavior, as well as thoughts and feelings about food, shape, and weight, it is hoped that the patient will begin to see the connections between thoughts and behaviors and recognize the consequences of the harmful activity.

Thoughts, Feelings, and Assumptions. The nurse helps patients to challenge their faulty thoughts, feelings, and assumptions by questioning the evidence supporting or challenging a particular belief. In the previous example, the nurse might ask the patient what specifically happened in the past

---

Box 26-6

Cognitive Distortions Related to Maladaptive Eating Regulation Responses

Magnification: Overestimating the significance of undesirable events. Stimuli are embellished with meaning not supported by objective analysis. "I've gained 2 pounds, so I can't wear shorts any more."

Superstitious thinking: Believing in the cause-effect relationship of noncontingent events. "If I eat a sweet, it will instantly be turned into stomach fat."

Dichotomous or all-or-none thinking: Thinking in extreme or absolute terms, such as that events can only be black or white, right or wrong, good or bad. "If I gain 1 pound, I'll go on to gain 100 pounds."

Overgeneralization: Extracting a rule on the basis of one event and applying it to other dissimilar situations. "I used to be of normal weight and I wasn't happy. So I know gaining weight isn't going to make me feel better."

Selective abstraction: Basing a conclusion on isolated details while ignoring contradictory and more important evidence. "The only way I can be in control is through eating."

Personalization and self-reference: Egocentric interpretations of impersonal events or overinterpretation of events related to the self. "Two people laughed and whispered something to each other when I walked by. They were probably saying that I looked unattractive. I have gained 3 pounds."

From Garner D et al: *Handbook of treatment for eating disorders*, New York, 1997, Guilford.

when she gained a pound. Did she gain 19 more pounds in the same week? If so, how often has it happened in the past? If not, why does the patient believe it will happen this time? It is also important for the nurse to ask the patient about the implications of this type of thinking. Do other people have the same problem if they gain a pound? If so, how do they

A Patient Speaks

Learning to separate my feelings from my eating has been the hardest part but the greatest benefit of treatment for my eating disorder. From early childhood, food had been my main outlet for almost every emotion. When I was sad, I comforted myself by eating. When I was happy, I celebrated by eating. Feelings of loneliness could be diminished by gathering up all my "food friends" and eating. Feeling angry at anyone other than myself was unacceptable, so I would eat and then had a "good reason" to be angry and focus it all on myself.

Discovering that everything in life is not black or white, good or bad, perfect or imperfect, or hungry or full has enabled me to be kinder to myself and more accepting of my imperfections and humanity. I now realize that shades of gray do exist when making a decision, performing a task, feeling an emotion, and even experiencing hunger. Another benefit of this insight is a decrease in my level of anxiety and in my feelings of worthlessness.

Each day is no longer a battle to control all aspects of my life, especially my food consumption. The struggle with food and my weight still remains, but now it doesn't completely overshadow everything else that happens in my life. Food is no longer the only friend and enemy life offers. I learned all of this from a nurse who took the time to get to know me and in turn helped me to get to know myself.

deal with it? The nurse can help the patient consider alternative explanations for his or her thoughts, thereby gradually modifying the irrational assumptions that underlie these beliefs. This is an example of the cognitive intervention of decentering. These and other cognitive behavioral techniques may be successfully used in patients with maladaptive eating regulation responses (see A Patient Speaks).

Eating Regulation Responses. The patient with an eating disorder needs help in solving problems and in making decisions. Rather than resorting to maladaptive responses, the patient must be helped to distinguish between adaptive and maladaptive coping responses and to find alternative solutions.

One way of doing this is to encourage the patient to make a list of high-risk situations that cue maladaptive eating and purging behaviors. The high-risk situation may be a certain day of the week, time of the day, season of the year, person, group, event, or emotional response, such as anger or frustration. The nurse can then help the patient to identify specific, alternative, and more adaptive ways of handling these high-risk situations.

Decision-making strategies may also need to be reviewed and modified. Many patients with eating disorders know what they need to do in a given situation but may feel inadequate or shy about carrying out a certain plan of action. These people may benefit from assertiveness training and role modeling sessions with the nurse.

Consequences. It is particularly important for the nurse and patient to explore the positive and negative consequences that result from cognitive distortions and maladaptive responses. These consequences can be biological, psychological, and sociocultural, with positive and negative consequences resulting from each behavior. Some of these consequences are presented in Table 26-3. A maladaptive behavior such as binging is maintained because the positive consequences are more immediate or are more valued than the negative consequences.

Strategies for change that focus on consequences involve the use of rewards that increase the likelihood of behavior

Table **26-3**

Consequences of Maladaptive Eating Regulation Responses		
	Positive Consequences	**Negative Consequences**
BIOLOGICAL	Reduced fear of fatness Reduced perception of hunger Avoidance of biological maturity	Weakness, fatigue, dizziness Poor concentration Electrolyte disturbance Dental problems
PSYCHOLOGICAL	Relief from tension, anger, and stress Relief from boredom Emotional anesthesia Feelings of nurturance or pleasure Thoughts about avoiding weight gain	Depression, guilt, shame Tendency to overreact emotionally Increase in negative self-reference or guilt-related behavior
SOCIOCULTURAL	Avoidance of interpersonal conflict Social reinforcement for not gaining weight Distraction from unpleasant tasks Avoidance of responsibility and independence	Social withdrawal Lying and lack of trust in relationships Occupational problems Financial problems Legal problems

change. In the example in which laxatives were taken in response to a 1-pound weight gain, rewards would be given if the person was able to resist taking the laxative. The reward should be received immediately following the desired behavior change. It should be something pleasurable and can be either a material item or a psychological reinforcer, but it should not involve food.

> *Should overweight nurses be assigned to care for patients with eating disorders? Why or why not?*

Body Image Interventions

Body image distortions are one of the most difficult-to-treat aspects of the eating disorder. This is partly because researchers disagree on what exactly constitutes a body image distortion. The only agreement is that body image distortion in the eating disorders involves perceptual, attitudinal, and behavioral features (Cash & Deagle, 1997) (Fig. 26-5). A distinction between body image distortion and body dissatisfaction must also be made. Body image distortion is a discrepancy between the patient's actual size and his or her perceived body size. Body dissatisfaction is the degree of unhappiness that a person feels in relation to his or her body size.

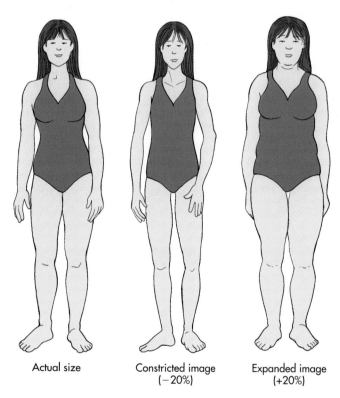

Actual size   Constricted image   Expanded image
(−20%)   (+20%)

Fig. 26-5 The perception of body shape and size can be evaluated through the use of special computer drawing programs that allow a subject to distort the width of an actual picture of a person's body by as much as 20% larger or smaller. Both anorectic and normal subjects adjusted the figures of other people's bodies to normal dimension. However, anorectic subjects consistently adjusted their own body picture to a size 20% larger than its true form, which suggests they have a major problem with the perception of self-image.

All people may express dissatisfaction with their bodies at some point in their lives, but such dissatisfaction is constant in persons with anorexia or bulimia. People with eating disorders place so much value on their appearance that it begins to define their self-worth to an exclusive degree. Behavioral features of body image disturbance are manifested in a lifestyle that revolves around a self-concern about the body. Examples of such behaviors include constantly measuring body weight, wearing baggy clothes, and avoiding social situations in which appearance might be scrutinized. Overestimation of body size or of a body part is a common perceptual distortion in anorexia and bulimia.

When intervening in body image problems, the nurse should first determine whether the patient has problems with perception, attitude, or behavior and then devise a treatment program targeting the specific problem area. Cognitive behavioral interventions are effective, as are dance and movement therapies, which create pleasant body experiences and can enhance the integration of mind and body, clarify body boundaries, and modulate negative feelings about the body (Thompson, 1996). Other therapeutic approaches include the use of imagery and relaxation, working with mirrors, and depicting the self through art.

Family Involvement

Families should be engaged from the beginning of treatment and included in family meetings and treatment planning sessions. The nurse should gather information about the family system and explore how the maladaptive eating response might serve a specific function within the family. Questions the nurse might ask include the following:

- What part does the eating disorder serve in stabilizing the family system?
- How has the family attempted to deal with the eating disorder?
- What is the central theme surrounding the eating behavior?
- What would be the consequences of change for each family member?
- What is the underlying therapeutic issue from a family perspective?

Many young patients need intensive family therapy after successfully completing the refeeding stage. The initial issue of such therapy is centered on the separation and individuation of the patient within the context of the family. This process requires much openness on the part of the family, and not every family may be able to complete the process. However, the nurse should work with identified family strengths and help involved family members work toward change (see A Family Speaks). Family therapy is described in more detail in Chapter 34.

Group Therapies

Many models of group therapy are used for patients with eating disorders, including cognitive-behavioral, psychoeducational, psychodynamic, and interpersonal models. Reality testing, support, and communicating with peers are essential therapeutic factors provided by group intervention. In addition, outpatient support groups may be helpful if they reinforce social alliances and encourage members to identify and express feelings. Therapeutic groups are described in detail in Chapter 33.

Medications

Patients with anorexia often resist medication, and no drugs have been found to be completely effective for this disorder. Medications should not be used as the sole or primary treatment for anorexia. The role of antidepressants is usually best assessed following weight gain, when the psychological effects of malnutrition are resolving (American Psychiatric Association, 2000a). An antidepressant medication may be helpful with comorbid depression, mood swings or irritability, and obsessions about food and fat.

In the treatment of bulimia, studies have shown that antidepressant medications have a therapeutic benefit in many patients. Medication-induced benefits include decreases in the frequency of binge eating and weight regulatory behaviors such as vomiting. Antidepressants such as the tricyclic antidepressants (TCAs) (imipramine, desipramine), selective serotonin reuptake inhibitors (SSRIs) (fluoxetine), and monamine oxidase inhibitors (MAOIs) (phenelzine) have demonstrated efficacy in the treatment of eating disorders (Mayer & Walsh, 1998; Jimerson et al, 1996). Chapter 28 discusses these medications in detail. They are most effective when used in combination with other psychotherapeutic interventions (see Citing the Evidence). Most of the medications that have been used in the treatment of bulimia have also had some success in treating binge eating disorder (Grilo, 1998).

The Nursing Treatment Plan Summary for patients with maladaptive eating regulation responses is presented on p. 544.

EVALUATION

Patients with maladaptive eating regulation responses present special challenges to psychiatric nursing care. The evaluation of their care should begin with a focus on the therapeutic nurse-patient relationship. Nurses should determine whether they provided effective role modeling, emotional support, biological monitoring, and reinforcement of the patient's attempts to explore and experiment with new cognitive and behavior patterns (George, 1997). Evaluation activities can then address three specific aspects of care:

- Have normal eating patterns been restored?
- Have the biological and psychological sequelae of malnutrition been corrected?
- Have the associated sociocultural and behavioral problems been resolved so that relapse does not occur?

In answering these questions, the nurse should review each aspect of the nursing process and modify care as needed to achieve the identified outcomes.

A Family Speaks

We have a 19-year-old daughter who has had an eating disorder for 8 years. These past 8 years have been most painful for our family—we went from doctor to doctor, counselor to counselor, and therapist to therapist, all with little or no results. What clinicians don't realize is how hard the day-to-day struggle is for families who want so much for their child to be healthy and happy but who feel so helpless in how to make this happen.

Then we were referred to a nurse who specialized in eating disorders, and slowly our lives began to change. Clearly, this nurse knew about our daughter's illness, and together we went about treating it. We went through individual and family therapy, all in an attempt to help our daughter recover. At times it was painful and even frustrating. In the family sessions the nurse helped family members be aware of the part they had to play in our daughter's struggle and helped us realize that it would take a family team effort to help her get well. The most important part is that all of the hard work of our daughter, each family member, and our nurse has been worth it. Our daughter now knows how to control her eating disorder. She has had very few problems in the last 6 months, and our family has become even closer as we look back on the past with relief and into the future with hope.

Citing the Evidence on

Treatment of Bulimia

BACKGROUND: Two treatments for bulimia nervosa have established efficacy: cognitive-behavioral therapy and antidepressant medication. This study addressed (1) how the effects of a psychodynamically oriented supportive psychotherapy compared to that of cognitive-behavioral therapy; (2) whether a two-stage medication intervention, in which a second antidepressant was used if the first was not effective, added to the benefit of psychological treatment; and (3) if the combination of medication and psychological treatment was superior to a course of medication alone.

RESULTS: Cognitive-behavioral therapy was superior to supportive psychotherapy. Patients receiving medication in combination with psychological treatment had greater improvement in binge eating and depression than patients receiving a placebo and psychological treatment. Finally, cognitive-behavioral therapy plus medication was superior to medication alone, but supportive psychotherapy plus medication was not.

IMPLICATIONS: Cognitive-behavioral therapy is the psychological treatment of choice for bulimia nervosa. A two-stage medication intervention adds modestly to the benefit of cognitive-behavioral therapy.

Walsh T: Medication and psychotherapy in the treatment of bulimia nervosa, *Am J Psych* 154(4):523, 1997.

NURSING TREATMENT PLAN *Summary* *Eating Regulation Responses*

NURSING DIAGNOSIS: Altered nutrition
EXPECTED OUTCOME: The patient will restore healthy patterns and normalize physiological parameters related to body weight and nutrition.

SHORT-TERM GOAL	INTERVENTION	RATIONALE
The patient will engage in treatment and acknowledge having an eating disorder.	Help the patient to identify maladaptive eating responses. Discuss the positive and negative consequences of maladaptive eating responses. Contract with the patient to engage in treatment.	The first step of treatment is for the patient to acknowledge the illness and see the need for help.
The patient will be able to describe a balanced diet based on the five food groups.	Complete a nutritional assessment, including eating-related behaviors and preferences. Teach, clarify, and reinforce the patient's knowledge of proper nutrition.	Knowledge of healthy nutrition is essential to establishing and maintaining adaptive eating responses.
The patient's nutritional status will be stabilized by a specified date.	Monitor physiological status for signs of compromised nutrition. Administer medications and somatic treatments for the management of symptoms. Monitor and evaluate the patient's response to somatic treatments. Implement nursing activities as specified in the program contract and protocol.	Weight stabilization must be a central and early goal for the nutritionally compromised patient. Medications may assist the appetite regulation center and neurochemical responses to feeding and satiety.
The patient will participate in a balanced exercise program on a daily basis.	Review established exercise routines. Modify exercise patterns, focusing on physical fitness rather than on weight reduction. Reinforce new exercise and fitness behaviors.	The focus of a balanced exercise program should be on physical fitness rather than on caloric reduction to lose weight.

NURSING DIAGNOSIS: Body image disturbance
EXPECTED OUTCOME: The patient will express clear and accurate descriptions of body size, body boundaries, and ideal weight.

SHORT-TERM GOAL	INTERVENTION	RATIONALE
The patient will correct body image distortions.	Modify body image misperceptions through cognitive and behavioral strategies. Use dance and movement therapies to enhance the integration of mind and body. Use imagery and relaxation interventions to decrease anxiety related to body perceptions.	Body image distortions involve perceptions, attitudes, and behaviors that place so much emphasis on appearance that they define self-worth.
The patient will modify cognitive distortions about body weight, shape, and eating responses.	Help the patient to identify cues that trigger problematic eating responses and body image concerns; the thoughts, feelings, and assumptions associated with each cue; the connections between these thoughts, feelings, assumptions, and eating regulation responses; and the consequences of the eating responses.	Cognitive distortions result in lowered self-esteem. Behavioral change results from an increased awareness of feelings and faulty cognitions.
The patient will identify social support systems that will reinforce accurate body perceptions and adaptive eating responses.	Include family members in the evaluation and treatment planning process. Assess the family as a system and the impact of the eating disorder on family functioning. Initiate group therapy to mobilize social support and reinforce adaptive responses.	Patients with eating disorders benefit from the involvement of family members and supportive group work.

Summary

1. Adaptive eating regulation responses include balanced eating patterns, caloric intake, and weight. Maladaptive responses include anorexia nervosa, bulimia nervosa, and binge eating disorder.
2. The majority of maladaptive eating disorders occur in females and may range from 1% to 4% of adolescent and young adult women.
3. Patient behaviors related to eating regulation responses include binge eating, fasting or restricting, purging, and related medical and psychiatric complications.
4. Predisposing factors for eating regulation responses are described from biological, psychological, and sociocultural perspectives. Precipitating stressors that affect eating responses include peer pressure, interpersonal rejection, and daily solitude.
5. The patient's level of motivation to change his or her behavior is an important coping resource to assess. A variety of maladaptive coping mechanisms may be used, including avoidance, intellectualization, isolation of affect, and denial.
6. Primary NANDA nursing diagnoses are anxiety, body image disturbance, fluid volume deficit, risk for self-mutilation, altered nutrition, powerlessness, and self-esteem disturbance.
7. Primary *DSM–IV–TR* diagnoses are anorexia nervosa, bulimia nervosa, and binge eating disorder.
8. The expected outcome of nursing care is that the patient will restore healthy eating patterns and normalize physiological parameters related to body weight and nutrition.
9. Planning activities involves decisions related to choice of treatment setting and the formulation of a nursing care plan contract.
10. Interventions include nutrition stabilization, exercise, cognitive behavioral interventions, body image interventions, family involvement, group therapies, and medications.
11. The nurse and patient should evaluate whether normal eating patterns have been restored and whether associated biopsychosocial problems have been resolved.

Competent Caring A Clinical Exemplar of a Psychiatric Nurse

DEBRA L. DAVIS, RN

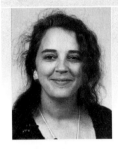

It seemed like a typically busy but uneventful day on our adult inpatient unit. After lunch, patients who had been participating in a group therapy session began returning to the unit. However, one patient was not with the group. Upon inquiring I discovered that Miss G, a 22-year-old patient with an eating disorder, had failed to attend the group session. I told the charge nurse of her absence and, almost simultaneously, the phone rang informing us that someone had been spotted standing on top of our building. I went outside and encountered a security officer, whom I followed to the site of the report. Sure enough, there on top of the three-story building was Miss G, who was saying she intended to jump.

As a staff nurse, I instantly assessed the situation as an emergency and knew that someone had to assume immediate crisis management. I also realized that my considerable tenure as a mental health technician, licensed practical nurse, and now registered nurse, would lend itself to the task. Certainly I had faced many crises during my years in the mental health field, but none was more perilous than this one, and none had begged for quicker or more decisive action.

In horror, I fixed my gaze on the patient, her toes draped over the edge of the building some 60 feet above the ground. Her precariously positioned frame was teetering, and her state of mind seemed to be of similar disposition. Miss G again threatened to jump and continued to repeat her desire to "end it all."

I yelled up to her and asked what could I do to reduce her distress. She asked to see Shelley, a staff member who had established a therapeutic relationship with Miss G and was someone she obviously trusted. I successfully bargained with the patient to step back from the edge of the building and sit down while I ran inside to get Shelley. I then directed the security officers to summon the mobile crisis unit to help. In the interim, I knew we had to continue efforts to retrieve the distressed patient. "Someone's got to go in the building and try to reach that roof," I said to Drew, another staff member on the scene. He agreed and quickly hurried off to find a way up. Extremely anxious that Miss G would either jump or accidentally fall, Shelley and I, along with some security personnel, dragged mattresses outside and placed them beneath where Miss G was standing.

Shelley began to communicate with the patient via a bullhorn, talking about the progress that Miss G had made and the plans she was looking forward to as they had previously discussed. Suddenly, as we watched, a pair of arms wrapped around Miss G and pulled her back from the edge of the building. Drew had found access to the roof and had snatched the patient back to safety. Applause erupted on the ground, and with the help of the mobile crisis unit and the security officers, Miss G was lowered to the ground and escorted back to the unit.

Those of us involved in the crisis removed ourselves from the scene, and uninvolved staff began postcrisis management interventions on the unit. I breathed deeply and felt the muscles in my neck relax for the first time in hours. So much for a typically busy but eventful day in psychiatric nursing.

MERLIN Visit **MERLIN: www.mosby.com/MERLIN/Stuart** to find these additional materials and student activities.

- **Worksheets**
- **"Drug of the Month" Updates**
- **"Citing the Evidence" Updates**
- **Critical Thinking Activities and Exercises**
- **Annotated Suggested Readings**
- **Web Links**
- **More!**

Chapter Review Questions

1. Match each term in Column A with the correct definition in Column B.

Column A

_____ Maladaptive eating regulation responses

_____ SSRIs

_____ Adaptive eating regulation responses

_____ Predisposing factors

_____ Serotonin

Column B

A. Balanced eating patterns, caloric intake, weight

B. Neurotransmitter implicated in eating disorders

C. Anorexia, bulimia, binge eating

D. Treatments for eating disorders

E. Biological, psychological, environmental, sociocultural

2. Fill in the blanks.

A. The majority of eating disorders occur in _____, and they may range from _____% to _____% of adolescents and young adults.

B. _____ is the rapid consumption of large quantities food in a discrete period of time.

C. Maladaptive coping mechanisms that may affect motivation for change in eating patterns and therefore must be assessed by the nurse include

_____,

_____, and

_____.

D. Several primary NANDA nursing diagnoses for a patient with an eating disorder are _____, _____, and _____.

E. The most effective treatment for eating disorders is _____.

3. Provide short answers for the following questions.

A. What are the differences in obese nonbingers, obese bingers, and nonobese bulimic patients regarding amount of binging, purging, and mood disturbance?

B. What is the expected outcome of nursing care for the patient with an eating disorder?

C. Keep a food diary for 1 week and list your thoughts about each meal. Ask a friend/classmate to evaluate it.

D. Design an eating disorder treatment contract that would help to improve your eating patterns and one that you think would be helpful for one of your friends or colleagues. What are the essential differences between the two?

E. How would you explain the differences in cultural support and stigma for the person with obesity and for the person with anorexia nervosa?

REFERENCES

American Psychiatric Association: Practice guidelines for the treatment of patients with eating disorders (revision), *Am J Psych* 157(1):1, 2000a.

American Psychiatric Association: *Diagnostic and statistical manual of mental disorders,* Fourth Edition, Text Revision, Washington, DC, American Psychiatric Association, 2000b.

Andersen A, Holman J: Males with eating disorders: challenges for treatment and research, *Psychopharmacol Bull* 33(3):391, 1997.

Barber N: The slender ideal and eating disorders: an interdisciplinary "telescope" model, *Int J Eat Disord* 23:295, 1998.

Brewerton T: Toward a unified theory of serotonin dysregulation in eating and related disorders, *Psychoneuroendocrinology* 20:6, 1995.

Brewerton T et al: The nature and prevalence of binge eating disorder in a national sample of women. In Widiger T et al, editors: *DSM-IV sourcebook,* vol 4, Washington DC, 1998, American Psychiatric Association.

Brink P et al: Childhood memories about food: the successful dieters project, *J Child Adolesc Psychiatr Nurs* 12(1):17, 1999.

Carlat D et al: Eating disorders in males: a report on 135 patients, *Am J Psychiatry* 154(8):1127, 1997.

Cash T, Deagle E: The nature and extent of body-image disturbances in anorexia nervosa and bulimia nervosa: a meta-analysis, *Int J Eat Disord* 22:107, 1997.

Chally P: An eating disorders prevention program, *J Child Adolesc Psychiatr Nurs* 11(2):51, 1998.

Erickson B, Yager J: The assessment and treatment of bulimia nervosa, *J Pract Psych Behav Health,* 4:76, 1998.

Fairburn CG et al: A cognitive behavioural theory of anorexia nervosa, *Behav Res Ther* 37:1, 1999.

Freund K et al: Detection of bulimia in a primary care setting, *J Gen Intern Med* 8:236, 1993.

George L: The psychological characteristics of patients suffering from anorexia nervosa and the nurse's role in creating a therapeutic relationship, *J Adv Nurs* 26:899, 1997.

Greeno C et al: Binge antecedents in obese women with and without binge eating disorder, *J Consult Clin Psychol* 68(1):95, 2000.

Grilo C: The assessment and treatment of binge eating disorder, *J Pract Psych Behav Health* 4:191, 1998.

Jansen A: A learning model of binge eating: cue reactivity and cue exposure, *Behav Res Ther* 36:257, 1998.

Jimerson D et al: Medications in the treatment of eating disorders, *Psychiatr Clin North Am* 19(4):739, 1996.

Jimerson D et al: Decreased serotonin function in bulimia nervosa, *Arch Gen Psychiatry* 54:529, 1997.

Keel P et al: Long-term outcome of bulimia nervosa, *Arch Gen Psychiatry* 56:63, 1999.

Lilenfield L et al: A controlled family study of anorexia nervosa and bulimia nervosa, *Arch Gen Psychiatry* 55:603, 1998.

Mayer L, Walsh T: The use of selective serotonin reuptake inhibitors in eating disorders, *J Clin Psychiatry* 59(S15):28, 1998.

McGilley B, Pryor T: Assessment and treatment of bulimia nervosa, *Am Fam Physician* 57(11):2743, 1998.

Pollice C et al: Relationship of depression, anxiety, and obsessionality to state of illness in anorexia nervosa, *Int J Eat Disord* 21:367, 1997.

Sanftner JL, Crowther JH: Variability in self-esteem, moods, shame, and guilt in women who binge, *Int J Eat Disord* 23:391, 1998.

Srinivasagam N et al: Persistent perfectionism, symmetry, and exactness after long-term recovery from anorexia nervosa, *Am J Psychiatry* 152:1630, 1995.

Strober M et al: Controlled family study of anorexia nervosa and bulimia nervosa: evidence of shared liability and transmission of partial syndromes, *Am J Psych* 157(3):393, 2000.

Taylor C et al: Factors associated with weight concerns in adolescent girls, *Int J Eat Disord* 24:31, 1998.

Thompson J: *Body image, eating disorder and obesity: an integrated guide for treatment,* Washington DC, 1996, American Psychological Association.

Vitousek K et al: Enhancing motivation for change in treatment-resistant eating disorders, *Clin Psychol Rev* 18(4):391, 1998.

Wade T et al: Anorexia nervosa and major depression: shared genetic and environmental risk factors, *Am J Psych* 157(3):469, 2000.

Weltzin T et al: Acute tryptophan depletion and increased food intake and irritability in bulimia nervosa, *Am J Psychiatry* 152:1668, 1995.

White J, Litovitz G: A comparison of inpatient and outpatient women with eating disorders, *Arch Psychiatr Nurs* 12(4):181, 1998.

Whittal M et al: Review: medication and cognitive behaviour therapy control symptoms of bulimia nervosa, *Behav Ther* 30:117, 1999.

Wilson G et al: Psychological versus pharmacological treatments of bulimia nervosa: predictors and processes of change, *J Consult Clin Psychol* 67(4):451, 1999.

Wonderlich S et al: Relationship of child sexual abuse and eating disorders, *J Am Acad Child Adolesc Psych* 36:1107, 1997.

Visit **MERLIN** for *Your Internet Connection*
to websites that are related to the content in this chapter.
www.mosby.com/MERLIN/Stuart

27 Sexual Responses and Sexual Disorders

Susan G. Poorman

LEARNING OBJECTIVES

After studying this chapter the student should be able to:

- Describe the continuum of adaptive and maladaptive sexual responses and the four phases of the nurse's growth in developing awareness of human sexuality
- Identify behaviors associated with sexual responses
- Analyze predisposing factors, precipitating stressors, and appraisal of stressors related to sexual responses
- Describe coping resources and coping mechanisms related to sexual responses
- Formulate nursing diagnoses related to patients' sexual responses
- Examine the relationship between nursing diagnoses and medical diagnoses related to sexual responses
- Identify expected outcomes and short-term nursing goals related to sexual responses
- Develop a patient education plan to promote adaptive sexual responses
- Analyze nursing interventions related to patients' sexual responses
- Evaluate nursing care related to patients' sexual responses

TOPICAL OUTLINE

Continuum of Sexual Responses
  Adaptive and Maladaptive Sexual Responses
  Self-Awareness of the Nurse
Assessment
  Behaviors
  Predisposing Factors
  Precipitating Stressors
  Appraisal of Stressors
  Coping Resources
  Coping Mechanisms
Nursing Diagnosis
  Related Medical Diagnoses
Outcome Identification
Planning
Implementation
  Health Education
  Sexual Responses within the Nurse-Patient Relationship
  Maladaptive Sexual Responses
  Dysfunctions of the Sexual Response Cycle
Evaluation

I locked myself away from you Too long, Tossing aside my feelings For you. Looking for a way out, an excuse Not to touch you; Because I want to, Inciting a riot within me. To reach out for you Is difficult, But less difficult Than turning away.

LESLIE BERTEL

Sexuality broadly refers to all aspects of being sexual and is one dimension of the personality. It includes more than the act of intercourse and is an integral part of life. It is evident in the person's appearance and in beliefs, behaviors, and relationships with others. Four aspects of sexuality are as follows:

- **Genetic identity**, which is a person's chromosomal gender
- **Gender identity**, which is a person's perception of his or her own maleness or femaleness
- **Gender role**, which is the cultural role attributes of one's gender, such as expectations regarding behavior, cognitions, occupations, values, and emotional responses
- **Sexual orientation**, which is the gender to which one is romantically attracted

Accepting a broad concept of sexuality allows nurses to explore ways in which people are sexual beings and understand more fully their feelings, beliefs, and actions. Nurses are often called on to intervene in the sexual concerns of patients when providing holistic patient care. Therefore it is important to develop skills and competence in addressing sexual issues by increasing awareness through education.

As nurses become educated in the basic principles of sexuality, they will better understand sexual needs and problems. If nurses are comfortable with sexual issues, they will convey this to the patient, who will feel more comfortable in discussing these issues. Patients are often experiencing pain and change as a result of threats to health or even as a part of normal growth and development. Thus it is important that the nurse-patient relationship allow for honest discussions about sexuality.

In answering the question, What do nurses need to know about sexuality?, several factors emerge. First, nurses need to know themselves and be aware of their feelings and values regarding sexuality. If nurses are not aware of their feelings, they cannot help patients meet their needs. Second, nurses need to understand that other people's feelings and values about sexuality are different from their own. Third, all nurses can become educated about sexual health and use sound counseling methods with patients. Specifically, nurses can:

- Develop confidence in their ability to discuss sexual issues with patients
- Learn interviewing skills for sexual assessment and history taking
- Counsel or refer patients for counseling

Education can be gained through nursing courses and continuing education programs. Some nurses pursue additional education and may become sex educators in schools, outpatient clinics, and planned parenthood agencies. Nurses prepared at the graduate level may become sex therapists through postgraduate work in human sexuality and extensive clinical supervision.

CONTINUUM OF SEXUAL RESPONSES
Adaptive and Maladaptive Sexual Responses

Experts in sexuality do not agree on what is normal sexual behavior. For years many people believed that only sexual relations between married heterosexual partners for procreation were normal. Today people view sexual behavior with a wider range of attitudes. Sexuality, on a continuum, ranges from adaptive to maladaptive (Fig. 27-1). The most adaptive responses meet the following criteria: between two consenting adults, mutually satisfying to both, not psychologically or physically harmful to either, lacking in force or coercion, and conducted in private.

Sometimes, however, sexual behavior can meet the criteria for adaptive responses but may be altered by what society deems acceptable and unacceptable. Unfortunately, society often decides this based on fear, prejudice, and lack of information rather than on data and facts (see Critical Thinking about Contemporary Issues). For example, the homosexual person may have the potential for healthy responses but be impaired by anxiety about societal disapproval.

Maladaptive sexual responses include behaviors that do not meet one or more of the criteria for adaptive responses. The degree to which these behaviors are maladaptive varies. Some sexual behaviors may not meet any of the criteria mentioned. For example, incest may include force and be psychologically harmful. However, other sexual responses may meet four of the five criteria for adaptive responses but still be maladaptive.

Caution must be used when attempting to label sexual behaviors as adaptive or maladaptive. There will always be disagreements and exceptions to the rule. The continuum shown in Fig. 27-1 is free of moral judgment and was developed to help the nurse in developing self-awareness and in understanding the range of sexual responses.

? CRITICAL THINKING about CONTEMPORARY ISSUES

Does Sex Education in Schools Promote Teenage Promiscuity?

Some people believe that teenagers are sexually active because they are taught sex education in their schools. The issue of sex education for youth in this country has raised a storm of questions and controversy. Unfortunately, much of it is based on values, beliefs, and personal opinion instead of facts. People who oppose sex education fight against comprehensive sex education programs in public schools. In contrast, many parents believe that their children are receiving sex education in school when they often are not.

Research provides some answers to this controversial question. Studies have demonstrated that comprehensive sex education programs can delay the initiation of first intercourse, reduce unprotected intercourse, and decrease unwanted teen pregnancy. Based on these findings, along with the rising incidence of teen pregnancy and sexually transmitted diseases, the more important question this country faces is whether we can afford not to provide comprehensive sex education in our schools.

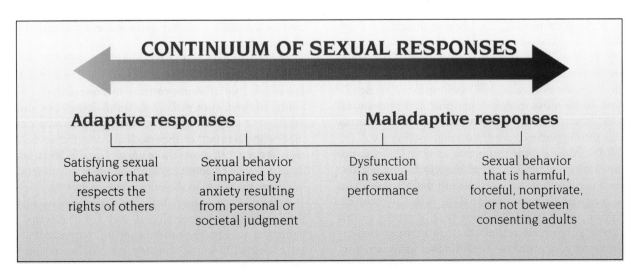

CONTINUUM OF SEXUAL RESPONSES

Adaptive responses		Maladaptive responses	
Satisfying sexual behavior that respects the rights of others	Sexual behavior impaired by anxiety resulting from personal or societal judgment	Dysfunction in sexual performance	Sexual behavior that is harmful, forceful, nonprivate, or not between consenting adults

Fig. 27-1 Continuum of sexual responses.

Self-Awareness of the Nurse

The nurse's level of self-awareness is critical in discussing sexual issues with patients. The first step in developing self-awareness involves clarification of values regarding human sexuality. Fig. 27-2 illustrates four phases of the nurse's growth: cognitive dissonance, anxiety, anger, and action (Foley & Davies, 1983).

Cognitive Dissonance. The first phase of growth in developing sexual self-awareness is cognitive dissonance, which arises when two opposing beliefs exist at the same time. For example, nurses grow up learning what society, family, and friends believe about sexual issues. If a nurse is raised in an environment that teaches that "it is impolite to talk about sex; it's too personal a subject," the nurse will carry that belief into nursing practice. When a patient wants to discuss a sexual concern, the nurse may feel two opposing reactions simultaneously: "I should not ask questions about such a personal subject as sex" and "As a professional, I should be able to discuss any problem, including sexual problems, with my patient."

These opposing thoughts, based on the different role expectations, make the nurse uncomfortable. However, the discomfort can be positive because it forces the nurse to examine feelings about the issue. The nurse resolves the cognitive dissonance in one of two ways: by continuing to believe that sexual concerns are too personal to discuss with patients or by examining the fact that sexuality is an integral part of being human.

Both of these beliefs have consequences for how the nurse relates to patients who voice sexual concerns. If the nurse continues to believe that sex is too personal to discuss with the patient, the nurse may become uncomfortable and choose not to follow up on sexual issues. This discomfort may be projected onto the patient, with the nurse stating, "The patient seemed too upset to talk about that right now." In this case the nurse should explore personal values and beliefs about sexuality and ask, "Do I believe these ideas about discussing sexual concerns because I have researched the facts and have accurate, current information?" Only when the nurse has examined the available information and made an informed choice on values will clarification of those values occur. If the nurse examines personal and professional values and believes that sexuality is an integral part of being human, a second phase of growth occurs.

Anxiety. Most people think that anxiety is a negative emotion. However, a mild level of anxiety can be positive because it can promote an awareness of danger, give extra energy, or stimulate professional growth by creating enough discomfort to initiate some type of action. In this second phase the nurse realizes that uncertainty, insecurity, questions, and problems regarding sexuality are normal. The nurse begins to understand that everyone is capable of a variety of sexual feelings and behaviors and that

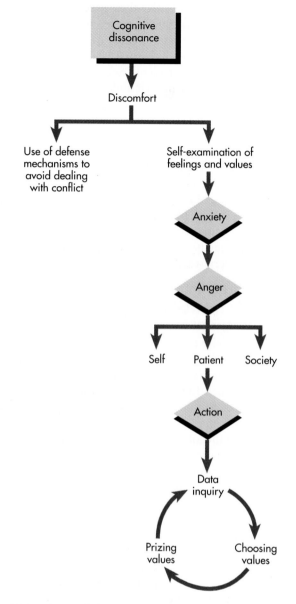

Fig. 27-2 Phases of the nurse's growth in developing awareness of human sexuality.

anyone can have a sexual dysfunction or question sexual identity.

The nurse experiencing anxiety may exhibit behaviors that hinder the discussion of sexual issues, such as talking too much (not allowing patients to express their feelings), failing to listen (not picking up on patients' cues and messages), and diagnosing and analyzing (becoming preoccupied with facts rather than feelings). As the anxiety level rises, the nurse becomes more uncomfortable and tries to reduce it. Learning about sexuality and facing conflicting values bring the nurse to the third phase of growth.

Anger. Anger generally arises after anxiety, fear, and shock subside. It is generally self-directed or directed to the patient or society. The nurse begins to recognize that issues associated with sex or sexuality are emotional and sometimes highly volatile. Rape, abortion, birth control, equal rights, child abuse, pornography, and religious issues all are related to sexuality and give rise to controversy and debate. This realization often breeds anger and contempt in the nurse. For example, the nurse may become angry at a colleague or a friend who makes judgmental remarks about pro-life or pro-choice activists.

During this phase of anger the nurse tends to choose words and actions that may be as judgmental as the attitudes the nurse is fighting against. The nurse may lecture other nurses about the need for sex education or critically judge a teenager who does not fear the consequences of having unprotected sex with someone known to be human immunodeficiency virus (HIV) positive. The nurse may also be angry with society for perpetuating ignorance about sexuality. Toward the end of this phase the nurse begins to understand that blaming self or society for lack of proper awareness does not help patients with sexual concerns. This realization helps defuse the anger, and the nurse is ready for the final phase.

Action. The final step in the growth experience is the action phase. Several behaviors emerge during this final phase of the growth experience: data inquiry, choosing values, and prizing values. Data inquiry occurs when the nurse seeks out additional information about sexual issues. Once the information is obtained, the nurse may discuss and debate the issues. These are healthy ways of exploring and deciding what to believe, and the nurse will eventually make some choices about a value position.

The final behavior is prizing the value position, which is an awareness and cherishing of feelings and values and being willing to share them publicly. Although prizing values is the final step in a positive growth experience, it does not mean that what is valued will not change. Values are never static; they evolve and shift as a person changes, grows, and acquires new experiences. Thus a person who once opposed abortion may later become understanding and empathetic toward women who have abortions.

The following clinical example shows the growth health professionals experience while increasing their awareness about sexuality. Chapter 2 has additional content on developing self-awareness and the nurse's therapeutic use of self.

 ## CLINICAL EXAMPLE

Carol was a new staff nurse at a rehabilitation hospital. At the monthly staff meeting the nursing supervisor asked whether there were any concerns the staff would like to discuss. Carol offered, "I wonder if any of you could help me with a suggestion. Over the past several weeks I've seen a number of patients masturbating. One patient was in the lounge and another was in his room when I came in to give him his meds. I was so embarrassed I didn't know what to do. I just ignored it both times, but part of me wanted to say 'stop that you dirty old man—that's not appropriate for a hospital!' I guess I could use some help with this one." Another staff nurse followed up and said "That's what I feel like saying when I see that kind of behavior." Several other staff in the room began to snicker. The nursing supervisor interrupted and asked, "Can anyone give Carol some suggestions on how to handle this situation therapeutically?" After several moments of silence, other staff

members admitted that they too were uncomfortable dealing with patients who were masturbating.

With the help of the supervisor, the staff began to brainstorm about how to handle this situation. Staff agreed that dealing with patients who are masturbating is a difficult issue for many nurses, and that the problem is most often the nurses' rather than the patients' because masturbation is a normal form of sexual expression. They decided that when they observe a patient masturbating in a public area, an appropriate nursing response would be to have the patient return to his or her room for privacy. If a nurse walks in on a patient masturbating in his or her room, the nurse should ensure the patient's privacy by excusing himself or herself and telling the patient he or she will return at a later time.

 In which phase of growth are you in relation to the development of awareness of human sexuality?

ASSESSMENT

Any basic health history must include questions about sexual history. A nurse who is comfortable discussing sexuality conveys the message that it is normal to talk about sexual health in a health assessment interview. If nurses can be composed and professional, they can ask questions about patients' sexual health naturally. The patient can then discuss sexual matters openly and without embarrassment.

Effective interviewing skills are an essential part of a sexual assessment. At times, nurses may be uncomfortable when addressing sexual issues. However, the principles of effective interviewing are the same for addressing sexual issues. Open-ended questions are one of the most effective ways of promoting a discussion on sexual issues, although some nurses report that direct questions can also be helpful in opening up the subject. Regardless, it is important to remember that questions must be asked at the patient's level of understanding, with sensitivity to the patient's cultural background, because each person is unique.

The time and number of questions needed to discuss a problem vary depending on the patient. Often just a few questions during an interview will obtain the relevant information. Examples of questions nurses may ask related to a patient's sexual health include the following:

- Tell me what you understand about (menstruation, intercourse, sexual changes with aging, menopause).
- Since you've been diagnosed, what questions have you had regarding your sexuality?
- Are there any changes you've noticed in your sexual patterns since becoming ill?
- Have you noticed any differences or problems in your sexual responses since taking this medication?
- Often people have questions about (masturbation, sexual frequency, safe sex, alternate positions).
- Sometimes it is uncomfortable to talk about sexual issues with your partner. How is this for you and your partner?

Behaviors

There are many modes of sexual expression. In a classic work, Kinsey (1953) identified a seven-point rating scale to examine sexual preference (Fig. 27-3); 0 represents exclusively heterosexual experiences, 6 represents exclusively homosexual experiences, and 2, 3, and 4 indicate a bisexual orientation. He suggested that most people are not exclusively heterosexual or homosexual. His studies indicated that a substantial percentage of men and women had experienced both heterosexual and homosexual activity.

Heterosexuality. Heterosexuality can be defined as sexual attraction to members of the opposite sex. It is the predominant sexual orientation among people in American society. The coupling of a man and a woman in a sexual partnership has both legal and religious sanctions. As such, it influences the culture, values, and norms of contemporary American life.

Homosexuality. Homosexuality can be defined as sexual attraction to members of the same sex. The term **gay** is used to refer to both male and female homosexuals; however, some use the term to refer only to male homosexuals and use the term **lesbian** to refer to female homosexuals. A person's attraction to people of the same sex, opposite sex, or both sexes is called sexual preference or sexual orientation. Some prefer the term **sexual orientation** over **sexual preference** because **preference** implies that homosexuals choose to be homosexual. Although sexual behaviors do involve choice, sexual orientation includes emotion and erotic attraction and may be genetically determined rather than a matter of free will (Cabas & Syein, 1996).

It is difficult to estimate the actual incidence of homosexuality in this country. The estimates have ranged from 3% to 10% of the population (King, 1999). However, many people have had a sexual experience with a member of the same sex at one time in their lives, and this is typically not identified when surveys are taken. One of the reasons that it is difficult to obtain an accurate incidence of homosexuality is that there is still considerable social stigma attached to labeling oneself as homosexual, so it is possible that many individuals do not report their true sexual identity.

Throughout history there have been many theories postulated concerning the origin of homosexuality. Although there is no conclusive evidence to support any one specific cause, most researchers agree that both biological and social factors influence the development of sexual orientation. Some sexuality experts question our need to find a cause for homosexuality rather than simply accepting the fact that it exists. If current estimates of homosexuality are accurate, nurses come into contact with homosexuals daily but often know little about homosexuality and often assume that all patients are heterosexual.

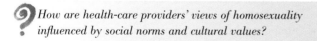

How are health-care providers' views of homosexuality influenced by social norms and cultural values?

Bisexuality. Bisexuality is defined as a sexual orientation or attraction to both men and women. Many studies on bisexuality include homosexuals in their research samples, and this has made the understanding of bisexuality more difficult. However, the studies that identified bisexuals separately found that data supported basic differences among heterosexuals, homosexuals, and bisexuals. Research in this

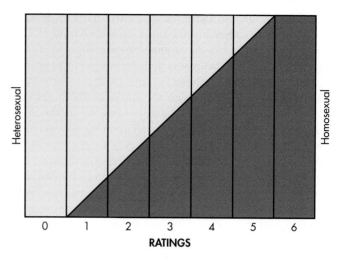

Fig. 27-3   Heterosexual-homosexual rating scale. Definitions of the ratings are as follows: *0,* Entirely heterosexual; *1,* largely heterosexual but with incidental homosexual history; *2,* largely heterosexual but with a distinct homosexual history; *3,* equally heterosexual and homosexual; *4,* largely homosexual but with distinct heterosexual history; *5,* largely homosexual but with incidental heterosexual history; *6,* entirely homosexual. (From Kinsey AC, Pomeroy WB, Martin AC: *Sexual behavior in the human female,* Philadelphia, 1953, WB Saunders.)

area showed heterosexuality to be the most common sexual orientation, followed by homosexuality and then bisexuality. Bisexuals reported experiencing stronger orgasms and were more sexually adventurous. They also described higher levels of eroticism and the increased incidence and enjoyment of masturbation (Van Wyk & Geist, 1995).

There has been an increased interest in the behavior and characteristics of bisexual men in light of the acquired immunodeficiency syndrome (AIDS) epidemic and the need to design effective preventive interventions for HIV infection. One problem that has been identified with bisexual orientation is that the sexual risk behaviors of bisexual men are quite high. However, their lack of identification with and participation in the homosexual community make them unlikely to be reached by the gay community's safe sex and AIDS prevention programs.

Transvestism. Transvestism is defined as cross-dressing, or dressing in the clothes of the opposite sex. Most often the transvestite who seeks treatment is a male; very little is known about female transvestism. No reliable statistics concerning the incidence of transvestism are available, but many professionals believe it is more common than generally assumed.

Transvestites tend to be married men who report heterosexual behavior. Although they occasionally or frequently dress in female clothes, they do not want hormonal or surgical sex change. Many transvestites try to find willing partners, and typically their activities of cross-dressing do not prevent sexual relationships with others.

Transsexualism. The term transsexual simply implies going from one sex to another. A transsexual is an individual with a gender identity disorder. They experience a mismatch between their biological sex and their gender identity. This person lives as a member of the opposite sex either part- or full-time and may seek to change his or her sex through hormone therapy and sex reassignment surgery.

Many times the transsexual patient describes himself or herself as "feeling trapped in the wrong body." Transsexuals genuinely believe that they belong to the other sex. Many experience intense emotional turmoil because of stigma from society. There are no accurate estimates of the incidence of transsexualism; however, postoperative transsexuals in the United States now number in the thousands.

Transsexuality is different from homosexuality in that homosexuals are comfortable with their anatomical identity and do not want to change their sex. Many transsexuals are heterosexual and express distaste for homosexual activity. Transsexuals are essentially heterosexual, not homosexual, but are often mistaken by others or themselves as homosexual, as seen in this clinical example.

 ## CLINICAL EXAMPLE

Mr. L is a 21-year-old biological male who was admitted to the psychiatric unit for evaluation after a serious suicide attempt. Mr. L told his nurse that he tried to kill himself because he has been "sexually mixed up for years" and is tired of feeling like a freak of nature. He said that his friends make fun of him and tell him he is a homosexual. Although he does feel sexually attracted to other men, he does not believe he is a homosexual. "I guess I don't feel like a man, I feel like a woman inside a man's body, and as a woman I am attracted to men."

Selected Nursing Diagnoses

- Altered sexuality patterns related to conflicting sexual feelings, as evidenced by verbalizations of confusion and happiness
- Risk for self-directed violence related to sexual identity confusion, as evidenced by suicide attempt

Think of a patient you took care of last week. How would your care have been different if you knew this patient was a homosexual, bisexual, transvestite, or transsexual?

The Sexual Response Cycle. In addition to modes of sexual expression or sexual orientation, the physiological and psychological responses to sexual stimulation can also be described. Masters and Johnson (1970) were the first to report the physiological changes that occur in men and women during sexual activity. They described the sexual response cycle as consisting of four phases: excitement, plateau, orgasm, and resolution. Kaplan (1979) also identified three stages of the sexual response cycle: desire, excitement, and orgasm. Currently, the accepted stages of the sexual response cycle are a combination of those defined by Masters and Johnson and those of Kaplan; they are listed in Box 27-1.

Sexual dysfunctions are more prevalent in women (43%) than men (31%). They are highly associated with negative experiences in sexual relationships and overall well-being (Laumann et al, 1999). Impairment in sexual response may occur in any one of the phases of the sexual response cycle.

For example, when the orgasm stage of the sexual response cycle is disrupted, premature or retarded ejaculation in males or orgasmic inhibition in females may result. If the excitement phase is inhibited, it may produce erectile dysfunction in males and a general sexual dysfunction in females. If the desire phase is absent, it may be evidenced by hypoactive sexual desire disorder or sexual arousal disorders. Although sexual dysfunction can occur when any phase is disrupted, resolution phase inhibition is rarely responsible for specific sexual dysfunctions.

The etiology of sexual dysfunction is varied and complex. Emotional and stress-related problems can increase the risk of sexual dysfunction in all phases of the sexual response cycle for both men and women. Sex therapists agree that many sexual dysfunctions are caused by psychological factors ranging from unresolved childhood conflicts to adult problems, such as performance anxiety, lack of knowledge, or failure to communicate with a partner. Sexual dysfunction can also be caused by physiological factors. Medical problems such as circulatory, endocrine, or neurological disorders as well as medication side effects can contribute to sexual problems. The interaction between physiological illness and the psychosocial aspects of that illness can also lead to sexual problems in the adult.

Predisposing Factors

No one theory can adequately explain sexual development or predisposing factors of maladaptive sexual responses. Several theories have been proposed, however, and are now briefly described.

Biological. Biological factors are initially responsible for the development of gender, that is, whether a person is genetically male or female. Somatotype includes chromosomes, hormones, internal and external genitalia, and gonads. Sex differentiation is determined by the Y chromosome. Research in humans confirms the general rule that

---

Box **27-1**

Stages of the Sexual Response Cycle

STAGE 1: DESIRE
Sexual fantasies and the desire for sexual activity.

STAGE 2: EXCITEMENT
Subjective sense of sexual pleasure along with physiological changes, including penile erection in the male and vaginal lubrication in the female.

STAGE 3: ORGASM
Peaking of sexual pleasure and the release of sexual tension accompanied by rhythmic contractions of the perineal muscles and pelvic reproductive organs.

STAGE 4: RESOLUTION
Sense of general relaxation, muscular relaxation, and well-being. Females may be able to respond to additional stimulation almost immediately during this stage; however, most males need some time before they can be restimulated to orgasm.

maleness and masculinity depend on fetal and perinatal androgens.

A biological female typically has XX chromosomes, with estrogen as the predominant hormone, appropriate internal and external genitalia, and ovaries. A biological male typically has XY chromosomes, with androgen as the predominant hormone, appropriate internal and external genitalia, and testicles. However, each of these typical configurations may vary. A person may have triple chromosomes, such as XXX, XXY, or XYY, or a single chromosome, XO. There is no YO chromosomal pattern. The triple pattern XXX and the single pattern XO (Turner's syndrome) result in a female body, whereas the triple patterns XXY (Klinefelter's syndrome) and XYY result in male bodies. Assuming no variation occurs, the biological factors result in a single, fully developed gender, either male or female.

Based on family studies and DNA samples of homosexual brothers, it has been suggested that a gene may be related to homosexuality. Early work in the field suggested that homosexuality may be inherited from the maternal side of the family through the X chromosome. Before such research is accepted as definitive, however, it will have to be validated by replication, and similar studies of lesbians have not yet been completed. In addition, such findings cannot account for all cases of homosexuality, but they do support a possible biological basis.

Psychoanalytical. Freud saw sexuality as one of the key forces of human life. In *Three Essays of the Theory of Sexuality* (1905) he proposed that sexuality began before puberty and that sexuality during infancy was central to personality development. He also believed that a person's choice of sexual expression depended on a mix of heredity, biology, and social factors.

The child, according to Freud, passes through a series of developmental stages in which a different erogenous zone is dominant. The first is the oral stage (birth to 12 or 18 months), in which the infant's chief sense of pleasure is derived from stimulation of the lips and mouth, that is, sucking. In the second, or anal, stage (ages 1 to 3 years), the child's attention is focused on elimination functions and control over body sphincters. The phallic stage follows (ages 3 to 5 years), in which the child's focus is on the genitals. An important occurrence in this stage is the development of the Oedipus complex in boys and the Electra complex in girls.

In the Oedipus and Electra complexes the child experiences sexual feelings for the parent of the opposite sex and resents the parent of the same sex. According to Freud, the boy fears retaliation from his father for desiring the mother and fantasizes that the father will cut off his penis (castration anxiety). This fear is the impetus for the young boy's eventually giving up the resentment of the father and identifying with him and the male gender role. The girl, on the other hand, has no penis to fear losing. She believes that at one time she had a penis but it was cut off, and she blames her mother for this.

After the resolution of the Oedipus or Electra complex, the child enters a prolonged stage where sexual impulses are repressed (latency stage). This stage lasts until adolescence, when the child enters the genital stage and sexual urges reawaken. The reemergence of Oedipal or Electra feelings and the need to assert themselves with parents also occur during this phase of development. The adolescent then makes the final transition into mature genital sexuality.

In recent years there has been much criticism of Freud's theory of psychosexual development. Feminists argue that psychoanalytical theory is male centered and views women as anatomically inferior to men (because they have no penis). Lack of scientific evidence is one of the major problems with Freud's theory. Other criticisms include that Freud was a victim of the Victorian era, a time of sexual repression, and that his thoughts and writings were bound by the period in which he lived. Finally, Freud's data were collected from observations of his patients, who were probably not representative of the total population since they were emotionally ill.

What impact has Freud's theory of psychosexual development had on society's view of women?

Behavioral. For the behaviorist, sexual reactions are the observable responses to overt, measurable stimuli. Behaviorists are not concerned with the intrapsychic process of early childhood and adolescence; rather, they view sexual behavior as a measurable physiological and psychological response to a learned stimulus or reinforcement event. Behaviorists consider the sexual behavior of adults who care for children as important in the children's later sexual development. They are thus interested in sexual difficulties that result from sexual abuse in childhood.

A number of studies suggest that many women who have been sexually abused as children experience physical and emotional problems in adult life. It is not unusual for these women to have frequent interpersonal, relationship, and sexual adjustment problems. The most common problems found in these women are depression, self-destructive behavior or suicidal attempts, anxiety, and panic attacks. They also report eating disorders and substance abuse problems (Roberts, 1996).

Sexual difficulties can also be seen in adult men who were abused as children. A survey of 1410 men and 1749 women conducted to examine sexual behavior in the United States found that women who experience sexual victimization were more likely to have arousal disorders and men who were sexually victimized as children were three times as likely to experience erectile dysfunction and twice as likely to experience premature ejaculation and low sexual desire. Both men and women who were victims of unwanted sexual activity showed long-term effects on sexual functioning (Laumann et al, 1999). The care of people who have experienced abuse and violence is described in detail in Chapter 41.

Precipitating Stressors

Physical Illness and Injury. Physical illness may alter sexuality. The patient may find that hospitalization alone changes sexual feelings and behavior. Nurses often care for patients with sexual dysfunctions or altered sexuality patterns; they need to discuss and therapeutically intervene in patients' responses to these changes. A person with rheumatoid arthritis may have body disfiguration and a change in body image caused by swollen areas around joints. The same patient may have decreased sexual interest because of joint pain during intercourse. People who have had a myocardial infarction may have decreased sexual interest because they fear sexual arousal may cause a heart attack.

Psychiatric Illness. Psychiatric illness affects a person's sexuality as well as the sexual behavior and satisfaction of the person's partner (see A Family Speaks). Depression can be either the result or cause of sexual dysfunction. As many as 70% of depressed patients have decreased sexual desire and decreased frequency of intercourse. Most often, depressed men engage in intercourse less often; depressed women may participate in sex but with less enjoyment. In contrast, hypersexuality may be the first symptom of a manic episode. People with bipolar illness have decreased sexual inhibitions, often impulsively choose sexual partners or begin extramarital affairs, display inappropriate sexual behavior, or act seductively or flirtatiously.

The sexual expression of patients with psychotic illnesses may be inappropriate and at times intrusive. Delusions and hallucinations may present with sexual content. Mental illness can interfere with one's ability to think coherently and express oneself in a clear and direct manner. Thus a patient's capacity for intimate relationships and sexual expression may be altered.

Although having a psychotic illness such as schizophrenia does not imply sexual dysfunction, sexual expression can be affected. The patient may not be able to understand or control sexual thoughts or impulses. For example, a patient may openly masturbate on an inpatient unit or inappropriately touch others. Thinking and judgment may also be impaired, resulting in sexual behavior that may be detrimental to the patient's health, such as unsafe sexual practices (see Citing the Evidence).

Questions have also been raised about the sexual lives of persons with serious and persistent mental illness who live in residential treatment facilities. It has been suggested that each facility and group of staff caring for residents need to identify ways to acknowledge and respect the normal sexual needs of these individuals and balance this with the need to keep the residents safe from sexually transmitted diseases,

A Family Speaks

Our daughter was diagnosed with schizophrenia 5 years ago when she was 17 years of age. Since that time we have received very good care for her. While we understand that she may never be completely well, she has her illness under control and has even started taking some courses at the local community college. She has also met some people her age and seems to enjoy their company.

But ever since she began doing better, we have had the added concern about her sexual needs and activities. As involved parents, we raised this issue with the different health-care providers who were managing her care over the years. In each case, almost without exception, we were told "Don't worry about such things; be grateful your daughter is as healthy as she is." While their intentions may have been good, they didn't help resolve our questions or fears. But then our daughter was assigned a nurse who we were told would be her case manager. The first time they met, the nurse took a detailed history and asked our daughter the unthinkable: What sexual feelings did she have and how was she managing her sexual needs? It was as if the floodgate had opened for all of us, and that session marked the beginning of an ongoing discussion we would all have about the very topic we had worried so much about. For the question of that nurse we will always be grateful, and if we could share one thought with future nurses in training, it would be to remember that patients are whole people and that sexuality is as important to those with psychiatric illness as it is to people everywhere.

Citing the Evidence on

Unsafe Sexual Behaviors Among Psychiatric Patients

BACKGROUND: Acute psychiatric inpatients were interviewed about whether they used substances just before or during sex and whether they engaged in unsafe sexual behaviors while using substances.

RESULTS: Nearly 40% of male patients and 36% of female patients reported using alcohol at least once during sex in the previous 6 months. Among male patients a significant association was found between using crack during sex and two high-risk behaviors: inconsistent condom use and sex with a high-risk partner. Among female patients the use of alcohol before or during sex was associated with the practice of receptive anal sex.

IMPLICATIONS: The demonstrated relationship between drug and alcohol use and unsafe sex practices among acute psychiatric patients suggests that AIDS prevention education efforts about safer sex targeted at this population should include information about risks of combining sexual activity with alcohol and drug use.

Menon A, Pomerantz S: Substance use during sex and unsafe sexual behaviors among acute psychiatric inpatients, *Psychiatr Serv* 48(8):1070, 1997.

unwanted pregnancies, and nonconsensual sexual advances or assaults (Torkelson & Dobal, 1999).

The nurse must therefore assess a psychiatric patient's sexual behavior carefully and intervene if there are inappropriate or dangerous sexual expressions. The nurse can help the patient identify and express needs related to sexuality. This includes helping the patient form healthy relationships with others, learn about safe sex practices, engage in healthy sexual expression, and decrease potentially dangerous sexual encounters.

Medications. Some medications contribute to sexual dysfunction, and nurses need to be knowledgeable about the medications they administer. The most common side effect of medication is diminished sexual desire, which occurs fairly equally in both sexes.

For men the most frequent problem is erectile difficulties followed by orgasmic difficulties. For women the most common problem is delayed orgasm (Crenshaw & Goldberg, 1996). The sexual side effects of psychiatric medications including neuroleptics and benzodiazepines are well documented, but side effects are even more frequently associated with antidepressants (Murray, 1998). Sexual dysfunctions are a common side effect of the selective serotonin reuptake inhibitors (SSRIs). These antidepressants can cause problems in any phase of the sexual response cycle. Men commonly complain of anorgasmia or ejaculatory difficulties. The most common complaint in women is delayed or absent orgasm (Moore & Rothschild, 1999). Psychiatric medications and their side effects are described in detail in Chapter 28.

Nurses should be familiar with the sexual side effects of medications, educate their patients about them, and encourage patients to notify a health professional when these effects occur. For example, a man may not be aware that his medication can cause impotence, yet he may be embarrassed and hesitant to talk with the physician or nurse about the problem. Often the medication itself or the dosage can be changed to correct the problem. Abuse of alcohol or nontherapeutic drugs may also have a debilitating effect on sexuality. Although many people believe alcohol is a sexual stimulant, prolonged use can cause erectile difficulty and other dysfunctions.

> *Consider two medications that you commonly administer to patients. Do you know whether they have sexual side effects, and have you talked about this possibility with your patients?*

HIV/AIDS. Fear of contracting a sexually transmitted disease (STD) may create change in sexual behavior. The most frightening STD is acquired immune deficiency syndrome (AIDS), which is caused by the human immunodeficiency virus (HIV). HIV/AIDS is a leading worldwide health problem despite the attempts by health-care professionals to educate society about safe sex practices. These practices include the following:

- Using condoms
- Reducing the number of sexual partners
- Promoting sexual behaviors that decrease the exchange of body fluids

Although in the United States the majority of those infected with HIV are men (80%), HIV is spreading most rapidly among women. Heterosexual contact has surpassed intravenous (IV) drug use as the most common mode of transmission in women (Wortley & Fleming, 1997). In 1998 the Centers for Disease Control and Prevention (CDC) reported that 38% of women with AIDS acquired it by heterosexual contact and 29% acquired it by IV drug use. The number of young people with AIDS is also alarming. In 1998 41% of persons diagnosed with HIV were under age 30 years at diagnosis. Although the number of young people with AIDS is beginning to decline, their represented proportion to all people with AIDS is significant. Sixteen percent of men and 21% of women with AIDS are in their twenties (CDC, 1998). While the success of treatment for AIDS is promising, the effects of this illness have a significant impact on all aspects of society. HIV/AIDS is discussed in more detail in Chapter 42.

The Aging Process. In the past researchers suggested that sexual activity decreased with aging. More recent studies indicate that patterns of sexual activity remain stable over middle and late adulthood years with only a small decline in later life. In 1999 the American Association of Retired Persons (AARP) conducted a sexual survey of 1384 adults over age 45 years. They found that overall seven in 10 of those with partners reported engaging in intercourse at least once a month. In addition, the majority of respondents felt good about their lives now and felt that a satisfying sexual relationship was important to the quality of their lives (Jacoby, 1999).

There is nothing in the biology of aging that automatically shuts down sexual functioning; however specific physiological changes do occur. In postmenopausal women the breasts may become less sensitive. Vaginal functioning changes in two ways. There is a reduced elasticity in the walls of the vagina and decreased vaginal lubrication. The decrease in vaginal lubrication is the result of decreased blood flow to the vagina, which is caused by low estrogen levels. In men several physiological changes occur in sexual response. Greater time and more direct stimulation is often needed for the penis to become erect, and erections tend to be less firm. The amount of semen is reduced, ejaculation is less intense and the physical need to ejaculate is diminished. The refractory period also becomes greater with age (Drench & Losee, 1996; Duffy, 1998).

In Western culture the myth of the older adult as asexual still prevails. Therefore, when health professionals care for older people who express an interest in sex or are sexually active, the professional often judges the older adult to be an exception to the rule. Older adults themselves may accept society's false beliefs about sexuality and aging. Many deny sexual attractions and feelings because they have been socialized to believe that sexual behavior in older people is abnormal or perverted. Older adults are influenced by cultural values of Western society that prize youth and vitality and often disapprove of an elderly person doing anything other than sitting in a rocking chair.

One important variable affecting sexuality in older adults is the lack of knowledge about the normal changes that occur with the aging process. Often nurses and older adults mistake a side effect of a medication or a symptom of a chronic medical illness for an expected part of the aging process. It is important for the nurse to understand the normal changes that occur with aging so that he or she can teach patients about these changes. This allows patients to learn what to expect and how they might compensate for the normal changes related to aging and sexual behavior.

It is equally important for nurses to realize that organic illness can affect sexual functioning. Many of the disease states seen in the elderly can interfere with sexual expression. People with arthritis have limited range of motion capabilities. Persons with chronic obstructive pulmonary disease (COPD) can experience dyspnea on exertion. A stroke can cause problems with nerve pathways that can lead to erectile dysfunction in men and anorgasmy in women, and can also change one's body image leading to feelings of unattractiveness and worthlessness. Medications taken by the elderly can lead to difficulties with sexual functioning as well. Beta-blockers and diabetes can contribute to impotence in men, and testosterone deficiency can create anorgasmy in women. These can be significant problems, and they often can be successfully treated.

Psychological factors, such as self-esteem, can also influence sexual activity in older adults. Older adults may be less inclined to be sexually active if they believe the physical changes that occur with aging make them unattractive. Marital status can influence sexuality. Because men die at younger ages than women, women are more likely to be widowed and live the last part of their lives alone. Because there are fewer men in the population, it is more difficult for older women to find partners than it is for older men.

Opportunities for sexual activity may also be limited for individuals who become dependent on others for their care. Older adults who must move in with their adult children, a personal care facility, or a nursing home may find it difficult to engage in any form of sexual expression. Many nursing homes restrict physical activity, so residents lack privacy from staff, who tend to care for older adults in a parental way. Physical contact between nursing home residents is often discouraged by nursing home staff, and many residents may feel restricted in their sexual expression.

However, nurses are becoming more sensitive about the sexual needs of nursing home residents. By recognizing their sexual needs, nurses can act as advocates and help residents with sexual expression by encouraging discussion of sexual concerns, closing doors to ensure privacy, and allowing socialization with sexual partners.

> *While working in a long-term care facility you walk into a patient's room and see two patients engaged in sexual relations. How would you respond?*

Appraisal of Stressors

Feelings of oneself as a sexual being change throughout the life cycle, and they are influenced by a person's appraisal of the stressful situation. Sexual identity cannot be separated from self-concept or body image. Therefore, when bodily or emotional changes occur, sexual responses change as well.

Coping Resources

It is important for the nurse to assess the patient's coping resources because these can have a significant impact on sexual health. Resources may include the person's knowledge about sexuality, positive sexual experiences the patient has had in the past, supportive people in the patient's environment, and social or cultural norms that encourage healthy sexual expression. It is also helpful to include the person's sexual partner whenever possible. This allows the nurse to evaluate the quality of this relationship and to frame all nursing interventions within the context of a supportive, loving partnership.

Coping Mechanisms

Coping mechanisms related to sexual response may be adaptive or maladaptive, depending on how and why they are being used. Fantasy is a coping mechanism used to enhance sexual experiences. Men and women may escape to erotic fantasies with unknown lovers during sex with their spouse. Although many people fear that fantasies about people other than their sexual partner indicate that they are unsatisfied or unattracted to their partner, this is typically not the case. Fantasies are often a creative way to increase sexual excitement and enjoyment and do not usually indicate dissatisfaction with a current partner. However, excessive fantasy can be maladaptive when used as a replacement for actual sexual expression or the development of intimate relationships with others.

Maladaptive coping mechanisms may result from problems with self-concept. Often one member of a sexually dysfunctional couple may use projection in blaming his or her partner for the total problem, absolving himself or herself from any responsibility: "I never had a sex problem with any of my previous lovers; I think you are the problem." Projection is also the coping mechanism used when a person's thoughts and feelings are unacceptable and anxiety producing. For example, a wife constantly accuses her husband of wanting to have an affair when actually the wife is contemplating an affair. Because her feelings are unacceptable to her, she projects them onto her husband and accuses him.

Denial and rationalization are also common coping mechanisms. Both allow the person to avoid dealing with sexual issues. The following are maladaptive examples:

- **Denial:** "I don't have a problem with sex" or "I never feel sexual."
- **Rationalization:** "I don't need sex; I'm fine without it. Besides, a good marriage is a lot more than just sex."

To cope with unacceptable feelings about becoming vulnerable and the resulting ambivalent feelings about intimacy, some people withdraw from any form of sexual behavior. Others may engage in increased sexual behavior with multiple partners to protect themselves from one intimate relationship.

NURSING DIAGNOSIS

When developing nursing diagnoses for variations in sexual response, the nurse should consider all the information gathered in the assessment phase and the components of the Stuart Stress Adaptation Model (Fig. 27-4). The identified nursing diagnoses serve as a foundation for future problem solving. There are two primary NANDA nursing diagnoses concerned with sexual response. The first is **altered sexuality patterns**, which include difficulties, limitations, or changes in sexual behaviors or activities. The second is **sexual dysfunction**, which includes lack of sexual satisfaction, alterations in perceived sex role, and conflicts involving values.

Other related nursing diagnoses that address additional behavioral problems may also need to be included. For example, a patient may be sexually functional but sexual identity may be unclear. Nursing diagnoses related to the range of possible maladaptive responses and related medical diagnoses are identified in the Medical and Nursing Diagnoses box on the opposite page. The primary NANDA diagnoses and examples of complete nursing diagnoses are presented in the Detailed Diagnoses box on p. 560.

Related Medical Diagnoses

Many people who have transient variations in sexual response do not have a medically diagnosed health problem. Those with more severe or persistent problems are classified into one of three categories of variations in sexual response according to the *DSM–IV–TR*: sexual dysfunctions, paraphilias (sexual perversions or deviations), or gender identity disorders (American Psychiatric Association, 2000). The medical diagnoses and the essential features of each of these diagnostic classes according to the *DSM–IV–TR* are described in the Detailed Diagnoses box.

OUTCOME IDENTIFICATION

Goals must be formulated realistically, remembering the uniqueness of each person. The expected outcome for patients with maladaptive sexual responses is the following:

The patient will obtain the maximum level of adaptive sexual responses to enhance or maintain health.

This outcome can be made more specific through the use of short-term goals. These goals must be mutually identified with the patient, priorities must be established, and criteria

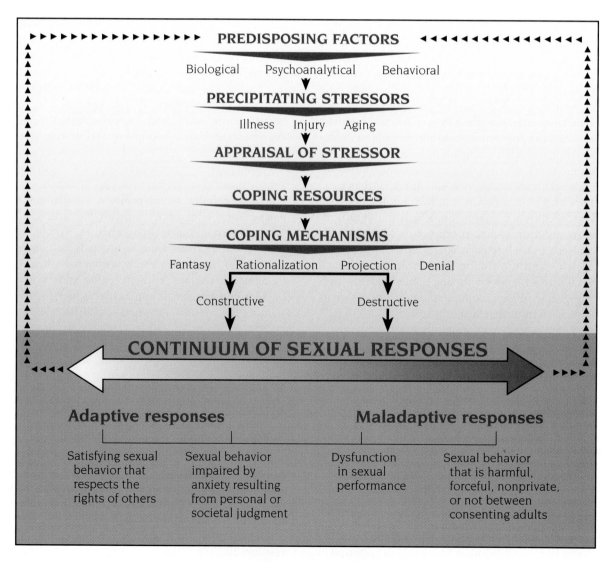

Fig. 27-4 The Stuart Stress Adaptation Model related to sexual responses.

used to measure progress toward the goals must be defined. Examples of short-term goals include the following:

- The patient will describe personal values and beliefs regarding sexuality and sexual expression.
- The patient will identify sexual questions and problems.
- The patient will relate accurate information about sexual concerns.
- The patient will implement one new behavior to enhance sexual functioning.
- The patient will report decreased anxiety and greater satisfaction with sexual health.

After identifying goals in partnership with the patient, the nurse begins to implement the appropriate nursing interventions.

PLANNING

The nurse's level of expertise determines the degree of planning. The planning phase can simply involve reviewing assessment data, exploring options, and making referral sources known and available. This phase can also include sexual instruction for the patient or the patient and partner together. The nurse and patient can discuss a specific sexual issue and approaches that will provide the needed information.

IMPLEMENTATION
Health Education

Primary prevention strives to promote health and prevent problems through specific methods such as teaching and planning, described in Chapter 13. Before engaging in health education or counseling, however, nurses must examine their values and beliefs about sexual behavior. This can be facili-

tated by exploring commonly held myths regarding human sexuality. Table 27-1 lists some common sexual myths, the results of believing them, and the facts related to each one.

Education is the most common method of primary prevention of sexual problems. The content and methods of sex education have changed little over the past several decades. Many people receive most of their sex education from friends, who may not provide accurate information. Too few parents discuss sexual issues with their children, and school sex education programs, to avoid discussion of controversial subjects, often focus only on biological factors, which is insufficient for the needs of today's youth.

Recently, because of the epidemic rates of teenage pregnancies and abortion and the spread of AIDS, many experts are suggesting more comprehensive sex education programs, and some are suggesting that these programs begin as early as preschool and kindergarten. Sex education is a lifelong process with the primary goal of promoting sexual health. This includes helping people develop positive views of sexuality, gain information and skills about taking care of their sexual health, and acquire decision-making abilities regarding sexual issues. A comprehensive sex education program has the following four goals (SIECUS, 1997):

- Communicating accurate information about sexuality
- Providing an opportunity to develop values, beliefs, and attitudes about sexuality
- Helping patients develop relationships and interpersonal skills
- Encouraging the exercise of responsibility in sexual relationships

It is also clear that teaching information about sex and sexuality is not enough. For a sex education program to be ef-

 Medical and Nursing Diagnoses *related to* Variations in Sexual Response

RELATED MEDICAL DIAGNOSES (DSM–IV–TR)*	RELATED NURSING DIAGNOSES (NANDA)†
Hypoactive sexual desire disorder	Anxiety
Sexual aversion disorder	Body image disturbance
Sexual arousal disorder	Decisional conflict
Orgasmic disorder	Fear
Premature ejaculation	Grieving, dysfunctional
Dyspareunia	Health maintenance, altered
Vaginismus	Health-seeking behaviors
Sexual dysfunction due to a general medical condition	Pain
Substance-induced sexual dysfunction	Personal identity disturbance
Exhibitionism	Powerlessness
Fetishism	Role performance, altered
Frotteurism	Self-care deficit
Pedophilia	Self-esteem disturbance
Sexual masochism	Sensory/perceptual alteration
Sexual sadism	**Sexual dysfunction‡**
Voyeurism	**Sexuality patterns, altered‡**
Transvestic fetishism	Social interactions, impaired
Gender identity disorder of childhood, adolescence, or adulthood	Spiritual distress (distress of the human spirit)

*Reprinted with permission from the *Diagnostic and statistical manual of mental disorders*, Fourth Edition, Text Revision. Copyright 2000. American Psychiatric Association.
†From North American Nursing Diagnosis Association: *Nursing diagnosis: definitions and classifications, 1999-2000*, Philadelphia, 1999, The Association.
‡Primary nursing diagnosis for variations in sexual response.

Detailed Diagnoses *related to* **Sexual Responses**

NANDA DIAGNOSIS STEM	EXAMPLES OF COMPLETE DIAGNOSIS
Sexual dysfunction	Sexual dysfunction related to prenatal weight gain, as evidenced by verbal statements of physical discomfort with intercourse
	Sexual dysfunction related to joint pain, as evidenced by decreased sexual desire
Sexuality patterns, altered	Altered sexuality patterns related to financial worries, as evidenced by inability to reach orgasm
	Altered sexuality patterns related to mastectomy, as evidenced by statements such as "My husband won't want to touch me" and "I don't feel like a woman"
	Altered sexuality patterns related to fear of pregnancy, as evidenced by stopping before penetration

DSM–IV–TR DIAGNOSIS	ESSENTIAL FEATURES*
Hypoactive sexual desire disorder	Persistent or recurrent deficit or absence of sexual fantasies and desire for sexual activity
Sexual aversion disorder	Persistent or recurrent extreme aversion to and avoidance of genital sexual contact with a sexual partner
Sexual arousal disorder	Persistent or recurrent partial or complete failure to attain or maintain the physiological response of sexual activity or persistent or recurrent lack of a subjective sense of sexual excitement and pleasure during sexual activity
Orgasmic disorder	Persistent or recurrent delay in or absence of orgasm following a normal sexual excitement phase during sexual activity that is judged by the clinician to be adequate in focus, intensity, and duration, taking into account the person's age
Premature ejaculation	Persistent or recurrent ejaculation with minimal sexual stimulation before, on, or shortly after penetration, before the person wishes it
Dyspareunia	Recurrent or persistent genital pain before, during, or after sexual intercourse
Vaginismus	Recurrent or persistent involuntary spasm of the musculature of the outer third of the vagina that interferes with coitus
Sexual dysfunction due to a general medical condition	Clinically significant sexual dysfunction etiologically related to a general medical condition
Substance-induced sexual dysfunction	Clinically significant sexual dysfunction that developed during significant substance intoxication or withdrawal
Exhibitionism	A persistent association, lasting at least 6 months, between intense sexual arousal, desire, acts, or fantasies, and exposing one's genitals to an unsuspecting stranger
Fetishism	A persistent association, lasting at least 6 months, between intense sexual arousal, desire, acts, or fantasies, and nonliving objects (such as female undergarments)
Frotteurism	A persistent association, lasting at least 6 months, between intense sexual arousal, desire, acts, or fantasies, and rubbing against a nonconsenting person
Pedophilia	A persistent association, lasting at least 6 months, between intense sexual arousal, desire, acts, or fantasies, and one or more children, aged 13 years or younger
Sexual masochism	A persistent association, lasting at least 6 months, between intense sexual arousal, desire, acts, or fantasies, and being humiliated, beaten, bound, or otherwise being made to suffer (real or imagined)
Sexual sadism	A persistent association, lasting at least 6 months, between intense sexual arousal, desire, acts, or fantasies, and the affliction of real or simulated psychological or physical suffering (including humiliation)
Voyeurism	A persistent association, lasting at least 6 months, between intense sexual arousal, desire, acts, or fantasies, and observing unsuspecting people who are either naked, in the act of disrobing, or engaging in sexual activity
Transvestic fetishism	A persistent association, lasting at least 6 months, between intense sexual arousal, desire, acts, or fantasies, and cross-dressing
Gender identity disorder of childhood, adolescence, or adulthood	Persistent and intense distress about being a male or a female, with an intense desire to be the opposite sex, a preoccupation with the activities of the opposite sex, and a repudiation of one's own anatomical structures

* Reprinted with permission from the *Diagnostic and statistical manual of mental disorders*, Fourth Edition, Text Revision. Copyright 2000, American Psychiatric Association.

fective it must promote behavioral change. The most effective sex education programs are comprehensive and skill based. For example, it is not enough to teach individuals to say no to sex, but they must be taught how to say no. This could be done by teaching decision-making and assertiveness skills and by role playing potentially difficult sexual situations.

Which sexual myth from Table 27-1 did you believe before reading this chapter? How will knowing the truth affect your nursing practice?

Table **27-1**

Ten Common Myths and Facts about Human Sexuality

Myth	Result of Myth	Fact
Patients become embarrassed when nurses bring up the subject of sexuality and would prefer that nurses not ask questions about sex.	If nurses believe this, they deny the patient the opportunity to ask questions and clarify concerns related to sexual issues.	Patients prefer that nurses initiate discussions of sexuality with them.
Excessive masturbation is harmful.	People often feel guilty or ashamed about masturbating; some people deny themselves this experience because of uncomfortable feelings perpetuated by society.	There is no evidence that masturbation causes physical problems. If masturbation leads to satisfaction and pleasure, it is unlikely to be a problem.
Sexual fantasies about having sex with a partner other than a lover or spouse indicate relationship difficulties.	People may become uncomfortable about having a fantasy with a different partner. They may feel guilty and view the fantasy as a sign of infidelity.	Imagining sex with a different partner is a common sexual fantasy and does not necessarily indicate a desire to act out the fantasy.
Sex during menstruation is unclean and harmful.	Women often view their bodies as unclean and even unfit or inferior during menstruation. Women use menstruation as an excuse to avoid intercourse rather than simply saying no without a "good reason."	Medically, menstrual flow is in no way harmful or dirty. If women desire, there is no reason to abstain from intercourse during menstrual flow.
Oral and anal intercourse is perverted and dangerous.	Many people refrain from these behaviors or indulge in them only to feel ashamed and guilty afterward.	Oral and anal intercourse is not harmful if certain precautions are taken when performing anal intercourse, such as avoiding contamination of the vaginal tract and wearing a condom to prevent the transmission of disease.
Most homosexuals molest children.	Known homosexuals are often fired from teaching jobs, and many parents do not allow their children to spend any time with anyone who is homosexual.	Research shows that the adult heterosexual male poses a far greater risk to the underage child than does the adult homosexual male.
Homosexuals are sick and cannot control their sexual behavior.	Homosexuals are denied jobs and are sometimes jailed for their homosexuality. Children may be taken away from homosexual parents by courts.	Most homosexuals' social and psychological adjustment is the same as the heterosexual majority, and objectionable sexual advances are far more likely to be made by a heterosexual (usually male to female) than by a homosexual.
Because of sex education programs, most adolescents and young adults are aware of the risks of getting sexually transmitted diseases and practice safe sex.	When health educators believe that young adults have adequate knowledge about sexually transmitted diseases, they may not take the time to assess, add to this knowledge, and correct any misperceptions.	A study of over 500 first-year students at a large university reported that of those who had multiple partners, fewer than 50% used condoms to lower the risk of disease.
Advancing age means the end of sex.	Many older adults become victims of this myth not because their bodies have lost the ability to perform, but because they believe that they have lost the ability to perform.	Sexually, men and women in good health can function effectively throughout their lives.
Alcohol ingestion reduces inhibitions and therefore enhances sexual enjoyment.	Many people use alcohol in the hope that it will increase their sexual pleasure and performance. Alcohol ingestion can also provide an excuse for engaging in sexual behaviors—"I would never have gone to bed with him if I hadn't had all that wine."	Data do not support the belief that alcohol ingestion reduces inhibitions and enhances sexual enjoyment.

Sexual Responses within the Nurse-Patient Relationship

Sexual Responses of Nurses to Patients. A clinical situation in which a nurse feels sexual attraction to a patient is a problem that has received little attention in the nursing literature. One reason for this is that nurses often deny sexual feelings for their patients. However, sexual attraction and sexual fantasies are part of the human experience. If these feelings are not examined, they can interfere with the quality of care by shifting the focus from the patient's needs to those of the nurse.

First, nurses must acknowledge their feelings without judging them. Often nurses try to ignore or deny these feelings because they are uncomfortable and frightening. They make judgments about themselves, such as, "What's wrong with me? I shouldn't feel this way about my patients. I must be really weird" and "I'm sure I'm the only nurse who ever had these feelings." The nurse who admits these feelings without judging them is able to deal with them.

One of the best ways to begin to deal with these feelings is to seek consultation from a more experienced nurse. A nurse should not tell the patient about these feelings, as it will only further complicate the issue. It is not the patient's responsibility to respond to the nurse's feelings. Rather, it is always the nurse's responsibility to preserve professional boundaries. The nurse needs to be aware of behaviors exhibited by the patient. The nurse should avoid flirtatious gestures or sharing personal information during interactions. Finally, it is never acceptable for a nurse to engage in sexual behavior of any kind with a patient. Such activity can lead to allegations of sexual misconduct, litigation, and loss of the nurse's license to practice (Stevens, 1998).

Sexual Responses of Patients to Nurses. One of the most common sexual behaviors of hospitalized patients is seductive behavior toward the nurse. This includes making passes and sexual comments, inappropriate touching, asking for a phone number and requesting a date. Nurses are often extremely uncomfortable with such behaviors. One study examining nurses' responses to sexual harassment by patients revealed that often the quality of care given to both the harassing patients and other patients was negatively affected. Many of the nurses in this study used avoidance as a defense mechanism (Lobell, 1999).

The first step in intervening in such a situation is to let the patient know that the behavior is unacceptable. The nurse needs to respond in a firm, matter-of-fact manner that clearly states what limits are being set, such as "Mr. Moore, I am uncomfortable when you suggest that I get into bed with you. Please stop saying that" or "Mr. Dean, take your hand off my breast."

Nurses are sometimes embarrassed or afraid to confront patients and attempt to laugh it off or ignore it. Patients do not have the right to be verbally offensive or to touch nurses' bodies without permission. Nurses are taught to be accepting of patients' behavior, and this principle is difficult to dispute. However, when the behavior violates nurses' rights, limits must be set.

Nurses have a responsibility as professionals to attempt to understand sexual behaviors and analyze their possible meanings. Patients may show seductive behaviors for various reasons, which may or may not include a serious desire for sex with the nurse. Seductive behavior is often a way of getting the nurse's attention. Hospitalized patients can also feel unattractive or insecure about themselves sexually; thus seductive behaviors may be a request for reassurance. Sometimes patients confuse their gratitude for and appreciation of the nurse with sexual attraction. These feelings may in turn generate thoughts such as, "Wouldn't my nurse make a wonderful wife? She's so giving and understanding all the time." In this case the patient views professional behavior and concern as self-sacrificing and altruistic.

Finally, patients may have difficulty understanding the difference between a professional and a social relationship. In many ways the nurse-patient relationship is idealized for the patient. The patient receives all the attention and caring and is not expected to give anything in return. It is easy to see how the patient could be confused about his or her relationship with the nurse. The clinical example that follows illustrates this point. Table 27-2 summarizes nursing considerations in sexual responses of patients to nurses.

 CLINICAL EXAMPLE

Mr. P has been hospitalized for an exacerbation of a chronic illness for the past 3 weeks. Ms. S has been his primary nurse during this hospitalization. The following is a conversation between the nurse and patient the day before his discharge.

Mr. P: I wish my wife were more like you, Ms. S.

Ms. S: Mr. P, I'm not sure I understand what you are saying.

Mr. P: Well, it's just that you are always so concerned about me. You always try to make me feel good and want to help me all the time. Sometimes my wife's a grouch; she's so wrapped up in her job and the kids she doesn't always pay as much attention to me as you do.

Ms. S: I'm glad you feel taken care of, but it's impossible to compare my role as your nurse with your wife's role.

Mr. P: I'm not sure I follow you.

Ms. S: They are very different types of relationships. It's nice to have someone take care of us when we can't take care of ourselves, but when we are healthy, we don't need someone to take care of us all the time. Your relationship with your wife is more of a sharing one with mutual benefits. You take care of her needs, and she takes care of your needs in return. If you feel that your relationship with your wife is not a satisfying one, perhaps you need to talk this over with her.

Maladaptive Sexual Responses

Illness. Stress, physical and emotional illness, injury, and aging can lead to changes in sexuality and sexual functioning. These changes and related nursing interventions differ based on whether the illness is acute or chronic. It is important for the nurse to obtain complete information on the nature and course of the illness, the types of medications used in its treatment, the patient's appraisal of the impact of the

Table **27-2**

Summary of Nursing Considerations in Sexual Responses of Patients to Nurses		
GOAL: Maintain a professional nurse-patient relationship that will enable the nurse to provide therapeutic nursing care		
Principle	**Rationale**	**Nursing Considerations**
Establish a trusting relationship.	An atmosphere of trust allows for open, honest communication between patient and nurse; this enables the nurse to aid the patient in discovering the underlying issues related to sexual feelings and behavior.	Express nonsexual caring and concern for the patient. Be a responsive listener, especially to feelings and needs that the patient may not be able to express directly. Reinforce the purpose of the therapeutic nurse-patient relationship.
Gain awareness of nurse's own feelings and thoughts.	Being aware of his or her feelings and thoughts enables the nurse to understand how they influence his or her behavior; with increased self-awareness the nurse can increase the effectiveness of his or her interactions with patients.	Recognize own feelings and thoughts. Identify any specific patient interaction or behavior that influences the nurse's feelings and thoughts. Identify the influence of the nurse's feelings and thoughts on one's behavior in an attempt to increase the effectiveness of nursing interventions.
Decrease patient's inappropriate expressions of sexual feelings and behaviors.	If the nurse is able to help the patient see that his or her sexual interactions and behaviors are being expressed to an inappropriate partner (the nurse), the sexual acting out will usually decrease; this allows the nurse to help the patient begin to identify the reasons for his or her behavior.	Set limits on patient's sexual behavior. Use a calm, matter-of-fact approach without implying judgment. Reaffirm nonsexual caring for the patient. Explore the meaning of the patient's feelings and behaviors.
Expand patient's insight into sexual feelings and behaviors.	Once the patient begins to identify the reasons for his or her sexual feelings and behaviors, he or she can see that the nurse is not an appropriate outlet for these feelings and behaviors and can move toward a more appropriate and therapeutic relationship.	Clarify misconceptions regarding any feeling patient may have about the nurse as a possible sexual partner. Point out the futile nature of the patient's romantic or sexual interest in the nurse. Redirect patient's energies toward appropriate health-care issues.

illness, and any physical limitation imposed by the illness that affects the patient's sexual health.

Several nursing interventions can then be implemented to facilitate the patient's adaptive sexual responses. The first is for the nurse to act in a supportive way and to help the patient express feelings, fears, and problems. Open communication between the patient and partner should also be encouraged. The nurse can reinforce the positive attributes of the patient, prevent social isolation, mobilize coping resources, and support adaptive coping mechanisms that have helped the patient deal with stressors in the past.

The nurse can also offer anticipatory guidance and give accurate information about the illness or injury, including what the patient may expect from medical or psychiatric treatment and its impact on sexual health (see A Patient Speaks). The nurse can also initiate counseling about sexuality and alternative means of sexual expression. Relaxation techniques, autoerotic activities, and variations in movement and positions may be suggested. The nurse should em-

phasize that pleasure can be obtained in a variety of ways and stress the importance of a loving relationship. Finally, if the problem is complex and of a long duration, the patient should be referred for psychotherapy or sex therapy from a qualified professional. A Patient Education Plan for patients recovering from an organic illness is presented on p. 564.

Should sexual behavior be permitted among patients who are residents of a long-term psychiatric facility? If so, what issues must be addressed by staff? If not, how will the sexual needs of these patients be met?

Sexual Orientation. Most heterosexuals, homosexuals, and bisexuals accept their sexual orientations, although some have difficulty and seek professional help. For example, it is possible that one's sexual behavior may not match one's sexual desire. Someone in a heterosexual relationship may wish to be in a homosexual one, or vice versa, and feel constrained to act because of personal, sociocultural, legal, economic, or religious reasons. This can create internal conflict and distress and the person may seek counseling. Although homosexuality is not a disorder or mental illness, research has suggested that homosexuals are at increased risk for suicidal behavior and certain mental health problems (Fergusson et al, 1999; Herrell et al, 1999). Although the reasons for this increased risk are complex, it is reasonable to assume that society's lack of acceptance of homosexuals is a contributing factor.

A Patient Speaks

It's bad enough to be depressed, but how's a person supposed to feel when the people taking care of him don't give him all the information he needs? From what I can see from talking to other patients in my group, my story is not that unusual.

For about 6 months I felt myself slipping deeper and deeper into the black hole of depression. I saw some ads on television and decided that maybe I needed some outside help, since I clearly wasn't getting better by myself. So off I go to a nearby clinic where I see someone who diagnoses me with depression and gives me some pills to take. In the beginning the drugs made me kind of jittery, but gradually I got over it. In a couple of months I actually almost felt like my old self again (all except for sex, that is). In that one area of my life I simply couldn't experience the satisfaction I used to have and didn't know what was going on. Well, it turns out that the pills I'm on limit my sexual performance, but nobody ever bothered to mention this to me. I guess they thought it wasn't important or something, but they were really wrong.

Now that I understand what's going on I can work around it, since the drugs have helped me in almost every other way. But still, it would be nice if the people that you turn to for help could give you all the information you need and not just talk about the parts that they think are important or limit themselves to the topics they're comfortable talking about.

Negative societal attitudes toward homosexuals affect everyone, including nurses who provide care and homosexuals, who can become victims if they internalize these negative attitudes. The literature has discussed the issue of the nursing profession and homophobia, which is an irrational fear of homosexuals along with a negative attitude and hostility to them. Questions have been raised about the impact homophobia among nurses has on providing competent nursing care to homosexual patients. It has also been suggested that perhaps nursing's commitment to caring may exclude caring for the homosexual patient (Misener et al, 1997). These concerns require serious self-analysis by each and every nurse.

Great sensitivity must be displayed by the nurse to acknowledge and accept the fact that patients may display a range of sexual responses. Replacing the term **spouse** with **partner** when addressing patients is a good place to start. Committing to this simple change is a daily reminder that not all patients are heterosexual. Other strategies that may increase the homosexual's comfort with health-care providers are allowing partners to be involved in decision making regarding patients' care, ensuring confidentiality and gaining knowledge of the coming out process (Taylor, 1999). **Coming out** simply refers to the process of disclosing one's homosexual orientation. Because of the homosexual element of bisexuality, bisexuals often encounter many of the same difficulties stemming from societal attitudes as homosexuals. Another factor that may present a problem for the bisexual is isolation from a support group. Because bisexuals are often accused of fence-sitting, they can be rejected by heterosexuals and homosexuals. Bisexuals may lack social support, and friends and family may pressure them to decide on one sexual orientation (usually heterosexual) so that they will be accepted by society.

An important step in working with homosexual patients who are attempting to come to terms with their homosexuality is to help them explore their beliefs about homosexuality, where they came from and whether they are based in fact or fiction. The patient may have internalized some of society's prejudices, such as "Homosexuality is a sick and abnormal behavior; because I am a homosexual, I am sick and ab-

 PATIENT EDUCATION PLAN *Sexual Responses after an Organic Illness*

CONTENT	INSTRUCTIONAL ACTIVITIES	EVALUATION
Describe the variety of human sexual response patterns.	Discuss the range of sexual desires, modes of expression, and techniques.	The patient identifies personal sexual orientation and typical level of sexual functioning.
Define the patient's primary organic problem.	Provide accurate information regarding the disruption caused by the organic impairment.	The patient understands the specific organic illness.
Clarify relationship between the organic problem and patient's level of sexual functioning.	Reframe distorted or confused perceptions regarding the impact of the illness on patient's sexual functioning.	The patient accurately describes the impact of the illness on sexual functioning.
Identify ways to enhance patient's sexual functioning and improve interpersonal communication.	Describe additional experiences that would add to the sexual satisfaction and the relationship between the patient and patient's partner.	The patient and partner report reduced anxiety and greater satisfaction with their sexual responses.

normal and should not act on my sexual feelings because they are wrong." Responses can be varied and include denial, confusion, and sexual promiscuity, especially among those trying to prove to themselves that they are not gay. It is helpful to have patients list their beliefs about homosexuality and bisexuality and to discuss each one. However, a review of beliefs about sexuality may not be sufficient. Encouraging the person to read about homosexuality and bisexuality is also helpful. Throughout this process the patient will be extremely sensitive to the nurse's acceptance or rejection.

Confidentiality is also a central issue. It is helpful for the nurse to demonstrate an appreciation for patients' concerns about unwanted exposure of their homosexuality to family members, friends, or co-workers. The nurse should not encourage or discourage the patient's disclosure of homosexual concerns but rather help the patient to explore and process the choice of disclosure or lack of disclosure with others, as in the following clinical example.

CLINICAL EXAMPLE

Ms. A, a 25-year-old single female, came to the mental health clinic with the complaint of a "sexual problem." Her history revealed that she had been sexually inactive for the past 5 years. At the age of 20, Ms. A had a brief sexual encounter with a man she had been dating for 2 years. She ended the relationship shortly afterward because she had no interest in maintaining a sexual relationship with the man. Recently she became involved in a relationship with a woman that was very satisfying to her. She felt she had to end the relationship because she would not tolerate thinking of herself as a homosexual. During one of the initial counseling sessions, Ms. A told the nurse that she must end the relationship before "it" happens again.

Nurse: What are you afraid will happen?

Ms. A: I'm afraid I'll feel attracted to her again.

Nurse: What about that frightens you?

Ms. A: (becoming upset) That will mean I'm homosexual!

Nurse: What does being homosexual mean for you?

Ms. A: It means I'm sick. It's a sin. I couldn't go to church anymore.

Nurse: Are all homosexuals sick?

Ms. A: Yes.

Nurse: How do you know this?

Ms. A: Everybody knows that homosexuality is morally wrong. Homosexuals have a lot of emotional problems.

Nurse: Do you know any homosexual people?

Ms. A: Well, not exactly.

Nurse: What have you read about homosexuality?

Ms. A: Nothing.

Nurse: Then it looks to me like you are basing all of your conclusions on hearsay and not real knowledge. I think that you and I need to explore your beliefs in more detail, then you can do some reading to find out the facts.

Selected Nursing Diagnoses

- Altered sexuality patterns related to questions about sexual preference related to recent interpersonal relationship
- Spiritual distress related to conflicting values, as evidenced by questions about religious beliefs

In the preceding clinical example the nurse and Ms. A developed a plan often used in sexual counseling to explore homosexuality. Some of the interventions included the following:

- Ms. A described her beliefs about homosexuality and homosexuals.
- The nurse encouraged Ms. A to explore the literature on homosexuality and suggested readings to help dispel the myths.
- The nurse then discussed these with Ms. A and suggested that she attend a social gathering for gay people to test out her new knowledge. The nurse suggested the social gathering because many people struggling with a homosexual identity are frightened to test out situations that would dispel the myths.
- Finally, the nurse helped Ms. A. explore her responses to these activities and integrate them into a positive view of self.

Gender Identity. Gender identity is a person's perceptions of his or her maleness or femaleness. Gender identity disorder or gender dysphoria is a profound discomfort with one's sex and a strong and persistent identification with the opposite gender. It can be experienced along a continuum of responses, with transsexualism being the most severe form of this disorder. Treatment of the transsexual person has been a controversial subject in recent years. In a 5-year follow-up study of people in the process of changing their sex, 70% of the subjects experienced a positive outcome. The authors attribute this to careful selection, close observation over long periods of time, and supportive follow-up treatment. They suggest that sex reassignment surgery is the treatment of choice for true transsexualism (Bodlund & Kulgren, 1996).

Standards of care for gender identity disorders provide guidelines for health professionals who work with patients who have gender problems (Harry Benjamin International Gender Dysphoria Association, 1998; Levine, 1999). These standards were developed because of the serious consequences of available treatments. Patients who believe they are transsexual and request surgical reassignment must meet these standards. They require that two therapists agree that the reassignment is appropriate; that the patient be at least 18 years old; and that the patient live in the role of the preferred gender for at least 1 year. The standards also require that follow-up care be provided.

Professionals who care for transsexual patients must be educated in sexuality. The assessment phase of treatment is especially important. The patient and therapist must be certain that implementing the treatment plan is the best approach because the surgery is not reversible.

A Nursing Treatment Plan Summary for maladaptive sexual responses is presented on p. 566.

Dysfunctions of the Sexual Response Cycle

Treating sexual dysfunctions is beyond the scope of the nurse generalist. However, the nurse should be aware of the principles involved and should know creditable sex therapists in the community for referral of patients. Two common models of sex therapy are briefly discussed here: the Masters and Johnson and the Helen Singer Kaplan models. They have been reported to be useful for several types of sexual

NURSING TREATMENT PLAN *Summary* *Maladaptive Sexual Responses*

NURSING DIAGNOSIS: Altered sexuality patterns
EXPECTED OUTCOME: The patient will obtain the maximum level of adaptive sexual responses to enhance or maintain health.

SHORT-TERM GOAL	INTERVENTION	RATIONALE
The patient will describe values, beliefs, questions, and problems regarding sexuality.	Listen to sexual concerns implied and expressed. Help the patient explore sexual beliefs, values, and questions. Encourage open communication between the patient and partner.	An accepting therapeutic relationship will allow patients to be free to question, grow, and seek help with sexual concerns. Communicate respect, acceptance, and openness to sexual concerns.
The patient will relate accurate information about sexual concerns.	Clarify sexual misinformation. Dispel myths. Provide specific education about sexual health practices, behaviors, and problems. Give professional "permission" to continue sexual behavior that is not physically or emotionally harmful. Reinforce positive attitudes of the patient.	Accurate information is helpful in changing negative thoughts and attitudes about particular aspects of sexuality. It can also prevent or limit dysfunctional behavior. Giving permission allows the person to continue the behavior and alleviates anxiety about normalcy. It allows patients to incorporate sexual behavior in a positive and accepting self-concept.
The patient will implement one new behavior to enhance sexual response.	Set clear goals with the patient. Identify specific behaviors that can be carried out focusing on enhancing self-concept, role functioning, and sexuality. Encourage relaxation techniques, redirection of attention, positional changes, and alternative ways of sexual expression as appropriate. Become familiar with the sex therapy resources available in the community. Refer the patient to a qualified sex therapist as needed.	Giving a patient direct behavioral suggestions can help relieve a sexual problem or difficulty and is a useful intervention when the problem is of recent onset and short duration. While all nurses need to screen for maladaptive sexual responses and provide basic nursing care, complex problems should be referred to qualified sex therapists for further treatment.

dysfunction, and some long-term follow-up studies have shown the positive sustained effect of therapy on individuals' and couples' sense of sexual satisfaction.

Masters and Johnson Model. Masters and Johnson began their pioneering research in sexuality in the 1950s. Before their work, patients with problems in sexuality were generally referred to a psychiatrist for psychotherapy or psychoanalysis, since health professionals incorrectly assumed that anyone who had a problem with sexuality was emotionally disturbed. Masters and Johnson's (1970, 1986) treatment includes short-term education with step-by-step instructions regarding the physical aspects of sexual activity and supportive psychotherapy. They believe that attitudes and ignorance are responsible for most sexual dysfunctions.

Their approach to patients begins with obtaining a detailed sexual and background history. Then the couple is instructed to carry out a sensate focus exercise in which each partner instructs the other in specific ways of caressing for sensual pleasure without involving the breasts or genitals. The next day the exercise is repeated, including breasts and genital areas, but without coitus. The exercise's purpose is to alleviate performance anxiety and to enhance warm, comfortable feelings between partners. After the sensate focus exercises are completed, the therapy is directed to the sexual dysfunction. The Masters and Johnson model emphasizes education, communication, and cooperation between partners.

Helen Singer Kaplan Model. Kaplan's (1975) method of treating sexual dysfunctions combines specific tasks with psychodynamic insights, dream interpretations, and gestalt and transactional techniques. Treatment begins with an extensive evaluation, including marital, psychiatric, sexual, medical, and family history from both partners. If serious intrapsychic or interpersonal difficulties are found, the couple may be referred to individual or conjoint therapy and is not accepted for sex therapy at that time.

Like Masters and Johnson, Kaplan uses sensate focus exercises and variations, such as showering together, to begin sex therapy or to further evaluate a person's suitability for sex therapy. Therapy itself consists of erotic tasks performed at home plus weekly or semiweekly meetings with the therapist. Couples and the therapist explore feelings experienced during the erotic exercises. The exercises take into account the motivations and dynamics of the relationship. The role of the therapist includes education, clarification, and support. Both Kaplan and Masters and Johnson emphasize communication between partners and exploration of the relationship and emotional concerns.

Pharmacological Treatment. One of the greatest advances in treating men with erectile disorders has been in understanding its medical etiology and therefore being able to treat it with drugs, devices, or surgery. The introduction of the drug sildenafil (Viagra) has been the first user-friendly medical treatment for this dysfunction (McCarthy, 1998). This drug acts by blocking the enzyme PDE5, which breaks down cyclic guanosine monophosphate, boosting relaxation of the smooth muscle in the penis and allowing it to become erect (Rosenstock, 1998).

Viagra is taken in pill form 1 hour before sex and requires sexual stimulation to be effective. Viagra has been effective for many men suffering from erectile dysfunction; however, sex therapists caution that although Viagra may eliminate a physical cause for erectile dysfunction, it is not a magic pill that will cure all. Relationship issues must also be addressed for satisfactory treatment of this dysfunction. The use of Viagra is also being explored for treatment of female sexual dysfunction. It is suspected by some researchers that Viagra may increase the blood flow to the pelvic region and may be useful in treating desire problems in women. Additional research is needed in this area.

EVALUATION

In the evaluation phase the nurse works with the patient to evaluate the effectiveness of the sexual counseling or intervention. Factors to consider include the following:

- **Sense of well-being.** How does the person feel about himself or herself? Have these feelings improved during the treatment?
- **Functioning ability.** If the person was dysfunctional, is functional ability restored? Somewhat improved? What about the person's ability to function within primary relations at work? With friends?

- **Satisfaction with treatment.** Does the patient believe that the treatment was helpful? Were the patient's goals adequately met?

Evaluation of any form of sexual counseling or intervention should be ongoing. The nurse and patient should work together on goals, problems, and alternatives.

Summary

1. Sexuality is defined as a desire for contact, warmth, tenderness, and love. Adaptive sexual behavior is consensual, free of force, performed in private, neither physically nor psychologically harmful, and mutually satisfying.
2. Patient behaviors related to sexual responses include heterosexuality, homosexuality, bisexuality, transvestism, transsexualism, and physiological and psychological responses to sexual stimulation.
3. Predisposing factors for variations in sexual response are described from biological, psychoanalytical, and behavioral perspectives. Precipitating stressors that may change sexuality include physical illness and injury, psychiatric illness, medications, and HIV/AIDS.
4. A variety of coping mechanisms are used with expressions of sexuality: fantasy, projection, denial, and rationalization.
5. Primary NANDA diagnoses are sexual dysfunction and altered sexuality patterns.
6. Primary *DSM–IV–TR* diagnoses are categorized as sexual dysfunctions, paraphilias, and gender identity disorders.
7. The expected outcome of nursing care is that the patient will obtain the maximum level of adaptive sexual responses to enhance or maintain health.
8. Interventions include sex education and preventive counseling and intervening in sexual feelings and behaviors within the nurse-patient relationship, maladaptive sexual responses, and dysfunctions of the sexual response cycle.
9. The nurse and patient should consider the following factors in evaluating nursing care: the patient's sense of well-being, functioning ability, and satisfaction with treatment.

Competent Caring   A Clinical Exemplar of a Psychiatric Nurse

DONALD RIBELIN, RN, C

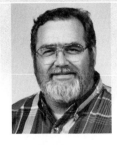

Having worked in nursing for over 20 years, I tend to have certain defined responses to almost any given situation. This works well until something comes along that doesn't fit into those preconceived notions of how things should be. I was working as evening charge nurse on an adult acute care psychiatric unit when one of the mental health assistants came to the desk to report that he had seen Mr. B and Mrs. G sneaking into the solarium and that they appeared to be "getting it on." Almost every nurse has had to confront patients, visitors, or both in a sexual situation of one type or another. We'd had our share of such encounters in the past, but the staff reacted very differently this time.

To begin with, Mr. B was a 72-year-old "street" person who had been admitted with a diagnosis of rule-out dementia, and

Ms. G was a lovely 70-year-old widow with a diagnosis of situational depression. Mr. B's apparent dementia had proven to be secondary to malnutrition and vitamin B₁₂ deficiency. Once he had received treatment for these, we had found him to be a remarkable person whose ready sense of humor lightened many an evening group. Ms. G had been admitted with one of the flattest affects I had ever seen. Her family reported that she had been increasingly depressed since her husband's death 3 years ago. This depression increased dramatically around the anniversary of Mr. G's death, which was right around this time of the year. Over the past week, Ms. G's depression had lifted noticeably. She could be seen talking, laughing, and joking with Mr. B during any free moment. They seemed to always be together, sitting next to each other during groups or meals or walking side by side on outings. We had all commented on how much they had helped each other and what a nice couple they made. Suddenly Mr. B and Ms. G had stopped being a nice

Continued

Competent Caring A Clinical Exemplar of a Psychiatric Nurse—cont'd

"old" couple and had become two psychiatric patients sneaking off to have "sex."

I found myself torn between several reactions to this news. The empathic nurse in me responded, "This is great: Two lonely people in their twilight years of their lives have found love and companionship." The analytical nurse in me wondered whether this relationship would really be therapeutic for Ms. G given Mr. B's background. The cautious nurse in me wondered whether Mr. B could simply be trying to ensure he had somewhere to stay after discharge. But the administrative nurse in me won out, thinking that I don't let other patients behave in this manner, so I have to intercede. Somewhat loudly I walked down the hall and into the solarium, taking a very long time fumbling for the light switch. The lights revealed Ms. G and Mr. B sitting side by side, holding hands and red faced. Ms. G's blouse was only partially buttoned, and she was obviously upset. I apologized to them, explaining that I had planned to spend my break in the solarium and hadn't meant to startle them. As they quickly stood up and headed toward their rooms, I could see a look of sadness and possibly shame replacing the happy smile that we had been seeing the past few days on Ms. G's face. Mr. B also looked sad, and for a moment I thought I saw the return of the shuffling gait he had at admission. By doing the "right" thing, I now felt like I had done the very worst thing possible.

During my shift report, I gave the incident only brief comment. Talking more about the possible therapeutic benefits of the relationship, I didn't mention the sexual aspects at all. Guilt can be a great censor and rewriter of history, and I was obviously really feeling guilty. Well, time may heal all wounds, but it only gives rumors time to grow. I was very surprised when, upon returning to work the next evening, my nurse manager asked for the incident report on Mr. B and Ms. G having sex in the solarium. She also wanted to know why I hadn't documented the incident in my nursing notes. By the time I had explained the previous evening's happenings, what had started out as two people wanting to be together had become a major event. Damage control began with a meeting of all unit staff, where we discussed what had and had not happened. It didn't stop there. A psychiatric unit is often like a small town where there are no secrets. That evening, in group, the patients brought up our hapless couple's "making out." Again I found myself in a position where I felt anything I said could and probably would be wrong. After careful thought I responded by first reminding them that this was a hospital and there were certain rules of conduct that had to be adhered to, even when we might personally disagree with them. Members of the group were asked to share their feelings about these rules and why they were or were not necessary. As the group proceeded, I kept a careful eye on Ms. G and Mr. B. They were sitting about as far from each other as possible and both were very quiet. As the patients talked, I kept trying to think of something to say or do to alleviate the obvious pain and embarrassment of our elderly, who were now the center of attention. Suddenly Mr. B stood up, smiled at the group, and said, "You know, I've been feeling real bad today. I felt like I had done something wrong and that I was just waiting for my punishment to come." Then he stated, "Yeah! I was feeling real bad until just a moment ago, when I remembered a button I saw once. It said, 'Old people need love, too,' and you know that's right because everyone needs to know that someone cares about them, needs them, and loves them. So it really doesn't matter what any of you think because I've found someone to love me and for me to love." I'll always remember that moment as a time that patients and staff clapped, cried, and laughed together.

 Visit MERLIN: www.mosby.com/MERLIN/Stuart to find these additional materials and student activities.

- **Worksheets**
- **"Drug of the Month" Updates**
- **"Citing the Evidence" Updates**
- **Critical Thinking Activities and Exercises**
- **Annotated Suggested Readings**
- **Web Links**
- **More!**

Chapter Review Questions

1. Match each term in Column A with the correct definition in Column B.

Column A
___ Bisexuality
___ Gender identity
___ Gender role

Column B
A. A person's chromosomal gender
B. A person's perception of his or her maleness or femaleness
C. Condition in which there is a profound discomfort with one's own sex and a strong and persistent identification with the opposite gender

___ Genetic identity

___ Heterosexuality

___ Homophobia

___ Homosexuality

___ Orgasm

___ Sexual orientation

___ Transsexualism

___ Transvestism

D. Condition in which usually a male has a sexual obsession for or addiction to women's clothing

E. Peaking of sexual pleasure and the release of sexual tension accompanied by rhythmic contractions of the perineal muscles and pelvic reproductive organs

F. Irrational fear of homosexuals along with a negative attitude and hostility toward them

G. Sexual attraction to members of the opposite sex

H. Sexual attraction to members of the same sex

I. Sexual attraction to persons of both sexes

J. The cultural role attributes attributed to one's gender, such as expectations regarding behavior, cognitions, occupations, values, and emotional responses

K. The gender to which one is romantically attracted

2. Fill in the blanks.

A. When a nurse holds two opposing beliefs at the same time it is called _____.

B. A biological female typically has _____ chromosomes, whereas a biological male typically has _____ chromosomes.

C. According to Freud, in the _____ complex the child experiences sexual feelings for the parent of the opposite sex and resents the parent of the same sex.

D. Behaviorists believe that _____ may predispose one to sexual difficulties later in life.

E. _____ is the most common method of primary prevention of sexual problems.

F. The nurse's first step in working with a patient in relation to maladaptive sexual responses is to communicate _____.

3. Provide short responses for the following questions.

A. Identify five criteria for adaptive sexual behavior.

B. Design a sex education program for adolescents that includes a focus on safe sex practices.

C. Critique the assessment form used in your treatment center for its inclusion of information related to a patient's sexual responses.

D. Describe specific ways in which culture defines a society's view of "normal" sexual behavior.

REFERENCES

American Psychiatric Association: *Diagnostic and statistical manual of mental disorders,* Fourth Edition, Text Revision. Washington, DC, American Psychiatric Association, 2000.

Bodlund O, Kullgren G: Transsexualism: general outcomes and prognostic factors: a five-year follow-up study of nineteen transsexuals in the process of changing sex, *Arch Sex Behav* 25:315, 1996.

Cabas R, Stein T: *Textbook of homosexuality and mental health,* Washington, DC, 1996, American Psychiatric Press.

Centers for Disease Control and Prevention: *HIV/AIDS surveillance—general epidemiology report,* Atlanta, GA, 1998, US Department of Health and Human Services.

Crenshaw T, Goldberg J: *Sexual pharmacology: drugs that affect sexual function,* New York, 1996, WW Norton.

Drench ME, Losee RH: Sexuality and sexual capacities of elderly people, *Rehab Nurs* 21:120, 1996.

Duffy L: Lovers, loners and lifers: sexuality and the older adult, *Geriatrics* 53:S68,1998.

Fergusson D et al: Is sexual orientation related to mental health problems and suicidality in young people? *Arch Gen Psychiatry* 56(10):876, 1999.

Foley T, Davies M: *Rape: nursing care of victims,* St Louis, 1983, Mosby.

Freud S: *Three essays of the theory of sexuality,* ed 3, London, 1962, Hogarth Press (originally published 1905).

Harry Benjamin International Gender Dysphoria Association: Standards of care for gender identity disorders (5th version), Dusseldorf, 1998, Symposium Publications.

Herrell R et al: Sexual orientation and suicidality: A co-twin control study in adult men, *Arch Gen Psychiatry* 56(10):892, 1999.

Jacoby S: Great sex: what's age got to do with it? *Modern Maturity* 42R:43,1999.

Kaplan HS: *The illustrated manual of sex therapy,* New York, 1975, New York Times Book Co.

Kaplan HS: *Disorders of sexual desire and other new concepts and techniques in sex therapy,* New York, 1979, Brunner/Mazel.

King B: *Human sexuality today,* ed 3, Upper Saddle River, NJ, 1999, Prentice-Hall.

Kinsey A et al: *Sexual behavior in the human female,* Philadelphia, 1953, WB Saunders.

Laumann E et al: Sexual dysfunction in the United States: prevalence and predictors, *JAMA* 281:542, 1999.

Levine S: The newly revised standards of care for gender identity disorders, *J Sex Educ Ther* 24:121, 1999.

Lobell S: Registered nurses' responses to sexual harassment, *Pelican News* 55:14, 1999.

Masters W, Johnson V: *Human sexual inadequacy,* Boston, 1970, Little, Brown.

Masters W et al: *Masters and Johnson on sex and human loving,* Boston, 1986, Little, Brown.

McCarthy B: Integrating Viagra into cognitive-behavioral couples sex therapy, *J Sex Educ Ther* 23:303, 307, 1998.

Misener T et al: Sexual orientation: A cultural diversity issue for nursing, *Nurs Outlook* 45:178, 1997.

Moore B, Rothschild A: Treatment of antidepressant induced sexual dysfunction, *Hosp Pract* 34:89,1999.

Murray JB: Physiological mechanisms of sexual dysfunction side effects associated with antidepressant medication, *J Psychol* 132:412, 1998.

Roberts S: The sequalae of childhood sexual abuse: A primary care focus for adult female survivors, *Nurse Pract* 21:44, 1996.

Rosenstock H, McGreer G: Viagra! *Contemp Sexuality* 32:2,11, 1998.

SIECUS Fact Sheet, Guidelines for comprehensive sexuality education: kindergarten-12th grade, *SIECUS Rep* 25:24, 1997.

Stevens J: When patient care gets too personal, *RN* 61:72, 1998.

Taylor B: 'Coming out' as a life transition: Homosexual identity formation and its implications for health care practice, *J Adv Nurs* 30:523, 1999.

Torkelson D, Dobal M: Sexual rights of people with serious and persistent mental illness: gathering evidence for decision making, *J Am Psychiatr Nurs Assoc* 5:150, 1999.

VanWyk PH, Geist CS: Biology of bisexuality: critique and observations, *J Homosexuality* 28:369, 1995.

Wortley PM, Fleming PL: AIDS in women in the United States: recent trends, *JAMA* 278:914, 1997.

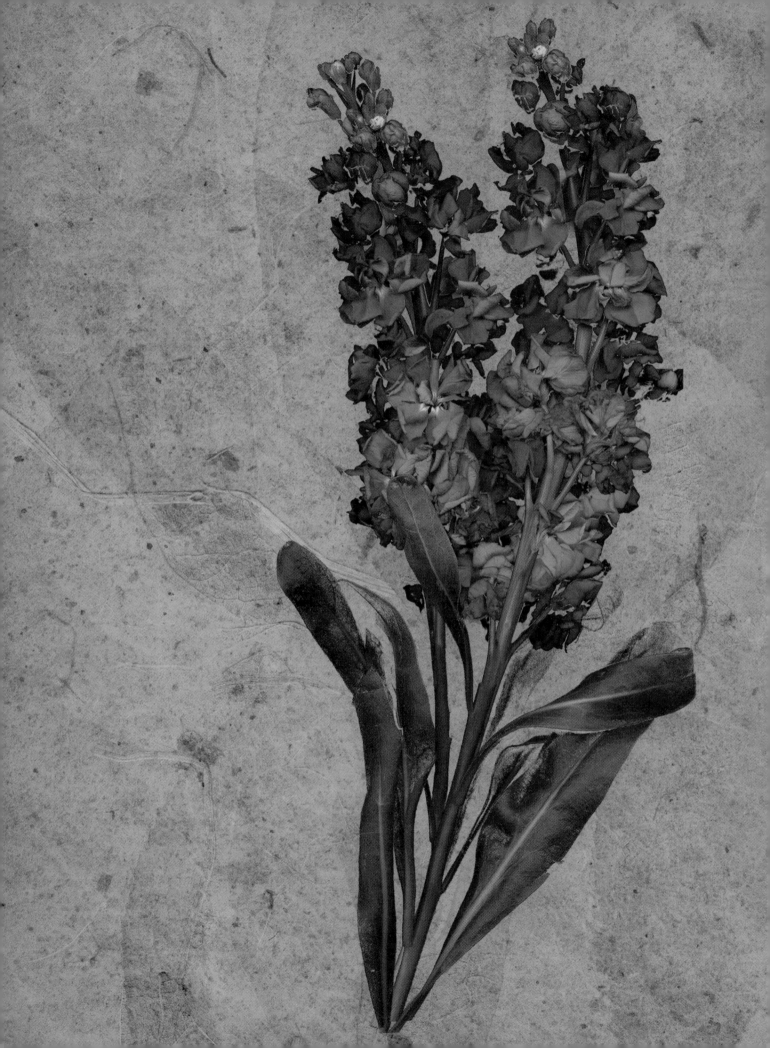

Unit 4
Treatment Modalities

Maybe there have been times when you felt that the problems people experience are truly overwhelming and you wondered how you could ever really help. Sure you are a nurse, but how can one person reduce the world's stress, illness, and social injustice? Although it is true that societal problems are great, it is also true that the contribution of each person is like a ripple in a pool that can eventually turn the tide of life. But to be effective you need to have the right tools for the task, tools that will allow you to help people think about their life situation and change their behavior, tools that will help you work therapeutically with individuals, families, and groups.

In this unit you will be exposed to a wide range of treatment tools, but do not think that these strategies will apply only to patients with psychiatric illnesses. The fact is that many people take psychotropic medications, and nurses deal with people who struggle with issues of control, aggression, and violence in almost all clinical settings. Also, strategies to change negative thinking patterns and problematic behavior can apply to children and adults throughout their experiences with health and illness. And finally, are not groups an essential part of every health-care delivery system, and do not all patients have families? As you can see, the skills you will learn in this unit will enhance your nursing practice regardless of setting. So grab your highlighters and get ready to add to your growing repertoire of nursing skills and competencies, because you can and will make a difference.

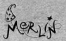
Visit **MERLIN** for *Your Internet Connection*
to websites that are related to the content in this chapter.
www.mosby.com/MERLIN/Stuart

28 Psychopharmacology

Michele T. Laraia

Medicines are nothing in themselves, if not properly used, but the very hands of the gods, if employed with reason and prudence.

HEROPHILUS

This chapter introduces the nurse to psychopharmacology and describes important principles of drug therapy in the treatment of patients with neurobiological brain disorders or mental illnesses. The pharmacological agents described in this chapter are all approved by the Food and Drug Administration (FDA). Dietary supplements, herbal preparations, and hormones used to treat the symptoms of mental illness are described in Chapter 30. The theoretical framework for psychopharmacology in this chapter is one of integration in that drug therapy complements other evidence-based therapies, such as cognitive-behavioral, psychosocial, interpersonal, psychodynamic, and complementary and alternative interventions. Drug therapy is not viewed as a quick fix or miracle pill. Psychopharmacological agents treat specific symptoms of neurobiological illnesses with significant effectiveness, although side effects and adverse reactions of drug therapy require expertise and sound clinical judgment on the part of the nurse. Psychopharmacology is the "gold standard" in the treatment of neurobiological illness, but drugs alone do not treat the patient's personal, social, or environmental responses to these illnesses, underscoring the need for an integrated approach to the treatment of persons with mental illness.

ROLE OF THE NURSE

Psychopharmacological treatment should be integrated with the principles of psychiatric nursing practice presented throughout this book. The psychiatric nurse has a wealth of knowledge and competencies that make nursing unique in the care of people with psychiatric disorders. Following are some examples of the nurse's role in psychopharmacological treatment of persons with neurobiological illness.

Patient Assessment

Psychoactive drugs treat specific symptoms of neurobiological brain disorders. However, not all patient behaviors are treated by drug therapy, and not every identified personality trait is a symptom of illness targeted for treatment with drugs. It is essential to do a thorough patient baseline assessment, including history, physical and laboratory examination (see Chapter 6), psychiatric evaluation (see Chapter 7), sociocultural assessment (see Chapter 8), and a medication history for each patient before any treatment interventions are initiated. This information helps distinguish aspects of the psychiatric illness from the patient's personality before the illness. As a result of baseline assessment, a diagnosis is made, psychiatric symptoms are identified as appropriate targets for drug treatment, and an integrated treatment plan is developed. Residual symptoms of the patient's illness may need specific interventions to enhance treatment effectiveness, and dysfunctional personality characteristics not related to the psychiatric disorder can be addressed by nonpharmacological treatments if appropriate. In addition, drug side effects that emerge after treatment has begun can be identified and appropriately treated as they appear. Symptoms of organ system dysfunction caused by drug treatment can also be identified and treated. Current nonpsychiatric diagnoses and treatments are also documented at baseline, as well as over-the-counter remedies the patient may be taking. Finally, careful baseline assessment of each patient can help identify undiagnosed medical illnesses that are concurrent with psychiatric illness or that possibly cause psychiatric symptoms. Box 28-1 provides a medication assessment tool to guide the nurse in taking a drug and substance history.

Coordination of Treatment Modalities

The nurse has an important role in designing a comprehensive treatment program. The most appropriate treatment choices should be individualized for each patient and reflected in the treatment plan. The coordination of treatment modalities is often the primary responsibility of the nurse who works with the patient in an ongoing therapeutic alliance as part of the health-care team. The nurse is in a position to integrate drug treatments with the wide range of nonpharmacological treatments in a manner that is knowledgeable, safe, effective, and acceptable to the patient.

Psychopharmacological Drug Administration

No one on the health-care team has a greater daily impact on the patient's experience with psychopharmacological agents than the nurse. In some settings the nurse administers each medication dose, works out a dosing schedule based on drug requirements and the patient's needs and preferences, and is continually alert for and treats drug effects. This role defines the nurse as a key professional in maximizing therapeutic effects of drug treatment and minimizing side effects in such a way that the patient is a true collaborator in the medication regimen.

Monitoring Drug Effects

The nurse has the important role of consistently monitoring the effects of psychopharmacological drugs. This includes making standardized measurements of drug effects on baseline target symptoms of illness, minimizing side effects, treating adverse reactions, and noting the often subtle effects

---

Box 28-1

Medication Assessment Tool

For each of the following categories of drugs taken by the patient:
- Prescribed psychiatric medications ever taken
- Prescribed nonpsychiatric medication taken in the past 6 months or taken for major medical illnesses if more than 6 months ago
- Over-the-counter medication taken in the past 6 months
  - Obtain the following information from the patient and other sources:
    - Name of the drug
    - Reason taken
    - Dates started and stopped
    - Highest daily dose
    - Who presecribed it?
    - Was it effective?
    - Side effects or adverse reactions
    - Was it taken as directed?
    - If not, how was it taken?
    - History of drug taken by first-degree relative
    - Drugs taken prescribed by others

For each of the following categories of drugs taken by the patient:
- Alcholol
- Tobacco
- Caffeine
- Street drugs
  - Obtain the following information from the patient and other sources:
    - Name of substance
    - Dates and schedule of use
    - Summarize effects
    - Adverse reactions/withdrawal symptoms
    - Attempts to stop/treatments to stop
    - Impact of substance on:
      - Quality of life
      - Relationships/spouse/children
      - Occupation/education
      - Health/productivity
      - Self-image
      - Expense

on the patient's self-concept and sense of trust. A drug should be given within the recommended dose range and for the appropriate amount of time before it can be determined if the drug has had an adequate therapeutic trial for a particular patient. Therapeutic drug monitoring is also important because some drugs have a narrow therapeutic range (such as lithium), can have sudden serious adverse reactions (for example, neuroleptic malignant syndrome), and are frequently co-administered, altering drug metabolism and clearance (such as cytochrome P-450 problems).

Medication Education

The nurse is in a pivotal position to educate the patient and the family about medications. This includes teaching complex information to the patient so that it is understood, discussed, and accepted. The patient should be well informed about each drug, be well educated about the expected benefits and potential risks, understand additional potential treatments for his or her condition, and know what to do and who to contact if there is a question or problem. Medication education is the key to the effective and safe use of psychotropic drugs, to patient collaboration in the treatment plan, and to patient adherence with drug treatment regimens.

Drug Maintenance Programs

For some patients the drug maintenance program may last many months and perhaps even a lifetime. The nurse can assume the important role of continuing a therapeutic alliance with a patient on drug maintenance. The nurse is often the contact for patients who may have ongoing questions about their current drug regimen, drug effects on lifestyle and concurrent illnesses, and new treatments as they become available.

Clinical Research Drug Trials

As a member of the interdisciplinary research team the nurse can contribute to the body of scientific knowledge, often adding a nursing perspective to team research efforts. The nurse can be included on many levels, from research data collector and principal investigator to funding agency monitor and consultant (Laraia, 1999). The nurse's roles in interdisciplinary clinical research drug trials continue to evolve. Nurses involved in psychopharmacological randomized controlled trials can enhance the research experience for the patient, who will need significant information about informed consent, double-blind randomization, experimental treatments, and, in particular, the risk-to-benefit analysis required for the use of placebos (see Citing the Evidence).

Prescriptive Authority

Legislation has been passed in almost every state in the United States authorizing advanced practice registered nurses (APRNs) to prescribe medications. Psychiatric nurses who are qualified under their state nurse practice acts are thus able to prescribe pharmacological agents to treat the symptoms and improve the functional status of patients with psychiatric illnesses. Specific psychopharmacological agents can be prescribed by APRNs based on diagnostic cri-

---

Citing the Evidence on

Placebo-Controlled Psychopharmacological Clinical Trials

BACKGROUND: This article reviews psychiatric drug treatment trials and examines the role of placebos in drug and in psychotherapy trials, their effect on drugs, the relevance of active placebos, and the ethics of using placebos in human research.

RESULTS: Evidence that placebos are required in clinical trials to prevent false conclusions about drug efficacy and to keep ineffective drugs off the market are presented.

IMPLICATIONS: Because psychiatric illnesses have a fluctuating course and the psychiatric diagnostic system is inexact, a large proportion of patients may experience a placebo effect. There is clinical benefit in being able to identify patients who are experiencing a placebo effect that may be helpful in planning the treatment of all patients, but particularly those who have a contraindication to continuing a psychopharmacological regimen.

Quitkin FM: Placebos, drug effects, and study design: A clinician's guide, *Am J Psychiatry* 156:829, 1999.

---

teria, clinical practice guidelines or medication prescribing protocols, and, in some states, supervision. Thus the role of nurses in psychopharmacological treatments has been expanded to encompass medication prescriptive authority in order to capitalize on the expertise of APRNs and to increase patient access to quality and cost-effective health care.

Does your state grant medication prescriptive authority to psychiatric–mental health APRNs? If so, what are the requirements for prescriptive practice?

PHARMACOLOGICAL PRINCIPLES
Pharmacokinetics

Pharmacokinetics is the study of how the body affects a drug. It answers the question: How does the body get drugs to and from where they are going? Body functions such as absorption (how the drug is moved into the blood stream from the site of administration), distribution (how much drug is moved into various body tissues), metabolism (how the drug is altered, usually by liver enzymes, into its active and inactive parts), and elimination (how much of the drug is removed from the body in a particular amount of time) are pharmacokinetic properties. The time course and location of drug concentrations in the body can be predicted, appropriate dosing schedules can be designed, side effects can be anticipated, and the time it takes a drug to be effective can be estimated by using pharmacokinetic models. Additional pharmacokinetic properties that assist in understanding psychopharmacological agents and how the body affects a drug include variables described here.

Bioavailability (how much of the drug reaches systemic circulation unchanged) is an estimate used to compare drug preparations, particularly if the same generic drug is made by different manufacturers. In general, generic instead of trade names of drugs are used to be more accurate, since trade names can differ; to take advantage of price differences; and to prevent confusion when a drug becomes generic (when the patent runs out and the drug can be made by any company, usually at a lower cost). Once a drug becomes generic, the patient should be taught to use the same company brand of a drug because the bioavailability of psychoactive drugs may vary significantly from one company to another, thus affecting drug dose and steady state. The patient can be taught to use one pharmacy regularly and ask the pharmacist to use the same company when filling generic prescriptions of a particular drug.

A drug's half-life is the time it takes for the amount of drug in the body to decrease by 50%. For example, the benzodiazepine alprazolam has a half-life of approximately 11 hours, so it takes about 2.5 days for nearly all traces of the drug to be eliminated from the body after a single dose. Half-life determines how long it takes to achieve steady state. Steady state means that the plasma drug concentration remains relatively constant between doses because the amount of drug excreted equals the amount ingested, and this equilibrium occurs in approximately five half-lives. Until steady state is reached the drug level continues to fluctuate, accounting for some acute side effects. Prior to steady state, the optimum dose for a particular patient cannot be determined, a blood level is not accurate in determining a proper dose range, and the daily dose may have to be divided. Termination of drug treatment is also affected by half-life. The effects of drugs with a long half-life or with active metabolites, can last a long time (sometimes weeks) after the last dose. Drugs with a shorter half-life usually must be tapered (discontinued gradually) over several days or weeks. In general, most psychoactive drugs should be tapered to avoid uncomfortable discontinuation symptoms.

Drug interactions can be the result of pharmacokinetic properties. A drug may interfere with the absorption, metabolism, distribution, and elimination of another drug, thus raising or lowering the levels of that drug in the blood and tissue. Some drugs inhibit and others induce the activity of liver drug-metabolizing enzymes, affecting the liver's ability to keep levels of psychopharmacological drugs stable. For example, co-administering classes of antidepressants must be done cautiously. Some antidepressants (such as fluoxetine and other drugs in its class) can inhibit drug-metabolizing liver enzymes, potentially causing toxic levels of other classes of antidepressants (such as imipramine), when these drugs are used together (co-administration).

Pharmacodynamics

Pharmacodynamics is the study of the effects of the drug on the body and, in particular, the interaction of the drug on the receptor that is its targeted site of action. Pharmacodynamics answers the question: What does a drug do once it

gets where it's going? The time course and intensity of drug effects on the body can be determined, drug interactions can be better understood, and safety profiles can be developed that affect clinical decision making by using pharmacodynamic models. Several pharmacodynamic properties related to how drugs affect the body include the areas listed here.

Receptor Mechanisms. Receptors are the gatekeepers of brain communication. They recognize and respond to molecules (messengers) that affect their biological function. Thus receptors are targets for drug actions acting as messengers that modify their biological activity, bringing a dysfunctional system back toward normal. A drug modifies a receptor by attaching (binding) to one (like a key to a single lock) or many (like a master key to many locks) subtypes of receptors in several ways: A drug can stimulate the receptor to fully (in this case, the drug is an agonist) or partially (partial agonist) open its channel; it can inhibit or block (antagonist) another chemical agonist from stimulating the receptor to open its channel; or it can directly close (inverse agonist) the receptor channel. For example, benzodiazepines are agonists for the gamma-aminobutyric acid (GABA) system (they enhance the activity of GABA, an inhibitory neurotransmitter), and most antipsychotic drugs are antagonists at dopamine receptors (they inhibit the activity of dopamine).

The Dose-Response Curve. If the concentration of the drug is plotted against the effects of the drug on a graph, the curve produced is a measure of drug potency. Potency is the amount of dose required to achieve certain effects. It answers the question: How much of this drug is needed to get these results? This concept is helpful when comparing the actions of one drug to another. For example, atypical antipsychotics differ in potency-risperidone is more potent than clozapine, requiring lower doses to achieve a therapeutic effect.

The Therapeutic Index. The therapeutic index is a relative measure of the safety and toxicity of a drug. The ratio produced by measuring the amount of drug necessary for 50% of patients to experience a therapeutic effect (median effective dose) and the highest amount of drug before 50% of patients experience a toxic effect (median toxic dose) is called the therapeutic index. It answers the question: What is the lowest dose of this drug needed to begin to produce a therapeutic effect, and what is its highest dose before it produces a toxic effect in the average patient? A low therapeutic index means that the difference between the amount of drug needed to begin to take effect and the amount that would cause toxic effects has a narrow range (like a window with a narrow opening). For example, the mood-stabilizer lithium has a low therapeutic index and requires frequent blood levels and careful monitoring and stabilizing measures to be used safely. On the other hand, the typical antipsychotic haloperidol has a high therapeutic index and thus is safely prescribed in a wide range of doses (like a window opened very wide). Individual patient differences such as age, gender, and race can also affect the therapeutic index of a specific drug.

The Development of Tolerance, Dependence, and Withdrawal Phenomena. Some patients become less responsive to the same dose of a particular drug over time (tolerance), often requiring higher doses of that drug to obtain the same therapeutic effect. The development of tolerance to some drugs like benzodiazepines (BZs) or opioids may also be associated with physical dependence on the drug, requiring tapering (gradual dose reduction) during discontinuation to avoid withdrawal symptoms. BZ withdrawal symptoms can be quite uncomfortable and, rarely, even fatal.

Drug Co-Administration

Once generally discouraged, the use of more than one psychopharmacological drug in the same patient at the same time is rapidly becoming standard clinical practice under specific circumstances. Patients prescribed multiple medications or taking over-the-counter medications in addition to their prescribed medications can potentially receive benefits from these combinations, but also may be at risk for drug interactions, lack of clarity about which drug is causing which effect, and higher costs of treatment. Box 28-2 lists guidelines for drug co-administration. Box 28-3 alerts the nurse to patients at higher risk for drug interactions. Table 28-1 is a reference list for the more common interactions of psychotropic drugs. The following list of drug co-administration principles will guide the nurse when multiple medications are prescribed (Weiden, 1999).

Primary Medication. The medication used to treat the target symptoms of the patient's primary diagnosis is the primary medication in a drug treatment regimen. For example, antidepressants are the primary medications in treatment of a primary diagnosis of major depression.

Combination Drug Therapy. Combination drug therapy refers to simultaneous use of two or more psychopharmacological drugs in the same class for long-term treatment. For example, in a patient who has only partial relief from a mood stabilizer for bipolar disorder, a second mood stabilizer may be added to increase the treatment effect in long-term treatment.

Augmentation or Adjunctive Therapy. Adding another class of medication to supplement the efficacy of the primary medication is becoming a widely accepted clinical practice. This is done when the primary medicine falls short of expectation and needs to have its efficacy augmented, or boosted. An example is the addition of lithium to the primary antipsychotic drug for persistent positive symptoms of schizophrenia. This is also done when the primary drug treats target symptoms effectively, but other symptoms remain. For example, an antidepressant is added to the primary antipsychotic drug for persistent symptoms of depression in a schizophrenic patient.

Concurrent Pharmacology. Some patients with more than one illness need drug treatments for each illness. An example is the diabetic taking insulin who also needs an antidepressant for a concurrent depression. Efforts must be taken to integrate such a patient's care in order to optimize treatments and avoid incompatible therapies.

Polypharmacy. "Polypharmacy" implies that the use of multiple psychopharmacological medications for long-term treatment is considered to be outside the usual practice standards or clinical guidelines (although sometimes this term is mistakenly used to include all types of combined drug therapy). An example of polypharmacy is keeping a patient on two antipsychotics without ever having tried therapeutic doses of a single antipsychotic.

Why do you think patients often fail to report over-the-counter remedies when asked what medicines they are taking? How can you, as a nurse, be sure to obtain this information?

Special Populations

Although this chapter focuses on the adult patient, special populations such as children, the elderly, and members of various diverse groups are regularly given psychoactive drugs, even though these drugs are rarely tested in clinical trials on these groups. An understanding of relevant issues will help the nurse administer psychopharmacological agents safely to persons who are members of special populations.

Box 28-2

Guidelines for Drug Co-Administration

- Identify specific target symptoms for each drug.
- If possible, start with one drug and evaluate effectiveness and side effects before adding a second drug.
- Be alert for adverse drug interactions.
- Consider the effects of a second drug on the absorption and metabolism of the first drug.
- Consider the possibility of additive side effects.
- Change the dose of only one drug at a time and evaluate results.
- Be aware of increased risk of medication errors.
- Be aware of increased cost of treatment.
- Be aware of decreased patient adherence when medication regimen is complex.
- In follow-up treatment, eliminate as many drugs as possible and establish the effective dose of the drugs used.
- Patient education programs regarding concomitant drug regimens must be particularly clear, organized, and effective.
- Patient follow-up contacts should be more frequent.
- If a patient has more than one prescriber, integration of care is required.

Box 28-3

Increased Risk Factors for Development of Drug Interactions

- Drug co-administration
- High doses
- Geriatric patients
- Debilitated/dehydrated patients
- Concurrent illness
- Compromised organ system function
- Inadequate patient education
- History of nonadherence
- Failure to include patient in treatment planning

Table **28-1**

Interactions of Psychotropic Drugs and Other Substances

Psychotropic Category	Possible Interactions
ANTIANXIETY AGENTS	
Benzodiazepines With:	
Central nervous system (CNS) depressants (alcohol, barbiturates, antipsychotics, antihistamines, cimetidine)	Potential additive CNS effects, especially sedation and decreased daytime performance.
Selective serotonin reuptake inhibitors (SSRIs), disulfiram, estrogens	Increased benzodiazepine effects.
Antacids, tobacco	Decreased benzodiazepine effects.
Sedative-Hypnotics With:	
CNS depressants (alcohol, antihistamines, antidepressants, narcotics, antipsychotics)	Enhancement of sedative effects; impairment of mental and physical performance; may result in lethargy, respiratory depression, coma, death.
Anticoagulants (oral)*	Decreased coumarin plasma levels and effect; monitor and adjust dose of coumarin.
ANTIDEPRESSANTS	
Tricyclics (TCAs) With:	
Monoamine oxidase inhibitors (MAOIs)*	May cause hypertensive crisis.
Alcohol and other CNS depressants	Additive CNS depression; decreased TCA effect.
Antihypertensives* (guanethidine, methyldopa, clonidine)	Antagonism of antihypertensive effect.
Antipsychotics and anti-parkinsonians	Increased TCA effect; confusion, delirium, ileus.
Anticholinergics	Additive anticholinergic effects.
Antiarrhythmics (quinidine, procainamide, propranolol)	Additive antiarrhythmic effects; myocardial depression.
SSRIs*	Increased TCA serum level/toxicity through inhibition of cytochrome P-450 system.
Anticonvulsants	Decreased TCA effect; seizures.
Tobacco	Decreased TCA plasma levels.
SSRIs With:	
Clomipramine, maprotiline, bupropion, clozapine	Increased risk of seizures.
MAOIs*	Serotonin syndrome.
Barbiturates, benzodiazepines, narcotics	Increased CNS depression.
Carbamazepine	Neurotoxicity: nausea, vomiting, vertigo, tinnitus, ataxia, lethargy, blurred vision.
MAOIs With:	
Many drugs and foods	Hypertensive crisis.
MOOD STABILIZERS	
Lithium With:	
Diuretics,* marijuana	Increased lithium levels/toxicity.
SSRIs	Lithium toxicity; enhanced therapeutic effect.
Nonsteroidal antiinflammatory agents*	Increased lithium blood levels/toxicity.
Antipsychotics	Increased CNS toxicity.
Tetracyclines	Lithium intoxication.
Acetylcholinesterase (ACE) inhibitors	Confusion, ataxia, dysarthria, tremor, electrocardiographic (ECG) changes.
Carbamazepine With:	
Lithium	Lithium intoxification; increased effect; inhibits lithium-induced polyuria.
Haloperidol	Decreased effect of either drug.
Calcium channel blockers	Neurotoxicity; dizziness, nausea, diplopia, headache.
Valproate	Decreased valproate serum concentration.
Cimetidine, erythromycin, isoniazid	Somnolence, lethargy, dizziness, blurred vision, ataxia, nausea.
Valproate With:	
SSRIs, erythromycin, cimetidine	Increased valproate serum concentrations.

*Potentially clinically significant.

Continued

Table **28-1**

Interactions of Psychotropic Drugs and Other Substances—cont'd	
Psychotropic Category	**Possible Interactions**
ANTIPSYCHOTICS WITH:	
Antacids, tea, coffee, milk, fruit juice	Decreased phenothiazine effect.
CNS depressants (narcotics, antianxiety drugs, alcohol, antihistamines, barbiturates)	Additive CNS depression.
Anticholinergic agents (levodopa)*	Additive atropine-like side effects and increased anti-Parkinson effects.
SSRIs	Increased neuroleptic serum level and extrapyramidal side effects (EPS).
ANTIPSYCHOTICS **Clozapine With:**	
Carbamazepine*	Additive bone marrow suppression.
Benzodiazepines*	Circulatory collapse, respiratory arrest.
SSRIs*	Increased risk of seizures.

*Potentially clinically significant

Children. There are few systematic studies of psychotropic drugs in children, yet they can experience quite severe psychiatric illnesses. Generally children metabolize drugs more rapidly than adults and therefore do not usually need lower doses than adults just because they may weigh less and have a smaller body size. Children and young adolescents exhibit a variable response to these drugs and thus need vigilant monitoring.

Geriatric Patients. For the elderly, drug distribution, hepatic metabolism, and renal clearance are all affected by age. This often results in a slower metabolism and elimination of drugs and an increased susceptibility to side effects. It is important to begin with a lower than recommended adult dose and titrate up slower than the recommended adult rate. Geriatric patients often take multiple medications, so the nurse should be aware of the increased risk for drug interactions.

Pregnant and Nursing Women. If a pregnant woman takes psychoactive drugs, the unborn infant may experience drug effects in utero and even withdrawal symptoms at birth. Since pregnant women are excluded from randomized clinical trials, experience with a drug in animal studies and in human anectodal reports are very useful. A careful risk-to-benefit analysis of the psychiatrically symptomatic mother should include these possible risks: inattention to prenatal care, poor maternal health, adverse effect on mother-infant bonding, increased stress levels on the fetus and infant, history of adverse drug effects on the fetus (teratogenesis), and blood levels of a particular drug measured in breast milk (Wintz, 1999). When the benefits outweigh the risks, some psychotropic drugs may be given during pregnancy and breast-feeding. For example, the selective serotonin reuptake inhibitors (SSRIs) have been reported anecdotally to be safe during pregnancy and breast-feeding, and the SSRIs that have been on the market longest usually have the largest human database from which to obtain information and thus are usually considered safest. Unless a bipolar woman is severely symptomatic, mood stabilizers are usually contraindicated in pregnancy and breast-feeding due to an increased risk for adverse effects on the fetus and infant.

Cross-Cultural Perspectives. Various racial and ethnic groups can differ in the way in which members seek help for illness, express symptoms of illness, relate to health-care professionals of different backgrounds, and believe in the effectiveness of treatments. This diversity can complicate the communication necessary for accurate diagnosis and successful treatment outcomes. Race, ethnicity, and gender can also affect biological response to medications. Genetic differences can affect how psychotropic drugs can be used by an individual or a group with common genetic ancestry. For example, 9% of Caucasians have a genetic mutation in the liver enzyme system that metabolizes some antidepressants and some antipsychotics, requiring lower doses of these drugs. Dietary substances such as grapefruit juice, more commonly used in some cultures than others, can inhibit the metabolism of some antidepressants and some benzodiazepines, resulting in higher than normal blood levels. While there is a little systematic study of these issues, they are becoming more important as the population becomes more diverse as a result of increasing geographical mobility and as newer psychopharmacological agents become available (Pi & Grey, 1998).

Medically Ill Patients. Medically ill patients with concomitant psychiatric illness may have an increased sensitivity to the adverse effects of psychotropic drugs, changes in metabolism and excretion, and interactions with co-administered medications. Patients with liver disease are extremely sensitive to most psychoactive drugs, and patients with renal impairment are particularly sensitive to lithium. As with children and the elderly, good clinical practice is to begin with lower doses and titrate slowly while evaluating frequently for both clinical benefit and adverse effects.

Biological Basis for Psychopharmacology

All communication in the brain involves neurotransmission, or neurons "talking" to each other across synapses at receptors. Neurons are the basic functional unit of the brain struc-

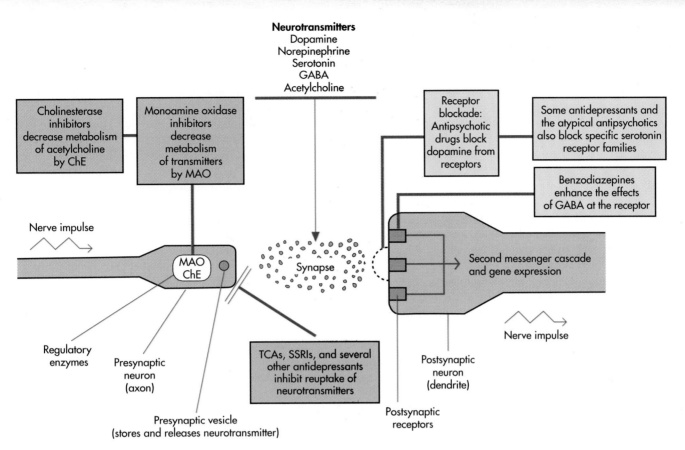

Fig. 28-1   Neurotransmission and drug effects at the synapse.

tures of the nervous system, and the study of this communication process forms the basis of much of the neurosciences (see Chapter 6). The following description is a basic frame of reference from which to view the complexity of neuropharmacological mechanisms. The synapse is a narrow gap separating two neurons: the presynaptic cell and the postsynaptic cell (Fig. 28-1). Most receptors, organized into many subtypes, are three-dimensional "gates" (channels) located on cells (neurons) that are targets for chemical first messengers (neurotransmitters, peptides, drugs, etc.). Depending on the message it receives, the receptor opens or closes its channel, allowing or stopping a flow of electrolytes (ions) into and out of the neuron, affecting the electrical nerve impulse of the neuron (stimulating or inhibiting its biological activity). This process causes a cascade of activity by the chemical second messengers in the neuron, activating the neuron's genetic code (gene expression). Gene expression is what tells the neuron how to respond and continue the process of communication to the next neuron. This genetically determined communication within and between neurons controls how the brain functions and ultimately how the person behaves.

Neurochemical messengers are synthesized (manufactured) from certain dietary amino acids (called precursors) by a chain of enzyme activity within the cell. These messengers are then stored in the presynaptic cell waiting to be released into the synapse. After neurotransmission takes place at a synapse, neurochemicals remaining in the synapse are either reabsorbed (reuptake) and stored by the presynaptic cell for

later use or are metabolized (broken down) by enzymes, such as monoamine oxidase (MAO) and cholinesterase (chE).

Many psychiatric disorders are thought to be caused by a dysregulation (imbalance) in the complex process of brain structures communicating with each other through neurotransmission. For instance, psychosis is thought to involve excessive dopamine and serotonin neurotransmission. Mood disorders are thought to result from disruption of normal patterns of neurotransmission of norepinephrine, serotonin, and other transmitters. Anxiety is thought to be a dysregulation of GABA and other transmitters. Alzheimer's disease is thought to result from a dysregulation of acetylcholine and other transmitters.

If a particular psychiatric illness is known to result from a dysregulation or imbalance of neurotransmission in a particular neurotransmitter system, and if the mechanism of action of psychiatric drugs is understood, then some order in the various pharmacological strategies used in psychiatric treatment can be recognized. This process of cell-to-cell communication at the synapse resulting in brain function can be affected by drugs in several important ways:

- **Release:** More neurotransmitter is released into the synapse from the storage vesicles in the presynaptic cell.
- **Blockade of postsynaptic receptors:** The neurotransmitter is prevented from binding to the target receptor.
- **Blockade of alpha-2 presynaptic autoreceptors:** This negative feedback system is prevented from turning off the release of norepinephrine into the synapse.

- **Receptor sensitivity changes:** The receptor becomes more or less responsive to the neurotransmitter.
- **Reuptake inhibition:** The presynaptic cell does not reabsorb the neurotransmitter well, leaving more neurotransmitter in the synapse and therefore enhancing or prolonging its action.
- **Interference with storage vesicles:** The neurotransmitter is either released again into the synapse (more neurotransmitter) or released to metabolizing enzymes (less neurotransmitter).
- **Precursor chain interference:** The process that makes the neurotransmitter is either facilitated (more is synthesized) or disrupted (less is synthesized).
- **Synaptic enzyme inhibition:** Less neurotransmitter is metabolized, so more remains available in the synapse and the presynaptic neuron.
- **Second messenger cascade:** A chemical chain reaction within the cell is initiated by neurochemical effects at the receptor during neurotransmission, activating genetically determined brain function.

Not all of these strategies have yielded clinically relevant treatments to date. Those that have are emphasized in this chapter (see Fig. 28-1): Antipsychotic drugs block dopamine from the receptor site; antidepressants block the reuptake of norepinephrine and/or serotonin and regulate the areas of the brain that manufacture these chemicals; monoamine oxidase inhibitors (MAOIs) decrease enzymatic metabolism of norepinephrine and serotonin; cholinesterase (ChE) inhibitors decrease the metabolism of acetylcholine; benzodiazepines potentiate (enhance the effects of) GABA; and some antidepressants block specific subtypes of serotonin receptors (thought to be responsible for serotonin side effects), thereby enhancing serotonin transmission at serotonin receptors implicated in depression.

Understanding synaptic and cellular functions has led to various treatment approaches in pharmacotherapy that attempt to modify one or more of the steps in neurotransmission. It has also led to research to develop drugs with more specificity (drugs that go to areas in the brain specifically targeted for their action, such as the brain regions implicated in mental illness, rather than to nonspecific or untargeted areas, causing drug side effects). The future of psychopharmacology holds much promise as new drugs are developed and new theories are proven. Drug effects on receptor function are most likely the basis of psychopharmacological efficacy in the treatment of psychiatric disorders. It is also likely that future diagnostic conceptualizations of the etiology of psychiatric disorders may be organized by neurotransmitter activity and dysregulation rather than the current *DSM–IV–TR* (American Psychiatric Association, 2000) symptom cluster approach (Keltner, 2000).

ANTIANXIETY AND SEDATIVE-HYPNOTIC DRUGS

Anxiety is a normal emotion under circumstances of threat and is part of the fight-or-flight instinct necessary for survival. The diagnosis of anxiety (symptoms of anxiety that are disproportionate to the circumstances) is based on the patient's description, the nurse's observation of behaviors and

assessment of *DSM–IV–TR* diagnostic criteria, and the elimination of alternative diagnoses. The possibility of a nonpsychiatric cause for anxiety symptoms must also be considered. Hyperthyroidism, hypoglycemia, cardiovascular illness, severe pulmonary disease, and a variety of medications and substances are often associated with high levels of anxiety. In addition to a careful physical assessment and a review of laboratory tests, the patient should be asked about the use of prescription and over-the-counter drugs, as well as "recreational" substances such as alcohol, caffeine, and nicotine. Anxiety also accompanies many psychiatric disorders. For example, depression and anxiety are often comorbid illnesses (existing together). In general, the primary disorder should be treated with the appropriate medication. For example, anxiety associated with psychosis or a mood disorder often goes away when the target symptoms for the primary disorder are treated successfully.

This section divides antianxiety and sedative-hypnotic drugs into two categories: the benzodiazepines and several nonbenzodiazepine antianxiety drugs. The benzodiazepines are the most widely prescribed drugs in the world, and their popularity is related to their effectiveness, prompt onset of action, and wide margin of safety. Concerns that are largely unfounded (Möller, 1999) regarding physiological dependance, withdrawal, and abuse potential have limited their use. While benzodiazepines have almost entirely replaced barbiturates in the treatment of anxiety and sleep disorders, they recently have been considered second-line agents after the antidepressants in the long-term treatment of anxiety disorders such as panic disorder and social phobia. Antidepressants are discussed in detail in the next section.

What sociocultural factors may help to explain why benzodiazepines are the most commonly prescribed medications in the United States?

Benzodiazepines

The BZs are thought to reduce anxiety because they are powerful potentiators (receptor agonists) of the inhibitory neurotransmitter GABA. A postsynaptic receptor site specific for the BZ molecule is located next to the GABA receptor. The BZ molecule and GABA bind to each other at the GABA receptor site. The result is an inhibition of neurotransmission (a decrease in the firing rate of neurons), resulting in a clinical decrease in the person's level of anxiety.

Clinical Use. The major indications for the use of BZs include anxiety, insomnia, alcohol withdrawal, anxiety associated with medical disease, skeletal muscle relaxation, seizure disorders, the anxiety and apprehension experienced before surgery, and substance-induced (except amphetamines) and psychotic agitation in emergency rooms (Ballenger, 2000). Used in higher doses, the high-potency BZs, alprazolam and clonazepam have been effective in the treatment of panic disorder and social phobia (see Citing the Evidence). The target symptoms for use of BZs are listed in Box 28-4.

Another clinical indication for the use of BZs is as a sedative-hypnotic to improve sleep (Stimmel, 1999). Insomnia includes difficulty falling asleep, difficulty staying asleep, or awakening too early with an inability to go back to sleep. It is a symptom with many causes and often responds to nonpharmacological strategies such as talking about problems, increased daytime exercise, elimination of stimulants such as caffeine, and physical comfort measures at night (see Chapter 18). When used as hypnotics the BZs should induce sleep rapidly, and their effect should be gone by morning. Any BZ can be an effective sedative-hypnotic when administered at bedtime, although the choice of drug should be tailored to the patient's complaints. For example, BZs with a short half-life are effective for patients with trouble falling sleep, but may make insomnia worse for patients with early morning wakening.

Because the BZs are in the same pharmacological class as alcohol, they can be used to suppress the alcohol withdrawal syndrome and are the treatment of choice for this indication. The ingestion of these two substances together is contraindicated, particularly for the patient using dangerous equipment or driving a car because it can produce extreme sedation.

The BZs have no significant clinical advantages over each other, although differences in half-life (Table 28-2) can be

---

Box 28-4

Target Symptoms for Antianxiety and Sedative-Hypnotic Benzodiazepines

PSYCHOLOGICAL

Vague sense of irritability and uneasiness
Sense of impending doom or panic
Insomnia

PHYSICAL

Flushed skin
Hot or cold flashes
Sweating
Dilated pupils
Dry mouth
Nausea or vomiting
Diarrhea
Tachycardia, palpitations
Dizziness
Shortness of breath
Hyperventilation
Paresthesias
Tremor
Restlessness
Headache
Urinary frequency

Citing the Evidence on

Clonazepam in Panic Disorder

BACKGROUND: The purpose of this study was to evaluate the high-potency BZ, clonazepam, in the short-term treatment of panic disorder and to assess the tolerability of a schedule for gradual discontinuation.

RESULTS: Clonazepam proved superior to placebo in the treatment of panic disorder during a 6-week therapeutic phase of treatment. Also, the gradual tapering of clonazepam over a 7-week discontinuation phase was well tolerated and was not associated with withdrawal symptoms or rebound effects, although patients experienced an increase in the number of panic attacks compared to baseline.

IMPLICATIONS: Clonazepam is a safe and effective BZ treatment of panic disorder, and discontinuation during and after slow tapering was well tolerated.

Moroz G, Rosenbaum J: Efficacy, safety, and gradual discontinuation of clonazepam in panic disorder: a placebo-controlled, multicenter study using optimized doses, *J Clin Psychiatry* 60:604, 1999.

Table 28-2

Antianxiety and Sedative-Hypnotic Drugs: Benzodiazepines

Generic Name (Trade Name)	Active Metabolites	Half-life (hr)	Equivalents (mg)	Usual Adult Dosage Range (mg/day)	Preparation
ANTIANXIETY DRUGS					
Alprazolam (Xanax)	Yes (not significant)	6-20	0.25	0.5-10 bid to qid	PO
Chlordiazepoxide (Librium)	Yes	6-100	10	10-150 bid to qid	PO, IM, IV
Clonazepam (Klonopin)	No	>20	0.5	0.5-10 bid	PO
Clorazepate (Tranxene)	Yes	>20	7.5	7.5-60 bid or qid	PO
Diazepam (Valium)	Yes	>20	5	2-40 bid	PO, SR, IM, IV
Halazepam (Paxipam)	Yes	>20	20	60-160 tid or qid	PO
Lorazepam (Ativan)	No	6-20	1	1-6 tid	PO, IM, IV
Oxazepam (Serax)	No	6-20	15	15-120 tid or qid	PO
Prazepam (Centrax)	Yes	>20	10	10-60 tid or qid	PO
SEDATIVE-HYPNOTIC DRUGS					
Estazolam (ProSom)	Yes	6-20	0.33	1-2 HS	PO
Flurazepam (Dalmane)	Yes	<6	5	15-30 HS	PO
Temazepam (Restoril)	No	6-20	5	7.5-30 HS	PO
Triazolam (Halcion)	No	>6	0.25	0.125-0.5 HS	PO
Quazepam (Doral)	Yes	>20	5	7.5-50 HS	PO

IM, Intramuscular; *IV,* intravenous; *PO,* oral tablet or capsule; *SR,* oral slow-release tablet.

Table **28-3**

Benzodiazepine Side Effects and Nursing Considerations	
Side Effects	Nursing Considerations
COMMON	
Drowsiness, sedation	Activity helps; use caution when using machinery.
Ataxia, dizziness	Use caution with activity, prevent falls.
Feelings of detachment	Discourage social isolation.
Increased irritability or hostility	Observe, support, be alert for disinhibition.
Anterograde amnesia	Inability to recall events that occur while on drug.
Cognitive effects with long-term use	Interference with concentration and memory of new material.
Tolerance, dependency, rebound insomnia/anxiety	Short-term use; discontinue, using a slow taper; contraindicated with drug or alcohol abuse.
RARE	
Nausea	Dose with meals, decrease dose.
Headache	Usually responds to mild analgesic.
Confusion	Decrease dose.
Gross psychomotor impairment	Dose related, decrease dose.
Depression	Decrease dose; antidepressant treatment.
Paradoxical rage reaction	Discontinue drug.

clinically useful. For example, patients with persistent high levels of anxiety should take a drug with a long half-life. Patients with fluctuating anxiety might do better with short-acting drugs. Drugs with a long half-life (longer than 18 to 24 hours) can be given once a day. Drugs with a short half-life (8 to 15 hours) need to be given more often; they can be taken as needed for increased symptoms of anxiety as such symptoms occur. The rate of absorption of the different BZs from the gastrointestinal tract varies considerably, thus affecting the rapidity and intensity of onset of their acute effects. Antacids and food in the stomach slow down this process when these drugs are taken by mouth. The injectable BZs (lorazepam and midazolam) have been proven reliable when administered in the deltoid muscle. Diazepam results in predictable and rapid rises in the blood level when used intravenously. When given intravenously, administration should be slow (over 1 minute) and direct, not mixed in an intravenous (IV) infusion, because plastic tubing absorbs the drug and the drug can precipitate when mixed with saline or dextrose. Concentrations of BZs in the blood have not yet been firmly correlated to clinical effects, so blood levels are not clinically helpful.

Some patients may need to take antianxiety drugs for extended periods. Due to the disadvantages of BZs, they should always be used with nonpharmacological treatments for the patient with chronic anxiety or insomnia. Psychotherapy, behavioral techniques, environmental changes, stress management, sleep hygiene, and an ongoing therapeutic relationship continue to be important in the treatment of anxiety disorders and insomnia.

Most experts believe that treatment with benzodiazepines should be brief, used during a time of specific stress or specific indication. The patient should be observed frequently during the early days of treatment to assess target symptom response and monitor side effects so that the dose can be adjusted. Some patients, such as those with

Box **28-5**

Benzodiazepine Withdrawal Syndrome		
Agitation	Generalized	Irritability
Anorexia	seizures	Nausea and
Anxiety	Hallucinations	vomiting
Autonomic	Headache	Sensitivity to
arousal	Hyperactivity	light and
Dizziness	Insomnia	sounds
		Tinnitus
		Tremulousness

panic disorder, may require regular daily dosing and long-term BZ treatment.

Side Effects and Adverse Reactions. BZ side effects are common, dose related, usually short-term, and almost always harmless. Table 28-3 summarizes these reactions and nursing considerations. The BZs generally do not live up to their reputation of being strongly addictive, especially if they are discontinued gradually, if they have been used for appropriate purposes, and if their use has not been complicated by other factors such as chronic use of other central nervous system depressants such as barbiturates or alcohol.

Tolerance can develop to the sedative effects of BZs, but it is unclear whether tolerance also develops to induced sleep or antianxiety effects. These drugs should be tapered to minimize withdrawal symptoms (Box 28-5) and rebound symptoms of insomnia or anxiety. If these symptoms occur, the dose should be raised until symptoms are gone and then tapering is resumed at a slower rate. Because the BZs have a very high therapeutic index, overdoses of BZs alone almost never cause fatalities. The BZ antagonist, flumazenil (Romazicon) can reverse all BZ actions and is marketed as a treatment for BZ overdose.

Elderly patients are more vulnerable to side effects because the aging brain is more sensitive to sedatives. Dosing ranges from one half to one third of the usual daily dose used for

Table 28-4

Newer Nonbenzodiazepine Antianxiety and Sedative-Hypnotic Agents

Generic Name (Trade Name)	Dose (mg)	Half-Life (hr)
ANTIANXIETY AGENTS		
Azaspirone		
Buspirone (BuSpar)	10-40	2-5
Beta-adrenergic blocker		
Propranolol (Inderal)	10 qid	3
SEDATIVE-HYPNOTIC AGENTS		
Imidazopyridine		
Zolpidem (Ambien)	10	2.5
Pyrazolopyrimidine		
Zaleplon (Sonata)	5-10	1
Antihistamines		
Diphenhydramine (Benadryl)	50	Unknown
Hydroxyzine (Atarax)	100 tid	Unknown
Antidepressant		
Trazodone (Desyrel)	50-200	4

adults. The BZs with no active metabolites (see Table 28-2) are less affected by liver disease, the age of the patient, or drug interactions. BZs during pregnancy have been rarely associated with palate malformations and intrauterine growth retardation, especially when used during the first trimester. When used late in pregnancy or during breast-feeding, these drugs have been associated with floppy infant syndrome, neonatal withdrawal symptoms, and poor sucking reflex.

Nonbenzodiazepine Antianxiety Agents

Buspirone, a nonbenzodiazepine anxiolytic drug, is a potent antianxiety agent with no addictive potential (Table 28-4). Buspirone is effective in the treatment of anxiety and does not exhibit muscle-relaxant or anticonvulsant activity, interaction with central nervous system depressants, or sedative-hypnotic properties. It is not effective in the management of drug or alcohol abuse or panic disorder. Generally it takes several weeks for its antianxiety effects to become apparent. It probably is most effective in patients who have never taken BZs and therefore are not expecting immediate effects from drug treatment.

Propranolol blocks beta-noradrenergic receptors centrally and in the peripheral cardiac and pulmonary systems. Beta-blockers probably decrease certain physiological symptoms of anxiety, especially tachycardia, rather than centrally acting on anxiety. Propranolol is used in the treatment of performance anxiety found in some forms of social phobia and in panic disorder if rapid heart beat is a significant deterrent to the patient's ability to function, even after appropriate treatment.

Nonbenzodiazepine Sedative-Hypnotic Agents

Zolpidem is the first of a new class of compounds for short-term treatment of insomnia. Structurally unrelated to BZs, it binds more selectively to neuronal receptors involved in inducing sleep (benzodiazepine-1 receptors on the BZ/GABA receptor complex) and has fewer of the BZ side effects. It is well tolerated and appears to have little antianxiety, anticonvulsant, or muscle-relaxant properties. Side effects can include daytime drowsiness, dizziness, and diarrhea. Zolpidem is a schedule IV controlled substance.

Zaleplon is another new nonbenzodiazepine sedative-hypnotic similar to zolpidem in that it binds to the BZ-1 receptor, but with a half-life of only 1 hour. It has a very rapid onset of action, can be taken even if the patient has only 4 hours before he or she must awaken, and has no morning hangover effects. It also has sedative, anxiolytic, muscle-relaxing, and anticonvulsant properties, and is a schedule IV controlled substance (Gelenberg, 2000).

Antihistamines are sometimes used as sedative-hypnotic agents for their sedating effects. They usually are not as effective as the BZs but do not cause physical dependence or abuse. A disadvantage of the antihistamines is that they lower the seizure threshold and cause anxiety in some people.

Trazodone is an antidepressant with significant sedating effects and is the preferred antidepressant used for insomnia. It is not well studied for this use, but is popular because it offers sedation with few cholinergic effects, has a much greater safety profile in overdose compared to tricyclic antidepressants, and shows no evidence of dependence or withdrawal. Side effects include orthostatic hypotension, anxiety, and a rare but very serious adverse effect, priapism (sustained and painful penile erection), can occur with daily doses as low as 50 to 200 mg, the doses recommended for sleep.

Barbiturates and Older Antianxiety and Sedative-Hypnotic Drugs

Barbiturates and the many older nonbenzodiazepine antianxiety and sedative-hypnotic agents have many disadvantages that have led to their greatly decreased use. The barbiturates (such as secobarbital and pentobarbital), propranediols (meprobamate), alcohols (ethchlorvynol), and chloral derivatives (chloral hydrate) have numerous disadvantages: tolerance develops to their antianxiety and sedative effects; they are very addictive; they cause serious, even lethal withdrawal reactions; they are dangerous in overdose; they cause central nervous system depression; and they can cause a variety of dangerous drug interactions, particularly when mixed with central nervous system depressants such as alcohol.

ANTIDEPRESSANT DRUGS

Research on the biology of depression has led to many new discoveries and even more hypotheses. It has been proposed that serotonin and norepinephrine and other neurochemicals are dysregulated in mood disorders. The biological understanding of antidepressant drug actions supports this theory. Antidepressants enhance the neurotransmission of these transmitters by several actions: they block the reuptake of neurotransmitters at the presynaptic neuron, inhibit their metabolism and subsequent deactivation, and/or enhance the activity of receptors. Thus antidepressant drugs regulate neurotransmitter systems and their balance with each other, enhancing communi-

Table 28-5

Indications for Antidepressant Drugs

PRIMARY INDICATIONS

Major depression	Acute depression, maintenance treatment of depression and prevention of relapse, bipolar depression, atypical depression, and dysthymic disorder
Anxiety disorders	Panic disorder, obsessive-compulsive disorder (COCD), social phobia, generalized anxiety disorder, post-traumatic stress disorder

EVIDENCE FOR OTHER ANTIDEPRESSANT CATEGORIES

Selective serotonin reuptake inhibitors (SSRIs)	Strong evidence:	Bulimia, premenstrual dysphoric disorder (full- and half-cycle administration)
	Moderate evidence:	Obesity, substance abuse, impulsivity, and anger associated with personality disorders, pain syndromes
	Preliminary evidence:	Body dysmorphic disorder, hypochondriasis, anger attacks associated with depression, attention deficit–hyperactivity disorder (ADHD)
Other newer antidepressant agents	Moderate evidence:	Trazodone: insomnia, dementia with agitation, minor sedative-hypnotic withdrawal
		Bupropion: ADHD, sexual side effects of antidepressants
Tricyclic antidepressants	Strong evidence:	Panic disorder (most), OCD (clomipramine), bulimia (imipramine, desipramine), enuresis (imipramine)
	Moderate evidence:	Separation anxiety, ADHD, phobias, generalized anxiety disorder (GAD), anorexia, headaches, diabetic neuropathy and other pain syndromes (amytriptyline, doxepin), sleep apnea (protriptyline), cocaine abuse (desipramine)
Monoamine oxidase inhibitors (MAOIs)	Strong evidence:	Panic disorder, bulimia
	Moderate evidence:	Other anxiety disorders, anorexia, body dysmorphic disorder

Modified from Mendelowitz A et al: Antidepressants. In Lieberman J, Tassman A, eds: *Psychiatric drugs*, Philadelphia, 2000, WB Saunders.

Table 28-6

Antidepressant Drug Synaptic Activity

Antidepressant Drug	Primary Synaptic Activity
ALL TCAs	Receptor blockade: H_1, ACh, alpha$_1$, 5HT$_2$
Particularly tertiary amines	Reuptake inhibition: 5HT
Particularly secondary amines	Reuptake inhibition: NE
MAOIs	Receptor blockade: ACh
	Enzymatic inhibition: MAO
SSRIs	Reuptake inhibition: 5HT
OTHER ANTIDEPRESSANTS	
Amoxapine	Reuptake inhibition: 5HT and NE
	Receptor blockade: D_2, ACh, H_1
Bupropion	Reuptake inhibition: NE and DA
Maprotiline	Reuptake inhibition: NE
	Receptor blockade: H_1, ACh
Mirtazapine	Presynaptic autoreceptor inhibition: alpha$_2$
	Receptor blockade: 5HT$_2$ and 5HT$_3$
Nefazodone	Reuptake inhibition: 5HT and NE
	Receptor blockade 5HT$_2$, Alpha$_1$
Reboxetine	Reuptake inhibition: NE
Trazodone	Reuptake inhibition: 5HT
	Receptor blockade 5HT$_2$, H_1, alpha$_2$, alpha$_1$
Venlafaxine	Reuptake inhibition: 5HT, NE, and DA

ACh, Acetylcholine; *alpha$_1$*, and *alpha$_2$*, norepinephrine receptors; *DA*, dopamine; *H$_1$*, histamine receptor; *5HT*, serotonin; *5HT$_2$*, serotonin receptor; *NE*, norepinephrine.

Table 28-7

Possible Clinical Effects of Synaptic Activity by Psychotropic Drugs

Synaptic Activity	Possible Clinical Effects
Serotonin (5HT) reuptake inhibition	Reduced depression, antianxiety effects, gastrointestinal disturbances, sexual dysfunction
Norepinephrine (NE) reuptake inhibition	Reduced depression, tremors, tachycardia, erectile/ejaculatory dysfunction
Dopamine (DA) reuptake inhibition	Reduced depression, psychomotor activation, anti-Parkinsonian effects
5HT$_2$ receptor blockade	Reduced depression, reduced suicidal behavior, antipsychotic effects, hypotension, ejaculatory dysfunction
Dopamine D_2 receptor blockade	Extrapyramidal movement disorders
Muscarinic/cholinergic (ACh) receptor blockade	Anticholinergic side effects (blurred vision, dry mouth, constipation, sinus tachycardia, urinary retention, cognitive dysfunction)
Histamine (H_1) receptor blockade	Sedation/drowsiness, hypotension, weight gain
Alpha$_1$-adrenergic receptor blockade	Postural hypotension, dizziness, drowsiness, memory dysfunction, reflex tachycardia, potentiation of antihypertensive effect of prazosin and terazosin
Alpha$_2$-adrenergic receptor blockade	Priapism, blockade of the antihypertensive effects of clonidine and α-methyldopa

Table **28-8**

Antidepressant Drugs

Generic (Trade Name)	Usual Adult Daily Dose (mg/day)	Preparations
SSRIs		
Citalopram (Celexa)	20-50	PO
Fluoxetine (Prozac)	20-80	PO
Fluvoxamine (Luvox)	50-300	PO
Paroxetine (Paxil)	20-50	PO
Sertraline (Zoloft)	25-200	PO
OTHER NEWER ANTIDEPRESSANT DRUGS		
Amoxapine (Asendin)	200-300	PO
Bupropion (Wellbutrin)	150-450*	PO and SR
Maprotiline (Ludiomil)	50-200*	PO
Mirtazapine (Remeron)	15-45	PO
Trazodone (Desyrel)	50-600	PO
Serotonin Antagonist and Reuptake Blocker (SARI)		
Nefazodone (Serzone)	200-600	PO
Serotonin-Norepinephrine Reuptake Inhibitor		
Venlafaxine (Effexor)	25-375	PO and XT
Selective Presynaptic Noradrenergic Reuptake Inhibitor		
Reboxetine (Vestra)	4-10	PO
TRICYCLIC DRUGS		
Tertiary (parent)		
Amitriptyline (Elavil)	50-300	PO, IM
Clomipramine (Anafranil)	50-250	PO
Doxepin (Adapin, Sinequan)	50-300	PO, L
Imipramine (Tofranil)	50-300	PO, IM
Trimipramine (Surmontil)	50-300	PO
Secondary (metabolite)		
Desipramine (Norpramin)	50-300	PO, L
Nortriptyline (Pamelor)	50-150	PO
Protriptyline (Vivactil)	30-60	PO
MONOAMINE OXIDASE INHIBITORS		
Isocarboxazid (Marplan)	20-60	PO
Phenelzine (Nardil)	45-90	PO
Tranylcypromine (Parnate)	20-60	PO

IM, Intramuscular; *L*, oral liquid; *PO*, oral tablet/capsule; *SR*, sustained release; *XT*, extended release.
*Antidepressants with a ceiling dose due to dose-related seizures.

Table **28-9**

Antidepressant Drug Target Symptoms

Middle and terminal insomnia
Appetite disturbances
Anxiety
Fatigue
Poor motivation
Somatic complaints
Agitation
Motor retardation
Dysphoric mood
Subjective depressive feelings (anhedonia, poor self-esteem, pessimism, hopelessness, self-reproach, guilt, helplessness, sadness)
Suicidal thoughts

cation in brain structures responsible for mood and emotion.

These actions at the synapse are immediate, but it takes several weeks for antidepressants to affect mood. This delay of clinical efficacy is the subject of considerable research. One proposal is that depression occurs when a depletion of neurotransmitters in the synapse causes the post-synaptic receptors for these transmitters to increase in number (up-regulation), as if they were adjusting to too little available transmitter. As the antidepressants make more transmitter available again in the synapse, it takes the receptors several weeks to return their numbers back to normal (down-regulation), allowing a normalization of synaptic activity. This time frame matches the several weeks it takes to see clinical improvement after initiation of antidepressant therapy (Delgado & Moreno, 1999).

The primary clinical indications and other suggested uses for antidepressant drugs are listed in Table 28-5. In addition to depressive disorders, several of the anxiety disorders are indications for treatment with antidepressant drugs. Table 28-6 presents antidepressant synaptic activity and receptor binding actions. Table 28-7 lists possible clinical effects of synaptic activity. Table 28-8 lists the antidepressant drugs. Table 28-9 lists the antidepressant drug target symptoms. Table 28-10 presents comparative side effect profiles of antidepressants.

Patients who respond to the initial course of treatment with an antidepressant should continue taking the drug at the same dosage for a continuation phase of 4 to 9 months afterward. If they are symptom-free during this time, they can then be tapered off the medication. Patients who have relapses after the continuation treatment is ended may require long-term maintenance medication of 1 or more years to prevent recurring depression (Depression Guideline Panel, 1993). Patients who have had three or more episodes of major depression have a 90% chance of having another and are therefore potential candidates for long-term maintenance medication. Patients who have a history of suicide attempts, severe disability when depressed, or a history of depression in first-degree relatives may also be candidates for long-term antidepressant treatment. The maintenance medication is generally given at the same dose that was effective in the acute phase of treatment.

When treating anxiety disorders with antidepressants, dose ranges are usually the same as those used for the treatment of depression, although the initial dose usually is lower, titration up to a therapeutic range may be slower, and, for some patients, doses may have to be higher for the treatment of anxiety disorders such as obsessive-compulsive disorder. Patients who have recurrent severe anxiety disorders, history of suicide attempts, and first-degree relatives with an anxiety disorder may also need long-term maintenance treatment with antidepressants.

Your patient who has been taking antidepressant medication for 2 months tells you that he feels better and wants to stop taking it. How would you respond?

Table **28-10**

Comparative Side Effect Profiles of Antidepressant Medications

	Central Nervous System			Cardiovascular			Other
	Anticholinergic*	Drowsiness	Insomnia/ Agitation	Postural Hypotension	Cardiac Arrhythmia	Gastrointestinal Distress	Weight Gain (over 6 kg)
Amitriptyline	4+	4+	0	4+	3+	0	4+
Clomipramine	4+	4+	1+	3+	3+	1+	3+
Desipramine	1+	1+	1+	2+	2+	0	1+
Doxepin	3+	4+	0	2+	2+	0	3+
Imipramine	3+	3+	1+	4+	3+	1+	3+
Nortriptyline	1+	1+	0	2+	2+	0	1+
Protriptyline	2+	1+	1+	2+	2+	0	0
Trimipramine	1+	4+	0	2+	2+	0	3+
Amoxapine	2+	2+	2+	2+	3+	0	1+
Maprotiline	2+	4+	0	0	1+	0	2+
Mirtazapine	1+	4+	1+	2+	0	1+	2+
Nefazodone	1+	3+	1+	2+	0	3+	0
Venlafaxine	1+	1+	3+	0	0	3+	0
Trazodone	0	4+	0	1+	1+	1+	1+
Bupropion	0	0	2+	0	1+	1+	0
Fluoxetine	0	0	2+	0	0	3+	0
Paroxetine	0	0	2+	0	0	3+	0
Sertraline	0	0	2+	0	0	3+	0
Fluvoxamine	0	0	2+	0	0	3+	0
Citalopram	0	1+	2+	0	1+	3+	0
MAOIs	1+	1+	2+	2+	0	1+	2+

Modified from Depression Guideline Panel: *Depression in primary care*, vol 2, *Treatment of major depression. Clinical practice guideline, Number 5* (AHCPR publication no. 93-0551), Rockville, MD, 1993, US Department of Health and Human Services, Public Health Service, Agency for Health Care Policy and Research.
*Dry mouth, blurred vision, urinary hesitancy, constipation.
0, Absent or rare; *1+, 2+*, in between; *3+, 4+*, common.

Antidepressants have no known long-term adverse effects, tolerance to therapeutic effects does not usually develop, and persistent side effects often can be minimized by a small decrease in dose without loss of effectiveness. Because antidepressants do not cause physical addiction, psychological dependence, or euphoria, they have no abuse potential. Their long half-life (24 hours or longer) allows most of them to be conveniently administered once a day after steady state is reached. If the patient experiences drowsiness, the drug should be taken at night. If the patient is activated, it should be taken in the daytime. Patients with bipolar illness may be switched into mania by antidepressants, thus they should be watched closely for increased activity, greater difficulty concentrating and eating, and decreased sleeping patterns if an antidepressant is added to their drug regimen.

Several of the antidepressant categories (SSRIs, TCAs) have been given throughout pregnancy when necessary without harmful effects on the fetus and should be considered after a careful risk-to-benefit assessment is done when a pregnant woman is severely depressed.

Selective Serotonin Reuptake Inhibitors (SSRIs)

All the SSRIs inhibit the reuptake of serotonin at the presynaptic membrane. This results in an increase of available serotonin in the synapse and therefore at receptors, promoting serotonin neurotransmission. While their actions and effectiveness are similar, they are structurally different from each other, accounting for some variation in their side effect

profiles and some differences in efficacy in some patients. Many initial side effects are short term and tolerance may develop, although some may last for as long as the patient takes the drug. Thus if a patient cannot tolerate one of the SSRIs (due to side effects) or receives only minimal effectiveness (the patient is an SSRI nonresponder), there are several choices to consider. For problems with SSRI side effects (Table 28-11), choices include lowering the dose, at least temporarily, to see if there is an improvement in side effects without a loss of efficacy; waiting for tolerance to develop for the side effect; using one of the nursing strategies to decrease side effects (Table 28-12); using drug co-administration strategies to treat the side effect (such as sildenafil for sexual dysfunction in men and women [Nurnberg et al, 1999]); and switching the patient to another antidepressant with a different side-effect profile. For SSRI nonresponders, choices include raising the dose to the limits of the therapeutic range (and the patient's tolerance); augmenting the primary antidepressant with another drug (such as lithium, thyroxine, another antidepressant, a stimulant, or buspirone) to increase efficacy; and switching to another SSRI or other antidepressant (Howland & Thase, 1999).

The SSRIs also have antidepressant effects comparable to those of the other classes of antidepressant drugs, yet without significant anticholinergic, cardiovascular, and sedative side effects. SSRIs usually do not cause weight gain, thus making them more acceptable to many patients. In addition, they are fairly safe in overdose. These properties have made them very popular, even though they cost more than the

Table 28-11

Antidepressant Drug Side Effects

	Receptors/ Neurotransmitters	Side Effects
ANTIDEPRESSANTS		
TCAs	H_1	Sedation/drowsiness, hypotension, weight gain
	ACh	Anticholinergic side effects: blurred vision, dry mouth, constipation, tachycardia, urinary retention, cognitive dysfunction
	Alpha$_1$	Postural hypotension, dizziness, tachycardia, memory dysfunction
	5HT$_2$	Hypotension, ejaculatory dysfunction
	5HT	Gastrointestinal (GI) disturbances (nausea, diarrhea), sexual dysfunction
	NE	Tremors, tachycardia, erectile/ejaculatory dysfunction
MAOIs	ACh	Anticholinergic side effects
SSRIs	5HT	GI disturbances (nausea, diarrhea), sexual dysfunction
OTHER ANTIDEPRESSANTS		
Amoxapine	NE	Tremors, tachycardia, erectile/ejaculatory dysfunction
	5HT	GI disturbance (nausea, diarrhea), sexual dysfunction
	D$_2$	Extrapyramidal symptoms and tardive dyskinesia (rare)
	ACh	Anticholinergic effects
	H$_1$	Sedation/drowsiness, hypotension, weight gain
Bupropion	DA	Psychomotor activation
	NE	Tremors, tachycardia, erectile/ejaculatory dysfunction
Maprotiline	NE	Tremors, tachycardia, erectile/ejaculatory dysfunction
	H$_1$	Sedation, drowsiness, hypotension, weight gain
	ACh	Anticholinergic effects
Mirtazapine	H$_1$	Sedation, drowsiness, hypotension, weight gain
	ACh	Anticholinergic side effects
Nefazedone	5HT	GI disturbances (nausea, diarrhea), sexual dysfunction
	NE	Tremors, tachycardia, erectile/ejaculatory dysfunction
	5HT$_2$	Hypotension, ejaculatory dysfunction
	Alpha$_1$	Postural hypotension; dizziness, tachycardia, memory dysfunction
Trazedone	5HT	GI disturbances (nausea, diarrhea), sexual dysfunction
	5HT$_2$	Hypotension, ejaculatory dysfunction
	H$_1$	Sedation/drowsiness, hypotension, weight gain
	Alpha$_1$	Postural hypotension, dizziness, tachycardia, memory dysfunction
	Alpha$_2$	Priapism
Reboxetine	NE	Tachycardia, decreased libido and sexual dysfunction
	ACh	Dry mouth, constipation, tachycardia, urinary retention
Venlafaxine	NE	Tremors, tachycardia, erectile/ejaculatory dysfunction
	5HT	GI disturbances (nausea, diarrhea), sexual dysfunction
	DA	Psychomotor activation

Additional side effects and adverse reactions of antidepressant drugs less clearly related to receptor/neurotransmitter effects:

TCAs	ECG changes, dizziness/lightheadedness
	TCA withdrawal syndrome (malaise, muscle aches, chills, nausea, dizziness, coryzia), hallucinations, delusions, activation of schizophrenic or manic psychosis, excessive perspiration
MAOIs	Hypertensive crisis, lightheadedness, drowsiness, insomnia, weight gain, sexual dysfunction
SSRIs	Nervousness, activation, headache, cytochrome P-450 inhibition, serotonin syndrome, insomnia
Venlafaxine	Sweating, nausea, constipation, vomiting, somnolence, dry mouth, dizziness, anxiety, blurred vision, headache, hypertension, insomnia
Reboxetine	Headache, nausea, insomnia, excessive perspiration

older tricyclic compounds. Particular care must be taken when combining SSRIs with other serotonin drugs and with drugs that are metabolized by liver enzymes that SSRIs may inhibit. For instance, combining serotonergic drugs can cause serotonin syndrome, a life-threatening crisis. Also, because the SSRIs may inhibit the cytochrome P-450 family of liver enzymes, which are responsible for the metabolism of many other drugs, care also has to be taken to monitor patients on multiple medications for signs of toxicity. See Table 28-12 for side effects of antidepressant drugs.

Other Newer Antidepressant Drugs

A growing number of other newer antidepressant drugs differ chemically from each other and from other classes of

Table 28-12

Nursing Considerations for Antidepressant Drug Side Effects

Side Effect	Nursing Care and Teaching Considerations
Anticholinergic side effects	
Blurred vision	Temporary; avoid hazardous tasks.
Dry mouth	Encourage fluids, frequent rinses, sugar-free hard candy and gums; check for mouth sores.
Constipation	Increase fluids, dietary fiber and roughage, exercise; monitor bowel habits; use stool softeners and laxatives only if necessary.
Tachycardia	Temporary, usually not significant (except with coronary artery disease), but can be frightening; eliminate caffeine; beta-blockers might help; supportive therapy.
Urinary retention	Encourage fluids and frequent voiding; monitor voiding patterns; bethanecol; catheterize.
Cognitive dysfunction	Temporary; avoid hazardous tasks, adjust lifestyle; supportive therapy.
*Cytochrome P-450 inhibition	SSRIs inhibit the liver isoenzyme cytochrome P-450, which is instrumental in the metabolism of a variety of drugs (TCAs, trazodone, barbiturates, most benzodiazepines, carbamazepine, narcotics, neuroleptics, phenytoin, valproate, verapamil). This effect can be potentially life-threatening because it increases serum concentrations as well as therapeutic and toxic effects of these drugs.
Dizziness/lightheadedness	Dangle feet; adequate hydration, elastic stockings; protect from falls.
ECG changes	Careful cardiac history; pretreatment ECG for patients over 40 and children; ST segment depression, T wave flattened or inverted, QRS prolongation; worsening of intraventricular conduction problems; do not use if recent myocardial infarction or bundle-branch block.
Ejaculatory dysfunction	Dose after sexual intercourse, not immediately before.
GI disturbances (nausea, diarrhea)	Take with meals or at HS; adjust diet if indicated.
Hallucinations, delusions, activation of schizophrenic or manic psychosis	Change to another antidepressant class of drug, initiate antipsychotics or mood stabilizers if appropriate.
*Hypertensive crisis	See Box 28-6.
Hypotension	Frequent BP; hydrate; elastic stockings; may need to change drug. For postural hypotension: lying and standing BP, gradual change of positions, protect from falls.
Insomnia	Dose as early in the day as possible; sleep hygiene, decrease evening activities; eliminate caffeine; relaxation techniques; sedative-hypnotic therapy.
Memory dysfunction	Temporary; encourage concentration, make lists, provide social support, adjust lifestyle.
Perspiration (excessive)	Frequent change of clothes, cotton/linen clothing, good hygiene; increase fluids.
Priapism	Change dose, change drug.
Psychomotor activation	Take drug in morning rather than HS, adjust lifestyle.
Sedation/drowsiness	Administer drug at HS, avoid hazardous tasks.
*Serotonin syndrome (SS)	SS is a life-threatening emergency resulting from excess central nervous system 5HT caused by combining 5HT-enhancing drugs or administering SSRIs too close to the discontinuation of MAOIs. Symptoms are confusion, disorientation, mania, restlessness/agitation, myoclonus, hyperreflexia, diaphoresis, shivering, tremor, diarrhea, nausea, ataxis, headache. Discontinue all serotonergic drugs immediately; anticonvulsants for seizures; serotonin antagonist drugs may help; clonazepam for myoclonus, lorazepam for restlessness/agitation, other symptomatic care as indicated; do not reintroduce serotonin drugs.
Sexual dysfunction	Dose after sexual intercourse, use lubricant if vaginal dryness is present; antidotes such as sildenifal, bupropion, or bethanecol.
Tachycardia	See anticholinergic side effects.
TCA withdrawal syndrome	Symptoms: malaise, muscle aches, chills, nausea, dizziness, coryzia; when discontinuing drug, taper over several days or weeks.
Tremors	Temporary; adjust lifestyle if indicated.
Weight gain	Increase exercise; reduced calorie diet if indicated; may need to change class of drug.

NOTE: Always educate the patient, consider decreasing or dividing drug dose, use the techniques in this table, and consider changing the drug only if necessary.
*Potentially life-threatening.

antidepressants and differ significantly in their effects at the synapse. They therefore have varying side effect profiles, although their efficacy is generally the same as that of other antidepressants, as is the length of time required for efficacy to occur (several weeks at optimal dose). Like SSRIs, the other newer antidepressants are safer than TCAs and MAOIs in side effect profiles and overdose. Some of these drugs appear to have more specificity than many of the other antidepressants. Several examples follow.

Bupropion is a norepinephrine and dopamine reuptake blocker (NDRI). Venlafaxine is a "dual" reuptake inhibitor because it inhibits both norepinephrine and serotonin reup-

Box 28-6

Signs and Treatment of Hypertensive Crisis on MAOIs

WARNING SIGNS

Increased blood pressure
Palpitations
Headache

SYMPTOMS OF HYPERTENSIVE CRISIS

Sudden elevation of blood pressure
Explosive occipital headache
Head and face and flushed and feel "full"
Palpitations, chest pain
Sweating, fever, nausea, vomiting
Dilated pupils, photophobia

TREATMENT

Hold MAOI doses
Do not lie down (elevates blood pressure in head)
IM chlorpromazine 100 mg, repeat if necessary
  (*mechanism of action:* blocks norepinephrine)
IV phentolamine, administered slowly in doses of 5 mg
  (*mechanism of action:* binds with norepinephrine
  receptor sites, blocking norepinephrine)
Manage fever by external cooling techniques
Evaluate diet, adherence, and teaching

take (SNRI). Nefazodone and trazodone block (antagonize) a subtype of the serotonin $5HT_2$ postsynaptic receptor that is thought to be associated with side effects and block serotonin reuptake (and norepinephrine to a lesser extent), thus are serotonin antagonists and reuptake inhibitors (SARIs). Mirtazepine has several complex actions: it blocks presynaptic alpha$_2$ autoreceptors, increasing levels of norepinephrine (which also increases serotonin) in the synapse; it serves as an agonist to the serotonin $5HT_1$ postsynaptic receptor, which is thought to be the serotonin receptor implicated in mood disorders; it antagonizes the $5HT_2$ receptor (thought to cause side effects); and it has fewer receptor actions in other neurotransmitter systems than some other antidepressants, so it is marketed as having a lower side-effect profile.

A newly approved antidepressant, reboxetine is the first truly selective norepinephrine reuptake inhibitor (NRI). It is comparable in efficacy for depression and side effects to the other newer antidepressants and is also expected to be effective against anxiety disorders such as panic. Because of its short half-life, the manufacturer recommends that it be taken twice daily. As with all newly approved drugs, it remains to be seen how well it will be accepted in daily clinical practice, so the nurse should be alert for post-marketing updates and anecdotal reports on reboxetine as they become available.

Tricyclic Antidepressants

Although the class of TCAs includes some drugs that are structurally dissimilar, the TCAs are quite similar in their clinical effects and adverse reactions (see Table 28-11). To varying degrees, TCAs all have the same primary actions, such as serotonin and norepinephrine reuptake inhibition (therapeutic effects); blockade of three receptors not implicated in depression: muscarinic cholinergic receptors (anticholinergic side effects), histamine H_1 receptors (sedation and weight gain), and alpha$_1$ noradrenergic receptors (orthostatic hypotension and dizziness). TCAs can also have dangerous cardiac side effects, requiring electrocardiograms in adults over age 40 years, all children, and any patient with cardiac conduction problems. Since TCAs are lethal in overdose, careful baseline and ongoing suicide assessment is important. Elderly patients and patients with a medical illness may require lower doses of these drugs than healthy adults and careful assessments for side effects while they are taking the drugs. Several TCAs (such as imipramine and nortriptyline) have clinically relevant blood levels, making monitoring therapeutic doses more precise if necessary. TCAs are as effective as the newer drugs, and since they have been on the market for many decades, many of them are less expensive than most drugs used to treat depression and anxiety, so they may be a good choice for some patients.

Monoamine Oxidase Inhibitors

MAOIs are very effective antidepressant/antipanic/antiphobic drugs and were the first clinically effective antidepressants to be discovered. The MAOIs used in psychiatry are listed in Table 28-8. MAOIs work by inhibiting both types of the enzyme (MAO A and B) that metabolize serotonin and norepinephrine. This inhibition is irreversible and lasts until the body is able to manufacture new MAO after the drug is discontinued. MAO A is linked to depression because it metabolizes the transmitters most closely linked to depression, but it is also linked to the control of blood pressure due to its inhibition of norepinephrine. Thus patients taking these drugs must avoid norepinephrine agonists (such as its dietary precursor, tyramine). A dangerous elevation in blood pressure can result from high levels of norepinephrine not metabolized by MAO. A hypertensive crisis can result (which can cause intracerebral hemorrhage and death) when tyramine-containing foods (such as cheese) and certain medicines (such as meperidine, SSRIs, and sympathomimetic agents) are taken along with these drugs.

Careful health teaching of a reliable patient is a critical component of nursing care when administering MAOIs. The patient must know the warning signs, symptoms, and treatment of a hypertensive crisis (Box 28-6), must avoid certain foods, drinks, and medicines (Box 28-7), and must be taught the more common side effects of MAOIs (see Table 28-11). The patient should be on the restricted diet several days before beginning the medication, while on the medication, and, because MAOIs have a long half-life, for 2 weeks after stopping the medication. Patients should not take contraindicated medications for 2 weeks before taking a MAOI (6 weeks for fluoxetine because of its long half-life), while on the MAOI, and for 2 weeks after stopping the MAOI. No more than one MAOI should be given at a time.

In general, these drugs should not be used along with other antidepressants. Because of the side-effect profile of

MAOIs, they are not usually considered as first- or second-line treatments, but are important to consider for patients who are nonresponders to the other classes of antidepressants. MAO B is thought to convert some amines into toxins that may cause damage to neurons. Drugs that are selective inhibitors of MAO B have no antidepressant properties, have no risk of hypertension, and are used to prevent progression of neurodegenerative diseases such as Parkinson's disease.

A novel class of MAOI not yet available in the United States with antidepressant efficacy comparable to that of other antidepressants is reversible and selective inhibitors of MAO A, called RIMAs (such as moclobemide and brofaromine). Unlike the irreversible and nonselective MAOIs, RIMAs are short-acting drugs, allowing the recovery of enzyme activity in hours rather than weeks. Thus they have fewer side effects specifically the absence of severe hypertensive interaction) and do not require the low-tyramine diet. RIMAs may prove to be valuable additions to the list of antidepressant drugs in the future.

MOOD-STABILIZING DRUGS
Lithium

Lithium, a naturally occurring salt, is the only drug with FDA approval as a first-line treatment for patients with acute mania (particularly those with a clear-cut, noncomplicated bipolar disorder) and the long-term prevention of recurrent episodes. Lithium also has a role in the treatment of recurrent unipolar depression, aggressive behaviors, conduct disorder, and schizoaffective disorder. Box 28-8 lists the target symptoms of mania and depression for mood-stabilizing drug therapy for patients with bipolar disorder. Table 28-13 lists the mood-stabilizing drugs. The exact mechanism of action of lithium is not fully understood, but many neurotransmitter functions are altered by the drug. It has been suggested that lithium may correct an ion exchange abnormality in the neuron; normalize synaptic neurotransmission of norepinephrine, serotonin, dopamine, and acetylcholine; and regulate second-messenger systems during neurotransmission (Hopkins et al, 2000).

Before treatment with lithium, a complete history and physical examination are required, with special attention to the function of the kidneys (lithium is excreted by the kidneys) and the thyroid (lithium inhibits several steps in thyroid hormone synthesis and metabolism). During the maintenance treatment phase, regular lithium blood levels and other laboratory values are monitored and the dose is adjusted as necessary (Box 28-9). Careful health teaching is necessary so that the patient taking lithium can differentiate between side effects and toxic effects (Box 28-10) and understands what can cause a toxic increase in lithium levels and how to maintain a stable lithium level (Box 28-11). Lithium toxicity is a life-threatening adverse event requiring emergency medical intervention (Box 28-12).

In acute manic episodes lithium is effective in 1 to 2 weeks, but it may take up to 4 weeks or even a few months to treat the symptoms fully. The addition of a benzodiazepine or other sedating drug may be necessary to help during the acute phase of treatment. In a maintenance regimen lithium decreases the number of affective episodes, their severity, and the frequency

Box 28-7

The MAOI Diet			
CATEGORY	**CONSUME WITH CAUTION**	**AVOID**	**AVOID COMPLETELY (CONSERVATIVE)**
Cheeses	Mozzarella, cottage, ricotta, cream, processed	Aged cheeses (Roquefort, camembert, blue, brie)	Any cheeses except cream or cottage
Meats and fish	Fresh: chicken liver, meats, liver, herring	Aged/cured meats (sausage, pastrami, salami), pickled fish, meat extracts, protein dietary supplements, shrimp paste	Any fish or meat that is not fresh
Fruits and vegetables	Raspberries, bananas (including the peel) Small amounts: avocado, spinach	Broad bean pods, fermented bean curd (tofu), soy bean paste	Banana peels
Alcoholic beverages	Wine	Alcohol-free beers, tap beers	Ale, all beer, chianti, liqueurs, vermouth, whiskey
Other	Monosodium glutamate, pizza Small amounts: chocolate, caffeine, nuts, dairy products	Sauerkraut, soy sauce, yeast extracts, soups (especially miso)	Ginseng All spoiled, nonfresh foods All foods prepared by someone else
Drugs	Insulin, oral hypoglycemics, oral anticoagulants, thiazide diuretics, anticholinergic agents, muscle relaxants	Other antidepressant drugs, nasal and sinus decongestants, allergy, hayfever and asthma remedies, narcotics (especially meperidine), epinephrine, stimulants, cocaine, amphetamines	

Modified from Gelenberg A: The MAOI diet, *Biol Ther Psychiatry Newsletter* 21:2, 1998.

of occurrence. However, mild mood swings or the recurrence of depressive, manic, or psychotic symptoms are not uncommon while on lithium maintenance. While lithium is an effective treatment for many patients with bipolar illness, it is only partially effective for some even at therapeutic doses, and some patients experience coexisting depression, anxiety, or psychosis. In addition, its side effect profile makes it difficult to tolerate, making some patients unable to reach a lithium level necessary for full efficacy. Therefore, when necessary, it is common clinical practice to cautiously augment the effectiveness of lithium with additional agents such as another mood stabilizer, an antidepressant, a benzodiazepine, or an antipsychotic agent, depending on the target symptoms (see Citing the Evidence on p. 593).

Lithium has a narrow therapeutic index, and toxic levels can quickly become fatal without appropriate intervention.

Because lithium is a salt, the sodium and fluid balance of the body affects lithium regulation. The nurse working with a patient on lithium needs a sophisticated understanding of the principles of lithium administration in order to keep lithium blood levels within the therapeutic range, side effects minimized, quality of life maximized, and the bipolar patient adherent to the treatment regimen. Intensive medication management and ongoing patient education and psychotherapeutic support are the gold standard for the long-term treatment of the patient with bipolar illness.

Lithium therapy usually is started with 300 mg tid until steady state is reached, usually in 7 days. Then a blood level is drawn in the morning, 12 hours after the last dose. In general, the serum concentration of lithium should be between 0.6 and 1.4 mEq/L. In geriatric patients or those with medical illness or kidney disease, a serum lithium level of 0.6 to 0.8 mEq/L is recommended. Use of lithium in pregnancy is not recommended, particularly during the first trimester, due to reports of various congenital abnormalities attributed to lithium.

> *Your patient's wife calls you and is upset. Her husband says he enjoys his manic highs and does not want to take his medication, which dulls his enjoyment of life. How would you help this family?*

Box 28-8

Target Symptoms for Mood-Stabilizing Drug Therapy

MANIA	DEPRESSION
Irritability	Irritability
Expansiveness	Sadness
Euphoria	Pessimism
Manipulativeness	Anhedonia
Lability with depression	Self-reproach
Sleep disturbance (decreased sleep)	Guilt
Pressured speech	Hopelessness
Flight of ideas	Somatic complaints
Motor hyperactivity	Suicidal ideation
Assaultiveness/threatening behavior	Motor retardation
Distractibility	Slowed thinking
Hypergraphia	Poor concentration and memory
Hypersexuality	Fatigue
Persecutory and religious delusions	Constipation
Grandiosity	Decreased libido
Hallucinations	Anorexia or increased appetite
Ideas of reference	Weight change
Catatonia	Helplessness
	Sleep disturbance (insomnia or hypersomnia)

Box 28-9

Prelithium Work-Up

Renal: urinalysis, blood urea nitrogen (BUN), creatinine, electrolytes, 24-hour creatinine clearance; history of renal disease in self or family; diabetes mellitus, hypertension, diuretic use, analgesic abuse
Thyroid: thyroid-stimulating hormone (TSH), T_4 (thyroxine), T_3 resin uptake, $T_4 I$ (free thyroxine index); history of thyroid disease in self or family
Other: complete physical, history, ECG, fasting blood sugar, complete blood count (CBC)

MAINTENANCE LITHIUM CONSIDERATIONS

Every 3 months: lithium level (for the first 6 months)
Every 6 months: reassess renal status, lithium level, TSH
Every 12 months: reassess thyroid function, ECG
Assess more often if patient is symptomatic

Table 28-13

Mood-Stabilizing Drugs

Generic (Trade Name)	Peak Plasma Levels (hr)	Half-Life	Usual Adult Daily Dose (mg/day)	Preparations
Lithium carbonate (Eskalith, Lithobid, lithium citrate, etc.)	1-4	18-36	600-2400	PO; SR; L
Carbamazepine (Tegretol)	1.5-6	25-65; 8-29	200-1600	PO; Ch
Valproic acid (valproate, Depakote, divalproex, etc.)	2-4	9-16	750+	PO; L
Lamotrigine (Lamictal)	1-5	26	12.5-150+	PO
Gabapentin (Neurontin)	3	5-7	300-1800+	PO
Topiramate (Topamax)	2	21	25-200+	PO

PO, Oral tablet/capsule; *SR*, oral slow-release tablets; *L*, liquid; *Ch*, chewable tablets.

Box **28-10**

Lithium Side Effects and Toxicity

Body image	Weight gain (60% of patients)
Cardiac	ECG changes, usually not clinically significant
CNS	Fine hand tremor (50% of patients), fatigue, headache, mental dullness, lethargy
Dermatological	Acne, pruritic maculopapular rash
Endocrine	Thyroid dysfunction: hypothyroidism (5% of patients); replacement hormone Diabetes mellitus: diet or insulin therapy
Gastrointestinal	Gastric irritation, anorexia, abdominal cramps, mild nausea, vomiting, diarrhea (dose with food or milk; further divide dose)
Renal	Polyuria (60% of patients), polydipsia, edema Nephrogenic diabetes insipidus: decrease dose; drink plenty of fluids; thiazide diuretics paradoxically reduce polyuria Microscopic structural kidney changes (10% to 20% of patients on lithium for 1 year); does not cause clinical morbidity

LITHIUM TOXICITY/USUALLY DOSE RELATED

Prodrome of intoxication (lithium level $\geq$ 2.0 mEq/L): anorexia, nausea, vomiting, diarrhea, coarse hand tremor, twitching, lethargy, dysarthria, hyperactive deep tendon reflexes, ataxia, tinnitus, vertigo, weakness, drowsiness

Lithium intoxication (lithium level $\geq$ 2.5 mEq/L): fever, decreased urine output, decreased blood pressure, irregular pulse, ECG changes, impaired consciousness, seizures, coma, death

Box **28-11**

Stabilizing Lithium Levels

COMMON CAUSES FOR AN INCREASE IN LITHIUM LEVELS

Decreased sodium intake
Diuretic therapy
Decreased renal functioning
Fluid and electrolyte loss, sweating, diarrhea, dehydration, fever, vomiting
Medical illness
Overdose
Nonsteroidal antiinflammatory drug therapy

WAYS TO MAINTAIN A STABLE LITHIUM LEVEL

Stabilize dosing schedule by dividing doses or use of sustained-release capsules.
Ensure adequate dietary sodium and fluid intake (2 to 3 L/day).
Replace fluid and electrolytes lost during exercise or gastrointestinal illness.
Monitor signs and symptoms of lithium side effects and toxicity.
If patient forgets a dose, a dose may be taken if less than 2 hours have elapsed; if longer than 2 hours, the dose should be skipped and the next dose taken; never double up on doses.

Anticonvulsant Mood Stabilizers

Growing evidence indicates that a variety of anticonvulsant drugs have beneficial effects in the treatment of bipolar disorder. Although they do not have FDA approval for this indication and have not been systematically tested in double-blind studies, these drugs are considered second-line treatments after lithium by many clinicians. Carbamazepine and valproate are the best studied of these agents and have acute antimanic and long-term mood-stabilizing effects in some bipolar patients, including patients intolerant to or inadequately treated with lithium. They also are reportedly better than lithium in the treatment of mixed or dysphoric bipolar states and in patients who are rapid cyclers. It is thought that the anticonvulsant mood-stabilizing drugs work in bipolar disorder by enhancing the effects of the inhibitory neurotransmitter GABA and by desensitizing the "kindling" effect in bipolar illness (see Chapter 6). Kindling is the process by which the brain apparently becomes sensitized by neurochemical reactions to events, such as stressors or injuries or drugs (such as alcohol and cocaine), and eventually seems to spontaneously respond in a dysfunctional manner in the absence of the precipitating events. Kindling is a model used to theorize about cyclical illnesses such as bipolar illness and intermittent symptoms of other illnesses such as panic attacks or the craving of substances of abuse.

As with lithium, side effect profiles, adverse effects, and contraindications require a sophisticated clinical approach for the safe and effective use of anticonvulsant mood-stabilizing drugs in patients with bipolar illness. The nurse is advised to frequently refer to current prescribing updates when treating patients on mood-stabilizing drugs.

Carbamazepine has its peak effects within 10 days of administration and is used either alone or in combination with other drugs in the treatment of bipolar disorder. Other psychiatric applications of carbamazepine can include the treatment of borderline personality disorder, schizophrenia, and schizoaffective disorder. The most common side effects in the first few weeks of treatment also tend to decrease over time. These include drowsiness, dizziness, ataxia, double vision, blurred vision, nausea, and fatigue. Less common are gastrointestinal upset and a variety of skin reactions, occasionally requiring discontinuation of the drug. A temporary benign 25% decrease in the white blood cell count does not require discontinuation.

A rare but serious side effect is carbamazepine-induced agranulocytosis, a significant decrease in the white blood cell count that does not return to normal. Blood cell and platelet counts and hepatic and renal function tests are taken at baseline and are monitored again several times during the first few months of treatment, and then only when the well-educated reliable patient reports petechiae, pallor, weakness,

Box 28-12

Management of Serious Lithium Toxicity

- Assess quickly; obtain rapid history of incident, especially dosing; offer support and explanations to patient.
- Hold all lithium doses.
- Check blood pressure, pulse, rectal temperature, respirations, and level of consciousness. Be prepared to initiate stabilization procedures, protect airway, and provide supplemental oxygen.
- Obtain lithium blood level immediately; obtain electrolytes, BUN, creatinine, urinalysis, CBC when possible.
- Electrocardiograph; monitor cardiac status.
- Limit lithium absorption; if acute overdose, provide an emetic; nasogastric suctioning.
- Vigorously hydrate: 5 to 6 L/day; balance electrolytes; IV line; indwelling urinary catheter.
- Patient will be bedridden: range of motion, frequent turning, pulmonary toilet.
- In moderately severe cases:
    - Implement osmotic diuresis with urea or mannitol.
    - Increase lithium clearance with aminophylline and alkalinize the urine with IV sodium lactate.
    - Ensure adequate intake of sodium chloride to promote excretion of lithium.
    - Implement peritoneal or hemodialysis in the most severe cases (serum levels between 2.0 and 4.0 mEq/L) with decreasing urinary output and deepening CNS depression.
- Ascertain reasons for lithium toxicity, increase health teaching efforts, mobilize postdischarge support system, arrange for more frequent clinical visits and blood levels, assess for depression and suicidal intent.

Citing the Evidence on

Augmentation of Lithium in Bipolar Depression

BACKGROUND: This randomized clinical trial was designed to clarify the appropriate treatment of bipolar depression by comparing the addition of an antidepressant versus a second mood stabilizer for inpatients being treated with lithium or divalproex (valproate) for bipolar disorder.

RESULTS: Both groups showed significant improvement in depressive symptoms over 6 weeks. There were significantly more side effects causing patients to drop from the study in the group taking two mood stabilizers compared to the group taking one mood stabilizer and one antidepressant.

IMPLICATION: Augmentation of a mood stabilizer for treatment of bipolar depression with either another mood stabilizer or an antidepressant is effective. However, the addition of an antidepressant rather than another mood stabilizer may be more tolerable and just as effective, thus may have more clinical utility in the treatment of bipolar depression.

Young LT et al: Double-blind comparison of addition of a second mood stabilizer versus an antidepressant to an initial mood stabilizer for treatment of patients with bipolar depression, *Am J Psychiatry* 157:124, 2000.

fever, or infection. Carbamazepine induces the cytochrome P-450 system and could cause a decrease in serum concentrations of drugs such as other anticonvulsants, benzodiazepines, anticoagulants, and oral contraceptives, causing a decrease in effectiveness of these drugs. Carbamazepine can be lethal in overdose. It is not recommended in pregnancy, and it should not be used (or used with caution) in patients with generalized seizures, heart block, blood disorders, bone marrow depression, cardiac damage, diabetes, and glaucoma.

Valproate has been effective in the manic phase of bipolar disorder and schizoaffective disorder, even in patients who did not respond to or were unable to tolerate lithium. Response usually occurs in 1 to 2 weeks. It can be used in long-term maintenance alone or with other drugs such as lithium, antipsychotics, or antidepressants. Valproate is well tolerated in general. The most common side effects include gastrointestinal complaints such as anorexia, nausea, vomiting, and diarrhea; neurological symptoms of tremor, sedation, headache, dizziness, and ataxia; increased appetite, and weight gain. Thrombocytopenia, with bruising, petechiae, hematoma, and bleeding, may necessitate a decrease in dose or discontinuation of the drug.

Very rare but serious side effects include pancreatitis and severe hepatic dysfunction. A thorough baseline examination should include liver and renal function and hematology panels, serum ammonia concentrations, and bleeding time determinations, which are repeated every 1 to 4 weeks for the first 6 months and then every 3 to 6 months. Valproate is not recommended in patients with hepatic disease, blood dyscrasias, organic brain disease, or renal function impairment. Valproate is not safe for use during pregnancy, and it can be lethal in overdose.

Three newer anticonvulsants are becoming popular in the treatment of bipolar disorder. They are lamotrigine (Lamictal), gabapentin (Neurontin), and topirimate (Topamax). Although very few systematic double-blind studies to date have assessed the safety and efficacy of these drugs in the treatment of bipolar disorder, they have been successful in treating mixed states and rapid cycling in people who have not received adequate benefit from or who are intolerant to lithium, carbamazepine, or valproate. Gabapentin may be more effective in treating anxiety and agitation than carbamazepine and valproate, and lamotrigine may have more of an antidepressant effect than the other anticonvulsant mood stabilizers. Approximately 0.1% of patients taking lamotrigine develop a serious rash requiring hospitalization. The risk for this reaction is increased in children and in patients taking lamotrigine and valproate in combination. Topirimate is the only anticonvulsant mood stabilizer not associated with weight gain. More studies are needed to document the safety and efficacy profiles of these drugs in the treatment of bipolar disorder.

ANTIPSYCHOTIC DRUGS

The original drugs used to treat psychosis are called "typical" or "conventional" neuroleptic drugs. Since their discovery in the 1950s, these drugs revolutionized the treatment of schizophrenia and other psychotic disorders. With the discovery of the newer antipsychotic drugs (called "atypical" antipsychotic drugs) in the 1990s, the treatment of these debilitating brain disorders has been revolutionized again. While there are advantages and disadvantages to both classes of these antipsychotic drugs, the atypicals offer a different pharmacological mechanism of action, an expanded spectrum of therapeutic efficacy, and a more acceptable side effect profile. Thus they are considered first-line therapy by most clinicians for the treatment of persons with psychosis.

The major uses for antipsychotic drugs are in the management of schizophrenia, schizoaffective disorder, organic brain syndrome with psychosis, and delusional disorder, in both acute and maintenance regimens. Their short-term use may be indicated in severe depression with psychotic features, the manic phase of bipolar illness, and substance-induced psychosis. They also treat the aggressiveness and behavioral problems seen in pervasive developmental disorders and in elderly patients with dementia and delirium with agitation and psychosis, and they decrease the vocal tics in Tourette's syndrome. Nonpsychiatric uses for antipsychotic drugs include treatment of vomiting, vertigo, and to increase effects of analgesics for pain relief. The antipsychotic drugs are listed in Table 28-14.

The clinical symptoms of psychosis that are considered the major target symptoms for pharmacotherapy with the antipsychotic drugs are listed in Box 28-13. The initial nursing treatment plan should address target symptoms, selection of drug, dose, response, and observed side effects and their treatment, along with patient safety, education, and reassurance. Although the relationship the nurse establishes with the patient who is very psychotic forms the basis for an ongoing therapeutic alliance, active nonpharmacological treatment of the residual symptoms of psychosis is more successful when the patient's behavior, mood, and thought processes begin to show improvement with pharmacotherapy.

Atypical Antipsychotics

All the atypical agents exert both dopamine receptor subtype 2 (D_2) and $5HT_2$ (serotonin receptor subtype 2) receptor blocking action (since they inhibit the reception of the

Table 28-14

Atypical Antipsychotic and Typical Neuroleptic Drugs

Generic Name (Trade Name)	Therapeutic Equivalent (Potency, mg)	Half-Life (hr)	Usual Adult Daily Dose: Range (mg)	Preparations
ATYPICAL ANTIPSYCHOTIC DRUGS				
Clozapine (Clozaril)	50	8-12	25-600 (+)	PO
Risperidone (Risperdal)	1-2	3-24	2-8	PO, L
Olanzapine (Zyprexa)	2-3	27	5-20	PO
Quetiapine (Seroquel)	50-100	7	150-750	PO
TYPICAL NEUROLEPTIC DRUGS				
Phenothiazines				
Chlorpromazine (Thorazine)	100	23-37	200-1000 (+)	PO, IM, L, Sup
Thioridazine (Mellaril)	100	24-36	200-600*	PO, IM, L
Mesoridazine (Serentil)	50	24-42	100-400	PO, IM, L
Perphenazine (Trilafon)	10	9	8-65	PO, IM, L
Trifluoperazine (Stelazine)	5	24	5-30	PO, IM, L
Fluphenazine (Prolixin)	2	22	2-20	PO, IM, L
Fluphenazine decanoate (Prolixin Decanoate)	12.5-50	q 2-3 weeks	2.5-50 q 2-4 weeks	L-A
Thioxanthene				
Thiothixene (Navane)	5	34	5-30	PO, L
Butyrophenone				
Haloperidol (Haldol)	2	24	2-20 (+)	PO, IM, L
Haloperidol decanoate (Haldol Decanoate)	50-300	3 weeks	50-300 q 3-4 weeks	L-A
Dibenzoxazepine				
Loxapine (Loxitane)	15	4	20-100 (+)	PO, IM, L
Dihydroindolone				
Molindone (Moban)	10	1.5	20-100 (+)	PO, L
Diphenybutylpiperidine				
Pimozide (Orap)	2	55	2-16	PO

IM, Intramuscular injection; *PO*, oral tab, capsule; *Sup*, suppository; *L*, oral liquid, elixir, suspension, concentrate; *L-A*, long-acting injectable preparation.
*Upper limit to avoid retinopathy.

neurotransmitters dopamine and serotonin at specific post-synaptic sites, they are DA and 5HT **antagonists**). Like the typical neuroleptic antipsychotics, these newer atypical drugs improve the positive symptoms of schizophrenia. Additionally, the atypical drugs also exert therapeutic action in treating the negative symptoms of schizophrenia without significant extrapyramidal symptoms (EPS) (one of the major causes of patient nonadherence to the typical neuroleptic antipsychotic drugs). Atypical agents are also reported to treat mood symptoms, hostility, violence, suicidal behavior, and the cognitive impairment seen in schizophrenia. Atypical antipsychotic drugs provide new hope for patients with psychosis, particularly those who are experiencing their first episode of psychosis (first-break patients) or those who have not responded well to typical antipsychotics or have suffered dose-limiting side effects from these drugs. The biggest disadvantage to the atypical drugs is the increase in cost over the typical agents. It is hoped that a cost-benefit analysis for each patient will show that their cost will be significantly outweighed by the improved efficacy and quality of life experienced by patients on these drugs.

While the atypical drugs are similar in their effectiveness, compared to each other, they differ in side effects due to their different receptor-binding profiles. For example, risperidone and olanzapine are associated with an elevation in plasma prolactin levels, and some cases of EPS have been reported at higher doses. These problems do not seem to occur with quetiapine. Table 28-15 lists the side-effect profiles of atypical antipsychotic drugs. Clozapine was the first of the newer atypical antipsychotics and has been shown to be more effective than typical antipsychotic drugs for patients with refractory symptoms (its major indication in the United States). In addition to the side effects listed in Table 28-15, clozapine may cause tachycardia, weight gain, and a paradoxical hypersalivation, especially during sleep. There is a seizure risk that increases with too rapid a titration and with increased dosage (up to 5% of patients taking 600 to 900 mg/day). Often a rapid return of psychotic symptoms occurs when the drug is discontinued.

The most serious adverse effect of clozapine is agranulocytosis, which occurs in approximately 1% to 2% of patients (this is 10 to 20 times greater than the risk for standard antipsychotic drugs). This risk continues to increase during the first 5 months of treatment, then declines substantially, but it never entirely disappears. Risk for clozapine-induced agranulocytosis increases with older age, female gender, and Ashkenazic Jewish ancestry. Patients taking clozapine must be entered in a national registry, and in the United States have their white blood cell (WBC) count monitored weekly for the first 6 months of treatment, then biweekly for as long as they are taking the drug. If there is a drop of 3000/μL in the WBC count or if the WBC count falls below 5000/μL, then counts should be perormed two or three times weekly. If the WBC count falls below 3500/μL or the absolute neutrophil count falls below 1500/μL, then clozapine should be discontinued and a hematologist should be consulted for further blood testing.

Agranulocytosis is almost always reversible after drug discontinuation, although while immunocompromised, the patient is vulnerable to infections. Clozapine prescriptions 1 to 2 weeks at a time are recommended. Once a patient has had an episode of agranulocytosis, rechallenge is contraindicated, as is the use of a phenothiazine because this group of drugs also has an increased risk of agranulocytosis. While on clozapine, carbamazepine is contraindicated due to its increased risk for agranulocytosis. Obviously, vigilant clinical care and regular laboratory examinations add a significant cost to the treatment of patients taking clozapine. For the schizophrenic patient who needs this drug, can be monitored as required for agranulocytosis, can afford the additional burden of cost, and does not need concomitant drugs that also lower WBC count, clozapine may make a significant difference in treatment outcome. The other atypical drugs thus far do not have an increased incidence of agranulocytosis, so they do not require frequent laboratory work.

Finally, although the atypical drugs reduce the negative as well as the positive symptoms of schizophrenia, patients taking these medications still need help with other aspects of their psychosocial functioning. Psychoeducation, social skills training, group support, and other rehabilitative interventions are beneficial in improving their overall level of functioning and quality of life (see Chapter 22).

 How would you help a family evaluate the risk/benefit ratio for clozapine treatment of their relative?

Typical Antipsychotics

The conventional neuroleptic drugs are predominantly dopamine (DA) antagonists, thus they block postsynaptic

---

Box 28-13

Antipsychotic Drug Target Symptoms

POSITIVE SYMPTOMS: AN EXCESS OR DISTORTION OF NORMAL FUNCTION*

Psychotic disorders of thinking
- Delusions (somatic, grandiose, religious, nihilistic, or persecutory themes)
- Hallucinations (auditory, visual, tactile, gustatory, olfactory)

Disorganization of speech and behavior
- Positive formal thought disorder (incoherence, derailment, illogicality)
- Bizarre behavior (catatonic motor behaviors, disorders of movement, deterioration of social behavior)

NEGATIVE SYMPTOMS: A DIMINUTION OR LOSS OF NORMAL FUNCTION†

Affective flattening: limited range and intensity of emotional expression

Alogia: restricted thought and speech

Avolition/apathy: lack of initiation of goal-directed behavior

Anhedonia/asociality: inability to experience pleasure or maintain social contacts

Attentional impairment: inability to mentally focus

*Responsive to traditional and atypical antipsychotics.
†Unresponsive to traditional antipsychotics, responsive to atypical antipsychotics.

Table **28-15**

Comparison of Typical, Atypical, and Newest Antipsychotic Drugs					
	Typical Neuroleptic	Clozapine	Risperidone	Olanzapine	Quetiapine
CLINICAL EFFICACY					
Dosage (mg/day)	Various	25-600+	2-8	5-20	150-750
Acute psychosis overall	+++	+++	+++	+++	+++
Acute positive symptoms	+++	+++	+++	+++	+++
Acute negative symptoms	+	+++	+++	+++	+++
Treatment-refractory psychosis	0	++	?	?	?
SIDE-EFFECT PROFILE					
Agitation	+ to ++	0	+/−	+	+
Agranulocytosis	Rare	+++	Rare	Rare	Rare
Anticholinergic effects	+ to +++	+++	+/−	++	++
EPS	+ to +++	0	+*	0	0
Dose-related increase in EPS	Yes	No	Yes	Yes	?
Nausea/dyspepsia	+	0	+/−	+	0
Orthostatic hypotension	+ to +++	+++	++	++	+
Elevation of prolactin levels	+ to ++	0	++	+	0
Sedation	++ to +++	+++	++	++	++
Seizures	+	+++	+	+	+
		(dose related)			
Tardive dyskinesia	+++	0	?	?	?

Modified from Jibson MD, Tandon R: A summary of research findings on the new antipsychotic drugs, *Psychiatr Nurs Forum* 2(Summer), 1996.
*Low risk for EPS for risperidone is associated only with low daily doses (<6 mg).
Efficacy: + = mild, ++ = moderate, +++ = marked, +/− = minimal, ? = uncertain, 0 = none.
Side effects: + = mild, ++ = moderate, +++ = severe, +/− = minimal, ? = uncertain, 0 = none.

Table **28-16**

Acute Side Effect Profile: Antipsychotic Drugs				
Drugs	Sedation	Extrapyramidal Symptoms	Anticholinergic	Postural Hypotension
LOW POTENCY				
Chlorpromazine	4	2	3	4
Thioridazine	4	1	4	4
Clozapine	4	1	4	3
Olanzapine	2	0	2	2
HIGH POTENCY				
Trifluoperazine	2	3	2	2
Thiothixene	2	3	2	1
Loxapine	2	3	2	2
Molindone	2	3	2	2
Mesoridazine	3	2	3	3
Perphenazine	2	3	2	2
Fluphenazine	1	4	2	1
Haloperidol	1	4	1	1
Risperidone	2	1	1	2

1, Lowest incidence; *4*, highest incidence.

D2 receptors in several DA tracts in the brain, although they have other synaptic effects as well. This action results in their two main effects: a decrease in the positive symptoms of schizophrenia, listed in Box 28-13, and the production of EPS. The typical drugs also bind to many other receptor sites in many transmitter systems, accounting for their broad side-effect profile. The typical antipsychotics are not different from each other in terms of overall clinical response at equivalent doses. Thus selection of a drug is determined by the extent, type, and severity of side effects produced, as well as effect of the drug in a first-degree relative.

For instance, a low-potency drug such as chlorpromazine can reduce the risk of EPS, or a high-potency drug such as haloperidol can minimize postural hypotension, sedation, and anticholinergic effects (Table 28-16). These drugs are equally effective in treating the positive symptoms, are equally less effective in the treatment of the negative symptoms of schizophrenia, and may even worsen these symp-

Table **28-17**

Nursing Considerations for Antipsychotic Drug Side Effects	
CNS Side Effects	Nursing Care and Teaching Considerations
Extrapyramidal symptoms (EPS)	General treatment principles: Tolerance usually develops by the third month. Decrease dose of drug. Add a drug to treat EPS, then taper after 3 months on the antipsychotic. Use a drug with a lower EPS profile. Patient education and support.
Acute dystonic reactions: oculogyric crisis, torticollis	Spasms of major muscle groups of neck, back, and eyes; occur suddenly; frightening; painful; medicate, parenteral works faster than PO; have respiratory support available; more common in children and young males, and with high potency drugs. Taper dose gradually when discontinuing antipsychotic drugs to avoid withdrawal dyskinesia.
Akathisia	Cannot remain still; pacing, inner restlessness, leg aches are relieved by movement; rule out anxiety or agitation; medicate.
Parkinson's syndrome: akinesia, cogwheel rigidity, fine tremor	More common in males and elderly; tolerance may not develop; medicate with DA agonist amantadine (must have good renal function).
Tardive dyskinesia (TD)	Can occur after use (usually long use) of conventional antipsychotics; stereotyped involuntary movements (tongue protrusion, lip smacking, chewing, blinking, grimacing, choreiform movements of limbs and trunk, foot tapping); if using typical antipsychotics, use preventive measures and assess often; consider changing to an atypical antipsychotic drug; there is no treatment at present for TD.
*Neuroleptic malignant syndrome (NMS)	Potentially fatal: Fever, tachycardia, sweating, muscle rigidity, tremor, incontinence, stupor, leukocytosis, elevated creatine phosphokinase (CPK), renal failure; more common with high-potency drugs and in dehydrated patients; discontinue all drugs; supportive symptomatic care (hydration, renal dialysis, ventilation, and fever reduction as appropriate); can treat with dantroline or bromocriptine; antipsychotic drugs can be cautiously reintroduced eventually.
*Seizures	Occur in approximately 1% of people taking these drugs; clozapine has a 5% rate (in patients on 600 to 900 mg/day); may have to discontinue clozapine.
OTHER SIDE EFFECTS OF ANTIPSYCHOTIC DRUGS	
*Agranulocytosis	This is an emergency; it develops abruptly, with fever, malaise, ulcerative sore throat, leukopenia. High incidence (1% to 2%) is associated with clozapine; must do weekly CBC and prescribe only 1 week of drug at a time; discontinue drug immediately; may need reverse isolation and antibiotics.
Photosensitivity	Use sunscreen and sunglasses; cover body with clothing.
Anticholinergic effects	Symptoms: constipation, dry mouth, blurred vision, orthostatic hypotension, tachycardia, urinary retention, nasal congestion; see Table 28-12 for nursing care.
Sedation, weight gain	See Table 28-12 for nursing care.

*Potentially life-threatening.

toms. Additionally, they have not been particularly effective in treating cognitive impairment and mood symptoms, the other symptom dimensions of schizophrenia.

Adverse Reactions of Typical Antipsychotic Drugs. The side effects of antipsychotic drugs are varied and require assessment, prevention, and intervention. Table 28-17 is a list of side effects and treatment considerations. Side effects can range from merely uncomfortable and easily treated to a life-threatening emergency. It is important to minimize the patient's fears, increased sense of stigmatization, and possible nonadherence with drug treatment through effective patient education and support and intensive medication management.

Most EPS side effects are common with the use of typical antipsychotic drugs (particularly with the high-potency drugs; see Table 28-16) and are often painful and disabling. They are also stigmatizing and can usually be prevented or minimized and effectively treated (tardive dyskinesia is the exception). Drug strategies to treat EPS include lowering the dose of the drug, changing to a drug with a lower incidence of that side effect, or administering one of the drugs in Table 28-18. If a high-potency drug such as haloperidol is prescribed, most clinicians also administer a course of prophylactic antiparkinson medication to decrease the incidence of EPS side effects. Because tolerance to most of these side effects usually occurs in the first 3 months, drugs to treat EPS are usually given for up to 3 months and then slowly discontinued. There is no effective treatment for tardive dyskinesia to date, although it is expected to decrease in incidence with the increased use of the atypical antipsychotic drugs, and clozapine has been reported to minimize it in some patients.

Another uncommon but potentially fatal (14% to 30% mortality) side effect of antipsychotic drugs is neuroleptic malignant syndrome (NMS). It is important for the nurse to

Table **28-18**

Drugs to Treat Extrapyramidal Side Effects		
Generic Name (Trade Name)	Adult Dosage Range (mg/day)	Preparations
ANTICHOLINERGICS		
Benzotropine (Cogentin)	1-6	PO, IM, IV
Trihexyphenidyl (Artane)	1-10	PO
Biperiden (Akineton)	2-6	PO
Procyclidine (Kemadrin)	6-20	PO
ANTIHISTAMINE		
Diphenhydramine (Benadryl)	25-300	PO, IM, IV
DOPAMINE AGONIST		
Amantadine (Symmetrel)	100-300	PO
BENZODIAZEPINES		
Diazepam (Valium)	2-6	PO, IV
Lorazepam (Ativan)	0.5-2	PO, IM
Clonazepam (Klonopin)	1-4	PO

Table **28-19**

Comparison of Serotonin Syndrome and Neuroleptic Malignant Syndrome		
Clinical Symptoms	Serotonin Syndrome	Neuroleptic Malignant Syndrome
Mental status	Confusion, disorientation, mania	Dazed mutism
Autonomic dysfunction*	50%-90%	>90%
Neuromuscular activity		
▪ Muscle rigidity	50%	90%
▪ Hyperreflexia	Common	Rare
▪ Myoclonic jerking	Common	Rare
▪ Ataxia	Common	Rare
▪ Extrapyramidal effects	Rare	Common
Hyperthermia	Mild-marked	Mild-marked
Leukocytosis	Rare	>80%
CPK elevation	Rare	Common
Acute renal failure	Possible	Possible

Modified from Bernstein JG: *Drug handbook in psychiatry*, ed 3, St Louis, 1995, Mosby.
*Tachycardia, labile blood pressure, diaphoresis, tremor, incontinence, dyspnea, shivering, restlessness.

assess for NMS and other serious drug side effects. Because many patients are taking more than one drug at a time, it can become confusing when symptoms of these side effects are similar. Table 28-19 compares the life-threatening side effects of serotonin syndrome with NMS.

Because of the importance in managing patients taking psychotropic medications and the problems they cause, medication-induced movement disorders are coded on Axis I of the *DSM–IV–TR* (American Psychiatric Association, 2000). Although they are labeled medication-induced, it is often difficult to establish the causal link between medication exposure and the development of the movement disorder because some of these disorders occur in the absence of medication exposure.

General Pharmacological Principles

A thorough baseline evaluation, including laboratory tests and ECG, should be performed before initiating treatment. Dosage requirements for individual patients vary considerably and must be adjusted as the target symptom changes and side effects are monitored. Initially, depending on the dosage recommendations for each drug, the patient receives several doses a day, and the daily dose can be titrated slowly until a standard dose is reached. Olanzapine (an atypical drug) is an exception, since a starting dose of 10 mg may be effective for the entire course of treatment. Some patients begin to respond to the sedating effects of the typical drugs in 2 to 3 days, and some take as long as 2 weeks. Full benefits from typical drugs may take 4 or more weeks. The atypical drugs may take several months to reach maximum efficacy. Thus the patient, family, and clinician must wait until the antipsychotic agent takes effect and not give in to the temptation to continue increasing the dose prematurely, since this strategy usually increases side effects and not efficacy. A brief course of a benzodiazepine may help the patient maintain control during this time.

When the patient's condition has been stabilized for several weeks, the daily dose can be lowered to the lowest effective dose. The half-life of antipsychotic drugs is greater than 24 hours, so the patient usually can be dosed once a day after steady state is reached. Bedtime dosing allows the patient to sleep through side effects when they are at their peak. After approximately 12 to 24 months of stable maintenance drug therapy, the patient can be slowly tapered from medication to assess the need for continued drug treatment. Some schizophrenic patients who have had more than three episodes in a 5-year period or who have chronic residual symptoms may require a lifetime of continuous medication management. A patient who is unresponsive to an adequate medication trial often responds to another chemical class of antipsychotic drug, so a second trial is given. Clozapine is usually considered after a second trial failure (at this point the patient is considered treatment resistant), particularly if the patient failed to respond to the other atypical drugs. When switching a patient from one antipsychotic to another, in order to avoid destabilizing the patient, cross-titration of the new and old drugs is the preferred method. This means that one drug is gradually decreased while the new drug is gradually increased, usually by 25% each every 2 to 4 days.

Several typical antipsychotic drugs have a short-acting injectable preparation and can be administered by intramuscular routes for use in acutely agitated patients. For long-term maintenance treatment there are two long-acting preparations. Fluphenazine comes in two depot injectable forms that can be given every 7 to 28 days. Haloperidol decanoate is an injectable preparation that has a 4-week duration of action. It is not appropriate to treat an acute psychotic episode with haloperidol decanoate alone because it takes 3 months to reach steady-state drug levels. The patient's ability to take these drugs should be tested by first

Box 28-14

Drug Treatment for Alzheimer's Disease

TACRINE (COGNEX)

Tacrine is the first drug to treat mild to moderate dementia related to Alzheimer's disease.

Tacrine prevents or slows the breakdown of ACh by inhibiting the action of the metabolizing enzyme acetylcholinesterase. An excessive loss of the neurotransmitter ACh is thought to cause the memory problems associated with Alzheimer's disease.

Dosing

10 mg qid PO for the first 6 weeks with weekly transaminase levels. Titrate by 10-mg increments to 40 mg qid, at 6-week intervals for each dose, given stable or slightly elevated transaminase levels and patient tolerability. If levels become extreme, stop tacrine until they return to normal and then carefully rechallenge. Measure transaminase levels every 3 months at maintenance doses.

Side Effects

Nausea, vomiting, diarrhea, dyspepsia, anorexia, muscle aches, and ataxia. Monitor patients for elevated transaminase levels and abnormal liver function, tacrine-induced bradycardia in patients with sick sinus syndrome, and symptoms of occult or active GI bleeding.

Drug Interactions

Can increase theophylline's half-life and plasma concentration. Cimetidine (Tagamet) increases and prolongs blood levels of tacrine. Synergistic effects are expected when given with succinylcholine and other cholinesterase inhibitors or cholinergic agonists.

Drug Limitation

Tacrine's beneficial effects diminish over time as Alzheimer's disease progresses.

DONEPEZIL HYDROCHLORIDE (ARICEPT)

In 1996 the U.S. FDA approved donepezil hydrochloride (Aricept) to treat symptoms of Alzheimer's disease. Aricept is only the second approved treatment for Alzheimer's disease.

Like Cognex, Aricept is a palliative that does nothing to slow the progressive neurodegeneration that ultimately leads to dementia and death. By helping the brain retain and use the neurotransmitter acetylcholine, however, both drugs slow the symptomatic progression of the disease, temporarily stabilizing or improving the cognitive state of those taking either drug.

Aricept has a major advantage in its low toxicity compared with Cognex, according to data submitted to the FDA. In addition to lack of liver toxicity, Aricept has a generally more benign side-effect profile than Cognex.

---

administering the oral form for several days. Long-acting injectables have been important in treating the outpatient who requires supervision with medication regimens.

There are no ceiling doses for these medicines, except thioridazine, which can cause pigmentary retinopathy when given in amounts over 800 mg/day. Abruptly stopping antipsychotic drugs can cause dyskinetic reactions and some rebound side effects. The drugs should be tapered slowly over several days to weeks. Antipsychotic drugs do not cause chemical dependency, nor is there tolerance to their antipsychotic effects over time. Because they do not produce euphoria, they also have a very low abuse potential. Due to their wide therapeutic index, overdoses of these drugs ordinarily do not result in death, so they have a low suicide potential. Antipsychotic drugs are not respiratory depressants but produce an added depressant effect when combined with drugs that produce respiratory depression. Therefore patients who also may be taking drugs such as benzodiazepines must be carefully observed. The effects of antipsychotics on the fetus are inconclusive, although what is best for a psychotic pregnant mother must be carefully considered.

DRUGS TO TREAT ALZHEIMER'S DISEASE

There has been a great deal of interest in medications reported to be effective in treating some of the symptoms of Alzheimer's disease. Drugs such as tacrine (Cognez) or donepezil (Aricept), both acetylcholinesterase inhibitors, have become available. These two drugs enhance the amount of acetylcholine in the brain, which in turn enhances memory and cognition in some people with Alzheimer's disease (Box 28-14). Two investigational cholinesterase inhibitors, rivastigmine and metrifonate also seem to have significant, although modest, effects on the cognition of patients with Alzheimer's disease. Stimulation of nerve growth with neurotropic factors, the neural protective effects of estrogen and nonsteroidal anti-inflammatory drugs, and the ability to enhance the sensitivity of neuronal receptors promise many future advances in the treatment of Alzheimer's disease.

FUTURE PSYCHOPHARMACOLOGICAL AGENTS

Based on current trends in psychoactive drug research, the nurse can expect to see new drugs approved for use in mental disorders. It is important to evaluate new drugs very carefully as they come into clinical use. The nurse should determine the advantages and disadvantages of a new drug as compared to the standard drugs in that class and in relation to the patient's reactions and preferences. The following list is a partial guide to help evaluate new drugs. Ask whether a new drug has the following:

- A different mechanism of action more specific to desired biological actions
- Quicker onset of action
- Fewer drug interactions
- A lower side-effect profile
- No addictive or abuse potential
- No long-term adverse effects

Table **28-20**

New Drugs in Development for Mental Illness			
Product Name	Indication	Development Status	Manufacturer
CGP 60829	Depression, anxiety	Phase II	Novartis
CI-1019	Depression	Phase II	Warner Lambert
Duloxetine	Depression	Phase II	Lilly
Fibanserin	Depression	Phase II	Boehringer Ingelheim
Flesinoxan	Depression, anxiety	Phase III	Solvay
MK-869	Depression, anxiety, bipolar disorder, schizophrenia	Phase II	Merck
SR 46349	Depression, anxiety, schizophrenia	Phase II	Sanofi
SR 58611	Depression, eating disorders	Phase II	Sanofi
Topiramate	Bipolar disorder	Phase II	RW Johnson
Olanzapine (Zyprexa)	Bipolar disorder (acute mania), bipolar depression and mood stabilization	Phase III	Lilly
Aripiprazole	Schizophrenia	Phase III	Otsuka
Iloperidone	Schizophrenia	Phase III	Novartis
SR 141716	Schizophrenia, dementia, eating disorders	Phase I/II	Sanofi
Risperidone (Risperdal IM Depot)	Schizophrenia	Phase II	Janssen
Cocaine vaccine	Cocaine dependence	Phase I	ImmuLogic
Dextromethorphan	Opiate dependence	Phase I	ALGOS
Lazabemide	Smoking cessation	Phase III	Hoffman-LaRoche
Nalmefene	Alcohol abuse/dependence	Phase II	Baker Norton
Subutex (buprenorphine)	Opiate dependence	Application submitted to FDA	Reckitt & Coleman

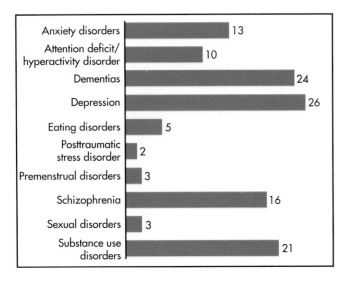

Fig. 28-2 Medicines in development for mental illness. (From Pharmaceutical Research Manufacturers of America, Washington, DC, 2000.)

- No suicide potential
- Permanent or curative effects on neurotransmitter regulation
- Several routes of administration, at least by mouth and intramuscularly
- A wide therapeutic index
- Fewer discontinuation problems
- Advantage in cost-effectiveness

Table 28-20 lists new drugs currently under review by the FDA or in Phase III (final phase) of clinical testing, soon to be submitted to the FDA for review and approval. There are over

Box **28-15**

Behavioral Rating Scales Related to Antipsychotic Medication Side Effects

- Abnormal Involuntary Movement Scale (AIMS)
- Barnes Akathesia Scale
- Simpson-Angus Extrapyramidal Symptoms Scale

85 psychotropic drugs in clinical trials in the United States (Fig. 28-2). Nurses can expect to see many of these medications approved for use with psychiatric patients in the future.

PSYCHIATRIC NURSING PRACTICE

The psychiatric nurse should make use of clinical guidelines and stay up to date on new, evidence-based theories and treatments for psychiatric illnesses. In addition, the safe practice of clinical psychopharmacology requires competencies in diagnosis, biological assessment, knowledge of available drugs, the design of medication regimens, and competent prescriptive practice at the advanced level (Bailey, 1999). An important part of the psychiatric nurse's role is to identify and intervene in side effects experienced by patients as a result of their medication regimens. Box 28-15 lists behavioral rating scales nurses can use to identify antipsychotic medication side effects in their patients.

Psychopharmacology Guidelines and Algorithms

Psychotropic medications are commonly used in the treatment of psychiatric disorders. It is therefore essential for psychiatric nurses to have a thorough understanding of psy-

Box 28-16

Psychopharmacology Guidelines for Psychiatric–Mental Health Nurses

NEUROSCIENCES

Commensurate with level of practice, the psychiatric–mental health nurse integrates current knowledge from the neurosciences to understand etiological models, diagnostic issues, and treatment strategies for psychiatric illness.

PSYCHOPHARMACOLOGY

The psychiatric–mental health nurse involved in the care of patients taking psychopharmacological agents demonstrates knowledge of psychopharmacological principles, including pharmacokinetics, pharmacodynamics, drug classification, intended and unintended effects, and related nursing implications.

CLINICAL MANAGEMENT

The psychiatric–mental health nurse applies principles from the neurosciences and psychopharmacology to provide safe and effective management of patients being treated with psychopharmacological agents. Clinical management includes assessment, diagnosis, and treatment considerations.

Assessment

The psychiatric–mental health nurse has the knowledge, skills, and ability to conduct and interpret patient assessments of psychopharmacological agents. Assessments include physical, neuropsychiatric, psychosocial, and psychopharmacological parameters.

Diagnosis

The psychiatric–mental health nurse has the knowledge, skills, and ability to use appropriate nursing, psychiatric, and medical diagnostic classification systems to guide the psychopharmacological treatment of patients with mental illness.

Treatment

The psychiatric–mental health nurse takes an active role in the treatment of patients with mental illness and integrates prescribed psychopharmacological interventions in a cohesive, multidimensional plan of care.

Modified from American Nurses' Association: *Psychiatric mental health nursing psychopharmacology project: ANA task force on psychopharmacology,* Washington, DC, 1994, The Association.

chopharmacology. The American Nurses' Association published a document (1994) that describes the skills and knowledge psychiatric nurses need to guide them in their work with psychopharmacological agents (Box 28-16). The document identifies specific areas that nurses can review to evaluate their ability to deliver competent nursing care.

In addition, various other professional organizations and groups have developed practice guidelines and psychopharmacology treatment algorithms (see Chapter 5). In particular, the Texas Medication Algorithm Project provides an evidence-based decision tree with information about how to make decisions regarding selection of medications, how and when to change medications, and how to augment medications (Rush et al, 1999). Fig. 28-3 presents an algorithm showing strategic recommendations for the use of psychopharmacological agents. Medication algorithms for specific psychiatric illnesses have also been included in the various clinical chapters of Unit 3 of this text.

Documentation

In addition to routine documentation of pharmacological activities, the nurse may have special documentation considerations in the pharmacological treatment of mental illness. The following issues are particularly important to document when working with psychiatric patients:

- Drugs administered outside usual recommended levels
- Rationale for medication or dose changes
- Drugs used for other than the indications approved by the FDA
- Continued use of a drug that is causing clinically significant side effects
- Polypharmacy rationale
- Patient and family knowledge, attitudes, and preferences

Patient Education

Patients taking psychotropic drugs must be knowledgeable about them. Serious consequences can result from what appears to be minor changes in some of the instructions for drug use, such as skipping medication one day, eating cheese, or failing to recognize certain side effects. A survey of 253 psychiatric patients discharged from a short-stay hospitalization reported that more than half did not know the name and dosage of the psychiatric medications prescribed for them and why they were taking them, even though they had received both group and individual medication instruction during hospitalization (Clary et al, 1992). Results suggest the need for more active forms of medication education, such as supervised self-administration in the final days of hospitalization.

Patients and their families need thorough and ongoing instruction on psychotropic drug treatment. Nursing programs focused on patient education need to address essential elements, such as missed medication doses, focus on self-management, and documenting effectiveness (Lakshman et al, 1995). Box 28-17 identifies specific nursing activities related to teaching a patient to take prescribed medications safely.

> *Many chronic mentally ill people have social workers as their case managers. What skills and knowledge would psychiatric nurses bring to this patient population that differ from those of social workers?*

Patient Assistance Programs

Because of limitations on health-care coverage for persons with psychiatric diagnoses and rising health-care

Step 1	**Patient with appropriate diagnosis and baseline psychiatric and medical history, physical, and evaluation.** Drug target symptoms Concomitant psychiatric and medical illnesses and treatments History of drug response in self and first degree relatives Contraindications, allergies, life-style issues, and cost considerations Coordination of treatments among patient's providers Patient education and inclusion in treatment plan
Step 2	**Choose monotherapy from primary first line medications for indication.** Drug has positive efficacy/side effect profile for patient Patient education and consent Non-medication therapy as appropriate
Step 3	**Wait appropriate time period to see response.** Side effects are minimized Dose is titrated/lab values as appropriate Target symptom rating is ongoing
Step 4	**Evaluate Response.** **(A) Good Response** *Is patient tolerating medication?* If yes, continue for appropriate time frame If no, adjust dose; add adjunctive treatment; change primary medication Repeat **Step 3** -- **(B) Partial Response** *Is dose adequate?* If no, adjust dose Repeat **Step 3** If yes, *is patient taking medication as prescribed?* If no, patient education and re-consent; initiate/increase non-medication therapy; re-evaluate patient's preference If yes, *has illness exacerbated or is there a concomitant illness?* If yes, adjust dose or begin concomitant treatment; initiate/increase non-medication therapy Repeat **Step 3** If no, *is diagnosis correct?* If no, repeat baseline diagnostic evaluation; consultation If yes, consider: augmentation; switch to another first line medication; switch to a second/third line medication; initiate/increase non-medication therapy; consultation. Repeat **Step 3** -- **(C) No Response** *Check:* Dose, patient adherence, diagnosis (see B, **Partial Response**) If diagnosis is correct, consider: Switch to another first line medication; switch to a second/third line medication; combination therapy with 2 agents with different mechanisms of action; triple medication combinations; other interventions as scientific data and clinical experience dictate. Repeat **Step 3** Repeat **Step 4** *Consider:* Referral.

Fig. 28-3 Medication algorithm: overview. (Modified from Rush et al: *J Clin Psychiatry* 60:284, 1999.)

costs, including the increased expense of newer drugs and long-term maintenance therapy regimens, patients are finding it more difficult to afford their medications. Additionally, many psychiatric patients are unable to earn a living unless they are on successful treatment regimens, including psychopharmacology. The nurse can assist the patient with this problem by educating him or her about the patient assistance programs (PAPs) offered by many pharmaceutical companies. Although each manufacturer has different requirements, most programs require an application documenting the patient's financial status. Patients who qualify for Medicaid, have private insurance, or exceed the income cap are usually ineligible. More detailed information can be obtained by calling the drug manufacturer or by going to the web at Needy Meds:

http://www. needymeds.com, or Directory of Prescription Drug Patient Assistance Programs: http://www. phrma.org.

Promoting Patient Adherence

Patients who do not take their medications as prescribed or who do not recognize warning signs of drug problems are at risk for unsuccessful results and adverse reactions. A review of research on medication compliance in psychiatric treatment identified patient nonadherence as a major problem. Specifically it found that patients receiving antipsychotics took 58% of the recommended amount of the medications, while patients receiving antidepressants took 65% of the recommended amount of the medications (Cramer & Rosenheck, 1998).

Box 28-17

Teaching Prescribed Medications

DEFINITION

Preparing a patient to safely take prescribed medications and monitor for their effects.

ACTIVITIES

Instruct the patient to recognize distinctive characteristics of the medications.
Inform the patient of both the generic and brand names of each medication.
Instruct the patient on the purpose and action of each medication.
Instruct the patient on the dosage, route, and duration of each medication.
Instruct the patient on the proper administration of each medication.
Evaluate the patient's ability to self-administer medications.
Instruct the patient to perform needed procedures before taking a medication (for example, check pulse and glucose level).
Inform the patient what to do if a dose of medication is missed.
Instruct the patient on which criteria to use when deciding to alter the medication dosage/schedule.
Inform the patient of consequences of not taking or abruptly discontinuing medications.
Instruct the patient on specific precautions to observe when taking medications (such as no driving or using power tools).
Instruct the patient on possible adverse side effects of each medication.
Instruct the patient on how to relieve or prevent certain side effects.
Instruct the patient on appropriate actions to take if side effects occur.
Instruct the patient on the signs and symptoms of overdosage or underdosage.
Inform the patient of possible drug/food interactions.
Instruct the patient on how to properly store medications.
Instruct the patient on the proper care of devices used for administration.
Instruct patients on proper disposal of needles and syringes at home, as appropriate, and where to dispose of the sharps container.
Provide the patient with written information about the action, purpose, side effects, and so on, of medications.
Assist the patient to develop a written medication schedule.
Instruct the patient to carry documentation of prescribed medication regimen.
Instruct the patient on how to fill prescriptions.
Inform the patient of possible changes in appearance or dosage when filling generic medication prescriptions.
Warn the patient of the risks associated with taking expired medication.
Caution the patient against giving prescribed medication to others.
Determine the patient's ability to obtain required medications.
Provide information on medication reimbursement.
Provide information on cost-saving programs and organizations to obtain medications and devices.
Provide information on medication alert devices and how to obtain them.
Reinforce information provided by other health-care team members.
Include the family/significant others as appropriate.

From McCloskey J, Bulechek G: *Nursing interventions classification*, ed 3, St Louis, 2000, Mosby.

The threats to patient adherence are many. Some of them come from the mental health team, others from the patient, and still others reflect a shared failure of the therapeutic alliance (Blackwell, 1997; Munetz, 1998). Nurses and patients should work together to minimize misunderstandings and unnecessarily complex medication regimens. Too often, however, clinicians blame patients for nonadherence without fully evaluating the treatment plan from the patient's perspective (Critical Thinking about Contemporary Issues). For example, the following are some common mistakes clinicians make in prescribing medication (Weiden, 1997):

- Incorrect prescribing as a result of misdiagnosis
- Excessive dosages of medications
- Too many drugs
- Downplaying side effects
- Providing inadequate patient education
- Overlooking the patient's expertise

- Not including family members in the treatment plan
- Inability of the prescriber to see the patient from a holistic perspective

In addition, a number of studies have explored reasons given by patients for nonadherence with their medication regimens (Chamberlain, 1998; Olfson et al, 1997). Risk factors for potential patient nonadherence are listed in Box 28-18. Understanding this issue from the patient's perspective will allow the nurse to anticipate problems and design nursing interventions that can target areas of potential difficulty.

For example, many patients decrease or completely stop taking their medications as soon as they start feeling better. If they have a bad day, they may take medication again for 1 or 2 days. Explaining to these patients how the medication works in the body and the need for therapeutic levels of the medicine in the blood stream may help patients better understand their illness and adhere to the treatment plan. Still

CRITICAL THINKING about CONTEMPORARY ISSUES

Is Nonadherence a Patient Problem or a Nursing Problem?

Every nurse and many patients and their families have had the difficult experience of facing relapse in psychopharmacologically treated psychiatric illness. An obvious problem-solving approach includes an assessment of compliance—is the patient taking the drug as prescribed? In the absence of concomitant medical illness, differences in bioavailability among generic brands of a drug, and increases in life stressors, the nurse and family return to the issue of compliance and wonder why the patient deviated from a previously effective drug regimen. Even if patients deny noncompliance, they usually carry the burden of blame for relapse, and their future relationships with mental health-care providers may be jeopardized.

The interactions of cultural belief systems and psychotropic drug effects are poorly understood. A relatively unacknowledged but well-documented fact is that the effects of pharmacoactive agents are not solely determined by their pharmacological properties. In the cultural context of care it must be recognized that psychotropic drugs affect diverse populations in diverse ways. Thus cultural differences must be considered in the patient and family medication education plan and in interactions with patients throughout the course of treatment.

The potential incompatibility between lay and professional values and between belief system and explanatory models of illness often determine patients' satisfaction with treatment, medication compliance, clinical outcome, and, most important, self-disclosure in the treatment setting (Cleaveland & Denier, 1998; Playle & Keely, 1998). The understanding, acceptance, and communication necessary to create a culturally competent and effective plan of care for the patient with mental illness rest with the nurse and the mental health team. If treatment planning is individualized and is a mutual and shared responsibility between the nurse and patient, then patient compliance or noncompliance must be viewed as a shared outcome of that responsibility.

Box 28-18

Risk Factors for Patient Medication Nonadherence

- Failure to form a therapeutic alliance with the patient
- Devaluation of pharmacotherapy by treatment staff
- Inadequate patient and family education regarding treatment
- Poorly controlled side effects
- Insensitivity to patient beliefs, wishes, complaints, or opposition to the idea of taking medication
- Multiple daily dosing schedule
- Polypharmacy
- History of nonadherence
- Social isolation
- Expense of drugs
- Failure to appreciate patient's role in drug treatment plan
- Lack of continuity of care
- Increased restrictions on patient's lifestyle
- Unsupportive significant others
- Remission of target symptoms
- Increased suicidal ideation
- Increased suspiciousness
- Unrealistic expectations of drug effects
- Concurrent substance use
- Failure to target residual symptoms for nonpharmacological therapies
- Relapse or exacerbation of clinical syndrome
- Failure to alleviate intrafamilial and environmental stressors that precipitate symptoms
- Potential for stigmatization

Summary

1. Psychopharmacology is the fastest growing treatment in the current practice of psychiatry, and the psychiatric nurse makes a unique contribution to the implementation of this treatment strategy.
2. Various principles of psychopharmacology relate to pharmacokinetics, pharmacodynamics, drug co-administration, and the role of neurotransmitters in the development of psychiatric disorders.
3. Benzodiazepines, the most widely prescribed class of drugs, have almost completely replaced other classes of antianxiety and sedative-hypnotic agents. They are therapeutic and have a wide margin of safety when taken alone. They can be mildly addictive, especially when taken in high doses over long periods of time or when used with alcohol or barbiturates. Common side effects include drowsiness, dizziness, slurred speech, and blurred vision.
4. Antidepressant drugs are effective and nonaddicting, and some can be lethal in overdose. Tricyclics, selective serotonin reuptake inhibitors, and newer drugs are more commonly used than monoamine oxidase inhibitors because they are safer in combination with other substances. Many of them are now first-line treatments for several anxiety disorders as well. Side effects of antidepressants are usually mild.
5. The mood stabilizer lithium is effective in the treatment of bipolar illness in short- and long-term treatment regi-

other patients may fear that the medications are addictive or may be embarrassed about the stigma of being on psychiatric medication. Clarifying the use of the medication and the positive impact it can have on all aspects of the patient's life may help to reframe the issue of taking medication in a way that promotes adherence. Most important, patients should be encouraged by the nurse to discuss their questions, fears, problems, and concerns about medication before treatment is altered. Finally, the nurse should realize that the quality of the nurse-patient relationship and the strength of the therapeutic alliance play an extremely important role in whether a patient will adhere to pharmacological treatment plan and affect the patient's recovery process.

mens. Lithium is not addictive but can be toxic. The therapeutic dose range is narrow and must be monitored by regularly assessing serum lithium levels. Several anticonvulsants also have mood-stabilizing effects.

6. The various classes of typical antipsychotic drugs have similar therapeutic effects but are dissimilar in side-effect profiles. Side effects are varied and can be disabling and life-threatening. Clozapine, risperidone, olanzapine, and quetiapine are newer, atypical antipsychotic agents with positive clinical effects and fewer movement disorder side effects. Patients taking clozapine must be closely monitored for agranulocytosis, which is its most serious side effect.

7. New psychopharmacological agents are being tested in clinical drug trials throughout the United States. Many of them will be beneficial to patients with psychiatric illness.

8. Important issues related to psychopharmacology and psychiatric nursing practice include following psychopharmacology guidelines, documentation, patient education, patient assistance programs, and promoting patients' adherence to their pharmacological treatment plan.

Competent Caring   A Clinical Exemplar of a Psychiatric Nurse

DIANA LAIKAM, MS, RN, CS

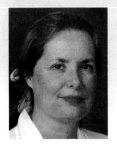

Henry David Thoreau wrote: "If one advances confidently in the direction of his dreams, and endeavors to lead the life which he imagined, he will meet with a success unexpected in common hours." Thirty years ago I confidently began my sojourn into the field of nursing. The journey has led to my role as a Psychiatric Clinical Nurse Specialist with prescriptive authority. When I began psychiatric nursing, hospital admissions lasted months instead of days. Lithium carbonate was still in clinical trials. Serotonin reuptake inhibitors were yet to be developed. Yet, from the beginning of my practice as a psychiatric nurse, I have known that working with the severely and persistently mentally ill was to be my life's work.

Psychotropic medications are the primary means of treating the symptoms of these illnesses. The medication treatment goals for my patients include management, reduction, and cessation of symptoms; establishment of an extended period of partial or complete remission; prevention of exacerbation or relapse symptoms; and prevention, identification, and treatment of side effects. I have learned over time that medication compliance is critical if the severely and persistently mentally ill patient is to avoid hospitalization. And I have had some success in this area.

One such success involved Mr. M., a 40-year-old man with a diagnosis of bipolar affective disorder, recurrent. Throughout his 20-year history of mood lability, he had been prescribed many antipsychotic and mood-stabilizing drugs. Most of his hospitalizations were as a result of medication noncompliance. He was referred to me on discharge from the inpatient psychiatric unit for medication monitoring, and I readily accepted the challenge.

My first glance at Mr. M. was as he sat in the waiting area before his appointment with me. He had a large, crumpled, brown paper bag at his feet. An anxious Mr. M. brought the brown bag into my office. The bag contained 22 bottles of assorted medications. He told me that he was feeling much better but that his medications had all been changed while he was an inpatient. He was confused regarding the names of the medications, the dosages he should take, and the times that he should take the medications. Some of the medicines were for his medical illnesses and some for his psychiatric illness. As the appointment progressed it became clear to me that even with sorting out the medications and explaining how to take them that he was still overwhelmed. With his involvement a plan evolved. Prescriptions were rewritten with medication names he recognized (brand rather than generic) and, whenever possible, prescribed at times convenient to his lifestyle. Medication information was transferred to a sheet of paper so he could read which medication to take and when to take it. He found this particularly helpful because he could not read the small print on the bottles. A medication reminder was to be filled weekly with my assistance until he could manage his own medication.

A year has passed. Medication treatment goals have been met. Mr. M is quite proud that he now takes his medication in an organized manner without a medication reminder. He is acutely aware of subtle changes in his mental status and knows how to observe for side effects. Most importantly, he has not required hospitalization. So each day Mr. M's spirit rejuvenates me in a very real way as I proceed in the direction of my dreams—practicing the profession I love.

Merlin **Visit MERLIN: www.mosby.com/MERLIN/Stuart** to find these additional materials and student activities.

- **Worksheets**
- **"Drug of the Month" Updates**
- **"Citing the Evidence" Updates**
- **Critical Thinking Activities and Exercises**
- **Annotated Suggested Readings**
- **Web Links**
- **More!**

Chapter Review Questions

1. Match each term in Column A with the correct definition in Column B.

Column A	Column B
____ Barbiturates	**A.** SSRIs with MAOIs
____ Selective serotonin reuptake inhibitors	**B.** Clozapine and risperidone
____ Antianxiety drugs	**C.** MAOIs with decongestants/cold remedies
____ Cytochrome P-450 inhibition	**D.** Triazolam (Halcion) and flurazepam (Dalmane)
____ Anti-parkinsonian drugs	**E.** Impramine (Tofranil) and amitryptiline (Elavil)
____ Tricyclics	**F.** Lithium and depakote
____ Serotonin syndrome	**G.** Chlorpromazine (Thorazine) and thiothixine (Navane)
____ Sedative-hypnotics	**H.** Fluoxetine (Prozac) and sertraline (Zoloft)
____ Atypical antipsychotics	**I.** Alprazolam (Xanax) and lorazepam (Ativan)
____ Hypertensive crisis	**J.** Secobarbital (Seconal) and pentobarbital (Nembutal)
____ Typical neuroleptic antipsychotics	**K.** SSRIs with various other drugs
____ Mood stabilizers	**L.** Benztropine (Cogentin) and trihexyphenidyl (Artane)

2. Match each term in Column A with the correct definition in Column B.

Column A	Column B
____ H_1 receptor blockade	**A.** Reduced depression, reduced suicidal behavior, antipsychotic effects, hypotension, sexual dysfunction
____ DA reuptake inhibition	**B.** Sedation/drowsiness, hypotension, weight gain effects
____ Alpha$_2$ receptor blockade	**C.** Reduced depression, antianxiety effects, GI disturbances, sexual dysfunction
____ NE reuptake inhibition	**D.** Postural hypotension, dizziness, tachycardia, memory dysfunction
____ ACh receptor blockade	**E.** Decreased depression, psychomotor activation, anti-Parkinson effects
____ 5HT reuptake inhibition	**F.** Priapism
____ Alpha$_1$ receptor blockade	**G.** Reduced depression, tremors, tachycardia, sexual dysfunction
____ 5HT$_2$ receptor blockade	**H.** Anticholinergic side effects

3. Fill in the blanks.

A. Patient assessment, coordination of treatment modalities, psychopharmacological drug administration and prescribing, medication education, monitoring and maintenance, and research are all within the _____.

B. Concurrent use of drugs, a frequently necessary and often complex practice in pharmacological interventions, is called _____.

C. _____ is the term used when one drug affects the absorption, metabolism, distribution, and excretion of another drug.

D. Many of the psychiatric disorders are thought to be caused by problems in the regulation of communication in the brain, such as an overresponse or an underresponse somewhere along the complex process of neurotransmission. This hypothesis of mental illness is called the _____.

E. The ANA Psychopharmacology Guidelines for Psychiatric Mental Health Nurses includes three broad categories that are essential content for nurses working with patients on psychotropic drugs. These categories are

_____, _____

and _____.

4. Identify whether the following statements are true (T) or false (F).

____ **A.** Serotonin syndrome is the enhancement of action of combinations of antidepressant drugs for better efficacy in patients with depression.

____ **B.** Neuroleptic malignant syndrome, a common side effect of antipsychotic drugs, responds well to increased doses of any of the psychotropic drugs used to treat mental illness.

____ **C.** Hypertensive crisis, a result of MAOIs and tyramine-rich foods, is treated by holding the next dose of drug, elevating the patient's head, and administering a dose of chlorpromazine.

____ **D.** Lithium toxicity occurs when blood levels of lithium are raised beyond the therapeutic window by fluid and electrolyte loss, decreased renal functioning, or overdose.

____ **E.** Tricyclic antidepressants should be avoided if possible, or prescribed in amounts for 1 week at a time, in patients who are at risk for suicide.

5. Provide short answers for the following questions.

A. List the positive and negative symptoms of schizophrenia, and note which respond better to atypical antipsychotics.

B. Briefly describe the difference between reuptake inhibition and receptor blockade. Identify a psychiatric disorder that might benefit from each of these strategies, and state why it is thought that this is so.

C. Discuss the reasons why suicide assessment should continue for several weeks after the depressed patient appears to be responding to antidepressants.

REFERENCES

American Nurses' Association: *Psychiatric mental health nursing psychopharmacology project: ANA task force on psychopharmacology,* Washington, DC, 1994, The Association.

American Psychiatric Association: *Diagnostic and statistical manual of mental disorders,* Fourth Edition, Text Revision. Washington, DC, American Psychiatric Association, 2000.

Bailey KP: Framework for prescriptive practice. In Shea C et al, editors: *Advanced practice nursing in psychiatric and mental health care,* St. Louis, 1999, Mosby.

Ballenger J: Benzodiazepine receptor agonists and antagonists. In Sadock B, Sadock V, editors: *Comprehensive textbook of psychiatry,* ed 7, Philadelphia, 2000, Lippincott Williams & Wilkins.

Blackwell B: *Treatment compliance and the therapeutic alliance,* Amsterdam, The Netherlands, 1997, Harwood Academic Publishers.

Chamberlain J: Confessions of a noncompliant patient, *J Psychosoc Nurs* 36:49, 1998.

Clary C et al: Psychiatric inpatients' knowledge of medication at hospital discharge, *Hosp Community Psychiatry* 43:140, 1992.

Cleaveland B, Denier C: Recommendations for health care professionals to improve compliance and treatment outcome among patients with cognitive deficits, *Issues Ment Health Nurs* 19:113, 1998.

Cramer J, Rosenheck R: Compliance with medication regimens for mental and physical disorders, *Psychiatr Serv* 49:196, 1998.

Delgado P, Moreno F: Antidepressants and the brain, *Int Clin Psychopharmacol* 14:S9, 1999.

Depression Guideline Panel: *Depression in primary care,* vol 2, *Treatment of major depression. Clinical practice guidelines no. 5* (AHCPR publication no. 93-0551), Rockville, Md, 1993, US Department of Health and Human Services, Public Health Service, Agency for Health Care Policy and Research.

Gelenberg A: Zaleplon: a new non-benzodiazepine hypnotic, *Biol Ther Psychiatry* 25:5, 2000.

Howland R, Thase M: What to do with SSRI nonresponders? *J Pract Psychiatr Behav Health* 5:216, 1999.

Hopkins H et al: Mood stabilizers. In Lieberman J et al, editors: *Psychiatric drugs,* Philadelphia, 2000, WB Saunders.

Keltner N: Neuroreceptor function and psychopharmacologic response, *Issues Ment Health Nurs* 21:31, 2000.

Lakshman M et al: Patient education in the drug treatment of psychiatric disorders: effect on compliance and outcome, *CNS Drugs* 3(4):291, 1995.

Laraia M: Scientific advancement through clinical trials. In Shea C et al, editors: *Advanced practice nursing in psychiatric and mental health care,* St Louis, 1999, Mosby.

Möller H-J: Effectiveness and safety of benzodiazepines, *J Clin Psychopharmacol* 19:2S, 1999.

Munetz M: Treatment compliance and the therapeutic alliance, *Psychiatr Serv* 49:1496, 1998.

Nurnberg G et al.: Sildenafil for women patients with antidepressant-induced sexual dysfunction, *Psychiatr Serv* 50:1076, 1999.

Olfson M et al: Medication noncompliance, *N Direct Ment Health Serv* 73:39, 1997.

Pi E, Grey G: A cross-cultural perspective on psychopharmacology, *Essential Psychopharmacol* 2:233, 1998.

Playle JF, Keeley P: Non-compliance and professional power, *J Adv Nurs* 27:304, 1998.

Rush J et al: Medication treatment for the severely and persistently mentally ill: the Texas Medication Algorithm Project, *J Clin Psychiatry* 60:284, 1999.

Stimmel G: Future directions in the drug treatment of insomnia, *Psychiatr Times Monog Pharmacol Manage Insomnia* Spring:1, 1999.

Weiden P: Polypharmacy: using adjuvant medications in the treatment of schizophrenia, *J Pract Psychiatry Behav Health* 5:165, 1999.

Weiden P: The road back: working with the severely mentally ill; psychosocial management of noncompliance, *J Pract Psychiatry Behav Health* 3:169, 1997.

Wintz CJB: Difficult decisions: women of childbearing age, mental illness, and psychopharmacological therapy, *J Am Psychiatr Nurs Assoc* 5:5, 1999.

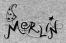

Visit **MERLIN** for *Your Internet Connection* to websites that are related to the content in this chapter.
www.mosby.com/MERLIN/Stuart

29 Somatic Therapies

Carol M. Burns

*Canst thou not minister to a mind diseas'd,
Pluck from the memory rooted sorrow,
Raze out the written troubles of the brain,
And with some sweet oblivious antidote
Cleanse the stuff'd bosom of the perilous stuff
Which weights upon the heart?*

WILLIAM SHAKESPEARE, MACBETH, ACT **V**

With the emergence of biological psychiatry and the growing knowledge bases in the neurosciences, interest has increased in somatic therapies for psychiatric illness. The limitations of psychotropic medications, increase in treatment-resistant psychiatric disorders, and refinement in treatment techniques have placed greater emphasis on evaluating the indications for and efficacy of somatic therapeutic interventions.

Psychiatric nurses are commonly involved in caring for patients who are receiving a somatic therapy. Thus it is essential that all nurses understand how these treatment modalities work and the nursing care that enhances their effectiveness. This chapter discusses five contemporary somatic therapies used for psychiatric illnesses: electroconvulsive therapy, phototherapy, sleep deprivation therapy, transcranial magnetic stimulation, and vagal nerve stimulation.

ELECTROCONVULSIVE THERAPY

Electroconvulsive therapy (ECT) was first described by Cerletti and Bini in 1938 as a treatment for schizophrenia. At that time it was believed that epileptics were rarely schizophrenic and therefore hypothesized that convulsions would cure schizophrenia. Later research did not support this hypothesis. Further experience with ECT showed that it is much more effective as a treatment for affective disturbances than it is for schizophrenia. It has also been noted that epilepsy and schizophrenia sometimes occur concurrently. ECT is now most often used as a treatment for severe depression (Fox, 1996b).

Electroconvulsive therapy is a treatment in which a grand mal seizure is artificially induced in an anesthetized patient by passing an electrical current through electrodes applied to the patient's head. Traditionally the electrodes have been applied bilaterally. More recently, alternative electrode placements have been used, including unilateral and bifrontal. It has been reported that patients have fewer cognitive side effects with these alternative placements, including less disorientation and fewer disturbances of verbal and nonverbal memory than bilateral placement (Bagby et al, 1996; Kellner & McCall, 1999). However, other data suggest that unilateral ECT may not be as reliably effective as bilateral ECT. Some preliminary information suggests that bifrontal placement may combine the efficacy of bilateral with the cognitive profile of unilateral (Bailine et al, 2000). Further studies are needed to clarify these issues. Fig. 29-1 illustrates the different electrode placements.

For ECT to be effective, a grand mal seizure must occur. The electrical stimulus is generally adjusted to the minimum level of energy that will produce a seizure. The number of treatments in a series varies according to the patient's presenting problem and therapeutic response. A usual course is 6 to 12 treatments. Patients with schizophrenia may require more. ECT is most commonly given two to three times a week, although it can be given daily (Shapira et al, 1998).

In some cases, after a successful initial treatment episode, continuation therapy with outpatient ECT may be recommended (Fox, 1996a). The precise timing of continuation ECT varies, but weekly treatment for the first month after remission, followed by a gradual tapering to monthly treatments, appears to be effective. Successful treatment with ECT may also be followed by antidepressant medication to prevent relapse.

 ECT is sometimes called "shock therapy." Describe how use of this term stigmatizes mental illness and its treatment.

Indications

The primary indication for ECT is major depression. ECT's response rate of 80% or more is equal to or better than response rates to antidepressant medications. It can be useful for people in most age groups who cannot tolerate or fail to respond to treatment with medication (Ghaziuddin, 1998; Hermann et al, 1999; Rey & Walter, 1997; Tew et al, 1999). Box 29-1 lists the primary and secondary criteria for the use of ECT as determined by the American Psychiatric Association (APA) Task Force on Electroconvulsive Therapy (2000).

The primary criteria are those in which ECT may play a life-saving role. Patients who meet these criteria may be extremely depressed and suicidal or, alternatively, so hyperactive that there is grave danger of self-harm, such as in acute mania. On occasion, ECT may be used for conditions other than affective disorders (see Citing the Evidence on p. 610). ECT is considered appropriate for schizophrenia in a few situations including when there is an exacerbation of the psychosis, when psychotic symptoms have an abrupt or recent onset, when the duration of illness is short, when catatonia is present, or when the patient has responded well to ECT in the past. Finally, ECT should be considered as an initial in-

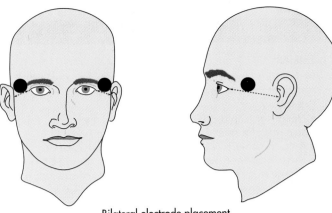
Bilateral electrode placement.

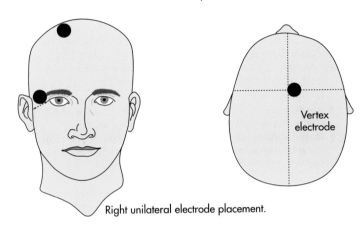
Right unilateral electrode placement.

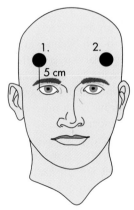
Bifrontal electrode placement

Fig. 29-1 Electrode placement in ECT.

tervention when its anticipated side effects are less than those associated with drug therapy, such as with the elderly, for patients with heart block, and during pregnancy. Box 29-2 summarizes behaviors for which ECT is and is not effective.

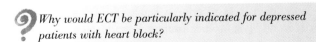 *Why would ECT be particularly indicated for depressed patients with heart block?*

Mechanism of Action

The specific way in which ECT works has been the subject of much research, but the precise mechanism of action is still not known. Most theories about the mode of action of ECT

Box 29-1

Criteria for the Use of ECT

PRIMARY USE

Situations where ECT may be used before a trial of psychotropic medications include, but are not limited to, the following:

- Need for rapid, definitive response owing to the severity of a psychiatric or medical condition
- Risks of other treatments outweigh the risks of ECT
- History of poor medication response or good ECT response in one or more previous episodes of the illness
- Patient preference

SECONDARY USE

In other situations, a trial of an alternative therapy should be considered before referral for ECT. Subsequent referral for ECT should be based on at least one of the following:

- Treatment resistance (taking into account issues such as choice of medication, dosage, duration of trial, and compliance)
- Intolerance or adverse effects with pharmacotherapy that are deemed less likely or less severe with ECT
- Deterioration of the patient's psychiatric or medical condition that creates a need for a rapid, definitive response

From American Psychiatric Association: *The practice of electroconvulsive therapy: recommendations for treatment, training, and privileging, second edition.* Washington DC, 2000, The Association.

Citing the Evidence on

Diagnoses of Patient Treated with ECT

BACKGROUND: This study assessed the extent to which patients treated with electroconvulsive therapy (ECT) had diagnoses for which ECT is an efficacious treatment according to evidence-based standards.

RESULTS: About 86% of the ECT treatments were for diagnoses within evidence-based indications. In about 14%, the diagnoses were outside the indications. Patients receiving ECT for diagnoses outside evidence-based indications were more likely to have been treated by psychiatrists who graduated from medical school between 1940 and 1980 than by those who graduated between 1981 and 1990.

IMPLICATIONS: Diagnoses of patients treated with ECT were mostly within evidence-based indications. Thus it appears that ECT is not used indiscriminately. Psychiatrists trained more recently were more likely to conform to evidence-based standards, suggesting an opportunity for targeted quality improvement.

Hermann R et al: Diagnoses of patients treated with ECT: a comparison of evidence-based standards with reported use, *Psychiatric Services* 50(8):1059, 1999.

---

focus on its efficacy with depressed patients. The following theories have been proposed (Kellner et al, 1997):

- Neurotransmitter theory suggests that ECT acts like tricyclic antidepressants by enhancing deficient neurotransmission in monoaminergic systems. Specifically, it is thought to improve dopaminergic, serotonergic, and adrenergic neurotransmission.
- Neuroendocrine theory suggests that ECT releases hypothalamic or pituitary hormones or both, which results in its antidepressant effects. ECT releases prolactin, thyroid-stimulating hormone, adrenocorticotropic hormone, and endorphins; but the specific hormones responsible for the therapeutic effect are not known.
- Anticonvulsant theory suggests that ECT treatment exerts a profound anticonvulsant effect on the brain that results in an antidepressant effect. Some support for this theory is based on the fact that a person's seizure threshold rises and the seizure duration decreases over the course of ECT and that some patients with epilepsy have fewer seizures after receiving ECT.

Despite unanswered questions regarding its mechanism of action, ECT is an effective treatment for many psychiatric disorders and is safe when properly administered.

Adverse Effects

The mortality rate associated with ECT is estimated to be the same as that with general anesthesia in minor surgery (approximately 1 death per 10,000 patients). Mortality and morbidity are believed to be lower with ECT than with the

administration of antidepressant medications despite the frequent use of ECT in patients with medical complications and in the elderly (American Psychiatric Association, 2000).

Medical adverse effects can, to some extent, be anticipated and prevented. Patients with preexisting cardiac illness, compromised pulmonary status, a history of central nervous system problems, or medical complications after anesthesia are likely to be at increased risk. Thus the work-up preceding ECT should include a thorough review of the patient's history, and may include a complete blood count, urinalysis, serum chemistry profile, chest and spinal radiographs, electrocardiography, and computed tomography scan of the head. Adverse effects can potentially occur in the following categories:

- Cardiovascular effects. Cardiovascular complications are the major cause of morbidity and mortality associated with ECT, so a cardiovascular evaluation before ECT is essential.
- Systemic effects. Headaches, nausea, muscle aches and soreness, weakness, drowsiness, and anorexia may occur after ECT; but they usually respond to supportive management and nursing intervention.
- Cognitive effects. ECT is associated with a range of cognitive side effects including a period of confusion immediately after the seizure and memory disturbance during the treatment course, although a few patients report persistent deficits. The onset of cognitive side effects varies considerably among patients. It is believed that patients with preexisting cognitive impairment,

Box 29-2

Target Behaviors for ECT

ECT EFFECTIVE	ECT INEFFECTIVE
Hyperemotionality	Severe character pathology
Hypermotility	Substance abuse and
Catatonia	dependence
Severe psychosis with	Sexual identification
acute onset	disorders
Life-threatening	Psychoneurosis
psychiatric conditions	Chronic illness without
Rigidity of parkinsonism	obvious psychopathology
or neuroleptic	
malignant syndrome	

From Fink M: Who should get ECT? In Coffey C, editor: *The clinical science of electroconvulsive therapy*, Washington, DC, 1993, American Psychiatric Press.

neuropathological conditions, and those receiving psychotropic medication during ECT may be at increased risk of developing more profound side effects. There is no evidence that ECT causes structural brain damage (Abrams, 1997).

NURSING CARE IN ELECTROCONVULSIVE THERAPY

The effectiveness and limitations of ECT have been the subject of considerable debate within the field of psychiatry (see Critical Thinking about Contemporary Issues). Because it is a somatic therapy for psychiatric illness, nurses have participated in both the debate and the implementation of ECT. Although sometimes thought to be a seldom-used form of therapy, the increasing number of ECT devices, the volume of recently published articles and books, and number of internet sites on the subject suggest that ECT usage may be rising.

Although psychiatric nurses have always had a role in assisting with the ECT procedure, nursing functions have historically been limited to supportive and adjunctive care. With the growing sophistication of nursing science and clinical practice, this role is evolving to include independent and collaborative nursing actions.

Education and Emotional Support

Nursing care begins as soon as the patient and family are presented with ECT as a treatment option. Initially, an important role of the nurse is to allow the patient an opportunity to express feelings, including any myths or fantasies about ECT. Patients may describe fear of pain, dying of electrocution, suffering permanent memory loss, or experiencing impaired intellectual functioning. As the patient reveals these fears and concerns, the nurse can clarify misconceptions and emphasize the therapeutic value of the procedure. Supporting the patient and family in their need to discuss, question, and explore feelings and concerns about ECT should be an essential part of nursing care before, during, and after treatment.

CRITICAL THINKING about CONTEMPORARY ISSUES

Is ECT a Therapeutic Treatment or a Primitive Form of Punishment?

ECT is still controversial. The controversy is not about its efficacy or safety, because these have been well established in numerous studies. Rather, it is about its presumed effects on the brain, public fears, and health-care professionals' lack of education about its beneficial effects. Some people regard ECT as a punishment, believing that it is inhumane. Still others are concerned that permanent brain damage could result.

The opposing view holds that it is more inhumane to allow a person to suffer a severe emotional disorder when ECT provides prompt relief. They believe that the stigmatization related to ECT does considerably more harm than the treatment. Part of the stigma associated with ECT stems from the fact that mental illness is seen as social deviance rather than a medical disorder. As a result, the treatment of mental illness is seen as a stigmatizing punishment (Fink & Tasman, 1992). The second major reason for the stigmatization of ECT is that few people understand the current administration of the procedure. Properly administered, ECT induces far less discomfort and medical complications than most surgical and many psychopharmacological treatments. The third reason rests in the language used to describe the treatment. The fact that it used to be called "shock therapy" conjures up the image of pain that further stigmatizes this treatment option.

It is up to each professional to reach a personal resolution on this issue. This decision should be based on objective data, observation of the treatment, and personal experiences in working with patients who have and have not received ETC.

After the patient has had an opportunity to express feelings, the nurse can begin ECT teaching, taking into consideration the patient's anxiety, readiness to learn, and ability to comprehend. Family teaching should occur at the same time as patient teaching, and the amount of information to be shared should be individualized. The nurse should review with the family and patient the information they have received from the physician regarding the procedure and respond to any questions they might have.

During this assessment process, the nurse should also attempt to define specific patient behaviors the family associates with the patient's illness and determine whether the patient or family member has received ECT in the past. Any information about the family's previous experiences with ECT helps the nurse identify familial beliefs about the patient's illness, ECT treatment, and expected prognosis. Both patient and family should also be asked what else they know about ECT, such as through friends who have received it or by reading about it or seeing ECT portrayed in movies. Open-ended questions may give the nurse the opportunity to identify and correct misinformation and address specific concerns the patient or family has about the procedure. These nursing actions may facilitate the family's ability to provide support to the patient during the treatment course and thus further alleviate the patient's anxiety.

Various media may also be used to supplement the teaching of the patient and family about ECT, including written materials and videotape presentations. A tour of the treatment suite itself may help familiarize the patient with the area, procedure, and equipment. Encouraging the patient to talk with another patient who has benefited from ECT may be worthwhile. Finally, the nurse should facilitate flexibility in family arrangements, particularly during the patient's first few treatments, allowing for family presence before and after ECT if the patient and family desire. This approach helps allay the family's anxieties and concerns about the treatment while encouraging the family to support the patient.

If the family cannot or does not want to be present, the nurse should contact the family after treatments to provide information and describe the patient's response. The nurse should also encourage the family throughout the course of treatment to discuss changes they observe or questions that arise. Providing emotional support and responding to the educational needs of both patient and family are essential components of the nursing role.

> *There are many misconceptions regarding ECT. Many of these are perpetuated by movies. Observe ECT in person, then watch the movies* One Flew Over the Cuckoo's Nest, Frances, *and* Ordinary People *and critique the way in which ECT is presented.*

Informed Consent for Electroconvulsive Therapy

Before ECT treatment begins, the patient should sign an informed consent form (see Chapter 10). If the patient does not have the capacity to give consent, the document can be signed by a legally designated person. This consent acknowledges the patient's rights to obtain or refuse treatment. Although it is the physician's ultimate responsibility to explain the procedure when obtaining consent, the nurse plays an important part in the consent process.

Informed consent is a dynamic process that is not completed with the signing of a formal document; rather, it continues throughout the course of treatment. As such, it suggests a number of nursing activities. First, it is helpful if a nurse is present when the information for consent is discussed with the patient. The most appropriate nurse is one who has established a trusting and therapeutic relationship with the patient and who is best able to assess whether the patient comprehends the explanation. The presence of a nurse at this time may enable the patient to feel comfortable asking questions, and the nurse may help to simplify the language if necessary. The nurse can also ensure that the patient has been provided with a full explanation of the treatment, including its nature, purpose, and implications; understands the option to withdraw consent at any time; and has had all questions answered before signing the consent form. After the informed consent is signed, but before the beginning of treatment, the nurse should again thoroughly review this in-

formation and discuss the treatment in an open and direct manner, thus communicating that this is an accepted and beneficial form of treatment.

Certain patients pose particular challenges to the nurse when obtaining informed consent. If a patient is unable to make independent judgments and meaningful decisions about care and treatment, the nurse is responsible for acting as a patient advocate. For example, concentration is often impaired in depressed patients, so they are less likely to comprehend and retain new information. For these patients it is essential that the nurse repeat the information at regular intervals because new knowledge is seldom fully absorbed after only one explanation. Then, throughout the patient's treatment course, the nurse should reinforce what the patient already understands, provide reminders of anything that has been forgotten, and be there to answer new questions.

Pretreatment Nursing Care

Providing optimal nursing care for the patient undergoing ECT includes evaluating the pretreatment protocol to ensure that it has been followed according to hospital policy. This involves completing appropriate consultations, noting that any abnormalities in laboratory tests have been addressed, and checking that equipment and supplies are adequate and functional. The treatment nurse is responsible for ensuring that the treatment suite is properly prepared for the ECT procedure. Box 29-3 provides a list of standard equipment needed to provide optimal patient care, as designated by the APA Task Force on ECT. Although not required to be in the treatment room itself, a crash cart with defibrillator should be readily available for emergency use.

Box 29-3

Equipment for Electroconvulsive Therapy

- Treatment device and supplies, including electrode paste and gel, gauze pads, alcohol preps, saline, EEG electrodes, and chart paper
- Monitoring equipment, including ECG and EEG electrodes
- Blood pressure cuffs (two), peripheral nerve stimulator, and pulse oximeter
- Stethoscope
- Reflex hammer
- Intravenous and venipuncture supplies
- Bite blocks with individual containers
- Stretchers with firm mattress and siderails with the capability to elevate the head and feet
- Suction device
- Ventilation equipment, including tubing, masks, Ambu bags, oral airways, and intubation equipment with an oxygen delivery system capable of providing positive-pressure oxygen
- Emergency and other medications as recommended by anesthesia staff
- Miscellaneous medications not supplied by the anesthesia staff for medical management during ECT such as labetalol, esmolol, glycopyrrolate, caffeine, curare, midazolam, diazepam, thiopental sodium (Pentothal), methohexital sodium (Brevital), and succinylcholine

Because ECT is similar to a brief surgical procedure, patient preparation is similar. General anesthesia is required, so fluids should be withheld from the patient for 6 to 8 hours before treatment to prevent the potential for aspiration. The exception to this NPO status is in the case of patients who routinely receive cardiac medications, antihypertensive agents, or H_2 blockers. These drugs should be administered several hours before treatment with a small sip of water. The patient should be encouraged to wear comfortable clothing, including street clothes, pajamas, or a hospital gown, provided that it can be opened in the front to facilitate the placement of monitoring equipment. The patient should also be reminded to remove prostheses before coming to the treatment area to prevent loss or damage. This may include dentures, glasses, contact lenses, and hearing aids. The patient's hair should be clean and dry for optimal electrode contact. Hairpins, barrettes, hair nets, and other hair ornaments should also be removed for placement of electrodes.

The patient should void immediately before receiving ECT to help prevent incontinence during the procedure and to minimize the potential for bladder distention and damage during treatment.

Nursing Care During the Procedure

The patient should be brought to the treatment suite either ambulatory or by wheelchair, depending on individual need, accompanied by a nurse with whom the patient feels at ease. If possible, the nurse should remain with the patient throughout the treatment to provide support. Because there will be a number of people in the room, including a psychiatrist, the treatment nurse, and the anesthesia staff, the patient should be introduced to each member of the treatment team and given a brief explanation of everyone's role in the ECT procedure.

The patient should then be assisted onto a stretcher and asked to remove shoes and socks. This allows for the placement of a blood pressure cuff on an ankle and clear observation of the patient's extremities during the treatment. Once the patient is positioned comfortably on the stretcher, a member of the anesthesia staff inserts a peripheral intravenous line while the treatment nurse and other members of the treatment team place leads for various monitors. One member of the treatment team should explain the procedure while it is occurring.

EEG monitoring consists of two electrodes, one on the forehead and one on the left mastoid (Fig. 29-2). A set of three-lead ECGs, connected to the oscilloscope, is placed on the patient's chest. A pulse oximeter is clipped to the patient's finger to monitor oxygen saturation. Blood pressure monitoring throughout the treatment is accomplished by a manual or automatic cuff. A peripheral nerve stimulator, preferably placed on the ankle over the posterior tibial nerve, serves to determine muscle relaxation.

The treating psychiatrist or nurse cleans areas of the patient's head with mild soap at the sites of electrode contact. This cleansing process facilitates optimal stimulus electrode contact during treatment, thus eliminating the potential for skin burns and minimizing the amount of electrical stimulus needed for the treatment. The areas being cleaned will be either the forehead, if bilateral or bifrontal electrode placement is to be used, or the right temple and top of the head 1 inch to the right of the midline, if unilateral placement is used.

Once the preparation is completed, an anticholinergic agent, such as glycopyrrolate (0.1 to 0.4 mg) or atropine (0.3 to 0.6 mg) may be administered intravenously to decrease oral secretions and minimize cardiac bradyarrhythmias in response to the electrical stimulus. Next an anesthetic, usually methohexital (usual dose approximately 1 mg/kg), is administered. When the patient is asleep, the blood pressure cuff on the ankle is inflated, allowing it to serve as a tourniquet. A muscle relaxant, succinylcholine (usual dose approximately 0.75 mg/kg), is then administered to minimize the patient's motor response to the ECT treatment. Because the tourniquet is in place on one ankle, the succinylcholine is not effective in that extremity. This is a desired effect because it is used in detecting a motor response of the seizure. Progressive muscle relaxation is monitored by the nerve stimulator, as well as by observing the patient for the cessation of fasciculations. As the muscle relaxant takes effect, the anesthesiologist provides oxygen by mask to the patient through positive pressure ventilation.

Although most muscles become completely relaxed, the patient's jaw muscles are stimulated directly by the ECT, causing the patient's teeth to clench. This creates the need for a protective device, or bite block, to be inserted in the patient's mouth by the treatment nurse before the electrical stimulus. This disposable or autoclavable device prevents tooth damage and tongue or gum laceration during the stimulus. The bite block should be placed between the upper and lower teeth. The nurse should then support the patient's chin firmly against the bite block during delivery of the brief electrical stimulus. After delivery of the stimulus, the bite block may be removed.

The electrical stimulus causes a brief generalized seizure, the motor manifestations of which can be observed in the cuffed foot. Characteristic EEG changes may also be observed. One member of the treatment team records the time elapsed during the seizure. A motor seizure lasting 30 to 60

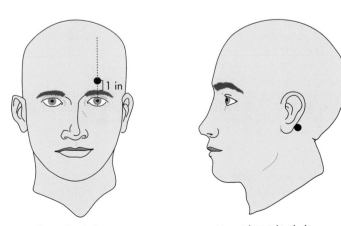

Frontal EEG lead placement   Mastoid EEG lead placement

Fig. 29-2 Electroencephalogram (EEG) electrode placement.

seconds is generally considered adequate to produce a therapeutic effect, and seizures lasting longer than 2 minutes should be terminated to prevent a prolonged post-ictal state. The seizure may be terminated by using a benzodiazepine, such as diazepam, thiopental sodium (Pentothal), or additional methohexital, given at half the induction dose. Anesthesia staff continuously ventilate the patient with pure oxygen during the procedure until the patient is able to breathe spontaneously. Vital signs should be monitored by the nurse both before and after the ECT treatment. Once the patient is stabilized, the anesthesiologist clears the patient for transfer to the recovery area.

Posttreatment Nursing Care

The recovery area should be adjacent to the treatment area to provide accessibility for anesthesia staff in case of an emergency. The area should contain oxygen, suction, pulse oximeter, vital sign monitoring, and emergency equipment. The area should be appropriately staffed and provide a minimal amount of sensory stimulation. Once in the recovery area with pulse oximeter in place, the patient should be unobtrusively observed by a staff member in close proximity until the patient awakens. At this time, the staff should be aware of the potential for falls from the stretcher caused by patient restlessness and maintain patient safety.

When the patient awakens, a nurse should discuss the treatment and check vital signs. Most patients do not remember receiving the treatment and may be confused and disoriented, similar to patients recovering from anesthesia. The nurse should provide frequent reassurance and reorientation and repeat this information at regular intervals until the patient retains it. Being post-ictal, the patient may have somewhat concrete thinking. Providing brief, distinct direction is most beneficial.

When the patient is awake and appears ready to return to the hospital room and has maintained a continuous oxygen saturation level of 90% or above, and when vital signs and mental status have returned to an acceptable level, the nurse should help to move the patient from the stretcher to a wheelchair for transport from the recovery area. When a wheelchair is used, the seatbelt should be securely fastened. The patient should be allowed to ambulate if desired.

At this time the ECT treatment nurse should convey as much information as possible about the patient's condition to the unit nursing staff. The most beneficial information includes medications given to the patient that may be evidenced in the patient's behavior or vital signs and any change in the procedure or the patient's response to treatment that may affect the patient's behavior on return to the unit. Table 29-1 identifies some common problems patients have at this time and related nursing interventions.

The nurse should assess the patient's condition to determine the level of observation required. If desired, the patient may return to bed and sleep, but the nurse should encourage eating breakfast and resuming normal activities as soon as possible. If the patient chooses to return to bed, the siderails should be in an upright position.

The patient should be observed at least once every 15 minutes; if the patient is agitated, confused, or restless, one-to-one observation may be required until the patient's condition has stabilized. Level of orientation should be assessed every 30 minutes if the patient is awake until mental status returns to baseline. If sleeping, the patient should remain undisturbed unless additional nursing intervention is warranted. Sleeping may help the patient return to baseline values more quickly.

The return of the gag reflex should be assessed before administering medication or offering breakfast to the patient. When fully awake, the patient should be observed when getting out of bed for the first time to ensure full muscle functioning after administration of muscle relaxants. Throughout the posttreatment interval, provision of support and reminders to the patient of having received ECT eliminate patient distress from posttreatment amnesia.

Potential side effects immediately after treatment that may be treated symptomatically include headache, muscle

Table **29-1**

Common Patient Problems and Nursing Interventions Related to ECT	
Patient Problem	**Nursing Interventions**
Pretreatment with beta-blockers may cause a decrease in blood pressure, pulse, or both.	Vital signs should be monitored frequently until they return to normal.
Lengthy seizures (more than 2 minutes) may increase the duration of disorientation or confusion.	Reorientation may need to be repeated for longer periods than usual.
If given a barbiturate or benzodiazepine to terminate the seizure, the patient may be more drowsy than usual.	Patient may need more time to rest after treatment.
Intensity of observation may need to be increased to prevent falls.	Nausea/vomiting creates potential for aspiration.
Increased Intensity of observation	Extended stay in the recovery area may be necessary to provide access to suctioning equipment.
Headache creates alteration in comfort.	After assessment for gag reflex return, an analgesic may be administered. If headache is a recurrent problem, a standing order for analgesia to be given as soon as possible after each treatment may be obtained. Change in activity schedule and environment to provide for a darkened room or quiet area may be necessary.

soreness, and nausea. Any confusion or disorientation is likely to be of short duration and may respond well to restricted environmental stimulation and frequent nursing contacts to remind the patient of ECT treatment and to provide reorientation. Memory loss affects primarily material that has been recently learned and information acquired during the time of the ECT treatments themselves.

Although memory loss may be distressing for the patient, the nurse should reinforce that such difficulty will pass within several weeks, with a minimal amount lasting up to 6 months. However, some information will not return, including the experience of the treatment itself and events that occurred just before the procedure, such as IV placement. In addition, events during treatment may be unclear. A summary of nursing interventions for patients receiving ECT is presented in Table 29-2.

What kind of post-ECT environment do you think would be most conducive to the patient's recovery?

Interdisciplinary Collaboration

The nurse is part of an interdisciplinary treatment team that not only administers the treatments but also collaborates to evaluate the effectiveness of ECT and recommend changes in the patient's treatment plan as appropriate. Within the team, the nurse identifies patterns of patient behavior and evaluates their implications of treatment. These include behaviors indicative of a positive treatment response such as improvement in activities of daily living; adaptive changes in social interactions with others; increases in energy, appetite, and weight; or other positive changes in target symptoms. The nurse might also report any adverse behaviors associated with ECT, including prolonged periods of confusion or disorientation, recurrent nausea or headaches, elevation in blood pressure that does not resolve within several hours after treatment, or an increase in the intensity or occurrence of target symptoms. In addition, the nurse's work with the patient's family provides information important for planning treatment.

With these clinical observations and judgments, the nurse becomes an active participant in the decision-making process regarding the patient's illness and proposed plan of care. Together the team evaluates such issues as the length of ECT treatment course, the need for alternative management strategies and adjustments in the frequency of treatments, considerations for maintenance ECT, indications for additional consultations, and other possible modifications in the treatment plan.

Give specific examples of ways in which the psychiatric nurse's role in ECT has evolved from the dependent function of implementing physicians' orders to more independent and interdependent areas of psychiatric nursing practice. How have patients benefited from this change?

Nursing Staff Education

Despite recent increases in the use of ECT and its effectiveness in the treatment of certain psychiatric illnesses, the procedure continues to elicit emotional responses from the public as well as the medical and nursing communities. Some of these responses may be positive. However, many people react negatively to ECT based on outdated ideas and procedures. It is critically important that when a patient is referred for ECT, the patient and family should be presented

Table **29-2**

Nursing Interventions for the Patient Receiving ECT		
Principle	Rationale	Nursing Intervention
Informed participation in the procedure	A patient who understands the treatment plan will be more cooperative and have less stress than one who does not; an informed family is able to provide the patient with emotional support.	Educate regarding ECT, including the procedure and expected effects; teach family about the treatment; encourage expression of feelings by patient and family; reinforce teaching after each treatment.
Biological integrity	General anesthesia and an electrically induced seizure are physiological stressors and require supportive nursing care.	Check emergency equipment before procedure; maintain NPO status several hours before treatment; remove potentially harmful objects, such as jewelry and dentures; check vital signs; maintain patent airway; assist to ambulate; offer analgesia or antiemetic as needed.
Dignity and self-esteem	Patients are usually fearful before ECT treatment; amnesia and confusion may lead to anxiety and distress; patient will need help to function appropriately.	Remain with the patient and offer support before and during treatment; maintain the patient's privacy during and after treatment; reorient the patient; help family members to understand behavior related to amnesia and confusion.

with information regarding treatment options in a balanced and unbiased manner. If a nurse has ambivalent or negative feelings about ECT, these feelings will probably be communicated to the patient and render the treatment course less effective. To function as patient advocates, nurses need to examine their attitudes and have as much information about the procedure as possible.

Educational efforts should be directed toward nurses who work on units where ECT is implemented as a treatment strategy. Programs should be developed that address both cognitive and attitudinal content because the more knowledge and clinical experience mental health professionals have with ECT, the more positive their attitude will be toward it.

Such programs might be initiated by asking staff to discuss their beliefs and feelings about ECT, including its potential therapeutic value, perceived risks, nature of the procedure itself, and ethical and legal issues concerning its use. The content can then progress to a discussion of factual material about ECT, including the rationale for the treatment, possible mechanisms of action, its efficacy relative to other treatment options, risks and side effects resulting from ECT, and current research on its indications and benefits. Time should be spent discussing the way in which the procedure has changed over the years, and all nurses should be encouraged to observe the ECT procedure as performed in their institution.

These discussions might be supplemented with written handouts, reference articles, and teaching videotapes about ECT. Finally, this information can be formalized and incorporated into the unit's daily nursing care by the establishment of nursing standards of care for patients receiving ECT and the development of a standardized nursing care plan that identifies appropriate nursing diagnoses, goals, and interventions.

In addition to informing nurses who care for patients undergoing ECT, there is a need to teach the larger nursing community about ECT. Psychiatric nurses who work with ECT can provide in-services to nurses in other clinical settings, such as geriatrics, neurology, or medicine, to dispel myths, clarify misconceptions, and provide current, accurate information.

What stereotypes did you have about ECT before reading this chapter? How have they changed, and how might this experience help you educate patients and colleagues about this treatment procedure?

PHOTOTHERAPY

Phototherapy, or light therapy, consists of exposing a patient to artificial therapeutic lighting about 5 to 20 times brighter than indoor lighting. Patients usually sit, with eyes open, about 3 feet away from and at eye level with a set of broad-spectrum fluorescent bulbs designed to produce the intensity and color composition of outdoor daylight. They then can engage in their usual activities such as reading, writing, or eating (Fig. 29-3). Light boxes currently cost between $350 and $500.

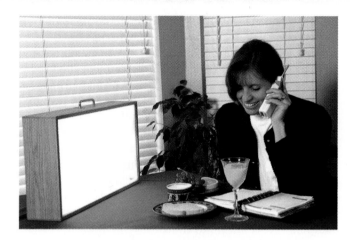

Fig. 29-3 Broad-spectrum fluorescent lamps like this one are used in daily therapy sessions from autumn into spring for people with SAD, who report feeling less depressed within 3 to 7 days. (Courtesy Apollo Light Systems.)

The most recently developed light therapy device is the light visor, a device shaped like a baseball cap and worn on the head, with the light contained in a visor portion suspended above and in front of the eyes. The obvious advantage to such a device is that it allows the person to move about while receiving treatments. However, the results of studies testing the device show great variability in effectiveness (Meesters et al, 1999; Teigher et al, 1995).

The timing and dosage of the light vary from person to person. Most literature indicates that light treatment administered in the morning is most effective (Lewy et al, 1998; Lingjaerde et al, 1998). The amount of light to which a person is exposed depends not only on the person but also on the intensity of the light source and duration of exposure. The brighter the light, the more effective the treatment per unit of time (Lee & Chan, 1999). For example, 2 hours of treatment with 2500 lux per day appears to have an antidepressant effect equal to that of 30 minutes per day at 10,000 lux (Fig. 29-4).

Light therapy appears to have important positive effects. Treatment is rapid and can be repeated. Most patients feel relief after 3 to 5 days, and they relapse equally rapidly after light treatment is stopped. Patients do not appear to develop tolerance to phototherapy, and many have used the treatment for years (Schwartz et al, 1996). Treatment can be received at home, and it need not disrupt daily routine. Light therapy also allows a person to actively participate in the treatment process, which enhances the patient's sense of control in recovering from illness (Rosenthal, 1993). However, the long-term efficacy of light therapy has not been fully evaluated.

Indications

Phototherapy has a 50% to 60% response rate in patients with well-documented, nonpsychotic winter depression or seasonal affective disorder (SAD) (Dalgleish et al, 1996). SAD is a cyclical mood disorder characterized by periods of depression that begin in October and subside in April (see

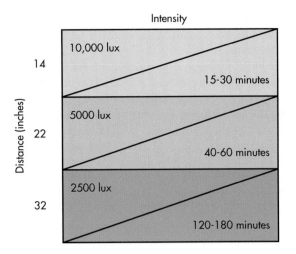

Distance versus intensity versus duration

Fig. 29-4 Timing, dosage, and exposure to light. All times are average durations and may vary with each person. *Lux,* Luminous flux density (unit of illuminance).

Chapter 20 for a full discussion of mood disorders). Although people in all latitudes can suffer from SAD, the prevalence of the disorder increases in the northernmost parts of the country. About 6% of the adult population in the United States, or 15 million people, suffer from the symptoms of SAD, which include sadness, irritability, increased appetite, carbohydrate craving, weight gain, hypersomnia, and decreased energy. In addition, 14% of Americans experience a more mild condition called "winter blues."

In a study examining predictors of response to light treatment, responders were characterized by atypical symptoms, especially hypersomnia, afternoon and evening slump, reverse diurnal variation (evenings worse), and carbohydrate craving. In contrast, nonresponders were characterized mainly by melancholic symptoms including retardation, suicidality, depersonalization, typical diurnal variation (mornings worse), anxiety, early and late insomnia, appetite loss, and guilt (Terman et al, 1996). Those with certain personality traits are also less likely to respond (Bagby et al, 1996; Reighborn-Kjennerur & Lingjaerde, 1996). Thus light therapy is a safe and satisfactory treatment for many, but may be insufficient for more severely ill patients (Ruhrmann et al, 1998; Thorell et al, 1999).

Light therapy should be administered by a professional with experience and training. It is a less conventional treatment that may be of value to patients who do not respond to drug therapy or prefer nonpharmacological treatments, or as an adjunct to drug treatments.

Mechanism of Action

Phototherapy is based on biological rhythms, particularly those related to light and darkness (see Chapter 6) (McEnany, 1996; Partonen et al, 1997) However, scientists are not sure exactly how phototherapy works. The therapeutic effect appears to be mediated primarily by the eyes, not the skin. Ongoing studies of the mechanism of phototherapy are exploring the eye itself, the way in which the eyes send messages to the brain, and the role of brain neurotransmitter systems such as serotonin and dopamine (Lee et al, 1997). It also appears that certain people may have a neurochemical vulnerability, possibly inherited, that causes them to develop SAD in the absence of adequate exposure to environmental light.

Do you think that people who experience common disturbances in body rhythms such as jet lag and shift work can be helped by phototherapy?

Adverse Effects

Side effects, when they occur, are generally mild. The most common adverse effects of phototherapy are eyestrain and headache. Others include irritability, insomnia, fatigue, nausea, and dryness of the eyes, nasal passages, and sinuses. These can usually be managed by decreasing the duration of therapy or increasing the patient's distance from the light. The long-term effects of phototherapy, if any, are currently unknown. Light therapy should be used with caution with specific ophthalmic conditions.

SLEEP DEPRIVATION THERAPY

It has been reported that as many as 60% of depressed patients improve immediately after one night of total sleep deprivation (Berger et al, 1997). Unipolar and bipolar patients appear to do equally well (Barbini et al, 1998). Although these findings have been reported in the literature, few randomized controlled clinical studies have been conducted on sleep deprivation. Furthermore, in the existing studies it is difficult to know the effect of the patient's expectations on the treatment outcome. Thus these findings should be considered with caution.

Unfortunately, many patients who respond to this therapy become depressed again when they resume sleeping even as little as 2 hours a night. This disadvantage has tended to discourage the use of sleep deprivation in clinical practice. However, there is some suggestion that improvement can be maintained if the sleep manipulation can be used repeatedly over time, such as by shifting the timing of sleep to earlier in the night, gradually advancing the time of sleep to a more acceptable schedule. For example, the patient can initially go to sleep at 5 PM and arise at 2 AM, and gradually shift those hours to 11 PM to 6 AM.

In addition, medications may help prevent relapse after sleep deprivation therapy (Kuhs et al, 1998). It is interesting to note that some antidepressants, especially the monoamine oxidase inhibitors, often interfere with sleep (see Chapter 28). This has led some researchers to wonder whether part of the efficacy of these drugs is a result of their ability to induce partial sleep deprivation.

How can a patient's expectations of a treatment influence its effectiveness? Can you think of a placebo treatment for sleep deprivation therapy that would control this problem?

Indications

Evidence suggests that depressed patients with symptoms of marked diurnal variation are most likely to improve after sleep deprivation. Patients who respond favorably to sleep deprivation also appear to have abnormally elevated night-time body temperatures. There is also some evidence that patients with seasonal affective disorder respond positively to sleep deprivation (Graw et al, 1998).

Mechanism of Action

The biological mechanisms of the antidepressant effects of sleep deprivation have not been identified. It has been hypothesized that sleep deprivation works by interrupting REM sleep (see Chapter 6). Another theory proposes that neuroendocrine changes accompanying sleep deprivation account for its antidepressant effects.

Adverse Effects

Unfortunately, sleep deprivation appears to induce mania in some patients with bipolar disorder. Thus, sleep deprivation, like some antidepressant medications, should be used with caution with patients who are susceptible to mania or have a family history of bipolar illness.

On the other hand, the knowledge that sleep deprivation may induce mania can have important preventive applications. For example, people who are biologically vulnerable to bipolar illness might monitor disruptions to their sleep caused by work schedules, travel, drugs, or other life events. Thus for vulnerable people, prevention of sleep loss at times of stress might help prevent mania.

TRANSCRANIAL MAGNETIC STIMULATION

Transcranial magnetic stimulation (TMS) is a noninvasive procedure in which a changing magnetic field is introduced into the brain to influence the brain's activity. The field is generated by passing a large electric current through a wire stimulation coil over a brief period. The insulated coil is placed on or close to a specific area of the patient's head, allowing the magnetic field to pass through the skull and into target areas of the brain (Fig. 29-5). The shape of the coil determines the properties and size of the magnetic field. A figure-of-8 shape is the most frequently used, since it is able to create a well-focused field (Fig. 29-6) (Hasey, 1999).

When the magnetic stimulus is given as a train of multiple stimuli per second, it is called repetitive transcranial magnetic stimulation (rTMS). Initially used to study various functions within the brain, such as attention, memory, and language, rTMS was also noted to change activity within the neurons. Therefore, in recent years, the technique has been studied as a potential therapeutic device for some neurological and psychiatric illnesses (George et al, 1999). When used for these indications, rTMS is administered at daily sessions. The number of sessions vary, depending on patient response.

At this point, rTMS is still experimental, and more work is in progress to determine its efficacy and safety. Studies to determine optimal treatment conditions are also underway. These include number of treatment sessions, most effective number of stimuli per second (i.e., "fast" [20 Hz] vs. "slow" [5 Hz], and modification of coil placement (i.e., left vs. right) for the treatment of specific conditions (Post et al, 1999).

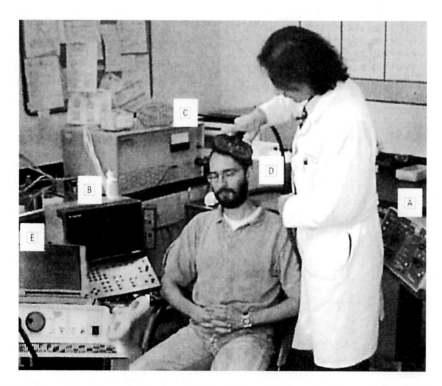

Fig. 29-5   Example of transcranial magnetic stimulation (TMS) application. (From *Arch Gen Psychiatry* 56:309-311, 1999.)

Indications

Since its inception, TMS has been studied for a number of indications. One early use of TMS was to "map" cortical areas of the brain to determine whether certain neurological functions are intact. For example, if the motor area was stimulated, a muscle movement was observed. Also, some TMS studies suggest improvement in motor symptoms of Parkinson's disease.

The most frequently cited indication in psychiatry has been the treatment of mood disorders. Imaging studies have found that depressed patients have reduced perfusion in the prefrontal cortex area of the brain, especially on the left side. The results of numerous small studies have suggested that rTMS, when administered at the left prefrontal cortex, may be an effective treatment for depression. Conversely, there is some suggestion that rTMS, administered at the right prefrontal cortex, can be helpful for mania. Additionally a few small studies have investigated the use of rTMS for the treatment of other psychiatric disorders such as schizophrenia, obsessive-compulsive disorder, and post-traumatic stress disorder. Although these studies reflect improvement for the above disorders, they have included only a small number of patients, and further work is needed in this area. At the present time there are no definitive studies describing the duration of improvement with rTMS.

Mechanism of Action

The mechanism of action of TMS is based on the principle of Faraday induction. According to this principle, when an electric current is passed through a coil, a magnetic field is generated. If another conductive material, such as a neuron in the brain, is exposed to a changing magnetic field, a second electric field is activated within that material. This activation may result in neurochemical changes based on alterations in gene expression, such as an increase in some receptor binding. Therefore, unlike ECT, in TMS the brain is **directly** stimulated to produce neurochemical changes; however, as in ECT, the exact changes that make the treatment effective are still under investigation.

Adverse Effects

The biggest concern when using rTMS is the potential for inducing seizures, even in patients with no preexisting epilepsy. Seven such cases have been described worldwide (Wasserman, 1998). Most occurred during early studies designed to test rTMS safety, and they appeared to be related to higher frequency pulses. Recommendations for treatment parameters have now been made, which should avoid further occurrences.

A second concern is the potential for tinnitus or even transient hearing loss caused by a high frequency noise produced by the treatment apparatus. This concern has prompted the routine use of ear plugs for both patient and investigator, which has minimized the occurrence of this adverse effect. The most common reported adverse effect from rTMS is the occurrence of headaches. The etiology appears to be contraction of scalp muscles during the stimulation. In most cases this discomfort resolves with standard analgesics.

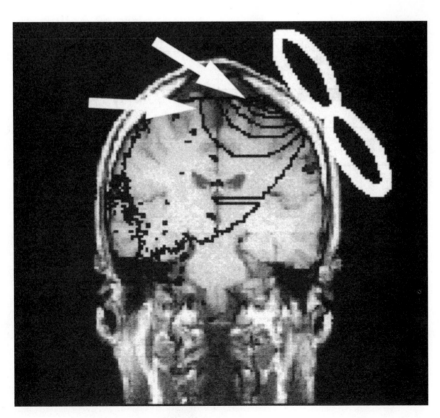

Fig. 29-6 Structural image of transcranial magnetic stimulation placement. (From *Arch Gen Psychiatry* 56:309-311, 1999.)

Mild, transient cognitive disturbances during the stimulation sessions have also been reported.

As a result of the strong (1 to 2 Tesla) magnetic fields involved in this treatment, some patients may not be candidates. These patients include those with metal objects such as screws, plates, or shrapnel anywhere in the body, unless it is known that the object will not create a problem. Patients with pacemakers or other implants that might create a low-resistance current path would also not be considered for rTMS. Patients with heart disease would be at increased risk, as would those with increased intracranial pressure because of their increased risk in the event of a seizure. Although one case of safe administration of rTMS in a pregnant woman has been reported (Nahas et al, 1999), in general, rTMS is not generally indicated in this group. Patients at increased risk for seizures owing to medication or a personal or family history of epilepsy should be considered with caution.

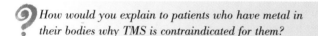

How would you explain to patients who have metal in their bodies why TMS is contraindicated for them?

VAGUS NERVE STIMULATION

Vagus nerve stimulation (VNS) is the newest of the somatic therapies currently under investigation. VNS was first studied in animals during the 1980s, when it was discovered that intermittent stimulation of the vagus nerve could be helpful in the treatment of seizures. In the 1990s, some epileptic patients receiving VNS via an implanted device reported improved mood. These reports stimulated interest in VNS as a treatment for depression. Results from a recent multicenter study, showing a 40% to 50% reduction in depressive symptoms using VNS, validates its potential as a promising new somatic therapy in psychiatry (Rush et al, 2000).

VNS involves surgically implanting a small (pocket watch-size) generator (Fig. 29-7) into the patient's chest. An electrode is threaded subcutaneously from the generator to the vagus nerve on the left side of the patient's neck. The end of the electrode is wrapped around the nerve (Fig. 29-8). Once implanted, the generator is programmed via computer for the frequency and intensity of the stimulus.

Indications

At the present time, VNS is approved only for clinical use in the treatment of epilepsy. The most compelling use in psychiatry is in the treatment of affective disorders, particularly depression. Given the multiple functions of the vagus nerve, VNS merits study in the treatment of other conditions including anxiety disorders, obesity, chronic pain syndromes, addictions, and sleep disorders (George et al, 2000). Clinical trials are currently being conducted to examine the efficacy of VNS with treatment-resistant, depressed patients.

Mechanism of Action

As with other somatic therapies, the exact mechanism of action of VNS is unknown, but thought to work via the neu-

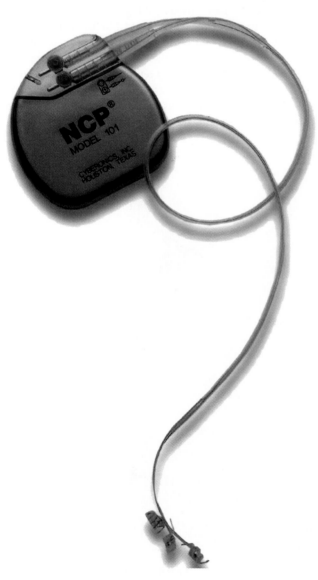

Fig. 29-7 Vagus nerve stimulation (VNS) generator. (Courtesy Cyperonics, Inc.)

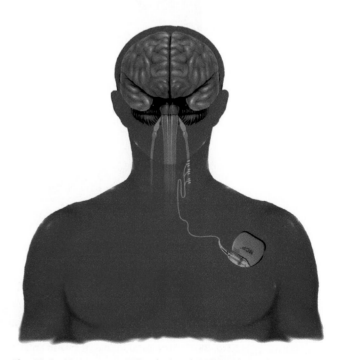

Fig. 29-8 Vagus nerve stimulation (VNS) implantation. (Courtesy Cyperonics, Inc.)

rotransmitter system. The vagus nerve has many functions; however, in this instance, the left vagus is chosen, as it is composed of mostly afferent sensory fibers. These fibers connect to brainstem and deep brain structures that are thought to be involved in epilepsy and some psychiatric disorders. Stimulation of these fibers is thought to cause changes in the function of some of these structures, as well as affecting the concentration of some neurotransmitters, such as γ-aminobutyric acid (GABA) and glutamate.

Adverse Effects

In general, reported adverse effects of VNS have been mild and tolerable. The most frequently reported adverse effect is hoarseness, which is most likely related to the stimulation. Other reported stimulation-related effects include throat pain, neck pain, headache, and shortness of breath. Other reported adverse effects are infection at the incision sites, coughing, and voice alteration. A few cases of vocal cord paralysis, lower facial muscle paresis, and an accumulation of fluid over the generator have been reported.

> *A patient with a history of chronic, severe depression asks you if she would be a good candidate for a new treatment she learned of on the Internet called vagus nerve stimulation. How would you respond?*

Summary

1. Electroconvulsive therapy (ECT) is an effective treatment for major depression, with an efficacy rate of 80% or more, which is equal to or better than response rates to antidepressant medications. It is particularly useful for people who cannot tolerate or fail to respond to treatment with medication.

2. Nursing care in ECT involves providing emotional and educational support to the patient and family; assessing the pretreatment protocol and the patient's behavior, memory, and functional ability before ECT; preparing and monitoring the patient during the actual ECT procedure; and observing and interpreting patient responses to ECT, with recommendations for changes in the treatment plan as appropriate.

3. Phototherapy, or light therapy, consists of exposing patients to bright, artificial lighting for a specified period each day. It is a treatment option for patients with nonpsychotic winter depression or seasonal affective disorder (SAD).

4. Sleep deprivation therapy has been reported to be effective with depressed patients; however, many become depressed again when they resume sleeping even as little as 2 hours a night.

5. Transcranial magnetic stimulation (TMS) consists of using a magnetic field to produce changes in brain chemistry. It is a promising new treatment for mood disorders, especially depression, and has a relatively low side effect profile.

6. Vagus nerve stimulation (VNS) is the newest of the somatic treatments. This procedure, still in experimental stages, involves surgically implanting a nerve stimulator into the patient's chest. An electrode is threaded from the generator to the vagus nerve on the left side of the patient's neck. Early studies have found this stimulation effective in relieving depressive symptoms.

Competent Caring A Clinical Exemplar of a Psychiatric Nurse

DEAN OLIVET, RN, MS, C

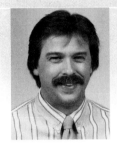

On this particular morning, I arrived at work as usual and performed all the morning rituals that a nurse does before venturing out on the clinical floor. After having several days off, I knew from reports and from listening to my co-workers that the acuity on the unit was high. Not only was the unit psychiatrically tense, but several geriatric patients had been admitted for evaluation and ECT. On a general psychiatric unit, these patients often elicit a variety of feelings from the staff, ranging from mild anxiety to downright fear. Therefore, I opted to take a few of the older, acute patients, including Mr. J, who was 80 years old.

Mr. J was newly admitted for evaluation of medications and a possible course of ECT. The staff who had contact with him described him as needy, confused, and wanting constant reassurance. At my first contact, Mr. J was asleep in his bed. He was disheveled, as was his room. I introduced myself to him and found out immediately why he seemed to have caused the staff to be anxious. He grabbed my arm and spoke to me in a high-pitched whine that anyone would want to avoid. My initial re-

action was a flight response. To resist this, I began to assess his level of independence, and it soon became clear that he was unable to make any choices with regard to planning his morning. In organizing my care, I decided to outline the morning routine for him in small time increments and assess his ability to make decisions with regard to his basic needs.

We began with his activities of daily living. Mr. J needed help to meet these physiological needs, and his anxiety level made it necessary for me to maximize his safety and security. He told me that his daughter and son had helped him the night before. He assured me that I was too busy and they would help him the next time they visited as well. My nursing pride was somewhat injured, and I was puzzled about the necessity for his family to perform what seemed to be a nursing responsibility. Nonetheless, I carried on with my care and convinced him to bathe while I cleaned up his room and made his bed. Implementing this minor intervention made me feel more comfortable in his room, and he didn't seem quite as overwhelmed.

Because his anxiety was still moderately high, I consulted with the nurse who was giving his medications and reviewed his chart. Here I learned that this was his second hospitalization, with many years free of symptoms of depression. During

Continued

Competent Caring A Clinical Exemplar of a Psychiatric Nurse—cont'd

his first hospital stay, he received a course of ECT that was very successful in helping him get well. I also learned that he was being cared for by his wife and daughter. Their treatment of choice was to medicate him until he slept. Learning this, I sensed the need to evaluate the quality of his experience with his last course of ECT, as well as the need for possible ECT and medication education for the family. These two educational needs became an ongoing process dependent on his and his family's readiness to learn.

My plan of care was quite simple. I would make sure that his activities of daily living were completed each morning, his environment kept orderly, and his introduction to the milieu made in short intervals. This was necessary to keep him safe from patients with less impulse control and avoid overwhelming him or the other patients. Mr. J needed some peer contact as well, and I introduced him to other patients as appropriate.

That afternoon his family came to visit, and I met with them to assess their need for information and their readiness to learn. I outlined Mr. J's day and apologized for his insistence that they perform his activities of daily living. I thought that perhaps they may be annoyed about this issue and was relieved when they expressed their appreciation for my interest in him.

They explained to me that I was the first person they had substantial contact with since he was admitted. In fact, they were quite upset with his condition the night before, and were considering raising the issue to staff. After listening to their concerns, I outlined my plan of care for Mr. J and explained that in my absence, the rest of the nursing staff would use the care plan to meet his daily needs. At this point, the family became an ally to the total hospital experience, and I became a resource to the patient and the family. This brought comfort to the family, which in turn allowed Mr. J to meet his basic needs and have the security to meet the challenge of recovering from his illness.

The family members were satisfied with my interventions, and a possible problematic hospital experience was averted. As nurses, we all can relate to experiences when we care for patients only to have family members complain about the care or lack of care their significant other received. We can also describe occasions when it was very rewarding to have a patient respond to our care and to have the family recognize this nursing effort. Given this dichotomy, which do you prefer? The answer really reflects the crux of good psychiatric nursing practice.

MERLIN Visit **MERLIN: www.mosby.com/MERLIN/Stuart** to find these additional materials and student activities.

- **Worksheets**
- **"Drug of the Month" Updates**
- **"Citing the Evidence" Updates**
- **Critical Thinking Activities and Exercises**
- **Annotated Suggested Readings**
- **Web Links**
- **More!**

Chapter Review Questions

1. **Identify whether the following statements are true (T) or false (F).**

____ **A.** For ECT to be effective a grand mal seizure must occur.

____ **B.** ECT cannot be followed by antidepressant medications or adverse reactions will occur.

____ **C.** There is evidence that ECT causes structural brain damage and permanent memory loss.

____ **D.** A seizure lasting 30 to 60 seconds is generally considered adequate to produce a therapeutic effect.

____ **E.** The timing and dosage of light therapy vary from person to person.

____ **F.** There is substantial research documenting the long-term effectiveness of light therapy.

____ **G.** Light therapy is particularly effective as a treatment for more severely ill patients.

____ **H.** Many patients who respond to sleep deprivation therapy become depressed again when they resume sleeping at night.

____ **I.** TMS is an invasive procedure that directly impacts the brain structures.

2. **Fill in the blanks.**

A. For affective disorders, _____ to _____ ECT treatments are normally administered.

B. For schizophrenia, as many as _____ to _____ ECT treatments may be administered.

C. The primary indication for ECT is

_____ .

D. ECT's response rate of _____ or more is equal to or better than response rates to antidepressant medications.

E. Preparation for ECT is similar to that implemented for any brief _____ procedure.

F. Potential side effects that may occur immediately after ECT that may be treated symptomatically include

_____ , _____ , and _____ .

G. Phototherapy has a _____ % to _____ % response rate in patients with winter depression or SAD.

H. Sleep deprivation appears to produce _____ in some patients with bipolar illness.

I. TMS is most frequently used for the treatment of _____ disorders.

J. _____ is the newest somatic therapy currently under investigation.

3. Provide short answers for the following questions.

A. You're talking with a nursing colleague and he asks you, "What exactly is ECT?" How would you respond?

B. ECT is often recommended for women with severe depression who are in their first trimester of a pregnancy. Why do you think this is?

C. Obtain the informed consent form used for ECT by your treatment facility. Review it for the elements described in this chapter. Try explaining the procedure to a friend or family member.

D. Review the incidence of depression among people geographically distributed in some of the most northern and southern states in the United States. Make a case for the impact of light and seasonal affective disorder among these populations.

REFERENCES

Abrams R: *Electroconvulsive therapy,* ed 3, New York, 1997, Oxford University Press.

American Psychiatric Association: *The practice of electroconvulsive therapy: recommendations for treatment, training, and privileging,* ed 2, Washington, DC, 2000, The Association.

Bagby RM et al: Seasonal and non-seasonal affective disorder and the five-factor model of personality, *J Affect Disord* 38(2-3):89, 1996.

Bailine S et al: Comparison of bifrontal and bitemporal ECT for major depression, *Am J Psychiatry* 157(1):121, 2000.

Barbini B et al: The unipolar-bipolar dichotomy and the response to sleep deprivation, *Psychiatry Res* 79:43, 1998.

Berger M, et al: Sleep deprivation combined with consecutive sleep phase advance as a fast-acting therapy in depression: An open pilot trial in medicated and unmedicated patients, *Am J Psychiatry* 154(6): 870, 1997.

Dalgleish T et al: Rhythm and blues: the theory and treatment of seasonal affective disorder, *Br J Clin Psychol* 35(pt 2): 163, 1996.

Fink P, Tasman A, editors: *Stigma and mental illness,* Washington, DC, 1992, American Psychiatric Press.

Fox H: Continuation and maintenance ECT, *J Pract Psychiatry Behav Health* 2:357, 1996a.

Fox H: Electroconvulsive therapy, an overview, *J Pract Psychiatry Behav Health* 2:223, 1996b.

George M et al: Transcranial magnetic stimulation: applications in neuropsychiatry, *Arch Gen Psychiatry* 56:300, 1999.

George M et al: Vagus nerve stimulation: a new tool for brain research and therapy, *Biol Psychiatry,* 47(4):287, 2000.

Ghaziuddin N: Use of electroconvulsive therapy in childhood psychiatric disorders, *Child Adolesc Psychopharmacol News* 3(2):1, 1998.

Graw P et al: Sleep deprivation response in seasonal affective disorder during a 40-h constant routine, *J Affect Disord* 48(1):67, 1998.

Hasey G: Transcranial magnetic stimulation: using a law of physics to treat psychopathology, *J Psychiatry Neurosci* 24(2):97, 1999.

Hermann R et al: Diagnoses of patients treated with ECT: a comparison of evidence-based standards with reported use, *Psychiatric Services* 50(8):1059, 1999.

Kellner C, McCall W: Novel electrode placements: time to reassess, *J ECT* 15(2):115, 1999.

Kellner C et al: *Handbook of ECT,* Washington DC, 1997, American Psychiatric Press.

Kuhs H et al: Repeated sleep deprivation once versus twice a week in combination with nortriptyline, *J Affect Disord* 47(1-3):97, 1998.

Lee T, Chan C: Dose-response relationship of phototherapy for seasonal affective disorder: a meta-analysis, *Acta Psychiatr Scand* 99(5):315, 1999.

Lee T et al: Pathophysiological mechanism of seasonal affective disorder, *J Affect Disord* 46(1):25, 1997.

Lewy A et al: Morning vs evening light treatment of patients with winter depression, *Arch Gen Psychiatry* 55:890, 1998.

Lingjaerde O et al: Dawn simulation vs lightbox treatment in winter depression: a comparative study, *Acta Psychiatr Scand* 98(1):73, 1998.

McEnany G: Phototherapy and sleep manipulations: an examination of two nondrug biologic interventions for depression, *J Am Psychiatr Nurses Assoc* 2:86, 1996.

Meesters Y et al: Prophylactic treatment of seasonal affective disorder (SAD) by using light visors: bright white or infrared light? *Biol Psychiatry* 46(2):239, 1999.

Nahas Z et al: Safety and feasibility of repetitive transcranial magnetic stimulation in the treatment of anxious depression in pregnancy: a case report, *J Clin Psychiatry* 60(1):50, 1999.

Partonen T et al: Suppression of melatonin secretion by bright light in seasonal affective disorder, *Biol Psychiatry* 42(6):509, 1997.

Post R et al: Repetitive transcranial magnetic stimulation as a neuropsychiatric tool: present status and future potential, *J ECT* 15(1):39, 1999.

Reighborn-Kjennerur T, Lingjaerde O: Response to light therapy in seasonal affective disorder: personality disorders and temperament as predictors of outcome, *J Affect Disord* 41(2):101, 1996.

Rey J, Walter G: Half a century of ECT use in young people, *Am J Psychiatry* 154:595, 1997.

Rosenthal N: *Winter blues: SAD—what it is and how to overcome it,* New York, 1993, Guilford.

Ruhrmann et al: Effects of fluoxetine versus bright light in the treatment of seasonal affective disorder, *Psychol Med* 28(4):923, 1998.

Rush A et al: Vagus nerve stimulation (VNS) for treatment-resistant depressions: a multicenter study, *Biol Psychiatry,* 47(4):276, 2000.

Schwartz P et al: Winter seasonal affective disorder: a follow-up study of the first 59 patients of the National Institute of Mental Health seasonal studies program, *Am J Psychiatry* 153:1028, 1996.

Shapira B et al: Cost and benefit in the choice of ECT schedule, *Br J Psychiatry* 172:44, 1998.

Teigher M et al: The phototherapy light visor: more to it than meets the eye, *Am J Psychiatry* 152:1197, 1995.

Terman M et al: Predictors of response and nonresponse to light treatment for winter depression, *Am J Psychiatry* 153:1423, 1996.

Tew J et al: Acute efficacy of ECT in the treatment of major depression in the old-old, *Am J Psychiatry* 156:1865, 1999.

Thorell L et al: Light treatment of seasonal affective disorder in combination with citalopram or placebo with 1 year follow-up, *Int Clin Psychopharmacol* 14 suppl 2:s7, 1999.

Wasserman E: Risk and safety of repetitive transcranial magnetic stimulation: report and suggested guidelines from the International Workshop on the Safety of Repetitive Transcranial Magnetic Stimulation, June 5-7,1996, *Electroencephalogr Clin Neurophysiol* 108:1,1998.

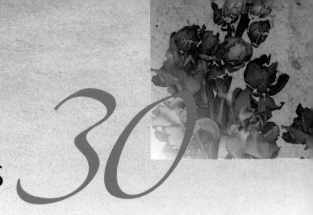

Complementary and Alternative Therapies

Therese K. Killeen

30

Through the like, disease is produced, and through the application of the like it is cured.

HIPPOCRATES, 4TH C. BC

Complementary and alternative medicine (CAM) is the term commonly used to describe a broad range of healing philosophies, approaches, and therapies that focus on the whole person, including biopsychosocial and spiritual aspects. CAM therapies are often used alone (often referred to as alternative), in combination with other CAM therapies, or in combination with other conventional therapies (sometimes referred to as complementary). Some therapies are consistent with principles of Western medicine, and others involve healing systems with a different origin. Whereas some therapies are outside the realm of accepted Western medical practice, others are becoming established in mainstream health care.

AN OVERVIEW OF CAM

People in the United States are increasingly utilizing and paying out of pocket for CAM therapies. This prompted the National Institutes of Health and Medicine (NIH) to develop a new branch called the Office of Alternative Medicine in 1992. This branch of the NIH became the National Center of Complementary and Alternative Medicine (NCCAM) in 1998. Use of CAM therapies has increased 65% from 1993 to 1997 (Eisenberg et al, 1998). Enhanced public health education has heightened health-care awareness and concern, prompting people to become more active in their health care and more willing to make lifestyle changes. CAM therapies often seem to be more available, accessible, and therefore more appealing to the health-care consumer. In addition, the benefits of CAM therapies may outweigh the barriers that are often associated with conventional therapies. For example, people identify many benefits of CAM therapy including less cost, more convenience, fewer side effects, more individualized care, and more contact with practitioners.

About 58% of all alternative therapies used in 1997 were for health promotion or disease prevention. A 1997 survey identified the most commonly used CAM therapies as chiropractic, relaxation techniques, and massage therapy. The largest increases from 1993 to 1997 were in the use of herbal medicines, massage, megavitamins, self-help groups, folk remedies, energy healing, and homeopathy (Eisenberg et al, 1998). However, the barrier between conventional and CAM therapies is a growing concern. In 1997 only 38% of people who used one or more CAM therapies discussed this with their traditional health-care provider (Austin, 1998).

This problem is an opportunity for intervention by nurses. Nurses can play an important role in educating consumers about the evidence supporting these new therapies, as well as the dangers involved in engaging in some of them, given the questions and limited information that is currently known about their safety, effectiveness, and interactions with other medications and body chemistry. But nurses can only educate consumers if they themselves have knowledge of the evidence base supporting these complementary and alternative therapies.

The NCCAM has developed a classification system of seven major categories for CAM therapies. Table 30-1 lists the seven categories, a description of each, and specific examples of CAM therapies that fall under each classification. Most CAM therapies use energy and system theories to support a rational approach to treatment. A proper balance of energy within the biopsychosocial and spiritual systems

must be maintained. The individual is an open system and exchanges energy with the environment to maintain balance and prevent illness. Illness is associated with an imbalance of energy, either deficiency or excess. The environment, as well as individual needs, are constantly changing throughout life; thus adaptation is synonymous with health.

Evidence Based Practice

Research in CAM continues to increase; however, studies with adequate scientific methodologies account for only a small amount of the research (see Critical Thinking about Contemporary Issues). Few CAM therapies claim to cure diseases; rather they propose to have therapeutic benefits on the reduction or relief of symptoms and the promotion of well-being.

Many problems occur because CAM is individualized, and thus people receive different treatments for similar

Table 30-1

NCCAM's Classification System for Complementary and Alternative Medicine		
Classification	Definition	CAM Therapy
Mind-body medicine	Involves behavioral, psychological, social, and spiritual approaches to health. Divided into four subcategories: mind-body systems, mind-body methods, religion and spirituality, and social and contextual areas.	Yoga, meditation, relaxation, imagery, hypnosis, biofeedback, spiritual healing
Alternative medical systems	Complete systems of theory and practice that have been developed outside of the Western biomedical approach. Divided into four subcategories: acupuncture and Oriental medicine, traditional indigenous systems, unconventional Western systems, and naturopathy.	Acupuncture, homeopathy
Lifestyle and disease prevention	Theories and practices designed to prevent the development of illness, identify and treat risk factors, or support the healing and recovery process. Concerned with integrated approaches for the prevention and management of chronic disease in general or the common determinants of chronic disease. Divided into three subcategories: clinical preventive practices, lifestyle therapies, and health promotion.	Exercise, stress management
Biologically based therapies	Natural and biologically based practices, interventions, and products. Many overlap with conventional medicine's use of dietary supplements. Divided into four subcategories: phytotherapy of herbalism; special diet therapies; orthomolecular medicine; and pharmacological, biological, and instrumental interventions.	Herbs, diet therapies, megavitamins
Manipulative and body-based systems	Systems based on manipulation and/or movement of the body. Divided into three subcategories: chiropractic medicine, massage and body work, and unconventional physical therapies	Chiropractic, massage, and body work, reflexology
Biofield	Systems that use subtle energy fields in and around the body for medical purposes.	Therapeutic touch, SHEN, Reiki
Bioelectromagnetics	Unconventional use of electromagnetic fields for medical purposes.	Electromagnets

symptoms. This makes it difficult to determine a specific intervention for an experimental or treatment group. Other methodological criticisms of CAM research include the small number of participants, high drop-out rates, self-report social response bias, maturation bias, selection bias, nonrandomization, and the possibility that placebo CAM therapies also produce some beneficial outcomes. Better methods of diagnosing or describing clinical characteristics of participants are also needed (Spencer & Jacobs, 1999).

There are only a modest number of well-designed CAM research studies in mental health. With the exception of certain herbal treatments such as St. John's wort for depression and kava-kava for anxiety, there are few high-quality studies of the main CAM treatments (such as acupuncture, homeopathy, herbal medicine, osteopathy, and chiropractic) for any of the major mental illnesses. Even when mental health outcomes are assessed, most research has not examined the psychiatrically ill. For example, although there are many trials showing a decrease in anxiety scores after massage, most have studied acute anxiety associated with cancer, intensive care, or surgery.

This creates a barrier for the transition of CAM outcome findings into psychiatric clinical practice. Considering that CAM interventions use mind-body approaches, it is quite surprising that research in this area is not being explored more aggressively. For example, it has been reported that 43% of survey participants used an alternative therapy for anxiety and 40% used an alternative therapy for depression. Aside from neck and back problems, more respondents used alternative therapies for depression and anxiety than for any other condition (Eisenberger et al, 1998). In another study that looked at the rates of psychiatric disorders in patients receiving complementary medical care, 69% met criteria for at least one lifetime *DSM–IV–TR* Axis I disorder, with major depression being the most common diagnosis (Davidson et al, 1998).

Still, with the increased usage of these therapies by the public and the establishment of NCCAM, more attention has been given and money made available to study the effectiveness of CAM therapies. Future research should continue to investigate and replicate promising CAM therapies using well-designed methodology.

> Many advocates of CAM therapies dispute the value of randomized controlled clinical trials and will not participate in such studies. How does this affect their acceptance by the larger community of health-care providers?

CRITICAL THINKING about CONTEMPORARY ISSUES

Does Science Play in a Role in Complementary and Alternative Health Care?

Critics of CAM claim that there is no scientific evidence to indicate that these therapeutic approaches work. This controversy is at an important juncture because it involves the potential acceptance or rejection of certain "healing" therapies by both health-care professionals and consumers. Opinions of many patients and providers are divided on whether these unproven treatments can or ever will be cost-effective, accessible, and medically useful and safe. Yet in recent years, this criticism has become somewhat outdated as research into these treatment modalities is increasing in the United States. In addition, much research in this area has been published in other countries, but this has often been discounted or ignored by the U.S. medical community.

It is important to differentiate between complementary approaches that truly represent alternatives and those that are simply unusual. From a cultural historical perspective, approaches that have no value probably would have died out a long time ago. Conversely, unusual approaches tend to have no cultural traditions. Typically, such approaches are associated with a few people who are unwilling or unable to scientifically replicate their results. To date, complementary approaches that have been validated by contemporary science are generally those with long cultural histories.

Finally, one of the most important ways CAM will be accepted and integrated into conventional medicine is through the use of an evidence based approach. This process assumes (1) that an adequate scientific methodology is in place, (2) that any treatment effects are measured and are clinically meaningful, and (3) that some application can be made to clinical practice (Spencer & Jacob, 1999). Evidence to enlighten and inform clinical practice is the starting point and ending point of this engaging controversy.

Ethical Issues

Ethical concerns about CAM therapies include issues of safety and effectiveness, as well as the expertise and qualifications of the practitioner. Of equal importance is the communication between CAM and traditional health-care providers. As cited in the Alternative Medicine Use National Survey, less than 40% of CAM therapies used were disclosed to the patient's physician. This is particularly dangerous with regard to drug and herb interactions. For example, it has been shown that the herbal product, St. John's wort, lowers blood levels of protease inhibitors, thereby decreasing their effectiveness by an average of 57%. This increases the chances that HIV-positive patients who are taking protease inhibitors would not respond to treatment (Piscitelli et al, 2000).

There is also the possibility that symptoms relieved by CAM therapies may mask signs of serious illnesses causing delays in seeking conventional, evidence based treatment. Other concerns are related to effective symptom management, potential for drug interactions, possible side effects, and the lack of regulation of herbal products for purity and potency. Because herbal products are unregulated, the consumer has no guarantee of the ingredients in the herbal product. This increases the likelihood of adverse effects and drug interactions. Finally, care needs to be taken when medications that affect absorption, distribution, metabolism, and elimination are used with herbal products. For example, ginkgo biloba may interact with aspirin or warfarin to prolong bleeding times, thus potentially placing the patient with bleeding disorders in jeopardy (Borins, 1998).

Given these concerns, the nurse who refers a patient to a CAM practitioner needs to explore the options, as well as the health risk-benefit ratios. Local and state regulatory boards, other health regulatory agencies, and consumer affair departments can also provide information about practitioner qualifications such as licensure, education, accreditations, and complaints that may have been filed. Table 30-2 provides information health consumers should consider when trying to decide on a complementary or alternative therapy (NCCAM, 2000).

The following sections describe the most common evidence based CAM therapies that have been used for some of the major psychiatric disorders.

DEPRESSION

Depression is one of the most common conditions for which people use alternative therapies (see Citing the Evidence). A review of the most beneficial CAM therapies for depression found there was evidence to support the use of exercise, herbal therapy, acupuncture and massage therapy (Ernst et al, 1998).

Herbal Products

One of the most widely researched herbal products is hypericum (St. John's wort). It is currently used throughout Europe and the United States to treat mild to moderate depression, anxiety, seasonal affective disorder, and sleep disorders. The herb's mechanism of action may involve monamine oxidase inhibition and possible serotonin, dopamine, and norepinephrine reuptake inhibition. There may also be some inhibitory effect on interleukin-6 activity, thereby reducing regulatory hormones.

The herb is available in tea, capsule, or tincture form, standardized to contain 0.3% hypericin (one of the purported active ingredients). The standard dose is 300 mg three times a day. Side effects are minimal and include dry mouth, dizziness, gastrointestinal symptoms, and photosensitivity. Drug interactions have been reported and hypericum should not be taken with other antidepressants. A 2-week wash-out period is recommended before initiating another antidepressant. In a recent small study a clinically significant drug interaction between hypericum and indinavir was discovered. Seven healthy males were given thera-

---

Citing the Evidence on

Comparing Therapies for Depression

BACKGROUND: This survey of subscribers to *Consumer Reports* was conducted to compare standard and complementary therapies for depression. A total of 46,806 individuals completed the survey.

RESULTS: In all, 85% of respondents with depression tried prescriptive medication, which was rated the most effective treatment. Exercise was seen as the second most effective treatment. Of the 30% of people who tried St. John's wort, most thought the herbal remedy helped only a little if at all. Exercise, diet, and meditation were said to be more helpful for depression than herbal therapy.

IMPLICATIONS: St. John's wort helped fewer patients for depression than expected, given the public and medical press attention given to this therapy. Diet, aerobic exercise, and resistance exercise, however, did appear to enhance mood.

The mainstreaming of alternative medicine, *Consumer Reports*, May: 17, 2000.

Table 30-2

Approaching Complementary and Alternative Therapies

- Ask a health-care provider about the safety and effectiveness of the desired therapy or treatment. Information can also be found in current publications and on the website of the NCCAM at the National Institutes of Health and Medicine.
- Contact a state or local regulatory agency with authority over practitioners who practice the therapy or treatment being sought. CAM usually is not as regulated as the practice of conventional medicine; but licensing, accreditation, and regulatory laws are increasingly being implemented. Check to see if the practitioner is licensed to deliver the identified services.
- Talk with those who have had experience with this practitioner, both health-care providers and other patients. Find out about the confidence and competence of the practitioner, and whether there have been any complaints from patients.
- Talk with the practitioner in person. Ask about education, additional training, licenses, and certifications, both conventional and unconventional. Find out how open the practitioner is to communicating with patients about technical aspects of methods, possible side effects, and potential problems.
- Visit the practitioner's office, clinic, or hospital. Ask how many patients are typically seen in a day or week, and how much time is spent with each patient. Look at the conditions of the office or clinic. The primary issue here is whether the service delivery adheres to regulated standards for medical safety and care.
- Find out what several practitioners charge for the same treatment to get a better idea about the appropriateness of costs. Regulatory agencies and professional associations may also provide cost information.
- Most important, discuss all issues regarding therapies and treatments with your usual health-care provider, whether a practitioner of conventional or alternative medicine. Competent health-care management requires knowledge of both conventional and alternative therapies for the provider to have a complete picture of your treatment plan.

peutic doses of indinavir, a protease inhibitor, sufficient to achieve a therapeutic blood concentration. When hypericum was added, blood concentrations of indinavir dropped an average of 57% below the therapeutic range (Piscitelli et al, 2000).

A meta-analysis of 23 randomized controlled trials using hypericum for depression compared it with placebo and tricyclic antidepressants. There was significantly greater improvement in the hypericum group compared with the placebo group and similar improvement with the antidepressant group (Ernst et al, 1998). Methodological flaws in this study were the variability of hypericum preparations used and the nature of the short-term clinical trial (4 to 8 weeks). No studies have yet been reported comparing St. John's wort to the selective serotonin reuptake inhibitors or other newer antidepressants, but the NCCAM is currently funding a large national 3-year study comparing hypericum with placebo and sertraline.

Other herbal products such as tryptophan, melatonin, and valerian have been used successfully to promote sleep in patients with depressive disorders. Tryptophan, an essential amino acid and precursor of serotonin, has been banned from sale in the United States after a contaminated batch was discovered.

Melatonin, a hormone secreted by the pineal gland, works by synchronizing circadian rhythms. In a recent small, double-blind, randomized controlled trial, improvement in sleep using slow-release melatonin (2.5 to 10 mg) plus antidepressant therapy (fluoxetine, 20 mg) was shown to be superior to antidepressant therapy plus placebo (Dolberg et al, 1998). Although research is scant, valerian may have a mild sedative effect by its action on γ-aminobutyric acid (GABA) receptors. The dosages used are 300 to 1200 mg at bedtime or 2 to 3 g of the dried root three times a day. Side effects are possible potentiation of other central nervous system depressants, blurred vision, headache, nausea, and excitability (Wong et al, 1998).

Another dietary supplement, s-adenosyl-methionine (SAMe), has been marketed in other countries for the treatment of depression and is now available in the United States Only a few small, older, short-term clinical trials have appeared in the literature. A meta-analysis of six placebo-controlled studies using SAMe concluded that SAMe was more effective than placebo and as effective as several tricyclic antidepressants for the treatment of major depression. The usual oral dose for the treatment of depression is 200 to 800 mg twice a day, with most studies using 1600 mg a day. The side effect profile was equivalent to that for placebo. A major drawback is that a month's supply of a 1600 mg per day dose cost $228 (*Med Lett*, 2000).

> *Conduct an informal survey of your friends and family. How many of them have taken St. John's wort? Were they aware that in a Los Angeles Times survey, 3 out of 10 brands of St. John's wort had no more than half the potency listed on the label? As a nurse, how would you advise them?*

Acupuncture

Acupuncture involves the insertion of needles into acupoints located along the body's meridians for the purpose of restoring energy balance. It is believed that acupuncture may stimulate the synthesis and release of endorphins, serotonin, and norepinephrine. In several randomized control trials, electroacupuncture was as effective in reducing depression as the tricyclic antidepressant, amitriptyline (Ernst et al, 1998). Another study using a double-blind procedure found that the group receiving specific or real acupuncture had significantly less depression after 8 weeks than the control groups given nonspecific acupuncture or no treatment (Allen, 1999). Finally, a randomized controlled study from China showed electroacupuncture to be as effective as amitriptyline, a tricyclic antidepressant, in reducing depression. Specifically, electroacupuncture produced significantly better changes in anxiety, somatization, cognitive processing, and reactive depression. In addition, electroacupuncture had a lower side effect profile (Luo et al, 1998). No studies currently exist comparing acupuncture to the newer antidepressants.

Exercise

Exercise has been investigated over the years for its positive benefits on mood. Physical exercise in the form of muscular strength training, flexibility training, and cardiovascular aerobic endurance has been associated not only with positive medical benefits but with improvement in mood and self-esteem, decreased tension, and a feeling of accomplishment and renewed energy. Numerous studies suggest that levels of depression are lower in exercise groups compared with control groups, and that this effect increases with the duration of therapy (Ernst et al, 1998).

Massage

Only a few controlled studies have evaluated the effects of massage therapy for the treatment of depression. One study looked at children and adolescents receiving either 30-minute back massages or watching a relaxing video for 5 days. The massage group had lower depression and anxiety ratings, improvements in sleep, less fidgety behavior, and lower saliva cortisol levels. However, these effects were short term.

Another study done by the same investigator randomized 32 depressed adolescent mothers to receive either massage therapy or relaxation therapy over 5 weeks. By the end of treatment, the massage therapy group reported less anxiety and depression, displayed less anxious behavior, and had lower cortisol levels than the relaxation group (Field et al, 1996). None of these studies compared massage with established medication or psychotherapy treatments.

> *What physiological changes are stimulated by massage therapy? How might these relate to one's thoughts and emotions?*

ANXIETY

Anxiety disorders are one of the major reasons people use CAM therapies (Astin, 1998). Anxiety disorders that have been investigated using CAM therapies include generalized anxiety disorders, social and specific phobias, panic disorder, obsessive-compulsive disorder (OCD), and posttraumatic stress disorder (PTSD).

Relaxation

Relaxation techniques are an accepted therapeutic strategy (see Chapter 32). Progressive muscle relaxation (PMR) uses a process of tensing and releasing groups of muscles starting from facial muscles and moving down the body to the muscles in the feet. Individuals learn the systematic technique and gain control over anxiety provoking thoughts and muscle tension.

PMR has also been used in conjunction with imagery, breathing retraining, autogenic training, and biofeedback. In a randomized, controlled study using PMR on medicated and nonmedicated individuals with insomnia, those receiving PMR experienced a significant improvement in anxiety and sleep efficiency and quality, and reduced their use of sleep medication by 80% (Lichstein et al, 1999).

Another relaxation technique, mindfulness meditation, has been found to be beneficial in generalized anxiety and panic disorders. Mindfulness meditation, a technique for gaining control over emotions, involves an intentional suspended awareness of the present-moment experience without reaction, judgment, or partiality. In a 3-year follow-up study of 18 patients who participated in an 8-week mindfulness medication group, significant improvement was maintained with regard to anxiety and depression scores, as well as severity and frequency of panic attacks (Miller et al, 1995).

Therapeutic Touch

Although not investigated in psychiatric populations, therapeutic touch has been shown to reduce anxiety in nonpsychiatric populations. Therapeutic touch involves the intentional exchange of energy between the practitioner and patient to promote healing and well-being. The use of the hands is the conduit for the energy exchange. This intervention is proposed to work by eliciting the relaxation response.

Therapeutic touch has been embraced by nursing in all areas of practice and is probably one of the most widely researched interventions in the nursing literature. More recent studies have shown some alterations in immunoglobulin levels and decreased percentage of suppressor T cells with the use of therapeutic touch (Clark, 1999).

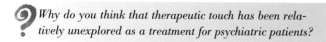

Why do you think that therapeutic touch has been relatively unexplored as a treatment for psychiatric patients?

Yoga

Several types of yoga have been used for stress and anxiety disorders. Yoga is a physical and emotional conditioning of the body through a series of postures, stretching exercises, breath control, and meditation. A randomized study using one type of yoga, kundalini yoga (KY), was found to have efficacy in treating OCD. This intervention consisted of eight primary and three nonmandatory KY techniques. One technique, requiring participants to perform left nostril breath-

ing, was suggested to be specific for OCD. At the end of 3 months, participants in the KY group had a significant improvement (38% reduction) in their symptoms compared with a control group receiving relaxation response and mindfulness meditation (14% reduction). When the groups were merged at 3 months and all participants received KY, a 15-month follow-up study showed a 71% reduction in obsessive-compulsive symptoms for all participants. Specifically after receiving KY, the original control group had a 44% reduction. The investigators also noted that these improvements were superior to several placebo-controlled, double-blind medication trials (Shannahoff-Khalsa et al, 1999).

Herbal Products

Several herbs are marketed for the relief of anxiety, but few have been empirically studied. Kava-kava is proposed to have anxiolytic, sedative, and muscle relaxant properties. A kava product standardized for 70% kava pyrone content was used in a randomized, placebo-controlled 25-week outpatient trial with 101 outpatients suffering various anxiety disorders. Statistically significant improvements in anxiety were seen in the kava group versus the control group at all follow-up assessments starting at 8 weeks. The only possibly related side effect reported was "stomach upset." Thus, kava may be better tolerated than other pharmacological agents presently used for anxiety disorders. The dosage used in this study was 90 to 110 mg of the 70% kava pyrone extract given three times a day (Volz & Kieser, 1997).

Eye Movement Desensitization and Reprocessing

Eye movement desensitization and reprocessing (EMDR) is a relatively new intervention that requires the patient to generate a number of rapid lateral eye movements while engaging in imaginal recall of significant aspects of a particular traumatic memory or feared stimuli. This therapy is based on the observations that spontaneous multiple eye movements combined with a number of traditional cognitive behavioral procedures is associated with attempts to diffuse negative emotions and cognitions.

A critique of EMDR studies for PTSD reported that four of ten studies revealed EMDR to be superior to no treatment in patient self-report behavioral rating scales, structured clinical interviews, and heart rate reactivity to combat-related sounds. Positive effects were also reported in panic disorder and public speaking anxiety. Two studies supported the effectiveness of EMDR compared with other therapies (i.e., relaxation with or without biofeedback, image habituation therapy, standard mental health care) in PTSD and anxiety symptom distress at follow-up assessment (Shapiro, 1999). However, another study found that a cognitive behavioral treatment called trauma treatment protocol (TTP) was significantly more effective than EMDR in the treatment of PTSD pathology, and these effects were more pronounced at 3-month follow-up evaluation (Devilly & Spence, 1999). One specific problem involved with conducting EMDR research includes maintaining treatment fidelity or making sure all parts of the procedure are implemented correctly.

SUBSTANCE USE DISORDERS

Acupuncture

One of the most widely researched CAM therapies for addiction is acupuncture. Many chemical dependency programs in the United States use acupuncture as an additional therapy. The National Acupuncture Detoxification Association has trained thousands of individuals on the standard auricular acupuncture procedure (Fig. 30-1). This procedure has been used with reported success in one New York clinic since 1975. In 1997 a consensus panel for the National Institutes of Health and Medicine stated that there was sufficient evidence to support the possibility that acupuncture may be effective for the treatment of addictions.

Although numerous studies have been done, acupuncture has the same methodological problems seen in other CAM research. Inconsistent dosage levels, high drop out rates, inability to keep the acupuncturist unaware of treatment groups and finding comparable control groups are but a few of the criticisms of acupuncture research for the treatment of addiction. Most studies on the use of acupuncture for cocaine and other substance use disorders have failed to detect differences between experimental (real) and control (sham) acupuncture groups.

Yoga

Only one study has compared hatha yoga with psychodynamic therapy. The interventions were delivered for 5 months in a group setting to methadone-maintained patients. Both groups showed reduction in both drug use and criminal activity (Shaffer et al, 1997).

Biofeedback

Some small studies have investigated the use of biofeedback for the treatment of addictions. Biofeedback is an intervention in which physiological responses such as heart rate, skin conductance, skin temperature, muscle activity, and neural activity are monitored for the purpose of teaching the patient to regulate these processes. Often patients engage in relaxation exercises to decrease activation of these physiological responses. One of the best designed studies randomized patients to receive transcendental meditation (TM), electromyographic biofeedback (BF), neurotherapy (NT), or routine therapy alone (RT) for the treatment of alcoholism. The NT and RT groups were the control groups. Outcome results 18 months after treatment showed significant increases in the number of nondrinking days for the TM and BF groups but not for the NT or RT groups (Taub et al, 1994).

EATING DISORDERS

Bulimia nervosa is a disorder of affect and anxiety dysregulation, and an inability to self-soothe. In a group of 50 patients who met criteria for bulimia nervosa, guided imagery interventions were significantly more effective in reducing binge and purge frequencies and eating disorder psychopathology, and improved ability to self-soothe at the end of 6 weeks of treatment (Esplen et al, 1998). More research is needed in this area.

DEMENTIAS

Gingko biloba is another herbal product that has been studied in psychiatric populations for its cognitive enhancing effects. Two well-designed studies using gingko biloba in patients with dementia of the Alzheimer's type, multi-infarct, or vascular dementias showed small but significant improvements in cognitive performance and social functioning (Wong et al, 1998). The dosage used was 40 mg three times per day in one study and 120 mg twice a day in the other. Side effects are rare but include headache, gastrointestinal tract upset, and skin allergy. There are some reports that gingko may potentiate the effects of anticoagulants.

NURSING IMPLICATIONS

CAM therapies can have an important impact on psychiatric nursing practice. They are beneficial, safe, cost-effective, and easily implemented throughout psychiatric settings. Confrontive interventions for the management of behavioral problems in the psychiatric population are often ineffective and frustrating for both patients and nurses. Yet nurses on psychiatric inpatient units using CAM therapies report better patient compliance, as well as a more relaxed, manageable milieu (Gurevich et al, 1996).

Most CAM therapies can be prescribed and implemented by nurses. Nurses should continue to follow the research literature to track the emerging evidence regarding the effectiveness of these therapies. Another valuable resource is the Cochrane Collaboration, which has an ongoing registry of randomized clinical trials related to CAM that can be accessed over the Internet. With its holistic framework, nursing is in an ideal position to gain ownership of many CAM therapies for the management of symptoms experienced by psychiatric populations. In addition, CAM therapies that empower the patient can play an important part in strengthening the nurse–patient partnership.

Summary

1. Complementary and alternative medicine is the term used to describe a broad range of nontraditional healing philosophies, approaches, and therapies. CAM can be de-

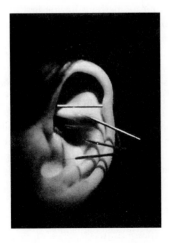

Fig. 30-1 Auricular acupuncture points.

livered alone or in combination with conventional therapies. Well-designed CAM research studies in mental health and psychiatric disorders are rare. Ethical concerns include issues of safety and effectiveness, the expertise and qualifications of the practitioner, and communicating the use of CAM therapies to the traditional health-care provider.

2. Evidence based CAM therapies for various psychiatric disorders include herbal products, acupuncture, exercise, massage, relaxation, therapeutic touch, yoga, eye movement desensitization and reprocessing, and biofeedback.

3. CAM therapies can be used by psychiatric nurses and potentially have a significant impact on their practice.

Competent Caring A Clinical Exemplar of a Psychiatric Nurse

PAULA E. JOHNSON, MSN, RN, CS

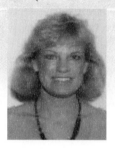

As a psychiatric nurse who has spent 15 years working in academic medical centers and 5 years in private psychotherapy practice, I have had the opportunity to study, personally experience, and offer to my patients many therapeutic modalities that are not commonly found in traditional or conventional health-care settings. I have come to appreciate the value and power of these practices commonly known as "alternative" therapies. I rarely use the term alternative therapy, however, because I do not see my work as precluding other forms of therapy. I believe that the most effective therapy incorporates an alternative perspective and includes rather than excludes the use of appropriate conventional treatments.

Early in my own personal quest for physical and mental wellness, I was drawn to the practices of yoga, meditation, and conscious breathing. Later in nursing school, I was given the opportunity to experience and investigate other holistic approaches to health care including therapeutic touch and guided imagery. After graduation, my interest and excitement in alternatives continued to grow. I pursued certification in reflexology, Reiki, transformational breathing, and the self-inquiry work of Byron Katie. With each of these alternative therapies, I first experience and apply it in my own life. Eventually, I bring those techniques that have a positive impact on my own health and wellness to my patients, the majority of whom enjoy similar results.

For example, after years of meditation practice, I began to incorporate the use of conscious breathing and mindfulness into my time with my patients. My intention is to pass onto them the healing effects of calmness, presence, and relaxation that I have experienced. In simple and clear ways, I talk with them about the power of conscious awareness and instruct them in how to use the breath to consciously bring themselves into the present moment and to increase their realization of what they are experiencing within their bodies. I have observed that when patients grow in their personal awareness of their internal experience, they are better able to express their feelings, are more likely to pay attention to early symptoms of distress and take appropriate action, and eventually are more comfortable in their body.

I recently worked with a woman who was experiencing marital and job-related stress and severe anxiety. I noticed that every sentence she spoke contained within it some projection into the future. "I won't be able to stand it if he doesn't change." "My boss will never appreciate what I do for him and the company." When I asked how she feels when she has these thoughts she said she felt tremendous fear. I suggested some homework in between sessions. I simply asked her to check in with herself throughout the day, notice her breathing, and for a few minutes practice being totally present in the moment. The following week she told me that she had never before realized just how little of her time is spent fully aware in the present moment. I observed her growing attention and even excitement as she learned to acknowledge and report her internal experiences. As she continued to apply this practice more and more in her everyday life, she reported that her husband seemed to be changing, she had started to ask her boss for what she wants, and she was feeling more in control of her own life.

Through this and many similarly powerful experiences with alternative modalities, I came to see that these practices to which I seemed to have been drawn were in fact not alternative to me but rather more closely resonating with my own nature than many of the conventional approaches. I am now able to distinguish more clearly between what is normal and what is natural, and to assist my patients in making that distinction for themselves.

More and more I find myself choosing to offer those alternative therapies that self-empower and give patients responsibility for their own healing and wellness. Through the practice of alternative therapies with my patients, I have come to know the tremendous benefits of shared common experience. Many of the patients I work with in private practice speak to me of the pain and suffering of anxiety, depression, mood swings, and addiction—all responses to life situations that I can find within myself. When I am able to recognize and acknowledge our common human condition, I no longer feel separate from them. This recognition never compromises our nurse–patient relationship. In fact, it actually creates an opening where we can truly communicate, perhaps for the first time.

Alternative therapies offer an approach to creating and maintaining health that is often not available in a conventional health-care setting. Yet this growing field of practices is perhaps nothing more than the manifestation of our growing conscious awareness of ourselves and how we exist in the universe. As I see it, the greatest benefit for patient and therapist is the opportunity to experience a relationship that honors and respects, listens and hears, and is open to all possibilities.

As nurses we can begin by looking within ourselves for the answers. To believe that we have reached the pinnacle of development in health care, that the physical world is all there is, or that we are separate from each other is to live in a myth. Whether it is an alternative therapy or a more conventional one, our full presence in the here and now makes the difference. This is where true healing begins.

MERLIN Visit **MERLIN: www.mosby.com/MERLIN/Stuart** to find these additional materials and student activities.

- **Worksheets**
- **"Drug of the Month" Updates**
- **"Citing the Evidence" Updates**
- **Critical Thinking Activities and Exercises**
- **Annotated Suggested Readings**
- **Web Links**
- **More!**

Chapter Review Questions

1. **Identify whether the following statements are true (T) or false (F).**

_____ **A.** In the United States fewer people are using CAM therapies because of rising concern over safety issues.

_____ **B.** There are relatively few scientific studies of CAM in patients with major psychiatric illnesses.

_____ **C.** Herbal products are not regulated for purity and potency.

_____ **D.** St. John's wort can be safely taken with other antidepressants.

_____ **E.** Mindfulness meditation has been found to be beneficial in generalized anxiety and panic disorders.

_____ **F.** Acupuncture has been found to be effective in treating cocaine and other substance use disorders.

2. **Fill in the blanks.**

A. _____ is the term used to describe a broad range of healing philosophies, approaches, and therapies that focus on the whole person.

B. The National Institutes of Health and Medicine (NIH) established the National Center of Complementary and Alternative Medicine (NCCAM) in _____.

C. _____ is the most common herbal alternative therapy used for depression.

D. A hormone secreted by the pineal gland that works by synchronizing circadian rhythms is called _____.

E. The process of tensing and releasing groups of muscles in the body is called _____.

F. _____ involves the intentional exchange of energy between the practitioner and patient to promote healing and well-being.

G. The most commonly used herbal product for anxiety is _____.

H. _____ is an herbal product that has been studied in psychiatric populations for its cognitive enhancing effects.

3. **Provide short answers for the following questions.**

A. Give three reasons why CAM therapies are seen as desirable by many people.

B. Identify four ethical concerns related to CAM therapies.

C. Describe the proposed mechanism of action of acupuncture.

4. **Critical Thinking Questions**

1. Why do you think there are relatively few scientific studies of CAM in patients with psychiatric illnesses? What strategies could be used to overcome this problem?

2. Analyze why it is dangerous for patients not to let their primary health-care provider know whether they are using CAM.

3. Why is it difficult to conduct a double-blind study using acupuncture?

4. Describe the physiology and neurobiology that may account for the antidepressant effect of exercise.

5. Why might the intervention of therapeutic touch be distressing to psychotic patients?

REFERENCES

Allen J: Innovative study shows acupuncture promising as depression treatment, *Psychiatric News,* August 6, 1999.

Astin J: Why patients use alternative medicine: results of a national study, *JAMA,* 279 (19):1548, 1998.

Borins M: The dangers of using herbs: what your patients need to know, *Postgrad* 104(1): 91, 1998.

Clark C: Concepts and issues. In Clark CC, editor: *Encyclopedia of complementary health practice,* New York:, 1999, Springer.

Davidson J et al: Psychiatric disorders in primary care patients receiving complementary medical treatments. *Compr Psychiatry* 39(1):16, 1998.

Devilly G, Spence S: The relative efficacy and treatment distress of EMDR and a cognitive-behavior trauma treatment protocol in the amelioration of posttraumatic stress disorder, *J Anxiety Disord* 13(1-2):131, 1999.

Dolberg O et al: Melatonin for the treatment of sleep disturbances in major depressive disorder, *Am J Psychiatry* 155(8):1119, 1998.

Eisenberg D et al: Trends in alternative medicine use in the United States, 1990-1997: results of a follow-up national survey, *JAMA* 280(18):1569, 1998.

Ernst E et al: Complementary therapies for depression: an overview, *Arch Gen Psychiatry* 55(11):1026, 1998.

Esplen M et al: A randomized controlled treatment of guided imagery in bulimia nervosa, *Psychol Med* 28:1347, 1998.

Field T et al: Massage and relaxation therapies' effects on depressed adolescent mothers, *Adolescence* 31(124):903, 1996.

Gurevich M et al: Is auricular acupuncture beneficial in the inpatient treatment of substance-abusing patients? *J Subst Abuse Treat* 13(2):165, 1996.

Lichstein, K et al: Relaxation to assist sleep medication withdrawal, *Behav Modif* 23(3):379, 1999.

Luo H et al: Clinical research on the therapeutic effects of the electroacupuncture treatment in patients with depression, *Psychiatry Clin Neurosci* 52(suppl):S338, 1998.

Miller J et al: Three-year follow-up and clinical implications of a mindfulness meditation-based stress reduction intervention in the treatment of anxiety disorders, *Gen Hosp Psychiatry* 17:192, 1995.

National Center for Complementary and Alternative Medicine: what is CAM? *http://altmed.od.nih.gov/nccam/what-is-cam,* 2000.

Piscitelli S et al: Indinavir concentrations and St. John's wort, *Lancet* 355:547, 2000.

SAMe for depression, *Med Lett* 41(1065): 107, 2000.

Shannahoff-Khalsa D et al: Randomized controlled trial of yogic meditation techniques for patients with obsessive-compulsive disorder, *CNS Spectrums* 4(12):34, 1999.

Shaffer H et al: Comparing hatha yoga with dynamic group psychotherapy for enhancing methadone maintenance treatment: a randomized clinical trial, *Altern Ther Health Med* 3(4):57, 1997.

Shapiro F: Eye movement desensitization and reprocessing (EMDR) and the anxiety disorders: clinical and research implications of an integrated psychotherapy treatment, *J Anxiety Disord* 13(1-2):35, 1999.

Spencer J, Jacobs J: *Complementary/alternative medicine: an evidence-based approach.* St. Louis, 1999, Mosby.

Taub E et al: Effectiveness of broad-spectrum approaches to relapse prevention in severe alcoholism: a long-term randomized, controlled trial of transcendental meditation, EMG biofeedback and electronic neurotherapy, *Alcoholism Treatment Q* 11(1-2):187, 1994.

Volz H, Kieser M: Kava-kava Extract WS 1490 versus placebo in anxiety disorders: a randomized placebo-controlled 25 week outpatient trial, *Pharmacopsychiatry* 30:1, 1997.

Wong A et al: Herbal remedies in psychiatric practice, *Arch Gen Psychiatry* 55:1033, 1998.

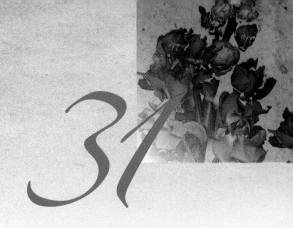

Preventing and Managing Aggressive Behavior

Christine Diane Hamolia

3

LEARNING OBJECTIVES

After studying this chapter the student should be able to:

- Discuss the prevalence of aggressive behavior among psychiatric patients and reasons for its increase
- Compare passive, assertive, and aggressive behavioral responses
- Describe five theories on the development of aggressive behavior
- Identify factors useful in predicting aggressive behavior among psychiatric patients
- Assess patients for aggressive behavioral responses
- Analyze nursing interventions for preventing and managing aggressive behavior
- Develop a patient education plan to promote patients' appropriate expression of anger
- Describe the implementation of crisis management techniques
- Evaluate the need for staff development related to educating staff, working with staff who have been assaulted, and understanding legal implications

TOPICAL OUTLINE

Dimensions of the Problem
Behavioral Responses
  Passive Behavior
  Assertive Behavior
  Aggressive Behavior
Theories on Aggression
  Psychological
  Sociocultural
  Biological
Predicting Aggressive Behavior
Nursing Assessment
Nursing Interventions
  Self-Awareness
  Patient Education
  Assertiveness Training
  Communication Strategies
  Environmental Strategies
  Behavioral Strategies
  Psychopharmacology
Crisis Management Techniques
  Team Response
  Seclusion
  Restraints
  Terminating the Intervention
Staff Development
  Education
  Staff Assault

Healthy children raised in decent conditions among loving people in a gentle and just society where freedom and equality are valued will rarely commit violent acts toward others.

RAMSAY CLARK, *A FEW MODEST PROPOSALS TO REDUCE INDIVIDUAL VIOLENCE IN AMERICA*

Nurses provide care for patients with many types of problems. People who enter the health-care system are often in great distress and may exhibit maladaptive coping responses. Nurses who work in settings such as emergency rooms, critical care areas, and trauma centers often care for people who respond to events with angry and aggressive behavior that can pose a significant risk to themselves, other patients, and health-care providers. Thus preventing and managing aggressive behavior are important skills for all nurses.

Psychiatric nurses in particular work with patients who have inadequate coping mechanisms for dealing with stress. Patients admitted to an inpatient psychiatric unit are usually in crisis, so their coping skills are even less effective. During these times of stress, acts of physical aggression or violence can occur. It is also true that nurses spend more time with patients on an inpatient unit than any other mental health

professional. Thus they are more likely to be involved in preventing and managing aggressive behavior and are more at risk for being victims of acts of violence by patients. For these reasons, it is critical that psychiatric nurses be able to assess patients at risk for violence and intervene effectively with patients before, during, and after an aggressive episode.

DIMENSIONS OF THE PROBLEM

High rates of assaultive behavior have been reported in a variety of health-care settings including outpatient clinics, nursing homes, and emergency departments. By far the highest rates of assault occur in psychiatric settings. Studies have found that 75% of all psychiatric nursing staff have been assaulted at least once in their careers (Poster, 1996). Although most assaults occur in inpatient settings, nurses in outpatient mental health settings are also at high risk for violence (Lewis & Dehn, 1999). Injury rates from violence in public sector psychiatric settings are alarmingly high across nursing employment categories, particularly among male technicians, male staff, and on-unit supervisory personnel (Love & Hunter, 1996).

There are many explanations for the increasing incidence of violent behavior in psychiatric settings. First, as more emphasis is placed on outpatient and partial hospital treatment programs in the community, an increasing number of patients referred for inpatient care are hospitalized because they display aggressive or dangerous behavior. Before patients can be committed to the hospital, most states require evidence that patients are dangerous to themselves or others (see Chapter 10). This results in a larger proportion of aggressive and violent patients on inpatient units (Tardiff et al, 1997). Second, the nature of the inpatient milieu has changed because of increasing patient acuity and shortened lengths of stay. In addition, economic constraints have resulted in fewer nurses assigned to inpatient units. Finally, evolving legal directives and perplexing ethical issues challenge the use of chemical and mechanical restraints and raise questions regarding patients' rights to refuse treatment and the nature of the least restrictive environment. This often results in conflict and confusion for inpatient staff, who try to manage patients effectively.

> *Members of different disciplines sometimes have different views on how to manage aggressive behavior. Talk with nurses and physicians who care for psychiatric patients about their personal experiences and clinical judgments regarding this problem.*

BEHAVIORAL RESPONSES

Within each person lies the capacity for passive, assertive, and aggressive behavior. In a threatening situation the choices are to be passive and fearful and to flee, to be aggressive and angry and to fight, or to be assertive and self-confident and to confront the situation directly. The situation and the characteristics of the people involved determine the appropriate response.

Passive Behavior

Passive people subordinate their own rights to their perception of the rights of others. When passive people become angry, they try to hide it, thereby increasing their own tension. If other people notice the anger by observing nonverbal cues, passive people are unable to confront the issue. This can also increase their tension. This pattern of interaction can seriously impair interpersonal growth. The following clinical example illustrates passive behavior.

 CLINICAL EXAMPLE

Ms. J was a staff nurse on a busy surgical unit. She enjoyed her work and liked the patients. She also placed a high value on getting along with her co-workers. Other staff members always spoke positively of her. Ms. C, the head nurse, valued Ms. J as an employee, stating particularly, "She's not like the rest of them. She never complains."

Ms. J made it a practice never to refuse a request made by a patient or another staff member. If a patient who was assigned to another nurse asked her to explain his diet or straighten his bed, she would do so, even if she was then behind in her own work. She never asked for help from others because she felt that her assignment was her responsibility. If a co-worker asked to change days off with her, Ms. J always agreed, even if she had plans, rationalizing that the other person probably had more important plans.

Ms. C began to sense a tenseness when she was around Ms. J. Because she could not think of any problem at work, she assumed that Ms. J must have been having a problem at home. She was concerned and asked Ms. J if she could help. To her amazement, Ms. J recited a long list of angry feelings related to the work situation. Ms. C then felt guilty when she realized that she and the other staff members had been taking advantage of Ms. J.

Although Ms. J had thought that she was acting in a healthy way, she was actually negating her own needs and diminishing her self-respect. Her co-workers, who superficially liked her, in reality felt uncomfortable with her because they were never allowed to reciprocate when she had been helpful. Ms. C's guilty response quickly changed to anger when she realized that she had been a victim of Ms. J's passivity. If Ms. J had informed Ms. C of her feelings, she would have treated her more equitably.

Passivity is also expressed nonverbally. The person may speak softly, often in a childlike manner. There is little eye contact. The person may be slouched in posture, with arms held close to the body.

Sarcasm is another indirect expression of anger. This usually provokes anger in the person who is the target. It is different from assertive behavior because it usually infringes on the rights of the other. A sarcastic remark generally conveys the message "You are not worthy of my respect." Sarcasm may be disguised as humor. Confrontation may then be responded to with a disclaimer such as "Can't you take a joke?" Humor that derogates another person is hostile and is indulged in for the purpose of self-enhancement. It tends to backfire because the joker is revealed as insecure.

Assertive Behavior

Assertiveness is at the midpoint of a continuum that runs from passive to aggressive behavior. Assertive behavior conveys a sense of self-assurance but also communicates respect for the other person. Assertive people speak clearly and distinctly. They observe the norms of personal space appropriate to the situation. Eye contact is direct but not intrusive. Gestures emphasize speech but are not distracting or threatening. Posture is erect and relaxed. The overall impression is that the person is strong, but not threatening.

Assertive people feel free to refuse an unreasonable request. However, they will share their rationale with the other person. They will also base the judgment about the reasonableness of the request on their own priorities. On the other hand, assertive people do not hesitate to make a request of others, assuming that they will inform them if their request is unreasonable. If the other person is unable to refuse, assertive people will not feel guilty about making the request.

Assertiveness also implies communicating feelings directly to others. As a result, anger is not allowed to build up, and the expression of feeling is more likely to be in proportion to the situation. If dissatisfaction is verbalized, the reason for the feeling is included. Assertive people also remember to express love to those to whom they are close. Compliments are given when deserved. Assertion also involves acceptance of positive input from others.

Aggressive Behavior

At the opposite end of the continuum from passivity is aggression. Aggressive people ignore the rights of others. They assume that they must fight for their own interests, and they expect the same behavior from others. Life is a battle. An aggressive approach to life may lead to physical or verbal violence. The aggressive behavior often covers a basic lack of self-confidence (Bushman & Baumeister, 1998). Aggressive people enhance their self-esteem by overpowering others and thereby proving their superiority. The next clinical example describes aggressive behavior.

 ## CLINICAL EXAMPLE

Suzy was a 9-year-old girl brought to the child psychiatric clinic by her mother on referral from the school nurse. She was described as a tomboy who loved active play and hated school. She was the first girl to make the neighborhood Little League baseball team and had proved her right to be there by beating up several male team members. Suzy was sent to the clinic after the teacher caught her forcing younger children to give her their lunch money.

When Suzy came to the clinic, she presented a facade of toughness. She did not deny her behavior and explained it by saying that the "little kids don't need much to eat anyway. I let them keep some of the money." Suzy was saving money for a new baseball glove. When she was asked about school, she said angrily, "I'm not dumb. I could learn that junk, but who needs it? I just want to play ball."

Psychological testing revealed that Suzy's IQ was slightly below average. She attended school with a group of upper-middle-class college-bound children. Even in fourth grade she was feeling insecure and unable to compete. She masked her insecurity with her bullying behavior, striving for acceptance in sports, where she did have ability. The medical diagnosis was conduct disorder, undersocialized, aggressive. When Suzy's problem was explained to her parents and the school, some of the pressure for academic achievement was alleviated. Her parents spent extra time helping her with her homework. Also, she was given genuine recognition for her athletic ability, demonstrated by the gift of a new baseball glove. Suzy gradually responded to the positive input from others by developing a sense of positive regard for herself. As she did so, she no longer needed to bully other children and began to grow into some real friendships.

Aggressive adults are not unlike Suzy. They try to cover up their insecurities and vulnerabilities by acting aggressive. The behavior is self-defeating because it drives people away, thus reinforcing the low self-esteem and vulnerability to rejection.

Aggressive behavior is also communicated nonverbally. Aggressive people may invade personal space. They may speak loudly and with great emphasis. They usually maintain eye contact over a prolonged period of time so that the other person experiences it as intrusive. Gestures may be emphatic and often seem threatening (for example, they may point their finger, shake their fists, stamp their feet, or make slashing motions with their hands). Posture is erect, and often aggressive people lean forward slightly toward the other person. The overall impression is one of power and dominance. Table 31-1 summarizes the major characteristics of passive, assertive, and aggressive behaviors.

> *Do you use passive, assertive, or aggressive behaviors most often in your personal life? How does this compare with your professional life as a nursing student?*

THEORIES ON AGGRESSION

It is useful for nurses to view aggressive and violent behavior along a continuum with verbal aggression at one end and physical violence at the other. Violence is the result of extreme anger (rage) or fear (panic). Specific reasons for aggressive behavior vary from person to person. Nurses need to communicate with patients to understand the events that

Table **31-1**

Comparison of Passive, Assertive, and Aggressive Behaviors

	Passive	Assertive	Aggressive
Content of speech	Negative Self-derogatory "Can I?" "Will you?"	Positive Self-enhancing "I can," "I will"	Exaggerated Other-derogatory "You always," "You never"
Tone of voice	Quiet, weak, whining	Modulated	Loud, demanding
Posture	Drooping, bowed head	Erect, relaxed	Tense, leaning forward
Personal space	Allows invasion of space by others	Maintains a comfortable distance; claims right to own space	Invades space of others
Gestures	Minimal, weak gesturing, fidgeting	Demonstrative gestures	Threatening, expansive gestures
Eye contact	Little or none	Intermittent, appropriate to relationship	Constant stare

they perceive as anger-provoking. In general, anger occurs in response to a perceived threat. This may be a threat of physical injury or, more often, a threat to the self-concept. When the self is threatened, people may not be entirely aware of the source of their anger. In this case, the nurse and patient need to work together to identify the nature of the threat.

A threat may be external or internal. Examples of external stressors are physical attack, loss of a significant relationship, and criticism from others. Internal stressors might include a sense of failure at work, perceived loss of love, and fear of physical illness. Anger is only one of the possible emotional responses to these stressors. Some people might respond with depression or withdrawal. However, those reactions are usually accompanied by anger, which may be difficult for the person to express directly. Depression is sometimes viewed as anger directed toward the self, and withdrawal may also be a passive expression of anger.

Anger often seems out of proportion to the event. An insignificant stressor may be "the last straw" and result in the release of a flood of feelings that have been stored up over time. Nurses need to be aware of this and not personalize anger expressed by a patient. The nurse may seem to be a safer target than significant others with whom the patient may also be angry.

A number of theories on the development of aggressive behavior have influenced the treatment of violent patients. They can be categorized as psychological, sociocultural, and biological. Current thinking in the field suggests that aggressive behavior is the result of the interaction among all three and that each of these factors must be considered when determining nursing care.

Psychological

One psychological view of aggressive behavior suggests the importance of predisposing developmental or life experiences that limit the person's capacity to select nonviolent coping mechanisms. Some of these experiences are listed in Box 31-1. They may limit a person's ability to use supportive relationships, leave the person very self-centered, or make the person particularly vulnerable to a sense of injury that can easily be provoked into rage. It has also been suggested that a disruption in the mother-infant bonding process can lead to the development of poor interpersonal behavior that may increase the likelihood of violent behavior. When combined with neurological deficits, the risk of violent behavior is increased (Rainee et al, 1997). Fig. 31-1 shows how these factors can contribute to an intergenerational transmission of violent behavior. Box 31-2 presents background information about the patient that may also be associated with violence.

Social learning theory proposes that aggressive behavior is learned through the socialization process as a result of internal and external learning. Internal learning occurs through the personal reinforcement received when enacting aggressive behavior. This may be the result of achieving a desired goal or experiencing feelings of importance, power, and control. For example, 4-year-old Johnny wants a cookie just before dinner. When his mother refuses, Johnny has a temper tantrum. If his mother then gives him a cookie, Johnny has learned that an aggressive outburst will be rewarded and he

will get what he wants. If similar situations occur, Johnny will continue to use an aggressive approach.

External learning occurs through the observation of role models such as parents, peers, siblings, and sports and entertainment figures. Sociocultural patterns that lead to the imitation of aggressive behavior suggest that violence is an acceptable way of solving problems and achieving social status. According to this view, activities such as violent crime, aggressive sports, and war depicted through the media or witnessed in person reinforce aggressive behavior.

Sociocultural

Social and cultural factors may also influence aggressive behavior. Cultural norms help to define acceptable and unacceptable means of expressing aggressive feelings. Sanctions are applied to violators of the norms through the legal system. By this means, society controls violent behavior and attempts to maintain a safe existence for its members. Unfortunately, this prohibition against violent behavior may also be extended to include any expression of anger. This can inhibit people from the healthy expression of angry feelings and lead to other maladaptive responses. A cultural norm that supports verbally assertive expressions of anger will help people deal with anger in a healthy manner. A norm that reinforces violent behavior will result in physical expression of anger in destructive ways.

Finally, a number of studies have attempted to explore the influences of race, culture, economics, and environmental factors on violent behavior. Physical crowding and heat appear to be related to violent behavior. Other social determinants of violence are linked in a cycle and include (Tardiff, 1996):

- Poverty and the inability to have basic necessities of life
- Disruption of marriages
- Production of single-parent families
- Unemployment
- Difficulty in maintaining interpersonal ties, family structure, and social control

Biological

Current neurobiological research has focused on three areas of the brain believed to be involved in aggression: the limbic system, the frontal lobes, and the hypothalamus (Fig. 31-2).

Box 31-1

Developmental Factors Limiting Use of Nonviolent Coping Techniques

- Organic brain damage, mental retardation, or learning disability, which may impair capacity to deal effectively with frustration
- Severe emotional deprivation or overt rejection in childhood, or parental seduction, which may contribute to defects in trust and self-esteem
- Exposure to violence in formative years, either as a victim of child abuse or as an observer of family violence, which may instill a pattern of using violence as a way to cope

From Menninger W: Management of the aggressive and dangerous patient, *Bull Menninger Clin* 57:208, 1993.

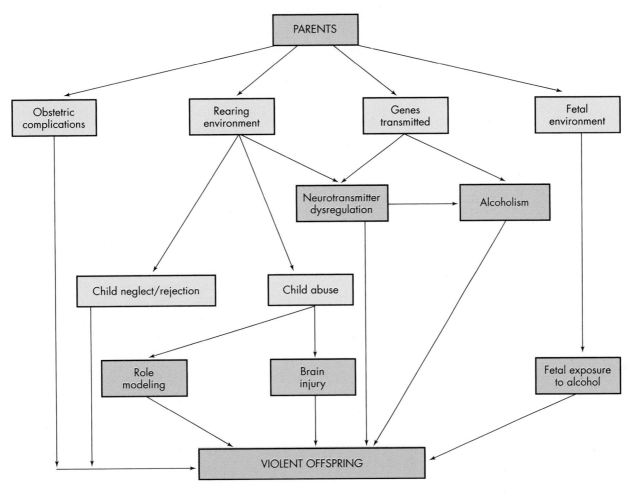

Fig. 31-1 Intergenerational transmission of violence. (From Volavka J: The neurobiology of violence, *J Neuropsychiatry Clin Neurosci* II(3):307, 1999.)

Neurotransmitters have also been suggested as having a role in the expression or suppression of aggressive behavior (Niehoff, 1999; Volavka, 1999). Each of these areas is described in more detail in Chapter 6.

The limbic system is associated with the mediation of basic drives and the expression of human emotions and behaviors such as eating, aggression, and sexual response. It is also involved in the processing of information and memory. Synthesis of information to and from other areas in the brain influences emotional experience and behavior. Alterations in functioning of the limbic system may result in an increase or decrease in the potential for aggressive behavior. In particular, the amygdala, part of the limbic system, mediates the expression of rage and fear. The surgical removal of this region makes aggressive wild rhesus monkeys docile and lethargic, unable to respond to threats to their safety. Perhaps in those prone to violence, the amygdala may be overresponsive, perceiving threats where there are none.

The frontal lobes play an important role in mediating purposeful behavior and rational thinking. They are the part of the brain where reason and emotion interact. Damage to the frontal lobes can result in impaired judgment, personality changes, problems in decision making, inappropriate conduct, and aggressive outbursts. The hypothalamus, at the base

Box 31-2

Background Information Associated with Violent Behavior

- Childhood cruelty to animals or other children
- Fire setting or similar dangerous actions
- Recent violent behavior toward self or others
- Recent accidents, threats, or poor judgment in potentially dangerous situations
- Altered states of consciousness
- Escalating irritability, sensitivity, or hostility
- Fear of losing control
- Efforts to obtain help
- Bothering family, neighbors, or police
- History of abuse of alcohol or other disinhibiting substances

From Menninger W: Management of the aggressive and dangerous patient, *Bull Menninger Clin* 57:208, 1993.

of the brain, is the brain's alarm system. Stress raises the level of steroids, the hormones secreted by the adrenal glands. Nerve receptors for these hormones become less sensitive in an attempt to compensate, and the hypothalamus tells the pituitary gland to release more steroids. After repeated stimulation, the system may respond more vigorously to all provocations. That may be one reason why traumatic stress in childhood may permanently enhance one's potential for violence.

Neurotransmitters are brain chemicals that are transmitted to and from neurons across synapses, resulting in communication between brain structures. An increase or decrease in these substances can influence behavior. Changes in the balance of these compounds can aggravate or inhibit aggression. There has been a suggestion that low levels of the neurotransmitter serotonin are associated with irritability, hypersensitivity to provocation, and rage. People who commit impulsive arson, suicide, and homicide have lower than average levels of 5-HIAA, the breakdown product of serotonin, in their spinal fluid.

Other neurotransmitters often associated with aggressive behaviors are dopamine, norepinephrine, and acetylcholine, and the amino acid γ-aminobutyric acid (GABA). For example, animal studies indicate that increasing brain dopamine and norepinephrine activity significantly enhances the likelihood that the animal will respond to the environment in an impulsively violent manner (Kavoussi et al, 1997)

Findings related to a gene associated with violent behavior are inconclusive. There is also conflicting evidence on whether men with high testosterone levels are more aggressive or prone to violence than others. Current understanding of the neurobiology of aggressive behavior is just beginning, and more research is needed on the delicate balance of neurotransmitters and the influence of environmental forces on neurochemistry and brain function.

PREDICTING AGGRESSIVE BEHAVIOR

Researchers have tried to determine which patients are more likely to become violent. Demographic variables such as age, sex, race, marital status, education, and socioeconomic level have not been useful in predicting violent behavior. In contrast, psychiatric diagnosis has often been correlated with assaultiveness. However, the ability of this variable to predict violence is complicated by the fact that many patients have more than one diagnosis. In addition, patients may have different clinical symptoms depending on the severity and acuity of their illness. Thus a patient's diagnosis is suggestive at best. In general, research indicates that two populations of patients are at increased risk of violence (Borum et al, 1996; Steinert et al, 1999):

- Patients with **active psychotic symptoms**, particularly those related to perceived threat or overriding of internal controls, such as delusions of thought control.
- Patients with **substance abuse disorders**. The prevalence of violence is 12 times greater for those with alcohol abuse or dependence and 16 times greater for those with other drug dependence compared with those with no psychiatric diagnosis. Comorbid substance abuse has an added effect in increasing the risk of violence for people with major psychiatric disorders.

Recent research efforts have focused on identifying clinical variables that are predictors of violence. The best single predictor of violence appears to be a history of violence (Tardiff, 1998). The quality of the initial therapeutic alliance may also be linked to the risk of violent behavior (see Citing the Evidence). Research also suggests that perhaps mental illness is not a risk factor for violence at all, and that mentally ill persons who commit acts of violence do so for the same reasons as persons without mental illness who become violent. In fact, psychopathic and antisocial personality traits are proving to be more predictive of violent behavior than mental illness (Harris & Rice, 1997; Nolan et al, 1999).

Situational and environmental factors can also be important in escalating patient behavior from dangerous to violent. These factors include aspects of the physical facilities and the presence of staff and other patients (Owen et al,

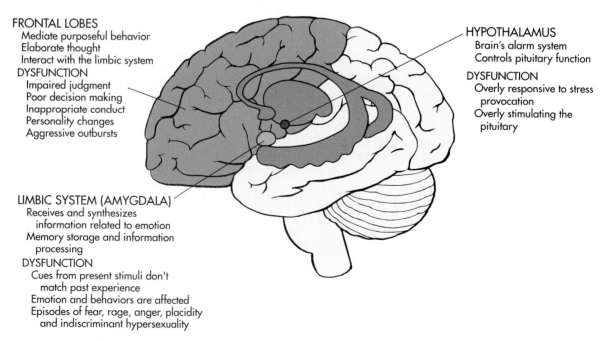

FRONTAL LOBES
Mediate purposeful behavior
Elaborate thought
Interact with the limbic system
DYSFUNCTION
Impaired judgment
Poor decision making
Inappropriate conduct
Personality changes
Aggressive outbursts

LIMBIC SYSTEM (AMYGDALA)
Receives and synthesizes
information related to emotion
Memory storage and information
processing
DYSFUNCTION
Cues from present stimuli don't
match past experience
Emotion and behaviors are affected
Episodes of fear, rage, anger, placidity
and indiscriminant hypersexuality

HYPOTHALAMUS
Brain's alarm system
Controls pituitary function
DYSFUNCTION
Overly responsive to stress
provocation
Overly stimulating the
pituitary

Fig. 31-2 Structures of the brain implicated in aggression.

1998; LePage et al, 2000; Lanza et al, 1997). For example, several studies have found that the number of violent incidents is greater when patients move or gather in groups, are overcrowded, lack privacy, or are inactive. Clinicians may also intentionally or inadvertently precipitate an outbreak of violence because staff attitudes and behavior have a powerful impact on patient behavior (Morrison, 1998; Ray & Subich, 1998). Staff provocation and inexperience, poor milieu management, close physical encounters, inconsistent limit setting, and a norm of violence may all negatively affect the inpatient environment (Lanza et al, 1994).

Finally, a patient's appraisal of the situation and level of perceived environmental, cognitive and communication stress also affect one's response. When an environment is interpreted as hostile, the response is likely to be hostile in return. Those suffering from psychiatric illness, substance abuse, past traumatic experiences, or brain damage may have distorted perceptions that can lead to aggressive responses. A model for the development of aggression in inpatient settings that incorporates these various factors is presented in Fig. 31-3.

 What role do you think culture plays in the expression and interpretation of aggressive behavior?

NURSING ASSESSMENT

Although researchers have made progress in determining reliable predictors of violence, a completely accurate predic-

---

Citing the Evidence on

The Therapeutic Alliance and Risk of Violence

BACKGROUND: Evaluation of patients' potential for violence is an important component of care in psychiatric emergency and inpatient settings. This study examined the interpersonal context in which violence occurs by assessing the quality of the initial therapeutic alliance between the psychiatrist and the patient.

RESULTS: Patients who had a poorer therapeutic alliance with their physician at the time of admission were significantly more ready to display violent behavior during hospitalization.

IMPLICATIONS: The results suggest a new class of situational-interactional variables, reflected in the quality of the therapeutic relationship, that may be useful in evaluating patients' potential for violence. Similar work should be done exploring the nurse-patient alliance.

Beauford J et al: Utility of the initial therapeutic alliance in evaluating psychiatric patients risk of violence. *Am J Psychiatry* 154(9):1272, 1997.

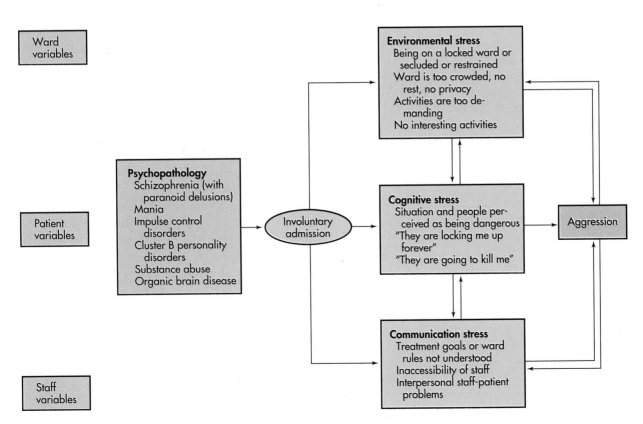

Fig. 31-3 Model of inpatient aggression. (From Nijman H et al: A tentative model of aggression on inpatient psychiatric wards, *Psychiatr Serv* 50[6]:832, 1999.)

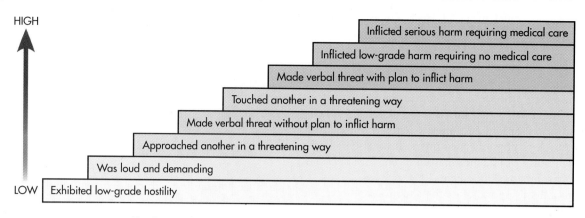

Fig. 31-4 Hierarchy of aggressive and violent patient behaviors.

Box 31-3

Behaviors Associated with Aggression

MOTOR AGITATION

Pacing
Inability to sit still
Clenching or pounding fists
Jaw tightening
Increased respirations
Sudden cessation of motor activity (catatonia)

VERBALIZATIONS

Verbal threats toward real or imagined objects
Intrusive demands for attention
Loud, pressured speech
Evidence of delusional or paranoid thought content

AFFECT

Anger
Hostility
Extreme anxiety
Irritability
Inappropriate or excessive euphoria
Affect lability

LEVEL OF CONSCIOUSNESS

Confusion
Sudden change in mental status
Disorientation
Memory impairment
Inability to be redirected

tion of patient violence is not possible (McNiel & Binder, 1995). For this reason it is important for psychiatric nurses to be alert for symptoms of increasing agitation that could lead to violent behavior (Haber et al, 1997). Using a hierarchy of aggressive behaviors by which to evaluate patients (Fig. 31-4) in which lower levels of aggression may lead to more violent behavior may be helpful. Some of these early behaviors include motor agitation such as pacing, inability to sit still, clenching or pounding fists, and tightening of jaw or facial muscles. There also may be verbal clues such as threats to real or imagined objects or intrusive demands for

attention. Speech may be loud and pressured, and posture may become threatening.

Another critical factor in the assessment of a potentially violent patient is the affect associated with escalating behaviors. Anger often is seen in patients who are imminently violent. Inappropriate euphoria, irritability, and lability in affect may indicate that a patient is having difficulty in maintaining control. Changes in level of consciousness may also be an indication of future violent behavior (Box 31-3).

In summary, psychiatric nurses should carefully assess all patients for their potential for violence. A screening or assessment tool such as the one presented in Fig. 31-5 can be useful. Other behavior rating scales used to assess aggressive behavior are listed in Box 31-4. Once completed, a violence assessment tool can help the nurse:

- Establish a therapeutic alliance with the patient
- Assess a patient's potential for violence
- Develop a plan of care
- Implement the plan of care
- Prevent aggression and violence in the milieu

Following the assessment, if the patient is believed to be potentially violent the nurse should:

- Implement the appropriate clinical protocol to provide for patient and staff safety
- Notify co-workers
- Obtain additional security if needed
- Assess the environment and make necessary changes
- Notify the physician and assess the need for PRN medications

NURSING INTERVENTIONS

The nurse can implement a variety of interventions to prevent and manage aggressive behavior. These interventions can be thought of as existing on a continuum (Fig. 31-6). They range from preventive strategies such as self-awareness, patient education, and assertiveness training to anticipatory strategies such as verbal and nonverbal communication, environmental changes, behavioral interventions, and the use of medications. If the patient's aggressive behavior escalates despite these actions, the nurse must implement crisis management techniques including seclusion and restraints.

ASSAULT AND VIOLENCE ASSESSMENT TOOL

Description: This tool is used if a patient
    a. Has a history of violence
    b. Is currently threatening violence
    c. Was threatening violence at the time of the referral

Directions: a. Assess each key factor.
    b. Circle one (of three) descriptor for each factor that best describes the patient.
    c. Add the points for each circled item to obtain the total score.

Key Factors	High Risk	Moderate Risk	No Precautions
History of Violence	Any single episode of violence with injury to others while hospitalized -OR- Multiple assaults with injury while outside hospital **2**	Destruction of property without injury to others while in hospital -OR- A single assault outside the hospital resulting in injury -OR- Multiple assaults outside the hospital not resulting in injury **1**	Violence only when using drugs or alcohol -OR- Destruction of property outside hospital -OR- No history of violence **0**
History of Recent Aggression	Physically threatening at time of referral/admission **2**	Verbally threatening at time of referral/admission **1**	Nonthreatening at time of referral/admission **0**
History of Aggression in Family of Origin	Victim or perpetrator of physical or sexual abuse **2**	Witness of physical or sexual abuse **1**	Witness or victim of verbal aggression -OR- No history of aggression in family **0**
Substance Abuse Status	Recent alcohol/substance abuse actively detoxing -OR- Currently under the influence of alcohol or drugs **2**	Recent substance/alcohol abuse with absence of withdrawal symptoms **1**	Rehabilitated abuser -OR- No history of alcohol/substance abuse -OR- Past history (>3 months ago) alcohol/substance abuse with no rehabilitation **0**
Paranoia/Hostility	Paranoia or hostility generalized to people in the immediate environment **2**	Paranoia or hostility generalized toward inaccessible people **1**	No apparent paranoia No apparent hostility **0**
Impulsivity	Physically impulsive **2**	Verbally impulsive -OR- History of physical impulsivity **1**	No apparent impulsivity **0**
Agitation	Psychomotor agitation with constant pressured physical activity **2**	Psychomotor agitation with intermittent bursts of hyperactivity **1**	No apparent psychomotor agitation **0**
Sensorium	Disoriented with impaired memory **2**	Oriented with impaired memory **1**	Oriented with intact memory **0**

Scoring Key
    9 or more   =   High-risk precautions
    3-8   =   Moderate-risk precautions
    0-2   =   No precautions

Total Score: _____

Assessed by (RN): _____

Date: _____

Time: _____

Fig. 31-5 Assault and violence assessment tool.

Self-Awareness

The most valuable resource of a nurse is the ability to use the self to help others. To ensure the most effective use of self, it is important to be aware of personal stress that can interfere with one's ability to communicate therapeutically with patients. If the nurse is tired, anxious, angry, or apathetic, it will be difficult to convey an interest in the concerns and fears of the patient. Furthermore, if the nurse is overwhelmed with personal problems, the energy available for patients is greatly reduced.

When dealing with potentially aggressive patients, it is important to be able to assess the situation objectively despite the positive or negative countertransference that might be present. Countertransference is an emotional reaction to some aspect or behavior of the patient (see Chapter 2). Negative countertransference reactions are a significant factor in the occurrence of violence in hospitals. To prevent this situation the nurse must demonstrate ongoing self-awareness and supervision with the goal of separating personal needs from those of the patient.

Patient Education

Teaching patients about communication and the appropriate way to express anger can be one of the most successful interventions in preventing aggressive behavior (see the Patient Education Plan). Many patients have difficulty identifying their feelings, needs, and desires and even more difficulty communicating these to others. Teaching patients that feelings are not right or wrong or good or bad can allow them to explore feelings that may have been bottled up, ignored, or repressed. The nurse can then work with patients on ways to express their feelings and evaluate whether the responses they select are adaptive or maladaptive. Providing patients with available choices in managing anger, such as those listed in Box 31-5, may be effective in reducing more restrictive interventions (Visalli et al, 1997).

Assertiveness Training

Teaching assertive communication skills is an important nursing intervention (see Chapter 32). Interpersonal frustrations often escalate to aggressive behavior because patients

Box 31-4

Behavioral Rating Scales Related to Aggression

- Brown-Goodwin Assessment for Life History of Aggression
- Buss-Durkee
- Hostility Inventory
- Hostility and Direction of Hostility Questionnaire
- Overt Aggression Scale

have not mastered the assertive behaviors. Assertive behavior is a basic interpersonal skill that includes the following:

- Communicating directly with another person
- Saying no to unreasonable requests
- Being able to state complaints
- Expressing appreciation as appropriate

For example, the nurse might discuss with the patient how, if the patient talks about angry feelings toward a co-worker with another noninvolved co-worker, it does nothing to solve the problem and may even create more negative emotions. If the patient pretends to not be angry, the anger is allowed to build up inside. It is likely that the anger will be misdirected at a later time or expressed out of proportion in another unrelated situation.

Patients with few assertive skills can learn them by participating in structured groups and programs. In these settings patients can watch staff demonstrate specific skills and then role play the skills themselves. Staff can provide feedback to patients on the appropriateness and effectiveness of their responses. Homework can also be assigned to patients to help them generalize these skills outside the group milieu. It is expected that aggressive behaviors will diminish as the patient learns new and more effective social skills (Aschen, 1997).

How can a nurse who has difficulty being assertive with peers and interdisciplinary colleagues effectively teach assertiveness skills to patients?

Communication Strategies

The psychiatric nurse can often prevent a crisis situation through the use of early verbal and nonverbal intervention. This is sometimes called "talking the patient down." Because it is much less dangerous to prevent a crisis than to respond to one, every effort should be made to carefully monitor patients who are at risk for violent behavior and intervene at the first possible sign of increasing agitation. Interventions aimed at strengthening the therapeutic alliance with the patient can decrease the need for aggressive behavior.

Speaking to the patient in a calm, low voice can help to decrease a patient's agitation. Agitated patients often speak loudly and use profanity. It is important that nurses not re-

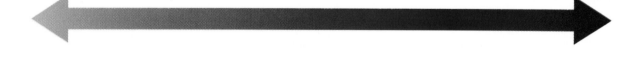

Preventive Strategies   Anticipatory Strategies   Containment Strategies

Self-awareness	Communication	Crisis management
Patient education	Environmental change	Seclusion
Assertiveness training	Behavioral actions	Restraints
	Psychopharmacology	

Fig. 31-6 Continuum of nursing interventions in managing aggressive behavior.

spond by raising their voices or by using profanity because this will probably be perceived as competition and will only further escalate the volatile situation. The nurse should use short, simple sentences and avoid laughing or smiling inappropriately.

The nurse can also help reduce a rising level of agitation by acknowledging the patient's feelings and reassuring the patient that the staff is there to help. It may be useful to allow the patient to communicate his or her concerns without interruption and engage the patient's participation in treatment decisions, providing the patient as much information about treatment as possible. Collaboration with patients can be enhanced, making it less likely that they will respond in an angry and aggressive manner.

It is also important that the nurse communicate expected behavior in a way that encourages the patient to maintain control of any violent impulses. At this early stage, some patients with encouragement may be willing to remove themselves from an overstimulating environment, thus facilitating their self-control.

The specific nonverbal communication used by the nurse can also greatly affect the outcome of the intervention. A calm and relaxed posture that does not tower over the patient is much less intimidating than a posture in which hands are placed on the hips and the nurse looms over the patient. Crossing the arms across the chest is another pos-

ture that communicates emotional distance and an unwillingness to help. The nurse's hands should be kept open and out of pockets. Threatening, nervous, and sudden gestures should be avoided. Altering position so that the nurse's eyes are at the same level as those of the patient allows the patient to communicate from an equal rather than inferior position.

Box 31-5

Ways of Managing Anger

- Positive self-talk
- Physical exercise
- Change of environment
- Write about your feelings
- Think of the consequences
- Listen to music
- Watch television
- Deep breathing exercises
- Take a walk
- Count to 50
- Comfort wrap with a blanket
- Relaxation exercises
- Talk about your feelings
- Use adaptive coping skills
- Read
- Being alone
- Medication

 PATIENT EDUCATION PLAN *Appropriate Expression of Anger*

CONTENT	INSTRUCTIONAL ACTIVITIES	EVALUATION
Help the patient identify anger.	Focus on nonverbal behavior. Role play nonverbal expression of anger. Label the feeling using the patient's preferred words.	Patient demonstrates an angry body posture and facial expression.
Give permission for angry feelings.	Describe situations in which it is normal to feel angry.	Patient describes a a situation in which anger would be an appropriate response.
Practice the expression of anger.	Role play fantasized situations in which anger is an appropriate response.	Patient participates in role play and identifies behaviors associated with expression of anger.
Apply the expression of anger to a real situation.	Help identify a real situation that makes the patient angry. Role play a confrontation with the object of the anger. Provide positive feedback for successful expression of anger.	Patient identifies a real situation that results in anger. Patient is able to role play expression of anger.
Identify alternative ways to express anger.	List several ways to express anger, with and without direct confrontation. Role play alternative behaviors. Discuss situations in which alternatives would be appropriate.	Patient participates in identifying alternatives and plans when each might be useful.
Confrontation with a person who is a source of anger.	Provide support during confrontation if needed. Discuss experience after confrontation takes place.	Patient identifies the feeling of anger and appropriately confronts the object of the anger.

The nurse should assume a supportive stance that is at least one leg length or 3 feet from the patient. It is helpful if the nurse remains at an angle to the patient and the patient's need for personal space is respected. It has been noted that violence-prone people need four times more personal space than non-violence-prone people. Intrusion into a patient's personal space can be perceived as a threat and provoke aggression.

Finally, when approaching potentially violent patients, nurses should carefully observe their behavior. Clenched fists, tightening of the facial muscles, and movement away from the nurse may suggest that the patient is feeling threatened. The nurse should respond by giving the patient as much distance as possible. These communication strategies are summarized in Box 31-6.

Why do you think that standing at an angle to the patient is less threatening than facing the patient full face? Try the two stances with a friend and describe your feelings about each one.

Environmental Strategies

Violent behavior is more likely to occur in a poorly structured milieu with undefined program rules and a great deal of unscheduled time for patients. Inpatient units that provide many productive activities reduce the chance of inappropriate patient behavior and increase adaptive social and leisure functioning. Both the unit norms and the rewards associated with such activities may reduce the amount of disorganized patient behavior and the number of aggressive acts.

In contrast, units that are overly structured with too much stimulation and little regard for the privacy needs of patients may increase aggressive behavior. For example, some psychiatric hospitals have patients eat in dining rooms that are crowded during mealtimes. Other hospital units restrict patients to a central day room to allow for better observation by staff and minimize patient isolation. In such situations, there is often one television and sometimes only one patient telephone. For patients who lose much of their privacy when they are admitted to a psychiatric unit, the lack of personal privacy and control over their lives can foster anger and hostility when their ability to cope is already challenged.

Aggressive behavior may be more effectively managed by allowing those at risk to spend time in their room away from the hectic day room rather than encouraging them to interact with others in a crowded milieu. The environment that may have been therapeutic in the days of extended hospital stays may no longer be suitable for patients who are hospitalized on short-term, acute inpatient units where the acuity of the patients is extremely high. Inpatient units should adapt the environment to best meet the needs of the patients they treat (see Chapter 35). The impact of the environment is seen in the following clinical example.

CLINICAL EXAMPLE

Mr. T was a 36-year-old man who was admitted for the third time to an acute care unit at a state psychiatric hospital. His medical diagnosis was bipolar disorder, manic. The nursing staff was apprehensive because the patient had a history of assaultive behavior on earlier admissions. At the time of this admission, the unit atmosphere was tense because one of the other patients had made a suicide attempt requiring emergency room treatment.

Mr. I was Mr. T's primary nurse from his previous admission. He was working when the patient arrived on the unit. During the nursing assessment, Mr. I discussed the nursing interventions that had seemed to be helpful in the past. He validated with Mr. T that he was usually able to maintain control of his behavior by participating in a structured physical activity when he was feeling upset. In addition, he recalled that the patient would begin to pace rapidly and sing when he was losing control. Mr. T agreed with these observations.

Mr. T responded very quickly to the tension on the unit. He began to pace up and down the hall and sing in a moderately loud tone of voice. Other patients also began to show signs of increased agitation. The nursing staff held a brief consultation. They decided that the charge nurse would gather the patients for a community meeting to discuss their feelings about the suicide attempt. Meanwhile, Mr. I would take Mr. T for a walk with one of the other staff.

The interventions were successful. More intensive nursing actions were not needed.

Room Program. In an inpatient setting, the use of a structured room program is another effective tool for the management of agitated patients. Research shows that removing patients from the stimulus is an effective strategy that greatly decreases the need for seclusion and restraint (Canatsey & Roper, 1997). A room program limits the amount of time patients are allowed in the unit milieu. For example, patients initially may be asked to stay in their rooms for a certain length of time, or conversely be allowed out of their rooms for a specific amount of time every hour. The amount of time in the milieu may then be increased by increments of 15 minutes as patients tolerate the environment. Another way of implementing a room program is to allow patients to come out of their rooms during certain

---

Box 31-6

Communication Strategies Used in Preventing Aggressive Behavior

- Present a calm appearance.
- Speak softly.
- Speak in a nonprovocative and nonjudgmental manner.
- Speak in a neutral and concrete way.
- Put space between yourself and the patient.
- Show respect for the patient.
- Avoid intense direct eye contact.
- Demonstrate control over the situation without assuming an overly authoritarian stance.
- Facilitate the patient's talking.
- Listen to the patient.
- Avoid early interpretations.
- Do not make promises you cannot keep.

designated hours, such as when the unit is quiet or when other patients are off the unit.

Such a structured program allows patients time away from situations that may increase agitation and provides a way to regulate the amount of stimulation patients receive. Its purpose is the prevention of a crisis that could result in more serious patient complications.

Cathartic Activities. Many clinicians support the use of cathartic activities as a way of helping patients physically release aggression. These strategies are based on the assumption that some physical activity can be useful in releasing aggression and can prevent more explosive or destructive forms of aggression or violence. However, research suggests that aggressive behavior exists on a continuum and that minor manifestations of aggression can lead to further aggressive behavior. These findings challenge the effectiveness of cathartic activities and call into question some traditional nursing interventions, such as encouraging patients to release tension through the use of punching bags or allowing patients to pace the halls in the expectation that their tension will decrease. Because these strategies are not supported by research and may increase the patient's potential for aggressive behavior, they are not recommended nursing actions. This is also an excellent example of the way in which nursing evidence can challenge traditional nursing interventions and help psychiatric nurses to base their practice on empirically based data rather than commonly held but untested assumptions.

Behavioral Strategies

Other interventions include applying principles of behavior management with the aggressive patient (see Chapter 32). Effective limit setting is one of the most basic interventions in this area.

Limit Setting. **Limit setting** is a nonpunitive, nonmanipulative act in which the patient is told what behavior is acceptable, what is not acceptable, and the consequences of behaving unacceptably. By explaining the rationale for the limit and communicating to the patient in a calm and respectful manner, potentially aggressive behavior can be avoided. When nursing staff communicate in an authoritarian, parental, controlling, or disrespectful manner, patients are more likely to respond in an angry, aggressive manner.

Research has shown that it is possible to prevent some of patients' anger by improving nurses' limit-setting styles (Lancee et al, 1995). The nurse does not assume responsibility for the patient's behavior, adaptive or maladaptive. It is recognized that the patient has the right to choose a behavior and understands its consequences. Limits should be clarified before negative consequences are applied.

Once a limit has been identified, the consequences must take place if the behavior occurs. Every staff member must be aware of the plan and carry it out consistently. If staff do not do so, the patient is likely to manipulate staff by acting out and then pointing out areas of inconsistent limit setting. Clear, firm, and nonpunitive enforcement of limits is the goal. It is also important for nurses to understand that when limit setting is implemented, the maladaptive behavior will

not immediately decrease; in fact, it may briefly increase. This is consistent with behavioral principles and testing behavior. If staff understand the dynamics of this intervention, they will be able to implement this strategy effectively and understand that patient behavior will eventually change.

Behavioral Contracts. If a patient uses violence to gain control and make personal gains, the nursing care must be planned to eliminate the rewards the patient receives while allowing the patient to assume as much control as possible. Once the rewards are understood, nursing care can be planned that does not reinforce aggressive and violent behavior. Behavioral contracts with the patient can be helpful in this regard. For example, head-injured patients with low impulse control can be told that staff will take them for a walk if they can refrain from using profanity for 4 hours.

To be effective, contracts require detailed information about the following:

- Unacceptable behaviors
- Acceptable behaviors
- Consequences for breaking the contract
- The nurse's contribution to care

Patients should also have input into the development of the contract to increase their sense of self-control. This negotiated process increases the mutuality of the therapeutic alliance and reduces the possibility of aggressive behavior.

Time-Outs. Time-out from reinforcement is a behavioral technique in which socially inappropriate behaviors can be decreased by short-term removal of the patient from overstimulating and sometimes reinforcing situations. Time-outs are most effective with patients who feel loss of social contact as a negative consequence. With time-out, patients have more control over the process, and thus this intervention offers an alternative that is less humiliating and has less risk of injury.

With implementation of this intervention, patients who appear to be escalating are prompted to enter time-out, which is usually a quiet, low-traffic area of the unit. They remain there until they have been nonaggressive for a couple of minutes. Patients who do not comply with time-out instructions may be asked to enter the seclusion room for further protection of themselves and others.

Token Economy. Another effective behavioral strategy is the implementation of a token economy. In this intervention, identified interpersonal skills and self-care behaviors are rewarded with tokens that can be used by the patient to buy items. Behaviors to be targeted are specific to each patient. Guidelines should clearly specify desired behaviors required to receive tokens, the number of tokens to be received for each behavior, and the length of time a desired behavior must be exhibited to receive tokens. Furthermore, in a token economy undesired behaviors can result in the loss of tokens.

Research has shown that inpatient units that have implemented token economies have significantly fewer aggressive episodes than more traditional settings (LePage, 1999). This strategy for managing aggressive behavior is particularly useful with chronic lower-functioning patient populations. The following clinical example describes the use of this intervention.

CLINICAL EXAMPLE

A regressed patient, Mrs. S, refused to get out of bed in the morning. She would not shower, dress, or wash her clothes. When encouraged to do these things, Mrs. S became agitated, swore, and threatened to hit anyone who tried to help her. A token store was set up with the number of tokens required to purchase each item. Under her contract, Mrs. S would receive two tokens for each of the following behaviors:

- Getting out of bed by 7:30 AM
- Showering before 8:00 AM
- Dressing before 8:00 AM
- Being at breakfast table by 8:15 AM
- Eating 100% of breakfast tray by 8:45 AM
- Arriving to community meeting by 9:00 AM

Her contract also included the following penalty:

- An episode of swearing will result in the loss of 4 tokens.

Psychopharmacology

Pharmacological interventions have proven effective in the management of aggressive behavior (Littrell & Littrell, 1998). They include a variety of therapeutic agents, all of which are discussed in greater detail in Chapter 28.

Antianxiety and Sedative-Hypnotics. These drugs are effective in the management of acute agitation. Benzodiazepines such as lorazepam are often used during psychiatric emergencies to sedate combative patients. Lorazepam in particular is frequently used because of its quick onset and because it can be administered either orally or intramuscularly. Antianxiety medications are not recommended for long-term use because they can result in confusion and dependency and may worsen depressive symptoms. Furthermore, some patients have experienced a disinhibiting effect from benzodiazepines that can result in increased aggressive behavior. Buspirone, an antianxiety drug that may be effective in the management of aggressive behavior associated with anxiety and depression, has also been shown to decrease aggression and agitation in patients with head injuries, dementia, and developmental disabilities.

Antidepressants. The selective serotonin reuptake inhibitors (SSRIS) appear to reduce the risk of violence associated with posttraumatic stress.

Mood Stabilizers. Studies have shown that lithium is effective in the treatment of aggression resulting from mania. Some evidence also shows that lithium may be useful in decreasing aggression resulting from other disorders such as mental retardation, head injuries, schizophrenia, and personality disorders, and in children with conduct disorder. In patients with temporal lobe epilepsy, lithium may actually increase the frequency of aggressive acts. Carbamazepine has been shown to be effective in managing aggressive behavior in patients with abnormal electroencephalograms (EEGs). There is also some evidence that carbamazepine may be effective in managing agitated behavior associated with dementia.

Antipsychotics. These drugs have been commonly used for the treatment of aggression. The atypical antipsychotics affect both dopamine and serotonin activity, and may have antihostility properties that the traditional antipsychotic medications lack. Because the drug action may take several weeks or months to take effect, the atypical antipsychotics are used in the intermediate and long-term treatment of the aggressive and psychotic patient.

In the acute management of the violent and psychotic patient, the sedating properties of conventional antipsychotics such as haloperidol are sometimes useful, although benzodiazepines such as lorazepam are preferred for acute sedation owing to their more favorable side effect profile. In some settings, neuroleptic medications such as haloperidol are used in combination with lorazepam, as the sedative properties act synergistically with each other and both can be given intramuscularly during emergency situations (Hughes, 1999).

Patients should be assessed for the occurrence of acute neuroleptic-induced akathisia, which can appear as worsening of agitation and acute dystonic reaction; this complication can be frightening and uncomfortable for patients. Finally, the atypical antipsychotic drugs clozapine and resperidol may be effective not only for patients with schizophrenia but also for people with dementia, brain injuries, and mental retardation.

Other Medications. Several case reports have suggested that naltrexone, an opiate antagonist, may reduce self-injurious behavior. This effect is particularly notable in patients with developmental disabilities.

Beta-blockers such as propranolol have also been shown to decrease aggressive behavior in children, adults, and particularly patients with organic mental disorder. Nurses should be aware of the side effects of beta-blockers including hypotension, bradycardia, and in some cases depression.

Psychostimulants are used to treat aggressive behavior in children with attention deficit hyperactivity disorder (ADHD). Lithium and the atypical antipsychotics are more effective than stimulants in the treatment of aggression in children and adolescents with conduct disorders.

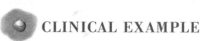

How do the strategies for managing aggressive behavior relate to the theories of aggression described earlier in this chapter?

CRISIS MANAGEMENT TECHNIQUES

There are times when attempts at early intervention are unsuccessful and more active intervention is necessary. If the patient is exhibiting behavior that is dangerous either to self or others, it may be unsafe to attempt a verbal intervention. This is evident in the following clinical example.

CLINICAL EXAMPLE

Mr. B was a 32-year-old man with a medical diagnosis of paranoid personality disorder. He was admitted to the locked ward of a psychiatric hospital because he had been arrested after his neighbors complained that he was letting the air out of their tires. He said that he did this because the neighbors laughed at him and talked about him when he was out walking his dog. He was angry about being arrested and wanted to leave the hospital, but he was held under commitment because he also threatened to burn down the house of the neighbor who had called the police.

Mr. B resisted the admission procedure. He belligerently demanded to be released, threatening to call the governor and "sue everybody in the place." When he was asked to prepare for a physical examination, he ran down the hall and barricaded himself in the dining room. As staff forcibly entered the room, he began to lash out. Several staff members removed him to a seclusion room, where he was given intramuscular medication and isolated until he regained control of his behavior. He paced the floor and pounded on the door for 30 minutes before he began to appear calmer.

Several days later, when Mr. B was used to the staff and felt more comfortable in the hospital, he related to a nurse, "I hope I didn't hurt you the other night, but I didn't know what you wanted to do to me. A man has to protect himself, you know."

Experience and wisdom are needed to determine when the time for verbal and other less restrictive interventions have failed. Nonviolent physical control and restraint should be used only as a last resort. Like medical emergencies, psychiatric emergencies require immediate action.

Team Response

Effective crisis management must be organized and should be directed by one clearly identified crisis leader (Box 31-7). Because psychiatric nurses are responsible for the management of patient care 24 hours a day, it is most appropriate that the crisis leader be a nurse. The leader may be the charge nurse, the primary nurse, nurse manager, or a staff nurse; however, the person should be decided in advance. Other staff members, including physicians, nurses, and counselors, can be used for support. The crisis leader must decide the intervention necessary to ensure the safety of both patients and staff. The decision can be a difficult one to make, especially when the acuity of the situation does not always allow adequate time to discuss all possible strategies with the entire treatment team.

Once the decision to intervene has been made, the crisis leader must obtain assistance to manage the crisis. All members of the crisis team should be trained in crisis management and have experience working as a cohesive group. The staff should be prepared to intervene under the direction of the crisis leader.

In many inpatient facilities, hospital security personnel are also notified when assistance is needed. It is the responsibility of the crisis leader to be acquainted with the security officers, give them a brief description of the situation, describe the intervention, and identify the role of security personnel in managing the crisis. Because security officers are not mental health professionals, their assistance should be used only when the patient cannot be physically managed by the nursing staff. Often, there is little time for planning, and the leader must balance the need to act quickly with the need to be organized so that the safety of the patients and staff is not jeopardized.

Box 31-7

Procedure for Managing Psychiatric Emergencies

- Identify crisis leader.
- Assemble crisis team.
- Notify security officers if necessary.
- Remove all other patients from area.
- Obtain restraints if appropriate.
- Devise a plan to manage crisis and inform team.
- Assign securing of patient limbs to crisis team members.
- Explain necessity of intervention to patient and attempt to enlist cooperation.
- Restrain patient when directed by crisis leader.
- Administer medication if ordered.
- Maintain calm, consistent approach to patient.
- Review crisis management interventions with crisis team.
- Process events with other patients and staff as appropriate.
- Gradually reintegrate patient into milieu.

The leader is also responsible for ensuring the safety of the other patients during a crisis. This can be accomplished by assigning a staff member to remove the other patients from the area. Quite often the other patients become more acutely distressed in response to a psychiatric emergency on the unit and require extra nursing attention both during and after the crisis. After the crisis has passed, allowing patients to verbalize their anxiety and concern about the crisis and processing it with them can be helpful. It is not appropriate to encourage this activity during a crisis intervention.

A room without furniture should always be readily available for an emergency. If restraints are necessary, they must be obtained from an easily accessible place. To protect the patient and staff, the leader must assess the situation quickly and devise a plan. This plan should include a brief explanation to the staff of the patient's behavior and the intervention necessary.

Staff members who will be directly involved in the intervention should each be assigned to secure one of the patient's limbs when directed to do so. The leader must also explain to the team what will be said to the patient and on what signal the staff should secure the patient's limbs. As the group approach within 6 to 8 feet from the patient, the leader should express concern for the patient's safety and the behavior demonstrated that has caused such concern. The patient should then be escorted to the appropriate room and informed of the necessary intervention. It should be emphasized that the intervention is not a punishment but is being provided to help ensure the safety of the patient and the rest of the unit.

If restraints are to be used, the patient should be asked to lie on the bed with arms at his or her side. Quite often, the presence of several staff is enough to enlist the patient's cooperation. If the patient is unable to cooperate, the patient should be told that the staff will be assisting. Patients often hesitate at this point in their attempt to remain in control. If patients cannot cooperate within several seconds, they may be unable to cooperate at all, and the leader must then direct the staff to restrain the patient as planned. This can be very frightening for patients, and they may need several reminders that they will not be hurt but that the staff will protect them from their impulses.

During this time it is critically important that the leader relate to the patient in a calm, steady voice and manner. Any anxiety or ambivalence will be conveyed to the patient and contribute to a feeling of insecurity. A leader who is anxious will be unable to think clearly about the situation. Many patients are afraid of losing control, and they become assaultive not because they want to frighten people but because they themselves are frightened. If the staff shows control of the situation, the patient's agitation is often defused. When the crisis team is overwhelmed by their own fears of the patient, they cannot be effective in reducing the patient's fear. Consistency is also important so that the patient cannot bargain with or manipulate staff members. If the leader is indecisive, inconsistent, or easily manipulated, the patient will not be assured that the staff can guarantee safety by controlling the situation.

After the crisis is over, the team should discuss any concerns they may have had during the crisis because this type of intervention can be stressful for both staff and patients. The patient's behavior may have evoked feelings of guilt, anger, or aggression in the staff. These issues should be discussed as a team so that care is consistent, interventions are therapeutic, and staff do not become discouraged, negative, or burned out. The final intervention is a reevaluation of the patient's status and the gradual reintegration of the patient into the milieu.

Seclusion

At times, secluding or separating the patient from others in a safe, contained environment is necessary after less restrictive measures have failed. Often staff members may have negative or conflicting views about using restrictive interventions such as seclusion and restraints. They may believe that they will betray the patient's trust and could jeopardize the relationships between staff and patient. Some staff may believe that it is unethical or nontherapeutic to restrict a patient's freedom. Because seclusion or restraints are the most restrictive ways to manage aggressive behavior, they should be used only as a last resort and only after less restrictive measures have been tried.

Seclusion and restraint have been the subject of much discussion in the field. A review of the literature on these interventions supports the following (Lendemaijer & Shortridge-Baggett, 1997):

- Seclusion and restraint can have negative physical and psychological effects on patients and staff and the psychiatric consumer/survivor movement has emphasized these effects.
- Nonclinical factors such as cultural biases, staff role perceptions, and the attitude of hospital administration have a great influence on rates of seclusion and restraint.

- Training in violence prediction and prevention, self-defense, and implementation of restraints or seclusion is valuable in reducing rates and untoward effects.
- Studies comparing well-defined training programs are potentially useful

Degrees of seclusion vary. They include confining a patient in a room with a closed but unlocked door or placing a patient in a locked room with a mattress but no linens and with limited opportunity for communication. Patients may be dressed in their clothes or in hospital clothing. A mattress and sheet or blanket are the minimally acceptable conditions for seclusion.

The rationale for the use of seclusion is based on three therapeutic principles:

- Containment
- Isolation
- Decrease in sensory input

Using the principle of **containment**, patients are restricted to a place where they are safe from harming themselves and other patients. **Isolation** addresses the need for patients to distance themselves from relationships that, because of the illness, are pathologically intense. Some patients, particularly those with paranoia, distort the meaning of the interactions around them. Their distortions create such psychic pain that seclusion may provide some relief and may be the only place they feel safe from their "persecutors." Seclusion also provides a smaller area for these patients to master, allowing for a gradual increase in their interactions with others. The third principle is that seclusion provides a **decrease in sensory input** for patients whose illness results in a heightened sensitivity to external stimulation. The quiet atmosphere and monotony of a seclusion room may provide some relief from the sensory overload. Nursing interventions related to seclusion are presented in Box 31-8.

Legal requirements for the care of the secluded patient vary from state to state. Good nursing care includes optimum fulfillment of basic human needs and concern for personal dignity. The nurse must help the patient to meet biological needs by providing food and fluids, a comfortable environment, and opportunity for use of the bathroom. Frequent observation and monitoring is essential. The room must be constructed so the patient can be observed without being unnecessarily exposed to those who are not involved in his or her care (see Critical Thinking about Contemporary Issues). Staff should be able to communicate with the patient. Careful records should include all nursing care and observation of the isolated patient. The need for continued isolation should be assessed on a regular basis. It may be necessary for the nurse to initiate this review of the patient's condition with other health team members.

There appears to be a gap between the understanding of staff and patients regarding each other's feelings and intentions related to seclusion. For example, many patients who have experienced seclusion or restraints find it to be a negative and often punitive experience and one that could have been avoided by interventions such as medication and increased interactions with staff to help them deal with their feelings and behaviors (Martinez et al, 1999; Johnson, 1998;

Box 31-8

Nursing Interventions Related to Seclusion

DEFINITION

Solitary containment in a fully protective environment with close surveillance by nursing staff for purposes of safety or behavior management.

ACTIVITIES

Obtain a physician's order, if required by institutional policy, to use a physically restrictive intervention.

Designate one nursing staff member to communicate with the patient and direct other staff.

Identify for patient and significant others the behaviors that necessitated the intervention.

Explain procedure, purpose, and time period of the intervention to patient and significant others in understandable and nonpunitive terms.

Explain to patient and significant others the behaviors necessary for termination of the intervention.

Contract with patient (as patient is able) to maintain control of behavior.

Instruct on self-control methods as appropriate.

Assist in dressing in safe clothing and removing jewelry and eyeglasses.

Remove all items from seclusion area that patient might use to harm self or nursing staff.

Assist with needs related to nutrition, elimination, hydration, and personal hygiene.

Provide food and fluids in nonbreakable containers.

Provide appropriate level of supervision/surveillance to monitor patient and allow for therapeutic actions as needed. Acknowledge your presence to patient periodically.

Administer PRN medications for anxiety or agitation.

Provide for patient's psychological comfort as needed.

Monitor seclusion area for temperature, cleanliness, and safety.

Arrange for routine cleaning of seclusion area.

Evaluate at regular intervals patient's need for continued restrictive intervention.

Involve patient, when appropriate, in making decisions to move to a more or less restrictive form of intervention. Determine patient's need for continued seclusion.

Document the rationale for use of restrictive intervention, patients response to the intervention, patient's physical condition, nursing care provided throughout the intervention, and rationale for terminating the intervention.

Process with the patient and staff, on termination of the restrictive intervention, the circumstances that led to the intervention, as well as any patient concerns about the intervention itself.

Provide the next appropriate level of restrictive intervention (such as physical restraint or area restriction) as needed.

From McCloskey JC, Bulechek GM: *Nursing interventions classification*, ed 3, St Louis, 2000, Mosby.

 CRITICAL THINKING about **CONTEMPORARY ISSUES**

Is Video Monitoring of Psychiatric Patients in Seclusion and Restraint Ethical?

Video monitoring of patients in seclusion and restraints to improve patient safety and to assist nursing staff to comply with policies and standards of care is a common practice in many psychiatric settings. However questions have been raised about the ethics of such a procedure. Specifically, does it violate a patient's sense of dignity given that the patient cannot leave the area and is often required to wear a hospital gown? Does it cause the patient distress due to lack of privacy and the inability to control self-presentation? Does it override patient autonomy and stimulate feelings of shame and embarrassment in the patient?

A decision to video monitor a patient should balance potential harm from loss of privacy, loss of human contact with nurses, breach of confidentiality, and feelings of shame and embarrassment with the potential good of increased safety and efficient use of staff resources, tempered by a clinical appreciation of individual patient fac-

tors. Thus, the following recommendations have been proposed (Olsen, 1998):

- Document a clinical justification for monitoring as loss of privacy at the same time seclusion or restraint is justified as a denial of liberty.
- Inform patients that they are being monitored.
- Place monitors where they can be viewed only by staff with direct clinical responsibility.
- Give careful consideration to who is responsible for watching the video monitor for changes in patient status.
- Viewing the monitor does not substitute for direct visual inspection and human contact with a nurse.
- Maintaining a personal relationship with the patient remains the most ethically appropriate action and the best liability protection.

Olofsson et al, 1998; Gillig et al, 1998). Therefore, it is recommended that staff spend more time talking with patients about the issues that led to seclusion and alternative methods of coping that might help the patient avoid seclusion in the future.

The nursing staff should always review the events that led up to the decision to isolate a patient. In particular, staff should be encouraged to give each other feedback about interpersonal relationships involving the secluded patient. Preventive measures that may help the patient to gain control in the future without requiring seclusion should be identified. It is also useful for staff to vent their own feelings following an episode of seclusion. Management of violent behavior is physically and emotionally stressful.

Restraints

Restraint involves the use of mechanical or manual devices to limit the physical mobility of the patient. Such an intervention may be indicated to protect the patient or others from injury, particularly if less restrictive interventions, such as environmental change and behavioral strategies, have failed.

The primary indication for restraints is the control of violent behavior, either self-directed or directed toward others, that cannot be controlled by medication or psychosocial techniques. Nursing interventions related to the use of restraints are presented in Box 31-9.

The patient in mechanical restraint may be confused or delirious and will probably be frightened at the limitation of movement. The nurse should not assume that the patient understands the need for restraint. Support and reassurance are essential. Restraints should be applied efficiently and with care not to injure a combative patient. Adequate personnel must be assembled before the patient is approached. Each staff member should be assigned responsibility for controlling specific body parts. Restraints should be available and in working order. Padding of cuff restraints helps to prevent skin breakdown. For the same reason, the patient should be positioned in anatomical alignment.

Privacy is important. If visitors are allowed, the nurse should explain the reason for restraints or seclusion before they see the patient. This may help them accept the situation. Physical needs must be included in the nursing care plan. Vital signs should be checked, and regular observation of circulation in the extremities is necessary. Fluids should be of-

Box 31-9

Nursing Interventions Related to Physical Restraint

DEFINITION

Application and monitoring of mechanical restraining devices or manual restraints to limit physical mobility of patient.

ACTIVITIES

Obtain a physician's order, if required by institutional policy, to use a physically restrictive intervention.

Provide patient with a private yet adequately supervised environment in situations where a patient's sense of dignity may be diminished by the use of physical restraints.

Provide sufficient staff to assist with safe application of physical restraining devices or manual restraints.

Designate one nursing staff member to direct staff and communicate with the patient during the application of physical restraints.

Use appropriate hold when manually restraining patient in emergency situations or during transport.

Identify for patient and significant others the behaviors that necessitated the intervention.

Explain procedure, purpose, and time period of the intervention to patient and significant others in understandable and nonpunitive terms.

Explain to patient and significant others the behaviors necessary for termination of the intervention.

Monitor the patient's response to procedure.

Avoid tying restraints to siderails of bed.

Secure restraints out of patient's reach.

Provide appropriate level of supervision to monitor patient and to allow for therapeutic actions as needed.

Provide for patient's psychological comfort as needed.

Provide diversional activities when appropriate (such as television, reading to patient, visitors, mobiles) to facilitate patient cooperation with the intervention.

Administer PRN medications for anxiety or agitation.

Monitor skin condition of restraint sites.

Monitor color, temperature, and sensation frequently in restrained extremities.

Provide for limited movement according to patient's level of self-control.

Position patient to facilitate comfort and prevent aspiration and skin breakdown.

Provide for movement of extremities in patient with multiple restraints by rotating the removal/reapplication of one restraint at a time (as safety permits).

Assist with periodic changes in body position.

Provide the dependent patient with a means of summoning help (such as a bell or call light) when caregiver is not present.

Assist with needs related to nutrition, elimination, hydration, and personal hygiene.

Evaluate, at regular intervals, patient's need for continued restrictive intervention.

Involve patient in activities to improve strength, coordination, judgment, and orientation.

Involve patient, when appropriate, in making decisions to move to a more or less restrictive form of intervention.

Remove restraints gradually (that is, one at a time if in four-point restraints) as self-control increases.

Monitor patient's response to removal of restraints.

Process with the patient and staff, on termination of the restrictive intervention, the circumstances that led to the use of the intervention, as well as any patient concerns about the intervention itself.

Provide the next appropriate level of restrictive intervention (such as area restriction or seclusion) as needed. Implement alternatives to restraints, such as sitting in chair with table over lap, self-releasing waist-belt, geri-chair without tray table, or close observation, as appropriate.

Teach family the risks and benefits of restraints and restraint reduction.

Document the rationale for use of restrictive intervention, patient's response to the intervention, patient's physical condition, nursing care provided throughout the intervention, and rationale for terminating the intervention.

From McCloskey JC, Bulechek GM: *Nursing interventions classification*, ed 3, St Louis, 2000, Mosby.

fered regularly and opportunities for elimination provided. Skin care is also essential. Restraints should be released at least every 2 hours to allow exercise of the extremities.

Despite explanations of the therapeutic purpose of the intervention, it is not uncommon for patients to perceive the use of restraints as a punishment. Thus every effort must be made to maintain a therapeutic alliance with the patient in restraints.

Compliance with the legal and clinical requirements for seclusion and restraint is problematic (Chandler et al, 1998). From 1988 to 1998, there were 142 deaths nationwide in psychiatric units, group homes, and residential facilities for troubled youth, and treatment centers and group homes for persons with mental retardation. These troubling statistics have attracted national concern from the media, consumer advocacy groups, and members of Congress. For the first time, federal legislation has been introduced regulating seclusion and restraint practices in the United States (Appelbaum, 1999). NAMI, the National Alliance for the Mentally Ill, has advocated three national policy responses (Ross, 1999):

- A single national standard on the use of seclusion and restraint should be established based on the premise that involuntary use of restraint or seclusion is appropriate only for emergency situations involving personal safety.
- All deaths and serious injuries resulting from the use of restraints or seclusion should be reported to a legal entity within the state for investigation.
- All Medicaid- and Medicare-funded facilities should use third-party, independent consumer, citizen, and family monitoring groups.

Furthermore, the Joint Commission on Accreditation of Health Care Organizations (JCAHO) has made the following recommendations to reduce the risk of restraint deaths (PSC Healthcare, 1999):

- Reduce the use of physical restraints and therapeutic holds through the use of risk assessment and early intervention.
- Revise procedures for assessing the medical condition of psychiatric patients.
- Consider the patient's age, sex, and gender in creating therapeutic hold policies.
- Continuously observe any patient who is restrained.
- Never place a towel, bag, or other cover over a patient's face as part of the therapeutic hold process.
- Discontinue use of certain types of restraints, such as high vests and waist restraints.

The adoption of such recommendations by psychiatric nurses will help to ensure that restraints are used safely and therapeutically.

Terminating the Intervention

The decision to terminate the use of seclusion or restraints should be well planned. Reviewing the behavior that precipitated the intervention and the patient's current capacity to exercise control over his or her behavior are key factors. Patients should be told which behaviors they need to exhibit

and which behaviors or impulses they need to control before the intervention can be discontinued. Communication and careful documentation are critical in making an accurate assessment of a patient's level of control.

Patients should be gradually reintegrated into the milieu. This allows them to test their control without feeling overwhelmed. Patients are initially reintegrated by reducing restraints from four points to three points and then to two points as soon as they begin to regain control. However, a patient should not be left in just a one-point restraint because the risk of injury is high.

Once restraints have been discontinued altogether, or once a patient no longer requires locked seclusion, the patient may be given a specified amount of time out of the room. This amount of time will be gradually increased as the patient is able to maintain control in the milieu. The primary nurse, in collaboration with the treatment team, can coordinate this into the interdisciplinary plan of care.

The success of the patient's reintegration into the milieu depends largely on the consistency of the staff. Some staff may wish to adhere to a structured room program only if the patient decompensates, but patients who are thrust back into a busy unit can be quickly overwhelmed with the sudden increase in stimulation. Sending them to their room after they have lost control again only reinforces their inability to stay in control and is more likely to be viewed by the patient as punishment. Thus, gradual reintegration into the milieu is more likely to ensure the ability of these patients to maintain control and increase their feelings of achievement.

Finally, debriefing is an important part of terminating the use of seclusion or restraints. Debriefing is a therapeutic intervention that includes reviewing the facts related to an event and processing the response to them. It provides staff and patients with an opportunity to clarify the rationale for the seclusion, offer mutual feedback, and promote more adaptive functioning.

Debriefing can be used after any stressful event. Describe how talking with your friends after an examination can be seen as a kind of debriefing.

STAFF DEVELOPMENT

Effective management of potentially dangerous patients requires highly skilled staff and attention to environmental and workplace factors (Levin et al, 1998). Nurses, physicians, and other support staff, including security personnel, must be trained in emergency psychiatric care and crisis management techniques. The use of least restrictive measures for de-escalating patients' behaviors have been found to be effective in decreasing patient assaults and staff injury and reducing the need for seclusion and restraints when staff receive training in nonviolent self-defense skills, alternative interventions, and crisis management techniques (see Citing the Evidence on p. 654).

Adherence to the 1996 JCAHO Standards (1996) on Restraint and Seclusion should also be an essential part of a

Citing the Evidence on

Staff Training

BACKGROUND: Rates of seclusion and restraint in an urban psychiatric hospital were compared during the 12-month periods before and after implementing the recommendations of a multidisciplinary quality improvement work group convened to reduce the hospital's use of physical containment. Interventions included a mandatory staff training session on the management of assaultive behavior, weekly discussion items during team meetings for each unit, and hospital-wide publicity charting the ongoing progress of the effort.

RESULTS: Total annual rates of restraint declined 13.8%. The average duration of restraint per admission decreased 54.6%. Staff injuries were reduced by 18.8% during the study period.

IMPLICATIONS: Mandatory training courses can be effective in increasing staff awareness of less restrictive alternatives and learning safer interventions with agitated and aggressive patients.

Forster P et al: Staff training decreases use of seclusion and restraint in an acute psychiatric hospital, *Arch Psychiatr Nurs* 13(5):269, 1999.

staff education program. Education should focus on assessment of the patient, particularly mental status, motor behavior, affect, and speech. Verbal intervention should be stressed as a way of defusing agitation, and helpful and nonhelpful responses should be reviewed.

Education

All nursing interventions should be grounded in theory and current research, and crisis intervention in psychiatric emergencies is no exception. The theoretical basis and supporting research for various intervention strategies should be discussed as part of the training. Pharmacological interventions should be reviewed, with particular attention given to the choice of medication, its purpose, and its potential adverse effects.

Ongoing practice sessions in crisis management should be required of all staff. These sessions should include basic self-protection maneuvers and strategies for restraining assaultive patients. Each member of the staff should be able to function as a leader in the event of a crisis, and the staff as a whole must be able to function smoothly as a cohesive emergency team. The nursing and medical care of these patients should be reviewed as well as the impact of countertransference issues. Finally, it is strongly recommended that current state laws regarding the civil rights of patients be discussed in staff meetings to ensure that care given to patients is proper and respectful of their rights.

Staff Assault

Unfortunately, nurses are sometimes assaulted by patients. It is impossible to predict and prevent all episodes of violent behavior in a psychiatric setting. If a staff member is assaulted, the support and assistance of colleagues are needed.

Poster and Ryan (1994) studied the beliefs and concerns of psychiatric nurses about patient assaults and the safety of the work environment. The majority of those surveyed thought that staff members working with mentally ill patients may be physically assaulted during their careers. In addition, 58% agreed that staff members have a right to take legal action against an assaultive patient. The decision to take legal action appears to be influenced by the degree to which the staff member believes that the patient was responsible for his or her actions and capable of controlling impulses.

Nurses who have been assaulted may experience symptoms such as anger, anxiety, helplessness, irritability, hyperalertness, depression, shock, or disbelief that the assault occurred. It is not unusual for nurses to blame themselves for the assault or to question their competence in managing potentially violent patients. Nurses can be supported by allowing adequate time off from work to address their physical and emotional needs. Discussing the event in a nonblaming manner can also be helpful. Validation from others that assaults occur despite clinical competence and appropriate interventions can help the assaulted nurse in healing.

Acknowledging the nurse's right to take legal action against the patient can also be helpful. In fact, many argue that it is therapeutic to bring criminal charges against assaultive patients. Legal action can help patients take responsibility for their behavior, and perhaps decrease future violent episodes. For the assaulted nurse, taking legal action articulates a position that the personal trauma of being physically assaulted should not be an accepted consequence of caring for others.

Another way of helping nursing staff members who have been assaulted is through a peer support group, which legitimizes staff responses and allows for the expression of feelings in a supportive setting (Flannery et al, 1998). Developing a staff action program made up of volunteers who work with staff in critical incident debriefing, run support groups, and offer specialized services such as family and community meetings is another effective strategy.

A final suggestion is the implementation of a nursing consultation support service that responds to the needs of assault victims and sets the tone for institutional attitudes of nonblaming concern. All of these programs have merit and each organization should select the best way to deal with the problem of staff assault based on the environment, group process, and institutional resources.

Summary

1. High rates of assaultive behavior have been reported in a variety of health-care settings including outpatient clinics, nursing homes, and emergency departments. By far the highest rates of assault occur in psychiatric settings.

2. Within each person lies the capacity for passive, assertive, or aggressive behavior. The situation and the characteristics of the person define the most appropriate response.

3. Theories on the development of aggressive behavior include psychological, sociocultural, and biological.

4. The best single predictor of violence is a history of violence. It is also important to assess the patient's current clinical condition and situation.

5. Nurses need to assess possible precipitants of violent behavior, issues related to provocation, and biological factors. A screening tool may be useful in this process.

6. Many nursing interventions may be helpful in dealing with aggressive behavior, including self-awareness, patient education, assertiveness training, communication strategies, environmental strategies, behavioral strategies, and psychopharmacology.

7. Effective crisis management must be organized and clearly directed by one team leader. Seclusion and restraint should be used only as a last resort.

8. Staff development issues include educating staff in crisis management techniques, working with staff who have been assaulted, and understanding the implications of possible legal action.

Competent Caring   A Clinical Exemplar of a Psychiatric Nurse

MARY BROWN, RN

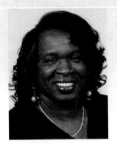

When I think about aggressive behavior, I think back to an incident that could have ended badly, but instead the people involved received the help needed. I was working as a case manager for an agency that provided intensive case management for chronically mentally ill people. The event took place on a weekend. Office hours were 9 AM to 5 PM during the week, and there was someone on call after working hours and on all weekends.

I was on call this particular weekend. One of the agency's patients had been hospitalized and was now ready for discharge. This patient was deaf, and I was to pick him up from the hospital and see that he was settled in his home. After I left the hospital with the patient, my beeper went off and I needed to call the answering service. I was close to the office, so I stopped there to use the phone. The building has two stories, and I had access only to the top floor. I climbed the stairs, the discharged deaf patient behind me, unlocked the door, and turned around to shut the door, but a large hand kept me from doing so.

The hand belonged to a man who was over 6 feet tall, weighed approximately 250 pounds, and appeared to be psychotic. He forced his way into the building with the patient and me. I was now terrified. He stated, "I came to get my money," in an angry and loud tone of voice.

I then recognized him as a patient I had worked with before and could see the changes in him, which made me feel unsafe to be alone with him. I tried very hard not to let him know how frightened I was of him. I told him the office was closed and he needed to come back Monday, when the appropriate people could help him. He shouted, "I want my money now!" I became increasingly frightened. There was no panic button to push for help. There were no other staff to distract him to allow me to get my deaf patient and myself to safety. I was the one who needed to protect us.

In a calm voice, I told him I couldn't help him get his money. I told him I would need to go to the staff room (he was aware that patients were not allowed in this room) to call someone to help him. He followed me into the room. I firmly told him that he was not allowed in the room and to please leave. He sat down anyway. I told him I was only at the office to return an emergency call. I called the service and the doctor who paged me was checking to see whether everything went okay with the discharged patient. I told him about the intrusion from the angry and irrational man who was insisting on staying until he got his money. The doctor said he would call the police. While waiting for the police, I kept trying to get the patient to leave the room. He repeatedly refused. He sat at one end of the table and I sat at the other end. The deaf patient was watching our interaction intensely.

The angry patient appeared to be responding to internal stimuli. He was looking at me and began to laugh. He stopped laughing and said, "Why won't you go out with me?" as he proceeded to my end of the table. I told him firmly that this behavior was not appropriate. I reinforced that I was his nurse and again asked him to leave the room. He stopped, looked at me unexpectedly, and said, "I'll be back on Monday to get my money."

When I heard the door slam, I quickly locked the door. The doctor called back to say that the police were on their way and asked whether everything was okay. While shivering, I said yes. The police picked the angry patient up downstairs and found that he was carrying a screwdriver. He told them that he was at the office before I arrived and intended to break into the office to take his money. The deaf patient who was watching all this communicated with me by writing on a piece of paper, "Are you all right? I can tell you were afraid of him." I was amazed. Nonverbal communication works both ways.

As a nurse, I am trained to look at what is not being said and make a determination. I realized that the deaf patient also could look at my nonverbal communication and make a determination. I also realized the value of setting firm limits and at all times giving clear, consistent, and nonthreatening messages when managing aggressive behavior.

Chapter Review Questions

1. Identify whether the following statements are true (T) or false (F).

_____ A. Patients who are mildly aggressive should be allowed to pace the halls to decrease tension.

_____ B. Overly crowded and stimulated environments may increase aggressive behavior.

_____ C. A patient's diagnosis is a good predictor of future violent behavior.

_____ D. A minority of psychiatric patients are responsible for a majority of the violent incidents.

_____ E. Failing to set effective limits with patients can lead to provocation and assault.

2. Match each term in Column A with the correct definition in Column B.

Column A

_____ Assertive behavior

_____ Debriefing

_____ Limit-setting

_____ Passive behavior

_____ Restraint

_____ Seclusion

_____ Token economy

Column B

A. Acting in a way that conveys a sense of self-assurance but also communicates respect for the other person nonpunitive, non manipulative behavior in which someone is told what is acceptable, what is not acceptable, and the consequences of behaving in an unacceptable way

B. Positive reinforcement in which patients are rewarded for performing desired targeted behaviors

C. Separating a patient from others in a safe, contained environment

D. Subordinating one's own rights to the perception of the rights of others

E. Therapeutic intervention that includes reviewing the facts related to an event and processing the response to them

F. Use of mechanical or manual devices to limit the physical mobility of the patient

3. Provide short answers for the following questions.

A. Identify the three areas of the brain that are believed to be involved in aggression.

B. Identify two preventive strategies, two anticipatory strategies, and two containment strategies for managing aggressive behavior.

C. A patient who appears agitated and potentially threatening approaches you. How should you physically position yourself when interacting with this patient?

D. Do you think that physical restraints are more or less restrictive than the use of chemical restraints (medications) with the aggressive patient? Defend your position.

REFERENCES

Appelbaum P: Seclusion and restraint: Congress reacts to reports of abuse, *Psychiatr Serv* 50(7):881, 1999.

Aschen S: Assertion training therapy in psychiatric milieus, *Arch Psychiatr Nurs* 11(l):46, 1997.

Borum R, Swartz M, Swanson J: Assessing and managing violence risk in clinical practice, *J Pract Psychol Behav Health* 2:205, 1996.

Bushman B, Baumester R: Threatened egotism narcissism, self-esteem, and direct and displaced aggression, *J Personality Social Psychol* 75(l):219, 1998.

Canatsey K, Roper J: Removal from stimuli for crisis intervention: using least restrictive methods to improve the quality of patient care, *Issues Mental Health Nurs* 18:35, 1997.

Chandler D et al: Performance improvement through monitoring seclusion and restraint practices, *Admin Policy Mental Health* 25(5):525, 1998.

Flannery R et al: Replicated declines in assault rates after implementation of the assaulted staff action program, *Psychiatr Serv* 49(2):241,1998.

Gillig P et al: A comparison of staff and patient perceptions of the causes and cures of physical aggression on a psychiatric unit, *Psychiatr Q* 69(l):45, 1098.

Haber L et al: Comparison of registered nurses' and nursing assistants' choices of intervention for aggressive behaviors, *Issues Mental Health Nurs* 18:1-3, 1997.

Harris G, Rice M: Risk appraisal and management of violent behavior, *Psychiatr Serv* 48(9):1168, 1997.

Hughes D: Acute psychopharmacological management of the aggressive patient, *Psychiatr Serv* 50(9):1135, 1999.

Johnson M: Being restrained: a study of power and powerlessness, *Issues Mental Health Nurs* 19:191, 1998.

Joint Commission on Accreditation of Healthcare Organizations: *Revised standards and scoring guidelines for restraint and seclusion*, Oakbrook Terrace, 1996, JCAHO.

Kavoussi R et al: The neurobiology of impulsive aggression, *Psychiatr Clin North Am* 20:395, 1997.

Lancee W et al: The relationship between nurses' limit-setting styles and anger in psychiatric inpatients, *Psychiatr Serv* 46:609, 1995.

Lanza M et al: Environmental characteristics related to patient assault, *Issues Mental Health Nurs* 15:319, 1994.

Lanza M et al: Staffing of inpatient psychiatric units and assault by patients, *J Am Psychiatr Nurses Assoc* 3(2):42, 1997.

Lendemaijer B, Shortridge-Baggett L: The use of seclusion in psychiatry: a literature review, *Scholarly Inquiry Nurs Pract* 11(4):299, 1997.

LePage J: The impact of a token economy on injuries and negative events on an acute psychiatric unit, *Psychiatr Serv* 50(7):941, 1999.

LePage J et al: The impact of the numbers of young adults on an inpatient psychiatric unit, *J Psychosoc Nurs* 3 8(l):33, 2000.

Levin P et al: Insights of nurses about assault hospital-based emergency departments, *Image*, 30(3): 249, 1998.

Lewis M, Dehn D: Violence against nurses in outpatient mental health settings. *J Psychosoc Nurs* 37(6):28, 1999.

Littrell K, Littrell S: Current understanding of violence and aggression: assessment and treatment, *J Pychosoc Nurs* 36(12):18, 1998.

Love C, Hunter M: Violence in public sector psychiatric hospitals, *J Psychosoc Nurs* 34:30, 1996.

Martinez R et al: From the other side of the door: patient views of seclusion. *J Psychosoc Nurs* 3 7(3):13, 1999.

McNiel D, Binder R: Correlates of accuracy in the assessment of psychiatric inpatients' risk of violence, *Am J Psychiatry* 152:901, 1995.

Morrison E: The culture of caregiving and aggression in psychiatric settings, *Arch Psychiatr Nurs* 12(l):21, 1998.

Niehoff D: *The biology of violence,* New York, 1999, Free Press.

Nolan K, et al: Psychopathy and violent behavior among patients with schizophrenia or schizoaffective disorder, *Psychiatr Serv* 50(6):787, 1999.

Olofsson B et al: Nurses' narratives about using coercion in psychiatric care, *J Adv Nurs* 28(i):45, 1998.

Olsen D: Ethical considerations of video monitoring psychiatric patients in seclusion and restraint, *Arch Psychiatr Nurs* 12(2):90, 1998.

Owen C et al: Violence and aggression in psychiatric units, *Psychiatr Serv* 49(11):1452, 1998.

Poster E: A multinational study of psychiatric nursing staff s beliefs and concerns about work safety and patient assault, *Ach Psychiatr Nurs* 10:365, 1996.

Poster E, Ryan J: A multiregional study of nurses and patient assault, *Hosp Community Psychiatry* 45:1104, 1994.

Rainee A et al: Interaction between birth complications and early maternal rejection in predisposing individuals to adult violence: specificity to serious, early-onset violence, *Am J Psychiatr* 154(9):1265, 1997.

Ray C, Subich L: Staff assaults and injuries in a psychiatric hospital as a function of three attitudinal variables, *Issues Mental Health Nurs* 19:277, 1998.

Restraint deaths cause JCAHO to release a sentinel event alert! *PSC Healthcare* 4(2):I, 1999.

Ross, E: Death by restraint, *Behavioral Healthcare Tomorrow* April, 21-23, 1999.

Steinert T et al: Aggressive behavior against self and others among first-admission patients with schizophrenia, *Psychiatr Serv* 50(l):85, 1999.

Tardiff K: *Concise guide to assessment and management of violent patients,* Washington, DC, 1996, American Psychiatric Press.

Tardiff K: Prediction of violence in patients, *J Practical Psychiatry Behavioral Health,* 4(l):12, 1998.

Tardiff K et al: Violence by patients admitted to a private psychiatric hospital, *Am J Psychiatry* 154:88, 1997.

Visalli H et al: Reducing high-risk interventions for managing aggression in psychiatric settings, *J Nurs Care Qual* 11(3):54,1997.

Volavka J: The neurobiology of violence: an update, *J Neuropsychiatry Clin Neurosci* II(3):307, 1999.

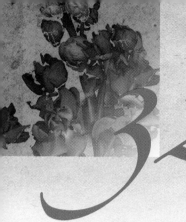

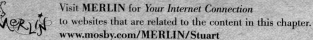

32 Cognitive Behavioral Therapy

Gail W. Stuart

But humanism stands for the whole person, the whole individual striving to become as conscious and responsible as possible about everything in the universe.

DORIS LESSING, *THE GOLDEN NOTEBOOK*

Cognitive behavioral therapy applies learning theories to problems of living, with the aim being to help people overcome difficulties in everyday life. These difficulties often occur along with a medical or psychiatric disorder (Deale et al, 1997; Esterling, 1996; Greenberger & Padesky, 1995). The techniques of cognitive behavioral therapy can also be applied to school, work, home, family, and leisure activities. In these situations cognitive behavioral therapy strategies can help people to achieve personal growth by expanding their coping skills. They can be used by nurses with any background and in any health-care setting to promote healthy coping responses and to change maladaptive behavior.

Cognitive behavioral therapy is problem focused and goal oriented, and it deals with here-and-now issues. It views the individual as the primary decision maker about goals and issues to be dealt with during treatment. This chapter reviews the key concepts of cognitive behavioral therapy, the treatment process, and specific strategies that can be used in nursing practice.

DEFINITION OF BEHAVIOR

Behavior is any observable, recordable, and measurable act, movement, or response. A behavior must be accurately described before it can be measured, and this is done in different ways. For example, the behavior of eating can be broken down into parts such as selecting the food items, preparing the meal, setting the table, eating the meal, and cleaning the dishes after the food is eaten. In contrast, this behavior can be more globally described as eating dinner.

This example shows that there can be several different and accurate definitions for what appears to be a single, simple behavior. It also points to the need to begin by describing what is seen or heard and then clarifying this information until the participants agree with the description.

A behavior is what is observed—not the conclusion, inferences, or interpretations drawn from the observation. For example, hyperactivity is not a behavior but is a conclusion drawn from a set of behaviors. Hyperactivity cannot be measured. What can be measured is the number of times a child gets out of his or her seat, interrupts a conversation, drops a book, or completes required homework assignments. Thus treatment for the child should focus not on hyperactivity but on the specific behaviors that interfere with the child's adjustment to school, home, or the community.

Other examples of inferences rather than behaviors are psychiatric diagnoses and the labeling of patients as uncooperative, aggressive, difficult, noncompliant, or hostile. These adjectives globally describe a person but do not reflect the specific behavior that led to such conclusions. Similarly, when formulating a nursing diagnosis it is essential that the nurse identify the specific defining characteristics of the nursing diagnosis that apply to the patient. In this way, the nurse will have recorded specific behaviors that can be measured over time. These can then be used to evaluate the patient's progress toward expected outcomes.

A clear definition of a behavior minimizes subjective interpretations. It is measurable, is not subject to interpretation, and states what the person does.

> *Think about your experiences in psychiatric–mental health nursing. In your view, how much treatment is based on inference rather than on behavior? What impact does this have on patient adherence with treatment plans?*

CLASSICAL CONDITIONING

Classical conditioning focuses on the process by which **involuntary behavior** is learned. It is derived from Pavlov's (1927) famous work in which he taught dogs to salivate at the sound of a bell by associating the bell with meat presented at the same time. The explanation is that one stimulus that is paired with another stimulus comes to produce the same response as that other stimulus. Other examples of classical conditioning include the following:

- Blinking in response to directing a puff of air to someone's eye
- Salivating at the aroma of cookies baking
- Automatically raising the leg when the patellar tendon is struck

A clinical example is when a person becomes conditioned to feel fear in neutral situations that have come to be associated with anxiety, such as heights or traveling in public places. Inconsistent pairings of the two stimuli lead to less reliable learning, and the response gradually disappears if the pairings are discontinued.

OPERANT CONDITIONING

Operant conditioning has been credited to the work of B.F. Skinner (1953) and his co-workers. It is concerned with the relationship between **voluntary behavior** and the environment. Operant behaviors are those that are influenced by the consequences of an action, and they are regarded as a more complex form of learning. Examples include correcting a spelling mistake when writing a letter or studying class notes before an examination. The basic idea is that behaviors are influenced by their consequences and that operant behaviors are cued by environmental stimuli. Behaviors that have a positive consequence will be stronger and are likely to be repeated. In contrast, behaviors that result in negative consequences will be weakened and are less likely to occur.

For example, if a person tells a joke and everyone who is listening to it laughs heartily, the person will probably repeat that joke in another social setting. However, if the person tells the joke and everyone stares blankly or appears quiet and embarrassed, the person will probably not repeat that joke in the future.

Unlike classical conditioning, operant conditioning is strengthened rather than weakened by inconsistent pairings of the behaviors and consequences. That is, a certain behavior is more likely to recur when it is followed unpredictably by positive or negative consequences.

Many of the techniques used in operant conditioning fall under the heading of behavior modification. They are based on the assumption that a high-frequency, preferred activity can be used to reinforce a low-frequency, nonpreferred activity. For example, if a boy enjoys playing with toy racing cars, this high-frequency preferred activity can be used to reinforce the low-frequency, nonpreferred activity of tidying his room. The terms **reinforcement** and **punishment** do not have the same meaning when used in operant conditioning as when used by most laypeople.

> *Give an example of classical and operant conditioning from your work in a psychiatric setting related to either patient or staff behavior.*

Increasing Behavior

Reinforcers are anything that increases the frequency of a behavior. By far the most commonly used form of reinforcement is positive reinforcement, or rewarding stimuli. An example is a teacher praising students for remaining in their assigned seats. Because of the praise, the students are likely to remain seated more often. However, what is regarded as a positive reward can be quite subjective, and many times people intending to decrease a behavior actually wind up reinforcing it. For example, when a father yells at his son for fighting with his sibling, the yelling may represent to the son a form of desired parental attention and thus may be interpreted as positive reinforcement. As a consequence, the son is likely to continue fighting with his sibling.

Negative reinforcement also increases the frequency of a behavior by reinforcing the power of the behavior to control an aversive, rather than a rewarding, stimulus. An example is putting on sunglasses in glaring sunlight. The sunlight is an aversive stimulus; putting on the sunglasses is the behavior; and escaping the sun's glare is the negative reinforcer. It is negative because it removes or subtracts something from the environment (sunlight), resulting in an increase in the desired behavior (wearing sunglasses). Other examples of negative reinforcement include the following:

- A child who is being scolded by his mother goes up to her and kisses her, and her scolding stops.
- An adolescent who is having trouble in school runs away from home, thus avoiding her parents' displeasure.
- Drivers maintain the speed limit to avoid receiving a traffic ticket.

Decreasing Behavior

Three techniques are used to reduce the frequency of behavior: punishment, response cost, and extinction. Punishment is an aversive stimulus that occurs after the behavior and decreases its future occurrence. An example is a child who must stay in from recess because he or she disrupted the class.

Response cost decreases behavior through the experience of a loss or penalty following a behavior. Examples include paying a fine for overdue library books, losing an allowance for not keeping a clean room, or not being able to attend the next school dance as a result of coming home after curfew.

Extinction is the process of eliminating a behavior by ignoring it or not rewarding it. For example, a child who has frequent temper tantrums is sent to summer camp. On the first day at camp, the child has a tantrum because he or she is not allowed to sleep in a specific bunk. The counselor ignores the child and continues to interact with the other campers. In the next 2 days the child has three more tantrums, and the counselor continues to ignore the outbursts. After the fourth day the child has no more temper tantrums.

The procedures of operant conditioning are summarized in Box 32-1. These procedures are incorporated in many cognitive behavioral treatment strategies, and they can be used by nurses in all areas of practice to help patients overcome a wide range of problems and resume productive lives.

> *Do you think the procedures of operant conditioning can be used by nurses working in medical-surgical settings? Give an example from your experience.*

ROLE OF COGNITION

Cognition is the act or process of knowing. Cognitive therapy proposes that it is not the events themselves that cause anxiety and maladaptive responses but rather people's expecta-

tions and interpretations of these events. It suggests that maladaptive behaviors can be altered by dealing directly with a person's thoughts and beliefs (Beck, 1976; Beck, 1995).

Specifically, cognitive therapists believe that maladaptive responses arise from cognitive distortions. Such distortions might include errors of logic, mistakes in reasoning, or individualized views of the world that do not reflect reality. The distortions may be either positive or negative. For example, someone may consistently view life in an unrealistically positive way and thus take dangerous chances, such as denying health problems and claiming to be "too young and healthy for a heart attack." Cognitive distortions may also be negative, such as those expressed by a person who interprets all unfortunate life situations as proof of a complete lack of self-worth. Common cognitive distortions are listed in Box 32-2.

The goal of cognitive therapy is to change irrational beliefs, faulty reasoning, and negative self-statements. Research has shown that cognitive therapy is an effective intervention for a wide range of clinical problems, particularly depression, anxiety, eating disorders, personality disorders, and schizophrenia (Wright & Beck, 1995). It can be used in inpatient, outpatient, and psychosocial rehabilitation treatment programs. Therefore interventions that include principles of cognitive therapy have much to contribute to psychiatric nursing practice (Blair, 1996; Stuart & Laraia, 1996).

> *Give an example from your personal experiences of each cognitive distortion listed in Box 32-2. What was the consequence of each distortion, if any?*

Box 32-1

Operant Conditioning Procedures

INCREASING BEHAVIOR

Procedure: **Positive reinforcement**

Definition: Adding a rewarding stimulus as a consequence of a behavior, thus increasing the probability that it will occur again

Example: Behavior → Rewarding stimulus → Behavior ↑

Procedure: **Negative reinforcement**

Definition: Removing an aversive stimulus as a consequence of a behavior, thus increasing the probability that it will occur again

Example: Aversive stimulus → Behavior → Aversive stimulus removed → Behavior ↑

DECREASING BEHAVIOR

Procedure: **Punishment**

Definition: Presentation of an aversive stimulus as a consequence of a behavior, thus decreasing the probability that it will occur again

Example: Behavior → Aversive stimulus → Behavior ↓

Procedure: **Response cost**

Definition: Loss or withdrawal of a reinforcer as a consequence of a behavior, thus decreasing the probability that it will occur again

Example: Behavior → Loss of reinforcer → Behavior ↓

Procedure: **Extinction**

Definition: Withholding a reinforcer as a consequence of a behavior, thus decreasing the probability that it will occur again

Example: Behavior → Reinforcement → Behavior → No reinforcement → Behavior ↓

COGNITIVE BEHAVIORAL THERAPY AND THE NURSING PROCESS

There are many misperceptions about cognitive behavioral therapy. One misperception is that it involves controlling the patient. Another misperception is that relationship factors are neglected in the treatment process. Neither of these perceptions is true. The major characteristics of cognitive behavioral therapy are listed in Box 32-3.

Cognitive behavioral therapy is totally patient centered. It views the person as a unique individual who has a problem of living rather than a psychopathological condition. Maladaptive behaviors, as well as adaptive coping responses, are believed to be acquired through the process of learning. Thus emphasis is placed on behavioral monitoring and on the completion of homework by the patient to reinforce the skills learned in therapy and to promote their use in real life. Rather than trying to remove problems by changing subconscious dynamics, the cognitive behavioral therapist works with the patient to plan experiences that encourage the development of new skills.

Another important characteristic is the high degree of mutuality in the treatment process. Cognitive behavioral therapists collaborate with the patient in defining the problem, identifying goals, formulating treatment strategies, and evaluating progress. Because the focus is on the patient's self-control, cognitive behavioral therapy is seen as educational and skill building rather than curative, with the therapist taking a facilitative role. Genuineness, warmth, empathy, and the therapeutic relationship are important, and full recognition is given to their significance in influencing the effectiveness of treatment.

Box 32-2

Cognitive Distortions

Distortion: **Overgeneralization**
Definition: Draws conclusions about a wide variety of things on the basis of a single event
Example: A student who has failed an examination thinks, "I'll never pass any of my other exams this term and I'll flunk out of school."

Distortion: **Personalization**
Definition: Relates external events to oneself when it is not justified
Example: "My boss said our company's productivity was down this year, but I know he was really talking about me."

Distortion: **Dichotomous thinking**
Definition: Thinking in extremes—that things are either all good or all bad
Example: "If my husband leaves me I might as well be dead."

Distortion: **Catastrophizing**
Definition: Thinking the worst about people and events
Example: "I'd better not apply for that promotion at work because I won't get it and I'll feel terrible."

Distortion: **Selective abstraction**
Definition: Focusing on details but not on other relevant information
Example: A wife believes her husband doesn't love her because he works late, but she ignores his affection, the gifts he brings her, and the special vacation they are planning together.

Distortion: **Arbitrary inference**
Definition: Drawing a negative conclusion without supporting evidence
Example: A young woman concludes "my friend no longer likes me" because she did not receive a birthday card.

Distortion: **Mind reading**
Definition: Believing that one knows the thoughts of another without validation
Example: "They probably think I'm fat and lazy."

Distortion: **Magnification/minimization**
Definition: Exaggerating or trivializing the importance of events
Example: "I've burned the dinner, which goes to show just how incompetent I am."

Distortion: **Perfectionism**
Definition: Needing to do everything perfectly to feel good about oneself
Example: "I'll be a failure if I don't get an A on all my exams."

Distortion: **Externalization of self-worth**
Definition: Determining one's value based on the approval of others
Example: "I have to look nice all the time or my friends won't want to have me around."

Box 32-3

Characteristics of Cognitive Behavioral Therapy

Empirically based. Extensive evidence supports cognitive behavioral methods for the treatment of many clinical problems.

Goal oriented. Explicit treatment goals are identified by the patient and therapist. They are then used to evaluate the patient's progress and treatment outcome.

Practical. The patient and therapist focus on defining and solving current problems of living. They discuss the here and now, not the history of the patient.

Collaborative. Collaboration with the patient and active participation by the patient in the treatment process are the norm. Cognitive behavioral therapy helps people to change.

Open. The therapeutic process is open and explicit. The patient and the therapist share an understanding of what is going on in treatment.

Homework. The patient is often given homework assignments for data collecting, skill practice, and reinforcement of new responses.

Measurements. Baseline measurements of the problem behavior are made during the assessment process. These measurements are repeated at regular intervals during and at the completion of treatment. Thus the treatment process is rigorously monitored.

Active. Change and progress in treatment must be meaningful to the patient and have a positive impact on the quality of the patient's life. Both the patient and the therapist are active in therapy. The therapist serves as a teacher and coach, and the patient practices the strategies learned in therapy.

Short term. Cognitive behavior therapy is a short-term treatment that usually lasts 6 to 20 sessions.

From this overview it is evident that cognitive behavioral therapy has many things in common with the nursing process. The steps of the nursing process closely resemble the steps involved in cognitive behavioral therapy. Similarly, both approaches are patient centered and strongly emphasize mutuality. Finally, cognitive behavioral therapy places a strong emphasis on an objective assessment process. Specifically, it uses standardized measurement tools, bases treatment strategies on research evidence, and values ongoing evaluation of patient progress.

These characteristics suggest that cognitive behavioral therapy can make a significant contribution to the therapeutic effectiveness of nursing care. Therefore it has relevance for psychiatric nurses practicing in any setting and with any patient population.

COGNITIVE BEHAVIORAL ASSESSMENT

Cognitive behavioral therapy places great importance on assessment. Cognitive behavioral therapists assess the patient's actions, thoughts, and feelings in particular situations. Assessment includes collecting information, identifying problems from the data, defining the problem behavior, deciding

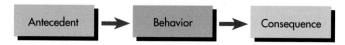

Fig. 32-1   Phases of behavior.

how to measure the problem behavior, and identifying environmental variables that influence the problem behavior. It also includes a review of the patient's strengths and deficits and minimizes the use of assumptions and unvalidated inferences.

> *Nurses form conclusions about the physiological problems of patients after using a variety of tools and tests to collect objective evidence. Why do you think nurses dealing with psychosocial problems often forget to use the scientific approach and instead frequently base their care on unsubstantiated inferences?*

It is important that the patient's problem be defined as clearly as possible. Initially the nurse addresses the following questions:

- What is the problem?
- Where does the problem occur?
- When does the problem occur?
- Who or what makes the problem occur?
- What is the feared consequence related to the problem?

The nurse can then assess the frequency, intensity, and duration of the problem.

The next step is to find out more about the patient's experience with the problem by using a behavioral analysis (Fig. 32-1). This analysis consists of three parts (**the ABCs of behavior**):

- Antecedent: the stimulus or cue that occurs before the behavior and leads to its occurrence
- Behavior: what the person does or does not say or do
- Consequence: what type of effect (positive, negative, or neutral) the person thinks results from the behavior

Antecedents can include the physical environment, the social environment, or the person's behavior, feelings, or thoughts. Behaviors can be broken down into discrete actions or a series of steps. Consequences can be viewed as powerful rewards or punishments of a person's actions. Thus each is a critical element of the assessment. An example of a behavioral analysis is as follows:

- Problem = Anxiety
- Feared consequence = Fear of losing control or dying
- Antecedent = Leaving the house
- Behavior = Avoiding stores, restaurants, and public places
- Consequence = Restriction of daily activities

Another way to assess a person's experiences is to consider the three systems (the **ABCs of treatment**) that are interrelated in this treatment framework:

- Affective: emotional or feeling responses
- Behavioral: outward manifestations and actions
- Cognitive: thoughts about the situation

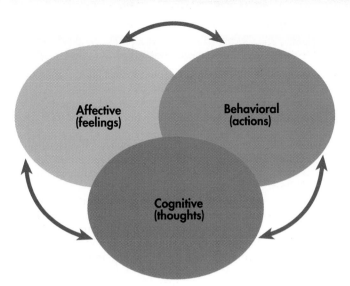

Fig. 32-2 Interacting systems in human behavior.

Fig. 32-2 shows that these three elements are interrelated in explaining human behavior because:

- Feelings influence thinking.
- Thinking influences actions.
- Actions influence feelings.

An assessment of each one of these areas has important implications for understanding the problem and treating it effectively.

Another aspect to be considered in the assessment process is whether the problem is expressed as an observable behavior and whether this behavior is current and predictable. Mutually agreed on treatment goals and strategies can then be determined. Finally, throughout the treatment process, cognitive behavioral therapists use various methods to measure problem severity. These may include case-specific measures as well as standardized rating scales. Chapter 7 discusses psychological evaluation and measurement issues in greater detail.

In your mental health setting, are standardized rating scales used by staff members who work with patients? If so, how are they used? If not, how could their use influence patient care?

TREATMENT STRATEGIES

Cognitive behavioral therapy is the most heavily researched form of psychotherapy and has proven effectiveness in the treatment of a wide variety of clinical problems. It is useful in working with children, adolescents, adults, elderly, and families and may be implemented both individually and in groups. In general, cognitive behavioral treatments include techniques aimed at the following:

- Increasing activity
- Reducing unwanted behavior
- Increasing pleasure
- Enhancing social skills

The three groups of cognitive behavioral treatment strategies are listed in Box 32-4. These techniques may be used

---

Box 32-4

Cognitive Behavioral Treatment Strategies

ANXIETY REDUCTION
Relaxation training
Biofeedback
Systematic desensitization
Interoceptive exposure
Flooding
Vestibular desensitization training
Response prevention
Eye movement desensitization and reprocessing

COGNITIVE RESTRUCTURING
Monitoring thoughts and feelings
Questioning the evidence
Examining alternatives
Decatastrophizing
Reframing
Thought stopping

LEARNING NEW BEHAVIOR
Modeling
Shaping
Token economy
Role playing
Social skills training
Aversive therapy
Contingency contracting

---

alone or in combination. They also require practical skills and efforts from both the nurse and the patient. This may include activities outside the clinical setting, such as taking a bus ride, riding an elevator, or going to a supermarket.

Anxiety Reduction

Relaxation Training. As a therapeutic tool, relaxation training effectively decreases tension and anxiety. It can be used alone, in combination with other cognitive behavioral techniques, or in addition to supportive or insight therapy. The basic premise is that muscle tension is related to anxiety. If tense muscles can be made to relax, anxiety will be reduced.

All relaxation procedures involve rhythmic breathing, reduced muscle tension, and an altered state of consciousness. Clinical experience suggests that there are individual differences in the experience of relaxation. Not everyone demonstrates all of the characteristics of a relaxed physiological state. The physiological, cognitive, and behavioral manifestations of relaxation are listed in Box 32-5.

Systematic relaxation training involves tensing and relaxing voluntary muscles in an orderly sequence until the body, as a whole, is relaxed. For this technique, the patient should be seated in a comfortable chair. Soft music or pleasant visual cues may be present. Before beginning the exercises, a brief explanation should be given about how anxiety is related to muscle tension. The relaxation procedure should also be described.

The patient begins by taking a deep breath and exhaling slowly. This is followed by a sequence of tension-relaxation

Box **32-5**

Manifestations of Relaxation

PHYSIOLOGICAL

Decreased pulse
Decreased blood pressure
Decreased respirations
Decreased oxygen consumption
Decreased metabolic rate
Pupil constriction
Peripheral vasodilation
Increased peripheral temperature

COGNITIVE

Altered state of consciousness
Heightened concentration on single mental image
Receptivity to positive suggestion

BEHAVIORAL

Lack of attention to and concern for environmental stimuli
No verbal interaction
No voluntary change of position
Passive movement easy

Box **32-6**

Sequence of Progressive Muscle Relaxation

Hands. First the fists are tensed and relaxed, then the fingers are extended and relaxed.
Biceps and triceps. These are tensed and relaxed.
Shoulders. They are pulled back and relaxed and then pushed forward and relaxed.
Neck. The head is turned slowly as far to the right as possible and relaxed, then turned to the left and relaxed. It is then brought forward until the chin touches the chest and relaxed.
Mouth. The mouth is opened as wide as possible and then relaxed. The lips form a pout and then relax. The tongue is extended out as far as possible and then relaxed, then retracted into the throat and then relaxed. It is pressed hard into the roof of the mouth and relaxed, then pressed hard into the floor of the mouth and relaxed.
Eyes. They are opened as wide as possible and relaxed, then closed as hard as possible and relaxed.
Breathing. The patient inhales as deeply as possible and relaxes, then exhales as much as possible and relaxes.
Back. The trunk of the body is pushed forward so that the entire back is arched, then relaxed.
Midsection. The buttocks muscles are tensed and then relaxed.
Thighs. The legs are extended and raised approximately 6 inches off the floor and then relaxed. The backs of the feet are pressed into the floor and relaxed.
Stomach. It is pulled in as much as possible and relaxed, then extended and relaxed.
Calves and feet. With legs supported, the feet are bent with the toes pointing toward the head and then relaxed. Feet are then bent in the opposite direction and relaxed.
Toes. The toes are pressed into the bottom of the shoes and relaxed. They are then bent to touch the top inside of the shoes and relaxed.

exercises. The patient is instructed to tense each muscle group for approximately 10 seconds while the nurse describes how tense and uncomfortable this body part feels. The nurse then asks the patient to relax this muscle group as the nurse comments, "Notice how all the hardness and tension is draining from your hands. Now notice how they feel—warm, soft, and calm. Compare this feeling to when they were tense and see how much better they feel now." The patient should be reminded to tense only the muscle group named. The patient then proceeds to the next muscle group in the sequence listed in Box 32-6.

The final exercise asks the patient to become **completely** relaxed, beginning with the toes and moving up through the body to the eyes and forehead. Once the patient has learned the procedure, these exercises can be performed only for the muscles that usually become tense. This is different for each person and may include the shoulders, forehead, back, or neck. Patients may also eliminate the tensing exercises and perform only the relaxation ones.

Meditation may also be used to evoke the relaxation response. It may follow or replace systematic relaxation. The basic components for meditation include the following:

- A quiet environment
- A passive attitude
- A comfortable position
- A word or scene to focus on

The first three components are necessary for any relaxation procedure. The fourth component refers to **visualization**—the process in which the patient selects a cue word or scene with pleasant connotations. The nurse then instructs the patient to close both eyes, relax each of the major muscle groups, and begin repeating the word silently at each exhalation.

Other relaxation techniques include guided imagery, centering, and focusing. Although each of these approaches varies slightly, the intent of all of them is to use the mind to get in touch with the inner self. As such, they have been found to promote relaxation, enhance sleep, reduce pain, and increase creativity (Hoffart & Keene, 1998).

Name four clinical settings in which nurses can use relaxation training with patients. Identify whether such training would be a primary, secondary, or tertiary prevention activity in each setting.

Biofeedback. Biofeedback uses a machine to reduce anxiety and modify behavioral responses. Small electrodes connected to the biofeedback equipment are attached to the patient's forehead. Brain waves, muscle tension, body temperature, heart rate, and blood pressure can then be monitored for small changes. These changes are communicated to the patient by auditory and visual means. The more relaxed the patient becomes, the more pleasant the sounds or sights that are presented. These pleasant sights and sounds stop when the patient stops relaxing, and they resume when the patient reachieves the relaxed state. After developing the ability to relax, the patient is encouraged to apply the technique in stressful situations.

Systematic Desensitization. Systematic desensitization was designed to decrease the avoidance behavior linked to a specific stimulus (e.g., heights, airplane travel). The goal of systematic desensitization is to help the patient change his or her response to a threatening stimulus. It involves combining deep muscle relaxation with imagined scenes of situations that cause anxiety. The assumption is that relaxation is incompatible with anxiety. Therefore if the person is taught to relax while imagining such scenes, the real-life situation depicted by the scene will cause much less anxiety.

With systematic desensitization the patient must first be able to relax the muscles. Next, a hierarchy of the anxiety-provoking or feared situations is constructed. These situations are ranked from 1 to 10 in order of difficulty, with 1 evoking little or no anxiety and 10 evoking intense or severe anxiety. Box 32-7 presents a sample hierarchy of a patient with agoraphobia.

With **in vitro**, or imagined, desensitization, the patient proceeds with the imagined pairing of the hierarchy items with the relaxed state, progressing from the least anxiety-provoking item to the most anxiety-provoking item. **In vivo** desensitization exposes the patient to real rather than imagined life situations. In vivo exposure is widely considered to be the treatment of choice for simple and social phobias and for obsessive-compulsive disorders.

This technique works through a combination of positive reinforcement for confronting anxiety-provoking stimuli and the extinction of maladaptive behavior by realizing that the feared negative consequences never occurred. It is helpful for the nurse to share the following thoughts with the patient during exposure therapy:

- Anxiety is unpleasant but is not dangerous; that is, the patient will not die or lose control.
- Anxiety does eventually decrease and does not continue indefinitely.
- Practice makes perfect; the more the patient repeats a particular exposure exercise, the easier it becomes.

For example, a boy may have a fear of spiders. His daily schedule may then include a series of planned activities involving reading about spiders. He may then begin gradual exposure to pictures and photographs of spiders, followed by looking at real spiders in his yard. Thus the exposure gradually leads to anxiety reduction and more adaptive behaviors.

Interoceptive Exposure. Interoceptive exposure is a technique used to desensitize a patient to catastrophic interpretations of internal bodily cues such as tachycardia, blurred vision, and shortness of breath. A hierarchy is made of the specific symptoms that increase the patient's anxiety. The patient is then asked to do the things that cause these symptoms in a gradually increasing, repetitive manner in order to desensitize him or her to these cues. Patients can be asked to jump in place, run up a flight of stairs, or spin in

Box 32-7

Sample Patient Hierarchy for Phobias

A hierarchy of phobias is a list of your fears and avoidances in order of severity. Your greatest phobia should be at the top of the list and your smallest fear at the bottom. In between, rank your other fears and phobias in order of severity. Try to list 10 but not more than 20 phobias. These activities should be convenient to do, because you will be doing them from several times a day to at least several times per week.

For example, think of yourself standing at the end of a football field marked off in 10-yard lines. Closest to you, at the 0-yard line, is something you are mildly fearful of or avoid doing sometimes but not always; the farthest end of the field is your biggest fear; at the 50-yard line is a medium fear; and on the 10-yard line is a minor fear but one that is stronger than at the 0-yard line.

Remember that everyone's hierarchy will be different. There are no "right" or "wrong" hierarchies. Your hierarchy is a tool to help you approach feared situations in a systematic and controlled way.

SAMPLE HIERARCHY

100	Driving alone across a high bridge in the rain
90	Driving alone on the interstate far from home
80	Driving alone on side streets that are unfamiliar
70	Speaking in front of groups of people
60	Using elevators alone
50	Eating in restaurants alone
40	Going to large public gatherings with safe people
30	Eating with friends or family in familiar restaurants
20	Driving more than several miles from home with a passenger in the car
10	Going shopping with a safe person in big stores and malls
0	Going shopping with a safe person in small stores near home

circles. This technique is especially helpful for patients who do not have agoraphobia but have spontaneous, unprovoked panic attacks that cause them increased worry and anxiety.

Flooding. Flooding is another form of exposure therapy in which the patient is immediately exposed to the most anxiety-provoking stimulus instead of being exposed gradually or systematically to a hierarchy of feared stimuli. If this technique uses an imaginary event instead of a real life event, it is called implosion.

Vestibular Desensitization Training. Vestibular desensitization training is an exposure therapy for patients whose panic attacks are provoked by environmental cues that cause them to have symptoms of motion sickness (e.g., dizziness, imbalance, vertigo, nausea, tinnitus, blurred vision, or headache). These environmental cues can include suddenly changing position, walking on floors with patterns, walking down a grocery store aisle that is stacked high with products on both sides, or riding in a car on a hilly road. A desensitization hierarchy is created to include activities that cause these symptoms, such as getting up suddenly from a prone position, making sudden head movements, or making sudden stop-and-go movements. Patients who get motion sickness when standing in a wide open space with no object to break the horizon are taught to turn in a full circle while keeping their eyes on a selected object for orientation, much like ballet dancers do when they turn repetitively.

Response Prevention. In response prevention the patient is encouraged to face a particular fear or situation without engaging in the accompanying behavior. This technique is based on the concept that repeated exposure to an anxiety-producing stimulus without the presence of the anxiety-reducing response will lead to anxiety reduction because the feared consequence does not occur (see Citing the Evidence).

For example, a patient may fear using a public restroom and engage in hand washing up to 20 times a day. With response prevention treatment, the patient's daily schedule would include using a public restroom, turning on the water faucets, and washing hands for only 30 seconds. Over time, the maladaptive behaviors would be reduced because the feared consequence of germs and illness did not occur.

Eye Movement Desensitization and Reprocessing. Eye movement desensitization and reprocessing (EMDR) is based on specific and repetitive rapid eye movements similar to those experienced naturally in rapid eye movement sleep. The principle behind this treatment is that

the brain lays down biological memory tracks during early traumatic experiences. These memory tracks are provoked later during seemingly unrelated events, causing anxiety and perhaps depression. With EMDR, the patient is asked to think about past traumatic events while the therapist moves his or her hand back and forth in front of the patient's face; the patient's eyes follow the therapist's hands. In this way, the neural tracks are hypothesized to become reprogrammed and less sensitized to anxiety-provoking experiences (Shapiro & Forrest, 1997).

EMDR is being used with a variety of psychological problems, including anxiety, stress, phobias, recurrent nightmares, substance abuse, and posttraumatic stress disorder (see Citing the Evidence). Special training and supervised practice are needed for the safe and successful application of EMDR (Barron et al, 1998).

> *Do you think a highly anxious nurse can effectively implement anxiety-reduction strategies with patients? Why or why not?*

Cognitive Restructuring

Monitoring Thoughts and Feelings. Changing cognitions begins with identifying what is reinforcing and maintaining the patient's dysfunctional thinking and maladaptive behavior. An important first step is for patients to become more aware of and monitor their own thinking and feeling. Patients can be helped to do this through the use of the Daily Record of Dysfunctional Thoughts Form (Fig. 32-3).

The patient uses this form by recording information in each of five columns, beginning with a brief description of a

---

Citing the Evidence on

Relapse Prevention

BACKGROUND: Although relapse prevention (RP) has become a widely adopted cognitive behavioral treatment intervention for alcohol use, smoking, and other substance use, outcome studies have presented an inconsistent picture of the efficacy of this approach. A meta-analysis was performed to evaluate the overall effectiveness of RP and the extent to which other variables may relate to treatment outcome.

RESULTS: Twenty-six published and unpublished studies with more than 9000 participants were included in the analysis. Results indicated that RP was highly effective when applied to alcohol or polysubstance abuse disorders and combined with the use of medication.

IMPLICATIONS: This analysis supports the overall efficacy of RP in reducing substance use and improving psychosocial adjustment. The outcome did not depend on treatment modality or on whether the setting was outpatient or inpatient. Given that this analysis was based on a current and complete body of literature, the findings should have great applicability for evidence-based clinical practice.

Irvin J et al: Efficacy of relapse prevention: a meta-analytic review, *J Consult Clin Psychol* 67(4):563, 1999.

Citing the Evidence on

EMDR

BACKGROUND: Controlled studies of treatments that are effective with victims of natural disasters are almost nonexistent. This is a small study conducted under difficult conditions to test the effectiveness of EMDR in treating trauma-related reactions following Hurricane Andrew.

RESULTS: EMDR produced significant improvement over wait-list controls in perceived posttraumatic avoidance behaviors and thoughts, and it produced significant improvement in subjective aversive reactions to representative experiences of the hurricane.

IMPLICATIONS: These results suggest that EMDR can be an effective intervention for trauma reactions. The study also highlights the difficulty in conducting research in the immediacy of a natural disaster.

Grainger R et al: An empirical evaluation of eye movement desensitization and reprocessing (EMDR) with survivors of a natural disaster, *J Trauma Stress* 10(4):665, 1997.

particular situation or event in the first column. The patient writes down his or her feelings or emotions, as well as the automatic thoughts in response to the situation; the strength of each is rated by the patient. The patient is then encouraged to think of a more rational response to the situation and record that in the fourth column. Finally, in the last column, the patient's reevaluates his or her level of belief in the automatic thought and subsequent emotions. By using such a form, patients are taught to distinguish between thoughts and feelings and to identify more adaptive responses to problematic situations. They also begin to recognize the connection between certain thoughts and maladaptive emotions and behaviors.

Questioning the Evidence. The next step is for the patient and therapist to examine the evidence that is used to support a certain belief. Questioning the evidence also involves examining the source of the data. Patients with distorted thinking often give equal weight to all sources of information or ignore all data except those that support their distorted thinking. Having patients question their evidence with staff, family, and other members of their social support network can clarify misinformation and result in more realistic and appropriate interpretations of the evidence.

Examining Alternatives. Many patients see themselves as having lost all options. This type of thinking is particularly evident in suicidal patients. Examining alternatives involves working with patients to generate additional options based on their strengths and coping resources.

Decatastrophizing. Decatastrophizing is also called the "what-if" technique. It involves helping patients to evaluate whether they are overestimating the catastrophic nature of a situation. Questions that the nurse can ask include, "What is the worst thing that can happen?" "Would it be so terrible if that really took place?" "How would other people cope with such an event?" The goal of this intervention is to help the patient see that the consequences of life's actions are generally not "all or nothing" and thus are less catastrophic.

Reframing. Reframing is a strategy that changes a patient's perception of a situation or behavior. It involves focusing on other aspects of the problem or encouraging a patient to see the issue from a different perspective. Patients who dichotomize events may see only one side of a situation. Weighing the advantages and disadvantages of maintaining a particular belief or behavior can help patients gain balance and develop a new perspective. By understanding both the positive and negative consequences of an issue, the patient can attain a broader perspective of it. For example, suggesting that a mother's overinvolvement with her son is actually a sign of her loving concern may help a family see the situation in a new light.

This strategy also creates an opportunity to help challenge the meaning of a problem or behavior; once the meaning of a behavior changes, the person's response will also change. For example, this strategy might involve helping a patient see an adversity as a potentially positive event. The loss of a job may be perceived as a stressor, but it can also be viewed as an opportunity for pursuing a new job or career.

Date	Situation	Emotion(s)	Automatic Thought(s)	Rational Response	Outcome
	Describe: 1. Actual event leading to unpleasant emotion, or 2. Stream of thoughts, daydream, or recollection, leading to unpleasant emotion	1. Specify sad, anxious, angry, etc. 2. Rate degree of emotion, 1-100.	1. Write automatic thought(s) that preceded emotion(s). 2. Rate belief in automatic thought(s) 0-100%.	1. Write rational response to automatic thought(s). 2. Rate belief in rational response 0-100%.	1. Rerate belief in automatic thought(s), 0-100%. 2. Specify and rate subsequent emotions, 0-100.

Explanation: When you experience an unpleasant emotion, note the situation that seemed to stimulate the emotion. (If the emotion occurred while you were thinking, daydreaming, etc., please note this.) Then note the automatic thought associated with the emotion. Record the degree to which you believe this thought: *0%*, not at all; *100%*, completely. In rating degree of emotion: *1*, a trace; *100*, the most intense possible.

Fig. 32-3   Daily Record of Dysfunctional Thoughts Form. (From Beck A et al: *Cognitive therapy of depression*, New York, 1979, Guilford.)

Think of a problem you encountered in the past year. How might you have used the technique of cognitive reframing to see the situation in a more positive way?

Thought Stopping. Dysfunctional thinking can often have a snowball effect on patients. What begins as a small or insignificant problem can, over time, gather importance and momentum that can be difficult to stop. The technique of thought stopping is best used when the dysfunctional thought first begins. The patient can picture a stop sign, imagine a bell going off, or envision a brick wall to stop the progression of the dysfunctional thought.

To begin, the patient identifies the problematic thought and talks about it as the problem scene is imagined. The nurse interrupts the patient's thoughts by shouting "STOP." Thereafter the patient learns to interrupt thoughts in a similar way. Finally, the patient converts the "stop" into an inaudible phrase or image and thus learns to use the technique quietly in everyday situations.

Learning New Behavior

Modeling. Modeling is a strategy used to form new behavior patterns, increase existing skills, or reduce avoidance behavior. The target behavior is broken down into a series of separate stages that are ranked in order of difficulty or distress, with the first stage being the least anxiety provoking. The patient observes a person modeling the behavior in a controlled environment. The patient then imitates the model's behavior. In participant modeling the model and patient perform the behavior together before the patient performs it alone. For the treatment to be most effective, it is particularly important that the model selected for this treatment be credible to the patient.

Shaping. Shaping induces new behaviors by reinforcing behaviors that approximate the desired behavior. Each successive approximation of the behavior is reinforced until the desired behavior is attained. Skillful use of the technique requires that the nurse carefully look, wait, and reinforce. The nurse needs to look for the desired behavior, wait until it occurs, and then reinforce it when it does occur. An example of this strategy is the nurse noticing that an aggressive child is playing cooperatively with a peer and then praising the child for this behavior.

Token Economy. A token economy is a form of positive reinforcement used most often on a group basis with children or psychiatric hospital inpatients (see Citing the Evidence). It consists of rewarding the patient in various ways (e.g., tokens, passes, or points) for performing desired target behaviors. These target behaviors might include performing hygienic grooming, attending classes, or verbally expressing frustration rather than striking out at others. Tokens may also be lost for inappropriate behaviors. If tokens or points are used, they may be cashed in periodically for rewards such as free time, off-unit outings, games, or sugarless candy.

Role Playing. Role playing allows patients to rehearse problematic issues and obtain feedback about their behavior. It can provide practice for decision making and exploring consequences. A related practice is role reversal, in which the patient switches roles with someone else and thus experiences the difficult situation from another point of view.

Social Skills Training. Smooth social functioning is central to most human activity, and social skill problems exist in many psychiatrically ill patients. Social skill training is based on the belief that skills are learned and therefore can be taught to those who do not have them. The principles of skill acquisition include the following:

- Guidance
- Demonstration
- Practice
- Feedback

These principles must be included in implementing an effective social skills training program, which is often a component of psychiatric rehabilitation programs (see Chapter 15). Guidance and demonstration are usually used early in the treatment, followed by practice and feedback. Treatment typically follows four stages:

1. Describing the new behavior to be learned
2. Learning the new behavior through the use of guidance and demonstration
3. Practicing the new behavior with feedback
4. Transferring the new behavior to the natural environment

Citing the Evidence on

Token Economy

BACKGROUND: Although the use of token economies has been shown to facilitate patient change and improve program functioning in many settings, they have received little attention in acute psychiatric settings. A token economy was introduced on an acute psychiatric care unit of a rural hospital, and the rates of negative events were compared before and after implementation.

RESULTS: The number of negative events fell significantly (a 43% reduction) after the token economy was introduced. Staff and patient injuries were also significantly reduced.

IMPLICATIONS: These findings support the use of the token economy in acute settings to improve the unit milieu by reducing negative events. An advantage of the token economy system for acute care settings is its encouragement of self-directed and self-motivational behavior toward goals. Planning and delay of gratification are central products of the token economy. Such factors are likely to be more relevant to returning patients to self-sufficiency than respite and medication adjustment alone.

LePage J: The impact of a token economy on injuries and negative events on an acute psychiatric unit, *Psychiatr Serv* 50(7):941, 1999.

The types of behaviors that are often taught in these programs include asking questions, giving compliments, making positive changes, maintaining eye contact, asking others for specific behavior changes, speaking in a clear tone of voice, and avoiding fidgeting and self-criticism. This treatment strategy is most often used with patients who lack social skills, assertiveness (assertiveness training), or impulse control (anger management), as well as with patients with antisocial behavior (Aschen, 1997).

Aversion Therapy. Aversion therapy helps to reduce unwanted but persistent maladaptive behaviors. Aversive conditioning applies an aversive or noxious stimulus when a maladaptive behavior occurs. An example is for a patient to snap a rubber band on the wrist when being bothered by an intrusive thought. Covert sensitization is an aversive technique in which patients imagine scenes that pair the undesired behavior with an unpleasant consequence. By imagining aversive consequences for a behavior such as overeating, the patient gains control by providing a form of punishment for his or her own behavior.

> *Aversive therapy has sometimes been criticized as unethical and detrimental to patients' well-being. Do you agree? If not, what conditions should be present before implementing aversive therapy with patients?*

Contingency Contracting. Contingency contracting involves a formal contract between the patient and the therapist, defining what behaviors are to be changed and what consequences follow the performance of these behaviors. Included are positive consequences for desirable behaviors and negative consequences for undesirable behaviors.

ROLE OF THE NURSE

Much of the history of behavioral therapy started in the United States. The first report of nurses functioning as behavioral therapists was from Ayllon and Michael (1959), who taught nurses to use operant skills in modifying the behavior of patients in long-term psychiatric institutions. It was believed that nurses were a natural choice because they made up the majority of the staff caring for the patients. Since that time, the practice of cognitive behavioral therapy nursing has been more dominant in Britain than in the United States.

In 1975 Isaac Marks, a psychiatrist and researcher in London, established the first program to prepare nurses to be cognitive behavioral therapists. This program continues today at the Institute of Psychiatry at the Maudsley in London. The clinical outcomes these nurses achieved were at least as good as those obtained by other professionals. Marks also calculated the cost-benefit ratio of employing nurses as therapists. He found that people treated by nurses used fewer health-care resources after treatment than before, resulting in a significant savings of resources (Ginsberg & Marks, 1977). These were impressive findings, and cognitive behavioral therapy became an increasingly important component of the nurse's role in England and Scotland in the years that followed.

CRITICAL THINKING about CONTEMPORARY ISSUES

Does Humanistic Nursing Care Embrace Cognitive Behavioral Treatment Strategies?

Humanistic care is highly valued in nursing. However, the definition and boundaries of such care are often vague and unspecified. Many believe in the primacy of psychodynamic psychotherapy, yet relatively little research specifies the clinical conditions and disorders for which it is effective. In comparison, there is overwhelming evidence in support of the effectiveness of cognitive behavioral therapy in treating a variety of psychiatric illnesses. This leads one to wonder why cognitive behavioral therapy is not incorporated to a greater degree into the practice of psychiatric nurses.

In fact, few nurses are skilled in the principles and techniques of cognitive behavioral therapy. There are several possible reasons for this. First, nurses may have little formal exposure to cognitive behavioral treatment strategies in the course of their education. Second, nurses have been traditionally reinforced for their unconditional nurturance of patients and their compliance with physicians' orders. In contrast, cognitive behavioral therapy requires the use of independent judgment, limit setting, reframing, and the selective use of rewards that may not be encouraged for nurses in clinical settings. Third, nurses place great emphasis on the therapeutic use of self, and this approach to nursing has sometimes created confusion between the concepts of caring and treatment. It incorrectly suggests that these are different events, with nurses responsible for caring and physicians responsible for treating. Fourth, myths continue to surround the field of cognitive behavioral therapy, and nurses have been slow to acknowledge the facts about this treatment modality (Heifner, 1998; Reilly, 1999).

Current changes in the scope and functions of contemporary psychiatric nursing practice underscore the need for all nurses to learn cognitive behavioral therapy skills (Wakefield & Pallister, 1997). Contemporary psychiatric nursing practice includes both caring and treating activities. The reality is that nurses have always been involved with helping patients reduce anxiety, change cognitions, and learn new behaviors. As influential agents of behavioral change, nurses need to be aware of their ability to promote adaptive or maladaptive responses and increase their skills and knowledge in effective treatment strategies.

In contrast, cognitive behavioral therapy must be more aggressively integrated into the role of the psychiatric nurse in the United States (see Critical Thinking about Contemporary Issues). Nurses are the front-line providers of care. They are the group called on most often to carry out selective reinforcement, modeling, extinction, skills training, shaping, and role playing. Because of their direct patient contact, nurses are best able to observe patients, assess problem areas, and recommend targets for cognitive behavioral intervention.

There are three basic roles for nurses involved in cognitive behavioral therapy. Each of these roles can be performed by all nurses at various levels of expertise—from novice through generalist and specialist:

- Providing direct patient care
- Planning treatment programs
- Teaching others the use of cognitive behavioral techniques

Psychiatric nurses provide direct patient care in both inpatient and community settings, and the value of cognitive behavioral therapy is evident throughout the continuum of care. Most treatments are ideally suited to community settings, and they can include interventions across the continuum of coping responses—from promoting health, to intervening in acute illness, to fostering rehabilitation. Nurses may also function as planners and coordinators of complex treatment programs, consultants, and teachers of other nurses, professionals, patients, and their families. It is clear that with the current emphasis on cost-effective treatment and documented outcomes of care, cognitive behavioral therapy will be a growing area of expertise for all psychiatric nurses in the next decade.

Summary

1. Cognitive behavioral therapy is aimed at helping people to overcome difficulties in any area of human experience. Behavior is any observable, recordable, and measurable act, movement, or response. It is what is observed—not the conclusions drawn from the observation.

2. Classical conditioning focuses on the processes by which involuntary behavior is learned.

3. Operant conditioning focuses on the processes by which voluntary behavior is learned, including increasing and decreasing behavior.

4. Cognitive therapists believe that maladaptive responses arise from cognitive distortions, and the goal of therapy is to correct the faulty thinking that underlies behavioral problems.

5. Cognitive behavioral therapy is similar to the nursing process in that both are patient centered, emphasize mutuality, and place a strong emphasis on the measurement of progress and evaluation.

6. Cognitive behavioral assessment includes collecting information, identifying problems, defining the problem, deciding how to measure the problem, and identifying environmental variables that influence the problem behavior.

7. A variety of cognitive behavioral treatment strategies may be used alone or in combination. They focus on anxiety reduction, cognitive restructuring, and learning new behavior.

8. Three basic roles for nurses involved in cognitive behavioral therapy are providing direct patient care, planning treatment programs, and teaching others the use of behavioral techniques. These roles may be enacted by all nurses in various practice settings.

Competent Caring   A Clinical Exemplar of a Psychiatric Nurse

DARCY O'NEILL, RN

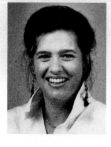

I first met A, a 13-year-old girl, when she was admitted by her mother to our combined child and adolescent psychiatric unit. Her mother reported that A was becoming increasingly oppositional, refusing to attend school, having sexual relations with multiple partners, running away from home for long periods, and exhibiting destructive outbursts when confronted. A was admitted to our unit following a 3-day runaway. She appeared tired and disheveled, somewhat older than her chronological age, and was extremely angry about hospitalization. However, despite her angry demeanor, it was rapidly apparent that A was a very bright and charming young girl. I was intrigued.

During this hospitalization A continued to have unpredictable violent outbursts. At times the most benign redirection would result in verbal threats, screaming, and cursing, which would often escalate into physical attacks on staff. At other times, a similar or more emphatic directive would be calmly accepted and performed. I was puzzled and rather frustrated by trying to balance this child's need to express some deeply felt anger while maintaining the safety of the milieu.

Our unit uses a token economy as part of a patient's treatment. Depending on the age and cognitive abilities, patients earn points or stickers for attending activities and participating in treatment. Points are earned as rewards and may be exchanged for special privileges. Although we specialize in short-term assessment and evaluation, many children quickly engage in this token economy and are able to address behavioral issues in a direct and timely fashion. Unfortunately, A was not one of these children. Her participation in the point system was as unpredictable and sporadic as her behavior.

The team began to discuss the therapeutic effectiveness of an individually designed behavioral program for A. As a new graduate nurse who knew little about the use of behavioral therapies, I balked. I felt that what A needed was more one-to-one time to process the strong emotions underlying her behavior. A and I were beginning to have regular but brief interactions in which she began to share some of her feelings. I feared that by making a more concrete program, obviously different from the program her peers experienced, we risked alienating a child who already had great difficulties with trust. I also feared that from a position of frustration we were falling into a punitive stance. Unfortunately, A was discharged to an outpatient program before the formulation of a new behavioral program. It seemed that many of my questions concerning the therapeutic value of special behavioral programs would remain unanswered.

After I had been on the unit for 6 months, A was readmitted. At this admission her mother reported an increase in the severity and frequency of the behaviors that had precipitated A's

Competent Caring   A Clinical Exemplar of a Psychiatric Nurse—cont'd

first admission. In the time that had passed since her first admission, I had had quite a few opportunities to work with individually designed behavioral programs. I had begun to appreciate this therapeutic approach and to understand that for many children these programs provided a sense of security and an opportunity to address their problem behaviors more concretely. What I had not understood at the time of A's first admission was that these programs increase the amount of one-to-one while helping children to take more control of their behavior. I had discovered that behavioral programs provided the framework for increased teaching and learning.

From the outset of her second admission, A was increasingly difficult to reach. She had become more physically and verbally threatening. I continued to try to engage her in the point system and had moderate success.

A was even more unpredictable. At one minute she was willing to discuss her emotions and was open to nurturance and support, and at the next she was isolated and violent, with no tolerance of any perceived frustration. I was quickly exasperated. I truly liked this charming, bright young girl who showed me through her behavior that she was in a great deal of pain. Many times after a violent or threatening outburst she would cry inconsolably, curled in the fetal position, appearing much younger than her 13 years. I agonized along with the team members on how to help this child out of a self-destructive, downward spiral.

The team quickly returned to the discussion of a special behavioral program. Almost as quickly the staff became divided on how to best design and implement this program. Individual philosophies, differing levels of appreciation for behavioral therapies, and personal limits and tolerances were shared in numerous discussions. With A's full participation and tenuous acceptance, a preliminary program was designed and implemented. Within 3 days some minor improvements were noted, but they were buried in continually violent and impulsive behavior. It took a great deal of painstaking discussion for staff to identify the positive behavior changes and suggest appropriate modifications in the behavior plan in an effort to increase these positive behaviors. Unfortunately, this was not effective for A, and within the next few days she needed seclusion to remain safe.

Again, the team reassessed the program and decided to adopt a more concrete contract with A. A could earn immediate rewards by either exhibiting new positive behaviors or by refraining from old negative behavior. The hope was to extinguish dangerous, self-destructive behaviors while replacing them with new coping strategies. Again, the changes were subtle and erratic and were surrounded by what appeared to be setbacks. This program necessitated hypervigilance on the part of staff to be aware of any positive change, no matter how slight.

I recall one time I was attempting to process with A after she was placed in open seclusion after threatening staff. I found myself desperately searching for positive feedback to offer her. All I could immediately identify was total frustration with her behavior and the program, in addition to my own feelings of inadequacy. Yet I was able to see a number of significant changes as I reviewed her behavioral contract. She had walked to seclusion independently; she needed only one directive to go to the seclusion room; and she was able to sit there without swearing at or threatening me. As soon as I realized all the changes I was witnessing, I became elated. Although she was still unable to talk with me, I continued to state how impressed I was by her ability to eliminate these behaviors. I made a point of sharing this information with passing staff, loud enough for A to hear. In time she was able to process what had happened and reintegrate into the milieu.

Through this trying, challenging experience I believe I was able to grow professionally and personally. I learned in a very deep way the therapeutic necessity of a fully functioning interdisciplinary team, as well as my integral role on that team. More important, I gained a new respect for behavioral programs and the opportunities they offer not only for patients but also for nurses. A well-designed behavioral program provides numerous opportunities for teaching, one-to-one relationship building, and a framework for continual assessment, planning, and evaluation. Although the desired outcomes may be slow in coming and the process difficult, I readily look forward to the next opportunity to use my skills creatively in designing and implementing a behavioral treatment program.

MERLIN **Visit MERLIN: www.mosby.com/MERLIN/Stuart** to find these additional materials and student activities.

- **Worksheets**
- **"Drug of the Month" Updates**
- **"Citing the Evidence" Updates**
- **Critical Thinking Activities and Exercises**
- **Annotated Suggested Readings**
- **Web Links**
- **More!**

Chapter Review Questions

1. Match each term item in Column A with the correct definition in Column B.

Column A	Column B
____ Behavior	**A.** An aversive stimulus that decreases behavior
____ Biofeedback	**B.** Any observable, recordable, measurable act or response
____ Contingency contracting	**C.** Combines deep muscle relaxation with imagined scenes of situations that cause anxiety
____ Extinction	**D.** Immediate exposure to one's most anxiety-provoking stimulus
____ Flooding	**E.** Induces new behaviors by reinforcing behaviors that approximate the desired behavior
____ Punishment	**F.** Involves a formal contract between the patient and the therapist, defining behaviors to be changed and the consequences
____ Shaping	**G.** Monitors brain waves and body activities, allowing a patient to modify behavioral responses
____ Social skills training	**H.** Process of eliminating a behavior by ignoring it or not rewarding it
____ Systematic desensitization	**I.** Strategy used to modify or change a person's perception of a situation or behavior
____ Reframing	**J.** Technique for learning new behavior; consists of guidance, demonstration, practice, and feedback

2. Fill in the blanks.

A. A person's pupil constricting when exposed to bright sunlight is an example of _____.

B. Putting on sunscreen lotion to avoid a sunburn is an example of _____.

C. The three operant conditioning techniques used to decrease behavior are _____, _____, and _____.

D. Cognitive therapy proposes that it is not the event itself but a person's _____ of the event that causes adaptive or maladaptive responses.

E. A list of a person's fears, avoidances, or maladaptive responses in order of severity is called a _____.

F. The three roles for nurses involving cognitive behavioral therapy are _____, _____, and _____.

G. In cognitive behavioral therapy, emphasis is placed on behavioral monitoring and the completion of _____ by the patient.

3. Provide short answers for the following questions.

A. Analyze the nursing assessment form you use in your clinical work from the perspective of a cognitive behavioral therapist. What changes would you make from this perspective?

B. Describe the ABCs of behavior and the ABCs of cognitive behavioral treatment.

C. For 2 days use the daily record of dysfunctional thoughts and evaluate its value for your work with patients.

D. Try the steps of relaxation training on yourself. Note your thoughts, feelings, and behaviors during the process.

REFERENCES

Aschen S: Assertion training therapy in psychiatric milieus, *Arch Psychiatr Nurs* 11:46, 1997.

Ayllon T, Michael J: The psychiatric nurse as a behavioral engineer, *J Exp Anal Behav* 2:323, 1959.

Barron J et al: Eye movement desensitization and reprocessing, *J Am Psych Nurs Assoc* 4(5):140, 1998.

Beck A: *Cognitive therapy and the emotional disorders,* Philadelphia, 1976, Center for Cognitive Therapy.

Beck J: *Cognitive therapy: basics and beyond,* New York, 1995, Guilford.

Blair DT: Cognitive behavioral therapies within the biological paradigm, *J Psychosoc Nurs* 34:26, 1996.

Deale A et al: Cognitive behavior therapy for chronic fatigue syndrome: a randomized controlled trial, *Am J Psychiatry* 154:408, 1997.

Esterling B: Coping with cancer: psychosocial problems and treatment approaches, *J Pract Psychiatry Behav Health* 2:350, 1996.

Ginsberg G, Marks I: Costs and benefits of behavioral psychotherapy: a pilot study of neurotics treated by nurse therapists, *Psychol Med* 7:685, 1977.

Greenberger D, Padesky C: *Mind over mood,* New York, 1995, Guilford.

Heifner C: Critique, *Perspect Psych Care,* 34: 35, 1998.

Hoffart M, Keene, E: The benefits of visualization, *Am J Nurs* 98(12):44, 1998.

Pavlov I: *Conditioned reflexes,* London, 1927, Oxford University Press.

Reilly C: A response to a response, *Perspect Psych Care* 35(3):38, 1999.

Shapiro F, Forrest M: *EMDR: the breakthrough therapy for overcoming anxiety, stress and trauma,* New York, 1997, Basic Books.

Skinner B: *Science and human behavior,* New York, 1953, Free Press.

Stuart G, Laraia M: Panic disorder with agoraphobia. In McBride A, Austin J, editors: *Psychiatric–mental health nursing,* Philadelphia, 1996, WB Saunders.

Wakefield M, Pallister R: Cognitive behavioral approaches to panic disorder, *J Psychosoc Nurs* 35:12, 1997.

Wright J, Beck A: Cognitive therapy. In Hales R et al, editors: *American Psychiatric Press Textbook of Psychiatry,* ed 2, Washington DC, 1995, American Psychiatric Press.

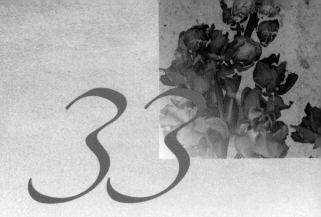

Therapeutic Groups

Paula C. LaSalle

Arthur J. LaSalle

33

Visit **MERLIN** for *Your Internet Connection*
to websites that are related to the content in this chapter.
www.mosby.com/MERLIN/Stuart

Self and world are correlated, and so are individualization and participation. . . . Participation means: being a part of something from which one is, at the same time, separated.

        Paul Tillich, *The Courage to Be*

A group provides nurses with a potentially more therapeutic modality than the two-person nurse-patient encounter. It offers its members a variety of relationships as they interact with each other and with the group leader. Group members come from many backgrounds and must deal with their likes, dislikes, similarities, dissimilarities, envy, timidity, aggression, fear, attraction, and competitiveness (Yalom, 1995). All of this takes place in the context of the dynamics of the group process in which, with careful leadership, members give and receive feedback about the meaning and effect of their various interactions with each other.

Groups can be conducted in a variety of settings, including inpatient units, community and university health centers, schools, churches, and places of employment. Families of people with serious mental illness may join a group for instruction, assistance with coping, mutual support, and crisis intervention. School nurses may lead groups for children who share developmental milestones or life problems, such as parental divorce or death. In each of these situations the format, setting, and goal of the group would vary. Thus group work is an important skill for all nurses to master, regardless of their practice setting or specialty area.

Think of some specific patient situations in which a group approach would be more effective than an individual nurse-patient encounter. Discuss the reasons for this. Describe other situations in which a group format would be less helpful.

DEFINITION

A **group** is a collection of people who have a relationship with one another, are interdependent, and may have common norms. Therapeutic groups have a shared purpose. For example, a group's purpose might be to help members who consistently enter destructive relationships identify and change maladaptive behaviors. Each group has its own structure and identity. The power of the group lies in the contributions of each member and the leader to the shared purpose of the group. These contributions are content and process oriented.

Content functions of the group are met when members share their experiences to help another member. When

673

members share the methods they used to solve a common problem, they are addressing the group's content functions.

Process functions allow the individual to receive feedback from other members and the leader about how the member interacts and is perceived within the group. The group is used as a laboratory or arena to see, experiment, and define relationships and behaviors. For example, a member who complains that his wife is always accusing him of being domineering may receive feedback from the group as to whether others see him acting similarly. Then he has the opportunity to work on changing his behavior in the group before risking the change in the outside world.

The group has primary and secondary tasks. The primary task is necessary for the group's survival or existence; secondary tasks may enhance the group but are not basic to its survival. An example of a primary task for a group of mothers might be to improve mothering skills; a secondary task might be to add to the mothers' social network. Relationships in the group may limit or enhance their willingness to share concerns about mothering.

COMPONENTS OF SMALL GROUPS

To be effective in therapeutic group work, it is necessary to understand the complex processes that occur and be able to use various approaches to increase the therapeutic potential of the group for its members. The components of small groups are summarized in Table 33-1.

Group Structure

Group structure is the group's underlying order. It describes the boundaries, communication and decision-making processes, and authority relationships within the group. The structure offers the group stability and helps to regulate behavioral and interactional patterns.

Group Size

The preferred size of an interpersonally oriented group is 7 to 10 members. The group must have enough people to give members the opportunity for consensual validation as well as the expression of different viewpoints. If the group has too many people, not all members will be given enough time to speak and some will feel excluded. There will also be insufficient time to analyze and discuss interactions. If the group has too few members, not enough sharing and interaction may occur.

Length of Sessions

The optimum length of a session is 20 to 40 minutes for lower-functioning groups and 60 to 120 minutes for higher-functioning ones. For the latter groups a few minutes are spent warming to the task of working, then most of the session is spent on group work, and finally the group summarizes and takes care of unfinished business from that session.

Communication

One of the group leader's primary tasks is to observe and analyze the communication patterns within the group. Using feedback, the leader helps members become aware of the group dynamics and communication patterns so that they may realize the significance of these patterns for the group and for themselves. The group or individual members may then experiment and change these patterns if they choose.

Observable verbal and nonverbal elements of the group's communication include the following:

- Individual member communications
- Spatial and seating arrangements
- Common themes expressed by the group
- How often and to whom members communicate
- How members are listened to in the group
- What problem-solving processes occur in the group

These behaviors help the leader assess resistance within the group, interpersonal conflict, the roles assumed by some of the members, the level of competition, and how well the members understand and are working on the task.

Group Roles

In studying groups it is important to observe the roles that members assume in the group. Each role has certain expected behaviors and responsibilities.

Table **33-1**

Components of Small Groups	
Components	**Characteristics**
Group structure	The group's underlying order; includes boundaries, communication, and decision-making processes, as well as authority relationships; offers stability and helps regulate behavior and interactional patterns.
Group size	Preferred size is 7 to 10 members.
Length of sessions	Optimum length of a session is 20 to 40 minutes for lower-functioning groups and 60 to 120 minutes for higher-functioning groups (divided into time for a brief warm-up, work time, and a brief wrap-up).
Communication	Feedback is used to help members identify group dynamics and communication patterns.
Roles	Determined by behavior and responsibilities assumed by the members of the group.
Power	Ability to influence the group and other members.
Norms	Standards of behavior in the group; influence communication and behavior; communicated overtly or covertly.
Cohesion	The strength of the members' desire to work together toward common goals; related to group's attraction and member satisfaction.

The role a member takes can be determined by observing communication and behavioral patterns. The following factors influence role selection: the member's personality, the interaction in the group, and the member's position in the group. Three types of roles people can play in groups are (Benne & Sheats, 1948) as follows:

- **Maintenance roles,** which involve group processes and functions
- **Task roles,** which deal with completing the group's task
- **Individual roles,** which are not related to the group's tasks or maintenance; they may be self-centered and distracting for the group

These roles are summarized in Table 33-2. A person who acts as a harmonizer and peacemaker would be taking a maintenance role. A person in the task role of questioner might clarify and seek new information.

Table **33-2**

Group Roles and Functions	
Role	Function
MAINTENANCE ROLES	
Encourager	To be a positive influence on the group
Harmonizer	To make/keep peace
Compromiser	To minimize conflict by seeking alternatives
Gatekeeper	To determine level of group acceptance of individual members
Follower	To serve as an interested audience
Rule maker	To set standards for group behaviors (such as time and dress)
Problem solver	To solve problems to allow group to continue its work
TASK ROLES	
Leader	To set direction
Questioner	To clarify issues and information
Facilitator	To keep the group focused
Summarizer	To state current position of the group
Evaluator	To assess performance of the group
Initiator	To begin group discussion
INDIVIDUAL ROLES	
Victim	To deflect responsibility from self
Monopolizer	To actively seek control by incessant talking
Seducer	To maintain distance and gain personal attention
Mute	To seek control passively through silence
Complainer	To discourage positive work and vent anger
Truant/latecomer	To invalidate significance of the group
Moralist	To serve as judge of right and wrong

Modified from Benne KD, Sheats P: *J Soc Issues* 4:41, 1948.

Members may experience a conflict when there is a difference between the role they seek or assume and the role given to them by the group. For example, a member may be expected to be a peacemaker because of having performed that role previously. Now, however, this member may be under additional stress or angry with someone in the group and may choose to start rather than resolve conflict. The group will often be confused and upset by this new role.

> *Consider the last group of which you were a member. Identify the roles that were taken by each group member. Which helped and which interfered with task accomplishment? Give an example of the behavior that was associated with each role.*

Power

Power is the member's ability to influence the group and its other members. The power structure in the group is usually resolved in its initial stages. To determine the power of various members, it is helpful to assess which members receive the most attention, which are listened to most, and which make decisions for the group.

Resolution of the power struggle does not necessarily mean that everyone will be satisfied with the arrangement. Sometimes a continual struggle for power occurs. This may be functional if the members are trying to gain new leadership that contributes to their therapeutic goals. It can be dysfunctional when it takes the group's energy and attention away from other tasks.

Norms

Norms are standards of behavior. They are expectations of how the group will act in the future based on its past and present experiences. It is important to understand norms because they influence the quality of communication and interaction within the group. The observance of norms results in conforming. The member who does not follow the norms may be considered rebellious or resistant by the other group members. Conforming to group norms is essential to being a fully accepted member. A member who is always late to meetings is not conforming to group norms. The group will decide to what extent it will tolerate this behavior.

Norms are created to:

- Facilitate accomplishment of the group's goals or tasks
- Control interpersonal conflict
- Interpret social reality
- Foster group interdependence

Norms may be communicated overtly or covertly. Overt expression of norms may be written or clearly stated. For example, members may tell a new member that smoking is not allowed in the group. Covert expression of norms may be implied through members' behavior. For example, a member who uses foul language may be ignored by the other members.

A highly cohesive group may have appropriate or inappropriate norms. For example, a group of patients may unite to help a patient sneak a cigarette when such behavior is contraindicated because of that patient's health problems. The group may also unite to do what it can to prevent that patient from smoking.

One area that is important for a group to address is confidentiality. For a group to be most effective, members will talk about issues that may be painful, embarrassing, or disturbing. The group members need to agree that whatever is discussed in the group belongs to the group. Group content will not be discussed outside of the group unless there is specific discussion and agreement about it. This norm should be communicated overtly, and some groups may even want members to sign an agreement of confidentiality.

> *Identify and describe group norms that you have observed in a selected clinical setting and in the classroom. Did anyone deviate from a norm? How did the group respond? How did the leader respond?*

Cohesion

Cohesion is the strength of the members' desire to work together toward common goals. It influences members to remain in the group. It is related to each member's attraction to and satisfaction received from the group. Cohesion is a basic fiber of any group because it affects its life span and success. Many factors contribute to the level of cohesion, including agreement of members on group goals, interpersonal attractiveness between the members, degree to which the group satisfies individual needs, similarities among members, and satisfaction of members with the leadership style.

Because cohesion is such an important dimension, some group leader interventions are aimed toward promoting it. These may include encouraging members to talk directly with each other, discussing the group in "we" terms, and encouraging all members to sit within the space reserved for the group. A leader can also promote cohesion by pointing out similarities among group members, helping members listen to each other, and encouraging cooperation among the members.

The group leader continually monitors the level of cohesion in the group. Group leaders might observe how much members express interest in each other and recognize each other for their individuality. Another way to measure cohesion is to find out whether members identify with the group and whether they want to remain in the group.

GROUP DEVELOPMENT

Groups, like individuals, have capacity for growth and development. Likewise, they have the ability to regress and resist working effectively. Every group develops according to a series of three interpersonal stages: inclusion, or being in or out; control, or being top or bottom; and affection, or being near or far. Each stage is characterized by members expressing various aspects of the same interpersonal issue or conflict.

In group development, phases may overlap, or a group may regress to a previous phase. For example, group regression can occur when a new member is added. Phases of group development can be thought of as a path that a group

takes to form and accomplish its objectives. The leader's task is to understand and assist the group as it moves along its growth path.

Pregroup Phase

An important factor to consider in starting a group is its goals. The group's purpose will greatly influence many of the leader's behaviors. There may be more than one group goal; if so, the primary goal should be clear. To guarantee success, the group's goals must be understood by all people involved, including the members and sponsoring agencies. It is the leader's role to clarify the task and help the group achieve it.

Once the purpose is established, the leader must be sure that the group has administrative permission. A written group proposal is one effective way to request this. Box 33-1 lists information to include in a group proposal. To avoid possible problems, the leader should explore any administrative limitations. For example, an agency may not permit a group to meet beyond its physical facilities or may prefer that the leader not use certain techniques in the group. Also, any potential cost to the agency should be clearly identified.

The leader is also responsible for finding physical space for the group. The leader identifies the room requirements of the group. For example, in a patient education group resources such as a blackboard or movie projector may be needed. A psychotherapy group may need space for comfortable chairs to be placed in a circle without a table. In a group that plans to use human relations exercises, a more spacious room will probably be needed. In all cases the group room should be comfortable, private, and quiet. The same room should be used for each meeting. Leaders often have to adapt inadequate space to fit the needs of the group. The session itself is more important than where it is conducted.

The next responsibility of the group leader is to select members. The selection is based on the purposes of the

---

Box 33-1

Group Proposal Guideline

List the group goals, primary and secondary.
List group leaders and their related expertise.
List theoretical frameworks used by the leaders to meet the group goals.
List criteria for membership.
Describe the referral and screening process.
Describe the structure of the group.
   Meeting place _____
   Meeting time _____
   Length of each meeting _____
   Number of members _____
   Length of group _____
   Expected member behaviors _____
   Expected leader behaviors _____
Describe the evaluation process for members and the group.
Describe resources needed for the group, such as coffee, a movie projector, or audiovisual equipment.
If pertinent, describe the expected cost and financial benefits incurred by the group.

group, referrals to the group, and interviews with potential members. The leader or the agencies must provide information about the group to potential sources of referrals. All information should clearly identify the group's purpose and state the criteria for membership eligibility and the time, place, and duration. The leaders' names and professional credentials should be provided.

Membership will greatly influence the group's outcome. In selecting members the leader should consider group cohesion and therapeutic problem solving. Selection criteria include problem areas, motivation, age, sex, cultural factors, educational level, socioeconomic level, ability to communicate, intelligence, and coping and defensive styles. Homogeneous groups will share preselected criteria (for example, all members will be women who suffered incest as children). Heterogeneous groups will include a mixture of people, such as a group for men and women who want to build their self-esteem.

If possible, the leader should decide whether the membership of the group will be closed or open before screening members. A group is closed if no new members are added once the group is started. In an open group, members leave and new members are added throughout the duration of the group. Open groups may maintain the same purpose, with both members and leaders changing. They usually continue indefinitely with no termination date. The closed group offers the advantage of consistency of leadership, norms, and expectations. The open group, on the other hand, continually brings fresh ideas and opportunities for learning to its members.

The screening interview's primary purpose is to determine the appropriateness of the potential member to the group. Secondary purposes accomplished during the screening interview include the following:

- Beginning to develop a relationship between the leader and the member
- Determining the motivation of the possible member
- Determining whether the candidate's goals are in agreement with the group goals
- Educating the candidate about the nature of the group

- Determining the type of group experience the person has had
- If appropriate, beginning to review the group contract

In addition to or instead of the screening interview, some clinicians use group intake meetings. Several new members meet in a group to learn about the group process and identify some possible treatment goals. This approach is less costly and has the same objectives as the screening interview.

As soon as possible a decision should be made about group membership. Candidates not selected should be referred to other treatment options. The reasons for not being selected should be explained to the candidate and, if appropriate, to the person who made the referral.

> *You are asked to develop a group treatment program for victims of discrimination. What membership characteristics will you list as necessary for inclusion in the group? What will you say to the patients who are not selected for inclusion in your group?*

Initial Phase

The initial phase includes meetings in which the group's members begin to settle down to work. This phase is characterized by anxiety about being accepted by the group, the setting of norms, and the casting of various roles. This phase has been subdivided into three stages by Yalom (1995): the **orientation**, conflict, and **cohesive** stages. These stages correspond to Tuckman's (1965) first three phases of group development: **forming**, **storming**, and **norming**. Table 33-3 summarizes Tuckman's and Yalom's stages of group development.

Orientation Stage. This stage corresponds to Tuckman's **forming** stage. The leader is more directive and active than in other stages. The leader orients the group to its primary task and helps the group arrive at a group contract. Some common factors that may be included in the group contract are goals, confidentiality, meeting times, honesty, structure, and communication rules (for example, only one person may talk at a time).

Table 33-3

Developmental Phases in Small Groups				
Yalom Phase	Tuckman Phase	Definition	Task Activity	Interpersonal Activity
Orientation	**Forming**	Group members concerned with orientation	To identify task and boundaries regarding it	Relationships tested; interpersonal boundaries identified; dependent relationship with leaders, other group members, or pre-existing standards established
Conflict	**Storming**	Group members resistive to task and group influence	To respond emotionally to task	Intergroup conflict
Cohesive	**Norming**	Resistance to group overcome by members	To express intimate personal opinions about task	New roles adopted; new standards evolved in group feelings; cohesiveness developed
Working	**Performing**	Creative problem solving done; solutions emerge	To direct group energy toward completion of task	Interpersonal structure of group becomes a tool to achieve its task; roles become flexible and functional

Because an important part of this phase is norm setting, the leader should ensure that the norms will help the group achieve its goals. Another task of the leader in this stage is to foster a sense of belonging or cohesion among the members. To accomplish this, the leader encourages interaction among members and maintains the group at a working level of anxiety. For example, the leader could refer to the group as "our" group and suggest how members can help each other. Members could be encouraged to state what they hope to learn from the group. The leader would then reinforce realistic expectations and give examples of how the group might meet them.

During the first stage the members are evaluating each other, the group, and the leader. They are deciding whether they are going to be a part of the group and how much they will participate. Some common conscious or unconscious concerns of members during this stage are fear of being rejected, fear of self-disclosure, and fear of not being seen as an individual. Social behaviors are important, and the members are attempting to develop their social roles. The roles members assume during this stage are often renegotiated during other stages.

The group is dependent, and members will often test out their dependency needs and wishes on the leader. They look to the leader for structure, approval, and acceptance and may try to please the leader with reward-seeking behaviors. The leader must not meet all the dependency wishes of the members but must encourage them to interact more with one another. This supports members in becoming more interdependent and less dependent on the leader. The dependency issue between the leader and the members may lead the group into conflict and thus into the second stage.

Conflict Stage. This stage of the group corresponds to Tuckman's **storming** stage of group development. Issues related to control, power, and authority become primary. Members are concerned about the pecking order or deciding who is top or bottom in control and decision making. The dependency conflict may be openly or covertly expressed, with members polarized between independent and dependent issues. This stage reflects a struggle between the counterdependent and dependent members, with the counterdependent members wanting to assume the leader's role. For example, a group may be divided over the issue of whether members can telephone each other. Some members may want the leader to decide, whereas others may think that the leader's statements are irrelevant. During this phase the counterdependent members might sit in the leader's chair and let the leader know that the directions have been unsuccessful or unheard. The dependent members might ask the leader for more directions. Other members who are neutral (neither dependent nor counterdependent) eventually may help the group resolve this conflict.

Subgroups usually form within the group, and hostility may be expressed. Often the hostility is directed toward the leader, but it may also be expressed toward other members. The leader's tasks are to allow expression of both negative and positive feelings, help the group understand the under-

lying conflict, and prevent or examine nonproductive behaviors such as scapegoating. This phase is usually the most difficult for the new leader because some members may lead the leader to believe that he or she has failed the group by not living up to its unrealistic expectations.

The leader must be careful not to avoid or suppress the group members' anxiety and, at times, should encourage the expression of hostility. If hostility toward the leader is expressed indirectly, such as anger toward other authority figures (staff members, teachers, or parents), the leader should help the group express its anger more directly. A useful technique is for the leader to give the group permission to discuss its anger by acknowledging that the group may be disappointed or angry at the leader.

By the end of the conflict stage the leader may be dethroned, and his or her omnipotent role, with its "magical" solutions, may be discarded. Slowly the leader becomes humanized. Members learn that responsibilities for the group are shared. Members may also learn that expressions of anger and disappointment do not destroy the leader and may help the group assess its resources and limitations more accurately. The group's resources can then be used to achieve its tasks. Members may realize that conflicts need not be avoided; instead, through discussion, conflicts may increase the group's maturity and usefulness.

Cohesive Stage. Tuckman's **norming** phase is closely related to the cohesive stage. Group members, after resolving the second stage, feel a strong attraction toward one another and a strong attachment to the group. Positive feelings toward one another and the group are often expressed, and negative feelings are usually not shared.

At this stage, members feel free to give self-disclosing information and share more intimate concerns. However, the group's problem-solving ability is restricted because negative communication is usually avoided in order to maintain the high group morale. The leader's task is to make a connection between the members' disclosures and the group's primary task. The leader should not interfere with the group's basic cohesion but should encourage the group to use its problem-solving ability. The leader shows how a group member can have individual concerns and values and still be productive within the group. In other words, the leader demonstrates that differing and opposite opinions may not destroy the group identity.

At the resolution of this stage, members may learn that self-discoveries and differences should not be feared. They also learn that similarities and differences between the members may help the group achieve its tasks. At the end of the cohesive stage the group begins to see task achievement as a reality. The members gain a more realistic and honest view of their ability to work together and accomplish their primary and secondary tasks.

Compare behaviors that would indicate that a group is in the orientation stage, the conflict stage, and the cohesive stage. Give specific examples. What leader interventions would be appropriate at each stage?

Working Phase

The working phase of a group can be compared with Tuckman's **performing** stage of group development. During this stage the group becomes a team. It directs its energy mainly toward completing its tasks. Although they are hard at work, this phase is enjoyable for both the leader and the members. Responsibility for the group is more equally shared, anxiety is usually decreased and tolerated better, and the group is more stable and realistic.

Therapeutic forces occur in group therapy. Eleven of these therapeutic or curative factors are presented in Table 33-4 (Yalom & Vinogradov, 1989). Although these factors were identified in relationship to therapy groups, they apply to experiences in all types of groups (Bender & Ewashen, 2000). Other therapeutic factors important in promoting positive change in short-term groups include self-responsibility and self-understanding.

The leader's major role is to help the group complete its tasks by maximizing effective use of its curative properties. Because the members are fully participating in the group's work, the leader's activity level decreases. The leader now acts more as a consultant to the group. The leader helps to keep the group goal-directed and tries to decrease the impact of anything that may regress or retard the group.

Because this phase is the group's creative problem-solving and resolution phase, there are few, if any, specific guidelines for the leader. The leader's interventions are based primarily on theoretical frameworks, experiences, personality, and intuition, as well as the needs of the group and its members. In addition to fostering group cohesion, maintaining its boundaries, and encouraging the group to work on its tasks, the leader may help the group solve specific problems. Because these problems are unique to the group, many are not predictable. Some of the more common problems are the formation of subgroups, the management of conflict, determining the optimum level of self-disclosure, and dealing with resistance.

Subgroups that conflict with the group's goals and are not acknowledged by the group can restrict its work. Other members may feel excluded, and loyalties will be divided between the subgroup and the whole group. For example, in a women's group, two of the members may become close friends, keeping secrets from the group and engaging in private conversations during the session. Other members may feel excluded from this pair and be ineffective in working with them. To decrease the negative impact of a subgroup, its consequences and the group's reactions should be openly discussed.

Conflict is unavoidable and can be used to foster growth. However, expression of conflict may need to be controlled so that the intensity does not exceed the group's tolerance. Examples of conflict are competition among members for the leader's attention and a disagreement between two members. A leader may manage conflicts by identifying the conflict, explaining that conflicts are natural and can lead to growth, and encouraging members to discuss the reasons for the conflict. Successful conflict resolution is related to the amount of group cohesion, trust, and acceptance among the members.

Self-disclosure in the group is usually related to the amount of acceptance and trust the member feels. Self-disclosure is always risky. If people give private information too quickly, they will feel vulnerable. On the other hand, if people disclose too little during the working phase they may not be able to form supportive interpersonal relationships. Their growth potential in the group may be decreased.

Resistance, or holding back the therapeutic process, can be expected in therapy groups. Resistance to working on the therapeutic goal can occur at both an individual and a group level. Group work can initially be anxiety producing, since working through interpersonal issues can be personally threatening and emotionally painful. The leader must actively structure the group to make it as nonthreatening as possible and to allow for some early successes for patients (Clarke et al, 1998).

Table 33-4

Yalom's Curative Factors	
Factor	**Definition**
Imparting information	Receiving didactic information and advice
Instillation of hope	Increasing hopefulness of group members
Universality	Realization that others experience similar thoughts, feelings, and problems
Altruism	Experience of sharing part of oneself to help another
Corrective re-enactment	Ability of members to alter learning experience previously obtained of primary family group in their families
Development of social interaction techniques	Opportunity to increase awareness of social interactions and develop social skills
Imitative behaviors	Opportunities to increase skills by imitating behaviors of others in group
Interpersonal learning	Ability to engage in wider range of interpersonal exchanges, thereby increasing each member's understanding of responsibility and complexity of interpersonal relationships and decreasing members' interpersonal distortions
Existential factors	Ability of group to help members deal with meaning of their own existence
Catharsis	Opportunity to express feelings previously unexpressed
Group cohesion	Attraction of member for group and other members

Modified from Yalom ID, Vinogradov S: *Group psychotherapy*, Washington, DC, 1989, American Psychiatric Press.

It is one matter to agree on goals and another to work on obtaining the actual therapeutic outcomes. Resistance by individual members may take many forms, such as avoiding discussion of a conflict, frequent or prolonged silences, attempting to become an assistant leader, absence from the group, pairing between two members, and prolonged or unusually intense expression of hostility. Resistance by the group or a majority of its members may be expressed in ways similar to those used by individuals. Other examples of group resistance include shared silence among the members, unusual amounts of dependency on the leader, scapegoating, subgroup formations, and the wish for magical solutions to resolve group conflict.

Resistance to group psychotherapeutic efforts can have a demoralizing effect on the therapist. With experience in handling resistance, it will become less threatening. The nurse should realize that resistance is a signal that treatment is progressing, that the therapist and the group members are getting close to crucial issues. Resistance may also occur due to increased anxiety related to conflict or change.

The management of resistance depends on the type of group, the group contract, and the therapist's theoretical framework. Some methods of decreasing resistance are to establish trust, make observations regarding the group process or individual behaviors, offer interpretations, counteract the resistant behavior, and demonstrate more adaptive behavioral patterns.

By the end of the second phase, members have made significant progress toward goal achievement. They have a sense of their own productivity and accomplishments. The need for the group or their involvement in the group is less apparent. The group must begin to deal more actively with its final task: separation.

Termination Phase

The work of termination begins during the first phase of the group. However, as the group or individual members approach termination, certain processes are more likely to occur. The termination phase is not always discussed as a definite phase in the literature. It is discussed as a separate phase here because of the significance it may have for the members.

There are two types of termination: termination of the group as a whole and termination of individual members. A closed group usually terminates as an entire group; in an open group, members (and perhaps the leader) terminate separately. Members and groups may terminate prematurely, unsuccessfully, or successfully.

Termination is a highly individual process. Members and groups will terminate in unique ways. If the group has been successful, termination may be painful and involve grieving or a sense of loss. It may cause the group to experience increased anxiety, regression, and a feeling of accomplishment. Permitting members to avoid discussing termination would deprive them of a possible growth experience. Leadership behaviors include encouraging an evaluation of the group or its terminating members, reminiscing about important events that occurred in the group, and encouraging members to give each other feedback.

Evaluation usually focuses on the amount of achievement of the group's or individual's goals. Leaders must be careful not to collude with members in denying termination; rather, they should encourage full discussion. Termination should be talked about several sessions before the final session to allow members time to work through issues that surface. Termination may lead to discussion of many related topics, such as other separations, death, aging, and the use and passage of time. If terminated successfully, members may feel a sense of resolution about the group experience and use these experiences in many other life situations.

Premature termination means that the group ends before its tasks are completed or a member leaves the group before his or her work is finished. Premature termination may occur for appropriate and inappropriate reasons. Appropriate reasons include moving to another city before the group is terminated. Inappropriate reasons might include a member's unwillingness to discuss an issue central to the group but painful to that person.

> As a staff nurse you are given the responsibility for developing a transition group for patients who are to be discharged from a day treatment program. Outline the points you will need to consider and the steps you would take to establish the group.

EVALUATION OF THE GROUP

Evaluation of the group and the group members' progress is an ongoing process that begins in the selection interview. Notes describing group sessions should be descriptive to help identify goal achievement. To make record keeping easy, it is usually helpful to have a group notebook. In this notebook leaders can write pertinent data on individual members such as their goals, their telephone numbers, their addresses, the screening note, any individual comments, and a termination summary note. In another section of the group notebook the leader can describe each group meeting. One format for quickly recording each group meeting is provided in Box 33-2. In most agencies summary notes are also included in individual members' clinical records.

In addition, it is helpful to determine each member's goal attainment periodically during the course of the group. This can be done using subjective ratings by the group leader and by obtaining individual members' perceptions on how they are meeting their goals. For a slightly more objective evaluation, members are asked to rate their goal achievement on a Likert scale (one that allows members to rate their response along a continuum, with 1 being low, 5 being high, for example). Members' goal achievement should always be evaluated at termination.

In addition, before, during, and at the end of the group the clinician should use behavioral rating scales to assess progress toward expected outcomes. The scales selected should be related to the expected changes in the group. For

Box 33-2

Group Session Note Outline

Date _____ Group Meeting No. _____

Membership:
  List members attending (state whether new member).
  List members who were late.
  List absent members.
List individual members' pertinent issues or behaviors discussed in the group.
List group themes.
Identify important group process issues (such as developmental stage, roles, and norms).
Identify any critical leadership strategy used.
List proposed future leadership strategies.
Predict member and group responses for the next session.

CRITICAL THINKING about CONTEMPORARY ISSUES

Do Computer Networks Provide a New Way for Nurses to Interact with Groups of Patients?

Interactions through computer networks and online groups are growing in popularity. Nurses have begun to identify opportunities to establish patient groups using this technology and have reported on the potential effectiveness of computer network groups and telecommunication in providing information and support (Cudney & Weinert, 2000). Advantages to the members include convenience, ability to relate to a variety of people in similar situations, and ready access to peer support. This approach also offers the option of anonymity to group members.

Psychiatric nurses also need to consider the possible disadvantages of therapeutic groups online (Finfgeld, 2000). The inability to perceive nonverbal communication removes an important dimension from the communication process. Because interaction may not be simultaneous, time gaps can occur between interventions and the responses of various members. Spontaneity may also be lost. The development of trust among group members could proceed differently than in traditional groups. Confidentiality may be even more of a concern to members than it is in face-to-face groups.

Identifying and exploring the dimensions of computer network groups offer a challenge to psychiatric nurses. Nurses who lead groups need to adapt their skills to enhance the advantages of the technology and minimize the disadvantages. As more people become computer-literate and accustomed to online relationships, the potential for this new form of group support will evolve.

---

example, an anxiety scale should be administered to members attending a group whose major goal is to reduce anxiety. Commonly used rating scales are identified in Chapter 7.

It is also essential to identify specific outcomes so that the impact and validity of nursing group interventions can be communicated to consumers and health-care organizations. For example, possible short-term outcome measures for nurse-led groups could include increased knowledge of coping skills and increased insight into the members' own effective and ineffective coping behaviors. Long-term outcomes may be related to a decrease in specific symptoms, such as anxiety or depression, as measured by specific behavioral rating scales. In contrast, a nursing staff support group might have as measurable outcomes the use of a problem-solving approach, the development of a unit communication tool, or the identification of strategies to negotiate staff conflict, seek assistance from each other when stressed, decrease patient complaints, or reduce staff turnover.

NURSES AS GROUP LEADERS

Nurses who are group leaders must be concerned about the many previously discussed factors regarding the group. The group leader must be able to study the group and participate in it at the same time. The leader must constantly monitor the group and, whenever necessary, help the group achieve its goals.

The qualities of an effective nurse leader are the same qualities that are important in the therapeutic relationship (see Chapter 2). In particular, these include the responsive and active dimensions of empathy, genuineness, and confrontation. In addition, creativity and opportunism are helpful qualities for leaders to possess. While they are listening to members' words, leaders also need to be aware of the group process. They must be alert to opportunities for the group to use themes and behaviors and see how these are related to individual issues.

Leaders may be likened to an orchestra conductor who seeks to focus on the sound of a particular instrument for the appreciation and reaction of the total orchestra. The leader may encourage examination of the music from different perspectives and look for possible variations that would create a new piece of music. Opportunities for creativity may also lead to the development of innovative group techniques (see Critical Thinking about Contemporary Issues).

Group leaders must make it safe for members to challenge their authority. In examining the interplay between the leader and the members, there are opportunities to practice conflict management, confrontation, and assertive communication. The leader needs to accept confrontation without taking it personally.

Leaders also need to have assertive communication skills so that they can foster independence in the group but also help the group focus to reach its goals. Achieving this balance requires a blend of skills and judgment that can be gained with practice in group leadership, supervision by an experienced group facilitator, and study of group process.

It is also critical for leaders to be able to organize a great deal of information and to identify themes for the session. Novice leaders usually need to review the group experience with a supervisor after the session so that they can identify and analyze the important events.

Finally, a nurse leader also needs a sense of humor. Laughter helps reveal truth and enables participants to share and empathize about serious matters without the high levels of tension that often accompany such discussions. For example, in a women's codependent group, humor and laughter were regularly used. The group adopted this technique to talk about their "rescuing" and controlling behaviors. This group was composed of fragile women who grew up in abusive families. They worked hard at seeing, understanding, and changing their contribution to the destructive relationships they developed. The members brought examples of their "setting themselves up" to the group weekly and laughed as they were able to find humor in recognizing behavior that was similar to their own. The humor also allowed the members to give feedback in a less confrontive manner.

Groups with Co-Leaders

For a group, the presence of co-leaders may have advantages and disadvantages. When two clinicians share the leadership, the breadth of observation and the choice of interventions are greater than with one. For example, a male and female team may represent the family and offer the group members an opportunity to deal with issues related to parents or other significant male and female figures.

A male-female team also offers group members opportunities to observe a man and a woman working together with mutual respect and without exploitation, sexualizing, or putting each other down. A variety of transference reactions are available with experienced co-leaders to assist in learning and the resolution of problems. Exploration of the members' fantasies regarding the relationship between the leaders can give them a chance to see conflict and resolution. This can contribute significantly to the group's openness and power.

Disadvantages of the leadership team are often related to difficulties between the leaders. When there is competition, a major philosophical difference, or great variance in strategy or style, the group will not work effectively. Differences in levels of experience are handled if both are comfortable with their roles of apprentice and senior leader. Conflict between co-leaders could lead to the splitting of the group or the group developing an alliance with one of the leaders, which could be very damaging. Splitting must be openly interpreted in the group and dealt with by the group members and leaders.

Nurse-Led Groups

Nurses lead groups in a variety of health-care settings. Some types of groups that may be led by nurses are task groups, self-help groups, teaching groups, supportive/therapy groups, psychotherapy groups, and peer support groups. The type of group intervention provided by an individual nurse is determined by the needs and goals of the patients and by the education and experience of the nurse.

Task Groups. Task groups are designed to accomplish a particular task. Nursing care planning meetings and com-

Citing the Evidence on

Empowerment Groups

BACKGROUND: The purpose of this study was to identify the issues and process faced by public health nurses facilitating empowerment groups with people with a chronic and persistent mental illness. Nurses kept field notes following each group session, and grounded theory was used to analyze the data.

RESULTS: The process of dismantling professional boundaries included three dimensions: experiencing the clash of worlds; joining the lives of people with mental illness; and an exploration of the professional self.

IMPLICATIONS: Working with others rather than doing for others is a shift in the traditional caring roles some nurses have assumed. This study highlights some of the issues nurses face when they move into an empowering role, including how to share responsibility and enter into a true partnership with patients.

Byrne C: Facilitating empowerment groups: dismantling professional boundaries, *Issues in Ment Health Nurs* 19:55, 1998.

mittees are examples of task groups. The emphasis of these groups is on decision making and problem solving. They often have specific goals to accomplish and a deadline for completion of the work.

Self-Help Groups. Groups organized around a common experience are labeled self-help groups. Some examples include smoking cessation groups, Overeaters Anonymous, Alcoholics Anonymous, Parents and Friends of Lesbians and Gays, Parents Without Partners, and numerous groups related to specific health problems. They may or may not receive consultation from a health-care provider, such as a professional nurse. Although some are established and organized by professionals, they are run by the members and often do not have a designated leader. Leadership evolves within the group depending on the need that arises. Nurses can support self-help groups by referring members and by offering advice and assistance if it is requested. They can also promote links between the self-help group and the health-care system (see Citing the Evidence). Self-help groups are discussed in Chapter 13.

Educational Groups. The goal of teaching groups is to provide information. Examples are childbirth preparation, parent education groups, and psychoeducation groups. In-service education groups for staff are also included in this category. The nurse leader is able to educate more people more efficiently using a group format. The members themselves often become co-teachers as they share their information and experiences (Webster & Austin, 1999). Psychoeducation groups are designed to teach symptom identification,

Citing the Evidence on

Nurse-Led Psychotherapy Groups

BACKGROUND: This quasi-experimental study assessed the effects of nurse-led cognitive and experiential group therapy on self-efficacy and perceptions of employability for 52 chemically dependent adult women, 98% of whom were African American. Therapy consisted of six 90-minute sessions held twice a week.

RESULTS: After the intervention the cognitive group had significantly higher levels than the experiential group of social self-efficacy and need for self-actualization, an indicator of aspiration for employment. Both groups increased their general self-efficacy and decisiveness, indicators of employability.

IMPLICATIONS: Interventions to enhance people's belief in their ability to successfully perform tasks and control outcomes, promote personal growth, teach responsibility, and enhance self-awareness could be used to develop employability skills that reduce recidivism.

Washington O: Effects of cognitive and experiential group therapy on self-efficacy and perceptions of employability of chemically dependent women, *Issues Ment Health Nurse,* 20:181, 1999.

symptom management, and recovery planning skills. They are discussed in Chapter 15.

Supportive Therapy Groups. The primary goal of supportive therapy groups is to help the members cope with life stress. The focus is on dysfunctional thoughts, feelings, and behaviors. Supportive therapy groups have value for patients of all ages and with both medical and psychiatric diagnoses (Bonhote et al, 1999; Samarel et al, 1998). Supportive therapy is discussed in Chapter 3.

Psychotherapy Groups. The goal of a psychotherapy group is the treatment of emotional, cognitive, or behavioral dysfunction. Group techniques and processes are used to help members learn about their behavior with other people and how it relates to core personality traits. The intent is for the members to change their behavior, not just understand or seek support for it (see Citing the Evidence). Members also learn that they have responsibilities to others and can help other members achieve their goals.

Brief Therapy Groups. Many managed care organizations are placing a new emphasis on group therapy as a cost-effective alternative to individual therapy. Most recently, the focus on cost containment and outcome evaluation in the treatment of health-related problems has been a major influence on the increasing importance of time-limited or brief therapy groups that are linked to individual treatment plans.

The purpose of brief therapy groups is to focus on the actions participants can take to improve their current situa-

Box 33-3

Planning Checklist for Time-Limited Psychotherapy Groups

Check for the following planning factors:

___ **Clear administrative mandate:** Establish achievable annual goals for the number of therapy groups and the number of patients seen in these groups in a particular setting.

___ **Clinical group coordinator:** Determine need for groups and guidelines for referrals, identify group therapists, conduct staff training, market the group, and establish pregroup and postgroup tests and outcome evaluations.

___ **Population-based approach:** Identify the main diagnostic categories to be included and the needs of the target population that could be met by group therapy.

___ **Group screening:** Pregroup orientation and screening ensure that patients understand how the group will operate and that the patient's needs will be addressed.

___ **Clear referral criteria:** Clearly written referral guidelines help reduce clinician resistance to making referrals, promote effective use of the group, and increase patients' acceptance of the referral.

___ **Regular status reports:** A weekly status report reminds referrers of the availability of groups. It should include the dates and times when groups meet, the types of groups, openings in groups, and the contact person.

___ **Testing and evaluation:** Pretesting and posttesting help clarify the patient's response to treatment and allow for assessment of the effectiveness of the group.

___ **Treatment models:** Use of a variety of group models (psychoeducational, social skills, relapse prevention, crisis intervention, cognitive-behavioral, and so on) matches patients with their presenting problems and increases patient receptivity.

___ **Training:** A group therapy apprenticeship (clinicians observe and assist the group and are observed by experienced therapists) increases clinician effectiveness, acceptance of group modality, and appropriateness of referrals.

___ **Adequate resources:** A reasonable fee schedule, adequate clinician time to develop and conduct groups, and appropriate physical space are essential for the group's success.

Modified from Crosby G, Sabin JE: A planning checklist for establishing time-limited psychotherapy groups, *Psychiatr Serv* 47:25, 1996.

tion. Far less importance is given to the causes of the patient's problems or the accompanying emotional reactions. These groups target what can be done now to change a patient's problem-solving approach and help the patient implement more adaptive coping skills. The establishment of a recognized and self-sustaining group program is greatly facilitated by advanced planning, well-thought-out structure, and clearly stated goals. A planning checklist for establishing time-limited psychotherapy groups is included in Box 33-3.

Intensive Problem-Solving Groups. Intensive problem-solving groups are designed for 6 to 10 patients, each working on the identification and resolution of specific target problems, goals, and problem-solving strategies related to an individual treatment plan. They are based on cognitive, behavioral, and interpersonal therapy models implemented in a structured problem-solving format. The goal is to identify and clarify the problem, explore alternative solutions, and get action-oriented commitments for change. The therapist acts as a leader, teacher, and coach, whose purpose is to teach group members the interpersonal skills needed to solve the problems identified in their treatment plans.

There are several keys to developing effective problem-solving groups (Gorski, 1996):

- Screen and match patients for entry into groups. Research shows that group members do best when they can easily relate to other members.
- Open each session with group members systematically reporting their reactions to the last session and their progress and problems in completing assignments.
- Use a standard group process. An example is one in which one patient presents a problem and the other members ask clarifying questions and give feedback.
- Use a standard closure procedure that identifies what members learned during the session, how this will help them solve their target problems, and the assignments they have given themselves to work on for the next session. This allows the therapist to identify progress made by members who did not directly work on their own issues, but developed insight into their own target problems by becoming involved in the problem-solving processes of other members.

Medication Groups. Clinical studies show that the combination of psychotherapy and psychopharmacology can often produce better results than the use of either treatment alone. A time-limited group can be an important modality for the combination of these therapies. Allowing patients to deal with their feelings regarding the taking of medication in a group setting not only facilitates compliance but also allows important psychodynamic issues to emerge, such as acting out, dependence, and authority conflicts, encouraging the resolution of these issues for all the patients in the group.

The prescription of medications can take place outside of the group setting for each patient or within the group itself. Having both a prescriber and a group leader in the group helps keep their roles from becoming blunted and confusing. The medication prescriber often fills an authoritarian or directive role, in contrast to the role of the group leader, which is more facilitative (O'Kelly & Piper, 1996).

Activity Groups. Activity group therapy is designed to enhance the psychological and emotional well-being of psychiatric patients. These patients often exhibit cognitive dysfunction, complacency, negativism, anxiety, disinterest, low self-esteem, poor interpersonal relationships, and isolation. Activity group therapy is a combination of group psychotherapy and remotivation therapy that stimulates interaction among members by focusing on simple tasks that encourage members to focus on group goals rather than their individual issues (Smith et al, 1996).

Tasks can include drawing, exercising to music, baking, community trips, arts and crafts, and reviewing current events. The benefits that have been reported from the participation of psychiatric patients in such activity groups include the expression of positive and negative feelings and the greater acceptance of oneself (McGarry & Prince, 1998). As mental health care continues to move away from the more costly inpatient setting toward community-based programs for the seriously mentally ill, nurses are in a good position to care for these patients with creative and effective interventions.

Peer Support Groups. Finally, peer support groups are an effective way for professionals to share the stresses and problems related to their work. An example of a peer support group is a group of advanced practice psychiatric nurses who meet monthly. Group purposes may include case consultation, sharing information about educational opportunities, providing information about management skills, and decreasing professional isolation. Another example is a group of nurses who work with people with HIV/AIDS. They meet regularly for nursing consultation and support in coping with the continual loss associated with this disease.

> *As a head nurse, you decide to form a staff support group. How would this differ from a therapeutic group? Discuss in terms of the roles of the leader and the members. Would there be any similarities?*

Summary

1. A group is a collection of people who are interrelated and interdependent and may share common purposes and norms.

2. Components of a small group, including structure, size, length of sessions, communication, roles of members, norms, and cohesion, were identified and described.

3. The phases of group development (pregroup, initial phase with orientation, conflict and cohesion stages, working phase, and termination) were presented.

4. Small group evaluation is based on accomplishment of individual goals and expected group outcomes. Careful documentation of each group session is required.

5. The responsibilities and qualities of nurse group leaders include empathy, nurturance, genuineness, creativity, acceptance of confrontation, assertive communication skills, organization, and a sense of humor. Types of nurse-led groups, including task, self-help, educational, supportive therapy, psychotherapy, brief therapy, intensive problem solving, medication, activity, and peer support groups, were described.

Competent Caring   A Clinical Exemplar of a Psychiatric Nurse

LYNN KLAIR, MS, RN

While I was working as a clinical nurse specialist in an inpatient psychiatric setting, I co-led a predischarge group. Five of the group members went to the same domiciliary care home. I was concerned about their adjustment to a community setting, so I arranged to continue providing group therapy in the community setting.

The group consisted of three women and two men. We met early in the morning, in part so I could stop on my way to work and in part so we could meet before the members became involved in their daily activities. All of the members attended the group on a fairly regular basis; two of them are particularly memorable to me because of the progress they made.

P was a former nurse who had depression and anorexia nervosa. One of her goals was to get some new clothes, but her finances were very limited. I obtained some used clothing that I brought to her to replace her old clothes, which were several sizes too large for her. It took her a long time to try the new clothes because she believed that they were too tight on her. This was evidence of her distorted body image. P's greatest accomplishment was to reestablish contact with her family, who lived in another state. The group provided support to her as she struggled with the decision to write to them. They all felt a sense of accomplishment when she wrote and then later talked to family members on the telephone. By the time the group terminated, P was beginning to gain confidence and had stayed out of the hospital longer than she had after any previous hospital discharge.

R was a middle-aged man who had been hospitalized for 15 years following an arrest for a serious assault. He was college educated and had been employed in the past. He was a very large man, and I thought of him as a "gentle giant." He was very kind to the other group members and was liked by all of them, even the most paranoid member. R needed to learn to manage money; he carried his money in his sock. He also needed new clothing, but resisted the group's encouragement to go shopping. When I brought some catalogs to the group, I discovered that R had great difficulty making choices. He finally decided that he would give me money to use to buy clothing for him. Although I felt somewhat uncomfortable with this, I agreed because I knew that it was difficult for him to develop this much trust in another person. When he wore his new clothing to the group, the other members complimented him and I could see his self-esteem improving. R eventually moved into a smaller group home. The group mourned his loss, but felt good about their role in helping him progress.

After several months of meeting at the house, we decided to have some of our meetings at a nearby fast-food restaurant. This was done to help members feel more comfortable out in the community, as well as to address their wish to have refreshments during the meetings. This change worked out well because we could work on socialization and community survival skills.

My experience leading this group was rewarding and resulted in professional growth for me. I gained a new understanding of what was required for patients to live successfully in the community and also developed an appreciation for the difficulties they face in doing this. I never stopped being impressed by their strength and courage as they met the challenges presented to them.

MERLIN Visit MERLIN: **www.mosby.com/MERLIN/Stuart** to find these additional materials and student activities.

- **Worksheets**
- **"Drug of the Month" Updates**
- **"Citing the Evidence" Updates**
- **Critical Thinking Activities and Exercises**
- **Annotated Suggested Readings**
- **Web Links**
- **More!**

Chapter Review Questions

1. Match each term in Column A with the correct definition in Column B.

Column A	Column B
___ Follower	A. Determines level of group acceptance of individual members
___ Moralist	B. Keeps the group focused
___ Truant	C. Serves as judge of right and wrong
___ Gatekeeper	D. States current position of the group
___ Encourager	E. Serves as an interested audience
___ Questioner	F. Discourages positive work and vents anger
___ Facilitator	G. Clarifies issues and information
___ Leader	H. Invalidates significance of the group
___ Complainer	I. Sets direction
___ Summarizer	J. Acts as a positive influence on the group

2. Fill in the blanks.

A. _____ is the member's ability to influence the group and its other members.

B. The stage of group development in which the leader is more directive and active than in other stages is the _____ stage.

C. The optimum length of a session is _____ for higher-functioning groups and _____ for lower-functioning groups.

D. The four phases of a group's development identified by Tuckman are _____, _____, _____, and _____.

E. According to Yalom, the realization that others experience the same thoughts, feelings, and problems is called _____ and the experience of sharing part of oneself to help another is called _____.

3. Provide short answers for the following questions.

A. Define a group and list eight components of small groups as described in this chapter.

B. Compare psychoeducational, intensive problem-solving, and activity groups.

C. Describe four functions that group norms serve.

D. Assess your own level of comfort working in groups. What roles do you usually assume? What additional skills would you need to be an effective group leader?

REFERENCES

Bender A, Ewashen C: Group work is political work: a feminist perspective of interpersonal group psychotherapy, *Issues Ment Health Nurs* 21:297, 2000.

Benne KD, Sheats P: Functional roles and group members, *J Soc Issues* 4:41, 1948.

Bonhote K et al: Altruism and creative expression in a long-term older adult psychotherapy group, *Issues Ment Health Nurs* 20:603, 1999.

Clarke D et al: Inpatient group psychotherapy: the role of the staff nurse, *J Psychosoc Nurs* 36:5, 1998.

Cudney S, Weinert C:Computer-based support groups: nursing in cyberspace, *Computer Nurse* 18:1, 2000.

Finfgeld D: Therapeutic groups online: the good, the bad, and the unknown, *Issues Ment Health Nurs* 21:241, 2000.

Gorski TT: Making group therapy work in the age of cost containment, *Treatment Today* 1:16, 1996.

McGarry T, Prince M: Implementation of groups for creative expression on a psychiatric inpatient unit, *J Psychosoc Nurs* 36:3, 1998.

O'Kelly JG, Piper WE: Group dynamics and medication in evening treatment, *Continuum* 3:85, 1996.

Samarel N et al: Women's perceptions of group support and adaptation to breast cancer, *J Adv Nurs* 28:6, 1998.

Smith M et al: Working with the patient with a chronic mental impairment: an activity group approach, *J Psychosoc Nurs* 34:28, 1996.

Tuckman B: Developmental sequence in small groups, *Psychol Bull* 63:384, 1965.

Webster C, Austin W: Health-related hardiness and the effect of a psychoeducational group on client symptoms, *J Psychiatr Ment Health Nurs* 6:3, 1999.

Yalom I, Vinogradov S: *Group psychotherapy*, Washington, DC, 1989, American Psychiatric Press.

Yalom I: *The theory and practice of group psychotherapy*, ed 4, New York, 1995, Basic Books.

Visit **MERLIN** for *Your Internet Connection*
to websites that are related to the content in this chapter.
www.mosby.com/MERLIN/Stuart

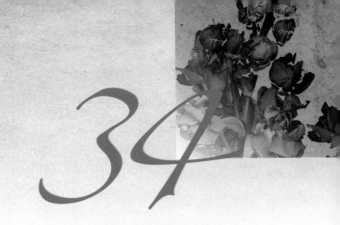

Family Interventions

Patricia E. Helm

We are truly heirs of all the ages; but as honest men it behooves us to learn the extent of our inheritance.

JOHN TYNDALL, "MATTER AND FORCE," IN VOLUME 2,
PRAYER AS A FORM OF PHYSICAL ENERGY

Psychiatric nurses work with families at all levels of functioning. Patients are or have been members of a "family" system. Thus past and present family relationships affect a patient's self-concept, behavior, expectations, values, and beliefs. Understanding principles of family dynamics and interventions is important for the nurse to make more acute observations of the individual patient as well as the family. Competence in this area will enhance the nurse's assessment of the individual and the families' needs and resources, selection of interventions to promote adaptive family functioning, and facilitation of a family's use of positive coping strategies. Skills in this specialty area can help the nurse more readily identify problems displayed by an individual and within family systems, intervene appropriately, and initiate appropriate referrals when necessary.

Clinical training programs in family therapy are open to psychiatric nurses and other health-care professionals across the United States. They vary in duration, theoretical framework used, and the level of knowledge and credentials required for participation. Usually they are limited to clinicians with graduate degrees in mental health. Although the nurse generalist needs knowledge of family systems in her everyday clinical work with patients, the nurse family thera-

pist should have a master's degree with didactic content and clinical seminars focused on formal family work. The nurse should also obtain individual or group supervision when doing family therapy in order to refine clinical skills and deepen theoretical understanding of family systems and interventions. It is important for the family therapist to be able to differentiate adaptive from maladaptive family functioning in order to appropriately identify target symptoms for change.

FAMILY FUNCTIONING

The concept of "family" has evolved from the "two married heterosexual parents with several children of their own" household of several decades ago to a variety of extended and creative nontraditional "family" systems. Nurses thus encounter many different types of families in their clinical work. Fig. 34-1 presents an overview of four dimensions of parent status that can be used to describe families in contemporary society. These include biological ties, marital status, sexual orientation, and gender roles. These various family configurations are the backdrop from which to assess and treat family dysfunction, and in and of themselves are not necessarily the cause of family dysfunction. Although these definitions have become more fluid in recent decades, a family is usually defined in terms of kinship: individuals joined by marriage or its equivalent, or parenthood. A **nuclear family** refers to parents and their children, while an **extended family** includes other people related by blood or marriage. A **household** is a residence consisting of an individual living alone or a group of people sharing a common dwelling and cooking facilities (Puri & Tyer, 1998). The many potential variations of family configurations provide challenges to the nurse's evaluation skills and perhaps to her own value system.

> *Examine the potential problems a nontraditional family may encounter regarding values held by their health-care providers, neighbors, employers, school system, church, and the legal system in your state.*

There are other ways in which families differ as well. Many families face special challenges because a member has experienced something out of the ordinary. This includes families with a mentally ill member, families who have a member with human immunodeficiency virus (HIV) or other significant health-related problem, families with genetically linked problems or birth anomalies, families affected by violence or abuse from within or outside of the household, natural disasters, poverty, or stigma. A well-functioning family can shift roles, levels of responsibility, and patterns of interaction as it experiences stressful life changes. A well-functioning family

may, under acute or prolonged stress or increased vulnerability, produce a symptomatic member, but should be able to rebalance as a system over time.

Characteristics of the Functional Family

A functional family can rebalance, even when faced with various life stressors, and function of all members is restored and symptoms fade. Ultimately, family members remain focused on healthy patterns and established values, and family relationships remain intact. Characteristics of such a family include (Walsh, 1993) the following:

- It completes important life cycle tasks.
- It has the capacity to tolerate conflict and to adapt to adverse circumstances without long-term dysfunction or disintegration of family cohesion.
- Emotional contact is maintained across generations and between family members without blurring necessary levels of authority.
- Overcloseness or fusion is avoided, and distance is not used to solve problems.
- Each twosome is expected to resolve the problems between them. Bringing a third person in to settle disputes or to take sides is discouraged.
- Differences between family members are encouraged to promote personal growth and creativity.
- Children are expected to assume age-appropriate responsibility and to enjoy age-appropriate privileges negotiated with their parents.
- The preservation of a positive emotional climate is more highly valued than doing what "should" be done or what is "right."
- Within each spouse there is a balance of affective expression, careful rational thought, relationship focus, and care taking; each spouse can selectively function in the respective modes.
- There is open communication and interactions among family members.

The functional characteristics just listed represent an ideal family that may be more fictional than real. Most families have some but not all of these elements and still operate with integrity and respect.

Cultural Components Affecting Families

Society has become more mobile and highly integrated, and the media have focused attention on alternate family configurations and practices. Additionally, the numbers of ethnic minority persons in the United States are increasing faster than Caucasian populations. These factors mean that the nurse will be caring for an increasingly diverse patient pool (Mohr, 2000). Thus there have been changes in the structure of U.S. society and in the subcultures within family systems. This has had a complex impact on the integrity of traditional family norms and culture over the past few decades. Many families maintain a structure that is at least partly mediated by a cultural continuum, affecting family function in a number of relevant ways. Nurses have a professional responsibility to be aware and sensitive to differential configurations of family structures that are attributable to culture and ethnic

---

Biological Tie
- Biologically both parents related
- One parent biologically related (artificial insemination, surrogate parenting, lesbian families, blended families)
- Neither parent biologically related (adoption)

Marital Status
- Single parent (by choice, heterosexual or insemination, or due to divorce)
- Married parents (parents married to each other, or stepfamily)
- Cohabiting parents (heterosexual or gay or lesbian)

Sexual Orientation
- Heterosexual
- Gay or lesbian

Gender Roles/ Employment Status
- Traditional
- Nontraditional

Fig. 34-1 Parent status in the contemporary family.

differences that are not necessarily appropriate as targets for treatment. Specifically, culture within a family determines the following:

- The definition of family
- The belief system governing family relationships
- The conflict and tensions present in a family and the adaptive or maladaptive responses to them
- The norms of a family
- How outside events are perceived and interpreted
- When, how, and what type of family interventions are most effective

Biological and nonbiological differences within cultures can cause differential responses to treatment.

Characteristics of Family Pathology

At the opposite end of the continuum are dysfunctional families. Some of the more common dysfunctional family patterns (conceptualized as "symptoms" within a pathology paradigm) include the following:

- The overprotective mother and distant father (distant through work, alcohol, or physical absence)
- The overfunctioning "superwife" or "superhusband" and the underfunctioning passive, dependent, and compliant spouse
- The spouse who maintains peace at any price and denies difficulties in the marriage but suddenly feels wronged and self-righteous when the mate is discovered to be in legal trouble or having an affair
- The child who evidences poor peer relationships at school while attempting to parent younger siblings to compensate for ineffective or emotionally overwhelmed parents
- The overly close three generations of grandparent, parent, and grandchild in which lines of authority and generational identity are poorly defined and the child acts out because of a lack of effective limit setting by an agreed-upon parental figure
- The family with a substance-abusing member
- The family subjected to physical, emotional, or sexual abuse by one of its members

> **?** *Describe the potential impact you might observe on family functioning between families that include a single parent, an interracial marriage, a homosexual partnership, and a family with several members with a severe mental illness.*

FAMILY ASSESSMENT

A family assessment is the first step in determining what interventions might bring the family unit to a level of functioning that has minimal conflict and is harmonious, organized, and satisfying (see Citing the Evidence). An assessment is also a good time to reframe family dynamics, since it is when family members are focusing time and energy on their relationships and may be the most open to change (Sherman, 2000). A relational problem is a situation in which two or more emotionally attached individuals (family members, romantic partners, etc.) engage in communication or behavior patterns that are destructive, unsatisfying, or both, to one or more of them. Relational problems tend to be enduring without intervention and can lead to other serious problems, such as individual family member symptoms (depression) or dissolution of the family (divorce) (Kay & Tasman, 2000). Five major evidence based constructs of the family are listed in Table 34-1. This is an ongoing area of research. Thus far, relational problems have been identified for two of these constructs (structure and communication).

Family History

Information about family history generally includes all family members across three generations. It is convenient to use a family genogram as the organizing structure for collecting this information. A three-generation family genogram is a structured method of gathering information and graphically symbolizing the factual and emotional relationship data in the initial interview and during subsequent family meetings (Jorde et al, 1999). A sample genogram is presented in Fig. 34-2. Drawing a family genogram in full view of the family on large easel paper or a blackboard broadens the family's focus and facilitates an understanding of the family constellation.

The genogram is designed around the proband, also called the index case, or patient, who is the first member of the family to become symptomatic, usually bringing the family to the attention of the health-care system. Included are all the relatives of the proband. First-degree relatives include parents, siblings, and children of the proband. Second-degree relatives include grandparents, uncles, aunts, nephews, nieces, and grandchildren of the proband. All family members by marriage or partnership, adoption, and step-family members are also included. The health status of each is noted, as are the

---

Citing the Evidence on

Importance of Interpersonal Relationships

BACKGROUND: Three bodies of empirical data were reviewed in support of the interpersonal school of psychotherapy and its selective focus on the role of relationships in health and illness.

RESULTS: Clinical experience and research findings suggest that clinicians treating couples and families may be helped by using techniques designed to both increase the intensity of the affectual bonds and repair the inevitable disruption of these bonds.

IMPLICATIONS: At a time of strong biological emphasis in psychiatry, it is important to emphasize that relationships with important others may play a crucial role in individual outcome.

Lewis J: For better or worse: interpersonal relationships and individual outcome, *Am J Psychiatry* 155(5):582, 1998.

Table **34-1**

Evidence Based Family Relational Constructs

Construct	Definition
STRUCTURE	Leadership and distribution of functions
Problem: over-involvement	Unclear boundaries; overdependence
COMMUNICATION	Amount and clarity of information exchange
Problem: communication deviance	Unclear, amorphous, fragmented, and/or unintelligible communication
Problem: coercion	Behavior control by use of aversive communication
EXPRESSION OF AFFECT	Implicit or explicit verbalization of affective tone
PROBLEM-SOLVING	Definition of problems, consideration of alternative lines of action, agreement to use optimal line of action
CONFLICT RESOLUTION	Process of resolving differences of opinion

From Kay J, Tasman A: Relational problems. In *Psychiatry: behavioral science and clinical essentials*, Philadelphia, 2000, WB Saunders.

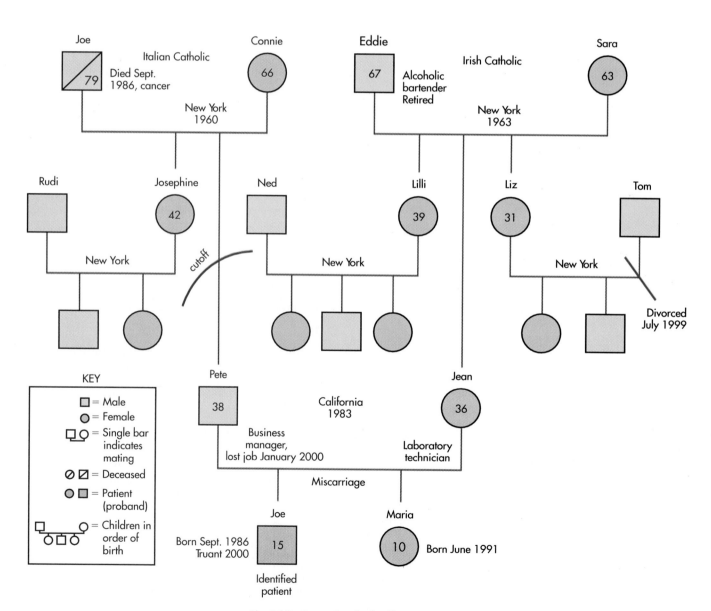

Fig. 34-2 Example of a family genogram.

current household configurations. Relationships between members are also recorded. The genogram provides an invaluable family map for both individual and family insights and discussions and can be updated by the family indefinitely.

 Do a genogram of your own three-generational family. Ask family members to join you in this project.

Family APGAR

Once the family structure is clear, the nurse should explore roles and relationships to determine who the patient is attached to and how family dynamics work. An evidenced based tool commonly used to assess the patient's satisfaction with relationships in the immediate family is the Family APGAR (Barkauskas et al, 1998). Functions measured by the Family APGAR include the following:

- How resources are shared, or the degree to which a member is satisfied with the assistance received when family resources are needed.
- How decisions are shared, or the member's satisfaction with mutuality in family communication and problem-solving.
- How nurturing is shared, or the member's satisfaction with the freedom available within the family to change roles and attain physical and emotional growth or maturation.
- How emotional experiences are shared, or the member's satisfaction with the intimacy and emotional interaction that exist in the family.
- How time (and space and money) is shared, or the member's satisfaction with the time commitment that has been made to the family by its members.

Family Relational Diagnosis

The nurse may find it useful to examine the family relational problems in terms of the categories described in the *Diagnostic and Statistical Manual for Mental Disorders (DSM–IV–TR)* (American Psychiatric Association, 2000). The *DSM–IV–TR* lists five relational categories (Table 34-2) under "Other Conditions That May Be A Focus Of Clinical Attention." Relational problems often necessitate clinical attention in order to avoid further family deterioration, individual symptoms, and decreased quality of life of family members. Many insurance and managed care companies may require a *DSM–IV–TR* psychiatric "diagnosis" before authorizing family therapy treatment that they will reimburse.

WORKING WITH FAMILIES

Contact with patients' families is an essential part of nursing care. Nurses have always made intuitive observations about functional and dysfunctional family dynamics. Although many nurses have additional information and training in formal family therapy techniques, all nurses use various nonclinical techniques, such as psychoeducational programs developed from a competence paradigm, in order to more competently work with families in everyday nursing practice.

Competence Paradigm

The competence paradigm provides a significant shift in how family interventions are thought about (Marsh, 2000). This approach was derived from the fact that older conceptual models tended to focus on pathological states and dysfunction rather than family strengths, resources, and competencies. The competency paradigm values empowerment instead of a dependency-producing helper-helpee ideology and stresses the importance of treating people as collaborators who are the masters of their own fate and capable of making healthy changes (see Table 34-3).

An empowerment model has been used increasingly as a framework for professional practice with families who are coping with a member who is mentally ill or mentally retarded. Its use is likely to increase the understanding of familial attributes that are relevant to coping with mental illness, facilitate the assessment of positive attributes among family members, offer a blueprint for designing effective interventions for families, and advance efforts to evaluate the outcome of family-oriented services. In addition, unlike

Table 34-2

Categories of Family Relational Problems in *DSM–IV–TR*

Problem	Essential Features
Relational problem related to a mental disorder or general medical condition	Focus of clinical attention is a pattern of impaired family interaction in the presence of a mental disorder or a medical condition in a family member
Parent-child relational problem	Impairment includes faulty communication, overprotection, or inadequate discipline. Clinically significant impairment or symptoms are present in an individual, in family functioning, or both
Partner relational problems	Pattern of interaction characterized by negative or distorted communication or noncommunication associated with clinically significant impairment in one or both partners
Sibling relational problems	Patterns of interactions associated with clinically significant impairment in individual or family members or the development of symptoms in one or more siblings
Relational problem not otherwise specified	Includes extra-family relational problems and difficulty with others, such as co-workers

Reprinted with permission from the *Diagnostic and statistical manual of mental disorders*, Fourth Edition, Text Revision. Copyright 2000. American Psychiatric Association

Table **34-3**

Paradigms in Working with Families		
	Pathology Paradigm	Competence Paradigm
Nature of paradigm	Disease-based medical model	Health-based developmental model
View of families	Pathological, pathogenic, or dysfunctional	Basically or potentially competent
Emphasis	Weaknesses, liabilities, and illness	Strengths, resources, and wellness
Role of professionals	Practitioners who provide psychotherapy	Enabling agents who help families achieve their goals
Role of families	Clients or patients	Collaborators
Basis of assessment	Clinical typologies	Competencies and competence deficits
Goal of intervention	Treatment of family pathology or dysfunction	Empowerment of families in achieving mastery and control over their lives
Modus operandi	Provision of psychotherapy	Strengthening of the relevant competencies
Systemic perspective	Family systems framework	Ecological systems framework

From Marsh D: *Serious mental illness and the family: the practitioners guide,* New York, 2000, John Wiley & Sons.

pathology models that may stigmatize and alienate families, a competence paradigm attempts to foster positive alliances between families and health-care providers and enhance the delivery of services. The competence paradigm emphasizes the following points:

- Focus is on growth-producing behaviors rather than on treatment of problems or prevention of negative outcomes
- Promotion and strengthening of individual and family functioning occurs by fostering the acquisition of prosocial, self-sustaining, self-efficacious, and other adaptive behaviors
- Definition of the relationship between the help seeker and help giver is a cooperative partnership that assumes joint responsibility
- Encouragement of assistance that is in line with the family's culture and congruent with the family's appraisal of problems and needs
- Promotion of the family's use of natural support networks

In this framework it is expected that families will play a major role in deciding what is important to them, what options they will choose to achieve their goals, and whether they will accept help that is offered to them. Chapter 16 describes some specific ways in which nurses can use this paradigm in working with families throughout the continuum of care.

Watch a popular television show that depicts a family situation. Evaluate the family's level of functioning in terms of "pathology," culture, and competencies.

Psychoeducational Programs

Psychoeducational programs for families are designed primarily for education and support. They are the result of the emergence of the family self-help movement in psychiatry. Due mainly to the efforts of National Alliance for the Mentally Ill (NAMI) and other family groups, a variety of psychoeducational programs have been developed for families of the mentally ill. Although these programs vary, they share

certain features. The program approach is mainly educational and pragmatic, and its aim is to improve the course of the family member's illness, reduce relapse rates, and improve patient and family functioning. These goals are achieved through educating the family about the illness, teaching families techniques to cope with symptomatic behavior, and reinforcing family strengths (McFarlane, 1995). Not all programs include the ill family member, but they do promote regular contact of the family with other affected families.

In general, a comprehensive program for working with families should include the following components (Marsh, 2000):

- A didactic component that provides information about mental illness and the mental health system
- A skill component that offers training in communication, conflict resolution, problem solving, assertiveness, behavioral management, and stress management
- An emotional component that provides opportunities for ventilation, sharing, and mobilizing resources
- A family process component that focuses on coping with mental illness and its sequelae for the family
- A social component that increases use of informal and formal support networks

Although no single program works equally well in all situations, it is possible to describe a general structure that can be modified to meet individual needs. The educational program outlined in Box 34-1 is time limited and didactic and is designed to primarily meet the cognitive and behavioral needs of families (Marsh, 2000). It is important that psychoeducational programs for families meet a range of needs and that there be an opportunity for families to ask questions, express feelings, and socialize with each other and mental health professionals.

Family Therapy Interventions: Overview

Family therapy has two essential principles that distinguish it from individual or group therapy and from nonclinical family interventions. First, the family is conceptualized as a behavior system with unique properties rather than as the sum of the characteristics of its individual members. Second, it is

Box 34-1

10-Week Educational Program for Families of the Mentally Ill

NATURE AND PURPOSE OF PROGRAM

Introductions of family members and staff
Purpose and scope of program
Description of treatment program, policies, and
  procedures
Brief, written survey of specific family needs and re-
  quests

THE FAMILY EXPERIENCE

Family burden and needs
The family system
Family subsystems
Life-span perspectives

MENTAL ILLNESS I

Diagnosis
Etiology
Prognosis
Treatment

MENTAL ILLNESS II

Symptoms
Medication
Diathesis-stress model
Recent research

MANAGING SYMPTOMS AND PROBLEMS

Bizarre behavior
Destructive and self-destructive behavior
Hygiene and appearance
Negative symptoms

STRESS, COPING, AND ADAPTATION

The general model
The stressor of mental illness
The process of family adaptation
Increasing coping effectiveness

ENHANCING PERSONAL AND FAMILY EFFECTIVENESS I

Behavior management
Conflict resolution
Communication skills
Problem solving

ENHANCING PERSONAL AND FAMILY EFFECTIVENESS II

Stress management
Assertiveness training
Achieving a family balance
Meeting personal needs

RELATIONSHIPS BETWEEN FAMILIES AND PROFESSIONALS

Historical context
New modes of family-professional relationships
Barriers to collaboration
Breaking down barriers

COMMUNITY RESOURCES

The consumer-advocacy movement
Accessing the system
Legal issues
Appropriate referrals

---

assumed that a close interrelationship exists between the way a family functions as a group and the emotional adaptation of its individual members. Family therapy has evolved from these principles in order to link the disorders of family living to the disorders of individual members of a family within one therapeutic approach. This approach, family therapy, assumes that individual emotional differences stem from disturbances in the overall interaction of the natural biopsychosocial unit, the family (Sadock & Sadock, 2000).

Deciding when family therapy is appropriate or indicated over individual or group therapy is not always easy. Resource availability is a factor; many settings do not have anyone trained in family therapy, and reimbursement issues have to be addressed. When the resources are available, the therapist's bias may have an influence on this decision. Some family therapists conceptualize all emotional problems within the family framework. Others recommend certain guidelines in determining which problems should be treated in family therapy. They suggest that family therapy is indicated in the following situations:

- The presenting problem appears in system terms, such as marital conflicts, severe sibling conflicts, or cross-generational conflicts (parents versus offspring, parents versus grandparents).
- Various types of difficulty and conflict arise between the identified patient and other family members.

- The family is experiencing a transitional stage of the family life cycle, such as beginning a family, marriage, birth of the first child, entrance of children into adolescence, the first child leaving home, retirement, or the death of a spouse or other family member.
- Individual therapy with one family member has resulted in symptoms developing in another family member.
- No improvement occurs with adequate individual therapy. Enlarging the conceptual field to include the family in therapy may produce therapeutic movement.
- The person in treatment seems unable to use individual therapy for personal understanding and change, but rather uses therapy sessions primarily to talk about or complain about another member.

Another important component of family therapy, as in all treatments, is to be clear about the targets for therapeutic change. A target list will help determine the type of family therapy interventions that might be most effective, as well as keep the sessions focused on the goals and expected outcomes of treatment. To produce an appropriate target list, the nurse should be up to date on research findings that affect practice and be familiar with behavioral rating scales related to family therapy (Box 34-2).

For instance, a surprising psychosocial research finding in the past two decades is the discovery that siblings raised

Behavioral Ratings Scales Related to Families

- Assessment of Strategies in Families Effectiveness Scale
- Conflict Tactics Scale
- Family APGAR
- Family Burden Interview Schedule
- Family Empowerment Scale
- Family Environment Scale
- Family Functioning Measures
- Zarit Burden Interview

together are almost as different in their personalities as people who grew up in separate families. Only 5% of the individual differences in personality traits can be attributed to the shared family environment, while 40% are attributed to environments outside the household that are not shared, and about 40% are genetic. Thus a shared family environment has little influence on personality (Sulloway, 1997). This information is important for the nurse who is in the process of deciding whether or not to target family dynamics as the focus of change for an individual member with dysfunctional personality characteristics that are not shared by other siblings in the family. The alternative in such a case might be to use family therapy to help understand the individual and to facilitate the education of the family and their support of the individual while he or she is in individual therapy for his problems.

This chapter provides an overview of three theoretical approaches to clinical interventions with families: family systems therapy, structural therapy, and strategic therapy. It describes some of the major techniques that are derived from each of these theories. The principles and strategies proposed by these theories are distinct and sometimes conflicting, yet each defines a theoretical framework developed from clinical research with families, and each has some utility in clinical practice.

Families of the mentally ill believe some family therapy theories stigmatize and blame families for their relatives' illnesses. Evaluate family systems, structural, and strategic therapies as presented in this chapter based on this criticism.

FAMILY SYSTEMS THERAPY

Family systems therapy was developed in the 1950s (Bowen, 1988) and continues to evolve as a major family therapy technique. A premise of this therapy is that a family is a homeostatic system. A change in the functioning of one family member results in a change in the functioning of other family members. It resembles a centerless web in which, when one strand moves, the tensions in the entire web readjust.

Systems therapy explains emotional dysfunction in human relationships, specifically in the family system. Symptoms in any member of the family, whether social (such as

child abuse or delinquency), physical (such as drug abuse, alcoholism, or chronic illness), emotional (such as depression or schizophrenia), or conflictual (such as marital conflict), are viewed as evidence of dysfunction in the family relationship process. Although the family is only one emotional system in which a person is involved, it is probably the most intense and influential one. Extrafamilial relationships rarely have the intensity of the family emotional system. The family system fosters or inhibits function but it does not totally determine behavior. Individuals are responsible for their own actions within the family system.

Family systems therapy identifies the functional facts of a relationship: what happened, when, where, how, and who was involved. These observable facts are more important than the reasons why the problematic behavior occurred. A systems therapist gathers from family members descriptions of behavior rather than feeling states.

A cornerstone of systems therapy is that some families fail to distinguish between the intellectual process of thinking and the more subjective process of feeling. It is as if the thinking processes are so flooded with feeling that members are unable to separate intellectual belief from subjective feelings. Routinely a person says, "I feel that . . ." when "I think that . . ." would be more accurate. The families focus on feelings in an attempt to foster togetherness and agreement. They avoid statements of opinion or belief that would make one member different or separate from the family "party line."

A key goal of systems therapy is to clarify and distinguish thinking and feeling in family members. The observation of this fusion between thinking and feeling led to the concept of the undifferentiated family ego mass. People with the greatest fusion between feeling and thinking function poorly. They inherit a high percentage of life's social, psychiatric, and medical problems.

Family systems theory consists of seven concepts. Three concepts apply to overall characteristics of family systems: differentiation of self, triangles, and the nuclear family emotional system. The remaining four concepts are related to the central family characteristics: the multigenerational transmission process, the family projection process, sibling position, and the emotional cutoff (Table 34-4).

Differentiation of Self

The concept of differentiation of self measures all human functioning on a continuum from the greatest emotional fusion of self-boundaries to the highest degree of differentiation or autonomy (Fig. 34-3, p. 696). A description of the differentiated person is one who is less anxious than the family system. This person is able to bring up emotion-laden issues in a nonassaulting way without anxiety. As the emotional intensity or fusion between two people increases and the self of one is incorporated into the other self, becoming enmeshed, the relationship is perceived to be uncomfortably close. This is usually followed by distance-creating behavior characterized by hostile rejection of the overly close feeling. The two people actively repel each other. Relationships can cycle through these phases because anxiety in the relationship ebbs and flows.

Table 34-4

Central Concepts of Family Systems Therapy

Concept	Definition
Differentiation	Sufficient separation between intellect and emotions so that one is not dominated by the reactive anxiety of the family's emotional system.
Triangle	A predictable emotional process that takes place when difficulty exists in a significant relationship, and a third entity is included.
Nuclear family emotional system	Patterns of interaction between family members and the degree to which these patterns promote emotional fusion.
Multigenerational transmission process	The assumption that relationship patterns and symptoms in a family have their origin several generations earlier; a four- or five-generation genogram reveals such patterns.
Family projection process	The projection of spouses' problems onto one or more children to avoid intense emotional fusion between the spouses.
Sibling position	Birth order and sex are seen as determining factors in a person's personality profile.
Emotional cutoff	A dysfunctional way in which some family members deal with intense family conflict by using either emotional isolation or geographical distance.

Relationships can also become fixed at an angry, repelling standoff. People who operate at the lower reactive end of the continuum are so fused that they are dominated by the automatic emotional system. These people are less adaptable, less flexible, and more emotionally dependent on those around them. They are easily stressed into dysfunction. People at the higher end of the continuum maintain a degree of separation between thought and emotion. In periods of stress they can retain intellectual functioning. They are more flexible, more adaptable, and more independent of the reactive emotionality around them.

The concept of differentiation eliminates the notion of normalcy. It has no direct connection to presence or absence of symptoms, although Bowen believes people at the lower end of the scale tend to inherit more of life's problems. People at the higher end of the continuum recoup rapidly after they are stressed into dysfunction (Bohlander, 1995).

How might a parent's level of self-differentiation affect the child's growth and development from infancy through adolescence?

Triangles

The triangle is the basic building block of an emotional system. It is a predictable emotional process that takes place in any significant relationship experiencing difficulty. The three corners of the triangle can be composed of three people; two people and a group, such as a religious affiliation or Al-Anon; two people and an issue, such as drinking or success; or two people and an object, such as a house or drugs. The possible list of groups, issues, or objects is endless, but it must have an emotional significance equal to that of a person.

All people seek closeness in emotional systems. Emotional closeness but separateness is difficult for two people to maintain; the tendency is to fuse, to lose self or parts of self, in the other. A natural urge exists to seek completeness of self by accumulating parts of the other. The old adage "opposites attract" reflects this assumption. It is difficult for two people to maintain sufficient emotional closeness without fusion.

The inevitable result is emotional distancing. The system is then ripe for the formation of a triangle. For example, the husband wants more expression of affection from an emotionally constricted wife. The more he pursues her, the more she withdraws, most often into preoccupation with her child. The husband starts working longer hours. Husband and wife then start arguing circularly: "You care more about making a new account than you do about your wife and children!" "You expect to have nice things and then blame me for working extra hours!" Triangles stabilize by maintaining the status quo while avoiding tension, conflict, or talking about sensitive emotional areas. The two people can then focus on the new issue (or person or object) and avoid discussing the painful issues between them. Feelings are thus drained off, and the focus is removed from the self and one's own part in the problem. Change in self is avoided.

The reciprocal function of a triangle and the idea of equal responsibility can be difficult to convey to a couple. This is especially true when the distancing mechanism used by one spouse is as emotionally charged as an extramarital affair. Suppose the wife distances from the painful issues in the relationship. By "triangling" his wife's affair, the husband makes it difficult to relinquish his self-righteous position of the "wronged husband." He does not see his behavior of working 14 to 16 hours a day as serving the same distancing function in the relationship. The nature of the distancing mechanism has meaningful content, whether it is overwork, extramarital affairs, homosexuality, psychotic symptoms, religious preoccupation, suicidal gestures, depression, or psychoanalysis. All serve the same function in a triangular relationship.

The concept of a family scapegoat originally broadened the individual pathological view to include the part the family played in the symptomatic behavior. However, the tendency was to view the scapegoat as the helpless victim of a persecuting family. For example, a husband and wife who are unable to settle their differences and wish to avoid their marital discord may focus on the "victim child." This leads to blaming the parents. In contrast, the concept of triangles from the systems view holds each person in the triangle responsible, as evident in Fig. 34-4. Father and mother avoid conflict by fo-

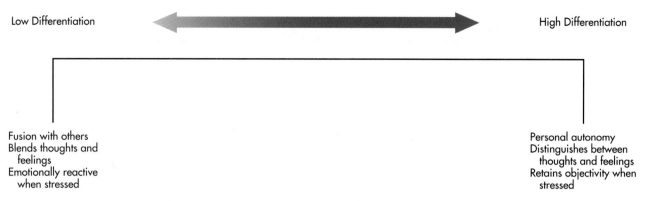

Fig. 34-3 Continuum of differentiation of self.

cusing on the son. Mother and son avoid dealing with their overcloseness by having a common enemy in the father. Father and son avoid awareness of their emotional distance by relating through the mother as go-between. Thus the "victim" is eliminated. All members of a triangle participate equally in maintaining the triangle, and no triangle can persist without the active cooperation of all its members.

It is not a problem to be in a triangle; in fact, it is impossible to stay out of all triangles. Triangles form and reform rapidly and are the daily way most people handle conflict or tension. Problems arise if a triangle becomes fixed and involves significant relationships of deep friendship, blood ties, or marriage. Triangles are not static but form and reform around emotion-laden issues such as money, sex, child rearing, religion, alcohol, and education. A person's position in a triangle changes depending on the issue. A mother and father may be distant on the highly charged issue of how to spend their money. They may be close and agree about their adolescent daughter's sexual activity. However, judgments about these issues are often based on emotion rather than careful thought.

 Many people marry thinking that they can change the parts of their spouse that they don't like after the honeymoon. What would a family systems therapist say about this?

Operating Principles. A person's operating principles are the laws that govern personal conduct. They must be inferred from what the person does in regard to an emotion-laden issue rather than what the person says. Operating principles vary from valuable ones based on conscious conviction to more immature, reactive, impulsive principles. Immature principles are other-focused rather than self-focused; they lead to a loss of freedom or self-determination. Any behavior that is predictable, such as behavior operated by a triangle, is not free. The loss of freedom impairs self-functioning, perpetuates problems, causes a deterioration in family functioning, and promotes symptom development (Kerr & Bowen, 1988).

Other-focused, triangle-promoting operating principles are reflected in various ways. These include declaring feelings "right" or "wrong"; using the plural pronouns **we** or **us** rather than **I**; accusing the other person, as in "You made me

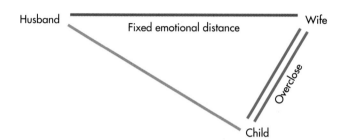

Fig. 34-4 Example of a family triangle.

do it"; stepping in to settle, side taking, or blaming in two other people's conflict; telling or holding secrets; telling the other person what to do; and assuming responsibility for the other person's feelings, for example, "I want to make her happy" or "I couldn't tell him because it would hurt him." These statements are typically interpreted as thoughtful or responsible. In fact, avoiding one's own feelings by focusing on the other person is irresponsible. Everyone falls into this pattern, especially in a marriage or parent-child relationship. When a person becomes anxious, it is more comfortable to project the problem onto the other person and then work to change the other. The implicit assumption here is, "I can't help my behavior, but he is behaving that way deliberately."

In more dysfunctional, closed family systems, interaction between family members is determined by fixed interactional patterns. These fixed triangles are an effort to maintain a homeostatic balance and avoid stress. When an additional stress occurs outside or within the family, such as a job change or the birth of a child, symptoms may arise in a dysfunctional attempt to reduce stress and restore balance. This is evident in the following clinical example.

CLINICAL EXAMPLE

Mr. and Mrs. D, who already had six children, had a seventh unplanned child. The family was financially strained, and Mr. and Mrs. D had a conflictual and distant relationship. When the last child was born, a middle sibling, 13-year-old Andy, developed symptoms and became school phobic. The school insisted that the child receive treatment. Late in the treatment the mother finally revealed that one of the reasons for the family's financial strain was the husband's work phobia and occasional gambling sprees. The wife had covered for him for years, calling his boss to make excuses and taking part-time work herself. Until the birth of the last child, the family was able to maintain a precarious, minimally functional balance. However, the additional stress produced symptoms that caused an outside agency, the school, to become involved.

Interventions. Treatment encourages key figures in key triangles to identify their emotional triggers. The person identifies the verbal or behavioral cues of the other person, to which he reacts with a predictable behavior. When the person pinpoints these cues, he can take control of his part in the process. Once one person takes control and changes his part in a triangle, the whole system changes.

An example of this was a mother who was overly close to her 16-year-old daughter. The daughter had become school phobic and stayed home from school for a year before the family sought treatment. The father would come home from work, see that the daughter had missed school another day, and angrily attack her with "shape-up speeches." The mother bitterly complained about the daughter being home all day doing nothing. However, when the father began his verbal attacks, she became protective of the daughter and launched an attack on the father: "How can you say those things to her? You know how upset she gets." When the mother was able to identify her emotional trigger (she had always been terrified of her "drill sergeant" father), she was able to step back and permit the father to become more effective with his daughter.

Nurses must identify key triangles in a family and the operating principles of its members. They must understand what sets off their emotional triggers and assume that the family will attempt to triangle them into its own emotional system to reestablish equilibrium. The nurse's job is to maintain sufficient emotional distance to watch the process unfolding between family members while maintaining emotional contact with each family member.

Therapist reactions that indicate that the therapist is part of a triangle include feeling sorry for or pitying the other, feeling angry at the system or member, being overly positive about the system, wanting to correct behavior, and finding oneself without questions or responses in the session. The nurse should limit the action to the two family members and avoid becoming involved. Once the therapist steps in to take sides, progress stops and status quo is reestablished. Side taking should be a planned strategy in which the nurse maintains the freedom to realign with specific family members.

Systems therapists do not believe they can change family members; change is possible only when it is generated within the self. Family members are encouraged to take responsibility for the self and not try to change the other. The therapist must avoid becoming part of a triangle in the system. To get out of an emotional process in the session, the nurse may elicit the members' responses. For example, if the nurse becomes irritated at a critical, intrusive husband, the nurse can ask the wife, "What happens to your insides when your husband interrupts with criticism?" This feeds the process back into the system, keeping it between the spouses.

CRITICAL THINKING about CONTEMPORARY ISSUES

Does a Strong Mother-Daughter Attachment Imply Low Self-Differentiation?

Much attention has been given to the impact of the mother-daughter relationship on the development of women, particularly focusing on issues related to mental health and self-efficacy. Some theorists emphasize self-differentiation and devalue interpersonal attachment as a feminine behavior. Others analyze the concepts of caring, intimacy, closeness, and emotional reciprocity only when their absence is evident in intergenerational conflict, delinquency, broken homes, or family violence.

However, research suggests that a daughter's attachment to her mother and her level of self-differentiation are not causally related, and that the concepts of self-differentiation and attachment appear to be separate variables in personality development (Davis & Jones, 1992). Specifically, these researchers found that daughters' levels of self-differentiation were positively related to positive energy, and women who were mentally healthy and functioning effectively also showed high levels of attachment. The findings from this research affirm the value of attachment behaviors and self-differentiation in adulthood, challenge the traditional bias against attachment behaviors of women, and provide psychiatric nurses with a focus for mental health promotion when working with women.

One area of controversy is the importance of the family therapist's working on his or her own family of origin. Systems therapists believe that it is a major aspect of training. "Working on" means that the nurse differentiates himself or herself in his or her own family of origin. The nurse identifies the issues in his or her own family that he or she is reactive to and with whom he or she is part of a triangle. The nurse then works to get out of the triangle by gaining control of reflexive distancing and fusing. This way the nurse has the freedom of emotional closeness and of some emotional distance with each family member (without using geographical distance to create emotional space). Unless a therapist is conscious of the triangles he or she is a part of in the family of origin, he or she will be vulnerable to the same roles and behaviors in the families being treated.

Nuclear Family Emotional System

The nuclear family emotional system refers to patterns of interaction between family members and the degree to which these patterns promote emotional fusion (see Critical Thinking about Contemporary Issues). These patterns of interaction are the ways the person behaves in most significant relationships. All marriage relationships reflect a balance, or complementarity, of operating principles and reciprocal function (Bowen, 1988). For example, the reasonable, object-oriented, and emotionally distant spouse is married to the affectively expressive, relationship-oriented, emotional pursuer. These differences provide the attraction and the balancing stability to the marriage relationship. One spouse is the object-oriented overfunctioner, the other the emotion-oriented overfunctioner. Difficulty arises when dependence on attributes of the spouse reduces acquiring those attributes in the self. The self borrows on the functioning of the spouse, and self-boundaries are blurred. This is called ego fusion. When there are fixed positions of overfunction-underfunction, symptoms can occur, such as chronic depression or physical illness. In such a relationship, to view one spouse as strong and independent and the other as weak and dependent fails to recognize the overfunctioner's dependence on the underfunctioning of the other spouse. The underfunctioner must be one-down for the other to appear one-up.

Emotional fusion operates in all marriages. When the relationship is unstressed, the reciprocal function works smoothly; however, when stress occurs, each spouse becomes more as one self. The distancer seeks space and objects (work, hobbies, alcohol); the pursuer seeks togetherness and expression of personal feelings. Both are efforts to avoid personal anxiety. The pursuer takes the distancer's withdrawal as personal rejection and reactively withdraws. No longer feeling crowded, the distancer then moves in emotionally, only to be met with, "Where were you when I needed you? Get lost." The distancer then pulls back, baffled and angry at the rejection. A fixed emotional distance sets in. These are the relationships often seen just before a couple decides on a divorce. These relationships are ripe for triangulation with an affair or with an unsuspecting therapist.

People tend to pick spouses who have similar levels of differentiation of self. The greater the undifferentiation, the greater is the tendency toward fusion and potential problems. If there is a high degree of ego fusion and intensity in the nuclear family, this intensity can be diffused and reduced through active contact with the family of origin. In periods of stress, contact with the extended family or family of origin can stabilize the nuclear family. Promoting such contact can be an effective therapeutic strategy.

There are two patterns in the nuclear family emotional system, labeled the explosive family and the cohesive family (Kerr & Bowen, 1988). Family units of a cohesive family are geographically close and in frequent contact and communication. The person who geographically separates from the family of origin because of the fusion or intensity of attachment may marry a spouse from a cohesive family. The person's unresolved attachments to his or her own family of origin lie dormant until ritualized contact (at a wedding or funeral) stirs them up. In a nuclear family in which both spouses are detached from their families of origin, the spouses tend to be more dependent on each other. The process between them is more intense, and these can be explosive families.

Bowen (1988) proposes three mechanisms by which spouses maintain sufficient emotional distance from each other to handle the anxiety associated with fusion. All three mechanisms may be used by the couple, or tension may be focused in one area. If tension is great enough, it will spill over into other social systems, such as mental health centers or school counselors. The three mechanisms used are marital conflict, dysfunction in one spouse, and projection of the problem onto one or more children.

How might the concept of emotional fusion explain why some people stay married to spouses who are physically or sexually abusive?

Marital Conflict. Conflictual marriages are built on a constant struggle between spouses. They want "their fair share" of needs met, freedom, love, attention, or control. Neither spouse is willing to compromise. A high percentage of the self is wrapped up in the "happiness" of the other. Functioning of the self is enmeshed in the function of the other. These relationships tend to be stable, whether positive ("Anything to make her happy") or negative ("I sacrificed the best years of my life helping him be a success; I'll never let him go now"). They endure predictable cycles of intense closeness, distance-creating conflict, making up, and then renewed closeness. It is commonly believed that this amount of conflict would harm the children of such marriages. However, Bowen believes that the children are protected because tension is focused between parents.

Intervention in conflictual marriages usually involves working with the most motivated spouse first. If both spouses are seen together, often the uproar between them is too great to tolerate. They are very reactive to each other. Limit setting, such as prohibiting interruptions, and strategies such as using a "listening chair" or turning one spouse's chair to the wall to listen are ineffective. In such situations spouses must be seen separately initially. The approach is to get the focus on the self and decrease efforts to change the other. The nurse focuses on what part the spouse plays in the situation. This spouse gains some self-control over reactive triggers. Once blaming is reduced, the spouse re-evaluates beliefs and values without the need to attack the other. Such re-evaluation entails contacting the family of origin by phone, letters, or planned visits. The goal is to understand better the source of the nuclear family conflict and to work to establish more personal relationships with the family of origin. This process is called "coaching." Usually, before this point is reached in the treatment, the absent, less motivated spouse seeks to join the sessions because of the changes that have occurred in the other spouse.

Significant changes in the marriage system occur when one spouse reduces overinvestment in the other and focuses on self. The spouse making changes must be warned of predictable efforts by the other to re-establish status quo. These efforts may include an escalation of anger-provoking behavior, threats to leave, and so on. If the spouse making changes can maintain a self-focused position through the resistance, both partners may become active in the treatment. While temporarily working with one spouse, nurses must guard against becoming part of a triangle. They may emotionally side with the spouse initially in treatment or become the spouse's only support. This can be especially difficult for nurses when the unexpressed plan of the unmotivated spouse is to deposit the husband or wife in treatment and obtain a divorce. Nurses may then be expected to "take care of" the spouse.

Spouse Dysfunction.   The second mechanism used by spouses to maintain emotional distance is the dysfunction of one spouse who may be emotionally, socially, or physically disabled to varying degrees. The degree to which the one underfunctions is the degree to which the other overfunctions. This ensures that emotional equilibrium is maintained because both partners are locked into a mutually dependent relationship. Interventions with such a relationship are similar to those used with the conflictual marriage. If the overfunctioning spouse is helped to pull back, the underfunctioning spouse then moves in to take up the slack, as seen in this clinical example.

 CLINICAL EXAMPLE

Mr. and Mrs. S sought treatment because the husband was missing many days at work. The couple had extensive arguments about Mr. S not wanting to work and Mrs. S feeling outraged at the financial stress he was creating. It became apparent that Mrs. S treated Mr. S as one of their adolescent boys. She overfunctioned to the point of cleaning up after her husband's destructive temper tantrums. Over time, with considerable coaching, she was able to pull back in several areas, refusing to wake her husband or clean up after him, leaving it up to him to pay the bills, and generally holding back her critical nagging. The first sign of progress was at Mr. S's next temper tantrum (he did delicate electrical work and had a low frustration tolerance). He carefully selected which objects he would throw or smash in his workroom, for example, not throwing a box of small nuts and bolts. He cleaned up his own workroom and began going to work regularly. As Mr. S's functioning improved, Mrs. S became depressed and began addressing unresolved issues in her family of origin. This couple demonstrated the reciprocity in the mechanism of underfunctioning and overfunctioning in a marriage.

Projection on Child.   The third distancing mechanism used by spouses to control the intensity of fusion between them is the projection of the problem to one or more of the children. How one child becomes a parental concern is a complex process. It may have its roots in several previous generations. Key triangles tend to repeat themselves over generations; thus the parent's natural tendency is to put one child in the parent's past position in the triangle. Nodal events are the normative events that occur in every family life but generate anxiety because change follows. These include such events as birth, death, sickness, marriage, job changes, school changes, divorce, and family relocation. The amount of stress generated around a nodal event depends on the amount of resultant change. If a significant developmental stage of the child (for example, in utero, birth, entering school for the first time, or adolescence) coincides with the occurrence of a nodal event, this child may be vulnerable to the focus of family stress and to impairment. The first-born and last-born children are also particularly vulnerable to family focus.

The primary goal of treatment is to remove the focus from the child and place the conflict between the parents where it belongs. The child's dysfunctions must be placed within the context of the family system by taking a family history and drawing a family genogram. The therapist's questions and comments are geared toward change of self rather than changing the child.

The therapist may identify problematic behavior in other family members to remove blame from the child. Another therapeutic strategy is to discuss how grandparents might handle the problem. With some families the nurse can coach the overly involved parent, such as the mother, to pull back from the focused child and send a note to her own mother telling her one thing about herself that she had not wanted her to know. This reveals the three-generational aspect of the presenting problem. It may also be helpful to work with the siblings at times, separately from the parents. This promotes a more positive support system among the siblings. Siblings often mimic their parents' negative behavior toward the focused child. They may also resent the excessive attention he or she receives from parents and act aggressively toward him or her.

Families with an acting-out child and two parents in the ineffective helpless position (or one parent set up as the "heavy" and the other as "the nice one") need a direct approach initially. The parents may have given up their authority to the child. This may be determined by asking them the following extreme questions: "If your child had third-degree burns, could you get her to take the horribly painful treatments?" or "If your child had heart disease, could you limit her activities?" Following are five guidelines for parents locked in a triangle with the acting-out child:

- The person who sets the rule must be present to enforce it.
- With two parents in the home, divide the areas of responsibility (such as allowance, bedtime, and nights out) so that when a dispute comes up, it is clear with whom the child must negotiate.
- Yelling is ineffective and inhibits thinking. Parents need to control their reactions and act as adults.
- Decide the logical consequences of repeated disobedient behavior and inform the child of them in advance. When the behavior occurs, without yelling, carry out the consequence even if the parents' personal plans must be changed to do so.
- Always give reassurance that the child is loved unconditionally.

As soon as the child focus is sufficiently reduced, the child is removed from the sessions. The therapist then becomes the third corner of the triangle, actively relating to both spouses without taking sides and thereby keeping any conflict focused on the spouses.

Multigenerational Transmission Process

The roots of the family emotional system extend back through generations. Drawing a three-generation family genogram as described earlier in this chapter often reveals certain relationship patterns otherwise believed to be peculiar to one nuclear family. For example, suicide of younger brothers, divorce among female siblings, or alcoholism might be a pattern across a family system when four or five generations are mapped out on a genogram. In family systems theory a symptom in one family member in one generation has its origin several generations before. This differentiates it from other forms of family therapy. However, families seeking treatment usually present symptoms as a nuclear family problem.

Family Projection Process

The family projection process is how anxiety about specific issues is transmitted through the generations. These are emotionally powerful issues, such as money, sex, child rearing, religion, work or school achievement, alcohol, politics, illness, and death, around which a rigid "party line" develops. Family members polarize around these issues, taking the family position or the direct opposite. Neither position allows freedom or flexibility of thought. Positions are reactive and fixed. Studying the family of origin helps identify a person's predictable position in family triangles involving specific issues. If individuals think about the issues they normally react to emotionally, they can plan strategies that will free them from triangled positions.

The family projection process also refers to the process that labels and assigns characteristics to certain family members. These labels may be overly positive ("Mary Sunshine," "The Genius") or overly negative ("The Crazy One," "Dummy"). They are equally unrealistic and confining. After years of family labeling, the labeled person will come to volunteer for the label and earn it.

> *Identify two emotionally powerful issues in your family of origin and think about your position related to them. Describe family labels you also heard while growing up.*

Sibling Position

The concept of personality profiles used in family systems theory is based on the belief that important personality characteristics are determined by the sex of one's siblings and one's birth order (Toman, 1993). For example, the younger brother of two older sisters is quite different from the older brother of a brother. The personality profiles developed can suggest marital discord or harmony on issues of rank or sex. For example, a younger brother of brothers may have more difficulty relating to his spouse than a younger brother of sisters. If this younger brother of brothers married a younger sister of sisters, they may both have discomfort with the opposite sex. In addition, they might struggle for juniority rights (who's going to take care of whom). The couple who recognizes sibling rank and each sibling's sex as a possible source of their conflicts can help each other to cope with their differences.

Emotional Cutoff

The emotional cutoff is a way to deal with intense unresolved attachment between children and parents. The cutoff is emotional isolation, although members may still live geographically close. It also may be physical distance from the family of origin. The cutoff creates the illusion of separation from parents. The more intense the emotional cutoff, the more likely it is that this problem will be reestablished in the next generation. Reconnecting emotionally with the cutoff family may prevent the same process from occurring with the parents and children of the next generation.

Modes of Therapy

Several modes of therapy have been mentioned thus far, including therapy with both spouses. Another mode of family therapy involves only one family member. This is most often used with the young adult who is single and self-supporting. This method includes learning about the functioning of family systems and triangles. It also involves keeping an active emotional relationship with important family members by planned phone calls, letters, and visits. This therapy requires developing an ability to control emotional reactiveness to avoid becoming part of an emotional triangle during visits with the family. The goal is to achieve more self-differentiation from the family of origin. The person must also develop a person-to-person relationship with important family members. This therapy is called coaching. Once the person is knowledgeable about triangles and methods of detriangling within the family, coaching sessions can be held as needed to supervise ongoing self-differentiation efforts.

The last mode of therapy is multiple family therapy (MFT) in which sessions are structured to ensure against emotional exchange between families. The idea behind MFT is as follows:

- To conserve teaching time of families
- To provide contact with a greater volume of families
- To allow the opportunity for families to learn from the efforts and experiences of other families

While other families observe, the nurse therapist works with each family as if only one family were receiving therapy. While the family answers detailed questions about its problem, the nurse defocuses feelings and addresses one spouse while the other spouse listens. Then the silent spouse is asked to share thoughts or reactions to what the other spouse has said. The family members observing can talk to the therapist about another family but cannot directly talk to the other family.

STRUCTURAL FAMILY THERAPY

Structural family therapy involves theory and techniques based on the individual within a social context that is clearly described by Minuchin (Minuchin & Fishman, 1981; Navarre, 1998). The assumption is that behavior is a consequence of the family's organization and the interactional patterns between members. Changing the family organization and the feedback processes between members changes the context in which a person functions. Thus the person's inner processes and behavior change.

The basic question of a structural family therapist is, "In what way is this family structure maintaining this maladaptive symptom?" Family structure is the invisible set of demands that determine how family members interact. A family is a system that operates through transactional patterns. Repeated transactions establish patterns of how, when, and to whom to relate, and these patterns determine whether the system is functional or dysfunctional.

> *What impact would sociocultural factors have on the effectiveness of a structural therapist's interventions with a family?*

Components

Family in Transition. In this model the family is a social system in transformation. The family system must maintain its continuity so that family members can grow. At the same time it must adapt to internal and external stresses to the system. Normal anxiety occurs during transitional stages.

 CLINICAL EXAMPLE

An elderly widow decided to move from her apartment where she had lived for 25 years because she came home one day and found it had been robbed. Soon after moving, she sought treatment from a psychiatrist. She complained that the people who moved her were trying to control her and had purposely lost precious possessions. They left sinister messages for each other on her furniture, and when she went outside, people followed her and signaled to each other. The psychiatrist diagnosed her as psychotic with paranoid delusions and prescribed tranquilizers. When this did not help, she sought a second psychiatrist, who recommended hospitalization. The third therapist she saw was a context-related therapist. He understood her symptoms as an ecological crisis. It was precipitated by feeling forced to move into an unfamiliar environment. He explained to her that she had lost her shell: the familiarity of objects in her apartment, the neighborhood, the neighbors. Like any crustacean that has lost its shell, she felt vulnerable and was experiencing reality differently than before. He instructed her to go home, unpack, and place her familiar objects, books, and pictures in the new apartment. He told her to do her daily chores routinely, go to the same shops and checkout counters, and for 2 weeks make no effort to meet neighbors. She was to visit old friends and family but not discuss her recent experiences. If anyone asked, she was to explain that those had just been the problems of an illogical, fearful old woman.

Structural family therapists change the relationship between a person and the familiar context in which the person functions. This changes the subjective experience and enables more functional behavior to emerge. In the preceding clinical example the therapist's interventions protected the woman from the unfamiliar and frightening environment until she could "grow a new shell." He blocked the environmental feedback that confirmed her paranoid fears as friends and family secretly discussed her frightening behavior. As her experience of her environment changed, her symptoms disappeared.

Stages of Family Development. Every family undergoes predictable stages of development over time. These stages require adaptive restructuring. Each stage involves a process of transition and requires changes in family functioning for adaptive growth and development. The stages of the family life cycle are presented in Table 34-5.

Family Structure. A third component of Minuchin's model of a functioning family relates to the family structure. The major elements of structure are as follows:

- Power and influence within the family
- Sets and family relationships, including subsystems
- Family boundaries that may be individual, sexual, or generational

Structure can become dysfunctional in any or all of these areas. First, as in any organization, the family system must have a power hierarchy with different levels of authority to function efficiently. Functions must be complementary because the family needs to work together as a team. Over the years, mutual expectations of particular family members evolve. These expectations may be openly negotiated but are often implicit, with patterns of behavior developing around minor daily events. Critics of this aspect of structural therapy point out that too often, restoring the parent-child hierarchy means restoring a traditional male authority structure, which supports damaging gender inequalities existing in the family and society. The nurse who focuses only on generational (parent-child) differences may ignore differences in power, resources, and needs among all family members. Thus the nurse could inadvertently promote gender-based power inequities that can result in destructive behavior. This dilemma highlights the need for family therapists to be particularly careful not to bring personal and sociocultural bias into their work with families.

> *Describe how wife abuse and childhood incest can arise from a family structure that is based on male power and authority and female dependence and submission.*

Second, the family system differentiates and functions through sets of relationships or subsystems. Subsystems can be made up of individuals or dyads. They are formed by generation, sex, interest, or function. Each person belongs to many subsystems. Each subsystem has different levels of power in which differentiated skills are learned.

Third, boundaries of a subsystem are the rules defining who participates in subsystem functions and how. Boundaries must be free of intrusion. Each subsystem has specific functions and interpersonal developmental tasks to be accomplished. Patterns of mutual accommodation and healthy competition cannot develop among siblings if parents or grandparents constantly interfere. Subsystem boundaries must be clear for proper family functioning but must also permit emotional contact among members.

Families with extreme boundary problems are either enmeshed or disengaged. Enmeshed boundaries are weak and fluid; personal space and subsystem boundaries rapidly change and affect all subsystems. This diffuseness of boundaries prevents the development of autonomy and competence.

Table 34-5

The Stages of the Family Life Cycle

Stage	Emotional Process of Transition: Key Principles	Second-Order Changes in Family Status Required to Proceed Developmentally
Leaving home: single young adults	Accepting emotional and financial responsibility for self	Differentiation of self in relation to family of origin Development of intimate peer relationships Establishment of self regarding work and financial independence
The joining of families through marriage: the new couple	Commitment to new system	Formation of marital system Realignment of relationships with extended families and friends to include spouse
Families with young children	Accepting new members into the system	Adjusting marital system to make space for children Joining in child-rearing, financial, and household tasks Realignment of relationships with extended family to include parenting and grandparenting roles
Families with adolescents	Increasing flexibility of family boundaries to include children's independence and grandparents' frailties	Shifting of parent-child relationships to permit adolescent to move in and out of system Refocus on midlife marital and career issues Beginning shift toward joint caring for older generation
Launching children and moving on	Accepting a multitude of exits from and entries into the family system	Renegotiation of marital system as a dyad Development of adult-to-adult relationships between grown children and their parents Realignment of relationships to include in-laws and grandchildren Dealing with disabilities and death of parents (grandparents)
Families in later life	Accepting the shifting of generational roles	Maintaining own or couple functioning and interests in face of physiological decline; exploration of new familial and social role options Support for a more central role of middle generation Making room in the system for the wisdom and experience of the elderly, supporting the older generation without overfunctioning for them Dealing with loss of spouse, siblings, and other peers and preparation for own death; life review and integration

From Carter E, McGoldrick M: *The changing family life cycle: a framework for family therapy*, ed 2, Boston, 1989, Allyn & Bacon.

Perceptions of self and others are poorly differentiated. A child in such a family might be so sensitized to conflict between parents that school performance may decline. The parents in such a family can become upset because the child refuses to eat vegetables at dinner. Such families flood with anxiety at times of stress and adapt poorly to change.

Disengaged families have rigid boundaries. Communication between subsystems is poor; supportive or protective contact is minimal. Members of such systems may function autonomously but have a skewed sense of independence. They lack feelings of loyalty and belonging and the capacity for interdependence. Some suggest that the product of a disengaged family is the sociopath. Because of the rigidity of subsystem boundaries, members may fail to respond adequately when one member is stressed. In such a family, a child's reading disorder might go unnoticed or a husband's suicidal behavior may be disregarded.

In this model of family therapy the nurse often functions as a boundary maker and may clarify diffuse boundaries by discouraging interruptions and encouraging shutting bed-

room doors. The nurse may also open overly rigid boundaries by recommending that a distant parent and child spend time together or by calling attention to a member's feeling that would otherwise go unnoticed by other members. The nurse's assessment of family subsystems and boundary functioning provides a rapid diagnosis of the family. It indicates the direction and goals of therapeutic interventions.

As mentioned earlier, each subsystem has specific functions and interpersonal developmental tasks to be accomplished. The spouse subsystem must develop patterns of mutual support. Couples must make decisions and settle arguments without domination or relinquishing of self by either spouse. Ideally, they will bring out the best in each other, with each promoting personal growth and creativity in his or her spouse.

Spouses typically engage in an "other-improvement program." They bring into the marriage certain expectations of their spouse and work hard to have the spouse meet them. Interpretations in this area should be directed to both spouses. The part each plays in the destructive process

Table 34-6

Methods of Joining the Family

Method	Description
Mirroring or mimicking	Matching the family's mood, pace, or communication patterns, such as becoming jovial, somber, fidgety, or terse in conversing with them
Respecting family values	Supporting family hierarchies, such as by addressing all communication through the spouse that appears to be the "central switchboard"
Finding common elements	Keying in culturally or establishing areas of kinship, such as by offering "I have an adolescent boy, too"
Searching for strength	Observing for the smallest positive aspect of each family member that the nurse can use to confirm that person's sense of self, such as by appreciating a clever phrase or a sense of humor
Supporting family subsystems	Confirming important family subsets, such as by giving small children toys to play with while talking with older ones, or by having parents sit together as they discuss their difficulty with the children
Tracking	Asking for elaboration with concrete details and examples of specific content in the family's discussion; this confirms people who are speaking and explores family structure, such as in tracking a mother's mentioning that she and her son are close by asking what time of the day and in which part of the house they are closest, thus learning that the mother and son sleep together while father sleeps in another room

should be pointed out. A mutual interpretation would be to say to the wife, "In your efforts to make contact with your husband, you are driving him away," and to the husband, "Your strong, silent style is alluring but elicits nagging." Balanced interpretations emphasize the complementarity of the system. Both positive and negative qualities are recognized in each spouse.

The parental subsystem socializes the children without sacrificing mutual support and accommodation between the spouses. Children must have access to each parent but be excluded from spouse functions. Parenting processes are different depending on the child's age. Part of promoting differentiation in the family is making the differentiation in ages clear. Adolescents have responsibilities and privileges that 12-year-old siblings do not. Children must learn to negotiate with their parents to live in a world of unequal power relationships.

Children first learn about peer relationships in the sibling subsystem. They learn to make friends, compete, negotiate, cooperate, and gain recognition of their skills. Knowledge of normal growth and development of children is valuable for the nurse, who at times must translate age-appropriate skills, needs, and values to parents. The nurse should support the child's right to growing autonomy and the parents' responsible authority at the same time.

Interventions

A vital part of structural family therapy is the process of joining the family (Navarre, 1998). Nurse therapists temporarily become part of the family system. They adapt their behavior to the particular family's rules and manner. The aim is to accommodate to the family to gain experiential entrance into the family system. Unless this is accomplished at the beginning, restructuring and change are impossible. Methods of joining the family are described in Table 34-6.

Another initial task of nurse therapists is to assume leadership in the session. They must join the family while still retaining the freedom to confront and challenge by presenting themselves as experts, gaining the family's confidence, and instilling hope. The nurse establishes the rules of the system by determining who attends the session, allowing no one to talk for another, and prohibiting interruptions. The nurse controls the flow and direction of communication.

At the beginning of the session, the nurse contacts each member. More than 15 to 20 minutes must not be spent with an individual or the nurse will become part of the system. Very soon the nurse asks two people to interact directly to enact a problem they have been describing. The nurse can now directly observe dysfunctional interactions. Rather than going from content issue to content issue, the nurse therapist can introduce the conflict inherent in small events and make conflictual events from nonevents.

Structural family therapy does not explore or interpret the past; it is active and immediate. Diagnosis in family therapy depends on the observation of how the family affects the nurse's behavior. It is also based on the nurse's impact on the family. The interactional diagnosis changes according to the family's acceptance or resistance of the therapist's restructuring interventions. It also varies depending on which family subsystem is active in the therapeutic situation at any one time. In this way, diagnosis and therapy are inseparable.

Intervention strategies transform the dysfunctional transactional patterns that maintain symptomatic behavior. The nurse is concerned about symptom removal and changes the family's organization to ensure that the symptom is not passed on. However, if an area of organization such as the parents' relationship does not contribute to the symptom, the therapist does not enter there. Therapy should be limited to the family's presenting symptom.

There are seven categories of restructuring operations: enacting family transactional patterns, marking boundaries, escalating stress, assigning tasks, using symptoms, manipulating mood, and supporting, educating, or guiding.

Enacting Transactional Patterns. Enacting transactional patterns involves family members actively discussing an event that they might otherwise be describing to the nurse. Instead, the nurse instructs specific members to discuss the matter between themselves. The nurse disengages from the interaction to observe nonverbal confirmation or contradiction of the content, patterned sequences, interruptions, distractions, alliances, and coalitions.

It may be difficult to stay outside these transactions, and the family may drag the nurse back into direct discussion. Going behind a one-way mirror after giving the family directions is a way to avoid this temptation. Manipulating space by rearranging seating or position can be an effective way of encouraging or intensifying dialogue. The seating pattern a family assumes when it first walks into a session provides clues to alliances, coalitions, centrality, and isolation. The nurse's manipulation of seating and space can be a diagnostic probe to see how flexible the family is to such change. It is also a graphic indication to the family of a therapeutic goal. For instance, the nurse may seat the spatially isolated father next to his son, where the mother was seated. The wife is placed next to the nurse. This encourages more direct involvement between father and son, with the mother outside that relationship.

Marking Boundaries. Boundaries must be marked in both individuals and subsystems. This promotes clarity in enmeshed families and reduces rigidity in disengaged families. Rules promote individual autonomy and include insisting that family members speak to each other and not about each other. No one speaks for another, no one may interrupt, and no one acts as another's memory bank. The nurse encourages subsystem boundaries by including or excluding various subsystems attending a session. She would ask children to leave or not attend a session about spouses' sex life. The nurse may assign tasks to promote subsystem boundaries. She might instruct the father and daughter to go out for a pizza once a week without the mother or younger siblings. Having the sibling subsystem interact in a session, with the mother behind a one-way mirror, helps the children find alternative ways to resolve conflicts normally interrupted by mother's interventions. At the same time, this lets mother identify more positive interaction among the children. Previously, she could only reflexively react to their anger, rebelliousness, and selfishness by intruding on their boundaries. Rigid triads involving cross-generational interactions can be especially resistant to boundary marking.

Escalating Stress. Increasing stress in a family forces members to develop more functional ways of resolving stress. In families seeking treatment, dysfunctional patterns have developed around the symptomatic member. To escalate stress, the nurse may block usual transactional patterns and emphasize differences the family ignores. Asking for the silent spouse's opinion following the dominant spouse's statements highlights unspoken family disagreements. Developing implicit conflict involves making covert conflict overt.

Families develop methods for diffusing conflict rapidly. For example, siblings may tease and shove each other noisily just before their parents argue. This prevents the parents' conflict from surfacing. Blocking the sibling conflict forces the parents to contact directly. The nurse can polarize conflict to increase stress. If the mother and father appear equally concerned about their son's delinquent activities, the nurse may ask the husband if he had ever tried telling his wife she was "messing up" with the son. The positions of the overprotective mother and the "reasonable" distant father develop.

The nurse can also produce stress by temporarily joining one member or subsystem. This operation must be carefully planned and requires the nurse's ability to disengage, which can be done serially to help members take differentiated positions. Also, a coalition can be formed, usually with a spouse, when the system rigidly resists open conflict. Joining a husband's attack on the wife makes the conflict too intense for the wife to diffuse stress onto the son; she is forced to address the conflict between herself and the husband.

Assigning Tasks. Task assignment structures the setting for alternative interactions and behavior. In designing tasks the nurse must have a clear idea of the family's structure and dysfunctional patterns. Specific interactional goals to accomplish through the task must be outlined. Tasks can be simple. The nurse may ask a husband and wife to sit next to each other as they discuss an issue. In a family in which the wife disciplines the children, the father is assigned the job. The mother handles only emergencies; otherwise, the father learns of infractions he does not directly observe. The wife may not interfere with her husband's disciplinary tactics. She takes notes. Both parents become active and effective.

In assigning tasks the nurse should give all critically involved members a portion of the task to complete. This reduces the likelihood of one member sabotaging another's new behavior if each member must remain self-focused. This also makes it easier to relinquish a fixed behavior if another behavior is assigned to replace it. Whether the task is completed or not, the family and nurse have new information about family patterns and progress.

Using Symptoms. Symptoms can be used in restructuring operations in various ways. Symptoms may be focused on, as in a family in which the daughter was a fire setter. The focus remained on the daughter, but the mother was instructed to spend time daily teaching the daughter how to light matches safely. This promoted a closer mother-daughter relationship, which was previously obstructed. A helpful focus remained on the symptom. Symptoms can be exaggerated to increase their intensity and mobilize family resources. A symptom can be relabeled, as in the case of a mother who continually nagged the son. Redefining her nagging as concern encouraged caring interactions. A new symptom shifts the family's focus onto another family member temporarily. For example, the husband fails to go to work and the wife alternately protects and threatens to leave him. Identifying her behavior as seriously depressed reduces her intense focus on the husband. A symptom's affect can also be changed, thereby altering interactions around it. For example, the mother who interacts positively with her fire-setting daughter evokes a new affect with the symptom.

Manipulating Mood. Manipulating the family's mood is another restructuring operation. For example, by exaggerating the common family mood, the family reacts by showing a wide range of expressions. The nurse can also model a more appropriate affect for the family, for example, by reacting with strong indignation to a young boy's criticism of his mother. This promotes respect and clarifies the boundaries of a passive, enmeshed parental subsystem.

Supporting, Educating, or Guiding. Support, education, and guidance can be a restructuring operation. They can take the form of modeling, assigning tasks, or sharing concrete information.

The goal of structural family therapy is not a change in behavior but a change in the whole family's organization. This allows individual members a new experience in the family. Using a model of an effectively functioning family, the therapist joins the family in a therapeutic system, hoping to restructure the family. The restructuring helps to maintain functional subsystems or form new subsystems that will promote healing and growth.

STRATEGIC FAMILY THERAPY

Strategic family therapy developed several decades ago out of communication theory (Watzlawick et al, 1967). Communication theorists contend that all behavior, not only verbal acts, is communication. They recognize that most communication consists of many levels between sender and receiver and that the significance of any message depends on how it is reinforced, contradicted, or framed by other messages. These, along with the setting and the relationship between sender and receiver, constitute the context that must be considered in interpreting any message (see Chapter 2).

Another basic tenet of communication theory is that communication is an ongoing process. There is no beginning point or end point in the stimulus-response-reinforcement pattern of human interaction. In most relationships the behavior of each participant depends on the other's behavior. In families, complex, highly patterned, repetitive interactions become established. When a two-person (or more) system is dysfunctional in its communication, the potential exists for problems. Three types of common communication problems are disqualification, disconfirmation, and incongruent communication.

Disqualification includes self-contradictions, inconsistencies, subject switches, incomplete sentences, misunderstandings, obscure mannerisms of speech, and literal interpretation of metaphor. An example of disqualification is a question an older brother used to baffle his younger sister: "Do you walk to school or carry your lunch?"

Disconfirmation involves ignoring or invalidating essential elements of a significant other's self-image. It involves saying that you do not feel the way you feel, need what you need, or experience what you experience. An example is when a spouse says, "I know you don't mean that. You're just upset and getting angry doesn't suit you."

Incongruent communication is delivering two conflicting messages at the same time. In responding to either message, the receiver will be charged with "badness or madness." This is the basis of the double bind. An example is the command "Be spontaneous!" or the direction to "Be assertive, and don't make waves."

Components

Strategic therapists make a distinction between difficulties and problems. Difficulties are either undesirable states of affairs that can be removed by a logical solution or undesirable, common life problems that must be lived with. Problems arise from small difficulties that escalate. They are maintained by mishandling attempts to solve them. Mishandling often occurs around adaptation to ordinary life events and ranges from ignoring or denying difficulties that require action to attempting to resolve an ordinary life difficulty that is unnecessary (such as a husband who would not talk to his wife before breakfast) or impossible to resolve (such as the generation gap), to difficulties where action is needed but the wrong kind is taken (Haley, 1996).

Strategic family therapists are not concerned with the history of the problem or the motivation behind it. They are not interested in characteristics of people, and they place no importance on insight. Little distinction is made between acute and chronic problems. Chronic problems are ones that have been mishandled longer. The presenting problem behavior and the problem-maintaining behavior are the primary focus of treatment.

Communication theorists have identified a positive feedback loop in human interaction. This is the vicious cycle that develops from efforts by family members, or the identified patient, to stop or "help" undesirable behavior. For example, the rebellious teenager, when faced with parental discipline, becomes increasingly rebellious. As discipline becomes harsher, the teenager's behavior escalates further. Thus the action that is meant to alleviate the behavior of the other party aggravates it. From this view, the cause and the nature of a problem are essentially the same process. People try to change behavior in the most logical way possible. Common sense suggests prevention or avoidance of undesirable behavior by means of opposite behavior. If this does not work, they try harder with the same behavior. The resolution of problems therefore requires changing the problem-maintaining behaviors. This interrupts the vicious positive feedback cycles.

Interventions

Intervention occurs with the identified patient, another family member, or both, depending on who is most concerned with the problem. This is the person most willing to change. Effective intervention can be made through any member of the system to break the positive feedback loop. This is illustrated in the following two clinical examples.

 CLINICAL EXAMPLE

A colonel was being militarily strict with his son, and the boy was becoming increasingly defiant. The therapist told the father that his son was "going to the dogs." The therapist suggested that the father hold back on his discipline to get a baseline measurement of how bad the boy's behavior would become. As pressure on the boy was reduced, his behavior improved.

CLINICAL EXAMPLE

A woman had problems with urinary frequency. She was isolated at home, feeling unable to leave the house to socialize. She was also isolated at work because she had her desk by the bathroom door where there were no co-workers. She worked from 12 to 8 PM. The therapist instructed her to urinate as many times as she felt she had to each morning before going to work but to use the toilet only three times; after that she was to urinate sitting in the tub. She was to make no effort to change her pattern at work. The next week the woman reported she had been in agony the first morning but was unable to urinate sitting in the tub. She then figured that if she could limit herself at home, she could do so at work and had no further problems with urinary frequency.

These examples demonstrate the use of reversal or symptom prescription. They stop the family or patient from trying to change. Persuading people to change behavior that they believe is correct often requires treatment strategies that appear weird, illogical, or paradoxical.

The nurse's first task is to obtain a statement from the patient of the presenting complaint in specific, concrete terms. After obtaining this statement, the nurse determines what about the behavior makes it a problem. The nurse asks what solutions the family has tried. This identifies which remedies to avoid and indicates the problem-maintaining behavior.

Next, the nurse asks what the family's or patient's minimum goal of treatment would be—that is, the smallest identifiable change that would signify progress or some success. General goals such as "improved communication" are not acceptable. Changes such as "feeling happier" or negative goals such as "stopping certain behavior" are equally unacceptable. Rather, the nurse seeks positive, specific behavioral goals that reflect an attitude or feeling change, such as "the father will engage in one positive activity with his son each

Table 34-7

Models of Family Therapy

	Family System (Bowen)	Structural (Minuchin)	Strategic (Haley)
View of normal family function	Differentiation of self in relation to others Balance between thinking and feeling	Generational hierarchy with strong parental authority Clear boundaries Flexibility of system for autonomy, interdependence, and adaptive change	Flexibility Large behavioral repertoire for problem solving and life cycle passage
View of symptoms/ dysfunction	Functioning is impaired by relationship with family of origin Poor differentiation Emotional reactivity Triangulation Emotional cutoff	Symptoms result from current structural imbalance and malfunctioning generational hierarchy or boundaries Enmeshed or disengaged style Maladaptive reaction to internal or external demands	Symptom is embedded in interaction pattern Origin of problem not significant Symptoms are maintained by unsuccessful problem solving Impasse at life cycle transition
Goals of therapy	Greater self-differentiation Increased thinking Decreased emotional reactivity Detriangulate self	Reorganize family structure to achieve strengthened parental hierarchy, clear, flexible boundaries, and more adaptive patterns	Interrupt rigid feedback cycle Change symptom-maintaining sequence to attain new outcome
Role of the nurse in change	Stays detriangulated Change can occur only within the self Change in one member can bring about systemic change	Joining the family is prerequisite for restructuring Nurse is responsible for change while crediting the family for beneficial changes	If treatment fails, the fault lies with the nurse Success is credited to the family, thus enhancing its confidence in future problem-solving skills
Interventions	Teach how family systems work Coach individual to establish person-to-person relationship with key members of family of origin Use genogram to track triangles, myths, and themes across the generations Ask factual who, what, when, where, and how questions to promote thinking and reduce emotionally reactive behavior	Joining Enacting Marking boundaries Escalating stress Assigning tasks Using symptom Manipulating mood Supporting Educating Advocacy	Detailed questions to track behaviors surrounding the problem Symptom prescription Reframing Strategies designed to interrupt self-reinforcing behavioral sequence maintaining the symptom

week." If a small but significant change can be made in what appeared to be a hopeless situation, a ripple effect may occur. That is, once a patient is mobilized and regains confidence in the ability to solve a small problem, sometimes other difficulties can be surmounted.

As soon as possible, the therapist attempts to grasp the patient's language and main ideas and values. Tuning in to the family's view and then extending that view is a critical step known as *reframing*. It precedes the therapist's strategic intervention. To reframe means to change the conceptual or emotional setting or viewpoint in which a situation is experienced. Using language common to the family's world view, the therapist places the experience in another frame that fits the "facts" of the same concrete situation equally well. The situation's entire meaning changes (Haley, 1996).

An example of reframing includes using hostility when it is present in a woman's frigidity. The therapist may reframe the problem as one produced by her overprotecting the male. Assuming that there is hostility and protecting the husband is the last thing the woman would want to do, the new frame to the problem uses hostility as an incentive to release her inhibited sexual feelings. Tom Sawyer reframed whitewashing the picket fence as an artistic, entertaining enterprise rather than a dreary chore. He used his friends' competitiveness to vie for the opportunity to whitewash. Reframing causes an attitudinal change and a change in emphasis of a situation's facts. This changes the situation's meaning to permit new behavior. The concrete facts remain unchanged.

The strategic therapist is an active and deliberate change agent. The therapist creates a strategy to bring about the change the patient wants to achieve. In this therapy the point at which termination takes place is clear. It occurs when the patient is satisfied with the improvement that has been made.

The theoretical views of family therapy presented in this chapter are summarized in Table 34-7. These models reflect current thinking in family therapy.

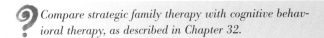

Compare strategic family therapy with cognitive behavioral therapy, as described in Chapter 32.

Summary

1. Family functioning was discussed, and functional, cultural, and dysfunctional characteristics were described.
2. Family assessment techniques were reviewed, including family history, the family APGAR, and the genogram.
3. Working with families included a review of the competence paradigm, psychoeducation, and family therapy.
4. Family systems theory conceptualizes all family systems on a continuum ranging from total dysfunction to high levels of functioning. Separating the thinking and feeling processes of family members is foundational to this therapy. The goal of systems therapy is for individual members to differentiate themselves from the family emotional "we-ness" system.
5. Structural family therapy assumes that behavior and the family's level of function are consequences of the family's organization and the interactional patterns between members. The major elements of a family structure that enable viable family functioning are a power hierarchy with different levels of authority, differentiated subsystems with different functions and levels of power, and subsystem boundaries sufficiently well defined to prevent intrusion but also able to allow emotional contact between members.
6. Strategic therapists are concerned with the removal of problematic behavioral patterns or symptoms. The goals of strategic therapy include obtaining a clear statement from the family of the presenting complaint in specific, concrete terms. The therapist reframes the problem, thereby changing the situation's meaning, permitting new behavior to occur.

Competent Caring   A Clinical Exemplar of a Psychiatric Nurse

CAROLE BENNETT, PHD, RN, CS

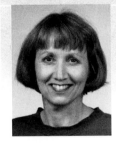

As a psychiatric nurse, I have always found it difficult to describe the rewards I experienced for the years of hard work I have dedicated to my profession. Sometimes the rewards elude even me. Then, quite unexpectedly, I have the opportunity to really help someone and I remember why I have been a psychiatric nurse for such a long time.

Recently a nurse working on our youth unit was having difficulty with teaching parenting skills to a mother. No matter how many times she demonstrated limit setting and reinforcement, this mother seemed unable to use these skills. The nurse asked me to see the mother and intervene using the family genogram and I agreed. The next day the family anxiously appeared: the mother, the father, and an aunt who flew down from New York. When I heard that the father's older sister from New York was waiting to be in family therapy, I thought that this would be a rough one. So I drew a deep breath, offered coffee all around, poured myself a big cup, and began the meeting. Yes, they all knew why they were there. Yes, they all knew it might get uncomfortable. Yes, they all wanted to stay.

The father and his sister began with their family. They grew up in the projects, had different fathers, described years of struggle, and related how the older sister was sent to New York to live with her natural father and how their mother managed all the while to raise them from a wheelchair. But she had done it; she had shown them how to do it, too.

Then the mother began. She too was raised in the projects, but by her grandparents. Her mother never really visited often, and her grandmother was an alcoholic. Yes, she had a grandfa-

Continued

Competent Caring A Clinical Exemplar of a Psychiatric Nurse—cont'd

ther, but he was an alcoholic, too. She also lived with other family members at various times, but they were all heavy drinkers. In fact, every adult in her childhood was an alcoholic. But it was hard for her to recall facts. Had she been sexually abused? Well, she remembers being told something about that but she couldn't remember any details. She does remember being beaten regularly by various people, but that didn't seem unusual to her.

Everyone was quiet. It was hard for me to know quite what to say. By this time the husband was patting his wife lovingly. He had known only parts of the painful story he just heard his wife describe. And his sister from New York moved closer to her sister-in-law on the couch. They were very supportive while I suggested that perhaps no one had ever shown the wife how to be a mother. No one had ever shown her what to do, and so she really didn't know how to take care of the seven boys she was now raising.

As a group, we continued to talk until we came up with a plan. The sister was leaving for home soon, but there would be two other sisters who could help. The father said he could shorten his workday, and perhaps the mother could look for a job, which was something she wanted to do. The unit nurse said she could arrange for the mother to spend entire days on the unit so that she could begin to learn how to do this thing called "child rearing." And finally, we discussed the issue of therapy. Well, no thank you. The mother didn't think she was ready to talk to someone about what had happened to her so long ago, but maybe she would be sometime in the future.

We all stood up and shook hands, smiling and sensing the partnership among us. The sister from New York gave my hand an especially firm squeeze and looked me right in the eye. I think she was saying she was glad I was there, and I was sending the same message back to her. At that moment I knew exactly why I have been a psychiatric nurse for such a long time.

MERLIN Visit **MERLIN: www.mosby.com/MERLIN/Stuart** to find these additional materials and student activities.

- **Worksheets**
- **"Drug of the Month" Updates**
- **"Citing the Evidence" Updates**
- **Critical Thinking Activities and Exercises**
- **Annotated Suggested Readings**
- **Web Links**
- **More!**

Chapter Review Questions

1. **Identify whether the following statements are true (T) or false (F).**

____ A. Triangles should be avoided at all costs.

____ B. Triangles distance a person from a painful issue and allow one to avoid change.

____ C. There is always a third person in a triangle willing to deflect emotional intensity.

____ D. Therapists can be most effective by becoming part of the triangle and thereby effecting change.

____ E. Participants of a triangle shift in a family depending on the emotional issue at stake.

2. **Fill in the blanks.**

A. Using the competency paradigm, a family's _____ are emphasized in therapy, as compared with older conceptual models, which emphasize a family's _____.

B. Psychoeducational interventions with families are designed primarily to _____ and _____.

C. The largest self-help and consumer advocacy group in the United States is _____.

D. Family systems therapy was developed by _____.

E. A basic premise of family systems therapy is that families fail to distinguish between _____ and _____.

F. When self-boundaries are blurred it is called _____.

G. Structural family therapy seeks to interrupt the sequence of _____.

H. To _____ means to change the conceptual or emotional setting or viewpoint in which a situation is experienced.

I. The first task of the strategic family therapist is to _____.

J. Two commonly used tools for family assessment are _____ and _____.

K. Individuals joined by marriage or its equivalent or by parenthood is the definition of a

_____.

3. Provide short answers for the following questions.

A. Discuss how a person with high differentiation of self differs from someone with low self-differentiation.

B. Define a genogram and sketch one for your own family.

C. Critique the adaptive and maladaptive family functioning portrayed in a novel by Pat Conroy (*Prince of Tides, Lords of Discipline*), Ann Tyler (*Accidental Tourist, Dinner at the Homesick Restaurant*), or another author of your choice.

D. Describe the two principles that distinguish family therapy from individual and group therapy.

REFERENCES

American Psychiatric Association: *Diagnostic and statistical manual mental disorders*, Fourth Edition, Text Revision. Washington, DC, American Psychiatric Association, 2000.

Barkauskas V et al: *Health and physical assessment*, St Louis, 1998, Mosby.

Bohlander J: Differentiation of self: an examination of the concept, *Issues Ment Health Nurs* 16:165, 1995.

Bowen M: *Family therapy in clinical practice*, ed 2, Northvale, NJ, 1988, Jason Aronson.

Davis B, Jones L: Differentiation of self and attachment among adult daughters, *Issues Ment Health Nurs* 13:321, 1992.

Haley J: *Learning and teaching therapy*, New York, 1996, Guilford Press.

Jorde L et al: *Medical genetics*, St Louis, 1999, Mosby.

Kay J, Tasman A: Relational problems. In *Psychiatry: behavioral science and clinical essentials*, Philadelphia, 2000, WB Saunders.

Kerr M, Bowen M: *Family evaluation: an approach based on Bowen theory*, New York, 1988, WW Norton.

Marsh D: *Serious mental illness and the family: the practitioners guide*, New York, 2000, John Wiley & Sons.

McFarlane W: Multiple family groups and psychoeducation in the treatment of schizophrenia, *Arch Gen Psychiatr* 52:679, 1995.

Minuchin S, Fishman H: *Family therapy techniques*, Cambridge, Mass, 1981, Harvard University Press.

Mohr W: Partnering with families, *J Psychosoc Nurs* 38(1):15, 2000.

Navarre S: Salvador Minuchin's structural family therapy and its application to multicultural family systems, *Issues Ment Health Nurs* 19:557, 1998.

Puri B, Tyer P: *Sciences basic to psychiatry*, ed 2, Edinburgh, 1998, Churchill Livingstone.

Sadock B, Sadock V: *Comprehensive textbook of psychiatry*, ed 7, Philadelphia, 2000, Lippincott Williams & Wilkins.

Sherman C: Assessment is good opportunity to change family dynamics, *Clin Psychiatr News* 3:25, 2000.

Sulloway F: *Born to rebel: birth order, family dynamics, and creative lives*, New York, 1997, Pantheon Books.

Toman W: *Family constellation*, ed 4, New York, 1993, Springer.

Walsh F: Conceptualizations of normal family processes. In Walsh F, editor: *Normal family processes*, ed 2, New York, 1993, Guilford.

Watzlawick P et al: *Pragmatics of human communication*, New York, 1967, WW Norton.

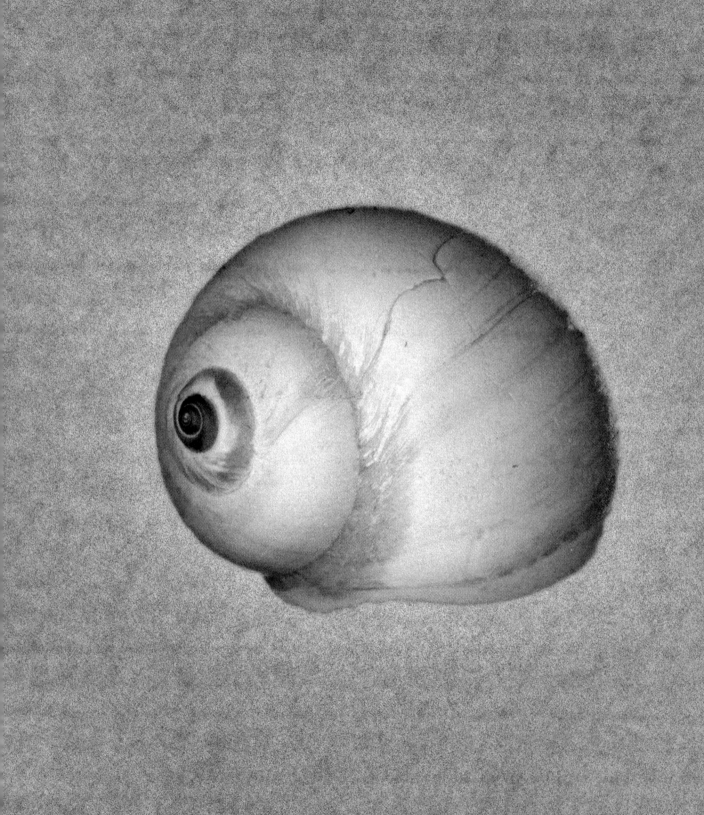

Unit 5

Treatment Settings

You may think that most people with emotional and psychiatric problems spend many days of their lives in an acute or long-term psychiatric hospital being cared for by specially trained staff. Years ago you would have been correct, but today most people with such problems live in the community and receive their mental health care in outpatient settings. These are the people you pass on the street, see at the mall, and laugh with at the movies. Today, we no longer try to separate and isolate the mentally ill in large, impersonal institutions. Rather, we ask our caregivers to reach out to these people and their families in the neighborhoods in which they live, love, and learn.

In this unit you will discover how contemporary psychiatric hospitals take care of patients. You will read how inpatient psychiatric nurses protect and stabilize people in crisis and then turn their care over to a variety of community-based mental health care providers. As psychiatric treatment grows in the community, new and expanded roles are opening up for psychiatric nurses. These tap into nurses' spirit of innovation, creativity, and resourcefulness. Finally, you'll learn about home care and how psychiatric nurses are returning to their roots in public health and crossing the hearths and homes of the patients they treat. So step up, step out, and step into the current practice settings of psychiatric care.

Visit **MERLIN** for *Your Internet Connection*
to websites that are related to the content in this chapter.
www.mosby.com/MERLIN/Stuart

35 Hospital-Based Psychiatric Nursing Care

Elizabeth G. Maree

"*We're all mad here. I'm mad. You're mad.*" "*How do you know I'm mad?,*" *said Alice.* "*You must be,*" *said the Cat,* "*or you wouldn't have come here.*" *Alice didn't think that proved it at all.*

LEWIS CARROLL, *ALICE'S ADVENTURES IN WONDERLAND*

The treatment of the mentally ill has always reflected social values and public policy. Before World War II, effective medications were largely unavailable, and the mentally ill were separated from the community and housed in institutions for the protection of patients as well as society. Nursing care for these patients was primarily custodial. With changing social perspectives and the move toward more humane treatment, the psychiatric hospital came to be seen as a possibly powerful force that could influence patient behavior and help people recover from mental illness. More recently, scientific advances have led to the use of effective medications and somatic therapies to treat symptoms of psychiatric illness. These, used in conjunction with therapeutic principles and management strategies of the treatment milieu, offer hospital-based psychiatric nurses valuable tools for the care of the mentally ill.

THE PSYCHIATRIC HOSPITAL IN TRANSITION

Health-care costs, changing reimbursement trends, and problems with accessibility of care among vast numbers of citizens have prompted major changes in how health care is delivered in the United States. As efforts to reduce the growth of health-care expenditures have shortened inpatient lengths of stay, less expensive treatment alternatives have emerged (Mechanic, 1997). Many hospital facilities have become integrated clinical systems and now provide a full range of services, including partial hospitalization, ambulatory, and even home care programs.

Inpatient Programs

In recent years the focus of psychiatric care has moved away from extended care in predominantly inpatient settings toward shorter lengths of inpatient stays and a wider choice among continuum of care options. For example, in 1988 the average length of stay for acute psychiatric inpatient treatment was about 25 days, as compared with 10.2 days in 1997 (Fig. 35-1). Many inpatient psychiatric settings now have an average length of stay of 5 to 10 days, and crisis stabilization inpatient programs may involve only a 2- or 3-day length of stay.

The major psychiatric diagnoses of patients admitted to inpatient and partial hospital programs are listed in Table 35-1. In previous years most patients with maladaptive cop-

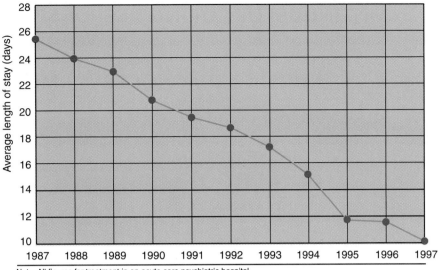

Note: All figures for treatment in an acute care psychiatric hospital

Fig. 35-1 Hospital stays for psychiatric patients.

ing responses entered the psychiatric hospital in the **acute** treatment stage and were able to stay in the hospital until the goal of symptom **remission** was attained (Fig. 35-2). Today, however, the majority of patients are admitted to hospitals in the **crisis** stage, with the treatment goal of **stabilization** rather than symptom remission (Hughes & Ashby, 1996; Goren, 1997; McGihon, 1999). The indications for inpatient hospital use have become more focused in recent years and include the following:

- Prevention of harm to self or others
- Stabilization to allow treatment at a less restrictive level of care
- Initiation of a treatment process with safety risks that must be monitored by specially trained personnel
- Management of severe symptoms resulting in significant confusion, disorganization, and inability to care for self
- Need for a rapid, multidisciplinary diagnostic evaluation that requires frequent observation by specially trained personnel

As the goals of hospitalization have shifted, treatment objectives have also become more focused and include the following:

- Rapid evaluation and diagnosis
- Decreasing behavior that is dangerous to self or others
- Preparing the patient and significant caregivers to manage the patient's care in a less restrictive setting
- Arranging for effective aftercare to facilitate continued improvement in the patient's condition and functional level

In some locations, brief admissions have been scheduled for patients with severe, persistent illness to prevent decompensation and maintain optimal functioning (see Citing the Evidence on p. 714).

The Role of the State Hospital

The history of mental health services reveals a debate over the best location of treatment. This "institution vs. commu-

Table 35-1

Major Diagnoses of Patients Admitted to Inpatient Programs and Partial Hospital Programs	
Diagnosis	Percentage
INPATIENT PROGRAMS	
Affective disorders	32
Schizophrenia	23
Substance use disorders	21
Adjustment disorders	7
Organic mental disorders	3
Personality disorders	2
PARTIAL HOSPITAL PROGRAMS	
Schizophrenia/affective	61
Personality	17
Disruptive behavior	4
Substance abuse	4
Developmental disability	1
Other	13

nity" controversy has driven policy and legal reforms for the past 50 years (Geller, 2000). A large part of this debate is the concern over **institutionalism**, which is described as "a pattern of passive dependent behavior observed among psychiatric inpatients characterized by hospital attachment and resistance to discharge" (Wirt, 1999). The prevention of this condition and the belief in the superiority of community treatment that would allow for the integration of family and social living lead to an advocacy movement away from the state hospital concept.

The philosophy of deinstitutionalization, changing health-care economics, and advances in the treatment of mental illness, especially psychopharmacology developments, were significant influences in the transformation of state mental hospitals. These were major factors in the

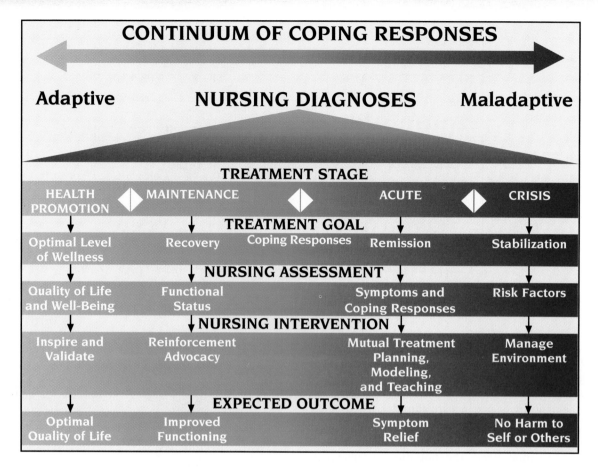

Fig. 35-2 Continuum of coping responses and treatment stages from the Stuart Stress Adaptation Model.

Citing the Evidence on

Scheduled Intermittent Hospitalization

BACKGROUND: The effect of scheduled intermittent hospitalization on hospital utilization, community adjustment, and self-esteem of persons with serious mental illness was examined in this experimental study. Patients were randomly assigned to either an experimental group prescheduled for four hospital admissions lasting 9 to 11 days per year or to a control group that had traditional access to hospital care.

RESULTS: The experimental group showed improvement in self-esteem, affect, and reports of physical symptoms at 1 year. No differences were found in hospital utilization, financial management, substance abuse, or psychological well-being.

IMPLICATIONS: Scheduled intermittent hospitalization may be an appropriate and promising alternative to traditional care for revolving-door patients. This intervention could maintain patients at a higher level of wellness than traditional care and reduce the recurrence of crises that precipitate hospitalization.

Dilonardo J et al: Scheduled intermittent hospitalization for psychiatric patients, *Psychiatr Serv* 49(4): 504, 1998.

downsizing and increasingly frequent closure of these facilities. Fifty-four state psychiatric hospitals closed between 1940 and 1999 (Ross, 1999/2000). Only 13 of these closures occurred before 1990 (Fig. 35-3). The period from 1970 to 1996 was a time of major downsizing with the total number of state and county psychiatric beds decreasing 50% (NASMHPD, 1996).

The downsizing and closing of psychiatric hospitals by state mental health agencies occurred along with funding shifts from hospital to community-based services. In 1993, for the first time, states spent more on community-based services than on state psychiatric hospitals. By 1998, community mental health spending was about $9 billion, far exceeding the $6.6 billion spent on state psychiatric hospitals (Ross, 1999/2000).

What is the role for state psychiatric hospitals in the next decade? Some states are eliminating them entirely. Others have created locked community-based facilities that have been termed "the new state mental hospital in the community" (Lamb, 1997). Although a majority of patients transitioning from state hospitals have been maintained in community services, there has been a rising concern for the population of persons with severe mental illness. Despite advancements, some patients continue to require long-term, highly structured care on a 24-hour basis. Safety of the patient and society, inconsistent patterns of appropriate and accessible services in the community, and prevention of the

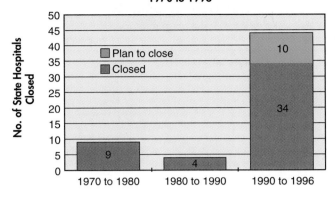

Fig 35-3 State psychiatric hospitals closed by decade, 1970 to 1996.

mentally ill becoming homeless or incarcerated are a few of the concerns and challenges in meeting the needs of the most severely mentally ill.

Some professionals argue that the debate over location has overshadowed the more important emphasis on delivery-based quality, humaneness, and effectiveness (Geller, 2000). With continued reforms based on these criteria, there is a belief by many that state hospitals are in the best position to provide long-term care to the most severely mentally ill (Belcher & DeForge, 1997). Extremely disruptive or dangerous behaviors, staffing demands, discharge complications, and funding problems all contribute to the difficulty this population has in using community services.

The nursing role in the state psychiatric hospital is also extremely challenging. The stigma of the population, the very real safety concerns, and even the high sound levels contribute to making it a stressful environment (Holmberg & Coon, 1999). Nurse researchers have explored a number of the dilemmas confronting state hospital nurses (see Citing the Evidence). They have also examined how nurses coped and developed meaning from their experiences. Direct relationships with patients, pride in their ability to cope, and gratification from the impact they made on patients were noted to be some of the factors in the nurses' ability to meet these challenges. Support for their contributions through opportunities to validate their experiences and expertise with others was also identified as a way to improve nurses' coping abilities (Thomas et al, 1999).

> Some say that state psychiatric hospitals have created a two-tiered (insured and indigent) system of mental health care that does not exist in general health-care settings. How would you respond to this?

Crisis Beds

Crisis beds have been developed as an alternative to traditional inpatient hospitalization. As the name implies, the focus is to assist the patient through a brief crisis period lasting 72 hours or less. After this brief, but intensive intervention phase, patients can usually be discharged back to the

Citing the Evidence on

State Hospital Nursing

BACKGROUND: The purpose of this study was to describe the meaning of work for nurses employed in two state psychiatric hospitals.

RESULTS: The interrelated dilemmas faced by nurses were identified as follows: (1) challenges in clinical decision-making due to inadequate or incorrect information, multiple simultaneous demands, and high noise levels; (2) challenges regarding control over the numbers and mix of patients on a unit, inability to impact the personnel system, the burden of paperwork, and the inflexibility of shift scheduling; and (3) challenges of maintaining professional standards, lack of role boundaries between nurses and paraprofessional nursing personnel, and concern for personal safety.

IMPLICATIONS: State hospital nurses provide care for some of the most disabled individuals in our society. Identifying and addressing ways in which they can be supported in their professional role is essential to maintaining quality care for these patients.

Thomas M et al: Meanings of state hospital nursing I: facing challenges, *Arch Psychiatr Nurs* 13(1):48, 1999.

community. For those who do not stabilize, transfer to inpatient hospitalization may be necessary.

The exact nature of the crisis bed concept is dependent on the structure of the behavioral health system in which it operates. Regardless of this structure, common goals underlie the development of a crisis program distinct from inpatient services. These goals include a focus on issues of suicidality, homicidality, and violence; assessment; a rapid resolution of the crisis; decreased dependency on the hospital; prevention of regressive behaviors; and improved functioning of the inpatient environment (Ash & Galletly, 1997).

The crisis bed concept is designed to decrease reliance on inpatient services, decrease costs, and improve clinical outcomes for patients appropriate for this kind of care. Concern regarding the consequences of severely reduced inpatient length of stay has generated studies on the characteristics and results of very brief inpatient and crisis-focused alternatives with interesting findings. Higher levels of suicidality and less severe psychiatric symptoms have been noted in studies of short-stay inpatient admissions (less than 48 hours). These patients demonstrated considerable improvement between crisis assessment and the first day of hospitalization. Dramatic improvement occurred during the brief stay (Yohanna et al., 1998).

Other researchers have suggested that the crisis bed alternative is especially useful in the treatment of personality and adjustment disorders (Ash & Galletly, 1997). The brief, focused nature of the intervention limits difficulties frequently seen in transitioning from inpatient to community treatment. The argument supporting this is that brief, focused intervention provides a normalizing experience that empowers patients, is comparable to inpatient hospitalization in effectiveness, and is more cost-effective (Rakfeldt et al., 1997).

Crisis beds require a differentiated role in the continuum of care to be successful. Defined admission and discharge criteria and expert coordination of all levels of care ensure appropriate utilization. Communications within the service, a structured environment, and staff trained in crisis intervention are all necessary components. When these conditions are present, crisis beds become an important addition to a behavioral health continuum of care. The ability to offer safety and continuity while minimizing costs and improving clinical outcomes is crucial in the development of mental health care delivery systems.

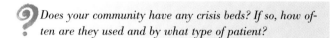 *Does your community have any crisis beds? If so, how often are they used and by what type of patient?*

Partial Hospital Programs

Partial hospital or day treatment programs have also become an important part of the continuum of care for mental health and chemical dependency treatment. Partial hospital programs are medically oriented, with a focus on providing specific treatments such as medication and individual, group, and family therapy in a highly organized, structured program. These programs are similar to inpatient programs without the room and board provided by hospitals. The services provided by partial hospital programs are listed in Table 35-2.

Partial hospital programs are designed to perform two major functions: crisis stabilization and intermediate-term treatment (Block & Lefkovitz, 1994), as follows:

- Crisis stabilization is used to avert psychiatric hospitalization or to offer transitional treatment back to the community in order to shorten an episode of acute inpatient care.
- Intermediate-term treatment provides more extended, daily, goal-directed service for patients at high risk for hospitalization or readmission because of the serious and persistent nature of their disorder.

Indications for the use of partial hospitalization are very similar to those for inpatient admission; the primary differences are related to the stability and supportiveness of the patient's living environment that are necessary to maintain safety during treatment. Length of stay is determined by the treatment team, in collaboration with the patient.

Typically, the patient is in treatment all day, every day for the first 1 or 2 weeks. As the crisis stabilizes and the level of functioning improves, there is a reduction in the number of days the patient attends. This allows the patient to gradually make the transition back to work, home, or school.

The partial hospital psychiatric team is multidisciplinary and generally includes a psychiatrist, psychiatric nurse, social worker, activity therapist, and vocational counselor. Each member of the team has discipline-specific functions as well as some overlapping ones. For example, group therapy is an important component of most partial hospital programs and

Table 35-2

National Profile of Partial Hospitalization Programs

Service	% Programs Providing
MENTAL HEALTH TREATMENT	
Group psychotherapy	85.5
Adjunctive therapy	82.1
Specialty group therapy	80.7
Life skills training	70.7
Individual psychotherapy	61.9
Family therapy	44.8
Psychological assessment	24.1
Speech and language	8.4
MEDICAL SERVICES	
Nutrition	57.6
History and physical examination	56.9
Psychiatric assessment	88.2
24-hour emergency services	60.8
Medication management	82.7
SERVICES TO FAMILIES	
Individual psychotherapy	40.3
Marital therapy	42.4
Multifamily group	33.3
Parent self-help or support	39.4
Parent and family education	70.1
EDUCATION SERVICES	
Assessment	44.7
Schooling	28.7
Prevocational	40.5
Vocational	21.2
Adult education	16.6
Transportation	50.1

n = 580.
From Culhane D, Hadley T, Kiser L: A national profile of partial hospitalization programs, *Continuum* 1:81, 1994.

psychiatric nurses, social workers, and activity therapists may all function as group psychotherapists or lead activity groups.

Unlike inpatient settings where the psychiatrist is expected to see patients daily, in most partial hospital programs the patient is usually seen weekly. The psychiatric nurse in most partial hospital programs assumes primary responsibility for assessing and identifying medical issues that may be contributing to the patient's psychiatric condition.

Partial hospital programs have been demonstrated to be an effective treatment modality for a variety of patient diagnoses and more cost-effective than inpatient care (Hoffman & Mastrianni, 1995; Hueller, 1996; Sledge et al, 1996). Studies combining inpatient care with an active, treatment-intensive partial hospital program can reduce symptoms and improve social functioning.

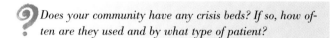 *How do you think the changes in hospital-based psychiatric care affect the families and support systems of the mentally ill? How can nurses help them with the problems they now face?*

Today the majority of psychiatric nurses work in inpatient and partial hospital psychiatric settings. Hospital-based psychiatric nursing practice is rich in history and tradition. Psychiatric nurses are the only group of mental health professionals who are responsible for meeting the needs of inpatients 24 hours a day, 365 days a year. In partial hospital programs, it is not uncommon for psychiatric nurses to be in contact with patients throughout the full day of treatment as other disciplines move in and out of the program to provide specific treatments.

To deliver cost-effective, high-quality inpatient or partial hospital care, psychiatric nurses must manage the one-to-one nurse-patient relationship within a complex social and organizational environment. The scope of contemporary psychiatric nursing practice requires knowledge and expertise in three broad areas:

- Managing the therapeutic milieu
- Implementing caregiving activities
- Integrating and coordinating care delivery

Through these three components, psychiatric nurses can improve a patient's overall treatment outcome.

All psychiatric nurses, regardless of education or experience, engage in these activities every day. To do so requires that the nurse be aware of and value the full range of psychiatric nursing activities (see Chapter 1) and know about the changing mental health-care delivery system (see Chapter 9). This chapter is organized around these three areas of functioning because they represent both the structure and the process of hospital-based psychiatric nursing care.

MANAGING THE THERAPEUTIC MILIEU

The basic difference between inpatient, crisis bed, partial hospital, and outpatient psychiatric care is the controlled environment, or milieu, in which it occurs. Hospital-based treatment facilities generally provide a milieu that physically shelters patients from what they perceive to be painful and frightening stressors. This respite, although brief, provides patients with an opportunity to begin to stabilize while being protected from factors that would interfere with their treatment progress. Similarly, partial hospital treatment provides structure and respite for part of the day and intensive support and intervention to promote a home environment that supports positive therapeutic outcomes.

Understanding the concepts of the therapeutic milieu is an essential part of effective psychiatric nursing care. The aim of the therapeutic milieu is to provide patients with a stable and coherent social environment that facilitates the development and implementation of an individualized treatment plan. Many people have studied different aspects of the inpatient psychiatric environment and identified structures and principles that make it helpful in treating the mentally ill.

The Therapeutic Community

Maxwell Jones (1953) first described the inpatient environment as a therapeutic community with cultural norms for behaviors, values, and activity. He saw patients' social interactions with peers and health-care workers as treatment op-

portunities. For example, he believed that interpersonal difficulties between patients provided fertile material for psychodynamic intervention. He also believed that the clinical staff should share community governance with the patient group on an equal basis. He further emphasized the benefit of mutual participation of patients in each others' treatment, predominantly through sharing of intimate information and feedback in group settings such as the community meeting.

Since its introduction, the concept of the therapeutic community seems to have lost some of its credibility and popularity (Delaney, 1997; Delaney et al, 2000). One reason for this is that its philosophy of democracy and egalitarianism among patients and clinical staff is not compatible with the medical model. Others point out that the concept of the therapeutic community was developed when patients spent months and even years in the hospital. This is in sharp contrast to the short-term nature of most current inpatient psychiatric hospitalizations.

> *The therapeutic community is an example of the social model of psychiatric care described in Chapter 3. Discuss how it differs from the medical model in the roles of patient and therapist and the therapeutic process.*

The Therapeutic Milieu

More than a decade later, the idea of the therapeutic milieu was introduced (Abroms, 1969). It serves two main purposes:

- It sets limits on disturbing and maladaptive behavior
- It teaches psychosocial skills

Five categories of disturbing behaviors and interventions that would help patients keep maladaptive behaviors under control and allow treatment to progress are listed in Table 35-3.

Once maladaptive behaviors are limited, the therapeutic milieu can be used to foster the development of four important psychosocial skills in mentally ill patients, as follows.

- **Orientation.** All patients could achieve a greater level of orientation and reality awareness. Orientation is the patient's knowledge and understanding of time, place, person, and purpose. Awareness of these elements can be reinforced through all patient interactions and activities. For example, introducing oneself, one's role, and the rationale for an interaction helps disoriented patients attend to their surroundings. Another intervention would be a "current events" group conducted with patients.
- **Assertion.** The ability to express oneself appropriately can be modeled and exercised in a variety of ways in the treatment setting. Supporting patients in expressing themselves effectively and in a socially acceptable manner on a specific topic or issue is the overall goal. Some sample interventions include assertiveness training groups, focus groups for lower-functioning patients, or any facilitated, interactive patient group.
- **Occupation.** Patients can feel a sense of confidence and accomplishment through industrious activity. Many

Table **35-3**

Managing Disturbing Behaviors in the Milieu	
Disturbing Behavior	Intervention
Destructiveness: Physically destructive behavior. It is a response to a variety of feelings, such as fear or anger.	In working with destructive behavior, the goal is to control or set limits on the maladaptive response but support the feeling underlying the behavior. Validation is essential to help the patient recognize the feeling and ultimately regain control of maladaptive behavior.
Disorganization: Distorted or unusual behavior a psychotic patient may exhibit as symptomatic of the illness. It may be triggered by elevated anxiety, profound depression, or organic dysfunctions.	Reassure and help the patient while reducing the degree to which these behaviors inhibit therapeutic processes.
Deviancy: Behaviors often described as acting out. They are the result of the patient expressing conflicts overtly in the environment. It is often difficult to determine precisely what acting out behavior is, as well as what is justifiable or even tolerable, because much of it may be influenced by sociocultural factors.	The therapeutic goal in working with deviancy is to analyze how the behavior affects the milieu and how it inhibits the patient's progress. Examining the behavior with the patient and identifying consequences and alternatives are useful approaches.
Dysphoria: Patients with mood alterations may be dysphoric, which is evident in maladaptive responses such as withdrawal from the environment, obsessional behaviors, intrusiveness, or hyperreligiosity.	Establishing a therapeutic alliance is the first task. From there, the nurse and patient can explore feelings and dysfunctional thoughts and begin to modify behavioral responses.
Dependence: Evidenced by patients who do not identify and meet their own needs despite being able to do so. The avoidant nature of dependency interferes with therapeutic progress.	The initial therapeutic goal is to work with the patient to draw on any remaining areas of independence and strength. Then, situations can be identified in which the patient can apply these independent behaviors successfully.

therapeutic opportunities are provided through completion of individual or group hands-on activities. Spending time working with patients on something as simple as a jigsaw puzzle can provide purposeful activity, physical skill development, and the added benefit of practiced social interaction.

- **Recreation.** The ability to engage in and enjoy constructive leisure activity is a beneficial outlet for pleasure and relaxation. Providing a variety of recreational opportunities helps patients apply many of the skills they have learned, including orientation, assertion, social interaction, and physical dexterity. Some examples include informal games such as cards, charades, or bingo and brief walks outdoors.

These are useful and practical ideas related to the therapeutic environment that continue to have value in both inpatient and partial hospital settings today. They support the use of some of the different therapies patients receive in structured settings, such as recreation therapy, occupational therapy, and art therapy. However, their appropriateness in short-term inpatient settings is being reevaluated given the acute nature of contemporary inpatient psychiatric care in many settings.

Perhaps the most important contribution to the concept of the therapeutic milieu came when Gunderson (1978) described five specific components of a therapeutic milieu: containment, support, structure, involvement, and validation. These components are commonly used to evaluate the therapeutic value of the treatment setting (Farkas-Cameron, 1998).

How would you respond to a patient's wife who asks you why her husband is spending time in a fitness program and attending a current events discussion group when he has only 5 days of insurance to pay for his hospitalization for severe depression?

Containment. Containment provides for the physical well-being of patients. It includes providing food, shelter, and medical attention, as well as the steps necessary to prevent the patient from harming self or others. Thus it includes a continuum of interventions, with the use of seclusion and restraints being the most extreme. It is intended to reinforce temporarily the internal controls of patients.

Containment is necessary to provide safety and foster trust. Therapeutic use of containment communicates to patients that the nurse will impose external controls as necessary to keep them and the environment safe. Appropriate and consistent limit setting is essential to meeting this goal. Nursing examples of therapeutic containment include the use of time-outs, room programs, specified observation periods, and seclusion (see Chapter 31).

Planning for containment in partial hospital settings poses additional challenges. The nurse must not only attend to the structured therapeutic milieu of the treatment program but also plan how containment can be enacted in the patient's living environment outside program hours.

The nurse must assess the patient's home environment, both physical and interpersonal, to identify supports and potential problems. This assessment may be based on data collected from interviews with the patient and family members or living companions or may be based on data collected by direct observation during a home visit.

The knowledge from the home assessment can then be analyzed with knowledge about the patient's triggers for disturbing behaviors and productive coping mechanisms that work best for the patient. In collaboration with the patient and others from the home environment, the nurse can develop an effective plan for reducing the triggers as much as possible and defining coping mechanisms for use in avoiding or managing disturbing behaviors.

Support. Support includes the staff's conscious efforts to help patients feel better and enhance their self-esteem. It is the unconditional acceptance of the patient, whatever his or her circumstances. The function of support is to help patients feel comfortable and secure and reduce their anxiety. It may take many forms, but it falls under the general heading of paying attention to the patient.

Support can be communicated through empathy, being available, appropriately offering encouragement and reassurance, giving helpful direction, offering food or beverages, and engaging patients in activities that they are reluctant to do. Other nursing examples include giving direction, suggestions, and education; promoting reality testing; and modeling healthy relationships and interactions.

To best accomplish this task, nursing staff activity must be coordinated, cohesive, and consistent with the patient's treatment goals. Supportive nurturance enhances self-esteem. Milieus that offer support also provide nurturance and encourage patients to become engaged in other therapeutic efforts.

In both inpatient and partial hospital programs it is essential to coordinate support with others in the home so that they understand the behavioral changes the patient is attempting, how difficult it is to make such changes, the improbability of complete success in initial attempts, and the importance of recognition and support for all attempts.

Structure. Structure refers to all aspects of a milieu that provide a predictable organization of time, place, and person. This dependability in activity, staff, and environment helps the patient feel safe. Having a predictable timetable of meetings, group sessions, and other activities is one feature of structure. Other nursing examples include the setting of limits and the use of contracts, token economies, and required meetings.

The more these uses of structure are planned with the patient according to shared ideas of what is adaptive and maladaptive, the more the structure becomes therapeutic in itself. For partial hospital programs this also involves planning with the patient how he or she will structure his or her activities while outside the hospital.

The patient can then begin to accept responsibility for behavior and its consequences. Providing structure helps the patient control maladaptive behaviors. The nurse uses appropriate consequences if the patient is unable, for whatever reason, to impose or honor effective limits. As natural consequences are consistently applied, the patient learns to delay impulsive and inappropriate responses through consistent expectations and behavioral responses.

Involvement. Involvement is a part of the structure that goes beyond compliance with rules and activities. It refers to processes that help patients to actively attend to their social environment and interact with it. The purpose is to strengthen a patient's ego and modify maladaptive interpersonal patterns. Interpersonal communication and shared activity provide patients with opportunities to interact with others in their community.

Nursing examples of involvement include the use of open doors and open rounds and facilitating patient-led groups, activities, and self-assertive experiences. Programs that emphasize involvement encourage the use of cooperation, compromise, and confrontation.

In addition, patients' patterns of involvement and interaction in their social environment can be identified. Progressively demanding opportunities for practicing these skills can then be planned and the results evaluated to help the patient to build the skills necessary to develop the level of social involvement needed to support continued therapeutic progress.

Through this involvement, patients learn appropriate interaction patterns and experience the consequences of unacceptable behaviors. For example, a patient who displays anger or offensive behavior that distances others can participate in activities that will help in verbalizing feelings, working out differences, and receiving feedback. This supportive experience strengthens the patient's sense of self, behavioral control, and social interactive skills. Thus encouraging involvement provides corrective experiences for the patient.

Validation. Validation means that the individuality of each patient is recognized. It is the act of affirming a person's unique world view. Validation can help patients develop a greater capacity for closeness and a more consolidated identity. The psychiatric nurse communicates this through individual attention, empathy, and nonjudgmental acceptance of the patient's thoughts, feelings, and perspective. Other nursing examples of validation include individualized treatment planning, showing respect for a patient's rights, and providing opportunities for the patient to fail as well as succeed.

Therapeutic listening and acknowledging the feelings underlying the patient's personal experience reinforce individuality. Clarification of these feelings helps the patient to understand and accept his or her own unique experience. This strengthens the patient's sense of individuality and encourages the integration of pleasant and unpleasant aspects of personal experience.

> *Visit an inpatient psychiatric unit. Which of the five components of a therapeutic milieu did you observe? Which ones were missing? What barriers prevented the unit from fully implementing this concept?*

Nursing Implications

One of the earliest advocates of the importance of the environment for nursing care was Florence Nightingale. She believed that the essential responsibilities of nursing included the provision of pure air and water, efficient drainage, cleanliness, and light. In addition, the "prudent" nurse prevented unnecessary noise and attended to the aesthetics and nutritional value of food and the comfort of bedding (Nightingale, 1960).

Since Nightingale's time, the inpatient environment and the therapeutic management of the milieu have continued to be important aspects of the role of all nurses and this has now been expanded to provide direction for nurses working in partial hospital settings.

Managing the therapeutic milieu remains the domain of the psychiatric nurse. It is essential that psychiatric nurses working in structured settings realize the potential impact that the environment can have on the patient and consciously use it for the patient's benefit (Melle et al, 1996). The challenge is for psychiatric nurses to adapt to changes in the patient population and the mental health delivery system by evolving new approaches to managing the milieu as needed.

Milieu management is a deliberate decision-making process. The psychiatric nurse should first identify what each patient needs from the therapeutic milieu, taking into consideration the needs of the larger patient group. Weighing individual needs against group needs can be difficult, but it is essential for the successful implementation of a therapeutic milieu. The nurse can then engage aspects of the therapeutic milieu to meet the patient's needs by providing the following:

- Limits and controls (containment)
- Education about the patient's illness and treatment plan (support)
- Therapeutic and predictable activity schedules (structure)
- Opportunities for social interaction (involvement)
- Acknowledgment of the patient's feelings (validation)

Activities related to each part of the therapeutic milieu can be incorporated in the nursing plan of care, thus maximizing the therapeutic effect of the environment.

Nurses have been challenged to better articulate the nursing component of the inpatient treatment program and what specifically they contribute to improving patient outcomes. The key processes of care should be centered on outcomes related to the stabilization of acute symptoms, the restoration of functioning, the establishment of a system of support and the formulation of a plan for symptom management. To that end, it has been suggested that inpatient nursing interventions be developed along four clinical functions: **safety, structure, support,** and **symptom management** (Delaney et al, 2000). Three of these functions are core functions identified by Gunderson, but an important fourth function, that of symptom management, has been added. This Four S model has been suggested to help nurses organize inpatient practice because it combines interventions that operate at both the individual and environmental levels of care. Table 35-4 outlines how a nurse might think about

Table 35-4

Six Processes and Outcomes of Inpatient Psychiatric Treatment

Outcome	Basic Process Label	Clinical Function
Resolve crisis	Increase patient's perception of control Increase supports to patient's system Decrease patient's symptom acuity	Support, safety, and symptom management
Normalize	Restore sleep pattern Re-engage in socialization	Structure
Thorough assessment	Comprehensive battery of diagnostic interviews and testing completed in a timely manner	Symptom management
Mutual goal setting	Ascertaining patient's goals Reaching understanding of what inpatient treatment can provide Assessing patient's attributions of illness and treatment	Support
Client understands presumed efficacy of medication cognitive/behavioral techniques and rationale for referrals	Outpatient treatment planning Guide patient and family through logic of basic cognitive/behavioral approaches Pharmacological recommendations and potentials of service agency referrals	Symptom management
Do no harm	Provide physical and psychologically safe milieu Handle milieu tension proactively Use least restrictive methods in handling dyscontrol Demonstrate persistent effort to develop collaborative relationship with patient Adequately train staff to maintain safety, sustain structure, affect-attune with client, and understand symptom management techniques	Safety structure

From Delaney K et al: Psychiatric hospitalization and process description: what will nursing add? *J Psychosoc Nurs* 38(3):7, 2000.

outcomes of inpatient care in relation to nursing process and these four clinical functions.

Compare the components of the therapeutic milieu with the responsive and action dimensions of the therapeutic nurse-patient relationship described in Chapter 2.

IMPLEMENTING CAREGIVING ACTIVITIES

Hospital-based psychiatric nurses must have clinical knowledge and skills and apply them for the benefit of patients and their families. The atmosphere created by the psychiatric nurse strives to provide patients with activities and interactions carefully designed to meet their needs. This includes both direct and indirect psychiatric nursing care functions as well as dependent, independent, and interdependent aspects of psychiatric nursing practice. A few of these caregiving activities in the hospital-based setting merit special discussion.

Assessing and Intervening in Potential Risks

One of the most important aspects of psychiatric nursing practice is physical safety for the patient and others. This process begins with a thorough assessment of risks at the time of admission and throughout the course of treatment. Common areas of risk for psychiatric patients include potential for aggression or violence, suicide attempts, elopement, seizures, falls, allergic reactions, and communicable diseases.

Based on assessment findings, the nurse is responsible for selecting and implementing the appropriate safety precautions or treatment protocols. Implementation includes not only enacting the prescribed nursing care but also explaining the assessed risk and nursing care plan to the patient, as well as notifying other members of the nursing staff and treatment team of the identified risk.

Patient and Family Education

Education of patients and significant others is essential for sustained therapeutic progress. The process of education must begin with an assessment of the patient's barriers to learning. Such barriers may include lack of insight or denial related to the illness, illiteracy, sensory deficits such as visual or hearing impairments, limited concentration and attention span, confusion, or impaired memory.

Once barriers have been identified, particular strategies can be incorporated in the teaching plan to help the patient retain and use the information. As with any learner, repetition of information, providing information through multiple sensory avenues, and opportunities for practice and feedback promote learning for psychiatric patients. Common topics for education include symptom recognition and management, desired effects and potential side effects of medication, relapse prevention, and importance of and plans for aftercare.

Almost every interaction provides an opportunity for informal education. For example, meal selection provides an opportunity to learn about nutrition as well as to practice decision making and communication skills. Conflicts between patients provide opportunities to learn about and practice problem solving, anger management, negotiation, cooperation, and assertive communication. In addition to these impromptu opportunities for learning, more formal educational activities may be structured into patient care.

Given that patients are admitted to psychiatric units in acute distress, how should a nurse structure his or her own approach to facilitate patients' participation in and retention of educational information presented to them?

Activities, Groups, and Programs

Therapeutic nursing activities, groups, and programs provide a wide variety of opportunities for the nurse to influence the patient's progress toward treatment goals. In providing these corrective experiences, the psychiatric nurse must be clear on the purpose of these activities.

They should be designed to accomplish specific nursing and patient goals in a constructive, efficient, and supportive way. The nurse's challenge is to plan these events to integrate the desired patient outcomes, the interests of the patients, and the ability of the patients to participate with feelings of pleasure and accomplishment.

Structured activities can accomplish several goals of the nursing process at the same time. For example, encouraging a cognitively impaired patient to play a common table game, such as cards, allows the nurse to assess the patient's concentration, orientation, memory, and abstract thinking. Based on these observations, the nurse can better understand the patient's learning needs and incorporate them in the plan of care. This same activity can help the socially withdrawn patient try out newly learned interactive skills, experience the role modeling of the nurse, and receive supportive feedback. In addition, the nurse can use these activities to evaluate the effect of nursing, somatic, and psychopharmacologic treatments. Thus planned nursing activities offer endless possibilities as supportive and corrective experiences for the psychiatric patient (McGarry & Prince, 1998).

Therapeutic nursing groups and programs provide a cost-effective way to implement psychiatric nursing care. Nursing interventions applied in a group allow one or two nurses to work with many patients at the same time. Such interventions are productive not only in hospital-based settings but across the continuum of care. For example, day treatment patients may join inpatients in the same groups or programs. This heterogeneity adds breadth of experience and perspective to the group. Each patient may accomplish a different goal within the same group or program, and such offerings can provide valuable structure to the therapeutic milieu. Some examples of psychiatric nursing groups are described in Box 35-1.

With the focus of psychiatric care shifting away from extended inpatient stays, opportunities for activity, group, and program development by psychiatric nurses are great. Nursing programs in social skills development, assertiveness, community-based support, crisis intervention, family preservation, and general health teaching are growing areas of psychiatric nursing responsibility.

Box **35-1**

Examples of Psychiatric Nursing Groups or Programs

MEDICATION EDUCATION GROUP

In this group, basic concepts related to medication can be discussed. Providing general information about taking medications, such as the influence of slight dosage or schedule changes, serum levels, the therapeutic window, or how some medication potentiates the effect of other medications, can help the patient and family understand the specifics of the prescribed regimen. Common problems encountered by patients taking psychotropic medication can be discussed, and strategies for dealing with these potential barriers can be shared.

COMMUNITY RESOURCE GROUPS

These can be ongoing groups with rotating topics. Topics should be selected based on the learning needs of the group members and their ability to share knowledge about and experiences with varied community resources. For example, a pertinent topic might be the public transportation system of the city. Using maps and information from the local transit authority, exercises can be constructed where patients go from destination to destination practicing getting around the area independently. Another topic may be how to use the newspaper, library, or telephone book to learn about and contact nonprofit, social service, health-care, philanthropic, or other agencies, thus teaching the patient how to mobilize resources after discharge.

NUTRITION GROUPS

Nutrition groups can be helpful in teaching patients the importance of balanced diets and how to recognize and prepare healthful and appetizing meals for themselves. Food ingredients also provide excellent topics for discussion with psychiatric patients. For example, caffeine can be discussed, pointing out its subtle but pervasive effects on the body and its ability to interfere with the effectiveness of some medications. Other topics can include the basic food groups, shopping strategies, and the role of exercise in promoting health and balanced body weight.

SLEEP IMPROVEMENT PROGRAMS

Sleep improvement programs are often needed by psychiatric patients. Relaxation techniques such as simple yoga positioning, progressive muscle relaxation, and deep breathing may be helpful for some patients. The importance of a healthy sleep-wake cycle can be discussed. Group members can be encouraged to share their sleep-inducing secrets. Commonly used ideas for encouraging sleep can be shared with the group, such as spending time in a soothing bath, sipping warm milk, or reading with a soft light. Behaviors and influences that inhibit sleep may be discussed as well. Group members can be encouraged to try out the ideas and report back to the group on their effectiveness.

Equally important are the nursing activities directed to involving the family in the treatment plan as soon as possible (see Chapter 16). From a clinical perspective, shorter lengths of inpatient stays mean that patients discharged to families are often still psychotic, thereby increasing the burden on families and increasing the importance of an alliance between professionals and families (Walkup, 1997). While this may present challenges to those working in inpatient settings, promoting family involvement needs to be a priority of every treatment setting (see Citing the Evidence on Mental Health Professionals' Involvement with Families).

Ask an inpatient psychiatric nurse whether you can "shadow" him or her for a day. Group the nursing functions you see performed as direct or indirect and as dependent, independent, or interdependent. Did this experience change your perception of the inpatient psychiatric nursing role?

Meeting Physical Needs

Studies have documented the prevalence of physical illness among psychiatric patients in both inpatient and outpatient treatment settings (Felker et al, 1996). Yet too often, physical illness is undetected in this patient population. Physical illness may:

- Be the causative factor in a patient's presumed psychiatric illness
- Exacerbate a psychiatric illness
- Have no direct relationship to the psychiatric illness but still require medical and nursing intervention for the patient's well-being

The increase in medical and psychiatric comorbidity among psychiatric patients emphasizes the need for psychiatric nurses to stay current with their physical assessment and medical-surgical nursing skills. It is not uncommon for patients in psychiatric programs to need dialysis, hyperalimentation, intravenous therapy, or dressing changes. Thus completing a physical assessment on admission and monitoring the patient's physical and psychological status throughout the hospitalization are essential functions of the psychiatric nurse.

Discharge Planning

The most obvious goal for inpatient or partial hospital care is to discharge the patient to outpatient status. Thus discharge planning must begin on admission and be a focused nursing activity throughout the patient's stay (Olfson & Walkup, 1997; Smith et al, 1998). The nurse must be knowledgeable about the patient's environment. Potential needs and resources should be identified on admission. Once the nurse has decided what knowledge, skills, and behaviors will help the patient adapt to the discharge environment, creative and purposeful activities can be planned to provide the needed resources (see Citing the Evidence on Teaching Inpatients to Re-Enter the Community).

Throughout this process the nurse should include family members, friends, significant others, and any other support system of the patient (Forchuk et al, 1998). Information regarding supportive resources and medications should be provided to patients and their families to encourage functional independence and decrease the chances of relapse

Citing the Evidence on

Mental Health Professionals' Involvement with Families

BACKGROUND: This study explored the impact of attitudinal, occupational, and organizational factors on mental health professionals' involvement with patients' families.

RESULTS: Providers' attitudes toward families had no significant effect on the frequency of their contact with them. Job and organizational factors were the strongest predictors. Specifically, being a social worker or therapist and working on day or evening shifts were associated with increased involvement with families. Staff members' perceptions of how well their unit functioned were also positively correlated with increased family contact. Psychiatrists had the most family involvement, followed by therapists, social workers, and then nurses.

IMPLICATIONS: The organizational environment in psychiatric hospitals has a significant influence on the extent to which professionals become involved with patients' families. In this study nurses, although present around the clock, had the lowest level of family involvement among the professional groups, raising questions about the ways in which nurses spend their time and the priority they give to family support.

Wright E: The impact of organizational factors on mental health professionals' involvement with families, *Psychiatr Serv* 48(7):921, 1997.

Citing the Evidence on

Teaching Inpatients to Re-Enter the Community

BACKGROUND: This study evaluated the effects of a brief manualized treatment program that taught patients skills to re-enter the community and actively follow through with their own care.

RESULTS: Patients in the community re-entry program significantly improved their knowledge and performance of the skills taught in the sessions, compared with patients in the occupational therapy group. Community re-entry participants were also significantly more likely to attend their first aftercare appointment than patients in the other group.

IMPLICATIONS: Not only can patients learn relatively complex material during a brief typical inpatient stay despite the acuity of their illness, but they can also meaningfully improve the continuity of their own care by participating in a brief and highly structured training program. The program fits well within the time and staffing constraints of typical inpatient facilities and should be considered for widespread adoption.

Kopelowicz A et al: Teaching psychiatric inpatients to re-enter the community: a brief method of improving the continuity of care, *Psychiatr Serv* 49(10):1313, 1998

---

once discharged. This can significantly influence patients' abilities to maintain adaptive coping responses.

Psychiatric discharge planning can be considered part of the psychiatric rehabilitation model that addresses biopsychosocial needs in a manner similar to the physical rehabilitation process. A discharge checklist can be used as an interdisciplinary tool to review the patient's discharge needs and include the patient in the planning process. Areas pertinent to discharge planning that should be included are medications, activities of daily living, mental health aftercare, residence, and physical health care. Special education and the need for financial assistance should also be reviewed with the patient and family.

Transitional care services for mentally ill patients leaving the hospital are often inadequate. Strong communication linkages between hospital-based and community-based providers are essential in order to ensure continuity of care, maximize the value of hospital-based services, and minimize future admissions (Behner, 1996). Some of the caregiving activities of hospital-based nursing practice can be seen in the following clinical example.

CLINICAL EXAMPLE

Ms. R was a 17-year-old, single high school student who was admitted to an inpatient psychiatric unit with the diagnosis of bipo-

lar disorder. She was admitted for uncontrollable behavior (sexual promiscuity, running away from home, hyperverbalization, and extreme irritability).

The initial nursing assessment provided a data base that revealed a chaotic family system with a long history of mental illness on both sides of the family, a social and cultural environment in which drug and alcohol abuse were prevalent, and a community that, because of its low socioeconomic status, had limited mental health resources. However, the patient was very bright, cooperative, and motivated to benefit from her hospitalization.

The initial nursing actions were to administer the prescribed medications, including lithium carbonate, and check blood levels three times a week until a therapeutic level was reached. The nurse assessed that there was an immediate need to protect the patient from her impulsive, uncontrollable behavior. The patient was placed under close nursing observation at all times until she was able to control her own behavior.

Once the patient's mood had stabilized, she was presented in nursing rounds. During this time the patient was able to identify a great need for the nurse to teach her and her family about bipolar disorder and the importance of continued lithium treatment. The patient and staff agreed that a home visit would explore the pressures that the family placed on the patient to function as a surrogate mother to her eight siblings. The patient also believed that it was important that her illness not be viewed in exactly the same manner as that of her sister, who was diagnosed as schizophrenic. The patient viewed her intellectual ability and the love that existed in her family system as her best resources. She thought that, with the help of the nursing staff, she and her family could develop more understanding of her illness and decrease the chaos within the family. After discharge the patient was followed up in outpatient therapy by her primary nurse.

INTEGRATING CARE DELIVERY

The integrative function of the hospital-based psychiatric nurse is very important, although it is often overlooked or taken for granted. It includes all activities involved in the coordination of patient care such as managing nursing resources, balancing costs and outcomes in decision making, evaluating nursing care delivery modalities, ensuring compliance with professional and regulatory standards, and encouraging communication, participative problem solving, and conflict resolution among mental health team members. In addition, the clinical practice of the nurse involves ongoing implementation of new ideas and approaches for improving quality and decreasing costs.

Teamwork and Coordinated Care

Almost all programs use a multidisciplinary team to deliver treatment. To integrate and coordinate patient care the psychiatric nurse must collaborate with professionals from other disciplines and manage a group of nursing care providers. If therapeutic outcomes are to be optimized, team members must work together to address targeted behaviors and treatment goals. To achieve this level of coordination, team communication must be open and active.

Psychiatric nurses can facilitate this process by organizing their observations and interactional data into useful assessment findings that reflect such things as the patient's responses to medications and other interventions, patterns of behavior indicating escalation, interventions that are found to be effective, and the patient's beliefs about what will help him or her progress toward treatment goals (Delaney et al, 1995).

The degree of cooperation and cohesion among disciplines may vary widely. Interdisciplinary problems have been identified that could interfere with the quality of psychiatric care (see Critical Thinking about Contemporary Issues). Problems between providers may involve poor communication, professional self-doubt, role confusion, and conflict, all of which may be increased by work-related stress.

Whenever multiple people, each with a unique perspective, are working together there is the potential for conflict. Handling conflict productively is an ongoing challenge for the psychiatric nurse. When poorly handled or avoided, conflict can interfere with the continuity of patient care and the management of a therapeutic milieu. However, effective management of conflict can facilitate stronger professional working relationships, model positive communication skills for patients, and contribute to the nurse's professional development.

Observe a multidisciplinary treatment team in the inpatient psychiatric setting. Did you see any areas of team conflict, role blurring, or turf struggles? If so, how did the team handle these issues?

CRITICAL THINKING about CONTEMPORARY ISSUES

Do Nurses and Psychiatrists View Patients in the Same Way?

It has been suggested that different members of the mental health-care team perceive patients differently and that this can create problems in developing cohesive treatment plans and maintaining a therapeutic milieu. One study compared characteristics attributed by nurses and residents to difficult-to-treat patients in a short-stay setting (Gallop et al, 1993). The researchers found that both groups identified self-harm behaviors, violence toward others, and treatment sabotage as characteristics of difficult patients, although these behaviors posed more problems for the nurses. Lack of response to medication and patient manipulation were the most important problems identified by the residents. Nurses found difficulty with patients who were unable to form therapeutic alliances.

The researchers suggest that this may be because psychiatric nurses have seen their role as shaping the therapeutic milieu. Thus their interventions center on providing opportunities within the unit for improving interpersonal and coping skills and maximizing healthy aspects of the patient's ego functions. If the patient fails to engage or withdraws, these treatment goals are thwarted and the nurse's role as a therapeutic agent is blocked. Such findings suggest that differing perceptions of difficult patients may create communication problems for the treatment team. If the different disciplines do not share common concerns, they may not recognize the significance of their observations and not respond to them.

Resource Allocation

Psychiatric nurses must be able to justify the type and level of personnel needed to provide high-quality nursing care. Allocation of numbers and types of personnel based on patient care needs is an essential consideration for achieving positive outcomes. Thus attention to the most appropriate and efficient use of personnel and other resources is an important part of the psychiatric nurse's role.

The assignment of nursing resources must be based on identified patient care needs, clinical competencies, and available resources. This requires that all nurses become actively involved in examining patient needs, identifying realistic outcomes of care, and assessing the strengths and weaknesses of available nursing personnel.

You report to work one evening and discover that you and one other staff member have been assigned to cover the 20-bed psychiatric unit. You realize that the hospital has been reducing costs, but you believe that this is unsafe staffing. How would you present your case for more staff to nursing and hospital administration?

Professional, Regulatory, and Accreditation Standards

Professional standards of the American Nurses' Association (ANA) for psychiatric-mental health clinical practice provide a basis for evaluating nursing care. In addition to the standards of care (see Chapter 11) and professional performance (see Chapter 12), other ANA standards are available to guide nursing activities in administrative and educational areas.

Regulatory and accreditation standards must also be considered by the hospital-based psychiatric nurse. These include the state laws and regulations governing nursing practice and facility licensure, the laws and regulations determining the payment of federal and state insurance funds (Medicaid and Medicare), and standards set forth by accrediting bodies. A health-care facility may be required to show how any of these standards are met, including those pertaining to the condition of the physical facility, credentialing of employees, or the documentation of patient care. Requirements vary depending on the type of facility, state regulations, and types of services offered.

The Joint Commission on Accreditation of Healthcare Organizations (JCAHO) has become a leading accrediting agency for many different types of health-care facilities. Their standards have served as a benchmark for many other regulatory agencies. JCAHO standards are a helpful and comprehensive guide for all aspects of health-care delivery in this country.

The Health Care Financing Administration (HCFA) is the federal agency that oversees the spending of Medicare and Medicaid funds. Each state has an identified agency that implements HCFA policies locally. Often, for the care and treatment delivered by health-care agencies to be reimbursed by Medicare or Medicaid, HCFA consultants or representatives of the state agency conduct surveys of the facility. They may review patient records, inspect the physical plant, interview staff, and evaluate programs to ensure that their specific regulations are met. Once the facility has shown that all required standards are met, it is eligible to receive payment for treating patients insured by Medicaid and Medicare. These standards are often similar to those of other regulatory and credentialing bodies and focus mainly on the sanitation and safety of the facility, competency of the personnel, and the adequacy and pertinence of the care delivered and documented.

> *Determine the bed charge for 1 day of care in your psychiatric inpatient unit. How does that compare with the bed charge in a medical-surgical unit? How much of that charge do you think is related to nursing services?*

Summary

1. The treatment goals, processes, expected outcomes, and length of stay related to hospital-based psychiatric care are changing. The majority of psychiatric nurses currently work in inpatient or partial hospital settings, but they must be ready and able to provide their services throughout the continuum of care.

2. The aim of the therapeutic milieu is to provide patients with a stable and coherent social environment that facilitates the development and implementation of an individualized treatment plan. Components of the therapeutic milieu include containment, support, structure, involvement, and validation.

3. Hospital-based psychiatric nursing includes both direct and indirect nursing functions as well as dependent, independent, and interdependent aspects of practice. Assessing and intervening in potential risks, providing patient and family education, implementing activities, groups, and programs, meeting patients' physical needs, and planning discharge are important caregiving activities.

4. The integrative function of the hospital-based psychiatric nurse includes all activities involved in the coordination of patient care such as those related to facilitating teamwork and coordinating care, managing nursing resources, and ensuring compliance with professional and regulatory standards.

Competent Caring   A Clinical Exemplar of a Psychiatric Nurse

SIMMY PALECKO, MSN, RN

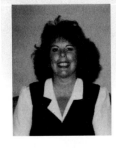

One of the true rewards of psychiatric nursing is that many patients get better and return to functional lives in which they can again experience pleasure and increased self-esteem. It is unbelievably fulfilling to see patients regain a sense of independence and renewed control over their own destinies. Ms. M was an example of how an intensive short-term psychiatric hospitalization can remarkably improve the quality of a patient's life. She was a 72-year-old woman who was admitted to our adult unit with electrolyte imbalance. She was psychotic and delusional, refusing to eat or drink, not sleeping, highly anxious, and refusing to perform her activities of daily living (ADLs). She believed that her body was rotting away. She was also extremely paranoid, insisting that the clients in the boarding home where she lived were plotting to kill her and that the staff were laughing and talking about her outside her door during the night. She complained of auditory hallucinations and how she felt tortured. Ms. M was extremely irritable and argumentative, as well as physically and verbally threatening. She refused to get out of bed and even ambulate. She insisted that we leave her alone so that she could die.

Ms. M was a recurrent patient on our unit. Her diagnoses were Axis I, bipolar affective disorder; Axis III, colon cancer

Continued

Competent Caring A Clinical Exemplar of a Psychiatric Nurse—cont'd

status postresection, hypertension, degenerative joint disease, peptic ulcer disease, neurogenic bladder, and recurrent urinary tract infections. She was a particular challenge to the nursing staff that we were more than willing to undertake. We were able to use our medical-surgical skills while drawing blood repeatedly, placing IVs, doing ECGs and urinary catheterizations for residual volumes, making accurate intake and output calculations, and carrying out range-of-motion activities. Safety and emotional support were also a major focus of our patient care. Ms. M was placed on fall precautions with continued teaching and reinforcement, even though she was minimally receptive. Within a few days of admission, her physical condition stabilized and she was scheduled for electroconvulsive

therapy (ECT), which had been successful for her in the past. The staff impatiently waited for Ms. M's mood to improve, her appetite to increase, her nighttime sleeping to improve, her interest in her ADLs to increase, and her auditory hallucinations, negativism, and anxiety to decrease. After the fourth ECT treatment, the staff began to see Ms. M's return to her baseline. She was smiling more and her humor was returning. She no longer stated that her body was rotting. She even began to joke with the nursing staff. Ms. M was discharged to the boarding home approximately 10 days after her admission. The change in the patient's mental and physical condition was remarkable, and I was again reminded of the intrinsic rewards of psychiatric nursing.

 Visit MERLIN: www.mosby.com/MERLIN/Stuart to find these additional materials and student activities.

- **Worksheets**
- **"Drug of the Month" Updates**
- **"Citing the Evidence" Updates**
- **Critical Thinking Activities and Exercises**
- **Annotated Suggested Readings**
- **Web Links**
- **More!**

Chapter Review Questions

1. Match each example in Column A with the correct component of the therapeutic milieu in Column B.

Column A

a. _____ Allows for predictable organization of time, place, and person

b. _____ Affirming the patient's world view

c. _____ Offering education and encouragement

d. _____ Promoting the patient's attention and interaction with the social environment

e. _____ Provision of food, shelter, medical care, and safety from harm

f. _____ Unconditional acceptance, nurturance, and promotion of self-esteem

g. _____ Use of contracts, token economies, and required meetings

Column B

A. Containment

B. Involvement

C. Structure

D. Support

E. Validation

h. _____ Use of individualized treatment plans and showing respect for patients' rights

i. _____ Use of open doors, open rounds, and patient-led groups

j. _____ Use of time-outs and room programs

2. Fill in the blanks.

A. Today the majority of patients admitted to psychiatric hospitals are in the _____ stage, with the treatment goal of _____.

B. A syndrome characterized by dependency on the hospital and resistance to discharge is known as _____.

C. The partial hospital psychiatric team is _____ in nature.

D. Maxwell Jones first described the inpatient environment as a _____ with cultural norms for behaviors, values, and activity.

E. One of the earliest advocates of the importance of the environment for nursing care was

_____.

F. _____ is the leading accreditation agency for hospital-based facilities.

3. **Provide short answers for the following questions.**

A. What are the two major functions of partial hospitalization programs?

B. Discuss characteristics of crisis bed programs.

C. Analyze the need for state psychiatric hospitals in the current mental health-care delivery system.

D. Describe how patient teaching would need to be modified in an inpatient setting where patients are in the most acute stages of their illnesses.

E. In many hospital-based facilities, psychiatric nurses rotate between inpatient and partial hospital programs. Discuss how this can benefit both patients and the nursing staff.

REFERENCES

Abroms G: Defining milieu therapy, *Arch Gen Psychiatry* 21:553, 1969.

Ash D, Galletly C: Crisis beds: the interface between the hospital and the community *Int J Soc Psychiatry* 43(3):193, 1997.

Behner N: Establishing linkages in a changing mental health practice environment, *Issues Ment Health Nurs* 17:51, 1996.

Belcher J, DeForge B: The appropriate role for the state hospital, *J Ment Health Admin* 24(1):64, 1997.

Block B, Lefkovitz P: *Standards and guidelines for partial hospitalization adult programs,* ed 2, Alexandria, Va, 1994, AABH Publications.

Delaney K et al: Seven days and counting: how inpatient nurses might adjust their practice to brief hospitalization, *J Psychosoc Nurs* 33:36, 1995.

Delaney K: Milieu therapy: a therapeutic loophole, *Perspect Psychiatr Care* 33(2):19, 1997.

Delaney K et al: Psychiatric hospitalization and process description: what will nursing add? *J Psychosoc Nurs* 38(3):7, 2000.

Farkas-Cameron M: Inpatient group therapy in a managed health care environment: application to clinical nursing practice, *J Am Psychiatr Nurs Assoc* 4(5):145, 1998.

Felker B et al: Mortality and medical comorbidity among psychiatric patients: a review, *Psychiatr Serv* 47:1356, 1996.

Forchuk C et al: Bridging the discharge process: staff and client experience over time, *J Am Psychiatr Nurs Assoc* 4(4):128, 1998.

Gallop R, et al: Residents' and nurses' perceptions of difficult-to-treat short-stay patients, *Hosp Community Psychiatry* 44:352, 1993.

Geller J: The last half-century of psychiatric services as reflected in *Psychiatric Services, Psychiatr Serv* 51:41, 2000.

Goren S: Pursuit of the ordinary: short-term inpatient treatment, *Arch Psychiatr Nurs* 11:82, 1997.

Gunderson I: Defining the therapeutic process in therapeutic milieus, *Psychiatry* 41:327, 1978.

Hoffman F, Mastrianni X: Partial hospitalization following inpatient treatment: patient characteristics and treatment outcome, *Continuum* 2:247, 1995.

Holmberg S, Coon S: Ambient sound levels in a state psychiatric hospital, *Arch Psychiatr Nurs* 13(3):117, 1999.

Hueller J: Partial hospitalization: a study of outcomes and efficiency, *Continuum* 3:59, 1996.

Hughes K, Ashby C: Essential components of the short-term psychiatric unit, *Perspect Psychiatr Care* 32:20, 1996.

Jones M: *The therapeutic community,* New York, 1953, Basic Books.

Lamb H: The new state mental hospitals in the community, *Psychiatr Serv* 48:1307, 1997.

McGarry T, Prince M: Implementation of groups for creative expression on a psychiatric inpatient unit, *J Psychosoc Nurs* 36(3):19, 1998.

McGihon N: Caring psychiatric nursing for the 21st century: the paced model, *J Psychosoc Nurs* 37(10):22. 1999.

Mechanic D: The future of inpatient psychiatry in general hospitals, *New Dir Ment Health Serv* 73:103, 1997.

Melle I et al: The importance of ward atmosphere in inpatient treatment of schizophrenia on short-term units, *Psychiatr Serv* 47:721, 1996.

NASMHPD: *State mental health agency profile system highlights: closing and reorganizing state psychiatric hospitals* (Contract No. 280-93-0006 & Contract No. 280-95-0013). Alexandria, Va, 1996, NASMHPD Research Institute, Inc.

Nightingale F: *Notes on nursing: what it is and what it is not,* New York, 1960, Dover.

Olfson M, Walkup J: Discharge planning in psychiatric units in general hospitals, *New Dir Ment Health Serv* 73:75, 1997.

Rakfeldt J et al: Normalizing acute care: a day hospital/crisis residence alternative to inpatient hospitalization, *J Nerv Ment Dis* 185(1):46, 1997.

Ross C: Role of state psychiatric hospitals as next century approaches, *NAMI Advocate* 11(Dec 1999/Jan 2000):2, 1999/2000.

Sledge W et al: Day hospital/crisis respite care versus inpatient care, part II: service utilization and costs, *Am J Psychiatry* 153:1074, 1996.

Smith L et al: Expertise in caring: a source of power, *J Psychosoc Nurs* 36(9):31, 1998.

Thomas M et al: Meanings of state hospital nursing II: coping and making meaning, *Arch Psychiatr Nurs* 13(1):55, 1999.

Walkup J: Family involvement in general hospital inpatient care, *New DirMent Health Serv* 73:51, 1997.

Wirt G: Causes of institutionalism: patient and staff perspectives, *Issues Ment Health Nurs* 20:259, 1999.

Yohanna D et al: Characteristics of short-stay admissions to a psychiatric inpatient service, *J Behav Health Serv Res* 25:337, 1998.

36 Community Psychiatric Nursing Care

Beth Gage Greco

Nancy K. Worley

Visit **MERLIN** for *Your Internet Connection* to websites that are related to the content in this chapter.
www.mosby.com/MERLIN/Stuart

LEARNING OBJECTIVES

After studying this chapter the student should be able to:

- Describe the goals of the community mental health movement
- Analyze the public health model of community mental health, including interventions and the role of the nurse
- Analyze the biological-medical model of community mental health, including interventions and the role of the nurse
- Analyze the systems model of community mental health, including interventions and the role of the nurse
- Analyze the patient-centered model of community mental health, including interventions and the role of the nurse

TOPICAL OUTLINE

Goals of Community Mental Health
Public Health Model
  Community Needs Assessment
  Identifying and Prioritizing High-Risk Groups
  Intervention Strategies
  Role of Nurses
Biological-Medical Model
  Deinstitutionalization
  Role of Nurses
Systems Model
  Community Support Systems
  Case Management
  Role of Nurses
Patient-Centered Model
  Homeless People with Mental Illness
  Mentally Ill People in Jail
  Rural Mentally Ill
  Intervention Strategies
  Role of Nurses

What life have you if you have not life together? There is no life that is not in community.

        T. S. Eliot, CHORUSES FROM *THE ROCK*

GOALS OF COMMUNITY MENTAL HEALTH

The Community Mental Health Centers Act of 1963 marked the beginning of a major federal effort to provide comprehensive community-based mental health services to all people in need regardless of income. Each community mental health center was mandated by law to provide five essential mental health services. Four of these services—inpatient, emergency, partial hospitalization, and outpatient—were to provide psychiatric care in the community to reduce the number of admissions to state hospitals. The goal of the fifth service, consultation and education, was to provide information about mental health principles to other community agencies, reduce the number of people at risk for mental illness, and increase community awareness of mental health practices through education. The dual nature of this mis-sion, care of those with diagnosed mental illness and prevention of mental illness, has led to controversy in defining the purpose of community mental health.

Four models have dominated the community mental health movement since 1963. Each one has been influenced by the political, social, and economic climate of the time. They have contributed much to the field, and the best parts of each model continue to be used today. They are summarized in Table 36-1.

PUBLIC HEALTH MODEL

Mental health professionals who believed in primary prevention through social change dominated the community mental health movement in its early years, using the public health model of service delivery. In this model the "patient" is the community rather than the individual, and the focus is on the amount of mental health or illness in the community as a whole, including factors that promote or inhibit mental health.

Table **36-1**

Models of Community Mental Health Services

Model	Conceptual Framework	Intervention Strategies	Nursing Role
Public health (1960-1970)	Focuses on prevention Community as patient Services target high-risk groups	Community needs assessment Identifies high-risk groups Consultation Education Crisis intervention	Some group and family involvement Caring for people with chronic mental illness Limited preventive work
Biological-medical (1970-1980)	Focuses on those with diagnosed mental illness Stimulated by deinstitutionalization Views mental illness as brain disease	Medical management Psychotherapy Aftercare programs	Medication administration and monitoring Coordination of aftercare programs Psychotherapy
System (1980-1990)	Focuses on the role of the biological, psychological, and environmental factors in rehabilitation Developed comprehensive systems of care	Community support systems Service coordination Case management	Coordination of community services Case management activities
Patient-centered (1990-present)	Focus on patients who overlap service systems Culturally relevant services Consumer participation	Assertive community treatment Multisystem therapy	Medication management New initiatives such as home health, outreach, collaborative practice, prevention, and family preservation

The emphasis in this model is on reducing the risk of mental illness for an entire population by providing services to high-risk groups. Use of the public health model required that mental health professionals be familiar with a range of skills that were not a traditional part of their training. These included community needs assessment, identifying and prioritizing target or high-risk groups, and intervening with new treatment modalities such as consultation, education, and crisis intervention.

 Do you believe it is possible to prevent mental illness in an individual or a community?

Community Needs Assessment

In the public health model services are developed and delivered based on a culturally sensitive assessment of community needs. Because it is not possible to interview each person in the community to determine mental health needs, four techniques are used to estimate service needs.

Social Indicators. Social indicators infer the need for service from descriptive statistics found in public records and reports, especially statistics that are highly correlated with poor mental health outcomes. Examples of statistics most commonly used are income, race, marital status, population density, crime, and substance abuse.

Key Informant Surveys. Key informants are people knowledgeable about the community's needs. Typical key informants are public officials, clergy, social service personnel, nurses, and primary care physicians.

Community Forums. In a community forum, members of the community are invited to a series of public meetings where they can express their ideas and beliefs about mental health needs in their community.

Epidemiological Studies. Epidemiological studies examine the incidence and prevalence of mental disorders in a defined population. Because they are expensive to carry out, most community needs assessments use results from previously published studies and apply these findings to their situation. For example, several large epidemiological studies have estimated that the impairment rate (the number of people with some form of emotional disorder) in the United States ranges between 15% and 30% (Regier & Kaelber, 1995). These studies have shown that high impairment rates in a population are correlated with certain demographic and socioeconomic characteristics such as poverty, low educational status, and a high number of people who are divorced, separated, or widowed.

Identifying and Prioritizing High-Risk Groups

When the data from the various community needs assessments are analyzed, specific high-risk groups begin to emerge. For example, socioeconomic data might show that a large number of elderly widows live in the community. Community forums and surveys of key informants may find that there are few services and programs for the elderly, and epidemiological studies might suggest that elderly widows living alone are at high risk for depression. Therefore elderly widows might become a target group for program development and intervention.

Demographic data might also show that a community has many preadolescent females, and socioeconomic indicators may suggest that many of these young women live in single-parent households and in poverty. Community forums and surveys of key informants may reveal few recreational and social services for children and adolescents. Finally, epidemiological studies may report high correlations among poverty, single-parent households, and adolescent pregnancy. Therefore community mental health administrators might consider adolescents in this community to be at risk for mental health problems and target them for intervention.

> *Describe the characteristics of a group that was at high risk for developing mental illness in the community in which you grew up.*

Intervention Strategies

Intervening with high-risk groups in the community can include primary, secondary, or tertiary prevention activities.

- **Primary prevention:** Targets people at risk for developing psychiatric illness and promotes their adaptive coping mechanisms
- **Secondary prevention:** Targets people who show early symptoms of an emotional disorder but regain pretreatment level of functioning through aggressive treatment
- **Tertiary prevention:** Targets those with mental illness and helps to reduce the severity, discomfort, and disability associated with their illness

The public health model of community mental health required the development of new interventions. Before the community mental health movement of the 1960s, most mental health outpatient services consisted of expensive, office-based, individual psychotherapy sessions. Although this may have been a good secondary prevention strategy, it did not promote mental health or prevent emotional problems on a community-wide basis. New treatment strategies that were developed to fulfill the goals of community mental health included mental health promotion (Chapter 13) and crisis intervention (Chapter 14).

Role of Nurses

The public health model had major consequences for the role of psychiatric nurses in community mental health. Social workers and psychologists who had years of experience in the public sector dominated administrative and management positions in this model. Theoretically, nursing should have been readily accepted as one of the mental health disciplines because of public health nurses' long-standing presence in community care; however, public health nurses were seen as closely allied with secondary and tertiary prevention activities, the medical model, and care of the sick.

Therefore, although patients with chronic mental illness were referred to public health nurses, few nurses were invited to join psychiatry, psychology, and social work as professional staff in most community mental health centers (De Young & Tower, 1971). A 1962 national survey of nurses' roles in outpatient psychiatric clinics found that fewer than 10% of these facilities included a nurse on the professional team (Glittenberg, 1963). The passage of the Community Mental Health Centers Act in 1963 did little to change that pattern. Specifically, the number of psychologists and social workers in community mental health centers increased between 1970 and 1980, while the number of psychiatrists and nurses declined.

In addition, nursing education was slow to revise curricula and change clinical practice to reflect this shift in care from the hospital to the community. As a result, nurses felt unprepared to function in the community and were unable to create a role for themselves. With few exceptions, the nurse's role in community mental health centers was limited to traditional nursing tasks such as medication monitoring and caring for patients with chronic mental illness.

BIOLOGICAL-MEDICAL MODEL

In the mid-1970s several events turned public attention to the second mission of the community mental health movement: the care of those with diagnosed mental illness. A new political administration, the waging of an expensive war in Vietnam, and a general economic downturn stimulated a national discussion regarding the best use of scarce healthcare resources. At the same time, public disillusionment with the deinstitutionalization of people with chronic mental illness led to questions about the cost-effectiveness of community mental health centers, with their focus on prevention rather than care of those who were already ill.

Families of people with mental illness had also become a political force in the late 1970s. Their agenda was to force as many resources as possible toward the care of those with severe and persistent mental illness and to direct federal research dollars toward finding a biological basis for the major mental illnesses. Psychiatrists, with their new focus on the biological model of psychiatry, and family groups thus became allies and formed a coalition that put biological psychiatry in a strong leadership position in the mental health field.

Financial pressures also brought about a change in the focus of mental health centers. At the beginning of the community mental health movement the federal government had promised to pay 75% of the cost of each center. Regulations stated that federal support would decrease by 15% each year; by the eighth year of their existence the centers were expected to be self-supporting through a combination of state funds and third-party reimbursement. By the early 1970s many centers faced the end of federal funding and state governments were unable or unwilling to take on the burden of funding them. The centers then had to rely heavily on third-party reimbursement through fee-for-service mechanisms, which were typically physician directed and illness oriented. Centers thus began to focus on the diagnosis and treatment of the deinstitutionalized people with severe and persistent mental illness, primarily through the reimbursable services of medication management and psychotherapy.

These factors led to major amendments of the Community Mental Health Centers Act in 1975, requiring centers to offer services for people with serious mental illness who had been discharged from the state hospitals. These services included screening admissions to inpatient services, aftercare services, and transitional housing. Because centers were not allowed to reduce the five original essential services and were not given sufficient funds to add these new services, decisions about priorities had to be made. Because of political and social pressure to care for those who were being discharged into the community in large numbers, the community mental health centers reluctantly decreased their preventive efforts and moved toward the increased use of the medical model and the care of people with diagnosed mental illness.

Deinstitutionalization

Between 1965 and 1975 nearly 500,000 patients were either discharged or diverted from state hospitals to care in the community. It was hoped that psychiatric treatment in community centers, combined with living arrangements provided by family or board and care homes, would allow these people to live more humane lives in their own communities. However, it rapidly became clear that policymakers had seriously miscalculated both the service needs of this population and the ability of communities to accommodate the large numbers of people with mental illness who had been discharged from the state hospitals (see Citing the Evidence). Often these former patients had to be readmitted to state hospitals. Others who could not meet the increasingly strict admission criteria of state hospitals drifted into the criminal justice system or into homelessness. Many who were elderly were admitted to nursing homes.

In reviewing the failures of this early attempt to move patients into community care, mental health experts agree that the following problems contributed to the lack of success:

- Poor coordination between state hospitals and community mental health centers

- Underestimation of the support systems needed to enable people with mental illness to live in the community
- Lack of knowledge about psychiatric rehabilitation
- Underestimation of community resistance to deinstitutionalization
- Shortage of professionals trained to work with this population in the community
- Reimbursement systems that rewarded hospitalization

It was apparent by the 1980s that the biological-medical model of community mental health might not be able to provide the psychological and social supports that were needed to allow people with severe and persistent mental illness to live successfully in the community.

Do you think that all psychiatric patients are better off living in the community rather than in public or private hospitals?

Role of Nurses

Nurses began to play a more important role in community mental health care during the 1970s and 1980s. This was partly because traditional nursing roles in the medical model were well known and readily accepted by physician team leaders and administrators of community mental health centers; also, the number of deinstitutionalized patients was growing. Initially, nurses worked in aftercare programs providing support, coordination of care, and health teaching. Gradually, those responsibilities grew to those of nurse therapists in individual, group, and family therapies with a variety of patients, not just those with chronic mental illness. Many psychiatric nurses with master's degrees opened private practices and initiated creative and innovative mental health services.

Nursing's expansion into less traditional roles in community mental health can be attributed to the influence of the National Institute of Mental Health (NIMH). In 1975 a NIMH task force examined the staffing needs in mental health and existing training programs. The result was a new NIMH policy mandating that to be eligible for NIMH training grants, educational programs had to address the needs of unserved and underserved populations including children, people with chronic mental illness, minorities, and women. By 1979, training grants were awarded only to educational programs that focused on one or more of these priorities, particularly those that focused on providing clinical training in community mental health centers.

The outcome of this mandate was that nursing school faculty began to reach out to community mental health centers to develop clinical placements for nursing students. In this process, faculty were able to educate center administrators about the scope of nursing practice and the variety of skills, in addition to medication administration and monitoring, that nurses could bring to the community setting. At the same time, curricula in nursing schools were revised to reflect this new practice setting. Crisis intervention, brief therapy, counseling, assessment, and diagnosis were emphasized as nurses began to take their place as members of the inter-

---

Citing the Evidence on

State Hospital and Community-Based Care

BACKGROUND: This study examines the service utilization and cost of treating individuals with serious mental illness in a community-based care system in which the state hospital was replaced with extended acute care beds in general hospitals and residential beds.

RESULTS: After the state hospital closed, the direct treatment cost of an episode of care per patient increased from $68,446 to $78,929, and the average annual cost of care per patient increased from $48,631 to $66,794 because of an increase in acute care hospitalization.

IMPLICATIONS: Seriously mentally ill patients need a mix of acute care, extended care, residential beds, and ambulatory services for cost-effective care to be delivered. Determining the appropriate allocation and supply of resources in different settings is essential if community mental health systems are to manage the seriously mentally ill outside of institutions.

Rothbard A et al: Cost comparison of state hospital and community based care for seriously mentally ill adults, *Am J Psychiatry* 155(4):523, 1998.

disciplinary teams in community mental health centers while striving to keep their unique identity.

> *Why is the role of the psychiatric nurse on an interdisciplinary mental health care team more difficult to define in community settings?*

SYSTEMS MODEL

The systems model of community mental health emerged in the 1980s and operated on the philosophy that all aspects of a person's life needed to be cared for—basic human needs as well as needs for psychiatric treatment and rehabilitation. The focus of this model was on developing a comprehensive system of care and coordinating needed services into an integrated package. This model of community mental health emerged as it became apparent that mental health treatment alone would not enable people with severe and disabling mental illnesses to live successfully in the community. A special federal initiative was launched to help states and communities develop comprehensive services for this population. This initiative was led by NIMH, which began to fund demonstration programs for community support systems in all states.

Community Support Systems

Community mental health centers were given primary responsibility for the development and implementation of community support systems for people in their service areas. In implementing these systems, case management became the primary means for ensuring that the components of the service system were available to every person with a chronic mental illness who needed them (Fig. 36-1). These components included client identification and outreach, mental health treatment, crisis response services, health and dental care, housing, income support and entitlement, peer support, family and community support, rehabilitation services, and protection and advocacy.

Case Management

Case management services are aimed at linking the service system to the consumer and coordinating the service components so that he or she can achieve successful community living (see Citing the Evidence). It includes problem solving to provide continuity of services and overcome problems of rigid systems, fragmented services, poor use of resources, and problems of inaccessibility. The six activities that form the core of case management are as follows:

- Identification and outreach
- Assessment
- Service planning
- Linkage with needed services

Citing the Evidence on

The Effectiveness of Case Management

BACKGROUND: This meta-analysis synthesizes the findings of 24 published studies dealing with the effectiveness of case management with the severe and persistently mentally ill.

RESULTS: Overall, case management interventions are effective—75% of the patients who participate in them do better than those who do not. The prevention of rehospitalization is also 30% greater for those receiving case management. Finally, various case management models do not differ significantly on effectiveness.

IMPLICATIONS: Case management is an evidence based intervention and should be implemented widely in community psychiatric care.

Gorey K et al: Effectiveness of case management with severely and persistently mentally ill people, *Community Ment Health J* 34(3):241, 1998.

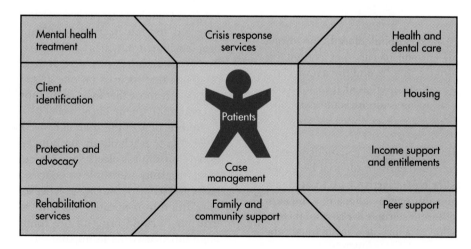

Fig. 36-1 Components of a community support system. (Department of Health and Human Services: *Toward a model plan for a comprehensive community-based mental health system,* Oct.1987.)

- Monitoring service delivery
- Advocacy

In addition, core components and specific interventions related to clinical case management are listed in Table 36-2.

Which interventions of clinical case management listed in Table 36-2 should be provided by a mental health professional and which ones, if any, can be carried out by a lay person?

Identification and Outreach. The federal government required that case management services be provided to every person with mental illness in a state that receives a significant amount of public funds or services (Parson, 1999). A comprehensive mental health service plan must have strategies to locate potential clients, inform them of available services, and ensure their access to these services. Establishing and maintaining close working relationships with potential referral sources such as public and community hospitals, community mental health centers, and social service agencies were essential to meeting this goal. Some case management agencies specialize in working with a particular target population, such as the homeless or those with a dual diagnosis of mental illness and substance abuse. These case managers establish contacts with potential clients in homeless shelters, soup kitchens, drug treatment centers, and emergency facilities.

Assessment. A thorough assessment of a person's strengths and deficits is required for an effective service plan. Assessments address all aspects of a person's life, including psychological, emotional, financial, medical, educational, vocational, social, and housing needs. Particular emphasis is placed on identifying patient strengths that can be used to compensate for weaknesses and understanding patients' cultural and health-related values and beliefs. The knowledge and skills needed for a comprehensive assessment are generally beyond the ability of one case manager and often require a multidisciplinary approach. The expected outcome of the assessment is a detailed outline of the person's present functioning, highest level of functioning, and needed services.

Service Planning. A comprehensive service plan guides all case management activities and must be carefully formulated with individual and family involvement. The goal of the service plan is to help the person to live in the community successfully. Because many of these people have histories of numerous psychiatric hospitalizations, the service plan should include new approaches that might interrupt the chain of events that previously led to rehospitalization. Treatment objectives and specific actions that will be taken should also be clearly stated.

Linkage with Needed Services. A major component of case management is linking the people with mental illness with the various social, medical, and rehabilitative services that they need to live successfully in the community. Once again, this activity often requires a team approach because the services needed are often diverse and span a broad range of agencies.

Mental health treatment. Clinical management of psychiatric disorders is an integral part of service delivery and may be provided on a long-term basis if needed. Clinical care should be directed at helping the patient manage symptoms, understand medications, recognize signs of relapse, and cope with daily living. Clinical care should also include diagnostic evaluation and ongoing monitoring of the patient's psychiatric condition. Supportive counseling and individual, family, or group intervention should be offered as appropriate.

An essential component of clinical management is medication management. Medication management services include prescribing medications, ensuring that needed medications are available, carefully monitoring medications to ensure maximal benefits and minimal side effects, and educating the patient and family about the medications.

Crisis response services. Despite the provision of ongoing clinical care, people with serious and long-term mental illness tend to have crises (see Chapter 14). The primary goal of crisis services is to help those in psychiatric crisis to maintain or quickly resume functioning within the community. Emergency services offered 24 hours a day must be provided by community mental health centers, and this can be accomplished in a variety of ways. It is common in large urban areas for this service to be provided by the emergency room of a local hospital. Other community mental health centers provide this service on site. In rural areas, where travel time and distance make a central crisis location unfeasible, mobile crisis outreach services visit the patient in the setting in which the crisis is occurring. Some community agencies provide 24-hour hotlines staffed by professionals or volunteers who offer crisis counseling or referral services over the telephone. However, when these services do not resolve the

Table 36-2

Components and Interventions of Clinical Case Management

Component	Intervention
Initial phase	Engagement
	Assessment
	Planning
Environmental interventions	Linkages with community resources
	Consultation with families and caregivers
	Maintenance and expansion of social networks
	Collaboration with physicians and hospitals
	Advocacy
Patient interventions	Individual psychotherapy
	Training in independent living skills
	Psychoeducation
Patient-environment intervention	Crisis intervention
	Monitoring

crisis, crisis residential services should be available in a residential nonhospital setting on a short-term basis.

Health and dental care. Psychiatric patients have been found to have higher mortality rates from both natural and unnatural causes than the general population. Numerous studies have also shown that psychiatric patients have higher rates of comorbid medical illnesses, which are largely undiagnosed and untreated (Farnam et al, 1999). These medical illnesses may cause or exacerbate psychiatric symptoms. Thus adequate health-care services for this population are very important (see Citing the Evidence).

Despite the fact that people with psychiatric illnesses also have serious medical problems, their use of general health-care services is often limited because of barriers to access and availability. Access problems often result from active psychiatric symptoms, such as hallucinations regarding body functions and paranoid or delusional thinking. These symptoms may prevent people from seeking appropriate health care or adhering to treatment. Another factor is that psychiatrically ill people who do seek medical care are sometimes regarded with fear, hostility, and suspicion by health-care professionals who are inexperienced in working with this population. Finally, access and availability of general health care are also affected by the current health-care delivery system, which is oriented toward specialization and episodic treatment of acute conditions rather than integrated primary care services (Gelberg et al, 2000).

Housing. An important goal of the community support system is to locate, secure, and maintain affordable housing for people with long-term mental illness. Group homes where three to six people with mental disabilities live together with minimal supervision are becoming available, as well as apartment complexes that have several units rented to people with mental illness scattered throughout the complex. Training, supports, and services are provided to allow people with mental illness to live as independently as possible. Commonly offered services include social and recreational activities, on-site crisis intervention, and client advocacy. A variety of more structured residential settings are being used for more disabled people. Finally, foster care homes that provide accepting, normalized settings for people with severe mental disabilities are also becoming more common.

Although great strides are being made to provide adequate and appropriate housing for people with severe mental illness, the greatest barrier continues to be community resistance to the placement of such people in residential settings. In many places the outcome of this resistance has been psychiatric ghettos in which large numbers of people with psychiatric impairment live in poorly supervised board and care homes in low-income areas or on the streets.

How would you and your family feel about a group home for people with mental illness being built in your neighborhood?

Citing the Evidence on

Medical Care of Persons with Mental Illness Living in the Community

BACKGROUND: The ability of the mentally ill in supervised living settings to manage their medical health care and the ability of the supervised living staff to help them in this process was assessed.

RESULTS: The supervised settings promoted routine health examinations and follow-up care. However, patients and staff alike lacked knowledge about health problems, medications, and ways to change unhealthy lifestyle practices. Although patients asked for information about sexually transmitted diseases, staff were not comfortable with this topic.

IMPLICATIONS: These findings suggest a role for nurses in informing and supporting the seriously mentally ill living in supervised settings and the staff in these settings in managing medical health-care functions.

Getty C et al: Capacity for self-care of persons with mental illness living in community residences and the ability of their surrogate families to perform health care functions, *Issues Ment Health Nurs* 19:53, 1998.

Monitoring Service Delivery. Monitoring is an important part of case management and is often difficult to implement. The monitoring function of case management has two basic purposes: It ensures that the objectives of the service plan are being met, and it provides the information necessary for an ongoing reevaluation of the plan. The case manager helps the patient obtain the services identified in the service plan. Because the needs of people with mental illness are usually complex and require the services of multiple agencies, the case manager must develop coordinating and facilitating skills. Periodic review of the person's progress with each of these service providers is part of the case manager's duties. Information gained from these contacts should also be documented in regular reviews of the overall service plan.

Advocacy. Helping people to receive the available services and influencing providers to improve existing services and develop new ones are important roles of the case manager. Psychiatric patients and their families struggle with issues of discrimination, stigma, compromised rights, and inadequate resources on a daily basis. Advocacy activities address these injustices proactively. They include political negotiation as well as consumer and professional collaboration. Finally, it is essential for advocacy efforts to be sensitive to the cultural background of the consumer and the norms and values of the community.

Managed Care and Case Management. At present, case management is an ambiguous concept without a clear base in any one professional discipline. Early definitions stressed the linking, brokering, and advocacy functions of the

Table 36-3

Qualifications and Functions of the Psychiatric Nurse Case Manager

Desired Skills/Qualifications	Functions
Certification in case management	Needs assessment
Baccalaureate/graduate/postgraduate education	Diagnosis
Physical and psychosocial assessment skills	Patient advocate
Empathy and enthusiasm	Family collaboration
Excellent communication skills	Liaison between physician, patient, and reimburser
Negotiation skills	Access community resources
Consultation skills	Treatment planning
Critical thinking skills	Crisis intervention
Knowledge of evidence-based treatments	Health promotion
Creativity and flexibility	Relapse prevention
Attention to detail	Implementation of treatment plan
Computer literacy	Documentation
Data management	Monitoring of care
	Outcome measurement

role. These roles evolved into a more clinically oriented definition. Furthermore, there are various models or types of case management, including service broker, therapist, intensive social support, collaborative, community advocate, and problem focused. There are also unresolved questions about the recommended case load of case managers (King et al, 2000).

The work of the case manager is very complex, covering a broad array of activities. Recently, with the advent of managed care, case management has come to reflect two basic but seemingly contradictory underlying goals: increasing access to services and limiting costs. In the public sector, case management is intended to increase access to care and make more services available to those eligible and underserved. In the private sector, case management has become synonymous with utilization review, where the emphasis is placed on cost control and limitation of resource use.

Clearly, functions resembling case management will be an increasingly prominent part of mental health care in the future as attempts are made to balance cost, access, and effectiveness. Resources of patients, families, providers, and society must be managed in order to carry out these complex goals. However, important questions remain, including what the tasks of case managers are, who should be doing case management (what personal qualities and training are needed), to whom the case manager is accountable, and how the work of case management should be organized (Sledge et al, 1995; Hall, 1998; Vallon et al, 1997).

Role of Nurses

The systems model of community mental health was based on a holistic approach that focused on the caring and the curative aspects of service delivery. Nurses, with a similar focus, thus had an opportunity to perform a variety of roles in this model. Case management, in particular, allowed nurses to assume direct care, supervisory, and consulting roles while working with patients and families by:

- Serving as their gatekeepers and facilitators in accessing the health-care system

- Helping them make informed decisions about their health-care needs
- Monitoring their health and human service plan of care
- Educating them to enhance their self-care ability

The American Nurses' Association (1993) states that:

Psychiatric and mental health nurses are highly qualified to function as both case managers and providers within managed care systems. Psychiatric and mental health nurses are positioned to have a maximum impact on the managed care of psychiatric clients because: They are committed to improving access, quality, and cost containment. They understand prevention and wellness and know how to educate patients to improve health. They know how to triage and assess the needs of patients. They know how to accurately evaluate the necessity for inpatient admissions and continued hospital stays.

There is great opportunity for nurses to expand their roles and develop new career directions by functioning as case managers who can address the physical and psychiatric needs of patients. This can include people with chronic mental illness as well as general psychiatric patients in outpatient settings (Rohde, 1997; Young et al, 1998). The desired skills and functions for the nurse case manager are listed in Table 36-3. The following clinical example illustrates the contributions a psychiatric nurse can make in providing case management services.

 CLINICAL EXAMPLE

Jane M is single, 33 years old, and has a history of multiple psychiatric admissions. She was referred to the community mental health center case management unit on discharge from a 6-month stay at the state hospital. She had a diagnosis of undifferentiated schizophrenia in remission and was discharged to the care of her family on risperidone 4 mg daily. Jane has occasional auditory hallucinations, is somewhat suspicious, and has a long history of disruptive family relationships and noncompliance with medications.

The psychiatric nurse case manager volunteered to take the case and made an appointment with the family for a home visit. When she arrived, the family was visibly upset and related that in the week since Jane had been home, she slept much of the day and roamed around the house during the night, taking long showers, slamming kitchen cabinet doors, and playing loud rock music. When she was awake during the day, she would disappear for hours at a time, causing great anxiety for the family. The mother was tearful and wringing her hands in an agitated manner while the father sat on the sofa with his head bowed. Jane sprawled in a chair and intermittently swore at her mother as the mother described these events.

The nurse recognized that Jane's illness dominated the household, essentially putting her in control of the rest of the family. The nurse worked intensely with this family to restore generational boundaries by supporting the parents in making mutually agreed upon rules about behavior that would be tolerated in their household. She helped the family identify ways to support Jane while setting limits that would promote adaptive family functioning. The family found this exchange to be very helpful, and they called on the nurse to validate their ideas and provide them with ongoing information on Jane's illness. The nurse also evaluated the impact of the medication on Jane's behavior and her compliance with taking it.

Over the next few weeks, Jane began to sleep at night. With continued support from the nurse, the parents became skilled and comfortable at presenting a united front. Although Jane initially resisted, she adapted rather quickly to the new norms in the house, and a family crisis that might have resulted in Jane's readmission to the hospital was averted.

Despite these expanding clinical services, the trend among psychiatric nurses with advanced training and education in the 1980s was to remain in inpatient settings rather than to work with people with serious mental illness in the community. Thus many challenges remained for nursing as the community mental health movement moved to the next model of care.

> *What factors influence whether psychiatric nurses work in inpatient settings or community-based psychiatric programs?*

PATIENT-CENTERED MODEL

Although the systems model of community mental health contributed to an improved and more coherent service delivery system, new problems and populations began to emerge (Williams & Siegmann, 1997). Many patients' problems did not fit well in any service system, but instead required intervention by more than one of these systems simultaneously. Examples of such groups include people with HIV/AIDS (discussed in Chapter 42) and patients who are dually diagnosed with both substance and psychiatric disorders (discussed in Chapter 25). Complex problems also emerged in three other groups: homeless people with mental illness, mentally ill people in jail, and the mentally ill in rural communities.

Homeless People with Mental Illness

Homeless people are an inescapable presence in American society, where they live in subway tunnels and on steam grates and die in cardboard boxes on windswept corners in communities throughout the country. To most Americans, homelessness seems neither invisible nor insurmountable (Box 36-1). People who are mentally ill and homeless reflect the tension between a mental health system that views housing as a social welfare problem and public housing agencies that believe that this population needs specialized residential programs provided by mental health agencies. Thus the needs of this population are underserved as services are fragmented and inaccessible (Walker, 1998).

However, a number of studies have shown that when homeless people with mental illness are given the opportunity to participate in treatment programs that address their needs for services in areas such as housing, health care, substance abuse, and income support, many can be helped to find homes and achieve substantial improvements in their lives (Goldfinger et al, 1999; Murray et al, 1995; Wolff et al, 1997). Thus mental health professionals have begun to explore the use of new approaches to providing treatment, rehabilitation services, and housing to homeless people with mental illness, who often avoid contact with traditional mental health programs because of past difficulty in gaining access to care, demands from clinicians for treatment compliance, or past involuntary hospitalization. Key compo-

---

Box 36-1

What Americans Say about the Homeless

A national survey conducted for *Parade* magazine in 1994 found the following:
- 70% saw homeless people in their own communities.
- 76% said something should be done to reduce homelessness in America.
- 36% can imagine a situation in which they might become homeless.
- 84% thought that at least half of the homeless could be helped enough to reenter society.
- 82% said the homeless should not be prohibited from public places.
- 77% thought homeless people are not adequately helped by the government.
- 69% did not want a legal procedure that would forcibly remove homeless people from the street.
- 7% thought homeless people were violent but 60% said the homeless contribute to the rising crime rate.
- 56% thought homeless people were not responsible for the situation they were in.
- 30% said a homeless person who is nonviolent but with a diagnosed mental illness should be institutionalized against his or her will.
- 16% said they would go out of their way to avoid homeless people.

nents of this new treatment approach have been identified as follows (Rowe et al, 1996):

- Frequent and consistent staff contact through assertive outreach
- Meeting the client where he or she is, both geographically and interpersonally
- Help with immediate survival needs such as food, emergency shelter, and clothing
- Gradual treatment through the development of trust
- An emphasis on client strengths
- Client choice of services and the right to refuse treatment
- The delivery of comprehensive services including mental health and substance abuse treatment, medical care, housing, social and vocational services, and help in obtaining entitlements

Access Program.　One particularly innovative program is the Access to Community Care and Effective Services and Supports (ACCESS) program. It was initiated in 1993 by the U.S. Department of Health and Human Services as part of a national agenda to end homelessness among people with serious mental illness. Demonstration projects have developed integrated systems of care for this population. The purpose of the ACCESS program is to determine whether integration initiatives implemented at the program, policy, and organizational levels will improve outcomes for the homeless people with mental illness beyond those obtained by integration at the direct service delivery level—that is, by case management (Calloway & Morrissey, 1998; Lam & Rosenheck, 2000; Randolph et al, 1997). Demonstration programs such as these hold hope for better care for this vulnerable population.

> *Should people be allowed to choose to be homeless if they are not dangerous to themselves or others?*

Mentally Ill People in Jail

One in six inmates in the nation's state prisons and local jails, and one in 14 federal inmates—nearly 284.000 persons altogether—said they currently had a mental condition or had spent at least one night in a mental hospital at some time according to the U.S. Department of Justice (Ditton, 1999). One in six persons in the community on probation gave similar histories. One in five reported being homeless in the year before being arrested, compared with one in 11 of the other inmates. Mentally ill inmates of both sexes reported higher rates of prior physical and sexual abuse than other inmates.

Six in 10 mentally ill persons in state and federal prisons and four in 10 in jails received some form of mental health care, most commonly prescription medication. Of all mentally ill populations, white female inmates were the most likely to receive care. They also related the highest rates of mental illness. Nearly four in 10 white female inmates age 24 years and under reported being mentally ill.

Clearly the presence of severely mentally ill persons in jails and prisons is an urgent problem (see Citing the Evidence). However, model programs attempting to deal with this problem are found in various parts of the United States (Project Link, 1999; Schnapp & Cannedy, 1998; Steadman et al, 1999). A community model for services (Fig. 36-2) has been proposed that includes methods for preventing incarceration of people with mental illness and intervening effectively when such a person is jailed. This model is based on the formation of a community board and includes both preventive and post-release interventions.

> *Have jails become today's substitute for yesterday's state hospitals for people with mental illness? If so, which alternative is better?*

Rural Mentally Ill

In the United States at least 15 million residents suffer with significant substance dependence, mental illnesses, and medical-psychiatric cormorbid conditions. Particularly in the more remote "frontier" areas, existing in 25 states and representing 45% of the land mass of the United States, barriers to care include insufficient access to multidisciplinary clinicians, crisis services, mental health and general medical clinics, hospitals, and innovative medicines and other therapies. More basic community services, such as transportation, electricity, water, and telephones, that are important to providing health care also may not be available.

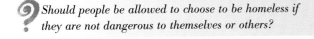

Citing the Evidence on

Persons with Severe Mental Illness in Jails

BACKGROUND: The literature since 1970 on mentally ill persons in jail was searched and analyzed.

RESULTS: Offenders with severe mental illness have acute and chronic mental illness and poor functioning. A greater proportion of mentally ill persons are arrested compared to the general population. Factors causing this include deinstitutionalization, more rigid criteria for civil commitment, lack of adequate community support for persons with mental illness, mentally ill offenders' difficulty gaining access to community treatment, and attitudes of police officers and society.

IMPLICATIONS: Recommendations to address this problem include training police in the field, careful screening of incoming jail detainees, assertive case management, and various social control interventions such as court-ordered treatment, psychiatric conservatorship, 24-hour structured care, involvement of and support for families, and provision of adequate mental health treatment.

Lamb H, Weinberger L: Persons with severe mental illness in jails and prisons: a review, *Psychiatr Serv* 49(4):483, 1998.

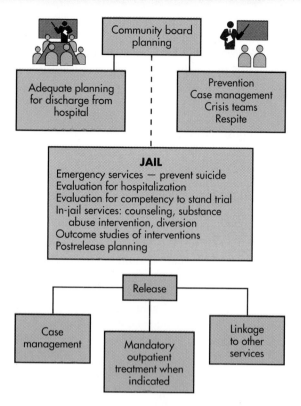

Fig. 36-2 Community model for services. (From Laben J, Blum J: Persons with mental illness in jail. In Worley N, editor: *Mental health nursing in the community*, St Louis, 1997, Mosby.)

Rural residents are at significant risk for substance use disorders and mental illness. Symptoms related to mood and anxiety disorders, trauma, and cognitive, developmental, and psychotic disorders appear to be as common among rural residents as among city dwellers, and rural suicide rates have surpassed urban suicide rates over the past 20 years. For these reasons mental health issues are among the most prominent health concerns faced in rural areas.

Many ethical dilemmas arise when practicing in the community (see Critical Thinking about Contemporary Issues), and some of these are unique to the rural setting. When there are limited numbers of providers in isolated settings, problems may arise due to overlapping social and professional relationships, altered therapeutic boundaries, challenges in protecting patient confidentiality, and differing cultural dimensions of mental health care. Ways to combat these dilemmas include the development of clinical support networks through electronic communications, attention to clinical ethics, and regular peer supervision or consultation (Roberts et al, 1999).

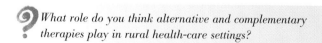 *What role do you think alternative and complementary therapies play in rural health-care settings?*

Intervention Strategies

Assertive Community Treatment. Assertive Community Treatment (ACT) was developed in Wisconsin in the early 1970s as a program originally called Training in Com-

CRITICAL THINKING about CONTEMPORARY ISSUES

What Ethical Issues Challenge Community Psychiatric Care?

Community psychiatric care is unique in three ways. First, the patients are some of the sickest, poorest, and overall least well-off members of the community. Second, community mental health-care delivery systems tend to be structured in ways that emphasize a multisystem, multidisciplinary approach to patient care. Third, the community mental health-care settings typically are underfunded and suffer from insufficient resources. One might question, therefore, whether these factors create unique ethical dilemmas as well.

Four general categories of ethical conflicts in community psychiatric care have been identified (Christensen, 1997). The first relates to the patient's ability to give valid informed consent or refusal of treatment, particularly when circumstances are complex and many parties may be involved. The second is related to paternalism in which there is a conflict between meeting a patient's **needs** versus respecting a patient's **rights** to self-determination. Issues here include forced medication, coerced outpatient treatment, and involuntary commitment (see Chapter 10). The third issue is that of resource allocation, as providers frequently find themselves in positions of deciding **who** receives **what** resources **when** and **how frequently**. Given scarce resources, these are often difficult decisions to make. The final problem arises around organizational relationships as the more systems that are involved in care, the greater the likelihood of differing treatment philosophies and priorities.

Unfortunately, the unique ethical conflicts in community psychiatric care have received little attention. Thus clinicians have little guidance in this area. More dialogue and study is needed to inform the field and assure quality, ethical community psychiatric care.

munity Living (TCL). It was created as a way of organizing outpatient mental health services for patients who were leaving large state mental hospitals and were at risk for rehospitalization. The original TCL model has been replicated in thousands of communities under names such as Continuous Treatment Teams (CTTs), Programs for Assertive Community Treatment (PACT), and Intensive Case Management (ICM). This model program provides a full range of medical, psychosocial, and rehabilitative services. The essential elements of Assertive Community Treatment are listed in Table 36-4.

ACT uses an interdisciplinary team-oriented approach that typically includes up to 10 staff members (nurses, psychiatrists, social workers, activity therapists) who meet regularly to plan individualized care for a shared case load of about 120 patients. More than 75% of staff time is spent in the field providing direct treatment and rehabilitation.

In a national survey of assertive outreach programs, it was found that 88% had a psychiatric nurse as an integral member of the treatment team (Deci et al, 1995). ACT teams func-

Table **36-4**

Essential Elements of Assertive Community Treatment (ACT)

ORGANIZATION AND DELIVERY OF SERVICES

1. Core services team
   a. Fixed point of responsibility
   b. Primary provider of services
   c. Continuity of care and caregivers across time and functional areas
   d. Low client-to-staff ratio
2. Assertive outreach and *in vivo* treatment
3. Individualized treatment
4. Ongoing treatment and support

TREATMENTS AND SERVICES PROVIDED

1. Direct assistance with symptom management
   a. Medications
   b. 24-hour crisis availability
   c. Brief hospitalization
   d. Long-term one-to-one clinical relationship
2. Facilitation of an optimally supportive environment
   a. Assistance with meeting basic needs
   b. Assistance with a supportive social environment
   c. Assistance with a supportive family environment (psychoeducation)
3. Direct assistance with instrumental functioning (work, social relations, activities of daily living)
   a. *In vivo* skills teaching
   b. *In vivo* support
   c. Environmental modifications

DESIRED PATIENT OUTCOMES

1. Reduced symptomatology and relapse
2. Increased community tenure
3. Enhanced satisfaction with life
4. Less subjective distress
5. Improved instrumental functioning
   a. Employment
   b. Social relations
   c. Activities of daily living

Adapted from Test MA: Training in community living. In Liberman RP, editor: *Handbook of psychiatric rehabilitation*, New York, 1992, Macmillan Publishing Co.

Box **36-2**

Nine Basic Principles of Multisystem Therapy

1. The primary purpose of assessment is to understand the fit between the identified problems and their systemic context.
2. Therapeutic contact should emphasize the positive, and interventions should use systemic strengths as leverage for change.
3. Interventions should promote responsible behavior and decrease irresponsible behavior.
4. Interventions should be present focused and action oriented, targeting specific and well-defined problems.
5. Interventions should target sequences of behavior within and among systems.
6. Interventions should be developmentally appropriate and fit the developmental needs of the young person.
7. Interventions should be designed to require daily or weekly effort by family members.
8. Intervention efficacy should be continuously evaluated from different perspectives.
9. Interventions should promote treatment generalization and long-term maintenance of therapeutic change.

Modified from Henggeler SW, Schoenwald SK, Pickrel SG, Brondino MJ, Borduin CM, Hall JA: *Treatment manual for family preservation using multisystemic therapy*, Charleston, 1994, South Carolina Health and Human Services Finance Commission.

tion as continuous care teams who work with patients with serious mental illness and their families over time to improve their quality of life. In effect, these programs function as a community-based "hospital without walls," providing a high-intensity program of clinical support and treatment.

Numerous controlled clinical trials have been conducted with a wide range of people with severe mental illness, including patients with schizophrenia, veterans, dually diagnosed patients, and homeless people. These studies report that patients spent less time in hospitals and more in independent community housing. Their symptoms were reduced, their treatment compliance was increased, and ACT costs were usually lower (Dixon et al, 1997; Lehman et al, 1999; Mueser et al, 1998).

The Program of Assertive Community Treatment (PACT) is recognized by the National Alliance of the Mentally Ill (NAMI) as the most effective service delivery model for community treatment of severe mental illness. As such, NAMI has launched a national grassroots effort called PACT Across America to educate people about PACT and to offer training, monitoring, certification, and management services to those mental health agencies wishing to implement the PACT model.

Multisystem Therapy. Multisystem therapy (MST) is a highly flexible treatment approach that addresses the multiple, interrelated needs of youths with serious behavioral and emotional problems and their families. It is usually delivered through the family preservation model of service delivery to provide interventions in home, school, and neighborhood settings.

The primary goal of family preservation has been to prevent out-of-home placement by providing home-based, intensive, and time-limited services to families whose children are at immediate risk of such placement. The goal of MST is to develop parent skills and resources needed to address the difficulties of raising teenagers and to teach youths to cope with family, peer, school, and neighborhood problems. At the peer or school level a goal of treatment is to decrease the youth's involvement with deviant peers and to increase involvement with prosocial peers.

MST uses pragmatic, goal-oriented treatment strategies, and interventions are guided by nine principles (Box 36-2). MST is usually delivered by master's-level clinicians with case load ratios of one staff to four to six families. Service duration usually ranges from 3 to 5 months, with an average of 40 to 60 hours of direct clinical contact over the course of treatment. Staff are available 24 hours a day, 7 days a week during the active treatment phase.

Controlled clinical trials provide strong support for MST as a viable approach to adolescents and their families who have traditionally been regarded as unresponsive to treatment. It has also been shown to improve communication in families of juvenile offenders and parent-child interaction in abusive or neglecting families. Other reported outcomes include improved family relations and peer relations and the prevention of expensive out-of-home placements (Henggeler et al, 1999; Randall et al, 1999).

> *ACT and MST programs are new models of psychiatric care. Determine whether they are being used in your community and the impact they may be having on vulnerable populations where you live.*

Assertive community treatment, used for adults with severe mental illness, and multisystem therapy, used for adolescents with serious emotional disorders, share common elements that differ from traditional systems and that have important implications for mental health policy (Table 36-5). They both use a social-ecological model of behavior applied to mental health patients. In addition, therapeutic principles emphasizing pragmatic (outcome-oriented) treatment approaches, home-based interventions, and individualized treatment goals are key elements of their success. Most importantly, both systems embody a therapeutic philosophy demanding therapist accountability, in which staff are rewarded for clinical outcomes and therapeutic innovation rather than for following a prescribed plan.

As evidence based approaches tested in multiple clinical trials using sound experimental designs, they provide a strong scientific foundation for continued mental health-care innovation. They also illustrate the critical elements needed in designing new community treatments for behavioral as well as medical conditions.

Role of Nurses

A number of new approaches are being implemented to deliver quality community psychiatric care. These represent unique opportunities and challenges for nursing, and the literature reflects the increasing participation of psychiatric nurses in community treatment initiatives (Atkinson, 1996; Guy, 1997). Psychiatric nurses are beginning to play pivotal roles in emerging treatment modalities. They are fulfilling vital functions in day treatment facilities, psychotherapy clinics, vocational and rehabilitation centers, psychopharmacology clinics, psychiatric emergency rooms, and other community settings that provide care for people with mental illness.

> *Describe an innovative psychiatric nursing service that you could provide to people with mental illness in your community.*

Forensic Nursing. Another frontier for nurses working in the community is the specialized area of forensic nursing. In relation to health care, the forensic process describes the stages in the management of the mentally disordered offender from precourt assessment through care, control, and custody to community supervision and discharge.

Forensic nursing has two very different and sometimes conflicting goals (Peternelj-Taylor, 1995). There is the goal of providing individualized patient care, and the goal of providing custody and protection for the community. The

Table 36-5

Differences between Traditional Mental Health-Care Systems, Assertive Community Treatment, and Multisystem Therapy			
Service Element	Traditional System	Assertive Community Treatment	Multisystem Therapy
Primary locus of care	Hospital, residential programs, day programs, offices	In the field (community, home, neighborhood, workplace)	In the field (community, home, neighborhood, school)
Provider of care	Individual clinician for individual outpatients, multidisciplinary teams for inpatients; treatment time highly variable; outpatient caseloads high, inpatient caseloads low; fragmented continuity of care across loci of care	Generalist teams share fixed case load; ratio of staff to patients = 1:10-15; treatment time unlimited; direct services continuously available	Generalist teams share temporary case load; treatment time averages 4 months; ratio of staff to patients = 1:6; continuous services and emergency response available around the clock for treatment period
Treatment approach	Specific individual or group psychosocial therapies and biological treatments provided mostly in a health-care facility; providers not held directly accountable for outcomes	Medication monitoring and social support (help with housing, health, basic needs) in natural community environment; providers held accountable for outcomes	Pragmatic approach addresses problems identified in the child, family, peer, school, and neighborhood; family taught to sustain benefits, providers held directly accountable for outcomes

From Santos A et al: Research on field-based services: models for reform in the delivery of mental health care to populations with complex clinical problems, *Am J Psychiatry* 152:1111, 1995.

forensic focus for nursing is the therapeutic targeting of any aspect of the patient's behavior that links his or her offending activity and psychiatric symptomatology. As such, the forensic nurse functions as a patient advocate, a trusted counselor, an agent of control, and a provider of primary, secondary, and tertiary health-care interventions to this incarcerated population. Interventions include crisis intervention, rehabilitation, suicide prevention, behavior management, sex-offender treatment, substance abuse treatment, and discharge planning.

Nursing is the backbone of correctional health care, and nurses are the major providers of health services. Yet forensic nursing has received limited professional recognition (Goldkuhle, 1999). Although advanced education is desirable, it is not widely available in this specialized role. Curriculum should be based on the public health approach with coursework covering medicolegal issues, criminal justice and psychopathology, family issues involving violence, and investigational techniques. Given the growing interest in forensic psychiatry, additional examination is needed related to the roles, functions, preparation, and work perceptions of forensic nurses.

Summary

1. The goals of community mental health are to care for those with diagnosed mental illness and prevent mental illness. There have been four models of community mental health.
2. The public health model (1960 to 1970) focused on the community and emphasized reducing the risk of mental illness for a population by providing services to high-risk groups. Intervention strategies included community needs assessment, identification of high-risk groups, consultation, education, and crisis intervention. The role of the nurse was minimal and often limited to caring for patients with chronic mental illness.
3. The biological-medical model (1970 to 1980) focused on people with diagnosed mental illness and viewed mental illness as brain disease. Interventions included medication management and psychotherapy. Nurses became more involved in community roles ranging from medication administration to coordinating aftercare programs and functioning as therapists for individuals, families, and groups.
4. The system model (1980 to 1990) focused on developing a comprehensive system of care and coordinated services. Interventions included community support systems, service coordination, and case management. Nurses began to assume roles as coordinators of community services and case managers.
5. The patient-centered model (1990 to the present) focuses on patients who overlap service systems and emphasizes consumer participation and culturally relevant services. Interventions include programs for assertive community treatment (ACT) and multisystem therapy (MST). Nurses are demonstrating the range and quality of their services in this system of care.
6. New psychiatric nursing roles are emerging with evolving models of community treatment, including those in forensic nursing.

Competent Caring   A Clinical Exemplar of a Psychiatric Nurse

SUZANNE SMITH, MSN, RN, CS

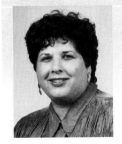

An experience I'll always remember involved a patient who was being discharged from the state psychiatric hospital and whom I interviewed for admission into an intensive case management program. R had been in and out of the state hospital for 3 years with the diagnosis of chronic schizophrenia. His frequent readmissions were related to the system's inability to place him in the community, which was due in part to his history of setting fires. Before this admission he had burned down his residence during a psychotic episode. However, his psychosis had resolved quickly after he was admitted to the hospital and started on a regimen of neuroleptics.

R was admitted into the intensive case management program, and his first 6 months had been very busy. He had been placed in an apartment with a roommate and became responsible for managing the apartment, cooking his own food, balancing his checkbook, and paying his bills. His adjustment to life in the community was progressing well. I was able to work with R on almost a daily basis, and all was going well.

On this specific day, I had called R to let him know that I would be coming to take him to the bank. We discussed in detail his checking account balance and financial obligations for that month. When I arrived at his home, R's roommate informed me that R had gone to the store to get a cup of coffee. While waiting, I walked into the hallway to check on a problem thermostat. As I glanced into R's room, I noticed that something was amiss. There were several cigarette burns in the carpet. On the bed there were a number of cigarette lighters. Propped on the pillows were cover photos from several women's magazines. The mouths on the models had been enlarged and a cigarette had been placed through the hole. In the bedside table I found several more cigarette lighters. I noted all of these things, as well as the fact that R did not smoke.

On his return, we discussed some problems R was having with his roommate and banking affairs. His conversation was calm and rational. I then talked with him about what I had seen in his bedroom. Initially he was silent and refused to discuss the matter. I realized that one of his greatest fears was returning to the state hospital to live for the remainder of his life, so I assured him that if something was wrong and he needed to go back to the hospital, it would be for a short-term hospital-

Continued

Competent Caring A Clinical Exemplar of a Psychiatric Nurse—cont'd

ization. At that point he began to explain that he had not taken his medication in a week and that recently he drank a six-pack of beer with several other patients in the program. Since then, he had been hearing messages from God in which she told him to smoke cigarettes because carbon monoxide was needed to clear all the pollution on the earth.

After a consultation phone call, I told R that I thought he was ill again and needed some time in the hospital. He agreed and we left in my car for an admission assessment at a local hospital. On the way, we stopped at the bank and R completed his banking business. When we arrived, several of my peers were astonished that I had let R ride in my car and go to the bank when he was obviously psychotic. They exclaimed that they would have certainly called for backup from the office or

the mobile crisis unit. I explained to them that I had assessed R and felt that this decision would not endanger him or me. My decision was based on my skills as a psychiatric nurse, my experience in working with psychotic patients for a number of years, and my evaluation of R, with whom I had worked closely for 6 months.

When I think back to this experience, I realize that it captured some of the critical essence of psychiatric nursing decision making. I believe that it is calculated thinking woven into a fabric of clinical experience that guides psychiatric nursing practice. For R it was also a nursing act that expressed both caring for and caring about. After 10 days in the hospital, R was stabilized once more and returned to the life he so wanted to live.

 Visit **MERLIN: www.mosby.com/MERLIN/Stuart** to find these additional materials and student activities.

- **Worksheets**
- **"Drug of the Month" Updates**
- **"Citing the Evidence" Updates**
- **Critical Thinking Activities and Exercises**
- **Annotated Suggested Readings**
- **Web Links**
- **More!**

Chapter Review Questions

1. Match each descriptor in Column A with the mental health model in Column B.

Column A

a. ____ Aimed at linking and coordinating needed services.

b. ____ Consumer participation and culturally relevant care were guiding principles.

c. ____ Defined the patient as the community.

d. ____ Developed and implemented community support systems.

e. ____ Emphasized preventive services to high-risk groups.

f. ____ Focused on programs for assertive community treatment.

g. ____ Shifted clinical priorities to treatment as a result of deinstitutionalization.

Column B

A. Public health model

B. Biological-medical model

C. System model

D. Patient-centered model

2. Fill in the blanks.

A. _____ studies examine the incidence and prevalence of mental disorders in a defined population.

B. Interventions that target those who have mental illness and help to reduce the disability associated with the illness are called _____ prevention.

C. _____ is a system in which services are aimed at linking the resources and coordinating care to achieve successful community living.

D. Interventions that target those at risk for illness and promote their adaptive coping are called _____ prevention.

E. _____ is a type of program that functions as a community-based hospital without walls to provide intensive clinical support and treatment.

F. Interventions that target people who show early signs of an illness and help them receive prompt treatment are called _____ prevention.

G. A treatment approach that addresses the needs of youth with behavioral and emotional problems and their families is called _____.

H. A relatively new specialty of nursing caring for the mentally ill in correctional facilities is called _____ nursing.

3. Provide short answers for the following questions.

A. Describe common elements of ACT and MST programs.

B. What groups are at high risk for developing mental illness in your community? How many resources are devoted to prevention activities with these groups? How can you help to better match community needs with community resources?

C. Most case managers in this country are social workers. Describe how you as a nurse and a social worker might differ in implementing the case manager role.

D. What new roles that you read about in this chapter appeal to you as a potential career option?

REFERENCES

Atkinson M: Psychiatric clinical nurse specialists as intensive case managers for the seriously mentally ill, *Semin Nurse Managers* 4(2):130, 1996.

American Nurses' Association: *Position statement on psychiatric mental health nursing and managed care,* Washington, DC, 1993, The Association.

Calloway M, Morrissey J: Overcoming service barriers for homeless persons with serious psychiatric disorders, *Psychiatr Serv* 49(12):1568, 1998.

Christensen R: Ethical issues in community mental health: cases and conflicts, *Community Ment Health J* 33(1):5, 1997.

De Young C, Tower M: *The nurse's role in community mental health centers: out of uniform and into trouble,* St Louis, 1971, Mosby.

Deci P et al: Dissemination of assertive community treatment programs, *Psychiatr Serv* 46:676, 1995.

Ditton P: *Mental health treatment of inmates and probationers,* Washington, DC, 1999, Bureau of Justice Statistics, US Dept of Justice.

Dixon L et al: Assertive community treatment and medication compliance in the homeless mentally ill, *Am J Psychiatry* 154(9):1302, 1997.

Farnam C et al: Health status risk factors of people with severe and persistent mental illness, *J Psychsoc Nurs* 37(6):16, 1999.

Gelberg L et al: The Behavioral Model for Vulnerable Populations: application to medical care use and outcomes for homeless people, *Health Serv Res* 34(6):1273, 2000.

Glittenberg J: The role of the nurse in outpatient psychiatric clinics, *Am J Orthopsychiatry* 39:713, 1963.

Goldfinger S et al: Housing placement and subsequent days homeless among formerly homeless adults with mental illness, *Psychiatr Serv* 50(5):674, 1999.

Goldkuhle U: Professional education for correctional nurses, *J Psychsoc Nurs* 37(9):38, 1999.

Guy S: Assertive community treatment of the long-term mentally ill, *J Am Psychiatr Nurs Assoc* 3:185, 1997.

Hall J: State of the art case management, *Occup Med* 13(4):705, 1998.

Henggeler S et al: Home-based multisystemic therapy as an alternative to the hospitalization of youths in psychiatric crisis: clinical outcomes, *J Am Acad Child Adolesc Psychiatry* 38(9):1118, 1999.

King R et al: The impact of caseload on the personal efficacy of mental health case managers, *Psychiatr Serv* 51(3):364, 2000.

Lam J, Rosenheck R: Correlates of improvement in quality of life among homeless persons with serious mental illness, *Psychiatr Serv* 51(1):116, 2000.

Lehman A et al: Cost-effectiveness of assertive community treatment for homeless persons with severe mental illness, *Br J Psychiatry* 174:346, 1999.

Mueser K et al: Models of community care for severe mental illness: a review of research on case management, *Schizophr Bull* 24(1):37, 1998.

Murray R et al: Components of an effective transitional residential program for homeless mentally ill clients, *Arch Psychiatr Nurs* 9:152, 1995.

Parson C: Managed care: the effect of case management on state psychiatric clients, *J Psychosoc Nurs* 37(10):16, 1999.

Peternelj-Taylor C, Johnson R: Serving time: psychiatric mental health nursing in corrections, *J Psychsoc Nurs* 33(8):12, 1995.

Project Link: Prevention of jail and hospital recidivism among persons with severe mental illness, *Psychiatr Serv* 50(11):1477, 1999.

Randall J et al: Neighborhood solutions for neighborhood problems: an empirically based violence prevention collaboration, *Health Educ Behav* 26(6):806, 1999.

Randolph F et al: Creating integrated service systems for homeless persons with mental illness: the ACCESS program, *Psychiatr Serv* 48:369, 1997.

Regier D, Kaelber C: The Epidemiologic Catchment Area (ECA) program: studying the prevalence and incidence of psychopathology. In Tsuang M, Tohen M, Zahner G, editors: *Textbook in psychiatric epidemiology,* New York, 1995, Wiley-Liss.

Roberts L et al: Frontier ethics: mental health care needs and ethical dilemmas in rural communities, *Psychiatr Serv* 50:4, 1999.

Rohde D: Evolution of community mental health case management: considerations for clinical practice, *Arch Psychiatr Nurs* 11(6):332, 1997.

Rowe M, Hoge M, Fisk D: Critical issues in serving people who are homeless and mentally ill, *Admin Policy Ment Health* 23:555, 1996.

Schnapp W, Cannedy R: Offenders with mental illness: mental health and criminal justice best practices, *Admin Policy Ment Health* 25(4):463, 1998.

Sledge W et al: Case management in psychiatry: an analysis of tasks, *Am J Psychiatry* 152:1259, 1995.

Steadman H et al: A SAMHSA research initiative assessing the effectiveness of jail diversion programs for mentally ill persons, *Psychiatr Serv* 50(12):1620, 1999.

Vallon K et al: Comprehensive case management in the private sector for patients with severe mental illness, *Psychiatr Serv* 48(7):910, 1997.

Walker C: Homeless people and mental health, *Am J Nurs* 98(11):26, 1998.

Williams R, Siegmann R: Community mental health centers for the new millennium, *J Pract Psychiatry Behav Health* 3(1):28, 1997.

Wolff N et al: Cost-effectiveness evaluation of three approaches to case management for homeless mentally ill clients, *Am J Psychiatry* 154:341, 1997.

Young A et al: The effect of provider characteristics on case management activities, *Admin Policy Ment Health* 26(1):21, 1998.

37 Home Psychiatric Nursing Care

Gail W. Stuart

Beth Gage Greco

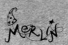 Visit **MERLIN** for *Your Internet Connection* to websites that are related to the content in this chapter. www.mosby.com/MERLIN/Stuart

*W*e shall not cease from exploration
And the end of all our exploring
Will be to arrive where we started
And to know the place for the first time.

T. S. ELIOT, *FOUR QUARTETS*

The first home care agencies were established in the United States in the 1800s by nurses who provided care to people in their community. Since that time, home care has undergone many changes. Rapid growth in home care occurred after initial Medicare legislation was passed in 1965 to allow reimbursement for home care services to the elderly. The number of home care agencies has increased dramatically, from 1100 in 1963 to more than 20,000 in 2000 (National Association for Home Care, 2000). However, psychiatric home care has had a slower start. Before 1987 there were few psychiatric home care programs in the United States. In 1987 a class action lawsuit against the Health Care Financing Administration (HCFA) resulted in the revision of the Medicare home care payment laws. This revision added to the growth of home care and led to the expansion of psychiatric home care programs.

GROWTH OF PSYCHIATRIC HOME CARE

Psychiatric home care is now available to a broad segment of the population. In addition to regulatory changes, other factors have contributed to the development of this treatment setting:

- A continued trend toward deinstitutionalization
- The availability of Medicare reimbursement for home care

- The growth of managed care, which focuses on cost, outcomes, and earlier hospital discharges
- Advocacy by consumer groups to find less restrictive and more humane ways of delivering care to people with mental illness

Psychiatric home care programs are changing rapidly in response to the competitive health-care market and to the increased numbers of acute psychiatric patients in the community. Most recently the growth of psychiatric home care has been limited as the result of the changes in Medicare home health reimbursement enacted as part of the Balanced Budget Act of 1997. Nonetheless, psychiatric home care programs have proven to be effective in meeting the needs of psychiatric patients in a cost-effective manner (see Citing the Evidence).

Perhaps the best argument for psychiatric home care is that it is a humane and compassionate way to deliver health care and supportive services. Home care reinforces and supplements the care provided by family members and friends and maintains the recipient's dignity and independence—qualities that are all too often lost in even the best institutions.

Psychiatric home care ranges from serving as an alternative to hospitalization to functioning as a single home visit

Citing the Evidence on

The Effectiveness of Psychiatric Home Care

BACKGROUND: Patients who are still recovering from depression are being discharged from the inpatient setting to their homes much sooner than before. Few studies of the effectiveness of home follow-up for patients with depression have been performed.

RESULTS: This study followed a total of 68 patients admitted to the mental health unit during a 30-day period. Patients received follow-up care only if it was prescribed by the physician. Twelve patients received psychiatric home nurse follow-up, and 56 received standard care. Both groups received similar outpatient care. Patients in the home nurse follow-up group had significantly fewer readmissions in 60 days. Specifically, no patients from this group were readmitted to the hospital compared with 33% of patients from the standard care group.

IMPLICATIONS: These findings provide support for psychiatric nurse home follow-up for patients with depression after discharge from an inpatient setting. Randomized and controlled clinical trials are needed to further document the clinical benefits and cost-effectiveness of psychiatric home care.

Barker E et al: The effect of psychiatric home nurse follow-up on readmission rates of patients with depression, *J Psych Nurs Assoc* 5(4):111, 1999.

for the purposes of evaluating a specific issue. Psychiatric home care programs receive and refer patients from general medical and mental health care services of the entire community. The advantages of home care in relation to inpatient treatment involve its ability to serve as the following (Soreff, 1994):

- An alternative to hospitalization by maintaining a patient in the community
- A facilitator of an impending hospital admission through preadmission assessment
- An enhancement of inpatient treatment through the integration of home issues in the inpatient treatment plan
- A way to shorten inpatient stays while keeping the patient engaged in active treatment
- A part of the discharge planning process by assessing potential problems and issues

Examples of other gains obtained by psychiatric home care include its outreach capacity and its emphasis on patient participation, responsibility, autonomy, and satisfaction.

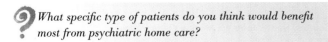

What specific type of patients do you think would benefit most from psychiatric home care?

Table 37-1

Sources of Payment for Home Care, 1997, National Home and Hospice Care Survey	
Source of Payment	**% Home Health Care**
Medicare	39.5
Medicaid	14.7
State and local government	7.0
Private insurance	11.4
Out-of-pocket	22.3
Other	12.2

Box 37-1

Medicare Guidelines for Psychiatric Home Care Nursing

PSYCHIATRIC EVALUATION, THERAPY, AND TEACHING

The evaluation, psychotherapy, and teaching activities needed by a patient with a diagnosed psychiatric disorder that requires active treatment by a psychiatrically trained nurse, as well as the costs of the psychiatric nurse's services, may be covered as a skilled nursing service. Psychiatrically trained nurses are nurses who have special training and/or experience beyond the standard curriculum required for a registered nurse. The services of the psychiatric nurse are to be provided under a plan of care established and reviewed by a physician.

Modified from Health Care Financing Administration, Publication 11, Washington, DC, 1996.

Reimbursement Issues

Reimbursement for psychiatric home care is largely provided by Medicare, Medicaid, managed care companies, and private insurance. Each payer has requirements for the services covered, and some require advance authorization for psychiatric nursing services in the home. The majority of home care is paid for by Medicare. The second largest source is out-of-pocket payments (Table 37-1). The Medicare population with mental illnesses falls into two broad categories. One group consists of patients over 65 years of age who may have a history of mental illness or a newly diagnosed mental illness, usually depression. The second group is composed of people under 65 years of age who qualify for Medicare because of their disability. The most common diagnosis in this second group is schizophrenia.

Medicare guidelines do not provide very specific information regarding the psychiatric nursing services that are covered on home visits (Box 37-1). However, they do require that the patient:

- Be homebound
- Have a diagnosed psychiatric disorder
- Require the skills of a psychiatric nurse

It is largely left up to the home care agencies to interpret the Medicare guidelines and apply them to psychiatric home care. This has created many problems in the field, and psychiatric home care programs continue to struggle with this reimbursement issue (Klebanoff, 1996).

Psychiatric homebound status is qualitatively different from medical homebound status. In determining psychiatric homebound status, a useful definition is a patient who is unable to access psychiatric follow-up independently and consistently. This definition is broad enough to include a person who is physically healthy and mobile but is too depressed to get out of bed. It also includes patients with agoraphobia and patients with psychotic thinking processes who are vulnerable in the community. Medicare considers a person to be homebound in the following situations:

- The condition restricts his or her ability to leave home without an assistive device or another person.
- The effort required to leave the home is considerable and taxing.
- It is medically contraindicated to leave the home.
- If the patient does leave home, the absences are infrequent, of short duration, or attributable to the need to receive treatment.

Box 37-2

Conditions That Might Make a Patient Psychiatrically Homebound

- Confusion, disorientation, poor judgment
- Immobilizing depression
- Severe anxiety that interferes with independence
- Agoraphobia with or without panic attacks
- Vulnerability in the community
- Psychosis or paranoid delusions that interfere with safety
- Need for 24-hour supervision

Each patient is individually evaluated with regard to homebound status. Box 37-2 lists some conditions that might make a patient psychiatrically homebound.

Medicare is a retrospective payer, with records reviewed by fiscal intermediaries to determine the necessity and appropriateness of psychiatric nursing care. Therefore when planning and delivering service, it is important that the psychiatric home care nurse concentrate on Medicare-recognized reimbursable skilled nursing services such as teaching, assessment, skilled management of the care plan, and direct care activities.

Managed care companies are beginning to control an increasing share of the market; in response, psychiatric home care programs are beginning to develop specific programs for these companies. Some examples are in-home substance abuse programs, crisis intervention programs, and hospitalization prevention programs. The requirements for psychiatric home care services vary among managed care companies, and preauthorization for services is the norm.

PSYCHIATRIC HOME HEALTH NURSING
Role Definition

More psychiatric nurses are choosing psychiatric home care as their practice setting, and conferences on psychiatric home care are held nationwide. To work in home care, the nurse must have a clear sense of his or her role in the patient's life and be able to articulate what help can and cannot be offered. The psychiatric home care nurse will be confronted with complicated social and economic situations as well as complex psychiatric and medical evaluations. The nurse must be able to identify the priorities for care, changes that can be accomplished realistically, and situations that

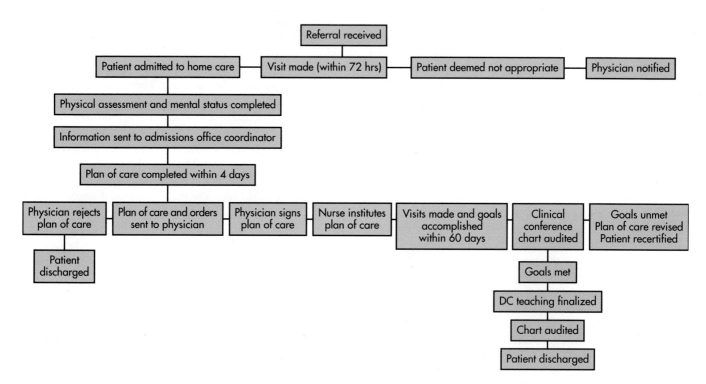

Fig. 37-1 Psychiatric nursing case management. (Courtesy North Mississippi Medical Center Home Health Agency.)

may be outside of the nurse's power or the patient's desire to change (Duffy, 1996).

One particularly effective role for the psychiatric home care nurse is case management (see Chapter 36) (Carson, 1995; Duckworth & Kitchens, 1996; Quinlan & Ohlund, 1995). Case management promotes self-care and encourages the cost-effective use of resources (Fig. 37-1). Other roles for the psychiatric home care nurse include teacher, counselor, therapist, resource coordinator, consultant, staff educator, supervisor, researcher, direct caregiver, and discharge planner. Participation in some role aspects requires advanced practice preparation (Iglesias, 1998). Other role aspects are part of the role of every psychiatric home care nurse and include assessment, direct care, patient-family education, supervision of home health aides, counseling, coordination of services, collaboration with multidisciplinary team members, and management of the care plan. Finally, psychiatric home care nurses function as members of an interdisciplinary treatment team and must have a clear understanding of the contributions each person can make to the comprehensive treatment plan of a patient (see Critical Thinking about Contemporary Issues).

Qualifications of the Psychiatric Home Care Nurse

Psychiatric home care is a subspecialty that calls for a nurse with certain types of skills, education, and experience. On any given day the nurse will be confronted with the extremes of the human condition and with multiple problems that have no obvious solution. The ability to laugh and find humor in the face of these realities is critical to maintaining perspective. Assertiveness, flexibility, curiosity, respect for

the patient's right to choose, and an awareness of one's own humanity are other important personal qualities needed by the psychiatric home care nurse. Medicare outlines the additional specific requirements for the psychiatric nurse practicing in the home care setting (Box 37-3).

> *Any nurse can be hired to work in an inpatient psychiatric unit, but Medicare has specific requirements for a psychiatric home care nurse. Discuss the implications of this from the point of view of the patient, the nurse, and the employing health-care organization.*

CONTEXT OF PSYCHIATRIC HOME CARE

Psychiatric home care nursing provides unique challenges and opportunities for the nurse. In an inpatient clinic or office setting the provider has the control and power that come with ownership. The patient is the guest and the nurse is the host. In the home setting, however, the nurse is the guest and the patient sets the rules. This raises four key issues for the nurse: cultural competence, flexibility in boundary setting, trust, and safety.

Cultural Competence

An awareness of the patient's ethnic and cultural background is critical to effective care in all settings, but nowhere is it more obvious to the attentive eye and more critical to treatment outcome than in the home care setting. The nurse is exposed to the patient's culture, and the patient will observe the nurse's reaction. Ways of addressing members of the family, views of health and mental illness, the role of the nurse (and of health-care providers in general), and the importance of alternative therapies are just a few of the issues that vary across cultures. All of these differences must be considered by the nurse who is planning care for the patient in the home. Recognizing and using the patient's cultural beliefs in the delivery of nursing care can positively influence the patient's participation in recovery (Spruhan, 1996).

CRITICAL THINKING about CONTEMPORARY ISSUES

Is There Conflict Between Social Workers and Psychiatric Nurses in the Field of Psychiatric Home Care?

Clinical territory can be a potential area of conflict among health-care providers. Medical social work, although somewhat focused on brief counseling, is primarily responsible for providing referrals for community resources, financial assistance, and transportation. In contrast, psychiatric nursing is focused on biopsychosocial interventions that include specific cognitive and behavioral strategies. The introduction of psychiatric nurses in a well-functioning home health agency may actually result in increased rather than decreased social work referrals, because psychiatric nurses can identify the people who need the services of the medical social worker.

The goal in home health is to provide care in a cooperative manner and to use the strengths of the various disciplines with minimal overlap. Overall, this collaborative approach can strengthen the home health agency and provide needed services to the most challenging psychiatric patients.

Box 37-3

Medicare Requirements for Psychiatric Nurses in Home Care*

- A registered nurse with a master's degree in psychiatric or community mental health nursing
- A registered nurse with a bachelor's of science in nursing (BSN) degree and 1 year of related work experience in an active treatment program for adult or geriatric patients in a psychiatric health-care setting
- A registered nurse with a diploma or associate degree and 2 years of related work experience in an active treatment program for adult or geriatric patients in a psychiatric health-care setting
- American Nurses Association (ANA) certification in psychiatric or community health nursing

*Other qualifications may be considered on an individual basis

It is also important that the nurse have an understanding of his or her own cultural background and prejudices related to socioeconomic status, gender, and family structure. Self-awareness gives the nurse the ability to step back from a judgmental stance and ask whether a certain behavior, opinion, or way of coping stands in the way of the patient's ultimate health.

> *Imagine yourself providing psychiatric home care to an individual with a cultural background very different from your own. How would this affect your assessment of the patient's biopsychosocial needs and your related nursing interventions? What resources would you draw on to provide culturally competent nursing care?*

Boundary Issues

Closely related to cultural issues are the differences in boundary issues. In the home setting it may be appropriate for the nurse to sit and share a cup of tea with the patient or to eat a piece of cake. If the patient's culture is one that sees hospitality as connected closely to the sharing of food and sees the refusal of food as an affront, then being willing to share in this ritual can build trust in the relationship between the nurse and the patient. Differing opinions exist regarding boundary issues in psychiatric home care (Daudell-Strejc & Murphy, 1995; Duffy & Miller, 1996; Brown, 1996), but the experienced psychiatric home care nurse knows that nursing care must be adapted to the needs and environment of each patient. This area requires further nursing research and clinical review.

Trust

The psychiatric home care nurse must consider many different factors when planning and implementing nursing care. Unlike nursing practice in the hospital or outpatient mental health center, psychiatric home care nurses have little control over their patients' environments. It is therefore essential to establish trust in the initial evaluation home visit. Trust then becomes a vital part of the nurse-patient relationship as the patient and nurse work together to solve problems and achieve goals. The nurse trusts the patient to be home for the scheduled visits, to take medications, and to participate fully in all aspects of the plan of care. The patient trusts the nurse to be reliable, clinically knowledgeable, competent, and caring. Methods to establish and build trust in home care patients include the following (Wendt, 1996):

- Cultivating the patient's trust with the first contact
- Establishing credibility with the patient
- Using an empathic, nonjudgmental approach
- Guarding the patient's privacy
- Expecting testing behavior from patients
- Learning to trust the patient
- Persevering with the nurse-patient relationship and demonstrating commitment to the patient despite any noncompliance or resistance

Safety

In general, psychiatric home care patients are not at greater risk for violence than the general home care patient population. However, an assessment of the environment should include issues of safety for the patient and the nurse. Strategies must be identified for dealing with suicidal or aggressive behavior. In this respect, home health nursing does have its limitations. The nurse and patient must work together to achieve an acceptable plan, given the reality of having intermittent visits. If the situation becomes unsafe, the nurse must leave the home. If the patient becomes dangerous, his or her family, caregivers, and other community resources should be urged to notify the police or to take him or her to the hospital for an evaluation.

NURSING PROCESS IN THE HOME SETTING

The nursing assessment of the home care patient is a comprehensive look at the many facets of an individual's life. Areas of assessment include physical, emotional, spiritual, environmental, economic, and cultural factors. All of these factors can affect a person's health and well-being. To gain a thorough understanding of the patient's problems, possible solutions, and available resources, the psychiatric home health nurse must be adept at interviewing the patient, family and, if indicated, friends, neighbors, and members of the patient's social support system.

Although policies differ among different home care agencies, the initial assessment should include standardized rating scales and tools to target and quantify symptoms and to allow easier identification of the patient's progress toward goals once nursing care has begun (Mayo, 1997). Other data gathered during the assessment visit include a health history; a full set of vital signs; history of present illness; current medication regimen; all concurrent medical diagnoses; patient's/family's understanding of psychiatric home care; home and patient safety issues; patient's functional status, social, spiritual, and financial needs; and patient's and caregivers' knowledge and skill level (Freed & Rice, 1997).

Careful attention is needed to identify patients with chaotic family or social situations or multiple medical diagnoses so early interventions by other disciplines can be planned at the start of care. The nurse must also be able to identify areas of possible or actual family violence or abuse and intervene appropriately (Freed & Drake 1999).

As patient problems and needs are identified, the psychiatric home health nurse formulates nursing diagnoses, collaborates with the patient's physician, and establishes an individualized plan of care. Home visit patterns are determined by the patient's needs and financial resources, with more frequent visits scheduled until the patient's condition stabilizes. Preauthorization for psychiatric home care may be required by some health insurance plans, and services could be limited to a few visits. In these cases it is critical that the nurse set priorities and plan obtainable goals.

With psychiatric home care, the plan of care must identify measurable and attainable outcomes. This is vital to attaining patient goals in a timely manner. Nursing interventions in the home include assessment, teaching, medication management, administration of parenteral injections, venipuncture for laboratory analysis, and skilled management of the care plan. Medicare recognizes all of these interventions as reimbursable skilled nursing services. In actuality, psychiatric home care nurses provide many other skilled nursing services (Box 37-4). They act as case managers and coordinate an array of services that include physical therapy, occupational therapy, social work, and community services such as home-delivered meals, home visitors, and home health aides. They collaborate with all of the patient's health-care providers and often facilitate communication among members of the multidisciplinary team (Gonzales et al, 1998).

Psychiatric home care nurses make appropriate referrals to community agencies and help their patients to access community resources independently. They educate families and patients, provide supportive counseling and brief psychotherapy, promote health and prevent illness and, above all, document everything in precise detail so their agency is reimbursed for the services they provide.

Box 37-4

In-Home Behavioral Health Services

In-home behavioral health services include, but are not limited to, the following:

- Direct patient care
- Development and implementation of specific mental health assessment tools
- Coordination of care or visits by other disciplines
- Joint visits with the primary nurses
- Consultation with the home care staff related to the psychosocial needs of patients

Services specifically include the following:

- Assessment of mental health status and evaluation of the patient's response to illness and treatment
- Assessment of the home environment
- Development and implementation of an individualized treatment/care plan through consultation with the primary psychiatrist or physician in regard to the following:
  - Therapeutic interventions
  - Safety issues
  - Medication compliance
  - Physical exercises
  - Education and support of the patient's caregivers
  - Medication instruction, monitoring, and administration
  - Provision of supportive psychotherapy
  - Development of individualized education plans regarding all aspects of the illness and how to develop coping skills
  - Collection of laboratory specimens and monitoring of results (e.g., lithium, carbamazepine [Tegretol], antidepressants)
- Referrals to and follow-up with community resources
- Support for patients with absent or inadequate family and community support to help prevent recidivism
- Provision of 24-hour on-call service for crisis intervention and referrals

From Lapierre E, Soileau J: In-home behavioral health services: establishing a program, *Caring* 7:7, 1995.

Documentation is one of the most challenging requirements of psychiatric home care. If the nurse's documentation does not reflect the skilled service given, the payment for that service can be denied by Medicare or other payers. Few guidelines are available for the documentation of psychiatric home care, but standardized coding and classification systems are preferred for the computer-based patient record (Parlocha & Henry, 1998). The psychiatric home care nurse must be very organized and detail oriented for successful management of the extensive and precise paperwork.

Finally, the psychiatric home care nurse continuously reviews the patient's progress toward goals and revises the care plan. The evaluation process is an ongoing collaborative task between the patient and the nurse. In addition, the patient's family and support system play a vital role in recovery. The patient moves increasingly closer to his or her highest level of functioning as goals are met or outcomes are achieved. Discharge from psychiatric home care is indicated when the patient reaches his or her maximum potential. Criteria for discharge include identification of the following (Freed & Rice, 1997):

- A reliable supportive other to assist with future health care needs
- Improved ability to perform activities of daily living and interact socially
- Follow-through with other health care contacts
- Optimal response to the treatment plan
- Adequate levels of independent living

A patient may be discharged to the care of the family, a day or partial hospital program, a skilled nursing facility, a personal care facility, or self-care. The psychiatric home care nurse terminates the relationship with the patient and caregivers and provides specific written instructions for follow-up care.

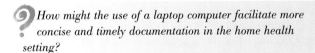

How might the use of a laptop computer facilitate more concise and timely documentation in the home health setting?

SPECIAL POPULATIONS

Many types of patients can benefit greatly from psychiatric home health care (Box 37-5). Chapters 38 to 42 address in more detail the nursing interventions related to some of these special groups.

Children and Adolescents

Psychiatric home care is often successful for children and adolescents. Children and adolescents have a unique set of needs that can be addressed by the psychiatric home care nurse. Providing care in the home gives the nurse immediate access to the family, the home environment, and the community surrounding the child or adolescent. This contextual understanding opens up new possibilities for intervention and new understandings of the complexity of the problem that the youth and family may be experiencing. Multisystem therapy, as described in Chapter 36, is one type of home-based intervention that is effective with youth.

Box 37-5

Who Can Benefit from In-Home Psychiatric Nursing Services?

- Patients with repeated inpatient or crisis unit admissions
- Patients with a history of medication or treatment plan noncompliance or lack of follow-through with aftercare plans
- Patients with combined diagnoses of a medical and psychiatric nature (e.g., elderly or HIV-positive patients)
- Patients with combined substance abuse and psychiatric diagnoses
- Patients receiving injectable medications who are homebound or do not follow through with scheduled outpatient appointments
- Patients in need of laboratory monitoring who are homebound or do not follow through with outpatient laboratory appointments
- Patients who are depressed and neglect self-care
- Patients who suffer from anxiety or panic and have difficulty leaving the home

Older Adults

Older adults make up the majority of the home care caseload and present many challenges to the psychiatric home care nurse. There is a high incidence of comorbidity in this group, and the nurse must often address both psychiatric and medical diagnoses in these patients (Felton, 1997). Care must be taken not to overlook the impact of the body on the mind and of the mind on the body (see Citing the Evidence).

Older adults often do not use available mental health services. They may be unable to access these services or may consider them embarrassing. Psychiatric home care overcomes these obstacles and can bring a much-needed service to the older adult. For the older adult living in an unsafe inner-city neighborhood, a visit from a psychiatric nurse can help bring order to chaos. For the older adult living in an isolated rural environment, a psychiatric home care nurse can provide support and education and decrease the impact of social isolation.

 CLINICAL EXAMPLE

Ms. P, a 78-year-old woman, was referred to psychiatric home care by a local hospital discharge planner. She had been hospitalized for an acute myocardial infarction (MI) and during her hospital stay developed depression with severe anxiety that resulted in her transfer to the inpatient psychiatric unit of the hospital. After 5 days on the inpatient psychiatric unit, Ms. P was discharged to her home.

Ms. P lived alone in a second-floor apartment and had functioned independently before her MI. However, her functional status on discharge from the hospital was much decreased. She could no longer climb a flight of stairs and became easily fatigued during activities of daily living (ADLs). She was taking several medications to improve her cardiac status and was also taking medication for her depression and anxiety. Her five children were supportive from a distance. She was also very determined to maintain her independent status and wanted very much to regain her previous lifestyle.

Citing the Evidence on

Therapy with Homebound Older Adults

BACKGROUND: The purpose of this study was to examine the process and outcomes of life review therapy provided by an advanced practice geropsychiatric nurse to older adults discharged from psychiatric hospitals to home health care.

RESULTS: 80 older adults over 65 years of age with a primary diagnosis of depression were treated at home with life review psychotherapy sessions. Themes that emerged included empowerment (connection, coping, efficacy, hope, and trust) or disempowerment (denial, despair, helplessness, isolation, loneliness, and loss). Findings showed a significant decrease in total disempowerment themes as a result of life review therapy.

IMPLICATIONS: This study provides evidence that psychosocial treatments developed specifically for older adults have a positive impact on their overall well-being and facilitate their ability to remain independent at home. Life review therapy may be an effective therapy for many homebound elderly with depression.

McDougall G et al: The process and outcome of life review psychotherapy with depressed homebound older adults, *Nurs Res* 46(5):277, 1997.

The psychiatric home care nurse completed an assessment and initiated a care plan with the patient and the physician. The patient's family was included in the planning process because it was necessary that they take an active role in their mother's care. Initial goals were established, with functional independence identified as the outcome of care. A physical therapist and a home health aide were provided by the home care agency.

Unfortunately, the patient fell during her second week of home care services. The focus of care changed as it became increasingly obvious that the patient would not regain independent function. The psychiatric nurse and the physician made a referral to the agency's social worker, and the process of locating appropriate placement for the patient began. The family was very supportive and helpful with the placement process, but Ms. P was not.

The nurse recognized that placement in a nursing home was a threat to Ms. P's self-esteem. She also knew that Ms. P was no longer safe alone in her own apartment. The nurse encouraged Ms. P to discuss her concerns, identify her fears, and participate in the placement process. Gradually, through tears and smiles, Ms. P grieved the loss of her health, her independence, and her home. The nurse discharged Ms. P to a local nursing home a few blocks from her home. Ms. P said, "At least I'll be in the same neighborhood" as she accepted her circumstances on that final visit.

Patients with Serious and Persistent Mental Illness

Patients with serious and persistent mental illness are particularly suited to home care interventions. This population often does not follow through with medications and scheduled outpatient appointments. Repeated hospitalizations are often needed to restart medications and stabilize symptoms. Noncompliance is a complicated issue but can be more readily addressed in the home setting. The nurse can create an alliance with the patient and family in the nonthreatening environment of the home (Morris, 1996). Assertive community treatment, described in Chapter 36, is one type of home-based intervention documented to be effective with patients who have serious and persistent mental illness.

The psychiatric home care nurse can identify obstacles to patient compliance, such as financial issues, transportation problems, and lack of knowledge. The nurse can work with the patient to find solutions to these and other problems and to help prevent relapse. The psychiatric home care nurse can also administer long-acting neuroleptic injections when the patient is unable to follow an oral medication administration schedule.

Many of the complications of living with a chronic mental illness can be helped with proper medication, patient-family education, and continued supportive therapy by a caring mental health professional. The psychiatric home care nurse can provide these services in the patient's home on a time-limited basis. The nurse can also act as the vital link between hospital and community services for patients with serious and persistent mental illness.

CLINICAL EXAMPLE

Sonia, a 49-year-old woman, was referred by a managed care company to psychiatric home care after a 2-week inpatient stay at a local psychiatric hospital. She had a long history of psychiatric admissions for stabilization of her schizophrenia. Most hospitalizations were preceded by the patient's noncompliance with her medication schedule and follow-up care at the mental health center.

Sonia lived with her sister and elderly mother in a small row house in the Hispanic section of a large city. The family's native language was Spanish; they spoke English as a second language and understood some written English. Sonia's sister was the family's caregiver. She cared for their bedridden mother and helped with Sonia's care. Sonia's sister could not understand why Sonia would be all right for long periods and then become "crazy" and not listen. Sonia agreed to psychiatric nursing visits but initially would not agree to treatment at the mental health center. Paranoia was a major component of her illness. Other barriers were financial concerns, a lack of knowledge about her illness, and cultural and language issues.

The psychiatric nurse's plan of care included educating the patient and her sister on the disease process, signs and symptoms of relapse, the importance of continued medical care, medication actions and side effects, and correct administration of the prescribed medication. As her care progressed and Sonia became stable, the nurse helped the patient and her sister to make and attend a follow-up appointment at the mental health center. Sonia was discharged from home care and agreed to go to the mental health clinic for her follow-up medical care.

Patients with Human Immunodeficiency Virus/Acquired Immunodeficiency Syndrome

Psychiatric disorders associated with HIV/AIDS include adjustment disorder, anxiety disorder, depression, and central nervous system dysfunction. Central nervous system dysfunction can include delirium symptoms, dementia, agitation, or confusion. Patients with HIV/AIDS have many mental health needs (see Chapter 42) and sometimes have chronic mental illnesses. They struggle with the stigma of AIDS and try to cope with the tremendous losses and grief. Psychiatric home care nurses can make a significant contribution by helping these patients with their many physical and emotional needs.

CLINICAL EXAMPLE

Mr. J was referred by an outpatient medical clinic nurse to the psychiatric home care program of the local Visiting Nurse Association. He had missed several of his scheduled appointments and was displaying increased anxiety about his health and future. He had been HIV positive for several years and was beginning to show symptoms of AIDS.

The psychiatric home care nurse arrived at the patient's home for the evaluation visit and was greeted by the patient, his brother, and his sister-in-law. Mr. J had just told his family of his AIDS diagnosis and was hoping the nurse could act as an intermediary for the family. Mr. J had not told the nurse of his intentions for her first visit. The nurse quickly sized up the family situation, intervened, and provided the family with essential education about HIV/AIDS.

Later home visits focused on teaching the patient about assertive communication, coping skills, and relaxation exercises to decrease anxiety. Brief cognitive psychotherapy was used to help Mr. J to identify his thoughts and feelings. Grief counseling was initiated, and the patient was encouraged to find a long-term therapist in his community who was sensitive to his needs. Mr. J made an appointment with a psychologist and attended his first session, but he canceled his final visit with the psychiatric home care nurse. The nurse was left to wonder about Mr. J's first visit with the psychologist. Did he have a surprise for that mental health provider, too?

Summary

1. Psychiatric home care programs developed in response to the changing health-care industry. Measures have been introduced to identify patient outcomes and to control the use of resources. Reimbursement for services is dependent on meeting medical necessity and appropriateness guidelines and on the demonstrated effectiveness of nursing services.

2. The home care setting offers autonomy and flexibility in nursing practice. Nursing roles in psychiatric home care are in part determined by the education, experience, and abilities of the nurse. Psychiatric nurses practice in the home care setting at both basic and advanced levels. All psychiatric home care nurses are required to have experience with psychiatric patients.

3. Issues of importance to psychiatric home care nurses include cultural competence, flexibility in boundary setting, trust, and safety.

4. Psychiatric home care patients may have comorbid illnesses, few support systems, inadequate housing and finances, and variable levels of motivation for change. Comprehensive assessment, outcomes identification, and case management techniques are important aspects of the nursing process in home settings.

5. Special populations that can benefit from psychiatric home care include children and adolescents, older adults, patients with serious and persistent mental illness, and patients with HIV/AIDS.

Competent Caring A Clinical Exemplar of a Psychiatric Nurse

ROYCE SAMPSON, MSN, RN, CS

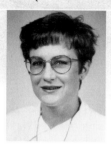

When I first saw this patient in his home, he was withdrawn and rarely spoke. He remained in his room all the time because he required total care and was incontinent of bowel and bladder. The medical history indicated that the patient had suffered a severe closed head injury several years before; he was aphasic and had a neurogenic bladder and bowel. His rehabilitation potential appeared poor. Through my multidimensional assessment of him and conversations with his family and home health aide, I identified multiple needs and strengths. By establishing a rapport with him and by gaining his trust, I was able to identify what he thought he needed to feel better. He wanted adequate food, care, security, and safety, and he wanted nursing home placement. I knew through my experience that many months would pass before nursing home placement could be obtained, if at all. After discussing all the alternatives with the patient and his family, we agreed on a few additional goals and selected a possible nursing home. I would help the family through the nursing home placement process and in the meantime would coordinate other services to meet his needs and maximize his ability to care for himself.

Through the assessment process, I identified that this patient was alert and oriented. He could communicate adequately and had through necessity (although unsafely) learned to transfer himself to his wheelchair. The home health aide also identified that the patient was capable of remaining continent if reminded. I talked to the patient about rehabilitation services in response to his remarks about his desire for increased independent mobility and function. He agreed that he would like to try these services. We decided that adult day-care services would be the best option to meet many of his needs with the limited community resources available.

Through negotiations with his physician and the other health-care providers, I arranged for the home health aide to get him ready for adult day care and for the bus to pick him up and take him to the center, where he would receive hot meals, group socialization, physical therapy, occupational therapy, and speech therapy. I also counseled his family about how they could better meet his needs at home. The patient had very limited social supports and financial resources and lived in a rural area, which complicated the process of meeting his needs. Home-delivered meals were unavailable, and the adult day-care bus did not usually travel to the patient's home.

Over the next few months the patient made tremendous progress. At day care, he met friends his own age from the boarding home that was attached to the center. These friends provided him with much-needed socialization. An added advantage was the motivation for self-care and independence that the peer group evoked in the patient. When he was with his peer group, he wheeled his wheelchair independently and toileted himself. Periodically, he stopped going to the day-care center, and the staff called me to intervene. The expense of my going to the patient's home when he refused to go to the center, as well as his loss in function when therapy was missed, might have led to the termination of all services. The recoordination of services was sometimes needed, but many times psychological support and counseling were indicated.

Therapy was painful, frustrating, and difficult for the patient. At times he was afraid of what his increasing independence would mean for him. If he became too independent, he would not be eligible for nursing home placement, and he did not want to remain in his home environment. We discussed the possibility of placement in a less restrictive environment, such as the boarding home where the day-care center and his friends were located, but the patient was afraid that he would not be able to maintain the level of independence the facility required. By spending much time counseling, by helping him to identify his abilities and the progress he had made, and by negotiating with the boarding home for a trial placement, I was able to help him gain enough self-confidence to try the boarding home placement. I maintained contact with the patient and the facility for the next month to ensure that he was appropriately placed and happy. The placement was a huge success.

Although I have always advocated maintaining a patient in his or her own home if possible, in this instance the patient's safety and security needs could not be adequately met at home. Boarding home placement not only met those needs but also helped him to obtain higher needs of socialization through his peer group, increased self-esteem through the confidence he gained by being able to function in a less restricted environment, and self-actualization through reaching for his maximum potential.

I learned a great deal from my involvement with this patient as I constantly reevaluated my own values and goals for him. I wanted the patient to reach his maximum potential, and I had faith in his ability. However, as he taught me time and time again, it was his goals on which I had to focus, and it was his belief in himself that I had to foster. My skills in collaboration, advocacy, coordination of services, counseling, and clinical nursing enabled me to attain a successful and satisfying outcome for my patient and a rewarding experience for me.

MERLIN Visit **MERLIN: www.mosby.com/MERLIN/Stuart** to find these additional materials and student activities.

- **Worksheets**
- **"Drug of the Month" Updates**
- **"Citing the Evidence" Updates**
- **Critical Thinking Activities and Exercises**
- **Annotated Suggested Readings**
- **Web Links**
- **More!**

Chapter Review Questions

1. **Identify whether the following statements are true (T) or false (F).**

____ A. The growth of managed care has contributed to the development of psychiatric home care programs.

____ B. As long as a patient is able to leave the house regardless of circumstances, he or she is ineligible for homebound status under Medicare guidelines.

____ C. Most managed care companies require preauthorization for psychiatric home care.

____ D. Medicare is a prospective payer.

____ E. If a home situation is identified as unsafe for the nurse, he or she must leave the home.

2. **Fill in the blanks.**

A. For Medicare to approve psychiatric home care, it is required that the patient _____, _____, and _____.

B. A patient who cannot access psychiatric follow-up independently and consistently can be described as _____.

C. One particularly effective role for the psychiatric home care nurse is that of _____.

D. The majority of home care is paid for by _____.

E. The two categories of the Medicare population with mental illness are _____ and _____.

F. The initial home health-care assessment should include the use of _____ to target and quantify symptoms and allow easier identification of progress toward goals.

G. The use of _____ can be one way to ensure the successful attainment of patient goals in a timely manner.

3. **Provide short answers for the following questions.**

A. Describe the advantages of home care in relation to inpatient psychiatric treatment.

B. Some people say that with home care, psychiatric nurses are "going back to their roots." Explain what is meant by this.

C. Many nurses believe there are few career options in psychiatry. Challenge this notion based on the expanding growth of psychiatric home and community care.

REFERENCES

Brown L: Legal and ethical issues in psychiatric home care, *Continuum* 3:187, 1996.

Carson V: Bay area health care psychiatric home care model, *Home Healthc Nurse* 13:26, 1995.

Daudell-Strejc D, Murphy C: Emerging clinical issues in home health psychiatric nursing, *Home Healthc Nurse* 13:17, 1995.

Duckworth C, Kitchens B: *An overview of psychiatric home health*, Tupelo, Miss, 1996, North Mississippi Medical Center Home Health Agency.

Duffy J: Beyond how to: theory-based management practice considerations for psychiatric home care, *Continuum* 3:163, 1996.

Duffy J, Miller M: Toward resolving the issue: in-home psychiatric nursing, *J Am Psychiatr Nurs Assoc* 2:104, 1996.

Felton B: The geropsychiatric clinical nurse specialist in home care, *Home Healthc Nurse* 15(9):635, 1997.

Freed P, Drake V: Mandatory reporting of abuse: practical, moral and legal issues for psychiatric home healthcare nurses, *Issue Ment Health Nurs* 20:423, 1999.

Freed P, Rice R: Managing mental illness at home. Part II: Clinical guidelines for psychiatric home health nurses, *Geriatr Nurs* 18(4):178, 1997.

Gonzales E et al: Management of psychiatric symptoms in medically ill patients in the homecare setting, *Crit Care Nurs Clin North Am* 10(3):315, 1998.

Iglesias G: Role evolution of the mental health clinical nurse specialist in home care, *Clin Nurs Spec* 12(1):38, 1998.

Klebanoff N: Mental health home care services: a review of current clinical issues, *Continuum* 3:147, 1996.

Mayo T: Mental health nurses in the home, *Home Healthc Nurs* 15(4):271, 1997.

Morris M: Patients' perceptions of psychiatric home care, *Arch Psychiatr Nurs* 10:176, 1996.

National Association for Home Care: *Basic statistics about home care*, Washington, DC, 2000, The Association.

Parlocha P, Henry S: The usefulness of the Georgetown Home Health Classification System for coding patient problems and nursing interventions in psychiatric home care, *Comput Nurs* 16(1):45, 1998.

Quinlan J, Ohlund G: Psychiatric home care, *Home Healthc Nurse* 13:20, 1995.

Soreff S: Psychiatric home care revisited: its scope and advantages, *Continuum* 1:71, 1994.

Spruhan J: Beyond traditional nursing care: cultural awareness and successful home healthcare nursing, *Home Healthc Nurse* 14:445, 1996.

Wendt D: Building trust during the initial home visit, *Home Healthc Nurse* 14:93, 1996.

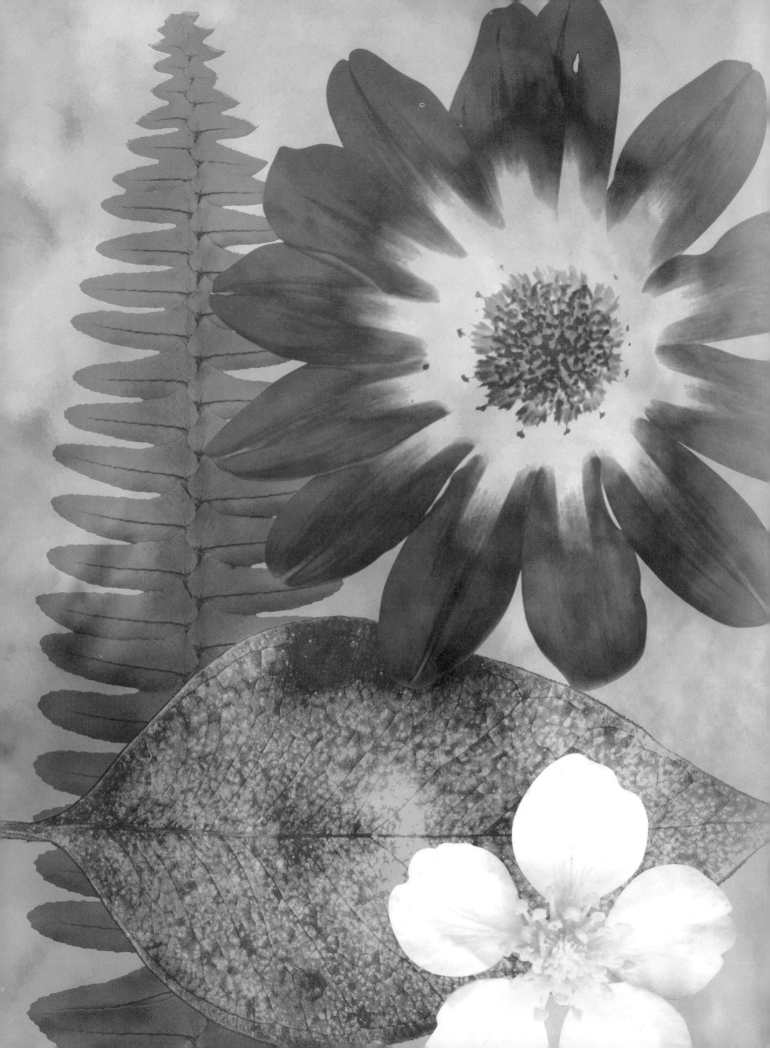

Unit 6
Special Populations in Psychiatry

Life is unfair. It is unfair that many people who are very young or very old may have to suffer in ways they are not even responsible for. But that is a reality of life that nurses, more than many others, need to understand and incorporate in their practice. It has been said that a society can be judged by how it treats its most vulnerable populations. Given that criterion, how would you rank American society? What level of compassion, protection, and caring is needed to make a society humane? What resources are given to health-care providers to educate, empower, and help heal these vulnerable groups? These are questions you may wrestle with the rest of your professional life.

In this unit you will enter the world of children, adolescents, and adults who are vulnerable to developing or being disabled by psychiatric illness. You will learn about their special needs and begin to search your heart and mind for ways to reach out and help them. In that sense, you have come to the end of your journey in this textbook. Your next passage as a professional nurse will be in other pages of your life. Good luck and godspeed.

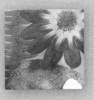

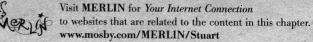

Visit **MERLIN** for *Your Internet Connection*
to websites that are related to the content in this chapter.
www.mosby.com/MERLIN/Stuart

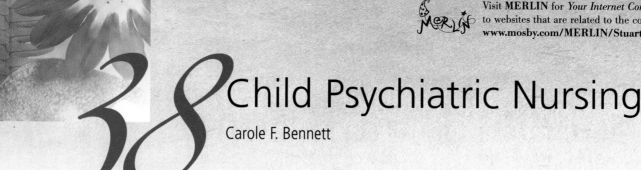

38 Child Psychiatric Nursing

Carole F. Bennett

Youth's love
Embracingly integrates
Successfully frustrates
And holds together,
Often unwittingly,
All that hate, fear, and selfishness
Attempt to disintegrate.

    R. Buckminster Fuller, *And It Came to Pass—Not to Stay*

In any given year, 9% to 13% of children suffer from clinically significant psychiatric disorders that should be treated, and suicide is the tenth leading cause of death among children ages 1 to 14 years (Weisz & Jensen, 1999; Workman & Prior, 1997). The Global Burden of Disease Study indicates that by the year 2020, childhood neuropsychiatric disorders will increase by more that 50% internationally to become one of the five most common causes of morbidity, mortality, and disability among children in the world. There is also evidence that alcohol and drug use begins by age 8 years in some children and can be a significant problem by age 12 years. Studies have found that 50% of eighth graders have used alcohol more than once, that marijuana has been smoked by 2% of eighth graders, and that increasing numbers of children are inhaling butane, glue, and gasoline (Finke & Bowman, 1997).

These statistics concerning psychiatric problems among children are alarming. Adding to this concern is the increase

in school-related shootings and other violent behavior displayed by young children in family and community settings. However, only 25% to 36% of children with mental disorders currently receive any form of treatment.

Another disturbing issue is the prognosis of a child who has been diagnosed with a psychiatric illness. For example, there is an established association between conduct disorder in a child and the development of antisocial personality disorder (Kasen et al, 1999). So, too, research suggests that prior anxiety, behavior, and mood disorders all increase the likelihood of the child having psychiatric problems as an adult (Shaw et al, 1998; Pine & Cohen, 1999).

Thus childhood disorders appear to set in motion a chain of maladaptive behaviors and environmental responses that foster more persistent psychopathology over time. These findings emphasize the importance of early identification and treatment of these children in order to reduce the risk for psychiatric disorders reaching into their adult lives (Seed, 1999).

PSYCHIATRIC ILLNESS IN CHILDREN
Systems of Care

Some states now offer psychiatric services to children in a wide variety of settings that together make up systems of care. Such systems are organized to be child centered and family focused, with the needs of the family dictating the types of services that are offered to each child. Systems of care for children are comprehensive and community based, offering a broad array of services. They are sometimes called "wraparound" services because they are meant to include all aspects of a child's life. The major goals of these treatment systems are as follows:

- Develop and provide a full array of community-based services for children with psychiatric illnesses and their families
- Reduce reliance on restrictive treatment environments and out-of-home placements
- Facilitate interagency coordination and collaboration in planning, developing, and delivering services
- Increase education to families and promote appropriate parenting skills
- Provide flexible, individualized services tailored to the unique needs of each child and family
- Contain costs and demonstrate the cost-effectiveness of systems of care for children

While conceptually sound, the evidence supporting this type of care is mixed. Some studies have found that while access to care, type of care, and amount of care were better in the comprehensive systems, many children who did not receive these enhanced services improved at the same rate as children who received these services (Bickman et al, 1999; Stroul et al, 1997). Thus more research is needed to demonstrate the efficacy and cost-effectiveness of these services.

In each of these settings, whether they are hospital based or community based, nurses are crucial members of the treatment team. Nurses function as team members, team leaders, milieu managers, case managers, therapists, prescribers, and program directors. They participate in assessment, treatment planning, and implementation of care in children's mental health services in all settings.

Etiology

Historically, discovering the cause of a mental illness in large part determined the approach to treatment. Etiological theories have proposed both genetic factors (nature) and childhood experiences (nurture) as predisposing and precipitating causes for the development of a psychiatric illness. It is now recognized that both nature and nurture play a role in the development of health and illness. With the current understanding of the roles of neurotransmitters and brain development, the effect of experience combined with genetic predisposition begins to explain the complexity of the development of child psychiatric illness (Keltner, 1996).

Traumatic events, for example, have been recognized to have a profound impact on children (see Citing the Evidence). The symptoms that are characteristic of posttrau-

---

Citing the Evidence on

Sexually Abused Children

BACKGROUND: This study examined the 5-year outcome of sexually abused children as compared to children who had not been abused.

RESULTS: The abused children displayed more disturbed behavior, had lower self-esteem, were more depressed or unhappy, and were more anxious than the controls. They also had higher levels of bingeing, self-injury, and suicide attempts.

IMPLICATIONS: It is clear that many children who have been sexually abused have ongoing problems. These problems may be indicative of false beliefs about themselves and the sexual abuse experience.

Swanston H et al: Sexually abused children 5 years after presentation: a case-control study, *Pediatrics* 100(4):600, 1997.

---

matic stress disorder (PTSD) in children are those of increased arousal, including hypervigilance, irritability, anxiety, physiological hyperactivity, impulsivity, and sleep difficulty. These symptoms are often also diagnosed as attention deficit–hyperactivity disorder (ADHD), conduct disorder, anxiety disorder, and mood disorder.

It is now also recognized that the particular constellation of symptoms a child experiences are often related to the family history. Specifically, if a family member has a history of anxiety disorder, the child may experience symptoms that are more anxious in appearance. However, if family members have a strong history of alcoholism and sociopathy, symptoms may pertain more to conduct disorder. Thus it is believed that there is a genetic predisposition to certain symptoms and that these symptoms can be stimulated as a response to an event in the environment.

After traumatic events, many factors are important in the development of the intensity of symptoms, including the nature of the trauma, the degree to which body integrity is threatened, the threat posed by the event to the child's self-system and security, and the nature of the family support system. The neurophysiology activated during acute stress is usually rapid and reversible. The brain has mechanisms that down-regulate the stress reaction after the threat has passed, returning the brain to its prior level of functioning. However, if the stress is prolonged, severe, or repetitive, the resulting increases in neurotransmitter activity are often not reversible.

This process has a significant impact on the development of the child's brain. A trauma-induced brain response would probably result in abnormal patterns, time, and intensity of catecholamine activity in the developing brain. Young children who are exposed to a high rate of stress-induced trauma are at risk for developing permanent changes in neuronal organization, making it more difficult for them to learn and to control their behavior.

Other psychiatric illnesses, such as ADHD, also illustrate the interplay of genetics and environment (Ludwikowski & DeValk, 1998; Glod, 1997). Children with ADHD usually have excessive activity and difficulty paying attention. These behaviors are often tolerated by a family. However, when these children begin school, they are identified as problematic because these behaviors interfere with the child's academic performance and peer relationships. As in PTSD, children with ADHD often have a range of symptoms, including symptoms that overlap with anxiety disorders, oppositional defiant disorder, and conduct disorder.

Although the precise etiology of ADHD remains unclear, it is believed that environmental factors such as lead ingestion, prenatal and perinatal complications, socioeconomic factors, genetic factors, and brain dysfunction resulting from brain damage may contribute to the development of the illness. No one finding has adequately explained this complex disorder, but there is agreement that it has a neurobiological basis. However, by the time a child and family seek treatment, the child may have developed secondary mental health problems such as low self-esteem and poor socialization. Thus the effect of this illness on the child is significantly mediated by its severity, the ability of the family to cope with the illness, and the secondary symptoms that result.

As these two examples show, psychiatric illness in children is complex and can be debilitating for both the child and the family. Treatment usually involves the combination of medication to improve brain function, social skills training to improve socialization, behavior management to learn impulse control, cognitive therapy to practice problem solving and communication, and parent education to integrate the new behaviors and skills into the child's life.

> *Do you think that the incidence of child abuse is increasing in the United States or that it is the same as in years before and is simply being discussed more openly?*

A Framework for Nursing Practice

To help organize this complex approach and individualize care to each child's needs, a skill development framework is presented in this chapter. This approach can be used in hospital, community, and home treatment settings. It is applicable to any psychiatric diagnosis that a child may have and includes the parents as partners in the treatment plan as they work with the child to incorporate these learning skills into family interactions.

Nurses are challenged to derive realistic, well-defined goals, respond to the complex social needs of the child, understand and advocate for the child, and develop a comprehensive treatment plan that identifies and integrates the child's needs and resources. All of this must be done with the realization that the behavior of children is largely culturally based and must be viewed from a sociocultural perspective.

Organizing child psychiatric nursing care around ego competency skills is an effective and culturally sensitive way of planning and implementing nursing interventions for children regardless of psychiatric diagnosis or setting. The nine skills that all children need to become competent adults include the following (Strayhorn, 1989):

- Establishing closeness and trusting relationships
- Handling separation and independent decision making
- Negotiating joint decisions and interpersonal conflict
- Dealing with frustration and unfavorable events
- Celebrating good feelings and experiencing pleasure
- Working for delayed gratification
- Relaxing and playing
- Cognitive processing through words, symbols, and images
- Establishing an adaptive sense of direction and purpose

Often a child's maladaptive responses are expressed differently from those of an adult. To develop the nursing plan the nurse must learn to recognize and describe symptomatic behavior in children. It is helpful to use a specific assessment form, such as the one presented in Fig. 38-1 (pp. 760-761), that identifies both competency skills and nursing diagnoses related to particular skill deficits to more fully describe the child's response or experience. Such a form would be used in addition to a standard nursing assessment tool completed by the nurse for each child.

The nurse should talk with the child about the child's strengths and then discuss the skills that need further development. Strategies used to teach these skills can be explained to the child and the parents, which allows them to become active participants in the planning of nursing care. Children will be more motivated to cooperate if they are encouraged to sign a copy of their care plan after it has been explained to them. Even if they cannot write, a mark that represents their name is sufficient to signify their participation in the process. Nursing interventions can then be designed to improve the maladaptive responses and teach the accompanying skill.

ASSESSING THE CHILD

Assessment of the child requires a biopsychosocial approach with attention given to the contribution of biological development, medical illness, cognitive and personality characteristics, cultural context, and the child's family, school, and social environment (AACAP, 1997). The components of a psychiatric assessment are shown in Box 38-1, p. 762. Behavior rating scales that can also be used with children are listed in Box 38-2, p. 762.

The nursing assessment focuses on the specific skills that all children need to become competent adults. Regardless of medical diagnosis, a child should be assessed for mastery of the nine ego competency skills that are now described (see Fig. 38-1).

Ego Competency Skills

Skill 1: Establishing Closeness and Trusting Relationships. A basic skill for positive growth and development is the child's ability to establish close and trusting relationships with others. Children with the medical diagnosis of generalized anxiety disorder may have difficulty establishing trusting relationships because they are very concerned about their perceived competency. The following questions are used to evaluate this skill:

- Does the child enjoy making friends?
- Does the child often feel picked on by other people?
- Does the child not know what to say when getting to know someone?

To reinforce this skill, nursing staff should encourage interaction and be attentive to the child without being intrusive. Talking with the child in a face-to-face position and offering nurturance are beginning nursing actions. Trust can then be demonstrated by the staff in their interactions with the child. If a child violates a trust, a discussion of the issue should take place, allowing trust to be reestablished. In this way children learn about acknowledging mistakes and the importance of forgiveness in developing trusting relationships.

Skill 2: Handling Separation and Independent Decision Making. Children who have separation anxiety have great difficulty tolerating separation from their mother or home. Yet individuation is an important mental health process. Being able to identify and express feelings and make independent decisions is critical to becoming a competent individual. The following questions are used to evaluate this skill:

- Does the child get upset or worry when away from his or her mother?
- Does the child get upset or worry if he or she thinks someone does not like him or her?
- When upset, is there something the child can do to feel better?

Nursing interventions that focus on helping the child identify and clarify aspects of the self are critical exercises for promoting individuation. This may be done in many ways, such as by encouraging children to draw self-portraits, interviewing staff members regarding their opinions on an issue, or identifying personality differences between themselves and others. Any experience that clarifies differences between individuals helps the child to identify himself or herself as a unique individual in a social context. In the therapeutic milieu, opportunities also can be provided for the child to make choices and decisions, further supporting the child's growing sense of individuality and ego competency.

Skill 3: Handling Joint Decision Making and Interpersonal Conflict. Children who have not been allowed to participate in joint decision making or who have not been rewarded for cooperating may be deficient in this skill. A child with oppositional defiant disorder may use aggression instead of negotiation to respond to interpersonal conflict. However, learning the skill of joint decision making is critical for success in interpersonal relationships. The following questions are used to evaluate this skill:

- When the child has a problem, can he or she usually think of several solutions?
- Does the child get angry if he or she does not get his or her way?
- Do other people make the child agitated or easily upset?

The therapeutic milieu can provide an opportunity for the child to learn and practice these skills. For example, the nurse can set up opportunities for problem solving. Exercises may be developed for making group decisions in which cooperation and collaboration are rewarded. The child should be helped to identify fears related to cooperating with others, and assertiveness can be modeled and taught. It is important that the nurse not resolve conflicts for the child. Rather, these situations should be used to teach negotiating skills and shape appropriate socialization through the use of reinforcement.

> *Games can be useful in teaching cooperation and compromise to children. What games can you identify that would be particularly helpful in teaching children this important skill?*

Skill 4: Dealing with Frustration and Unfavorable Events. Tolerating frustration, although difficult, is critical to becoming a competent adult. Children with conduct disorders often have difficulty understanding a situation from another's perspective. The following questions are used to evaluate this skill:

- Does the child feel bad if he or she has hurt someone's feelings?
- If someone disagrees with the child, does it make him or her angry?
- Does the child not like playing a game if he or she loses?

Children who have little frustration tolerance become angry easily and are often unable to complete tasks. Children typically learn this skill through cooperation and competition in playing childhood games. However, if a child has not had the opportunity to play games in this way and if tolerance has not been modeled for the child, he or she probably has not developed this skill. The child will experience numerous frustrations during the course of treatment. The nurse should use these opportunities to think through the process with the child and help increase the child's frustration tolerance and anger control.

> *Do you think that a child's ability to handle frustration and stressful events is influenced by biological makeup? If so, does biology excuse people from being responsible for their actions?*

Skill 5: Celebrating Good Feelings and Feeling Pleasure. Healthy children raised in a nurturing environment naturally experience good feelings and pleasure. However, children who are depressed or anxious are not able to celebrate good feelings or experience spontaneous pleasure. Also, in a maladaptive environment shame is often used to control children's behavior, with the result that they feel guilty for having angry or unacceptable thoughts. Consequently, they may lose the ability to celebrate life and feel pleasure. The following questions are used to evaluate this skill:

- Does the child worry about the future a lot?
- Does the child not like it when people say good things about him or her?
- Does the child feel good about the things he or she does well?

Questions used to evaluate competency skills are presented on the left. Nursing diagnoses related to these skills appear at the right. The screened response (N = 0 or Y = 1) represents the appropriate competency skill. A patient score of 2 or 3 indicates a skill deficit, and the nurse should then select an appropriate nursing diagnosis based on the child's history and presenting problem.

SCORE 1. _____	**Establishing Closeness and Trusting Relationships**	
N Y	1. I like making friends.	Fear
N Y	2. People pick on me a lot.	Anxiety
N Y	3. I don't know what to say when I am getting to know someone.	Posttrauma Response Family Processes Altered Growth and Development Altered

SCORE 2. _____	**Handling Separation and Independent Decision Making**	
N Y	1. I'm upset when I am away from my mom and worry about her.	Self-Esteem, Chronic Low
N Y	2. If I think someone does not like me, I worry and get upset.	Anxiety Thought Processes Altered
N Y	3. When I am upset, there is something I can do to feel better.	Coping, Ineffective Individual

SCORE 3. _____	**Handling Joint Decisions and Interpersonal Conflict**	
N Y	1. When I have a problem, I can usually think of several solutions.	Social Interaction Impaired
N Y	2. If I do not get my way, it makes me mad.	Communication Impaired, Verbal
N Y	3. Other people get on my nerves a lot.	Violence, Potential for Decisional Conflict

SCORE 4. _____	**Dealing with Frustration and Unfavorable Events**	
N Y	1. If I have hurt someone's feelings, I think about it and feel bad.	Social Interaction Impaired
N Y	2. If someone disagrees with me, it makes me mad.	
N Y	3. I do not like playing a game if I lose.	

SCORE 5. _____	**Celebrating Good Feelings, Feeling Pleasure**	
N Y	1. I worry about the future a lot.	Hopelessness
N Y	2. When people say good things to me, I don't like it for some reason.	Body Image Disturbance
N Y	3. There are things I do well, and it makes me feel good.	

SCORE 6. _____	**Working for Delayed Gratification**	
N Y	1. Most rules are reasonable and I don't mind following them.	Growth and Development Altered
N Y	2. I find it hard to be honest; sometimes, lying is the only thing I do.	Sexuality Patterns Altered
N Y	3. I get mad if my mother dosen't get me what I want.	

Fig. 38-1 Competency skills assessment form.

SCORE 7._____	Relaxing and Playing	
N Y	1. There are some things I really enjoy doing.	Social Isolation Grieving-Anticipatory Sleep Pattern Disturbance
N Y	2. I have lots of fun.	
N Y	3. I enjoy sitting around and thinking about things.	

SCORE 8._____	Cognitive Processing through Words, Symbols, and Images	
N Y	1. It is hard for me to describe how I feel to someone.	Growth and Development Altered Social Interaction Impaired Thought Process Altered Anxiety
N Y	2. I never know how something is going to turn out for me.	
N Y	3. I know what my strengths are.	

SCORE 9._____	An Adaptive Sense of Direction and Purpose	
N Y	1. I feel my life is going to get better.	Personal Identity Disturbance Family Coping, Potential for Growth Hopelessness
N Y	2. I am confused about growing up and don't know what to do about it.	
N Y	3. I know school is important and going is my job in life right now.	

Fig. 38-1—cont'd   Competency skills assessment form.

A healthy environment is one in which celebrating good feelings and feeling pleasure are natural, spontaneous occurrences. Celebrating and having fun are important nursing interventions. These activities should not be confined to holidays but should be part of the child's weekly activities. Children's families can be invited to participate in these celebrations, where nursing staff model having fun with the children. In this way, children and their families learn the skill of celebrating good feelings and feeling pleasure.

How often and in what ways did your family celebrate good feelings and experience pleasure when you were growing up? How do you incorporate this in your life today?

Skill 6: Working for Delayed Gratification. As children grow they are expected to delay needed gratification by following rules and waiting their turn. This skill is often difficult for impulsive children with ADHD or conduct disorder to achieve. The following questions are used to evaluate this skill:
- Does the child believe that most rules are reasonable and does he or she not mind following them?
- Does the child find it difficult to be honest and think that lying is the only thing to do?
- Does the child get angry if his or her mother doesn't give what he or she wants?

Delayed gratification can be taught by the nurse through the earning of points for daily expectations, such as tidying one's room or completing homework assignments. Children's games, such as Red Light, in which they respond to "stop" and "wait" commands, are also useful in teaching this skill to younger children. As a child's behavior improves, the reward for the points earned can require the accumulation of many points or tokens. Thus the child is given the opportunity to delay the reinforcer for a reward of higher value to be received at a later time. As the child learns greater self-control, he or she will be better able to delay gratification for longer periods of time.

Skill 7: Relaxing and Playing. Given the stressful environment of current family life, many children may have little opportunity to learn the skill of relaxing and playing. For children with mood, anxiety, or behavior disorders, learning to relax and play is an important skill. The following questions are used to evaluate this skill:
- Are there some things the child really enjoys doing?
- Can the child have lots of fun?
- Does the child enjoy sitting around and thinking about things?

Time should be devoted to learning this skill. Children should be given unstructured play time in which the staff participate with them in playing games. Having spontaneous talent shows or other forms of fun can contribute to a child's well-being. In this way, relaxing and playing become part of the therapeutic experience and children learn to value and master this skill.

Skill 8: Cognitive Processing through Words, Symbols, and Images. Children with psychiatric illnesses may not have developed the important skill of cognitive processing. The following questions are used to evaluate this skill:

- Is it difficult for the child to describe how he or she feels?
- Does the child feel as if he or she never knows how something is going to turn out?
- Can the child identify his or her strengths?

A responsive environment should be created to stimulate children's cognitive development. Furnishings and toys, communications and interactions, and group experiences should all be designed to support the child's cognitive processing. The nurse can help the child learn this skill by encouraging abstract thinking whenever possible, such as by asking "What is the moral of the story?" or "What point do you think the movie was trying to communicate?" Children who are encouraged to express themselves in a responsive environment will gain greater competency in this important area of development.

Skill 9: Adaptive Sense of Direction and Purpose. Children who experience symptoms of mental illness may feel hopeless about their purpose in life. As they view adult life from watching those around them, they begin to draw conclusions about themselves in the world. The following questions are used to evaluate this skill:

- Does the child feel that his or her life is going to get better?
- Is the child confused about growing up and doesn't know what to do about it?
- Does the child believe that school is important and see it as his or her job in life at present?

Having role models for healthy, meaningful adult experiences is essential to healthy growth and development. Feeling valued as an individual provides the child with an opportunity to learn to value others. Nurses should actively listen to children in their interactions, and even young children should be encouraged to express their needs and feelings. The child's importance as a person can be shown through the approach the nurse uses in providing basic care. Older children can benefit from more in-depth discussions and the use of journals to gain perspective on the direction of their lives. Above all, the nurse should actively help all children realistically assess their abilities and potential to contribute to a better world.

Box 38-1

Child Assessment Components

FAMILY INTERVIEW

Define the problem(s), developmental and family history (genogram), parental mental and physical health, family interactions (see Chapter 34)

INTERVIEW WITH THE CHILD

Mental state: Do they have a problem? School experiences, friendship, play, and teasing. Worries, fears, mood (including tears and suicidal ideas), expression of anger, sleep and appetite, habits and obsessions, and (when indicated) inquire about sexual/physical abuse, auditory hallucinations, and delusional ideas

Development of conscience and values, interests, hobbies, talents

Supplement the interview by play and drawing (ask the child to draw a person/family/dream)

Physical examination: including assessment of handedness, motor coordination, or clumsiness

STRUCTURED QUESTIONNAIRE RATING SCALES (see Box 38-2)

Provide an overall scale score and problem domain subscale scores

OTHER INVESTIGATIONS

Psychological tests (e.g., IQ profile)—indicated when there are learning problems, delayed or uneven development, cognitive or perceptual disturbances

Laboratory tests (e.g., chromosome analysis)—indicated when there is the possibility of an associated biological problem, such as fragile X syndrome or thyroid disease

Neuroimaging and electroencephalogram—indicated when there may be associated neurological disorder such as epilepsy

---

Box 38-2

Behavioral Rating Scales Related to Children

- ADHD Rating Scale-IV
- Ansell-Casey Life Skills Assessment 2.0 (ACLSA)
- Brief Psychiatric Rating Scale (BPRS) for Children
- Caregiver-Teacher Report Form for Ages 2-5 (C-TRF/2.5)
- Child and Adolescent Adjustment Profile (CAAP)
- Child and Adolescent Functional Assessment Scale (CAFAS)
- Child Assessment Schedule (CAS)
- Child Behavior Checklist (CBCL)
- Child Depression Inventory
- Children's Depression Rating Scale, R (CDRS-R)
- Children's Global Assessment Scale (CGAS)
- Columbia Impairment Scale
- Competency Skills Questionnaire (CSQ)
- Conners Parent and Teacher Rating Scale–Home and School Questionnaire
- Developmental Behavior Checklist
- Devereux Rating Scale School Form (DSF)
- Direct Observation Form and Profile for Ages 5-14 (DOF)
- Ohio Youth Problems, Functioning, and Satisfaction Scales
- Revised Behavior Problem Checklist
- Self-Control Rating Scale
- Severity of Psychiatric Illness: Child and Adolescent Version
- Tennessee Self Concept Scale: Second Edition (TSCS-2)
- Vanderbilt Functioning Inventory (VFI)
- Yale-Brown Obsessive Compulsive Scale (YBOCS) for Children
- Youth Outcome Questionnaire (YOQ)

Many people believe that youth in contemporary society lack a sense of hope, direction, and purpose in life. Do you agree with this, and if so, what sociocultural factors might influence the learning of this skill?

DIAGNOSES
Medical Diagnoses

Children with psychiatric illness experience disabling symptoms that are responses to biological alterations, traumatizing situations, and maladaptive learning. The *DSM–IV–TR* classifies disorders usually first evident in infancy, childhood, or adolescence by separating them into 10 major groups (American Psychiatric Association, 2000). These diagnostic categories and their essential features are listed in Table 38-1.

Children can also experience a number of psychiatric illnesses common to adults. Four of the most common psychiatric disorders in childhood are anxiety, depression, conduct disorder, and ADHD. There is a range of efficacious psychosocial and pharmacological treatments for each of these disorders (Weisz & Jensen, 1999; U.S. Department of Health and Human Services, 1999). Table 38-2 summarizes the symptoms, family factors, and management strategies for each of these disorders.

Anxiety Disorders. The most common sign of anxiety in children is fear of being separated from parents and home and refusal to attend school. The prevalence of anxiety is highest at times of transition: moving from preschool to primary school, and from primary to secondary school. Children who refuse to attend school are usually capable but self-critical students, and most have separation anxiety, being frightened to leave home. The prognosis is good with treatment, but persistent anxiety disorder predicts the development of panic disorder in adulthood (Silverman et al, 1999; Ollendick & King, 1998).

Depression. Contrary to earlier beliefs, persistent depression occurs in children and becomes progressively more common after puberty. Up to 14% of children will experience an episode of major depression before age 15 years. It seriously affects social, emotional and educational development and is the most important predictor of suicidal behavior in young people age 15 to 24 years.

Although the symptoms of depression in children are similar to those seen in adults, they also usually have irritable mood, may fail to make expected weight gain, and tend to keep secret their depressive thoughts and crying. Depression can also occur in combination with another disorder such as anxiety, conduct disorder, or ADHD. The prognosis is good when the depression is secondary to a life stress and responds to psychological treatment (Kaslow & Thompson, 1998). A positive family history of mood disorder and a good response to antidepressant medication indicate an increased risk of further depressive or bipolar disorder in adult life.

Table **38-1**

DSM–IV–TR Disorders of Infancy, Childhood, and Adolescence	
Disorder	**Essential Features**
Mental retardation	Significantly subaverage intellectual functioning with an IQ of approximately 70 or less. Mild retardation = 55-70 Moderate retardation = 40-55 Severe retardation = 25-40 Profound retardation = less than 25
Learning disorders	Functioning that is below that expected given the person's chronological age, measured intelligence, and age-appropriate education. May be evident in the areas of reading, mathematics, or written expression.
Motor skills disorder	Motor coordination is substantially below that expected given the person's chronological age and measured intelligence.
Communication disorders	Difficulty with receptive or expressive language or the articulation of speech.
Pervasive developmental disorders	Impairment in a variety of indicators related to normal growth and developmental milestones, including social interaction, communication, and the display of restricted, repetitive, and stereotyped patterns of behavior, interest, and activities (autistic disorder).
Attention deficit and disruptive behavior disorders	Behaviors related to inattention that are maladaptive and inconsistent with the child's developmental level (attention deficit or hyperactivity disorder); violation of the basic rights of others (conduct disorder); or negativism, hostility, and defiance (oppositional defiant disorder).
Feeding and eating disorders of infancy and early childhood	Behaviors related to eating of nonnutritive substances (pica), regurgitation and rechewing of food (rumination disorder), and failure to eat adequately (feeding disorder).
Tic disorders	An involuntary, sudden, rapid, recurrent, nonrhythmic, stereotyped movement or vocalization (Tourette's disorder).
Elimination disorders	Repeated passage of feces in inappropriate places after age 4 years (encopresis) or voiding of urine into bed or clothes after age 5 years (enuresis).
Separation anxiety disorder	Inappropriate and excessive anxiety concerning separation from home or from those to whom the child is attached.

Table **38-2**

Symptoms, Family Factors, and Management of Pediatric Disorders Common in Children			
Disorder	Symptoms	Family Factors	Management
Anxiety	Distress and agitation when separated from parent and home School refusal Pervasive worry and fearfulness Restlessness and irritability Timidity, shyness, social withdrawal Terror of an object (e.g., dog) Associated headache, stomach pains Restless sleep and nightmares Poor concentration, distractibility, and learning problems Reliving stressful event in repetitive play	Parental anxiety, overprotection, separation difficulties Parental (maternal) depression and agoraphobia Family stress: marital conflict, parental illness, child abuse Family history of anxiety	Cognitive-behavioral therapy Treat parental anxiety/depression Interpersonal psychotherapy Teacher support Drug therapy (tricyclic antidepressants or selective serotonin reuptake inhibitor) as adjunct to psychological interventions
Depression	Persistent depressed mood, unhappiness, and irritability Loss of interest in play and friends Loss of energy and concentration Deterioration in school work Loss of appetite and no weight gain Disturbed sleep Thoughts of worthlessness and suicide Somatic complaints (headache, abdominal pain) Comorbid anxiety, conduct disorder, attention deficit–hyperactivity disorder, eating disorders or substance abuse	Family stress (ill or deceased parent, family conflict, parental separation) Repeated experience of failure or criticism Family history of depression	Cognitive-behavioral therapy Family therapy for grief and conflict Interpersonal psychotherapy Success achievement school programs Antidepressant drug therapy
Conduct disorder	Persistent disruptive and antisocial behavior Hostile, defiant, spiteful, vindictive behavior Aggression toward people and animals Vandalism, fire lighting Truancy, lying, stealing Acting alone (about 20%) Acting with group (about 80%) Hyperactive (about 30%) and with learning problems (about 50%) Depression, low self-esteem (about 20%) Running away from home	Social disadvantage Inconsistent, hostile parenting Parental conflict Foster home/institutional care Parental criminality Child abuse and family violence Antisocial peer groups	Early intervention: parenting-skills training Cognitive problem-solving skills training Parent management training Functional family therapy Multisystem therapy (MST) Creating opportunities for success in sport and recreation Success achievement in educational programs Behavior treatment (social skills)
Attention deficit–hyperactivity disorder	Inattention Carelessness Does not listen Does not follow through Interrupts and cannot wait turn, talks excessively Avoids difficult tasks Fidgets, unable to sit still Forgetful, distractible, disorganized Impulsive Anxiety/depression (in about 20%) Difficult temperament Learning disabilities	Pregnancy and perinatal complications with soft neurological signs (brain impairment) (e.g., clumsiness) Family conflict and parenting problems (may be a reaction)	Parenting-skills training and home help Educational program for learning disabilities Environment modification to reduce distraction Tasks in small steps to channel energy Contingency management Behavior therapy Family therapy for conflict Stimulant drug therapy (good efficacy in the short-term; long-term benefits have not yet been assessed)

Table 38-3

Ego Competency Skills Summary

Competency Skill	Developmental Stage and Tasks	Related Nursing Diagnosis	Nursing Care for Skill Deficit
Trusting, closeness, relationship building	**Infancy** Trust Attachment Learning to walk, talk, and feed self	Anxiety Posttrauma response Altered family processes Altered growth and development	Encourage interaction. Use face-to-face positioning. Use touch (when appropriate) and nurturance. Offer food and transitional objects. Be attentive without being unnecessarily intrusive. Offer nurturance to the child's mother. Make attempts to connect family to child. Take time to develop relationship through play.
Handling separation and independence	**Toddlers** Autonomy Separation Toilet training Learning right from wrong	Chronic low self-esteem Anxiety Altered thought processes	Offer frequent exercise and motor activities. Allow child opportunities to make choices. Offer transitional object. Take control if child is out of control; otherwise let child have some control. Set limits and boundaries to help the child feel secure.
Handling joint decisions and interpersonal conflicts	**Preschoolers** Initiative Tolerance of others Sexual identity Socialization Developing a conscience	Social interaction, impaired Impaired verbal communication Violence, potential for Decisional conflict	Set up opportunities for problem solving and cooperative thinking. Help child to identify fears through books, art, play. Shape appropriate socialization using reinforcement. Become model for conflict resolution.
Dealing with frustration and unfavorable events Celebrating good things, feeling pleasure	**Middle childhood** Industry Physical skill development Peer relationships Learning to read, write, and calculate Development of morality and values	Social interaction, impaired Hopelessness Body image disturbance	Help the child to cope with frustration using stories and plays. Model cooperation and reinforce cooperative behavior. Do not use shame or humiliation to gain control. Have fun with the child. Use community meetings for peer support and modeling. Use positive reinforcement for child's strengths and abilities.
Working for delayed gratification Relaxing and playing	**Early adolescence** Identity Role acceptance New relations with peers of both sexes	Altered growth and development Altered sexuality patterns Anticipatory grieving Sleep pattern disturbance	Use daily expectations and games to teach delayed gratification. Encourage self-reinforcement. Encourage playfulness at appropriate times.
Cognitive processing Adaptive sense of direction and purpose	**Later adolescence** Emotional and economic independence from parents Preparation for occupation Civic responsibility	Altered growth and development Social interaction, impaired Altered thought process Anxiety Personal identify disturbance Family coping, potential for growth Hopelessness	Offer games that use cognitive processing. Discuss abstractions such as the moral of stories or movies. Actively listen to and encourage the expression of needs and goals. In community meetings discuss relevant issues and life events. Help the child to realistically assess his or her ability and potential.

Conduct Disorder. Serious and persistent patterns of disturbed conduct and antisocial behavior predominantly affect boys and comprise the largest group of childhood psychiatric disorders. Conduct disturbance may begin early in childhood, as oppositional, aggressive, and defiant behavior, becoming established during the primary school years and increasing after puberty. The presence of other psychological disorders is common in these children, with about 30% showing ADHD and learning problems. Clinical depression is also found in about 20% of young people with conduct disorder.

This group of childhood disorders requires vigorous early intervention, assessment, and management because, although about a third make a reasonable adjustment, there is evidence that at least half of the young people with serious conduct disorder will continue to experience mental health and psychosocial problems in adult life, such as personality disorder, criminality, and alcoholism (Brestan & Euburg, 1998).

Attention Deficit-Hyperactivity Disorder (ADHD). Controversy exists regarding the exact nature of this disorder. It is estimated that 3% to 5% of children have ADHD, and it is more common in boys than girls (National Institutes of Health, 1998). There is usually a history of difficult and uneven development from infancy. It is likely that the disorder has a neurobiological basis that is complicated by family interactions and the progressive consequences of related learning problems.

Evidence suggests that the young person does not necessarily grow out of the problem. Symptoms tend to persist, although adolescents usually become more goal directed and less impulsive, channeling activity into sport or work if the opportunity is possible (Cipkala-Gaffin, 1998; Pelham et al, 1998). The outcome is less favorable for those who have an associated conduct disorder. In these cases there is an increased risk of continuing to have mental health, personality, and social adjustment problems.

Nursing Diagnoses

Regardless of the child's medical diagnosis, nursing care must be focused on the child's response to illness and the nursing interventions designed to teach and model to the child and family more adaptive coping responses and improved methods of functioning. Thus nursing diagnosis and intervention proceed independently of and concurrently with medical diagnosis and treatment. Although nursing and medicine have collaborative roles, nursing has a critical and distinct contribution to make in the care of the child with psychiatric illness. Child psychiatric nurses should refer to the ANA *Standards of Child and Adolescent Psychiatric and Mental Health Nursing Practice* when implementing care (American Nurses' Association, 1985).

Once the nurse has completed the ego competency skill assessment, the appropriate nursing diagnosis should be formulated. Nursing interventions can then be identified for each competency skill deficit, developmental stage, and related nursing diagnoses as summarized in Table 38-3.

Altered Family Processes. The family should be included in the child's treatment process as soon as possible (Scharer, 1999). Psychiatric illness in any one family member affects all other family members. In addition, the most common problem that precipitates hospitalization in children is the inability of the family to control the child at home. When the need for hospitalization is identified, the parents have usually exhausted all immediately available resources. A combination of reflective thinking with the parents about their child, clarifying problems, and behavioral parent training provides the best results in reducing family stress (Elder, 1997).

The nurse should focus on the needs of each family and either promote family competence through education and support or engage the family in specific clinical interventions, such as family therapy (see Chapter 34). In addition, some children with psychiatric problems may not have had consistent nurturing or may come from families that display maladaptive responses. Therefore activities that are less threatening should be used initially to teach the child about family relationships. Pictures of families cut out from magazines can provide opportunities for a child to interpret emotional content in the picture and describe what he or she thinks is happening in the picture. The nurse can then describe a healthy family scenario for the child to learn about adaptive family functioning.

> *Many people believe that families are in crisis in the United States. Describe the evidence for this conclusion, and give specific ways to address these problems.*

Altered Growth and Development. Normal growth and development in childhood require a supportive, nurturing environment. A child with a psychiatric illness often has delayed physical and emotional development. However, through carefully planned nursing interventions, a child can be taught the skills that have not yet been developed. For example, for the child to achieve independence in dressing, grooming, and room cleaning, a checklist can be made using pictures instead of words. Points can then be given for each accomplished task. Using similar behavioral interventions (see Chapter 32), the nurse can help the child to make significant gains in the area of growth and development.

When considering altered growth and development, delays are often the presenting problem. However, many children who are unprotected by their parents and have early exposure to abuse or violence can develop a pseudomaturity. At times, they may have experienced a role reversal with their parents; the child may have become the more responsible person while the parent assumed the dependent role. These children appear to be overcompliant with adults. Although this behavior may seem well-adapted, it is inappropriate developmentally and should not be reinforced. Rather, the child should be encouraged to choose developmentally appropriate play activities and the parent encouraged to resume appropriate adult role responsibilities.

> *What special problems are experienced by a child who is unusually short or tall for his or her age? How could you, as a nurse, help the child with these growth and development issues?*

Altered Sexuality Patterns. Children who are exposed to sexual behavior prematurely may exhibit precocious sexuality. Those children who have been sexually abused may reenact the abuse experience by sexually acting out with other children. The nurse can provide the child with needed insight about his or her behavior, information about prevention, and protection from future abuse (see Chapter 41).

Reporting sexual abuse is a legal and ethical issue for nurses. Although they are required by law to report suspected abuse, nurses are not required to prove that the abuse actually occurred. Nurses are permitted to enter evidence and testify on behalf of the victim, especially if the abuse is harmful or traumatic to the child. However, frequent interviewing can retraumatize a child and distort the child's perception of what occurred and must be carefully considered. Because it is unclear during this process whether a child will be returned to a parent's custody, the nurse must be able to maintain a relationship with both the child and the parent. This process may be difficult for a nurse, who may experience a kind of vicarious trauma (Crothers, 1995). Therefore, when working with sexually abused children, it is critically important for the treatment staff to meet regularly to express their feelings and support each other in this difficult work.

Altered Thought Processes. Anxious and depressed children often have difficulty thinking, identifying options, and making decisions. Behaviorally disturbed children become easily frustrated and may respond to their frustration with aggressive behavior. The most effective intervention for school-aged children with these problems is to help them think through options in a nonthreatening way. This thinking process can be practiced by inventing a hypothetical situation that is potentially threatening and helping the child think through possible options. Through practicing identifying options and making decisions in nonstressful situations, the child can learn to respond more adaptively to stressful situations.

Although rare, children may have psychotic episodes. It is important that the psychiatric nurse be able to discriminate between normal and abnormal thought processes in children. Healthy preschool and school-aged children typically have vivid imaginations, and their normal fears can become quite intense; however, these responses should not be confused with psychotic delusions or hallucinations. Psychotic episodes are distinguished by their level of intensity, distress, and duration. They are terrifying and should be treated as psychiatric emergencies.

> *Cognitive-behavioral therapy is one of the most effective treatments for children with psychiatric problems. How would you adapt this intervention, as described in Chapter 32, to use it with children?*

Anticipatory Grieving. Children in chaotic families often experience many losses, including the loss of stability, the loss of security, and in many ways the loss of childhood. Children who have experienced repetitive losses begin to anticipate the future with grief. They may lose interest in play-

ing and become withdrawn. Children who are withdrawn can easily be overlooked. However, they need to be encouraged to actively express their grief. Rumination is discouraged, and participation is encouraged. Most importantly, the significance of their grief should not be minimized.

Anxiety. Children who are anxious may become very active and appear to be uncooperative, or they may withdraw from their environment. Gentle touch and redirection are often effective in restoring a child's self-control. If this is insufficient, a child may need to be moved to a less stimulating environment to reduce anxiety and regain self-control. Also, children may have separation anxiety related to particular people, often their parents. The child may have difficulty separating from a parent, and the parent may similarly be ambivalent about leaving the child. Each may require a great deal of reassurance to tolerate separation when needed.

The nurse in the inpatient setting can help the child reduce anxiety by providing some attachment object, such as a small cuddly toy or other object the parent brings from home. Often, drawing pictures of home, a family gathering, or the family's reaction to the hospitalization can be reassuring to a young child (Fig. 38-2). The nurse can also help the parent by having frequent telephone contact to report the child's progress. Nursing interventions are then planned to help the child and parent anticipate the future, reduce anxiety related to each other, and focus on further development of the child's sense of self.

Body Image Disturbance. Some children may have distorted ideas about their body and experience gender identity confusion. This is usually identified in drawings in which a child consistently deletes important body parts or covers them up by marking through them with dark colors. They may also draw gender-specific details that are incorrect, such as breasts on a boy or male genitalia on a girl. An effective nursing intervention is to have a child recline on a large piece of paper and draw a body outline. The child then draws in features, clothes, and other accessories. The child can separate himself or herself from the drawing and be more explicit about details and differences between boys and girls. At this time, open discussion can clarify any distortions or misperceptions. Also, children who have been sexually abused are often confused about body invasion for themselves and others. These children may be intrusive and need to be taught about appropriate and inappropriate touching and respect for body boundaries.

Chronic Low Self-Esteem. Children with psychiatric illness often have low self-esteem. It may be expressed by infrequent eye contact, lack of motivation, withdrawal, or the use of negative behavior to seek attention. Specific therapeutic activities can be planned to improve a child's self-esteem. Accomplishment of a goal, no matter how small, is very rewarding, and incremental goal setting can be an effective way to provide opportunities for success.

For example, a child who is a chronic complainer could be rewarded for refraining from complaining for 15 minutes. The time can then be gradually increased. At the same time, new methods of communication, such as initiating a conversation, can be taught and rewarded. A bedtime review of accomplishments of the day in which the child lists personal

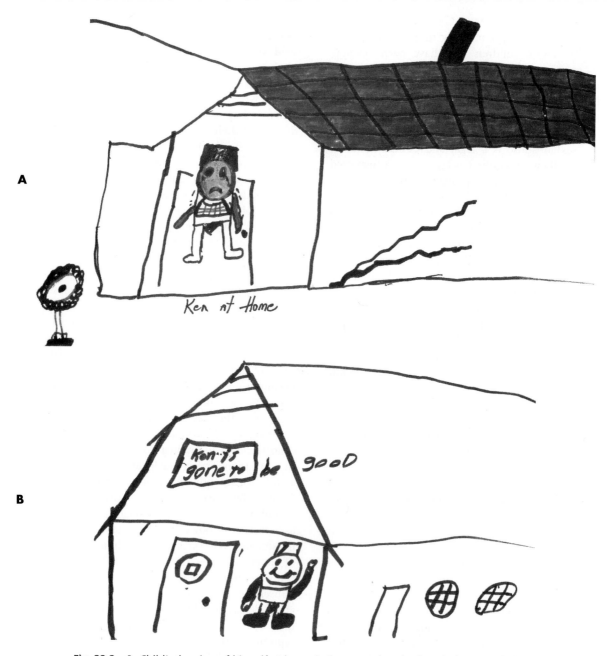

Fig. 38-2   A, Child's drawing of himself at home before entering the hospital: "I'm sad about the things I do and how people feel about me." **B,** Same child's drawing of himself entering the hospital.

strengths can also be positively reinforcing. Finally, the nurse can provide information and guidance to parents to help them enhance their child's self-esteem (Table 38-4).

Decisional Conflict. Children who have been abused or otherwise traumatized often respond to their experience by appearing defiant and oppositional. In evaluating a child's ability to handle interpersonal conflict, the child's developmental level should be considered. There are many tasks that are difficult for children to complete, particularly if they are developmentally delayed or anxious. Therefore, expectations must be carefully evaluated to determine whether they exceed a child's capability. An intervention should be planned to reward or positively reinforce a child's appropriate decision-

making ability. For example, a point system in which a child earns points and then exchanges them for privileges may be very helpful.

Family Coping: Potential for Growth. Each family has an extensive history that has shaped the development of each family member. This collective family history and its adaptability for change have a powerful influence on a child's prognosis for learning, practicing, and applying new skills. Therefore the family's willingness to participate in the therapeutic process and interest in making change should guide the nursing intervention for the child. During parent education a nurse models the effective use of reinforcement, communication, and behavior management techniques

Table **38-4**

Enhancing a Child's Self-Esteem

Targeted Area	Strategy
Caregiver expectations	Describe expectations for the child.
	Assess anticipated developmental milestones.
	Review family patterns and influences.
Personal value	Communicate confidence in the child.
	Structure situations to promote success of the child.
	Implement effective ways of praising the child.
	Role model self-value.
Communication	Listen attentively.
	Encourage openness to feelings.
	Avoid using judgmental statements.
	Elicit different points of view.
Discipline	Use effective methods of limit setting.
	Discuss and implement appropriate consequences.
	Review problem-solving techniques.
	Teach that physical punishment should not be used.
Guidance	Encourage open exchanges with the child.
	Know the child's activities away from home.
	Plan family time and activities together.
	Express interest in school events.
	Become familiar with the child's friends.
Autonomy	Demonstrate respect for the child.
	Promote the child's responsible decision making.
	Expect reciprocal respect.

Box **38-3**

Strategies for Behavior Management of Children

- Respond warmly to a child's positive behaviors.
- Communicate approval by facial expression, tone of voice, and touch.
- Express excitement around a child's accomplishments.
- Ignore negative behavior whenever appropriate.
- Refrain from giving unnecessary commands.
- Respond calmly but effectively to negative behaviors. (Example: "No yelling," stated in a calm tone of voice.)
- Use time-outs when necessary and appropriate (30 to 60 seconds per year of a child's age). This should be done in a nonpunitive manner and presented as a way to help the child gain control or use problem-solving techniques.
- Avoid making unrealistic demands of a child.
- Avoid negative remarks about the child.
- Communicate often, using the following techniques:
  - The parent or staff member telling about personal experiences.
  - The parent or staff member listening, paraphrasing, and asking follow-up questions.
  - Nightly review of positive behaviors noted during the day that the parent wants to be repeated. (Negative behaviors should not be mentioned at this time.)

identified in Box 38-3. The parents are then expected to practice these techniques with their child during the course of treatment.

Do you think the strategies for behavior management of children described in Box 38-3 are culture bound or culture free? Defend your position.

Hopelessness. Many children live in chaotic and dangerous environments. Communities are often unsafe, and schools may be plagued with violence. Children in these situations may feel very hopeless. Setting small goals that a child can accomplish may help to reduce feelings of hopelessness. Nurses also have an opportunity to teach these children and families about community helping agencies, to find advocates for the child, and to teach the child about self-protection. Trips to the police station, fire station, or community centers may help reduce the child's sense of hopelessness. Often a relative, teacher, guidance counselor,

or church member can provide the child with a concerned adult in the community. Contact with some individual or agency that can provide safety for the child is an essential nursing intervention.

Children who are frequently hospitalized or who live in foster care or residential facilities often experience hopelessness. It can be helpful to make a scrapbook about the child's life. It should begin with the child's birth and biological family. By drawing pictures or using pictures from magazines, the child can create a book. The current hospitalization should be included with a picture of the nursing staff. Accomplishments from the treatment program are featured as important life events. Autographs and words of encouragement may be written by staff members to the child. The child can then take this record to the next treatment facility or foster home. In this way the child begins to record life events so that hope for the future can be created.

Imagine you are taking one of your school-age patients on a trip to the community. What helping agency would you visit, and what would you like the child to learn from the experience?

Impaired Social Interaction. Children with emotional problems often have not learned basic social skills that help them relate to others (Fopma-Loy, 2000). The therapeutic nurse-patient relationship can be used to learn these skills. Group therapy (see Chapter 33) and cognitive-behavioral strategies (see Chapter 32) such as social skills training and modeling socially appropriate responses that demonstrate respect for other people are effective nursing interventions.

Through guidance, demonstration, practice, and feedback, social interaction can be improved.

Impaired Verbal Communication. Being able to describe personal experience and express feelings is important to a child's mental health. The nurse can model clear communication by starting a conversation with a child about a recent life experience, such as something that happened on the way to work. The nurse can then prompt the child to tell about some personal life experience. As the child begins, the nurse reinforces communication with a smile, nod, and touch.

After the child has mastered the skill of talking about external experiences, the nurse can change the intervention to talking about an internal experience or feeling. Once again, the nurse may begin by describing a feeling that has become associated with an event and then prompt the child, wait, and reinforce. A child who has never been encouraged to talk about feelings may require the use of therapeutic play involving dolls to express feelings or may be better able to talk about feelings by drawing. This is evident in the artwork shown in Fig. 38-3, in which a 6-year-old boy was able to draw his different feelings.

> *Have you ever tried to talk with a shy or unresponsive child? What techniques did you find to be effective in drawing the child out, and could these strategies be applied to a child in a psychiatric setting?*

Personal Identity Disturbance. As children approach adolescence they begin to struggle with an individual identity. Without role models for finding meaning in life, a child's personal identity formation becomes a crisis. If a child does not have successful adult models in life, people in the news or fictional characters can be used. The nurse may begin by discussing the skills and courage that the person showed in overcoming problems or adversity. This discussion can then flow into finding direction and purpose in life. Within the context of important discussions such as this, a child with personal identity disturbance can develop a competent identity of self and meet the challenges of the adult world.

Posttrauma Response. Children who have been traumatized may have sudden and dramatic mood changes (Lovrin, 1999). Often some unexpected event reminds them of a previous abuse episode, and they experience the anxiety associated with the earlier abuse. At that time their behavior may change without any identifiable cause. Nursing interventions such as art therapy and play therapy can be very useful in helping a child to cope with a previous abuse incident and reduce a posttrauma response. Through a guided process using play or drawings, a child may be able to identify the things that are associated with the trauma, such as certain types of weather, body features such as mustaches, or experiences such as hearing loud voices. With this awareness a child can learn to anticipate responses and may be able to gain some control over them.

Potential for Violence. Being able to handle conflict without becoming aggressive toward oneself or others is very important for children to learn (Modrcin-McCarthy et al, 1998). In contemporary American culture, violence is widespread, and children may perceive it to be an acceptable way of dealing with conflict. Also, with extensive media and television coverage of violent events, children may become numb to feelings related to violence. Therefore alternatives

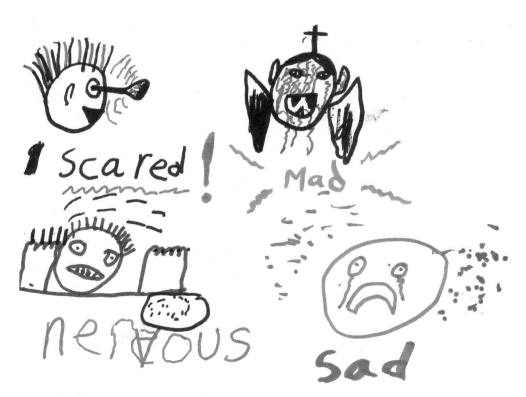

Fig. 38-3 Drawing by a hospitalized 6-year-old boy of his different feelings.

such as anger management must be taught so that a child will have a repertoire of solutions to use in conflict situations (see Chapter 31).

A brief time-out may be effective in interrupting behavior that is escalating or becoming out of control. During these periods alone it may be helpful for a child to read a story about a similar conflict or for an older child to write thoughts and feelings in a journal. Another useful strategy is to establish a contract with a child who is capable of understanding, writing, and adhering to it. Such a contract would identify the consequences that the child would face, based on the specific behavior. Contracts allow the child to play an active role in the treatment process and provide immediate and constructive feedback about the child's actions.

As a last resort, in an inpatient setting seclusion may be needed. Seclusion should never be used as punishment, for the convenience of staff, or as a substitute for individualized treatment (see Critical Thinking about Contemporary Issues). During seclusion the child should be encouraged to express feelings so that the nurse can help the child gain insight into the interconnectedness of emotions, actions, relationships, and alternatives to aggressive behavior.

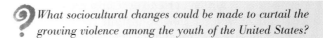

What sociocultural changes could be made to curtail the growing violence among the youth of the United States?

Sleep Pattern Disturbance. Children who are experiencing anxiety may have sleep disturbances and nightmares. If a child is receiving psychostimulants, such as methylphenidate (Ritalin), and has disturbed sleep, the medication should not be given in the evening if the child has insomnia. Sleep disturbances can also be treated with various nursing interventions. Back massage can be helpful in encouraging relaxation. Many children's stories that deal with nightmares and fears related to bedtime can be read and discussed. In general, however, the most effective way to make a successful transition to bedtime and subsequently to sleep is to develop a consistent, predictable bedtime ritual, such as taking a bath followed by quiet time and a bedtime story. The consistent application of these activities usually reduces this maladaptive response in children.

THERAPEUTIC TREATMENT MODALITIES

Once a thorough assessment has been completed and nursing diagnoses have been formulated, the nurse can implement a variety of individualized interventions that are effective in treating maladaptive responses in children.

Therapeutic Play

Because play is normal and fun for children, it is a very effective tool for nurses to use. Interventions that are enjoyable, arouse curiosity, and stimulate the imagination will capture the child's attention and interest. Many children with psychiatric problems may have lost interest in play or may have never experienced the joy of spontaneous play. Learning to play is critical not only to a child's development but also to mental health. Therapeutic aspects of play and their beneficial outcomes are listed in Table 38-5. The nurse should keep these elements in mind when incorporating play therapy into the plan of care.

CRITICAL THINKING about CONTEMPORARY ISSUES

Is the Use of Seclusion and Restraints with Children Therapeutic?

The use of seclusion and restraint in the care and treatment of children with psychiatric problems has been the subject of considerable debate. Advocates of these techniques cite the widespread problem of violent behavior among psychiatric patients, including children, and describe the clinical efficacy of these interventions. In fact, seclusion and restraint are used in inpatient settings by nurses who are the front-line professionals responsible for initiating emergency procedures and supervising the actions taken to prevent violent outbursts (Goren & Curtis, 1996). However, these interventions have also been associated with punishment, custodial care, and institutional abuse and neglect. Some even view seclusion as a violation of a patient's civil liberties.

There are a number of alternatives that nurses can use when dealing with dangerous, inappropriate behavior by children, including aggressive, destructive, and highly disruptive behavior (Fisher & Kane, 1998). First, nurses can teach and reinforce acceptable ways for children to express themselves and satisfy their needs. Second, nurses can use less restrictive interventions such as time-outs, therapeutic holding, room programs, or open-door seclusion to reduce inappropriate behavior (Delaney, 1999; Berrios & Jacobwitz, 1998). Third, nurses should evaluate the effect of these interventions on the child and continuously monitor the efficacy of these interventions in research studies using objective measures and experimental controls. As with all other nursing interventions, the therapeutic value of seclusion and restraints for children is determined by the treatment goals, context of care, and respect shown by the nurse for the needs of the child and family.

Table **38-5**

Therapeutic Aspects of Play	
Therapeutic Factor	**Beneficial Outcome**
Overcoming resistance	Working alliance
Communication	Understanding
Competence	Self-esteem
Creative thinking	Problem solving
Catharsis	Emotional release
Abreaction	Perspective on traumatic event
Role playing	Learning new behaviors
Fantasy	Compensation and sublimation
Teaching through metaphors	Insight
Relationship enhancement	Trust in others
Mastering developmental fears	Growth and development
Game play	Socialization

Modified from Schaefer C: *The therapeutic powers of play,* Northvale, NJ, 1993, Jason Aronson.

The first step is for the nurse to develop a therapeutic alliance and trust with the child so that life can be perceived from the child's perspective and the child's concerns can be anticipated. When a child feels understood and safe, participation in therapeutic play with the nurse is common. If the child is anxious, his or her developmental level may fluctuate rapidly, and this should be continuously assessed by the nurse. However, care must be taken to ensure that the child does not fail at the activity, either because the developmental level is too advanced or because of the severity of the child's symptoms. Children will become easily frustrated with play that is too difficult and thus feel a sense of failure when their self-esteem is already compromised.

Toys that are age appropriate and imaginative should be offered to a child. These may include blocks, a play house, family characters, soldiers, trucks, and rescue vehicles. The child is then encouraged to begin play without specific direction from the nurse. The nurse may ask the following clarifying questions:

- What is this person doing?
- How does this little boy feel?
- What is happening now?

The nurse can then follow up with some clarifying and validating statements such as, "This little girl looks afraid." The nurse refrains from guiding the play, making unnecessary remarks, or making interpretations that may link the play to the child's life experience. The play should continue until the child is no longer engaged. The nurse can then evaluate the play intervention by considering the following questions:

- What did the play activity communicate about the child's developmental level?
- What emotions and behavioral responses were evidenced by the child while at play?
- What information can be added to the child's assessment or treatment plan based on observations during play therapy?

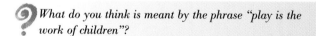 *What do you think is meant by the phrase "play is the work of children"?*

Art Therapy

Drawing is a valuable tool for children to use in describing an event or expressing a feeling. Children often do not have the vocabulary to express themselves, and they feel pressured to answer questions they do not understand. Through drawings, a child can provide information about behavior and developmental maturity that the nurse can then use to help the child in preparing for future change.

Art is particularly useful in assessing a child's therapeutic needs (Carpenter et al, 1997). Children may find drawing stressful if they have been criticized about it in the past. However, with some encouragement they will usually produce an interesting and often revealing picture. The nurse might ask the child what is happening in the picture or to name the people. The nurse should make notes about whatever the child reports the people are saying or thinking. This process can be continued until the child becomes disinterested in the activity or the child's anxiety level becomes too

great. In evaluating the effectiveness of this intervention, the nurse should consider the following:

- What was learned about the child's experience and perceptions from this intervention?
- What do the pictures reveal about the child's view of the world?
- Is there any gender confusion evident?
- Is there any distortion between the child's perception of personal experience and that which was reported?

Children's Games

Children with behavioral disorders often have difficulty with motor control. Games that teach motor control can be helpful to these children. Such games include Simon Says, Red Light, Musical Chairs, and many others. Games can also be used to increase a child's concentration and frustration tolerance. Games such as Candy Land, Hide and Seek, and Find the Button can be played with gradually increasing difficulty to teach these skills.

When initiating these activities the nurse should consider the child's motor development and level of anxiety and choose among games that engage large or small muscle groups. Thought should also be given to the child's tolerance for frustration and competition. Games may then be modified to meet the specific therapeutic needs of the child. Games can also be played with increasing demands placed on concentration and cognitive processing; however, it is important to stop playing a game that is too difficult or stressful for a child. The nurse should consider the following questions at the completion of the game:

- Was the game developmentally appropriate for the child?
- Was playing the game a pleasurable experience?
- If not, why not?
- Was the nurse's therapeutic goal met?
- How should the game be modified in the future to further the child's skill development and adaptive coping responses?

Bibliotherapy

Bibliotherapy is the use of literature to help children identify and express feelings within the structure and safety of the nurse-patient relationship. Because children actively engage in imaginary thinking, they can easily identify with the fictional characters in a story and gain insight into their own lives.

In implementing this activity the nurse should carefully consider the child's age and attention span. To be effective the story should have illustrations that capture the child's interest. The nurse should also think about the child's situation and try to select a book that describes a situation or issue relevant to the child's life situation. While reading the story the nurse should be sensitive to the child's response. If the text is wordy, the child may become bored or distracted. If this occurs, paraphrasing the story or asking what the child thinks is happening to the characters may be helpful. In this way the child's imagination becomes engaged and the experience will have value. It is also important to give the child an opportunity to reflect on the story and discuss any thoughts or feelings about the characters because it is often easier to talk about the feelings of the characters than one's own.

After reading the story the nurse should evaluate the usefulness of the intervention and assess the following:

- Was the story appropriate to the child's developmental age?
- Was the child engaged with the story?
- Did the child enjoy the experience?
- What was learned by the child and about the child as a result of this intervention?

Traditional fairy tales are based on and convey many gender stereotypes. Do you think this is a problem, and how might you go about dealing with this issue in working with children?

Storytelling

The therapeutic use of storytelling for relieving distress and teaching new coping skills is a valuable intervention. Because children do not separate imaginary experiences from real experiences, stories that teach appropriate problem-solving skills can serve as models for real situations.

Initially the nurse must identify a social skill that the child needs to learn, such as assertiveness. The nurse may make up a story about a character who needs that particular skill, giving the hero or heroine characteristics similar to those of the child. It is important to select an ending to the story that will guide the child in learning the skill. The story should be told using animated facial expressions and expressive voice inflections, and the child should be actively involved in the story as much as possible. At the end of the story the nurse should ask the child about the story and how it made the child feel. This may then lead to a broader discussion of other aspects of the child's life. In evaluating the outcome of the intervention, the nurse should consider the following questions:

- Could this character be used to teach this child other skills through other stories?
- Could the child add to the story or make up one of his or her own?
- What was the moral of the story, and how did it apply to the child?
- Could the story be used in other creative ways, such as by having the child enact the story or by including others?

Autogenic Storytelling

A similar version of storytelling is autogenic storytelling, a therapeutic activity in which the child participates in creating the story. Nurses may find this activity particularly valuable in helping children explore fears related to traumatic events. This intervention is particularly useful for a school-age child who has been traumatized or is having nightmares. A child will often reenact anxiety-related experiences in a story portrayed by animals or other fictional characters. Unlike real life, the child can have control over the experience if it is relived in play or storytelling.

Children often like audiotaping the story and then listening to their voice telling the story. The nurse should discuss the general structure of the story with the child, and together they can decide on the main characters and the beginning plot. The nurse should begin the story with the introduction and then stop, allowing the child to add the next event. The nurse picks up the storytelling when the child runs out of material or becomes anxious or overstimulated. At the end of the story, if the child has chosen an unhealthy ending, the nurse begins the storytelling intervention again. In the retelling, however, the nurse takes on a more active role and adds adaptive responses at important moments in the story. This allows the child to explore a traumatic event while learning healthy coping responses. At the conclusion the nurse should evaluate the following:

- What emotions and behaviors did the child portray in the story?
- What were the predominant themes?
- How did the child resolve the story, and what does it suggest about the child's ability to solve problems and resolve conflicts?

Pharmacotherapy

Many children with a psychiatric illness receive psychotropic medication as part of their treatment (Laraia, 1996; Lieberman & Tasman, 2000). Table 38-6 lists child and adolescent psychiatric disorders and drug treatments. Chapter 28 discusses these drugs in detail. The psychiatric nurse should consult child psychopharmacology resources and carefully calculate dosages based on the child's body weight.

Psychiatric nurses must be knowledgeable about these medications and develop interventions to monitor, educate, and evaluate medication effects with children and their families. Nurses should also be aware that promoting a child's knowledge of medications can have a positive effect on self-esteem and feelings of control and self-worth. Thus numerous therapeutic outcomes can be achieved by effective medication teaching.

This area allows for many creative nursing interventions. A variety of puppet play, art, graphics, and audiovisual materials can be used to successfully teach and prepare children for managing their medications and their illness. Peer group participation is particularly effective in helping children describe common experiences, decrease their sense of isolation, and enhance their responses to the teaching materials. Through imaginative but goal-directed nursing interventions, children can learn important information and experience greater control over the treatment of their illness and their future mental health.

Finally, it is important for nurses to realize that children metabolize and eliminate medications more rapidly than adults. Although initial doses may be low, doses can ultimately be as high as adults, requiring frequent clinical and laboratory follow-up. Psychopharmacological treatment is increasingly used in children with some reports of significant benefit, but there are still relatively few studies of these drugs in children and limited indications for their use with children approved by the Food and Drug Administration (FDA).

Explore the controversy that exists about medicating ADHD children with Ritalin. What is the scientific evidence supporting or not supporting its effectiveness as a treatment strategy?

Table **38-6**

Child and Adolescent Psychiatric Disorders and Drug Treatments

Disorder	Drug Class	Comments/Nursing Considerations
Affective disorders: depression, bipolar disorder	Antidepressants (clomipramine, imipramine, fluoxetine)	Careful diagnosis is necessary to differentiate depression from normal feeling states.
	Mood stabilizers (carbamazepine, lithium)	Some mood stabilizers require blood levels.
Anxiety, transient insomnia, acute extrapyramidal symptoms (EPS)	Antihistamines (Benadryl) Benzodiazepines	Tolerance to sedative effects may develop.
Attention deficit-hyperactivity disorder (ADHD)	Stimulants (dextroamphetamine, methylphenidate, pemoline)	Do not dose in the evening due to insomnia. Used when primary symptoms are manifest in school. Measure growth and cardiovascular parameters.
Conduct disorders (aggressive and nonaggressive)	Antipsychotics, stimulants, antidepressants, mood stabilizers	May improve a child's capacity to benefit from social and educational interventions.
Functional enuresis	Antidepressants (imipramine)	Used when an immediate therapeutic effect is necessary because of severe emotional distress.
Impulsivity	Antipsychotics, mood stabilizers	Help to increase behavioral control.
Mental retardation with psychiatric symptoms and behavioral problems	Antipsychotics	Used to control behavioral and psychiatric complications.
	Antidepressants	Treat affective symptoms.
	Stimulants	Treat ADHD.
	Lithium	Helps control aggression.
	Carbamazepine	Anticonvulsant that can help control aggression.
Obsessive-compulsive disorder (OCD)	Antidepressants (clomipramine, SSRIs)	Reduce OCD symptoms.
Panic and school phobia	TCA, MAOI, SSRIs	Concurrent behavioral interventions recommended. Dietary restrictions for MAOIs.
Pervasive developmental disorders (including autism)	Antipsychotics	Used to treat agitation, stereotypical movements, destructive behaviors.
	Antidepressants (clomipramine, SSRIs)	Stereotypical movements and OCD-like symptoms.
Psychosis	Antipsychotics	Assess for EPS and tardive dyskinesia.
Rage	Haloperidol, mood stabilizers	Require careful education and laboratory monitoring.
Schizophrenia	Antipsychotics	As with adults, choice of drug depends on prior efficacy and the spectrum of pharmacological properties.
Separation anxiety disorder	Antidepressants (imipramine, SSRIs)	Effective at high doses. Speculative: panic disorder symptoms.
Tic disorders: Tourette's disorder	Antipsychotics (haloperidol), SSRI	Stimulants are avoided because they worsen symptoms.
	Alpha-adrenergic agonist (clonidine)	Hypotension, dizziness, dry mouth, drowsiness.

Milieu Management

An important role of the child psychiatric nurse is the organization, management, and integration of multiple treatment interventions with the child throughout the continuum of care, such as in the inpatient setting, day treatment program, or intensive in-home intervention. The developmental needs of children in a psychiatric milieu are complex and dynamic. The design of the unit and treatment philosophy should provide the context of treatment within a safe, caring environment. A planned program of activities is essential for safe milieu management. Family participation and support from the staff are also essential for successful treatment outcomes (DeSocio et al, 1997; Lawson, 1998).

With escalating aggression among children, the management of a therapeutic milieu in any of these settings is very challenging (Goren et al, 1996). The child's day must be organized into manageable time units that are age appropriate, with specific but varied activities assigned to each time unit.

Citing the Evidence on

Child Psychotherapy

BACKGROUND: Few studies have evaluated the effectiveness of traditional child psychotherapy. This study used a randomized design to evaluate its effectiveness as typically delivered in outpatient settings. Patients were assigned to either traditional child psychotherapy or academic tutoring.

RESULTS: Both children receiving psychotherapy and academic tutoring reported significant improvement. Little support was found for the greater efficacy of traditional child psychotherapy.

IMPLICATIONS: The results suggest the need to revise traditional psychotherapy techniques or to replace or supplement them with techniques whose efficacy has been demonstrated by transporting empirically validated treatments to clinical settings.

Weiss B et al: The effectiveness of traditional child psychotherapy, *J Consult Clin Psychol* 67(1):82, 1999.

For example, younger children's development requires that they be assigned shorter time units and large motor activities should be scheduled to follow periods of sitting or after therapy sessions, which might produce anxiety.

Whenever possible, children should be assigned to a small group with specific staff members. A schedule should be set up in advance that is predictable from one day to the next. Consistency and predictability are very important. Transitioning from one activity to the next is often difficult for children; therefore a transitional object such as a reward sheet of stickers that is carried from one activity to the next can be helpful. Before leaving one activity, the child should be prepared for the next activity. Helping children to anticipate what is expected of them in the next time period will help them better manage their anxiety.

Anxiety and aggression in any setting can be contagious, and they can escalate abruptly. Nurses should be prepared to act quickly and decisively if a child becomes aggressive. If this occurs, the child who is aggressive or anxious must be separated from children who are in control of their behavior. When the child is isolated, the aggressive behavior will begin to de-escalate, the child can be brought under control, and the process of learning about why this occurred can begin.

These problems can be minimized by having a well-planned schedule and implementing it consistently. Whenever tension in the milieu begins to rise, the staff must be very visible and engage the children in activities while being vigilant for potential problems. A carefully planned milieu schedule anticipates problems, creates solutions, and capitalizes on the strengths and energy of the children. Keeping the milieu safe and therapeutic is a high priority for child psychiatric nursing intervention. Ongoing clinical supervision and peer review improve communication and collaboration among staff members. These activities allow staff to evaluate and refine their therapeutic skills and facilitate goal-directed interactions with children.

Psychotherapy

Structured child and adolescent psychotherapy, tested through controlled clinical trials, have produced beneficial effects in hundreds of studies (Weisz & Jensen, 1999). These include cognitive, behavioral, and interpersonal therapies, as well as contingency management. In contrast, the limited pool of research on traditional child psychotherapy raises doubts about its effectiveness (see Citing the Evidence). A graduate degree in nursing is required for the practice of psychotherapy. Additional research is needed that considers the developing child in context, the measurement of various domains of functioning and outcomes, and the inclusion of multiple sources of information (Mohr, 1999).

Summary

1. Today, 9% to 13% of children have some type of mental disorder, but only 25% to 36% of them receive treatment. Psychiatric services are offered to children in a wide variety of settings that together make up systems of care. Nurses function in these settings by assessing a child's competency skills and providing interventions to teach the skills that are deficient.
2. Assessment of the child requires a biopsychosocial approach with a focus on the nine ego skills that all children need to become competent adults.
3. Four of the most common medical diagnoses of childhood are anxiety, depression, conduct disorders, and ADHD. Nursing diagnoses relate to each ego competency skill deficit.
4. Psychiatric nurses implement a variety of therapeutic treatment modalities when caring for children, including therapeutic play, art therapy, games, bibliotherapy, storytelling, autogenic storytelling, pharmacotherapy, milieu management, and psychotherapy.

Competent Caring A Clinical Exemplar of a Psychiatric Nurse

EVELYN MIDDLETON, BSN, RN, C AND LEEANN WELSH, RN

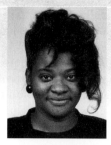

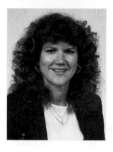

L, a 9-year-old African American girl, was admitted to our 25-bed combined child and adolescent psychiatric unit because of recent suicidal attempts and homicidal ideation. L was extremely depressed and had a difficult time talking about the situations that brought her to the hospital. Her family was dysfunctional. Her father was physically and sexually abusive to both her and her mother.

Early in her hospitalization, L didn't trust anyone. She had suffered numerous traumatic events. She would lie in a fetal position, suck her thumb, and periodically talk about wanting to jump off a large bridge in the downtown section of our city. Working as a team on the evening shift, we (with other members of the nursing staff) were able to assess the chronically low self-esteem and sadness this child was feeling. With a lot of one-to-one attention and the therapeutic use of touch, we developed a bond with this child, who viewed us as caregivers, and we were able to establish a trusting relationship with her. She asked questions about our childhoods and how we were brought up by our parents. She also asked about how we treated our children. From this conversation, she understood she was not to blame for the beatings and the sexual abuse she endured. L continued talking to us with tears in her eyes and her hands clenched while hitting her pillow in an effort to control her anger. She would talk about a dream she often had, and we encouraged her to vent her feelings about this dream. The more this child spoke, the clearer it became to us that it was not only her father who repeatedly violated her, but also her grandfather. She constantly referred to these memories as dreams because she did not want to believe a grandfather could do this to his own flesh and blood. We continued to sit with L at night, consoling and reassuring her that

she was not to blame and how great it was that she was finally able to release these ghosts.

During these conversations L had decided that she no longer wanted to be home with her father because she felt the beatings would continue. We prepared her for discharge by discussing different options for placement, her responsibility to keep herself safe, and other ways besides suicide to express her anger. At one point, the Department of Social Services failed to substantiate any sexual misconduct on the father's part toward L. It was their recommendation that she be returned to her father. This disappointment encouraged L to feel betrayed by the adults she had begun to trust. She cried, exclaiming that she told us everything and we had let her down. She stated she would kill her father if she went home. We again reassured her that we would help see that she not be returned home. Because of the time factor and lack of support from the Department of Social Services, L had to be prepared to go to the state hospital. With a team effort, we were honest and positive about this placement at the state hospital. L was informed as to how she would be transported. We then called the state hospital and gathered some general information to share with her about the facility and different activities that went on there.

On the day of discharge, L wanted to meet our children. LeeAnn brought her little boy in to have lunch with L. While interacting with us, L was able to see a healthy parent-child relationship. Once she was settled at the state hospital, she called the unit, requesting to speak to Evelyn and LeeAnn. We encouraged her to trust the staff there and mentioned that she was welcome to call us anytime to let us know how she was doing. Working as a team, we shared the hurt and love this child was feeling. As two experienced psychiatric nurses, we were able to assess, implement, and plan care for this suicidal patient. Together we established a trusting relationship and created a safe environment for her. Our expertise allowed this child to grow, develop self-esteem, and reclaim the will to live. For us, it truly reflected the essence of child psychiatric nursing practice.

Chapter Review Questions

1. **Indicate whether the following statements are true (T) or false (F).**

____ A. Mental disorders are rare in children averaging less than 1% of the population.

____ B. Nursing care of children with psychiatric disorders is focused on skill development regardless of psychiatric diagnosis.

____ C. Nurses who take care of children who have been abused can be traumatized vicariously.

____ D. Young children who exhibit overt sexual behavior should be ignored in order not to reinforce the behavior.

____ E. To avoid aggression in the milieu, the nurse should make strict rules and follow them without exception.

2. **Fill in the blanks.**

A. About _____ of the children who need psychiatric treatment in the United States currently receive it.

B. If a child becomes upset when away from his or her mother, it may indicate problems mastering the competency skill of _____.

C. If a child gets mad when he or she doesn't gets his or her way, it may indicate problems mastering the competency skill of _____ .

D. _____ is the use of literature to help children identify and express feelings.

E. A therapeutic activity in which the child participates in creating the story is called _____.

F. The most common problem that precipitates hospitalization in children is the _____.

G. Reporting child abuse is a _____ and _____ issue for nurses.

H. The four most common psychiatric illnesses among children are _____, _____, _____, and _____.

3. **Provide short answers for the following questions.**

A. What competency skills are associated with middle childhood?

B. Identify areas that parents can target to enhance a child's self-esteem.

C. Television networks are now rating television programs for violence and nudity, and new technologies are allowing parents to block the viewing of certain programs. Do you think this will have a significant impact on the upbringing of children? Why or why not?

D. It has been said that children have a low priority in contemporary American society. Learn about how two other countries provide for the health, education, and welfare of their children and compare them to the United States.

REFERENCES

AACAP: Practice parameters for the psychiatric assessment of children and adolescents, *J Am Acad Child Adolesc Psychiatry* 36(suppl):4S, 1997.

American Nurses' Association: *Standards of child and adolescent psychiatric and mental health nursing practice,* Kansas City, Mo, 1985, The Association.

American Psychiatric Association: *Diagnostic and statistical manual mental disorders,* Fourth Edition, Text Revision, Washington, DC, American Psychiatric Association, 2000.

Berrios C, Jacobwitz W: Therapeutic holdings: outcomes of a pilot study, *J Psychosoc Nurs* 36:14, 1998.

Bickman L et al: Long term effects of a system of care on children and adolescents, *J Behav Health Serv Res* 26(2):185, 1999.

Brestan E, Eyburg S: Effective psychosocial treatments of conduct-disordered children and adolescents: 29 years, 82 studies, and 5272 kids, *J Clin Child Psychol* 27(2):180, 1998.

Carpenter M et al: Indicators of abuse or neglect in preschool children's drawings, *J Psychosoc Nurs* 35:10, 1997.

Cipkala-Gaffin J: Diagnosis and treatment of attention-deficit/hyperactive disorder, *Perspect Psychiatr Care* 34(4):18, 1998.

Crothers D: Vicarious traumatization in the work with survivors of childhood trauma, *J Psychosoc Nurs* 33:9, 1995.

Delaney K: Time-out: an overused and misused milieu intervention, *J Child Adolesc Psychiatr Nurs* 12:53, 1999.

DeSocio J et al: Lessons learned in creating a safe and therapeutic milieu for children, adolescents, and families: developmental considerations, *J Child Adolesc Psychiatr Nurs* 10(4):18, 1997.

Elder J: Defining parent training for practice and research, *J Am Psychiatr Nurs Assoc* 3:103, 1997.

Finke L, Bowman A: Factors in childhood drug and alcohol use: a review of the literature, *J Child Adolesc Psychiatr Nurs* 10(3):29, 1997.

Fisher P, Kane C: Coercion theory: application to the inpatient treatment of conduct-disordered children, *J Child Adolesc Psychiatr Nurs* 11:129, 1998.

Fopma-Loy J: Peer rejection and neglect of latency-age children: pathways and a group psychotherapy model, *J Child Adolesc Psychiatr Nurs* 13:29, 2000.

Glod C: Attention deficit hyperactivity disorder throughout the lifespan: diagnosis, etiology, and treatment, *JAPNA* 3:89, 1997.

Goren S et al: Reducing violence in a child psychiatric hospital through planned organizational change, *J Child Adolesc Psychiatr Nurs* 9:27, 1996.

Goren S, Curtis W: Staff members' beliefs about seclusion and restraint in child psychiatric hospitals, *J Child Adolesc Psychiatr Nurs* 9:7, 1996.

Kasen S et al: Influence of child and adolescent psychiatric disorders on young adult personality disorders, *Am J Psychiatry* 156(10):1529, 1999.

Kaslow N, Thompson M: Applying the criteria for empirically supported treatments to studies of psychosocial treatments to studies of psychosocial interventions for child and adolescent depression, *J Clin Child Psychol* 27(2):146, 1998.

Keltner N: Neuroanatomy and physiology in modern child psychiatric nursing, *J Child Adolesc Psychiatr Nurs* 9:5, 1996.

Laraia M: Current approaches to the psychopharmacologic treatment of depression in children and adolescents, *J Child Adolesc Psychiatr Nurs* 9:15, 1996.

Lawson L: Milieu management of traumatized youngsters, *J Child Adolesc Psychiatr Nurs* 11(3):99, 1998.

Lieberman J, Tasman A: *Psychiatric drugs,* Philadelphia, 2000, WB Saunders.

Lovrin M: Parental murder and suicide: post-traumatic stress disorder in children, *J Child Adolesc Psychiatr Nurs* 12(3):110, 1999.

Ludwikowski K, DeValk M: Attention-deficit/hyperactivity disorder: a neurodevelopmental approach, *J Child Adolesc Psychiatr Nurs* 11:17, 1998.

Modrcin-McCarthy M et al: Childhood anger: so common, yet so misunderstood, *J Child Adolesc Psychiatr Nurs* 11(2):69, 1998.

Mohr W: Beyond cause and effect: some thoughts on research and practice in child psychiatric nursing, *J Child Adolesc Psychiatr Nurs* 12:118, 1999.

National Institutes of Health: Consensus statement on the diagnosis and treatment of ADHD, Washington, DC, 1998, NIH.

Ollendick T, King N: Empirically supported treatments for children with phobic and anxiety disorders: current status, *J Clin Child Psychol* 27(2):156, 1998.

Pelham W et al: Empirically supported psychosocial treatments for attention deficit hyperactivity disorder, *J Clin Psychol* 27(2):190, 1998.

Pine D, Cohen E: Relationships between psychiatric disorders in children and adults: behavior disorders as an example, *J Pract Psychiatry Behav Health* 5:121, 1999.

Scharer K: Nurse-parent relationship building in child psychiatric unit, *J Child Adolesc Psychiatr Nurs* 12:153, 1999.

Seed M: Identification and measurement of maladaptive behaviors in preschool children: movement toward a preventive model of care, *J Child Psychiatr Nurs* 12(3):61, 1999.

Shaw K et al: Behavioral problems in infants and toddlers were associated with later psychiatric disorders, *J Abnorm Child Psychol* 26:441, 1998.

Silverman W et al: Treating anxiety disorders in children with cognitive- behavioral therapy: a randomized clinical trial, *J Consult Clin Psychol* 76(6): 995, 1999.

Strayhorn J: *The competent child: an approach to psychotherapy and preventive mental health,* New York, 1989, Guilford.

Stroul B et al: State health care reforms: how they affect children and adolescents with emotional disorders and their families, *J Ment Health Admin* 24:386, 1997.

US Department of Health and Human Services: *Mental health: a report of the surgeon general,* Rockville, Md, 1999, SAMHSA, CMHS, NIH, NIMH.

Weisz J, Jensen P: Efficacy and effectiveness of child and adolescent psychotherapy and pharmacotherapy, *Ment Health Serv Res* 1(3):125, 1999.

Workman C, Prior M: Depression and suicide in young children, *Issues Comprehensive Pediatr Nurs* 20:125, 1997.

Adolescent Psychiatric Nursing

Audrey Redston-Iselin

Visit **MERLIN** for *Your Internet Connection* to websites that are related to the content in this chapter. www.mosby.com/MERLIN/Stuart

LEARNING OBJECTIVES

After studying this chapter the student should be able to:

- Identify the developmental tasks of adolescence
- Compare the various theoretical views of adolescence
- Discuss the major areas that should be included when assessing adolescents
- Examine maladaptive responses evident in adolescence
- Analyze nursing interventions useful in working with adolescents
- Evaluate nursing care provided for adolescents

I'm so mixed up and lonely Can't even make friends with my brain. I'm too young to be where I'm going But I'm too old to go back again.

JOHN PRINE, "ROCKY MOUNTAIN TIME"

Adolescence is a time of transition—an age when the person is not yet an adult but is no longer a child. The issues raised during adolescence are central to personal development. Psychiatric nurses treating adolescents focus on their movement toward adulthood, considering social, emotional, and physical aspects of their adjustment in their family, school, and peer groups.

DEVELOPMENTAL STAGE

Adolescence is a unique stage of development that occurs between ages 11 and 20 years, when a shift in growth and learning occurs. The developmental tasks that emerge during adolescence threaten the person's defenses. They can either stimulate new adaptive ways of coping or lead to regression and maladaptive coping responses. Old problems may interfere with the adolescent's coping abilities, and environmental factors may help or hinder the adolescent's attempts to deal with these issues. Previous coping skills, if used successfully, can promote healthy adaptation and integrated adult functioning.

An earlier, but still popular view of adolescence described it as a time of conflict and upheaval that was necessary for later personality integration. More recent research suggests that this is not true; the complex changes in biological, so-cial, and emotional development do not necessarily lead to psychological conflicts.

During adolescence major events occur, and attempts are made to deal with them. This results in behavior uniquely "adolescent." Tasks that should be accomplished during adolescence are as follows (Havighurst, 1972):

- Achieving new and more mature relations with age mates of both sexes

- Achieving masculine or feminine social roles
- Accepting physical build and using the body effectively
- Achieving emotional independence from parents and other adults
- Preparing for marriage and family life
- Preparing for a career
- Acquiring a set of values and an ethical system as a guide to behavior and developing an ideology

Different theories describe these developmental tasks and how their positive resolution moves the adolescent toward adulthood. They will be briefly reviewed and are summarized in Table 39-1.

THEORETICAL VIEWS OF ADOLESCENCE
Biological Theory

One of the fundamental features of adolescence is the series of biological changes known as puberty. These changes transform the young person physically from a child into a reproductively mature adult. This process is so basic to adolescent development that many people identify puberty as the beginning of adolescence. Puberty involves a set of biological events that produce changes throughout the body. The changes fall into two categories: hormonal and somatic. In both sexes, increases in hormone production lead to the development of reproductive capability and a mature physical appearance. Physical changes include pubic hair growth, breast development, and menarche in girls, and genital development, pubic hair growth, voice change, and the emergence of facial hair in boys. A spurt in height and weight occurs in both sexes. Although all adolescents experience the changes of puberty, there are large individual differences in the timing of these changes, as well as the pace at which they take place.

Brain growth continues into adolescence as well. Although the number of neurons does not increase, there is a proliferation of the support cells that brace and nourish the neurons. In addition, growth of the myelin sheath around nerve cell axons continues at least until puberty, enabling faster neural processing. Simultaneously, the number of interconnections between adjacent neurons decreases, probably reflecting the disappearance of redundant or inappropriate neural connections. This fine-tuning of the neural system coincides with the development of formal operational thought.

Psychoanalytical Theory

Freud believed that human development was biological and marked by stages. During puberty (age 13 to 18 years), Freud's genital stage, a reawakening of sexual interest occurs. The adolescent with new sexual urges looks for gratification outside the home. This renewal comes from physiological maturing, which results in sexual exploration. Increased drives or impulses due to hormones cause a personality reorganization as adolescents attempt to adjust to their new physical status. These increased impulses confront a weak ego. Adolescents therefore return to earlier coping skills in an effort to reestablish mastery over the environment

Psychosocial Theory

Erikson and Sullivan emphasized the effect of social factors on these developmental processes. Erikson (1963) described ego identity, or the relationship between a person's self-perception and how a person appears to others. To Erikson, adolescence represented an attempt to establish an identity within the social environment. He described this search as normal adolescent identity crisis and called this stage of adolescence "identity versus identity diffusion." This stage is followed in young adulthood by the stage of "intimacy versus isolation." He stressed that identity must be established before intimacy can occur.

For Sullivan (1953), psychological growth is driven by a desire to seek increasingly intimate personal relationships. He suggested that adolescents try to coordinate needs of self-security and self-esteem, closeness and intimacy, and general

Table 39-1

Summary of Theoretical Views of Adolescence	
Theory	**Description**
Biological	Emphasis is on physical growth, behavior, and the environment, which influence feelings, thoughts, and actions.
Psychoanalytical	Puberty is called the genital stage, in which sexual interest is awakened. Biological changes upset the balance between the ego and id, and new solutions must be negotiated.
Psychosocial	Adolescents attempt to establish an identity within the social environment. They seek to coordinate self-security, intimacy, and sexual satisfaction in their relationships.
Attachment	Focuses on the quality of attachments as defining one's vulnerability to developmental changes and sees insecure attachments as a risk factor that can result in maladaptive responses to loss or trauma.
Cognitive	Adolescence is an advanced stage of cognition in which the ability to reason goes beyond the concrete to more abstract thinking, described as formal thought.
Cultural	Views adolescence as a time when a person believes that adult privileges are deserved but withheld. This stage ends when society gives full power and status of an adult.
Multidimensional	Adolescence is seen as adaptation on a continuum of development. There is less emphasis on age and more on the developmental level and timing of biological, psychological, and environmental influences.

activity and satisfaction of sexual strivings. If these needs become conflicting rather than integrated, emotional problems may result.

Attachment Theory

In this theory, attachment is the prominent developmental issue in adolescence (Rosenstein & Horowitz, 1996). It views development as a process of reorganizing previous personality patterns and structures, and contends that the adolescent's attachments with others play a major role in defining one's vulnerability to developmental changes. Insecure attachment is a risk factor in the development of adolescents. Autonomous adolescents value attachment relationships and regard experiences with attachment as important. Adolescents who have difficulty with attachments may have experienced rejection in the past or may not have had caretakers who were physically and emotionally available to them. For example, adolescents in foster care may engage in self-protective strategies to deal with their perceived devaluation and lack of consistent attachments by keeping relationships superficial, maintaining an attitude of defensiveness, and distancing themselves from others (Kools, 1999). This may result in maladaptive responses.

> *What problems might adolescents face if they decide to get married as teenagers, and what resources may be helpful to them?*

Cognitive Theory

Cognitive theory views adolescence as an advanced stage of cognitive functioning in which the ability to reason goes beyond concrete objects to symbols or abstractions, or what Piaget (1968) called formal thought. He believed that the adolescent is able to deal with logic, metaphors, and rational thought. This develops continuously from the concrete thinking of childhood to about age 12 years, when the concern with realities, tangible objects, and action is transferred to ideas, allowing for conclusions to be made and for reflection to take place without the reality or object being present.

Cultural Theory

Anthropologists who have studied adolescents in different cultures report that primitive cultures have less stressful periods than those experienced by American teenagers and conclude that adolescent rebellion is culturally determined and not biologically based. They view adolescence as a period when the person believes that adult privileges are deserved but are being withheld. It ends when society gives the person the social status of an adult. Anthropologists see growth as a continuous process and a cultural phenomenon, with people reacting to social expectations. The more clearly defined these expectations, the less stressful and ambiguous is the adolescent period. The more culture changes, the greater the generation gap becomes.

Several issues in contemporary American society directly influence the support an adolescent can obtain from the environment. Blurring sexual roles is one such issue. Women have less traditional attitudes, expectations, and behaviors, while men have become more involved in functions that were previously believed to be women's, and vice versa. So too, adolescents have more overt exposure to sex and violence in society. Another social issue is the changing job market and the increased costs of higher education, which has resulted in the prolonged economic dependency of youth. Finally, the Internet has become a source of both information and recreation for adolescents, as well as giving them access to material that may not be appropriate to their developmental stage. All of these changes increase the complexity of society and add new pressures to adolescents, who are becoming adults and attempting to define their role in today's cultural milieu.

Multidimensional Theory

Multidimensional theory proposes that there is no one view of adolescent development. Rather, there are three main themes (Meeks, 1990):

- Profiles of ego and moral development are used to characterize adolescents for rates of progression, regression, and stability in age-related development.
- Attention is given to biological, sociological, psychological, and cultural integration. These variables change rapidly during adolescence and affect the adolescent's behavior and view of self.
- The developmental issues of both psychological and biological maturation are viewed as affecting the adolescent's adaptation and functioning. For example, the timing of the adolescent's physical development in relation to a peer group has a direct influence on the teenager's self-esteem.

These issues may vary widely, not only individually but also by culture and society.

The multidimensional view of adolescence sees adaptation on a continuum of development. Less emphasis is placed on specific age and more is put on developmental level and the timing of various biological, psychological, and environmental influences. This theory also proposes that severe family conflict need not necessarily occur. Rather, the degree and nature of conflicts change from childhood through adolescence and reflect both the diversity and the functional and dysfunctional aspects of family life.

ASSESSING THE ADOLESCENT

Nursing care of adolescents begins with a thorough assessment of their health status. Data collection by the nurse is based on current and previous functioning in all aspects of an adolescent's life (AACAP, 1997). A variety of approaches and tools may be used (see Chapters 6 to 8) but data collection should include the following information:

- Appearance
- Growth and development (including developmental milestones)
- Biophysical status (illnesses, accidents, disabilities)
- Emotional status (relatedness, affect, and mental status, including mood and evidence of thought disorder and suicidal or homicidal ideation)

- Cultural, religious, and socioeconomic background
- Performance of activities of daily living (home, school, work)
- Patterns of coping (ego defenses such as denial, acting out, withdrawal)
- Interaction patterns (family, peers, society)
- Sexual behaviors (nature, frequency, preference, sexually transmitted diseases)
- Use of drugs, alcohol, and other addictive substances (tobacco, caffeine)
- Adolescent's perception and satisfaction with health (functional problems or complaints)
- Adolescent's health goals (short- and long-term)
- Environment (physical, emotional, ecological)
- Available human and material resources (friends and school and community involvement)

These data are collected from adolescents and significant others through interviews, examinations, observations, and reports. Behavioral rating scales commonly used with adolescents are listed in Box 39-1. In addition, the nurse may ask the following questions of the adolescent's family:

- What concerns you about your adolescent?
- When did these problems start?
- What changes have you noticed?
- Have the problems been noticed in school as well as home?
- What makes the behavior better or worse?
- How have these problems affected your adolescent's relationship with you, siblings, peers, and teachers?
- Has your adolescent's school performance changed?

One outcome of the nursing assessment should be the identification of teenagers at high risk for problems (DiClemente et al, 1996). Nurses need to understand the difference between constructive and age-appropriate exploration and engagement in activities that are potentially dangerous and threaten the adolescent's physical and emotional well-being (see Critical Thinking about Contemporary Issues).

A profile of the high-risk adolescent is presented in Fig. 39-1. Teenage behaviors that contribute to death and injury include smoking, poor diet, lack of physical activities, alcohol and drug abuse, unprotected sex, violence, suicide, homicide, and automobile crashes (Centers for Disease Control and Prevention, 1999). A number of factors combine to impact adolescent risk-taking behavior, including age, socioeconomic status, education, race, gender, self-esteem, autonomy, social adaptation, vulnerability, impulsivity, and thrill-seeking activity (Brage et al, 1995). Nurses who work in schools and community settings can engage in screening and early nursing intervention with high-risk teenagers to promote adaptive responses and prevent the development of future problems.

In summary, an examination of typical adolescent behaviors reveals that adolescence is a time of change. The issues of body image, identity, independence, social role, and sexual behavior can produce adaptive or maladaptive responses as the adolescent attempts to cope with the developmental tasks at hand.

Box 39-1

Behavioral Rating Scales Related to Adolescents

- Adolescent Drinking Index (ADI)
- Adolescent Treatment Outcomes Module (ATOM)
- Ansell-Casey Life Skills Assessment 2.0 (ACLSA)
- Child and Adolescent Adjustment Profile (CAAP)
- Child and Adolescent Functional Assessment Scale (CAFAS)
- Devereux Scales of Mental Disorders (DSMD)
- Devereux Rating Scale School Form (DSF)
- Million Adolescent Clinical Inventory (MACI)
- Million Adolescent Personality Inventory (MAPI)
- Ohio Youth Problems, Functioning, and Satisfaction Scales
- Revised Behavior Problem Index (RAPI)
- Severity of Psychiatric Illness: Child and Adolescent Version
- Tennessee Self Concept Scale: Second Edition (TSCS-2)
- Vanderbilt Functioning Inventory (VFI)
- Youth Outcome Questionnaire (YOQ)
- Youth Self Report (YSR)

? CRITICAL THINKING about CONTEMPORARY ISSUES

Are All Adolescents at High Risk for Problems?

Although it is a commonly held belief that adolescence is a time of conflict and turmoil, some dispute the notion that teenagers must experience a difficult adolescence. Nonetheless, nurses should not underestimate the nature of adolescent high-risk behavior and the potential resulting problems. The 1999 Youth Risk Behavior Surveillance System conducted a national school-based survey of more than 16,000 students in 151 schools. The data reveal many threats to the health and well-being of teenagers, as follows:

- 19% of students had rarely or never worn seat belts when riding in a car driven by someone else.
- 37% had ridden one or more times with a driver who had been drinking.
- 17% had driven a vehicle one or more times after drinking.
- 88% had rarely or never worn a helmet when riding a bicycle.
- 46% of the male students and 26% of the female students had been involved in at least one physical fight in the past year.
- 28% of the male students and 7% of the female students carried a weapon at least once in the past month.
- 72% of the male students and 54% of the female students participated in vigorous physical activity in the past week.
- 4% of students had missed one or more days of school in the past month because they felt unsafe at school or traveling to and from school.

Each of these findings represents both an area of concern and an opportunity for health education and early intervention by psychiatric nurses.

Many nursing students are adolescents themselves. How might this positively and negatively affect their work with adolescent patients?

Body Image

Chronological age is not a true guide for physical maturation because growth often occurs in spurts and individual differences exist. Because school classes and extracurricular activities are usually grouped by age, the adolescent must face being with others who vary greatly in physical development and interests. This explains why adolescents often imitate behavior to keep within the expected range of conduct and be compatible with peers. The greater one's difference from the rest of the group, the greater is the adolescent's anxiety. The lack of uniformity of growth often puts great demands on physical and mental adaptability. Growth is uneven and sudden, rather than smooth and gradual, and causes a change in body image.

Adolescents reevaluate themselves in light of these physical changes, particularly the onset of primary and secondary sex characteristics, which are so pronounced. They tend to compare themselves and their physical development to their peers. They are very concerned about the normality of their physical status. The physical changes of puberty cause adolescents to be self-conscious about their changing bodies. Often they are reluctant to have medical examinations because they fear abnormalities will be found. Examinations may intensify masturbatory conflicts, sexual fantasies, and guilt feelings. The early and middle phases of puberty may also give rise to increased conflict, distance, and dissatisfaction in parental relationships.

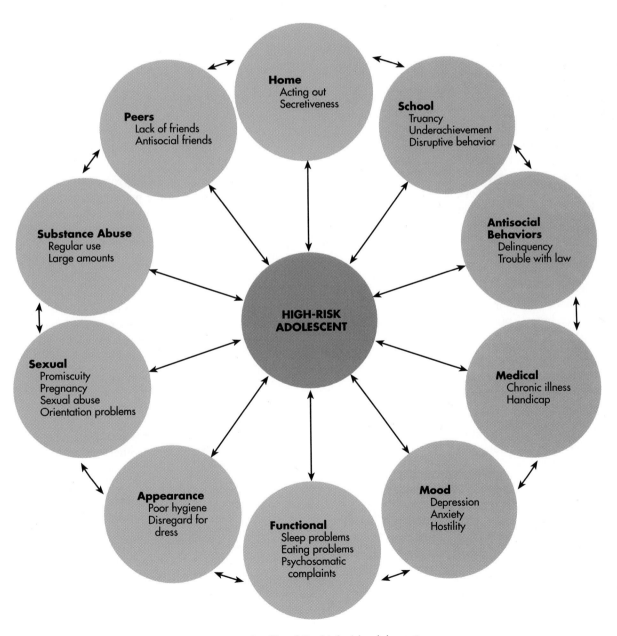

Fig. 39-1 Profile of the high-risk adolescent.

Identity

In response to the physical changes of puberty, adolescents experience heightened periods of excitement and tension. They use defenses against these feelings that were helpful in childhood and experiment with new, more adultlike attempts at mastery. Thus in their attempt to cope, adolescents sometimes act like adults and at other times behave like children. For example, adolescents show behavior marked with experimentation and test the self by going to extremes. This can be useful in establishing self-identity. The rebelliousness or negativism of the adolescent shows a movement toward individuation and autonomy that is more complex than but similar to the 2-year-old's "no." Adolescents may also assert themselves by acting in a negative or contrary manner when relating to parents and other authority figures who they believe are not allowing them to be separate and unique. This is seen in the following clinical example.

 CLINICAL EXAMPLE

Scottie, an avid football fan for several years, suddenly switched his interest to basketball. He quit his local football team despite his father's urgings to continue. His father, also a football fan, could not understand Scottie's sudden negative attitude toward football and newly found interest in basketball.

The individuation process of adolescence is accompanied by feelings of isolation, loneliness, and confusion because it brings childhood dreams to an end and attributes them to fantasy. This realization of childhood's end can create intense fears or panic. Many adolescents attempt to remain in this transitional stage. The awakening of emotional ties with the family also occurs in the establishment of new, more interdependent relationships. This fearful yet exciting entrance into adulthood is a profound experience that is not resolved in adolescence but is confronted throughout life. Adolescents mourn the loss of childhood, and the feelings of loneliness and isolation that accompany this loss create an intense need for closeness, love, and understanding. If they are unable to obtain support during this struggle, depression may result.

Exploratory behavior allows the adolescent to try on new roles and find what fits as identity is formed. Adolescents with poor identity formation are vulnerable for engaging in high-risk behaviors because there is a link between an adolescent's self-concept and the use of adaptive coping responses (McCaleb, 1995). Parenting styles that encourage individuality and relatedness to families are associated with support of adolescent identity exploration. Adolescents expressing high levels of identity exploration have parents who express mutuality and separateness, encourage member differences, and are aware of clear boundaries between themselves and their teenagers. These adolescents are also more likely to have competent approaches to peer and social relationships and more developed skills in initiating, diversifying, sustaining, and deepening peer friendships.

Independence

Adolescents have an unconscious longing to give in to their dependency needs. Adolescence is also a time of movement toward independence. Adolescents show this ambivalence by responding to petty annoyances and irritations with intense outbursts. They see the process of gaining independence as being free of parental control. They do not see gaining independence as a gradual learning process but as an emancipation accomplished by acting "differently." If one acts adult, then one is adult. Therefore they expose themselves to situations beyond their capabilities and then become overwhelmed and frightened. They seek reassurance in an attempt to reduce their anxiety by returning to childlike ways and being dependent on those with whom they feel most secure, usually their parents. This accounts for the inconsistency of adolescent behavior.

Well-adjusted adults usually use a problem-solving approach and do not feel as threatened when inexperience requires dependency on others. However, adolescents who are already tempted to give in to dependency needs feel as if they are regressing to childhood, which deflates their self-esteem. They must deny their need for their parents. Sometimes they criticize their parents for treating them as a child and then remark that their parents are not helpful enough. When adolescents seem to be rebelling against their parents, they may be rebelling against their own childhood conscience or superego. They project their ambivalence onto their parents because they were the original source of restrictions. This projection actually reveals a movement toward a more mature standard and also indicates their insecurity about giving up childhood standards. By blaming their parents for their childish actions, they can avoid blows to their fragile self-esteem and protest that their actions result from parental demands, not their own.

The interaction between adolescent changes in autonomy and family relationships is important. Three parenting styles have been described in relation to whether they help or hinder independent functioning in adolescence (Powers et al, 1989):

- Traditional parents tend to value a sense of continuity and order. They accept the value judgments that come from previous generations. Adolescents from these families tend to be more attached to their parents, conforming, and achievement oriented. Often they avoid major conflicts in their teenage years.
- Authoritarian parents are oriented toward shaping, controlling, and restricting the adolescent to fixed standards. Obedience is seen as a virtue. Power and responsibility are not shared with the adolescent. Harsh discipline is used to curb autonomous strivings that are viewed as willfulness. The approach here is often punitive and it can result in problems with the adolescent's development of autonomy.
- Democratic parents do not believe that their standards are always right. They tend to be supportive and respond to the specific situation with solutions that promote the adolescent's autonomy. They foster stimula-

tion and challenge. This parenting style combines limit setting with negotiation, thus encouraging the teenager's participation in the disciplinary process. It is shown to predict greater independent functioning in adolescents.

Did your parents have a traditional, authoritarian, or democratic parenting style, and what would you do differently in raising children of your own?

Social Role

Adolescents respond intensely to people and events. They may be totally invested in one interest and then suddenly change to something different. These intense and unstable feelings can account for their extreme sensitivity to the response of others. They are easily hurt, disappointed, and fearful of others. There is a tendency toward hero worship and crushes, but with little evaluation of the people to whom these feelings are directed.

Adolescent relationships serve many functions. Often adolescents relate to a friend as if neither person were a separate individual. They often mimic each other's dress, speech, language, and thoughts. These relationships help in the development of self-identity and establishment of a social role. The peer group is also very important because within the security of the peer group, adolescents can attempt to resolve conflicts. With peers they can test out their thoughts and ideas. Their thoughts may differ, but through mutual sharing, they can try to find an answer. The peer group can also explore other ways of dealing with problems and offer its members companionship, protection, and security. In the peer group, adolescents can accept dependency, not as a child but as one of the gang, testing out ideas and trying new values. Within the safety of the peer group, they can observe, comment on, and evaluate the activities of others. Adolescents usually are very loyal to their group of friends. Sometimes group security is so important that it is pursued at all costs, even if it involves destructive behavior.

Adolescents react to many stimuli and drain off the tension created by new drives and impulses by investment in many interests. They do this with great intensity, which is why adolescents are susceptible to fads. This is often seen in their dress, music, or hobbies. Close relationships with the opposite sex provide adolescents with security (often by "going steady") and a person with whom to discuss problems and evaluate solutions. Often the partner may take on similar characteristics. This reciprocal relationship enhances self-esteem by demonstrating sexual attractiveness to the self and to the world, and it indicates that one is lovable. It also allows for bisexual expression because the girl expresses her partner's feminine parts and her boyfriend represents her masculine parts.

Think about a current television program that is a favorite among adolescents and describe why it is popular, based on adolescent norms and developmental tasks.

Sexual Behavior

Adolescents use fantasy to discharge sexual tension. However, they may feel guilt and shame about sexual feelings or fantasies. Fantasies usually are an attempt to find solutions and evaluate consequences. They may indicate a disturbance if they continually occupy the adolescent's thoughts, are not converted into constructive actions, or are not modified by reality. Then they may disrupt other activities important to adolescent functioning and indicate a withdrawal from reality.

Masturbation is another way in which adolescents discharge sexual tension. The value of masturbation may be lessened if shame and guilt accompany it. Male adolescents often fear discovery of evidence of ejaculation, and females often fear changes in their genitalia as a result of masturbation. Fears are not limited to discovery by others. They may also result from the loss of ego boundaries experienced during orgasm. Mutual masturbation can serve the purposes of tension release and fusing of identity. It can help to dispel anxieties about sexuality by assuring adolescents that they are sexually adequate.

More teens are engaged in sexual activity, including intercourse and oral sex, than ever before and at an earlier age. Some believe that this is a result of increased parental divorce, inattentive parents, and early pubescence. However, most note that society gives very mixed messages to adolescents about sex. Whatever the cause, there is rising concern about the emotional and physical consequences of early sexual activity. Specifically, it is questioned whether the mechanical and dehumanized aspects of early sex may lead to troubled and detached relationships later in life.

Although 5% to 10% of American youth acknowledge homosexual experiences and 5% feel that they could be gay, homosexual experimentation is common during late childhood and early adolescence. Experimentation may include mutual masturbation and fondling of the genitals and does not by itself cause or lead to adult homosexuality. Theories about the cause of homosexuality include genetic, hormonal, environmental, and psychological models (see Chapter 27). Specifically, nurses need to be aware of the following:

- Not all homosexual adolescents are sexually active.
- Many homosexual adolescents are heterosexually active.
- Many heterosexual adolescents are homosexually active.
- The relationship between sexual identity and sexual behavior is variable during adolescence.
- Sexual issues produce stress and anxiety for adolescents of all sexual orientations.

Societal acceptance of homosexuality varies among cultures. The United States lags behind other nations in their attitudes towards homosexuality, often seeing it as "deviant" or "unacceptable." How adolescents cope with their emerging sexuality can be affected by these destructive views. Gay and lesbian adolescents may repress their desires, compartmentalize their experiences, or suppress their sexual impulses by withdrawing and becoming asexual. In such cases the developmental process of identity formation can be jeopardized and healthy emotional adjustment inhibited (Owens, 1998; Ryan et al, 1998).

MALADAPTIVE RESPONSES

Behaviors that impede growth and development may require nursing intervention. The nurse should consider the nature of the adolescent's maladaptive responses and the harm resulting from them. If the difficulty is significant and ongoing, intervention may be needed. Adolescents may also be diagnosed with the various *DSM–IV–TR* psychiatric illnesses described in Chapters 17 through 27 of this text (Parmelee, 1996). The nursing interventions described in these chapters can be implemented with adolescents, as well as the various treatment modalities described in Chapters 28 through 34. Evidence-based treatment strategies for adolescents have been identified that take into account the particular developmental issues and the unique challenges of establishing a therapeutic alliance with an adolescent (Weisz & Jensen, 1999).

Inappropriate Sexual Activity

Sexual behaviors can be the cause of many teenage problems. Some of these behaviors are described in Table 39-2. Sexual activity is often not as much an outlet for sexual passion as an attempt to achieve closeness with another person. Adolescents tend to use their sexuality to sublimate other needs, such as those of love and security, and personal anxiety about sexual adequacy and peer group pressure may lead the adolescent to have inappropriate sexual relations. For example, some adolescents engage in sexual relations as a means of punishing themselves. Their promiscuity elicits external control and criticism from others. This is especially true when there is an exhibitionistic quality and subtle efforts to "get caught" are seen. This is evident in the following clinical example.

 CLINICAL EXAMPLE

Isabel, a 14-year-old girl, had been sexually active since age 12 years. She was brought to the clinic by her parents when a neighbor told them Isabel had bragged of her sexual ventures. Two years before referral, her parents had placed her in a more controlled parochial school because they were concerned she was "acting wild." It became apparent that Isabel wanted her parents to know about and put limits on her behavior. She admitted to not enjoying sexual intercourse very much. She seemed to be trying desperately to get approval from her distant mother. She described her father, who was a policeman, as "a hopeless case," secretly wishing that he would be a better policeman for her.

However, it is important to differentiate between inappropriate behavior and defects in socialization that may result from the absence of an adequate parental role model, physical disabilities, sexual abuse, and personality temperament.

The additional risk of sexually transmitted diseases, including human immunodeficiency virus (HIV), makes sexual experimentation more problematic because of its potential short-term and long-term effects. Adolescents' needs for exploration and sexual gratification, as well as their feelings of invincibility, put them at great risk for HIV infection and other sexually transmitted diseases (see Citing the Evidence). Despite educational efforts, many adolescents are misinformed about the transmission of these illnesses and effective preventive strategies. Some believe "it can't happen to me" or think that having only one partner ensures their safety. Unprotected sex is the area of highest risk. Oral, anal, and vaginal contacts all pose a risk because they involve the transfer of body fluids that can contain viruses. Alcohol and drug use increases the risk potential of adolescents because they are more likely to have unplanned sex and not use a condom, and in the case of drug use, there is the additional risk from contaminated needles.

Table **39-2**

Adolescent Sexual Behavior—Report of a 1997 Survey
48% of students have had sexual intercourse
7% of students have had sexual intercourse before age 13 years
16% of students have had sexual intercourse with four or more partners
57% of currently sexually active students used a condom during their last sexual intercourse
17% of currently sexually active students used birth control pills before their last sexual intercourse
28% of currently sexually active students used drugs or alcohol during their last sexual intercourse
7% of students had been pregnant or gotten someone else pregnant
92% of students had been taught about HIV/AIDS in school
63% of students had talked about HIV/AIDS with parents or other adult family members

From Centers for Disease Control and Prevention: Youth risk behavior surveillance–US, 1997, *MMWR* 47(No. SS-3), 1998.

Citing the Evidence on

Youth Perception of Sexual Risk

BACKGROUND: The purpose of this qualitative descriptive study was to define college students' perceptions of AIDS risk for themselves, their friends, and their peers and to identify their risk behavior.

RESULTS: Most students appraised their risk as "nil" or "small" and their friends' risk similar to their own, but their peers' risk was seen as "great." Students "self-identified" certain sexual and drug use practices as AIDS risks. Yet they minimized the riskiness of their personal and their friends' behaviors while maximizing the riskiness of their peers' behavior.

IMPLICATIONS: Because college students tend to underestimate their AIDS risk given their sexual behavior, strategies are needed to help them appraise their AIDS risk based on the broadly accepted and evidence-based research on the riskiness of their behavior.

Brown E: College students' AIDS risk perception, *J Psychosoc Nurs* 36(9):25, 1998.

The nurse must explore the meaning of the adolescent's sexual behavior by asking the following questions:

- Does the adolescent desire sexual gratification or punishment?
- Do the adolescent's goals match the situation, or is self-deception present?
- Is the adolescent demanding adult privileges while acting irresponsible and dependent?
- To what extent is the sexual behavior experimentation, a defense against depression, or a way of expressing anger toward others?
- Is the sexual behavior a way to avoid anxiety-producing fantasies?
- How close is the relationship to a mature one?

Interventions related to sexual responses are discussed in Chapter 27 and care of the patient with HIV or acquired immunodeficiency syndrome (AIDS) is discussed in Chapter 42.

Unwed Motherhood

Pregnancy in adolescence is a complicated issue (Lesser et al, 1998). Some adolescent girls have low self-esteem and fears of inadequacy. To ease these fears, they may become pregnant. Sometimes pregnancy is an effort to escape a difficult family situation or to force the parents to agree to a marriage that may be inappropriate, as shown in the following clinical example.

 CLINICAL EXAMPLE

Susie, a 15-year-old girl, had run away for the second time, only to return home to the same chaos. She had tried to run away with her boyfriend. Her alcoholic mother and angry 19-year-old brother were making life unbearable. Her mother was surprised to learn about 3 months after her return that Susie was pregnant. Susie was delighted because she had hopes that she could get out of the house, knowing her mother would now approve of her marriage to her boyfriend.

Occasionally, emotionally deprived adolescents hope to give their child what they believe they have never received (or, perhaps more accurately, receive from the child what they have not received). Sometimes pregnancy appears to be a way to allow parents to give up parental responsibility for the adolescent. In other cases the adolescent has lived out a scapegoat role as the bad one in the family, thereby justifying parental neglect and hostility. The pregnancy can then improve family relationships because, with the adulthood the pregnancy implies, parents may be freed of guilt and may not need to encourage the adolescent to act in ways that make her unlovable.

Pregnancy in adolescence may have other origins. It can occur accidentally after sexual exploration. The adolescent may be unaware of contraceptive methods or may have delayed obtaining contraceptives. Research suggests that most teenage girls delay seeking contraceptives and become pregnant either because they are unwilling or unable to make conscious decisions about their sexual and contraceptive behavior or because they do not mind becoming pregnant

(DiClemente et al, 1996). Thus regular contraceptive use among sexually active adolescents requires that they believe that they can become pregnant and that using contraceptives is safe and the only way to prevent pregnancy. They must also have access to reliable, affordable contraceptives and must have a positive self-concept that allows them to make conscious decisions about their sexual and contraceptive behavior. Finally, they must want to postpone childbearing.

Pregnancy for unmarried adolescents may also be associated with sexual promiscuity. If it is, the girl may be ostracized. Sometimes pregnancy occurs within a close, caring relationship. Peer groups can be supportive to a girl who becomes pregnant as a result of a meaningful relationship but intolerant of one whose pregnancy is the result of promiscuity. Both the circumstances and the adolescent's level of maturity need to be assessed. In some cultures, out-of-wedlock pregnancies are an accepted part of adolescence.

Decisions involving abortion, placement of the baby, and marriage are difficult. Attitudes and laws influencing these decisions are diverse. Many believe that to force the adolescent to have the baby and then give the infant up is more traumatic for her than abortion. Others believe that abortion can be more disturbing. Marriage is another alternative. Forcing a marriage to avoid societal stigma usually adds to the adolescent's problems, but a mature couple might do well in marriage. All the alternatives should be presented to the adolescent, with the consequences clearly stated. The adolescent should make her decision with the aid and support of her partner, her family, the nurse, and other involved health-care professionals.

> *Pregnancy among adolescents is increasing in the United States. Why is this, and what, if anything, should be done about it?*

Depression and Suicide

The symptoms of depression in adolescence are somewhat different than those seen in adults (Box 39-2). Adolescents have difficulty describing their emotional or mood states. Young teenagers often do not complain about the way they feel and instead act moody and irritable. Between ages 11 and 15 years the rate of depression in girls rises rapidly, while only slightly in boys. Girls have been found to worry more than boys, feeling they have less control over their environment and what is happening in their lives. Boys tend to focus more externally on their actions and activities (Mohr, 1999). For both groups, however, symptoms of depression in adolescence strongly predict an episode of major depression in adulthood (Pine et al, 1999).

Suicide is the fourth leading cause of death among children age 10 to 14 years and the third leading cause of death among youth age 15 to 24 years. The suicide rate for people age 15 to 24 years has more than tripled in the past 30 years (Potter et al, 1998; Rosewater & Burr, 1998). Among high school students, 21% had seriously considered attempting suicide in the past year and 16% had made a specific plan to do so. Adolescents who successfully commit suicide use firearms, hanging, jumping, carbon monoxide, and drug

Box **39-2**

Symptoms of Adolescent Depression

- Frequent, nonspecific physical complaints
- Absences from school
- Poor school performance
- Talk or actions of running away
- Boredom or lethargy
- Outbursts of crying or moody behavior
- Irritable, angry, or hostile demeanor
- Lack of interest in friends
- Alcohol or drug use
- Decreased interaction and communication
- Fears of death
- Lack of interest in usual hobbies, sports, or recreational activities
- Sensitivity to rejection or failure
- Reckless risk-taking behavior
- Relationship problems

overdose. Males age 15 to 19 years are nearly five times more likely to kill themselves than females in the same age group, although female adolescents attempt suicide two to three times more often than their male counterparts.

Depression has been shown to be significantly related to suicidal behavior, as have diagnoses of conduct disorder, bipolar disorder, and substance abuse (Gould et al, 1998) . As adolescents move away from parental dependency, they increase their isolation and reduce their supervision. Peer problems often add to their sense of distress and alienation. The pressures to deal with intimate relationships, bodily changes, and an unstable sense of self can be overwhelming and lead to hopelessness and helplessness. One of the most common factors in adolescent suicide is lack or loss of a meaningful relationship. It has also been found that suicidal attempts and completion rates appear to be higher in gay, lesbian, and bisexual youth, based perhaps on the stress and loneliness they experience related to their sexual orientation (Remafedi et al, 1998; Fergusson et al, 1999).

Suicide is a bid for help that must be recognized. Subtle references, as well as attempts, should always be taken seriously and explored. Suicidal gestures are more often seen in girls, with boys expressing their depression by bravado that results in accidents, as in the following clinical example. It is often difficult to distinguish between risk-taking behavior, accidents, and suicidal gestures, thus requiring careful nursing assessment.

 CLINICAL EXAMPLE

John, a 12-year-old depressed adolescent, had just gotten a dirt bike. Six months earlier John's grandfather, his only friend, had died. John's father had died when he was 2 years old, and he had lived with his mother and grandparents ever since. John, feeling hopeless, had ridden his bike into a car. After medical treatment for his broken arm and rib and multiple bruises, John began to receive therapy. He described feeling helpless and lonely, especially without his grandfather.

Parent-adolescent relationships can influence suicidal behavior. For example, the adolescent may be prevented from acting on suicidal feelings by parental concern and the establishment of new relationships. In contrast, feelings of helplessness and worthlessness can be caused by threatened abandonment, being asked to take the adult role, and lack of opportunities to be dependent. Sometimes these adolescents perceive themselves to be expendable because they believe that the family unconsciously wishes them dead.

The nurse must make it clear to the adolescent that suicidal behavior is not confidential and that parents must be told. Family involvement is essential to avoid angry, hostile, and hopeless feelings of abandonment and to create support and caring.

In working with suicidal adolescents, the nurse should explore the following areas (Rudd & Joiner, 1998; Bloch, 1999):

- The seriousness of the attempt
- The mental status of the adolescent
- The extent of environmental stress, especially family problems
- The adolescent's wider social environment and the strength of support systems (social isolation, school performance, parental loss, disruption of friendship or romantic alliance)
- The likelihood of repeated suicidal attempts, especially if conditions remain the same

Nursing interventions related to depression are described in Chapter 20, and interventions related to suicide are described in Chapter 21. The next two clinical examples illustrate suicide attempts by adolescents.

 CLINICAL EXAMPLE

Maria, a 15-year-old girl, was referred to her local community mental health center from the neighborhood emergency room after ingesting pills. Maria had taken five of her mother's "arthritis pills" after an argument with her father about her 17-year-old boyfriend, José. Her father, who came home only on weekends, told her to stay away from him. After he left, the other family members noticed that Maria became sleepy while playing cards in the living room. Maria admitted to taking the pills and was rushed by her mother to the emergency room.

She had performed poorly in school in the year since her father had left the family. Maria had always been her father's favorite. When she reached puberty at age 13 years, that relationship changed. Maria's position as her father's favorite was delegated to a younger female sibling, causing Maria to feel angry and rejected. Her father left the family a year later and returned for weekend visits, during which he mainly disciplined the children. Maria's attempt to get close to José as a replacement for her father was sabotaged by her father as well. She thought her only recourse was to elicit her father's caring and concern through a suicide attempt.

 CLINICAL EXAMPLE

Donald, age 13 years, was brought to the emergency department after cutting his wrists one evening when he thought his family was asleep. His mother had awakened and found him bleeding. She rushed him to the local emergency room, where he received medical treatment. It was then revealed that this was Donald's second suicide attempt. The first attempt occurred a year ago, when he ingested pills. Donald had received therapy for about a month. It was then discontinued because the family moved to a new location, despite recommendations to continue with a new therapist. Donald was always an isolated child. He was never very close with anyone but had two friends. Since the move he had become more withdrawn. He had done well in school in the past but now had given up and was failing almost every subject. The youngest of nine children, Donald had little contact with his siblings, who were not at home much. Donald's parents, both approaching old age, seemed not to notice that he had become increasingly upset. Donald was hospitalized because the risk of his attempting suicide again was high.

Runaways

The number of adolescents who run away or are forced from their homes and become homeless is growing. Many of these young people have left or been forced from dysfunctional or abusive families only to face a life on the streets that can bring more problems such as poverty, substance abuse, physical and sexual assault, pregnancy, injury or illness, HIV infection, psychological and emotional problems, trouble with the law, and suicide. In addition, their prospects for a healthy and productive adulthood are reduced by the health risks they face and the lack of educational and employment opportunities for homeless youth.

Running away might be a cry for help or an attempt to escape from an unbearable living situation, including child abuse and family violence (Warren et al, 1997). It is sometimes a solution for an unmotivated youth who has little self-direction, drive, or ambition, and conduct disorder and severe aggression are common among runaway and homeless youth (Booth & Zhang, 1996). Finally, it is common in inner cities, where an unknown number of older children and adolescents move among the homes of friends or relatives, the streets, and abandoned buildings. Usually victims of poverty and overburdened single-parent homes, these teenagers may have had little opportunity to gain any sense of security or loving discipline or to have a vision of a hopeful future.

Adolescent runaways often have been rejected by their parents since birth, and the parent may alternate between extreme punitive measures and a laissez-faire attitude toward the adolescent. Adolescent runaways are often conflicted, especially regarding dependence and independence, and feel embarrassed, helpless, and defeated by their dependency wishes. This can result in a panic that motivates running away to prove autonomy and escape painful circumstances. They usually run away from disappointment toward something viewed as favorable and supportive. Parents often feel guilty and ashamed and have difficulty acting on practical issues, although some, relieved of their responsibility, are secretly pleased. Often the adolescent becomes involved in

dangerous activities after running away. Most runaway adolescents want to return home if they believe their parents really want them. The following clinical example illustrates home conditions that may lead to an adolescent's running away.

CLINICAL EXAMPLE

Karen, age 14 years, ran away from home to a friend's house. Her mother had often expressed a desire to leave; in fact, she had once left the family to the charge of Karen's father when Karen was 9 years old. Karen's mother had suddenly told her she could not see her boyfriend for a month because she had come in late the night before. This caused a tremendous scene because Karen had been out late every night the week before without her mother even noticing. Karen's friend's mother was different. She spent a lot of money on her children, talked to them, and never limited their activity; thus the friend's home appeared attractive to Karen.

 How would you design a community-based program to prevent adolescents from running away from home?

Conduct Disorders

Adolescents with conduct disorders display behavior that violates the basic rights of others or societal norms and rules. Examples include fighting, cruelty, lying, truancy, and destroying property. Conduct-disordered adolescents often have poor relationships with their parents. Antisocial acts allow the adolescent to express anger toward parents, who are often punished for the adolescent's acts. Children are socialized mainly by their parents and, it is hoped, learn from their parents' acceptable behaviors that become part of the internalized self or conscience. A good relationship between parent and child facilitates this process.

However, adolescents learn not only from their parents but also from others. The school and peer groups are influencing factors, as are the social, economic, and cultural environments. The self-destructive behaviors seen in conduct-disordered adolescents may indicate the need for punishment, anger at the family, peer group pressure, depression, feelings of self-defeat, a search for opportunities to take what they feel emotionally deprived of, and testing omnipotence through exciting experiences. Alignment with delinquents gives a defeated adolescent a feeling of self-respect and companionship through a sense of belonging to a subculture.

CLINICAL EXAMPLE

Levar, age 13 years, was referred by the juvenile court for therapy because he had been picked up for the second time after breaking into a store with another boy. Levar's parents were separated for the past 2 years, after his father served a sentence in jail for possession of drugs. Levar was extremely upset when his parents separated and rarely saw his father. His antisocial acts caused his father to become more involved with him because his father claimed he did not want his son to go through what he had experienced in prison. Levar gained his father's attention during these times, even though his father was angry. His delinquent actions enabled Levar to express his anger at his father's leaving, as well as to fantasize about having his father return.

This clinical example illustrates the many factors that may lead to adolescent delinquency. Adolescents may not differentiate between their stealing and their parent's business dealings. Stealing may also be an effective way to rebel against parents. Adolescents may perpetuate childhood by indulging in immediate gratification through stealing rather than working for things. Sometimes adolescents steal in hopes of getting caught and obtaining help. Parents may consciously or unconsciously condone stealing. Adolescents may also act out their anger with the justification that they deserve the stolen items.

Finally, the conflict of dependence and independence can be expressed in poor school adjustment. Some adolescents view teachers as parental surrogates who do not help or who merely apply rules of attendance and homework. Dependent feelings are sometimes elicited by these rules, and adolescents, in proving their independence, may become negative about learning. They may think that schoolwork is secondary to more important activities they are attempting to master. Daydreaming may interfere with schoolwork as adolescents concentrate on and fantasize about achieving independence.

Adolescents may drop out of school for financial reasons, or they may be rebelling against education laws. The adolescent may be part of a peer group that denounces school attendance and involvement. Parents may overtly or covertly discourage education. This is conveyed through lack of support and approval for education or by their making it difficult for the adolescent to follow through with school expectations, as illustrated by the following clinical example.

 CLINICAL EXAMPLE

Debbie, a 15-year-old girl, dropped out of school after several years of poor school performance and truancy. She occasionally went shopping with her mother on a school day. Her mother never knew the names of her teachers or guidance counselor and did not provide her with a place or time to study.

Violence

Violence among youth in America is on the rise (Box 39-3). Most adolescents displaying aggression have experienced frustration and have had violent role models during their childhood. Aggression is a human impulse that must be channeled constructively by a learned process that occurs within a supportive, loving relationship. Under favorable conditions a child learns the healthy expression of aggression by involvement in activities that result in pleasure and active problem-solving attempts. Under less favorable condi-

Box 39-3

Violence Fact Sheet

- In 1996 there were 969,018 reported cases of violent crimes committed against children.
- In 1996-1997 10% of all public schools reported at least one serious violent crime to law enforcement.
- Gunshot wounds to children age 16 years and under have increased 300% in major urban areas since 1986.
- According to the Federal Bureau of Investigation (FBI), 2900 juveniles were arrested for murder in 1996.
- As many as 5000 youth die each year as a result of mistreatment and abuse from parents and guardians.
- Everyday in America 16 youth are killed by firearms.
- Nearly 1 million students took guns to school during 1998.
- Each year 123,400 children are arrested for violent crimes in the United States.
- Persons under age 25 years make up nearly 50% of all victims of serious violent crime.

tions, aggression can result in destructive activities that are harmful to self and others (Modrcin-McCarthy et al, 1998).

The increase in school-related violence such as at Columbine High School in Colorado has encouraged the development of efforts by parents and school officials to be more aware of potentially violent children. The National School Safety Center has identified the behaviors listed in Box 39-4 that could indicate a youth's potential for harming himself or herself. In addition, parents can ask themselves the following questions:

- Do you know your children's friends?
- How are they spending their time?
- What movies, videos, and Internet sites are they watching?
- What music are they listening to?
- Who are their role models and why?
- How are they doing in academics and usual school activities?
- Have they made any threats about hurting another person?

Much anxiety of adolescents is related to the fear that they may be unable to control their destructive aggression. Adolescents often have violent dreams and fantasies that they express in threats, even though in some the potential for violence is minimal. Pointing out the harmlessness of these thoughts is helpful to adolescents because it shows them that these thoughts are not as powerful as they fear. However, some adolescents are genuinely fearful that they will be unable to stop their thoughts from becoming actions. They require the recognition of their fear and the reassurance of external limits. Pointing out to the adolescent the necessity for self-responsibility and control is very important. Their defenses against aggressive outbursts should be reinforced and supported. Focus should be on the behavior and feared loss of control, not on the roots of the anger. The following clinical example illustrates the management of a violent adolescent.

CLINICAL EXAMPLE

Ricky was a 14-year-old boy referred for treatment for violent outbursts at home. When frustrated, he would break and destroy objects in his path. Ricky was an only child, adopted shortly after birth by a couple in their forties who were unable to have children. Now Ricky's parents, who were about age 55 years, were increasingly frightened by his aggressive outbursts. They had also felt powerless with his childhood temper tantrums and had consistently responded to outbursts by attempting to limit frustrating situations. They felt guilty and inadequate about his being an adopted child and continually made attempts to reassure Ricky of their love for him. They consequently reinforced his lack of control by assuming that these outbursts were results of his fear of being unloved and would offer gifts and rewards to make peace. Ricky assumed he was omnipotent, successfully controlling his parents, but was afraid that he could not control his anger.

Acknowledging Ricky's fear of loss of control, applying external controls, and pointing out areas of Ricky's ability for responsibility and control resulted in a gradual decrease in outbursts.

Adolescents who have committed extreme acts of violence or homicide are often from families in which violence is condoned in some form. These adolescents may have experienced physical or sexual abuse, as described in Chapter 41, or they may have witnessed violence between their parents. Often these adolescents are encouraged to be violent by having guns in the home and by family members who extol the virtues of war, hunting or aggressive activities.

Sometimes parents can predict the adolescent's ability to injure or kill. Often there is a history of dangerous assaults on family members and pets. Other predictors of potentially violent behavior include drug abuse, poor school performance, and a history of fighting (Sege et al, 1999). In severely violent adolescents, violent acts can be followed by a calmness and lack of sorrow or guilt, or they may claim that outside forces provoked them. Many homicidal adolescents freely discuss their violent plans or fears. These should be explored and homicidal intent evaluated. Does the adolescent have a victim, weapons, or a plan? This information, along with the history, shows the level of success or failure in controlling feelings and delaying gratification.

 What do you think society can do to decrease gang violence among adolescents in this country?

Substance Use

Nationwide, substance use and abuse are significant problems for adolescents. They carry serious consequences, causing 50% of the deaths in youths age 15 to 24 years. Alcohol and drugs also contribute to assaults and rapes by adolescents.

Alcohol is the most commonly used and abused substance by youth. Nearly all high school seniors report some experience with alcohol. Although not all youth who drink have a drinking problem, nearly one third of seniors report being intoxicated in the past 30 days. Higher levels of adolescent

Box 39-4

Behavior Checklist for Potentially Violent Youth

_____ Has a history of tantrums and uncontrollable angry outbursts
_____ Characteristically resorts to name calling, cursing, and abusive language
_____ Habitually makes violent threats when angry
_____ Has previously brought a weapon to school
_____ Has a background of serious disciplinary problems at school and in the community
_____ Has a background of drug, alcohol, or other substance abuse or dependency
_____ Is on the fringe of his or her peer group with few or no close friends
_____ Is preoccupied with weapons, explosives, or other incendiary devices
_____ Has previously been truant, suspended, or expelled from school
_____ Displays cruelty to animals
_____ Has little or no supervision and support from parents or a caring adult
_____ Has witnessed or been a victim of abuse or neglect in the home
_____ Has been bullied or bullies or intimidates peers or younger children
_____ Tends to blame others for difficulties and problems caused by self
_____ Consistently prefers television shows, movies, or music expressing violent themes and acts
_____ Prefers reading materials dealing with violent themes and acts
_____ Reflects anger, frustration, and the dark side of life in school essays or writing projects
_____ Is involved with a gang or antisocial group on the fringe of peer acceptance
_____ Is often depressed or has significant mood swings
_____ Has threatened or attempted suicide

From National School Safety Center, Westlake Village, CA 91362.

alcohol use are associated with the three most frequent forms of mortality among adolescents: accidental deaths, homicides, and suicides. Nearly 9 out of 10 teenage automobile accidents involve the use of alcohol. Risk factors for adolescent alcohol use are presented in Table 39-3. Alcohol use has also been characterized as a gateway substance, preceding the use of marijuana and then other illegal substances such as cocaine and heroin.

The onset of drug use before age 20 years predicts more sustained use over time. From 70% to 90% of males and 50% to 60% of females who abused drugs in adolescence continue to do so in adult life. Chemical dependency is the result of a gradual process. Table 39-4 presents the stages of adolescent substance abuse. It is important for the nurse to remember that not all adolescents progress through these stages, but the younger the user, the greater the risk for chemical dependency. Specifically, first use of alcohol at age 11 to 14 years greatly increases the risk of the development of an alcohol disorder (DeWit et al, 2000). Substance abuse is discussed in detail in Chapter 25.

Table **39-3**

Risk Factor	Example
SOCIETAL-COMMUNITY	
Laws and normative behavior	Encouragement of youthful drinking in the media, absence of legal enforcement of underage drinking.
Availability	Easy access via the home or adults (such as siblings) purchasing liquor for minors.
Extreme economic deprivation	Escapist drinking to cope with harsh realities of everyday life.
Neighborhood disorganization	Undermine sense of security and purpose in life.
SCHOOL	
Low commitment to school	School expectations and career expectations very low.
Academic failure	Poor attendance, poor grades, underachievement.
Early persistent behavior problems	High aggression, attention problems.
FAMILY	
Family members alcohol users (abusers)	Role modeling influences.
Family management practices	Failure to monitor children; inconsistent parenting practices or harsh discipline.
Family conflict	Marital dysfunction or partner violence.
Low bonding to family	Lack of reciprocal nurturing and open communication.
PEERS	
Peer rejection in elementary grades	Rejection or neglect by peers undermines positive self-concept.
Associating with alcohol-using peers	Peer selection fosters cycles of negative behaviors.
Friends with attitudes favorable to alcohol use	Peer selection fosters cycles of negative attitudes and beliefs.
INDIVIDUAL	
Physiological	Genetic susceptibility to alcohol via enhanced tension reduction or misjudgment about level of intoxication.
Alienation and rebelliousness	Removed from normative attitudes and values of society and commitments toward societal goals.
Early-onset deviant behavior	Early-onset deviant behaviors consolidate and perpetuate negative spiraling cycles.
Problem-solving coping skills	Absence of strong problem-solving skills may contribute to adaptation of less desirable negotiating strategies (such as an aggressive coercive interpersonal style).

The meaning of drug use in adolescence is complex. The adolescent's motivation must be explored. The nurse must keep in mind that it may be an expression of rebelliousness with support of a peer group, as well as a way of obtaining gratification. It may also indicate an effort to come to grips with feelings of vulnerability and emptiness. Repeated and regular use of drugs for recreational purposes can lead to problems of anxiety and depression. Some teenagers use substances to decrease their anxiety, especially when socializing.

Adolescents often report a wish for closeness that is satisfied by sharing a drug experience with friends. Drug users can experience an illusion of closeness because drugs decrease anxiety and users can share anticipation of drug use. Some adolescents fill the void of isolated loneliness with drugs and would otherwise feel suicidally depressed. Drugs can be crippling and delay healthy maturity by promoting the avoidance of developing an adult identity in a real world, as illustrated in the following clinical example.

 CLINICAL EXAMPLE

Carlos was a 16-year-old boy who had been school phobic since age 10 years. He had been receiving home instruction since that age and was referred for a yearly assessment to obtain approval for a continuation of home instruction services. Carlos proudly spoke of his drug episodes. He and his small group of friends were close and had many exciting experiences induced by various hallucinogens and amphetamines. Carlos had little support in the real world because he had been isolated at home and developed interpersonal relationships primarily by obtaining drugs and experiencing their effects.

Finally, even though tobacco use has decreased among adults from 40% in 1965 to 25% today, teen smoking has increased. Over 3000 youth start smoking each year, and adolescents account for 85% to 90% of first-time smokers. Smoking usually begins in the sixth to ninth grades, and addiction typically occurs before age 20 years. It has been estimated that 35% of high school students are current tobacco smokers.

Tobacco can be the first drug adolescents use before expanding the experimentation to other substances. It has also been noted that smoking teens tend to fight more, carry weapons, and engage in risky sexual behaviors. However, simply telling young people the health hazards of smoking

Table 39-4

The Five Stages of Substance Abuse in Youth

Stage	Drugs	Sources	Frequency	Feelings	Behavior	Treatment
Curiosity	None	Available but not used	—	Curiosity	Risk taking, desire for acceptance	Optimal time, anticipatory guidance to develop good coping skills and strong self-esteem, clear family guidelines on drug and alcohol use, drug education skills and strong self-esteem, clear family guidelines on drug and alcohol-use, drug education
Experimentation	Tobacco, alcohol, marijuana	House supply, friends, siblings	Weekend use for recreational purposes	Excitement, pleasure, few consequences; learning how easy it is to feel good	Lying, little change	Drug education; attention to societal messages; reduction of supply; strict, loving rules at home; establishment of drug-free alternative activities
Regular use	As above, plus hashish or hash oil, tranquilizers, sedatives, amphetamines	Buying	Progresses to midweek use; purpose is to get high	Excitement followed by guilt	Mood swings, faltering school performance, truancy, changing peer groups; changing style of dress	Drug-free self-help groups (Alcoholics Anonymous or Narcotics Anonymous), family involvement, psychiatric counseling unhelpful unless family therapy and aftercare provided
Psychological or physical dependency	As above, plus stimulants, hallucinogens	Selling to support the habit, possibly stealing or prostitution in exchange for drugs	Daily	Euphoric highs followed by depression, shame, guilt, and perhaps suicidal thoughts	Pathological lying; school failure; family fights; involvement with the law over curfew, truancy, vandalism, shoplifting, driving under the influence, breaking and entering, violence	Inpatient or foster care programs that require family involvement and provide aftercare
Using drugs to feel "normal"	As above; any available drug, including opiates	Any way possible	All day	Euphoria rare and harder to achieve; chronic depression	Drifting, with repeated failures and psychological symptoms of paranoia and aggression; frequent overdosing, blackouts, amnesia; chronic cough, fatigue,	Inpatient or foster care programs that require family involvement and provide aftercare

Modified from MacDonald DI: *Pediatr Rev* 10:89, 1988.

does not appear to be an effective smoking cessation strategy. Instead, convincing them that they are being exploited by the tobacco industry seems to be a better approach. Much work remains to be done with this health issue, since only 3% of adolescents who attempt to quit are successful 12 months later.

> *You're concerned about your best friend's increasing use of drugs, but she denies that it is a problem. How can you best help her?*

Hypochondriasis

Adolescents are preoccupied with their bodies and body sensations. They are uncomfortable with their bodies because of the rapid changes in size, shape, and functioning. To establish their identity, adolescents try to become familiar with their changing bodies. They respond to sensations with increased intensity. When an adolescent appears overly concerned, it may indicate problems with self-image.

Hypochondriasis occurs when the adolescent has intense anxiety about personal health. This anxiety may be diffuse or directed toward one specific area. Adolescents may worry that their bodies are inadequate or that they will be rejected by others. Hypochondriasis may be a way of avoiding activities that expose these and other stressful fears. Fears such as inadequacy at school, either socially or in schoolwork, may be a projection of general fears of inadequacy. Lack of knowledge of normal body changes may be a simple precipitating factor. This can be helped by reassurance that these changes are normal. If reassurance does not relieve the anxiety, more intense fears may be involved.

It is important to communicate to adolescents that people are aware something is wrong and that their concerns will be taken seriously until the core problem is solved. Intense body concern is a signal that something is wrong and help is needed. Physical status must be assessed before one assumes that there is a psychological basis for concern. Sometimes body preoccupation is an effort to recreate childhood dependency by eliciting caregiving. This is particularly seen in adolescents who experienced early emotional deprivation, as shown in the following clinical example.

 CLINICAL EXAMPLE

John, age 12 years, was referred for treatment from the local hospital after having been seen for chest pains. The physician found no medical problems. John was embarrassed and angry about the episode, insisting that the physician was wrong. The chest pains had disappeared, but he now had injured his arm. He also was often plagued by attacks of tonsillitis and middle ear infections. John had experienced early emotional deprivation because he was often moved around in his living arrangements. He was born out of wedlock and lived occasionally with his mother, often with his maternal grandmother, and infrequently with his father. He generally had the feeling that no one really cared for him. Further exploration revealed that John's body concerns were vocalized to initiate

caregiving by those around him, who, he feared, really were not there for him. He performed well in school and had friends, but none of these compensated for his feelings of inadequacy.

Weight and Body Image Problems

Eating disorders are another group of problems often seen in adolescence. They include anorexia nervosa, bulimia nervosa, and obesity. The sociocultural milieu for female adolescents in the United States has precipitated identity and body image confusion and anxiety in this age group (see Citing the Evidence). The emphasis on thinness, athletics, and physical attractiveness suggests that these are highly valued achievements for young women. These traits demonstrate self-control and social success and are culturally rewarded. The result is that fear of fat, restrained eating, binge eating, and body image distortion are common problems among teenage girls.

Recent understandings suggest that eating disorders represent a complex of issues related to many possible causes. Psychosocial factors, family characteristics, physiology, and biochemical interactions all play a part in the development and treatment of these disorders. They are discussed in detail in Chapter 26. The following clinical example illustrates the development of anorexia nervosa in a young girl.

 CLINICAL EXAMPLE

Janet, age 15 years, was admitted to the hospital because it was feared that her extreme weight loss was endangering her life. Exploration revealed that Janet was afraid of her sexual feelings and the response of others to her budding sexuality. Her father, provocative and teasing toward Janet, was continually kid-

---

Citing the Evidence on

Weight Concerns in Girls

BACKGROUND: A community survey was conducted to assess the prevalence of the significant weight and shape concerns among adolescent girls.

RESULTS: Significant weight or shape concerns were present in 15% of the 11- to 14-year-olds and in 19% of the 15- to 16-year-olds. Only among those age 15 to 16 years was the presence of such concerns linked to disordered eating habits.

IMPLICATIONS: Concerns about weight and shape start early in adolescence and before the development of diagnosable eating disorders. Early preventive interventions could be targeted at the emergence of these early concerns.

Cooper P, Goodyer I: Prevalence and significance of weight and shape concerns in girls aged 11-16 years, *Br J Psychiatry* 171: 542, 1997.

ding her about her oncoming sexual attractiveness and implied that he really preferred her to her mother. This created panic, and Janet refused to eat. She liked her thinness, which was a protection from sexual desires. In the hospital the area of concentration was not the behavior of not eating, but rather the underlying feelings about her sexuality and her relationship with her father. This provided freedom for normal sexual growth and development.

Boys have body image problems as well. They respond to society's pressure to be muscular and virile, and many adolescent boys are ostracized from social groups for being short, overweight, or too thin. Boys may also evaluate their self-worth by the qualities of their bodies. Body dysmorphic disorder is a psychiatric illness common in male adolescents in which they are obsessively preoccupied with flaws they perceive in their appearance. Symptoms include continually checking mirrors and attempts to hide perceived, imaginary imperfections. The average age of onset is 15 years.

Parental Divorce

Nearly one fourth of all children and adolescents in the United States live in single-parent homes. Nearly half of all youngsters born in the past decade will experience a parental divorce. The effect of divorce on children varies with the child's age and developmental level. Adolescents are particularly vulnerable, and their initial reactions may include depression, anger, and identification of one parent as the victim and rejection of the other. Over time, adolescents may become anxious or pessimistic about their own future involvement in intimate relationships. However, some adolescents become more mature and independent in perceiving that they have helped their parents in this time of crisis.

The most favorable outcome of divorce is seen when the divorced parents are able to put aside old conflicts and anger and return to meaningful caretaking relationships with their children. The adolescent's adaptation is also influenced by the amount of relief the divorce provides from marital strife and the young person's own emotional strengths, vulnerabilities, coping resources, and support systems. The treatment of adolescents of divorced parents include helping the adolescent (Thompson, 1998):

- Grieve the loss of the family unit
- Maintain distance from parental conflicts
- Express age-appropriate involvement in developmental tasks
- Decrease anger, anxiety, depression, and acting out
- Assess both parents realistically
- Improve communication with both parents
- Continue the separation-individuation process
- Control overly aggressive and sexual drives

How might growing up in a single-parent household positively and negatively affect an adolescent?

WORKING WITH ADOLESCENTS

Knowledge of normal adolescent development is necessary to differentiate between age-expected behavior and maladaptive responses. When working with an adolescent, it is best if the nurse can have an initial contact directly with the adolescent. Many adolescents are concerned that the nurse is aligned with the parents. Other adolescents take a passive role, letting the adults straighten things out for them. By initiating contact with the adolescent, the nurse aligns with the patient's independent, mature aspects. Parents asking for advice on how to approach the adolescent about seeking treatment should be advised to be honest, stating the true nature of the visit and their reasons for requesting it. Family sessions can also be helpful in completing a thorough assessment, understanding family interactions, and establishing family support.

Health Education

The psychiatric nurse is in an excellent position to educate the adolescent, the parents, and the community. Basic health information can be given in such areas as smoking, drugs, sex and contraception, suicide prevention, and crime prevention. Adolescents want information about what activities are healthy and unhealthy, including facts about exercise, nutrition, dealing with anger, sexuality, conflict resolution, and where they can access help (Coggan et al, 1997; Hamburg, 1997). The nurse can also provide information on healthy emotional functioning, including coping with stress and anxiety and pursuing personally meaningful activities (Puskar et al, 1997). Coping with stress includes the following:

- Skills and motivation to manage acute, major life stressors and recurring daily stressors
- Skills to solve problems (problem-focused coping) and skills for emotion management (emotion-focused coping)
- Personal flexibility and the ability to meet the demands of varying types of stress

Involvement in personally meaningful activities includes:

- Skills and motivation to engage in instrumental and expressive activities that are personally meaningful
- Behaviors and activities that are experienced as autonomous and self-determined

By educating them on normal adolescent behavior and by interpreting the underlying conflicts, the nurse prepares parents, teachers, and other community members to support adolescents and encourage healthy independent functioning. Often parents and other adults become frustrated, angry, and confused by the independent strivings of adolescents. Encouraging independence and lessening power struggles can produce a positive change in adolescents' relationships with adults and in their feelings about themselves. However, adults should still set limits. Setting limits and providing structure can be done in a way that encourages the adolescent's independent functioning. Many parents are conflicted about their children becoming adults. This, together with the adolescent's own ambivalence and fears about independence, can create havoc.

One of the best ways to educate parents on adolescent development is through a parents' group. The nurse can inform parents on normal adolescent functioning and provide them with much needed support from other parents in the same situation. Sharing mutual experiences and searching for solutions in a supportive environment can be extremely helpful to parents. It is important to remember that parents have nurtured children to reach adolescence and many believe that "showing them how" is their primary parental responsibility. It is a difficult change for them to suddenly switch from the "how to" of the child to the "try to" of the budding adult. Parents can learn the process of providing increased responsibilities based on a gradual progression of independent functioning. Despite their fears of their teenagers getting into trouble, they can be educated to promote self-reliance. The next two clinical examples show the need to educate parents and community members.

 CLINICAL EXAMPLE

Mr. and Mrs. B came to the attention of the psychiatric nurse by their distressed calls to the community mental health center. Mrs. B tearfully explained that they had lost all control of their 14-year-old daughter. She had become arrogant and hostile, locking herself in her bedroom after an argument they had about her going to the movies with a 14-year-old boy she had met at school. Further exploration revealed that Emily was an honor student at school, maintaining a solid A average. She had many friends at school, was on the volleyball team, and baby-sat regularly on weekends for the neighbors' two children. She had always been pleasant, happy, and friendly. Suddenly this boy that the parents did not know called her at home. After many phone conversations he asked Emily to join him on a weekend evening at the movies. Mr. and Mrs. B felt that Emily was much too young to date, that she could get involved with drugs, sexual promiscuity, and so on. They were sad and worried that they had lost their little girl who always did what she was told. Emily was hurt and furious. She thought her parents were being totally unreasonable and that they did not trust her. It turns out that Mrs. B had gotten into trouble sexually as a young girl. She did not want Emily to make the same mistake. Mrs. B's parents had been very lenient, and she blamed their lack of guidelines for her error. Mrs. B became aware of her overreaction. After discussion with a psychiatric nurse, she was able to understand that dating was a normal part of adolescent development. A compromise was arranged when she recognized Emily's competent and responsible functioning. After Mr. and Mrs. B met the boy, Emily was able to go to the movies with him and two other friends on a Saturday afternoon.

 CLINICAL EXAMPLE

Lui Lee, an adolescent girl starting high school, had always functioned well. Beginning high school was a totally different experience. She became overwhelmed by the large building, increased academic responsibilities, and complex peer relationships. She began school in September with much anxiety. By October she began having numerous illnesses that prevented her from attending school. This came to the attention of the school guidance counselor, who noticed her increased absences. The guidance counselor saw her and, after no medical problems were found, invited Lui Lee to come to her office whenever she felt sick at school. When this did not help, she suggested that Lui Lee receive some home instruction until she felt less anxious. This suggestion validated Lui Lee's fears that she could not handle high school and its increased pressures. Her solution of retreat was supported. Fortunately, her parents sought the help of a psychiatric nurse, who encouraged immediate return to school with entry into a peer support group, with individual sessions initially as needed. This enabled her to talk out her fears and receive support from her peers. This also strengthened her confidence and fostered healthy functioning. She found she could handle high school after all. The nurse educated the guidance counselor on ways to be supportive while encouraging independent functioning.

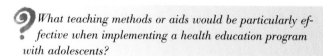

What teaching methods or aids would be particularly effective when implementing a health education program with adolescents?

Family Therapy

The nurse needs to assess the level of family functioning and determine how to best interact with and help the family of the adolescent. Family therapy is particularly useful when disturbed family interaction is interfering with the adolescent's development. Sometimes a series of family sessions may be enough, and the adolescent may benefit from either individual or group approaches to support the effort to separate emotionally from the family. Occasionally, after a few family sessions, it may become clear that the adolescent may not need the intervention directly. Engaging the parents may free the adolescent to progress on the developmental continuum.

The techniques used in family therapy are reviewed in detail in Chapter 34. Whatever modality is selected in working with the adolescent, a family orientation and the adolescent's attempt to separate from the family and become an independent adult should be considered.

Group Therapy

Group therapy addresses adolescents' need for peer support. The conflict between dependence and independence with adults becomes somewhat diluted by the presence of other adolescents. Conflicts, especially about authority, can be detected by peers rather than adults, making group therapy particularly helpful for adolescents. It is valuable in teaching skills in relating and dealing with others. Group therapy also helps fulfill the adolescent's need for a positive, meaningful peer group for ego identity formation.

Adolescent groups, in contrast to other groups, are difficult to manage because many adolescents react to peers defensively. Sibling rivalry often disrupts group cohesion. Many groups suffer from poor attendance, a high dropout rate, antisocial behavior, and a lack of group cohesion. However, group therapy with adolescents has proved to be successful in many community mental health centers, outpatient clinics, and hospital settings.

Often, beginning group sessions with some activity provides a stabilizing factor for young adolescents. The number of members to include in the group depends on the type. For example, it may not be feasible to limit an outpatient walk-in group. Because of the age spread among adolescents, it is usually preferable to form at least two groups. A possibility is an early adolescence group consisting of 13- to 15-year-olds who have conflicts of separation from parents. An older adolescent group, age 15 to 17 years, would probably consider issues such as the further establishment of identity, the beginning of dating, sex, experimentation with drugs, handling money, responsibilities of driving, and vocational plans.

Conflict between therapists, if there is an open and honest discussion, can provide a corrective experience because adolescents can see adults disagree without devastating consequences. If therapists are of the opposite sex, a parental similarity is often apparent; members often play on the therapist's feelings and try out tactics as they would with their own parents. Even if both therapists are of the same sex, one is usually more active, and a member may project a good or bad image onto each therapist that corresponds with how the parents are viewed. Group process with adolescents is often similar to that with adults, and specific aspects of working with groups are reviewed in Chapter 33.

When might a same-sex adolescent therapy group be most helpful? Compare this to the value of a mixed male and female group.

Individual Therapy

Individual therapy is done by the advanced practice psychiatric nurse. Once the decision to engage in individual therapy is made, a pact or contract between the nurse and adolescent is established and a therapeutic relationship is initiated (see Chapter 2).

Therapeutic Alliance. This contract is a therapeutic alliance in which a nurse aligns herself with the healthy, reality-oriented part of the adolescent's ego and moves toward an honest and critical understanding of the adolescent's thoughts and behaviors. The alliance is a central aspect of individual therapy. Once it is established, a feeling of working together is apparent. Specific ways to establish and maintain this alliance include the following (Meeks, 1990):

- Point out that behavior is motivated by feelings. Often, early in treatment, adolescents express feelings of impatience, helplessness, and failure at having to seek treatment. Defenses are often seen in rebelliousness, passivity, shyness, negativism, and intellectualization. Adolescents generally have a tendency to act out and avoid examining their feelings.
- Limit acting out by pointing out how it interferes with the therapeutic process and that it must be controlled to proceed. Maintain a neutral but interested attitude toward all behavior.
- Point out the adolescent's tendencies to be judgmental and self-critical. This is supportive and helps to encourage the adolescent to look for sources of behaviors, attitudes, and feelings.
- Establish that the adolescent's behavior is the result of automatic thoughts and inner feelings that are interfering with the adolescent's happiness. This knowledge strengthens the motivation for therapy and maintains an alignment with the adolescent's wishes for autonomy.
- Point out the adolescent's tendency to see things in extremes; the desire to be complete master opposes the feelings of total helplessness. Reveal areas of strength and competence that are often unrecognized. Avoiding exclusive focus on problems and weaknesses shows neutrality and is supportive. Giving the adolescent as much information as possible to make decisions helps the adolescent work toward self-direction.
- Distinguish among thoughts, feelings, and actions, discouraging impulsiveness. Encourage open expression of strong feeling but not strong action. For example, anger does not mean killing; sexual feeling does not mean intercourse. Adolescents sometimes confuse discussion with permission to experiment with action, especially with sexual issues.
- Encourage emotional catharsis in sessions by expressing interest in and acceptance of feelings involving the nurse and events outside the session. Point out the importance of feelings.
- Be alert to the defenses of denial and reaction formation. Maintain neutrality and encourage objectivity without directly attacking needed defenses.

Adolescents often act provocatively to force punishment by adults. This puts the nurse in alignment with the self-hatred aspect of the adolescent's conscience and should be avoided. The nurse provides support by continuing therapy even during these difficult periods.

The work of the nurse is to recognize the adolescent's anxiety and assist in finding ways to deal with emerging impulses. Accepting any healthy and adaptive responses of the adolescent strengthens the sense of ego mastery. Adolescents often have wishes that they regard as crazy and frightening. Open discussion of fears helps adolescents realize that these feelings are uncomfortable but harmless thoughts.

Transference. Transference often occurs in adolescent treatment. The nurse must point out that these projections originate in the adolescent's mind and not in reality and that they usually represent a meaningful person such as a parent. It often helps to mention this is a common response. Several common transference patterns include the following:

- **Erotic-sexual,** especially if the nurse is young and of the opposite sex. This transference typically is shown by awkward blushing and agitated confusion on the part of the adolescent. It is usually best to emphasize the mutual work of emotional growth while tactfully establishing the nurse's unavailability as a sexual object. Focusing on origins or encouraging elaboration of these feelings is not helpful and provokes anxiety.

- **Omnipotent,** expecting that the nurse will have answers to all questions. It is easy for the nurse to drift into this pattern because often the adolescent appears to be helpless. The adolescent's secret desire for personal omnipotence is somewhat fulfilled by granting it to the nurse.
- **Negative transference,** usually intense and pervasive. Negative feelings toward the nurse usually represent a negative attitude toward all adult authority figures. This transference is often defensive to cover feelings of shame, inadequacy, and anxiety, and it disappears as the adolescent respects the nurse's feelings. The adolescent tries to force the nurse's rejection. Open discussion to explore these feelings objectively and establish their origin is helpful. Sometimes interpretations arouse anger toward the nurse because of the anxiety they create. These are reactions to the realities of therapy and are not to be confused with negative transference.

A true negative transference occurs when situations reactivate early experiences of negative feelings toward important others. The nurse unavoidably will frustrate the adolescent, who often has trouble delaying gratification to reach long-range goals. Negative transference, like any other resistant behavior, is dealt with through objective exploration, which includes seeking causes of anger and pointing out irrationality. This is often followed by a period of regression and depression. Empathic understanding that the adolescent is mourning a loss is helpful, but it should be emphasized that what was lost was an illusion. Another common occurrence is for an adolescent to rebel against conscience and then respond to guilt through self-destructive behaviors. Pointing out this pattern helps the adolescent to eventually become aware of this.

Termination. Termination of therapy is an important part of the therapeutic process. Often, leaving therapy symbolizes the process of loosening bonds to parental images and giving up desires to be passive. One therefore expects defensive and regressive behaviors as the adolescent attempts to deal with the anxieties related to the termination process. This can mean the recurrence of emotional crises, symptoms, self-destructive fantasies, and even dependency behavior to provoke rescue.

Termination should be flexible and correctly timed. The decision should be made in line with adolescent norms, not adult ones. Often adolescents verbalize appropriate interest in termination. When this occurs, it is often helpful to open it to discussion without commitment to a set time. This implies that further work needs to be done in a definite time span, and it maintains a focus on the adolescent's responsibility to finish. Gradually supporting and approving of the adolescent's independence and mature functioning prepares for a positive termination.

Sometimes terminations occur prematurely because an alliance has not been established or some external event has occurred. Occasionally terminations are forced because of a nurse's change of location, death, or illness. The adolescent will express anger at the new therapist until the feelings about the lost therapist are accepted and resolved. In working out this attachment, a new therapeutic alliance can be established.

Pharmacotherapy

For adolescents, it is a particular challenge to determine which of the changing and often tumultuous behaviors are target symptoms for psychopharmacological interventions. This treatment strategy is more complex for this age group because of the following:

- The need for comprehensive family involvement (often optional in adults)
- Developmental differences that affect assessment, treatment alliance, management, compliance, and pharmacokinetics
- The difficulty in diagnosing emerging first episodes versus adjustment disorders in this age group
- The lack of controlled clinical drug trials in adolescents

In terms of medication management, adolescents are neither children nor adults. They have a metabolism more like adults than like children. Thus dosing regimens for adolescents are usually closer to those of adults (Lieberman & Tasman, 2000). Biologically, it cannot be assumed that drug response will be within the generally expected range for adults. The current state of the art in adolescent psychiatric practice is to carefully prescribe psychopharmacological agents when they are determined to be appropriate and necessary as part of a comprehensive treatment plan. The increased recognition of psychiatric disorders in adolescents and their resulting negative effects on social, psychological, and emotional development, the increasing efficacy and safety of these drugs in adults, and the increasing evidence of efficacy of these drugs in adolescents have contributed to this practice (Greenhill & Waslick, 1997).

The use of selective serotonin reuptake inhibitors (SSRIs) is generally preferred over tricyclic antidepressants (TCAs) in the treatment of adolescents because of their lower side effect profile and their relative safety in overdose. Additionally, there is increasing evidence that they are effective in the treatment of adolescent obsessive compulsive disorder and some anxiety disorders, such as panic disorder. The use of benzodiazepines for anxiety is generally not recommended in this age group because of the increase in drug experimentation by adolescents and the negative effects on learning and memory that these drugs may have. Lithium is generally well tolerated in this age group and is effective in the treatment of mania, aggression, and conduct disorder. The other mood stabilizers have not been well studied in adolescents. Antipsychotics are the standard treatment for psychotic symptoms in adolescents. Although few studies exist, it appears that children and adolescents respond to lower doses of antipsychotics than adults and are more likely to experience extrapyramidal side effects, particularly teenage males when conventional rather than atypical drugs are used. Finally, adolescents have a positive response to psychostimulants for ADHD, similar to that seen in younger children. Chapter 28 provides comprehensive information about psychopharmacology in general, and Chapter 38 contains a table specific to the psychopharmacological treatment of children and adolescents.

Talking with Adolescents

The following discussion focuses on some important considerations in communicating with adolescents.

Silence. Silence is often effective with adults but frightening to the adolescent, especially in the beginning stages of treatment or evaluation. This anxiety often reflects the adolescent's feelings of emptiness and lack of identity. Brief silences can be creative and productive when the adolescent is engaged in treatment; when the adolescent is able to tolerate them without anxiety, it indicates growth in self-confidence and acceptance of inner feelings. More often, however, silence is used defensively by adolescents to avoid discovery of hostile feelings or fantasies. Older adolescents may tolerate interpretive remarks, but with younger adolescents it is usually helpful to suggest an activity to help facilitate discussion and establish a relationship. For some adolescents, silence is a defense of inhibition and withdrawal because they have never learned to communicate in a positive way. In these cases the therapist must be responsible for dialogue.

Confidentiality. Confidentiality is a concern to many, but especially to the adolescent who is fearful of the nurse reporting to parents. A blanket promise to tell nothing to the parents is not advised because the nurse may need to contact the parents if the adolescent reveals suicidal or homicidal behavior or the use of illegal drugs. It is usually best to tell the adolescent that the nurse will not give out any information without informing the adolescent in advance. It is also helpful to explain that feelings are confidential but that actions considered dangerous to the adolescent or others must be shared.

> *You receive a call from the school guidance counselor of one of your adolescent patients asking what progress is being made in treatment. How would you respond?*

Negativism. Negative feelings are often expressed by adolescents, especially initially, because they are frightened of the implications of coming for treatment. The young adolescent's lack of objectivity and upsurge of impulses, as well as the tendency to confuse fantasy and action, make the discussion of feelings threatening. Usually, gently noting in a supportive way defensive techniques the adolescent uses during the session helps to gain cooperation.

Resistance. Often adolescents begin by testing nurses to see whether they will be authoritarian figures. The rebellious adolescent may deny the need for therapy or help. If the adolescent appears anxious, it is best to be supportive and sympathetic, expressing interest in getting to know the adolescent and then discussing a neutral area. A more angry, rebellious adolescent may require a direct approach, with the nurse saying openly that the adolescent is opposing the visit because of a false belief that no help is needed. This can lead to a further discussion of feelings about the visit (such as parental coercion to come to the session) or feelings about authority. Some adolescents are just baiting and testing to see whether the nurse is an anxious, defensive adult. If so, it is best to ignore their comments about not wanting treatment and move on. Often adolescents with an angry facade depend on their omnipotent control of the environment and are successful in manipulating their families. They are angry at attempts to disturb this power, and the anger is expressed in their lack of cooperation in the session.

Arguing. Adolescents often argue and, although they do not admit it, learn from arguments. Often the adolescent goes against the viewpoint of the nurse and then in the next session adopts the nurse's opinion. It is best not to comment on this and accept it as a harmless defense.

Testing. Adolescents often need and want limits. They are confused and cannot set their own limits. Often adolescents test nurses to see how firm and consistent they will be. Controls are effective if there is a basic positive relationship with the nurse. Limits should be set only when they are essential for current and future well-being. Adolescents will dare to be independent if it is conveyed that the nurse will serve as a control against carrying independence too far.

Dreams and Artistic Creations. Adolescents are often creative, and much can be learned from studying their works. As long as the discussion is relevant, it can be a productive source for exploring inner feelings. Along with dreams, these feelings can reveal valuable information about their real concerns, even when the adolescent attempts to avoid them.

Bringing Friends. The adolescent who brings a friend to a session may be attempting to avoid therapy. There is some benefit in sharing the experiences with the peer group because this lowers anxiety. Telling the adolescent that bringing friends is not allowed may not be successful because the nurse cannot always enforce such a rule. The reason for bringing friends may vary, but it should be explored and understood. Sometimes adolescents want to refer friends. This may be positive but may also focus attention away from the original adolescent. The nurse should insist on exploring motives behind the referral before accepting the new patient because the adolescent may think the nurse's acceptance of another is a betrayal of loyalty. If the friend clearly wants and needs therapy, referral to a colleague is usually best. If a friend is brought late in therapy, it may mean that the adolescent is preparing to terminate.

Embarrassment about Being in Therapy. Embarrassment may occur in any age group, but it is prominent in adolescents, especially during the early stages of treatment. It also can become an issue as therapy progresses because it often reveals the adolescent's embarrassment about a desire for dependency. Therefore adolescents may become uncomfortable in the therapeutic relationship. This is usually dealt with by indicating that these feelings are normal. Behind the fear of accepting help is the wish for care, and this can be dealt with by pointing out the adolescent's strengths and areas of independence.

Some adolescents, by expressing embarrassment about being in therapy, are actually revealing a fear or social stigma that they have heard from their parents. The adolescent who has feelings of inferiority often focuses these on the therapeutic process, blaming therapy for discomfort. It is best to encourage and support the adolescent, gently refusing to accept blame for this discomfort.

Requests for Special Attention. Some adolescents can develop intense dependency ties to the therapist. They reflect this in requests for additional appointments, extra time in appointments, frequent telephone calls, or social contact outside the therapeutic sessions. Focus should be on the exploration of feelings of inner emptiness, deprivation, and incompleteness that are responsible for these requests.

> *Do you think adolescents can benefit from treatment if their parents deny there is a problem, refuse to be involved, or are opposed to seeking help?*

Parents of the Adolescent

If group or individual treatment is selected for the adolescent, the nurse must still consider the family. Parents cannot help the adolescent's treatment if they do not understand and accept it. The nurse can work with the parents without revealing confidential material.

It is helpful for parents to have treatment if the adolescent is asked to assume an inappropriate role at home because this interferes with the adolescent's adaptive responses. If the parents are resistant, the nurse must usually begin with the adolescent until the parents are more receptive.

Telephone contact is a helpful way to ensure cooperation and support by having the parent call when necessary. Parents should tell the adolescent when they call. Parents should be told of normal adolescent behavior they can expect. The nurse should avoid advising the parents about specific actions and focus on attitudes and feelings, especially concerning discipline. Parents can be helped with understanding the purpose of limit setting. Some parents exclude themselves entirely from their adolescent's life. They have brought the adolescent to treatment to ease their guilt by doing all that is possible. They may want the nurse to take over parenting functions. This should not be permitted, especially during crises. If the adolescent is suicidal or homicidal, the parents are informed and helped to take responsibility for action.

Adolescents often need help in dealing with their parents. Parents should be discussed in an open exploratory way, with emphasis on them having their own feelings and reasons for their actions. Adolescents should be helped to see their parents realistically and to work on their own strengths and weaknesses.

Sometimes adolescents want to leave home because they hope they will feel more adult away from their parents. It is usually best to explore the wish to leave, emphasizing that it must be done in an adult way. If leaving is an impulsive thought with no feasible plan, it will result in failure, parental rescue, and continued dependency.

EVALUATING NURSING CARE

Problems presented by adolescents often activate the nurse's own unresolved conflicts. Thus evaluating nursing care must begin with nurses monitoring their responses, including countertransference reactions. The nurse should watch for alignment with the parents against the adolescent or the adolescent against the parents. Most adults are resistant to re-experiencing the feelings of adolescence and have repressed these experiences. As a result of anxiety, the nurse

occasionally may have trouble listening or may encourage the adolescent (because of unrecognized wishes) to do what the nurse never dared do. The adolescent may be acting as the nurse did during adolescence. The nurse, in an effort to deny this, may see this adolescent behavior as nondeviant.

Identification of the nurse with the adolescent can contribute to delays in exploring areas important for psychological growth. The nurse may relate well to the adolescent but because of unresolved, unrecognized conflicts or resentment toward the nurse's own parents, may be locked into adolescent rebellion. The nurse may overtly or covertly encourage adolescents to express rage toward their families. Both the adolescent and the nurse then avoid facing the reality of adult burdens.

Evaluation of psychiatric nursing care with adolescents also involves objective measurements of the adolescent's and the family's progress toward the goals of treatment. Specifically, the nurse may ask:

- Were the concerns of the adolescent and family addressed?
- Has the problematic behavior decreased and been replaced with more adaptive responses?
- Have the adolescent's relationships with others improved?
- Has school or work performance been enhanced?
- Are the adolescent and family satisfied with the treatment outcome?

By reviewing areas of growth and progress, the adolescent is able to integrate the learning that has been accomplished and gain from the experience a greater sense of self-efficacy and mastery.

Summary

1. Adolescence is a unique stage of development that occurs between ages 11 and 20 years and is accompanied by a shift in development and learning.

2. Various theories explain the adolescent's resolution of tasks, including biological, psychoanalytical, psychosocial, attachment, cognitive, cultural, and multidimensional.

3. Issues that are particularly problematic for adolescents include body image, identity, independence, social role, and sexual behavior.

4. Maladaptive responses impede growth and development and require nursing intervention. These are often related to inappropriate sexual activity, unwed motherhood, depression and suicide, running away, conduct disorders, violence, substance use, hypochondriasis, weight and body image problems, and parental divorce.

5. Nursing interventions useful in working with adolescents include health education, family, group, and individual therapy, and medication management. Special attention should be given to talking with adolescents and working with their parents.

6. Evaluation of nursing care requires special focus on countertransference issues and the need for objective measurements of the adolescent's and family's progress toward the treatment goals.

Competent Caring ## A Clinical Exemplar of a Psychiatric Nurse

KAREN M. MCHUGH, BSN, RN, C

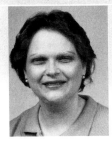

When I graduated with a bachelor's degree in nursing, I never imagined I would be interested in psychiatric nursing. After 1½ years in medical-surgical nursing, I decided I wanted more interpersonal time with my patients rather than being so skill and task oriented. One of my first experiences as a psychiatric nurse was on a 32-bed adolescent unit in North Carolina. There I encountered a 14-year-old girl, S, who was admitted to our inpatient unit for depression. At that time patients typically stayed for about 3 months, which is very different from the current length of stay for adolescents in the hospital, which is most often 5 days.

S had several problems, most occurring within the previous year. She had a history of running away, crying spells, skipping school, failing grades, and suicidal threats. She lived at home with her father and 9-year-old brother. Her mother was no longer involved in her life because she had left the family and given up custody of the children several years before.

S settled into the milieu but had a difficult time engaging with the staff. I began to spend time with her every day to establish a trusting relationship. The first few days we just sat in silence. Eventually we were able to talk about her history of oppositional behavior and low self-esteem. S trusted me more and more over time. Then, about 1 month after admission, she approached me and asked if we could talk again. S asked me if I could promise not to tell anyone (especially her father or doctors) if she confided in me about something. I knew then that something was troubling her, but I had to be honest with her. I told S that I couldn't make that promise because the treatment team works in the best interest of the patient and I would have to share pertinent information with them. She decided not to confide in me then, but the next day she approached me again.

S began to tell me that the past few months her father began to drink and had hit her several times, leaving marks on her legs and arms. She stated that one day she had to stay home from school because her legs were swollen and painful from the bruises. She said that her father always apologized once he was sober and promised that he would never hit her again. I gathered a few more details and was honest with her and informed her that I would have to collaborate with the treatment team and possibly seek help from the Department of Social Services. After meeting with the treatment team the next day, I told S that we had to report her father to Social Services. She began to yell and scream and blame me for telling everyone about her problems. Even though I had been honest with her, she couldn't understand that I was actually helping her.

At this point I had to examine my feelings, and I even questioned my judgment. I went home from work that evening quite upset. I began to ask myself, Did I do the right thing? Will S ever confide in me again or even talk with me? Despite feeling a little guilty, I knew that I had made the right decision because protecting S and her future was of utmost importance. After a few days of cooling off S approached me and was able to express her feelings of relief and even apologized to me. We began to work on identifying and expressing her feelings of guilt, relief, sadness, and concern over the situation with her father. Social Services found no evidence of abuse to her 9-year-old brother, so he remained at home with the father.

At discharge, an aunt assumed foster care of S temporarily until her father could obtain the therapy he needed. S was referred to outpatient therapy as well. Several weeks after her discharge, I saw her at the mall and she thanked me for helping and listening to her even though she didn't see it that way at first. She stated that she was happier now and was doing well in school and that she and her father were continuing therapy.

I had made the right decision. Being a young person's advocate and maintaining a patient's safety during an inpatient stay and after discharge are always a nurse's first priority. As I reflected on this experience, I learned not to take things in my personal life so much for granted, such as a loving and supportive family. I also realized that psychiatric nurses do provide excellence in nursing and that we truly can make a difference.

 Visit MERLIN: www.mosby.com/MERLIN/Stuart to find these additional materials and student activities.

- **Worksheets**
- **"Drug of the Month" Updates**
- **"Citing the Evidence" Updates**
- **Critical Thinking Activities and Exercises**
- **Annotated Suggested Readings**
- **Web Links**
- **More!**

Chapter Review Questions

1. **Identify whether the following statements are true (T) or false (F).**

_____ A. Brain growth ends before the beginning of adolescence.

_____ B. Chronological age is a good guide for physical maturation during adolescence.

_____ C. There is a link between an adolescent's self-concept and the use of adaptive coping responses.

_____ D. Masturbation can be an effective way for adolescents to discharge sexual tension.

_____ E. When working with adolescents it is best to have the initial contact with the family to obtain an accurate assessment of the adolescent's problem.

_____ F. Silence is a therapeutic technique that is often frightening to adolescents, especially in the beginning stages of treatment or evaluation.

2. **Fill in the blanks.**

A. Erikson called the task related to the stage of adolescence _____ .

B. Piaget described adolescence as characterized by the cognitive functioning of _____ .

C. More _____ than _____ are likely to die by suicide.

D. Drug use is responsible for _____ % of the deaths in youth age 15 to 24 years.

E. When a person is overly concerned with his or her body and body sensations it is called _____ .

F. Two dimensions of positive mental health for adolescents are _____ and _____ .

3. **Provide short answers for the following questions.**

A. Explain why teenagers delay seeking and using contraceptives.

B. Describe what is meant when tobacco and alcohol are called gateway drugs.

C. Identify the five stages of substance abuse in adolescence.

D. Give four reasons why medication as a treatment strategy is more complex for adolescents than for adults.

References

AACAP: Practice parameters for the psychiatric assessment of children and adolescents, *J Am Acad Child Adolesc Psychiatry* 36(suppl):4S, 1997.

Bloch D: Adolescent suicide as a public health trust, *J Child Adolesc Psychiatr Nurs* 12(1):26, 1999.

Booth R, Zhang Y: Severe aggression and related conduct problems among runaway and homeless adolescents, *Psychiatr Serv* 47:75, 1996.

Brage D, Campbell-Grossman C, Dunkel J: Psychological correlates of adolescent depression, *J Child Adolesc Psychiatr Nurs* 8:23, 1995.

Centers for Disease Control and Prevention: Youth risk behavior surveillance—US, 1997, *MMWR* 47(No. SS-3), 1998.

Coggan C et al: Suicide: qualitative data from focus group interviews with youth, *Soc Sci Med* 45(10):1563, 1997.

DeWit D et al: Age at first alcohol use: a risk factor for the development of alcohol disorders, *Am J Psychiatry* 157(5):745, 2000.

DiClemente R, Hansen W, Ponton L: *Handbook of adolescent risk behavior,* New York, 1996, Plenum.

Erikson E: *Childhood and society,* ed 2, New York, 1963, WW Norton.

Fergusson D et al: Is sexual orientation related to mental health problems and suicidality in young people? *Arch Gen Psychiatry* 56:876, 1999.

Gould M et al: Psychopathology associated with suicidal ideation and attempts among children and adolescents, *J Am Acad Child Adolesc Psychiatry* 37(9): 915, 1998.

Greenhill L, Waslick B: Management of suicidal behavior in children and adolescents, *Psychiatr Clin North Am* 20(3): 641, 1997.

Hamburg D: Toward a strategy for healthy adolescent development, *Am J Psychiatry* 154(6):7, 1997.

Havighurst R: *Developmental tasks and education,* ed 3, New York, 1972, David McKay.

Kools S: Self protection in adolescents in foster care, *J Child Adolesc Psychiatr Nurs* 12(4):139, 1999.

Lesser J et al: "Sometimes you don't feel ready to be an adult or a Mom": the experience of adolescent pregnancy, *J Child Adolesc Psychiatr Nurs* 11(1):7, 1998.

Lieberman J, Tasman A: *Psychiatric drugs,* Philadelphia, 2000, WB Saunders.

McCaleb A: Global and multidimensional self concept as a predictor of healthy practices in middle adolescents, *J Child Adolesc Psychiatr Nurs* 8:18, 1995.

Meeks J: *The fragile alliance,* ed 4, Malabar, Fla, 1990, Robert Krieger.

Modrcin-McCarthy M et al: Childhood anger: so common, yet so misunderstood, *J Child Adolesc Psychiatr Nurs* 11(2):69, 1998.

Mohr W: Beyond cause and effect: some thoughts on research and practice in child psychiatric nursing, *J Child Adolesc Psychiatr Nurs* 12:118, 1999.

Owens R: *Queer kids: the challenges and promise for lesbian, gay and bisexual youth,* New York, 1998, Harrington Park Press.

Parmelee D: *Child and adolescent psychiatry,* St Louis, 1996, Mosby.

Piaget J: *Six psychological studies,* New York, 1968, Vintage.

Pine D et al: Adolescent depressive symptoms as predictors of adult depression: moodiness or mood disorder? *Am J Psychiatry* 156(1):133, 1999.

Potter L et al: Suicide in youth: a public health framework, *J Am Acad Child Adolesc Psychiatry* 37(5):484, 1998.

Powers S et al: Adolescent mental health, *Am Psychol* 44:200, 1989.

Puskar K et al: Teaching kids to cope: a preventive mental health nursing strategy for adolescents, *J Child Adolesc Psychiatr Nurs* 10(3):18, 1997.

Remafedi G et al: The relationship between suicide risk and sexual orientation: results of a population based study, *Am J Public Health* 88(1):57, 1998.

Rosenstein D, Horowitz H: Adolescent attachment and psychopathology, *J Consult Clin Psychol* 64:54, 1996.

Rosewater K, Burr B: Epidemiology, risk factors, intervention, and prevention of adolescent suicide, *Curr Opinion Pediatrics* 10:338, 1998.

Rudd M, Joiner T: An integrative conceptual framework for assessing and treating suicidal behavior in adolescents, *J Adolesc* 21:489, 1998.

Ryan C et al: Helping our hidden youth, *Am J Nurs* 98(12):37, 1998.

Sege R et al: Ten years after: examination of adolescent screening questions that predict future violence-related injury, *J Adolesc Health* 24(6): 395, 1999.

Sullivan H: *Interpersonal theory of psychiatry,* New York, 1953, WW Norton.

Thompson P: Adolescents from families of divorce: vulnerability to physiological and psychological disturbances, *J Psychosoc Nurs* 36(3):34, 1998.

VanderMeer J, Gabert H: Psychiatric nursing admission tool for children and adolescents, *J Child Adolesc Psychiatr Nurs* 6:15, 1993.

Warren J et al: Runaway youths in a southern community: four critical areas of inquiry, *J Child Adolesc Psychiatr Nurs* 10(2):26, 1997.

Weisz J, Jensen P: Efficacy and effectiveness of child and adolescent psychotherapy and pharmacotherapy, *Ment Health Serv Res* 1(3):125, 1999.

Visit **MERLIN** for *Your Internet Connection*
to websites that are related to the content in this chapter.
www.mosby.com/MERLIN/Stuart

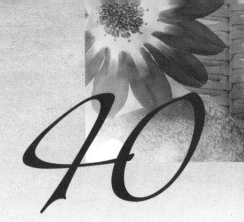

Geriatric Psychiatric Nursing

Georgia L. Stevens

Suzanne D. Friedman

*Y*outh is like a fresh flower in May. Age is like a rainbow
that follows the storms of life. Each has its own beauty.

DAVID POLIS

People age 65 years and older comprise the fastest growing age group in the United States. Changing mortality, fertility, and immigration patterns create some degree of uncertainty when predicting the future size of the elderly population. Therefore estimates for the year 2040 vary between 59 million and 92 million, whereas estimates for the "oldest old" (those 85 and older) range from 8.3 million to 20.9 million (Friedland & Summer, 1999).

The future elderly population will be especially diverse. Socioeconomic factors that will affect the elderly's status are changes in the labor force, family structure, and caregiver characteristics. Many of tomorrow's elderly will be better educated, healthier, and wealthier than cohorts at the end of the 20th century, resulting in a rethinking of our concepts of retirement and old age. Minority groups are projected to have the highest growth rates. Historically, minority groups have had lower socioeconomic status and less access to health care. Thus for many elderly there will be a disparity among health, income, and education levels, presenting public health and policy challenges (Friedland & Summer, 1999).

Since 1900 the elderly population has doubled approximately three times. While this group has increased by more than 100% since 1960, the general population has increased by only 50%. This increase in the elderly dependency ratio (the ratio of the elderly to the working-age population) will negatively impact the financial support of social programs, such as Medicare, Social Security, and other federal and state health-care and disability programs. By the year 2050, the "oldest old" segment of the elderly population is anticipated to increase between 24% and 30%. With projections of 10.8 million to 14 million people requiring long-term care, it is this segment of the population that will drive up the demand for services and programs that address chronic illness and disability. It is also projected that those 65 and older with potentially disabling serious mental illness will increase from 4 million in 1970 to 15 million in 2030. Mortality rates for younger mentally ill patients will decrease, resulting in many mentally ill individuals living into old age. It is also anticipated that aging baby boomers (those born between 1946 and 1964), who number 75 million in the United States, will be at greater risk for substance abuse, anxiety disorders, and depression than the current cohort of elders, and thus the need for these specialty services will increase (Patterson & Jeste, 1999).

Historically, older adults with mental health problems have relied on their primary care providers for management of all their health needs. The occurrence of mental illness may be underestimated in nonpsychiatric settings, as symptoms may be misattributed to cognitive impairment, physical disorders, normal aging, or the lack of age-appropriate diagnostic criteria. Illnesses such as depression are often misdiagnosed or undertreated. The comorbidity of somatic and psychiatric illnesses makes accurate diagnosis more difficult. Medicare's restrictive reimbursement policies are unsatisfactory for severely mentally ill elderly patients. As of the beginning of the 21st century, Medicare offered no prescription drug coverage, limited inpatients hospital days, and imposed restrictions on the number of visits to health-care providers. Similar problems for the elderly mentally ill exist in the recently developed models of managed mental health care. Older persons requiring intensive or long-term mental health care will not fare well in the coming decades (Jeste et al, 1999). Thus the economic and personal costs of mental disorders of older adults are considerable.

On the other hand, there have been impressive changes in academic and research interests in aging and the elderly in the past few decades. New scientific findings and hypotheses, such as a better understanding of normal aging and the discovery of a cholinergic deficit in Alzheimer's disease, have joined with the concepts of health promotion and preventive medicine to move studies beyond what aging **is**, to what **is possible** with aging. The importance of understanding **potential** in relation to aging is profound, because doing so will not only enable older people to access latent skills and talents in later life, but will challenge today's younger age groups to think about what is possible in their later years in a different way (Cohen, 2000).

Helping older adults to maximize their potential can be a challenging and rewarding experience for the nurse. Stereotypes and myths often depict the elderly as a homogeneous group. On the contrary, the older adult represents a combination of multiple biological, interpersonal, developmental, and situational experiences. The complexity and interaction of the needs and problems of old age are often understated and misunderstood. Mental health in late life depends on a number of factors. These include physiological and psychological status, personality, social support system, economic resources, and usual lifestyle. This chapter addresses selected aspects of the psychiatric-mental health needs of geriatric patients and their families.

ROLE OF THE GEROPSYCHIATRIC NURSE

The nurse who works with mentally ill elders is challenged to integrate psychiatric nursing skills with knowledge of physiological disorders, the normal aging process, and sociocultural influences on the elderly and their families. Many nurses who work with these patients find that it is useful to combine nurse practitioner and psychiatric nursing skills. Case management is a particularly effective approach to providing for the biopsychosocial needs of the elderly. Mental health services are provided to this population in a variety of settings, including general and psychiatric hospitals, nursing homes, assisted living residential centers, outpatient mental health clinics, adult day-care programs, senior centers, and the person's own home.

As a primary care provider, the geropsychiatric nurse should be proficient at assessing patients' cognitive, affective, functional, physical, and behavioral statuses, as well as their family dynamics. The nurse also needs knowledge of community resources and how to access them. Planning and nursing intervention may occur with the patient and family or other caregivers. Providing nursing care to these patients can be complex because they are often involved with a number of agencies, thus the need for coordination of services is great.

As a consultant, the geropsychiatric nurse helps other providers to address the behavioral, social, and cognitive aspects of the patient's care. For instance, a nurse may help nursing assistants understand how to respond to a patient who wanders or one who is aggressive. Advanced practice geropsychiatric nurses who have graduate education in this specialty may be employed by agencies to help the entire staff to develop therapeutic programs for seniors with psychiatric or behavioral problems.

Geropsychiatric nurses should be knowledgeable about the effects of psychotropic medication on elderly people. They often work closely with the physician and nurse medication prescriber to monitor complex medication regimens and help the patient or caregiver with medication management. They may lead a variety of groups, such as orientation, remotivation, bereavement, and socialization groups, whereas nurses with advanced degrees may provide psychotherapy and medication prescriptions.

Finally, the role of patient advocate is a critical one for the nurse caring for elders with mental illnesses, particularly those with concurrent physical illness. Because of cognitive changes or symptoms of acute or chronic health problems, elders may not be able to effectively voice their wishes or concerns. Sensitivity is required when addressing the families of the seriously mentally ill, as they may have had many years of "caregiving challenges." Reviewing legal options such as advanced directives or a living will helps in the promotion of the elder's wishes. In cases where conflict exists regarding the elder's care, particularly in long-term care settings, an ombudsman or guardian may be contacted to help resolve these issues. Information about ombudsman or other advocacy programs for the elderly may be obtained by contacting any local office on aging.

THEORIES OF AGING

Ways of defining aging and explaining the causes and consequences of the aging process are based on three major theoretical approaches: biological, psychological, and sociocultural theories of aging. The nurse should be well-acquainted with each of these theories of aging to best understand, evaluate, and care for geriatric patients. These theories provide the basis for a number of the evidence-based nursing interventions discussed in this chapter.

Biological Theories

Biological theories of aging are described as follows:

Biological programming theory: The life span of a cell, its "biological clock," is stored within the cell itself, thus the process of aging is programmed by deoxyribonucleic acid (DNA) and is inevitable and irreversible.

> *Give at least two examples that contradict the biological programming theory of aging. How do you feel about the idea of a biological clock determining life span?*

Cross-linkage theory: Collagen forms bonds between molecular structures with increasing rigidity over time.

Error theory: Errors during protein synthesis create error cells that then multiply.

Free radical theory: Free radicals damage cell membranes, causing physical damage and decline.

Gene theories: Harmful genes activate in late life; cell divisions are finite; or failure to produce growth substances, which stops cell growth and division.

Immunological theory: The immune system becomes less effective in surveillance, self-regulation, and response.

Stress adaptation theory: The positive and negative effects of stress on biopsychosocial development are emphasized; stress may drain a person's reserve capacity physiologically, socially, and economically, increasing vulnerability to illness or injury, accelerating the aging process.

Wear-and-tear theory: Cells wear out from internal and external causes; structural and functional changes may be speeded by abuse and slowed by care; this theory is the basis of many myths and stereotypes ("What can you expect from someone his age?").

> *Discuss how the wear-and-tear theory of aging compares with the present emphasis on nutrition and physical fitness in American culture.*

Psychological Theories

The following list details psychological theories of aging:

Erikson's stage of ego integrity: This developmental theory identifies tasks that must be accomplished at each of the eight stages of life. The last stage of development involves reflection about one's life and accomplishments. The result of resolving this conflict between ego integrity and despair is wisdom.

Life review: A universal process of examination and reintegration of memories, giving meaning to life and preparing one for death by relieving anxiety and fear.

Stability of personality: One's personality is established by early adulthood and remains fairly stable yet adaptable (rather than a developmental progression over the life span). Radical changes in personality in old age may be indicative of brain disease.

> *Can personality traits be altered in old age? If yes, how? If no, why are we interested in intervening in nonproductive behaviors of older adults?*

Sociocultural Theories

Sociocultural theories of aging are described in the following list:

Disengagement theory: Older adults and society mutually withdraw from active exchange with each other as part of the normal aging process (see Citing the Evidence). This controversial theory assumes this separation to be a sign of psychological well-being and adjustment and has reinforced many stereotypes (such as "older people only enjoy the company of people their own age").

Activity theory: Disputes about the reliability of disengagement theory led to the view that activity produces the most positive psychological climate for older adults and that the aged should remain active as long as possible. It emphasizes the positive influence of activity on the older person's personality, mental health, and life satisfaction.

> *What type of program would you design for older adults who must stop working or participating in community activities?*

Family theories: Focus is on the family as the basic unit of emotional development. Interrelated tasks, problems, and relationships are emphasized within the three-generational family. Physical, emotional, and social

---

Citing the Evidence on

Social Disengagement in the Elderly

BACKGROUND: This longitudinal cohort study examined the relationship between social engagement (the maintenance of many social connections and a high level of participation in social activities) and cognitive decline in 2812 non-institutionalized elderly persons.

RESULTS: Compared with persons who had 5 or 6 social ties, those who had no social ties were at increased risk for cognitive decline after adjustment for multiple factors (age, sex, ethnicity, education, income, housing, disability initial health and cognitive function, alcohol use, and smoking).

IMPLICATIONS: Social disengagement is a risk factor for cognitive impairment among elderly persons.

Bassuk S et al: Social disengagement and incident cognitive decline in community-dwelling elderly persons, *Ann Intern Med* 131:165, 1999.

symptoms are believed to reflect problems in negotiating the transitions of the family life cycle.

- Person-environment fit theory: This approach addresses the relationship of the personal competencies of older adults and their environments. If competencies decrease or change with age, one's capacity to relate to the environment may diminish. Frail older adults are especially vulnerable to perceiving the environment as threatening (environmental demand).

ASSESSING THE GERIATRIC PATIENT

Nursing assessment of the geropsychiatric patient is complex. The interplay of biological, psychological, and sociocultural factors related to aging sometimes makes it difficult to clearly identify nursing problems. For example, it can be quite difficult to sort out the behaviors related to the 4 D's of geropsychiatric assessment: depression, dementia, delirium, and delusions (see Chapter 24). The co-existence of simple medical problems such as a urinary tract infection or dehydration can exacerbate psychotic symptoms (Kim & Goldstein, 1997). Aside from major psychotic disorders, delusions are also characteristic of depression in the elderly, and those with dementia may seem delusional because of the trouble they have in interpreting the environment. Delirium may occur related to physical illness, medications, or sensory deprivation. Behaviors associated with delirium include hallucinations, delusions, confusion, disorientation, and agitation. Delirium may be mistaken for dementia, depriving the patient of treatment that could reverse the problem. Depressed elders often appear confused and cognitively impaired because of the lethargy and psychomotor retardation related to depression. Patients with dementia may also present with anxiety, agitation, and depression, especially if they are aware of their declining mental functioning. The first episode of depression in later life is associated with greater chronicity, relapse, cognitive dysfunction, and an increased rate of dementia (Bellelli et al, 1998).

Behaviors have been identified that help to differentiate between depression and dementia. Depressed patients are oriented and maintain socially appropriate behaviors. They are unlikely to undress in public or be incontinent. In contrast, patients with dementia will try to answer questions, but have trouble with logic and relevance. Depressed patients will be annoyed and reject the questioner with silence or short, unresponsive answers. Irritability and hostility are more characteristic of the depressed person.

Careful nursing assessment can be helpful in identifying the primary disorder. Nursing diagnoses are based on observation of patient behaviors and related to current needs. A comprehensive nursing assessment sets the stage for the rest of the nursing process (Table 40-1). Content and behavioral rating scales related to assessment of the elderly are found in the appropriate chapters of this book: cognitive responses, including Alzheimer's disease and related disorders, are discussed in Chapter 24; emotional responses, including depression, in Chapter 20; anxiety responses in Chapter 17; and suicidal behavior in Chapter 21.

Table **40-1**

Key Components of Geropsychiatric Nursing Assessment	
Component	Key Elements
Interviewing	Therapeutic communication skills
	Comfortable, quiet setting
Mental status	Mini-Mental State Examination
	Mental status examination
	Depression
	Anxiety
	Psychosis
Behavioral responses	Description of behavior and triggers
	Assessment of behavioral change
	Frequently observed problem behaviors
Functional abilities	Mobility
	Activities of daily living
	Risk for falls
	Physiological functioning
General health	Nutrition
	Substance abuse
Social support	Social support systems past and current
	Family-patient interaction
	Caregiver concerns

The Interview

Establishing a supportive and trusting relationship is essential to a positive interview with the geriatric patient. The elderly person may feel uneasy, vulnerable, and confused in a new place or with strangers. Patience and attentive listening promote a sense of security. Comfortable surroundings help the patient relax and focus on the conversation.

Therapeutic Communication Skills. The nurse shows respect by addressing the patient by his or her last name: "Good morning, Mr. Smith." The nurse opens the interview by introducing herself and briefly orienting the patient to the purpose and length of the interview. Occasionally reinforcing the amount of time left may help direct a wandering discussion and give the patient the security of knowing that the nurse is in control of the situation. Older people may respond to questions slowly because verbal response slows with age. It is important to give the patient enough time to answer and not assume that a slow response is due to a deficit in knowledge, comprehension, or memory.

The language used by the nurse is important since older people often are unfamiliar with new words, slang, colloquialisms, jargon, abbreviations, or medical terminology. Choice of words should also be based on knowledge of the person's sociocultural background and level of formal education. Questions should be short and to the point, particularly if the patient has difficulty with abstract thinking and conceptualization. Techniques such as clarification and summarization, described in Chapter 2, are important in validating information. The nurse should rephrase a question if the patient fails to answer appropriately or hesitates when answering.

Concentrated verbal interaction may be uncomfortable for the older person. The nurse can demonstrate interest and support by giving nonverbal cues and responses, such as direct eye contact, nodding, sitting close to the patient, and using touch appropriately. Touching the shoulder, arm, or hand of the patient in a firm, purposeful manner conveys support and interest. Avoid stroking or patting the patient. Cultural background and altered tactile perception may result in misinterpretation. The nurse's ability to collect useful data depends greatly on how comfortable she feels during the interview. Negative feelings toward the aged or ignorance about aging will surface in an interview. Older people are sensitive to others' disregard, lack of interest, and impatience.

Elderly patients have much to tell and may offer more information than the nurse needs at a particular time. The nurse should encourage this when possible. Reminiscence and life review may be an excellent source of data about the patient's current health problems and support resources. Even though keeping the patient focused on the topic at hand may be difficult, these formats allow the nurse to assess subtle changes in long-term memory; decision-making ability; judgment; affect; and orientation to time, place, and person.

Many geriatric patients are aware of changes in their physical or psychological functioning. They may hesitate to have their fears confirmed. They may minimize or ignore symptoms, assuming that they are related to age and not to current medical or psychiatric problems. Often these beliefs are reinforced by myths about aging and the false assumption of many health professionals that the problems of older people are irreversible or untreatable.

Contrary to popular myths, most older people do not dwell unrealistically on their health. However, some older people are preoccupied with the physical decline that occurs with age. The nurse should observe carefully for clues that help distinguish whether the patient's preoccupation reflects lifelong personality factors or current distress.

The geriatric patient may misunderstand the purpose of the nurse's questions. Questions regarding habits, previous life experience, or social supports may not seem to be related to current concerns. Careful and repeated explanations are necessary to gain the patient's cooperation. The nurse should never assume that the patient understands the purpose or protocol for the assessment interview. It is wiser to overstate than to increase the patient's anxiety and stress by omitting information. The nurse should take cues from the patient's responses by listening carefully and observing constantly.

> *What special challenges might you face in obtaining informed consent for treatment from a geriatric patient? How might you deal with them?*

The Interview Setting. The new and unfamiliar surroundings of the health-care agency may obstruct the initial interview by distracting the patient and increasing fear of the unknown. If possible, the nurse should assess the patient in a familiar environment to reduce the patient's anxiety.

The physical environment should promote comfort. Many older people are unable to sit for long periods because of arthritis or other joint disabilities. Chairs should be comfortable. Changing positions should be encouraged.

Most older people experience some form of sensory deficit, particularly diminished high-frequency hearing or changes in vision as a result of cataracts or glaucoma. The setting should be quiet and without distracting noises. The nurse should speak slowly and in a low-pitched voice. Because fatigue may contribute to diminished mental functioning, morning may be the best time for the interview, as patients may tire as the day progresses.

The reliability of the data obtained from the assessment interview should be carefully evaluated. If there are questions about some of the patient's responses, the nurse should consult family members or other people who know the patient well. The nurse should also consider the impact of the patient's physical condition at the time of the interview and other factors, such as medications, nutrition, or anxiety level.

Mental Status

Mental status should be part of any geropsychiatric assessment for a number of reasons, including the following:

- The increasing prevalence of dementia with age
- The close association of clinical symptoms of confusion and depression
- The frequency with which physical health problems present with symptoms of confusion
- The need to identify specific areas of cognitive strength and limitation

An in-depth discussion of the assessment of mental status and other cognitive functioning scales used with the elderly is included in Chapter 7.

Depression. Affective status is an essential part of geropsychiatric assessment. The need to include a depression assessment is based on the following:

- The prevalence of depression in the elderly
- The effectiveness of treatment for this disorder
- The potential negative outcomes of depression (such as suicide or neglect)
- Frequent misdiagnosis of depression as a physical problem
- The tendency to dismiss elders as complainers or demanding
- The necessity of accurately distinguishing between depressive and bipolar disorders
- The tendency for depression to recur with increasing age

General estimates of the prevalence of depression among the elderly are 15% to 20%. There is a higher incidence of depression among people of all ages who have disabilities. Because the number of physical disabilities tends to increase with age, this may account for some of the prevalence in the elderly. Prevalence rates for elders residing in the community and those in nursing homes range from 15% to 40% for depressive symptoms and from 1% to 16% for major depressive disorder (Mulsant & Ganguli, 1999).

Diagnosis of depression in the elderly is missed 85% of the time (Bair, 2000), perhaps because it differs in some ways from that in younger populations and thus is assumed to be part of the normal aging process. It may begin with decreased interest in usual activities and lack of energy. There may be increased dependence on others. Conversation may focus almost entirely on the past. There may be multiple somatic complaints with no diagnosable organic cause. The person may have pain, especially in the head, neck, back, or abdomen with no history or evidence of a physical cause. Other symptoms in the elderly include weight loss, paranoia, fatigue, gastrointestinal distress, and refusal to eat or drink, with potentially life-threatening consequences.

Physical illness can cause secondary depression (see Chapter 20). Some illnesses that tend to be associated with depression include thyroid disorders; cancer, especially lung, pancreas, and brain; Parkinson's disease; stroke; and Alzheimer's disease. Many of the medications routinely prescribed for older people can increase depression. Examples include antianxiety drugs and sedative/hypnotics, antipsychotics, cardiotonics (digoxin), and steroids. A medication history is an essential part of patient assessment, especially for the elderly, most of whom tend to take multiple medications.

Anxiety. A thorough assessment of anxiety levels, coping responses, and precipitating stressors provides the nurse with information necessary for planning effective nursing care for the elderly. Anxiety disorders are common and a serious public health concern. They lower the quality of life for many elderly people and increase the burden on family, care providers, and health services. All anxiety disorders affect the elderly: phobias (10% to 12%), generalized anxiety disorder (0.7% to 4.7%), and panic disorder and obsessive compulsive disorder (each less than 1%) (Krasucki et al, 1999). When combined, their symptom prevalence among older people may be even higher than rates of depression alone. Untreated or inappropriately treated anxiety among older people can also contribute to sleep problems, cognitive impairments, and decreased quality of life. Comorbid anxiety and depression are common in the elderly and complicate diagnosis and treatment outcome (see Citing the Evidence).

Psychosis. The prevalence of psychotic disorders increases with age and is estimated to be between 4% and 23% in the elderly (Targum & Abbott, 1999). Therefore, the nurse may frequently find prominent psychotic features during her assessment of older adults. Psychosis may be associated with delusions, delirium, dementia, depression with psychosis, hallucinations, substance abuse, or problems with reality testing. It is important for the nurse to be familiar with the clinical risk factors for developing psychosis in later life. These include cognitive impairment, sensory impairments (vision and hearing), social isolation, female gender, confined to bed with a conflictual caregiver relationship, somatic comorbidity, multiple medications, or underlying medical disorders (Kim & Goldstein, 1997). Patients with a psychiatric diagnosis of psychosis may respond to supportive therapy and low doses of atypical antipsychotic drugs (see Chapter 28).

Citing the Evidence on

Comorbid Anxiety Disorders in Depressed Elderly Patients

BACKGROUND: This cross-sectional study measured current and lifetime rates and associated clinical features of anxiety disorders in 182 depressed patients age 62 and older seen in primary care and psychiatric settings.

RESULTS: Thirty five percent of subjects had at least one lifetime anxiety disorder diagnosis, and 23% met criteria for a current disorder. Presence of a comorbid anxiety disorder was associated with poorer social functioning, increased somatic symptoms, and higher level of suicidality.

IMPLICATIONS: This relatively high rate of comorbid anxiety disorders were associated with a more severe presentation of depressive illness in elderly patients. This information is not generally appreciated in settings caring for depressed elderly patients, potentially resulting in decreased quality of life, increased disability, and increased mortality in the elderly.

Lenze E et al: Comorbid anxiety disorders in depressed elderly patients, *Am J Psychiatry* 157(5):722, 2000.

Behavioral Responses

A thorough behavioral assessment is especially important as a basis for planning nursing care for an elderly person. Behavioral changes may be the first sign of many physical and mental disorders. It is important to identify who is bothered by the behavior—the patient, the family, peers, or unrelated caregivers.

If possible, initial assessment should be completed in the home environment. This will capitalize on environmental factors that reduce the elder's anxiety. It will also give the nurse a chance to observe possible triggers of disruptive behavior. Family members or other caregivers can be asked about their usual responses to the patient's behavior, especially what is helpful and unhelpful. This may provide further clues about the source of the behavior.

It is also helpful to know why the behavior is bothersome. Elders and their families may be frightened by changes in behavior because they associate them with deterioration and the possible onset of dementia. Based on the assessment, the cause of the problem may be treated and the person returned to normal. For instance, a woman who is agitated because of an undiagnosed urinary tract infection returns to her normal, calm self after the infection is treated. In other cases it may not be possible to remove the cause of the behavior, but nursing intervention can help the patient and family adapt to it. For example, a man is irritable because he is becoming forgetful. Early Alzheimer's disease is diagnosed. The patient becomes less irritable after the nurse teaches him and his family

Box 40-1

Behavioral Excesses Observed in Geropsychiatric Patients

Agitation	Intrusiveness
Apathy	Isolating self
Biting	Kicking
Catastrophic reaction	Negativity
Complaining	Pacing
Confusion	Rapid speech
Constant talking	Refusal to eat/drink
Delusions	Repetitive movement
Disinhibition	Resistiveness
Emotional lability	Restlessness
Fatigue	Scolding
Forgetting	Sexual disinhibition
Hallucinations	Spitting
Hand wringing	Suspiciousness
Hitting	Swearing/racial slurs
Hoarding and hiding	Threats of harm
Incontinence	Throwing things
Indifference	Wandering

ways to maximize his memory. Behavioral changes related to declining cognitive functioning are often difficult to manage and necessitate creative treatment.

Behavioral assessment involves defining the behavior; its frequency; duration; and precipitating factors or triggers, including the environment. When a behavioral change occurs, it is important to analyze the underlying meaning. For instance, the person may be experiencing a threat to self-esteem or a change in sensory input. A complete physical examination is needed after any abrupt behavioral change. Caregiver response to behavior must also be assessed because it may reinforce or increase disturbed behavior. Common problem behaviors (behavioral excesses) in the elderly are listed in Box 40-1.

Mr. Jones, an elderly patient, strikes out at the staff every morning when he is approached to take his bath. Describe the steps you would take to assess this behavior. What questions might you ask his family? What advice would you give to the staff who work with him?

Functional Abilities

Assessment of the geropsychiatric patient is not limited to indicators of mental health. Rather, mental status can depend greatly on the older person's overall functional ability. This discussion emphasizes the aspects of the functional assessment that have the greatest impact on mental and emotional status.

Mobility. Mobility and independence are important to the elder's perception of personal health. Three aspects of mobility should be assessed:

- Moving within the environment
- Participating in necessary activities
- Maintaining contact with others

In assessing ambulation the nurse would address motor losses, adaptations made, use of assistive devices, balance, eyesight, and the amount and type of help needed. Factors that influence ambulation include restriction of joints caused by degenerative diseases, orthostatic hypotension, and the type and fit of footwear. Motor ability of the arms can be tested by observing the patient comb the hair, shave, dress, and eat.

Many medications taken by geriatric patients alter perception, making ambulation and mobility difficult and thus contributing to falls. This is particularly so with sedative-hypnotics, antianxiety, cardiovascular, and hypertensive drugs. Patients should be cautioned about side effects of medications and should be encouraged to take plenty of time when ambulating and moving from one position to another.

The incidence of falls and negative outcomes increases with age; 30% of people older than 65 fall every year, with women falling at twice the rate of men. Falls result in physical injuries, such as hip fractures, as well as psychological effects, such as fearfulness. Risk factors should be assessed and are summarized in Table 40-2.

Activities of Daily Living. The assessment of self-care needs and activities of daily living (ADLs) is essential for determining the patient's potential for independence. Activity may be limited because of physical dysfunction or psychosocial impairment. Although geriatric patients should be encouraged to become more independent in self-care, it is unrealistic to expect all patients to function independently. This is particularly so for people who are in a hospital or long-term–care setting. Conforming to the routines and procedures of the institutional environment fosters dependence in the patient. Since such behavioral deficits or excess disability are associated with premature comorbidity and mortality, institutional environments present the nurse with opportunities for creative intervention and care planning.

ADLs (bathing, dressing, eating, grooming, and toileting) are concrete and task-oriented. They provide an opportunity for purposeful nurse-patient interaction. Encouraging patients to be as independent as possible in performing their own ADLs is important. This helps elders meet their needs for safety, security, personal space, self-esteem, autonomy, and personal identity.

Physiological Functioning

Assessment of physical health is especially important with elderly patients because of the interaction of multiple chronic conditions, the presence of sensory deficits, the taking of many medications, and the behaviors presented by physical health problems. Diagnostic procedures that may be useful include blood and urine chemistry values; the electrocardiogram; and for some patients, the electroencephalogram, lumbar puncture, and brain visual imaging techniques, such as the computed tomography scan and magnetic resonance imaging. In addition to these physiological factors, nutritional status and substance abuse should be assessed. A complete medication profile that includes all prescription and over-the-counter drugs, drugs "borrowed"

Table **40-2**

Assessment of Risk for Falls	
Risk Factors	**Assessment Factors**
Environmental hazards	Excessive stimulation (noise)
	Poor lighting
	Slippery or wet surfaces
	Stairs (no handrails, steep, poorly lit)
	Loose objects on the floor
	Throw rugs
	Small pets underfoot
Patient variables	History of falls
	Diurnal alertness level
	Familiarity with surroundings
	Emotional state (agitated, angry, etc.)
	Willingness to request help
	Confusion
	Usual activity level
	Type of activity
Assistive devices	Presence and adequacy of:
	Eyeglasses
	Hearing aid
	Ambulation aids (cane, tripod, walker)
	Prostheses
	Environmental aids (grab bars, hand rails)
	Uncluttered surroundings
Medications	Taking medications (prescribed or over-the-counter) that cause:
	Drowsiness
	Confusion
	Orthostatic hypotension
	Incoordination
	Decreased sensation
	Polypharmacy
Physical or mental disorders	Cardiovascular
	Orthopedic
	Neuromuscular
	Perceptual
	Cognitive
	Affective
	Altered nutritional status
	Fatigue and weakness
	Unsteady gait/mobility problems

from another, and all herbal remedies (including teas) and dietary supplements is essential.

The latest research documents a direct relationship among stress, immune system functioning, and mood. Clinical observations have identified a failure-to-thrive syndrome, especially in the final phase of life. This includes weight loss, decreased appetite, poor nutrition, and inactivity. It is often accompanied by dehydration, depressive symptoms, impaired immune functions, and a low serum cholesterol level. Failure to thrive in the elderly occurs in both acute and chronic forms, leading to impaired func-

tional status, morbidity from infection, pressure sores, and increased mortality.

Nutrition. Many elderly patients do not require help to eat or plan a nutritious diet. However, many geropsychiatric patients do have psychosocial problems that create a need for help with eating and monitoring dietary intake. These problems include the following:

- Depression or loneliness, resulting in decreased appetite
- Changes in cognition, such as confusion, agnosia, or apraxia
- Suicidal tendencies
- Removal from familiar ethnic and cultural eating patterns
- Fear of institutional routines or procedures

The range of physical problems varies greatly. The following areas should be assessed:

- Whether the patient has enough mobility and strength to open cartons of milk, cut meat, and handle utensils
- The presence of neurological or joint conditions that interfere with hand and arm coordination
- The presence of vision problems
- Missing teeth and other losses of chewing ability
- Problems in swallowing or breathing
- The presence of ulcerations on the tongue or elsewhere in the mouth
- Periodontal disease
- Dry mouth because of medications

The nurse should routinely evaluate the patient's dietary needs. Nutritional deficiencies are one of the most significant problems of the institutionalized elderly and can cause other problems, such as skin breakdown, inadequate absorption of medications, and impaired wound healing.

Nutritional assessment should also explore personal preferences, including prior routines (such as largest meal at lunchtime), time of day for meals, portion sizes, and food likes and dislikes. Serum cholesterol and albumin levels provide additional information about the person's nutritional status.

Substance Abuse. Most studies of alcoholism have focused on a younger population, so the prevalence of alcohol abuse by elders has not been well-documented. There is a risk of developing alcoholism in later life if there has been habitual drinking in the past. A second group begins drinking in later life (Hirata et al, 1997). Significant loss and role changes or increased anxiety and concern over health add to the risk. Alcohol is the most commonly abused substance by the elderly because it is readily available and not usually perceived as a drug. The abuse of prescription drugs, particularly sedative-hypnotic and antianxiety medications, is also common and may not be seen as an addiction. Alcohol and substance abuse can lead to increased morbidity and mortality. Abuse of alcohol or any substance may be a means of attaining distance from painful issues such as loss and loneliness. Assessment tools for substance abuse are presented in Chapter 25.

Social Support

Positive support systems are essential for maintaining a sense of well-being throughout life. This is especially important for the geropsychiatric patient. With age, close family members and friends are lost. As a person's significant contacts decrease in number, it is important that the remaining support systems be consistent and meaningful.

Caring behaviors among elderly nursing home residents have been found to be a major way in which residents maintain their personal identity, sense of value, and continuation of personhood. This demonstrates that support systems that develop among patients are beneficial to those who give and receive care.

Health behaviors, such as acceptance of outside interventions and self-efficacy, are guided by cultural beliefs and life experiences. For example, access to services has been limited for the poor, frail, and members of ethnic minority groups. These groups may have depended more on informal caregivers, such as the extended and immediate family, and informal support networks. The nurse should be sensitive to the individual's belief system and should assess the support systems available to the patient while at home, in the hospital, or in another health-care setting. Family and friends can help reduce the shock and stress of hospitalization and offer reassurance and comfort to the distressed elder.

Family-Patient Interaction. Family demographics are changing. Increased life expectancy, declining birth rate, and higher life expectancy for women all affect the availability of family to participate in caregiving and support of the elder. The majority of elders have a minimum of weekly contact with their children.

> *Discuss the ways in which changing demographics in American society are affecting the social support systems of elderly people. What is the impact on their families?*

Family expectations about caring for older members vary. The decision to care for an aging member at home or to include extended family members in the household is discussed over time within the family unit. The majority of caregiving in the United States is provided by family members. Significant issues that affect families in late adulthood are retirement, widowhood, grandparenthood, and illness.

Nurses should become more comfortable and knowledgeable about dealing with issues of sexuality, marital discord, cohabitation, spousal abuse, and elder abuse. The cultural norms that previously placed elderly people in a position of respect as pivotal members of the community appear to have eroded in much of American society. Social and organizational structures have not developed supports to replace those previously available through extended family networks. There is a great deal of discussion in the literature concerning abuse of elderly people, but more research is needed to establish its prevalence and the factors related to it. The nurse should be aware of changing trends and be alert for the possibility of elder abuse, which is addressed in more detail in Chapter 41.

When assessing the older adult, the nurse should note previous success in dealing with life issues. The elder's adjustment to losses and changes associated with aging is affected by earlier life experiences. Behavioral problems in the elderly may result from the family's inability to deal with the losses and increasing dependence of an older member. Reliable and valid measurement tools, along with a careful diagnosis, help strengthen the nursing process, moving it from intuitive to evidenced based assessment.

DIAGNOSIS OF THE GERIATRIC PATIENT

Although older adults may experience a wide range of psychiatric problems, the nursing diagnosis of greatest significance to the nurse and patient in promoting a therapeutic outcome is altered thought processes.

Altered Thought Processes

Memory Impairment.   Memory loss is one of the most distressing and frustrating aspects of aging. Although memory loss may be caused by organic brain disease or depression, it is not necessarily related to a disease process. With age, loss of short-term memory (recall of recent events) is more likely to occur than loss of long-term memory (recall of events that occurred in the distant past). Speed of access appears to slow with increasing age. Failure in retrieval of information, original acquisition, or learning may cause memory impairment (Ebersole & Hess, 1998).

Many factors contribute to altered memory in older adults. Stress or crisis, depression, a sense of worthlessness, loss of interest in present events, cerebrovascular changes that affect cerebral function, loss of neural cells because of disease or trauma, and sensory deprivation or social isolation may all occur with advancing age. Impaired memory for recent events may actually be a result of decreased vision or hearing. This may lead the older person to seek comfort in old memories and experiences, which replace the need to remain in touch with the present.

Institutionalized elderly people appear to have more difficulty with memory than those who live at home or in other community settings. Psychosocial, functional, and environmental approaches to nursing intervention can counteract and often reverse decline and withdrawal in the elderly psychiatric patient. As the person becomes more comfortably involved in relationships and activities, memory and function may improve.

Confusion.   Confusion is a constellation of behaviors, including inattention and memory deficits; disruptive behaviors such as aggressiveness, combativeness, and delusions (called behavioral excesses); and inability or failure to perform ADLs (called behavioral deficits) (Davis & Burgio, 1999). Often, **confusion** is a nonspecific term used by staff to label apathetic, withdrawn, or uncooperative patients. Several categories of patients are likely to be labeled as confused: the problem patient, the patient with communication problems (slurred speech, expressive dysphasia), the patient who challenges staff members' personal values, the depressed patient, and the patient who does not get well. It is important for the nurse to be specific when referring to a patient as "confused."

Institutionalized elders are at particular risk of confusion. From 40% to 80% suffer from some degree of organic brain disease, with disorientation to time, place, and person; remote and recent memory loss; and inability to do simple calculations. In many long-term care facilities, more than 30% of the patients have severe confusion (Ebersole & Hess, 1998). The precipitating factors depend on both the physiological and psychological condition of the patient.

Early morning confusion, sometimes called sunrise syndrome, may result from the hangover effects of sedative-hypnotics or other nighttime medications that interact with drugs for sleep. Sleep problems and insomnia are common in the elderly. Adverse reactions to drugs prescribed for sleep often occur. Increasing disorientation or confusion at night, resulting from loss of visual accommodation and other factors, is known as **sundowning syndrome**. The nurse should take special precautions to prevent falls at these times.

The most logical cause of sundowning is the deterioration of the suprachiasmatic nucleus in the hypothalamus. This major pacemaker of circadian rhythms regulates the sleep-wake cycle (see Chapter 6) and has been found to be deteriorated in demented people. Assessing and then minimizing or eliminating any environmental and underlying physiological causes of afternoon or evening confusion or irritability would be important activities for the nurse. These include the following:

- Elimination of toxic, infectious, metabolic, or pharmacological causes of delirium
- Elimination of underlying physiological causes of agitation and confusion such as pain, febrile illnesses, and incontinence
- Minimization or elimination of daytime sleep
- At least minimal exposure to direct sunlight each day, particularly in the morning, to reset the circadian pacemaker
- Increase in mild activity, such as walking
- Increase in conversations and other social interactions with staff and others
- Assessing for appropriateness of short-term use of low-dose antipsychotic drugs

A nurse's aide tells you that a patient is "wandering down the hall, staggering, pajama top unbuttoned." It is early morning, and the other patients are asleep. What would you do in this situation?

The nurse should never assume that confusion and disorientation are natural results of changes in cognitive or physiological status. Confusion is reversible in more than half the patients who experience it. It is usually transient or short term. The nurse has primary responsibility for intervening in this problem. Well-planned nursing care can be a significant factor in preventing and intervening in this distressing condition.

Although the term **disorientation** is often used interchangeably with **confusion**, they are different. A disoriented patient is not necessarily confused, and a confused patient does not necessarily experience complete disorientation. Mental status tests differentiate disorientation to place, person, and time from components of confusion, such as alter-

ations in memory, judgment, decision making, and problem solving. Cognitive responses are discussed in detail in Chapter 24.

Paranoia. Some older people react to loss, isolation, and loneliness with paranoia and fear. Classic paranoia, involving a well-organized and elaborate delusional system, is rare in older people. Delusions and disturbances in mood, behavior, and thinking may be temporary conditions caused by sensory deprivation or sensory loss, social isolation, medications, deliriums, and dementias (Ebersole & Hess, 1998).

Paranoid symptoms may be general or specific. The geriatric patient may feel threatened by certain people (such as unfamiliar staff, or even by family, friends, or neighbors) or at certain times (such as night). Relocation to a new home, new room, or strange environment may cause fears; anxiety; and for some, paranoid ideation.

The personality of aging paranoid patients is characterized by withdrawal, aloofness, fearfulness, oversensitivity, and often secretiveness. As long as patients do not call attention to themselves or threaten themselves or others, their paranoia may remain hidden. Once they become a potential threat to themselves or others, institutionalization may be needed. Older people who have transient or chronic paranoia are at high risk for victimization by others as well as self-neglect and abuse (such as refusal to eat, take prescribed medications, or attend to hygiene needs).

Affective Responses

Disturbances in mood, mood swings, or oversensitive emotional reactions are common to people of all ages. An older person's reaction to physical limitations or disabilities, psychological loss (particularly of a spouse or other close person), or the possibility of institutionalization depends on past coping styles, support systems (especially family), and present psychological and physiological strength.

Extreme or sudden mood changes occur in response to stress or as inadequate coping mechanisms in people facing progressive loss or dependency. When this behavior is seen in elderly people who have been content and happy, physiological factors, including side effects of medications, should be considered. Reassurance and support are given to reduce the patient's anxiety and diminish the perceived threat.

Dysfunctional Grieving. Depression and sadness are sometimes viewed as a natural part of aging. In fact, depression, grief, and loss are common in later life. Prolonged grief and mourning over a real or imagined loss should be recognized and treated as depression. Common symptoms include weight loss; appetite loss; fatigue; apathy; loss of interest in friends, family, and usual activities; and psychomotor retardation. None of the symptoms is caused by increasing age; all are problems that can be effectively treated (see Chapter 20).

Death of a life partner can compound the cumulative loses of aging. Key points from research on grief responses in the elderly for the nurse to remember when caring for a grieving elder are (Hegge & Fischer, 2000):

- Elderly widow(er)s are likely to have multiple cumulative losses of aging, which complicate the grieving process

- Coping strategies of elderly widow(er)s include faith, flexibility, participation in activities, and support of family or friends
- Symptoms of grief such as disruptions in sleeping and eating patterns can lead to false labels of dementia
- Peaks and valleys of grief were less intense in the eldest widow(er)s because they were more at peace with their own mortality

The loss of hope expressed by some older people, particularly those with increasing disabilities, may cause or result from a depressive reaction. Undiagnosed depression may have serious effects on the elderly because depression always causes physical symptoms.

The person's attitude toward aging, dying, and death influences whether the depression can be treated successfully. The old differ from the young in their attitudes toward death in several ways: Older people tend to integrate attitudes toward death with their religious beliefs, to have experienced the death of significant others, to be more accepting of death, and to approach problems primarily from an internal focus. The state of the older person's health, in addition to what he or she has learned from seeing people die, may signal that his or her life may be ending. Awareness of the older person's "stage of dying" is important to understanding his or her needs and concerns.

Risk for Violence: Self-Directed. Intentional deaths among the elderly are common. Older people in the United States have the highest suicide rate of any age group. The suicide rate of white males older than 65 is especially high. Others at high risk include isolated elderly people who have lost family or friends through death; those with changes in body function and decreased independence because of pain, weakness, immobility, or shortness of breath; those with changes in body function because of surgery or stroke; and those who are terminally ill. Suicide in elderly people is strongly associated with depression, physical illness, loss of adaptive coping mechanisms, and neurobiological alteration.

Elderly suicide victims use more violent and lethal means to take their lives, resulting in a higher ratio of completed-to-attempted suicides, suggesting that effective treatment must include prevention. Sadly, the majority of elderly suicide victims have seen their primary care provider in the month before their death, but their suicidal intentions were not detected and they were not treated for their depression. Finally, other examples of intentional deaths include excessive risk-taking, lack of caution in the management of ordinary affairs; refusal to eat; overuse or misuse of alcohol or drugs; and noncompliance with life-sustaining medical regimens, such as refusal to take insulin or digoxin. Suicidal behavior is discussed in detail in Chapter 21.

> *Were you surprised to learn that the elderly have the highest suicide rate? How would you increase public awareness of this important public health problem?*

Situational Low Self-Esteem. Low self-esteem in the elderly is often expressed through preoccupation with physical and emotional health and expression of concern through body complaints. This may be labeled hypochon-

driasis but really represents the person's insecurity. One of the real problems encountered by elders with a history of somaticizing is health professionals' tendency to dismiss their complaints, assuming there is no real illness. All symptoms should be taken seriously and investigated thoroughly. Ways in which to promote self-esteem are discussed in Chapter 19.

As a sign of the geriatric patient's sense of deterioration, somaticism communicates the distress that accompanies decreased self-worth. The sick role is a legitimate and socially acceptable way to deal with stress and anxiety. The patient receives support, concern, and interest and experiences a sense of control. Unfortunately, caregivers may reinforce the elder's dependency by providing care that discourages the patient from doing for himself or herself. This vicious cycle sets the stage for behavioral deficits, excess disability, and decreased self-worth (Blair, 1999).

Somatic Responses

Sleep Pattern Disturbance. Insomnia may be a symptom or a problem in itself for the geropsychiatric patient. Many older adults experience chronic or intermittent sleep problems. Persistant insomnia, a risk factor for major depression, occurs among 5% to 10% of elders. Complaints of interrupted sleep; loss of sleep; or poor sleep, with frequent awakenings and morning exhaustion, are common. Daytime napping and drowsiness add to the problem. Nonetheless, sleep disorders in the elderly can be systematically diagnosed and treated (Beck-Little & Weinrich, 1998).

Opinions vary regarding normal sleep patterns in older adults. Some researchers suggest that people need less sleep as they age. However, chronic fatigue, physical illness, pain, and decreased mobility may cause a need for more sleep. Geriatric patients often express distress over their inability to sleep well. Perceived lack of sleep becomes a cyclical reaction. Worry about lack of sleep prevents falling asleep. Fatigue is the most common physical complaint of adults older than 75. Lack of exercise, limited mobility, and side effects of drugs may also contribute to insomnia.

Altered Nutrition: Less than Body Requirements. Appetite loss is common in patients with depression. Inadequate dietary intake also occurs in confused or disoriented patients. Forgetting to eat or being unable to prepare meals may add to the problem of appetite loss. Side effects of some drugs (such as dry mouth or change in taste) contribute to lack of interest in food. The toothless patient or someone with gum disease avoids chewing when possible. The interaction of appetite loss and emotional dysfunction should always be considered in the nutritional evaluation. Poor nutrition contributes to fatigue, listlessness, and immobility.

Stress Responses

Progressively Lowered Stress Threshold (PLST). Nurses should know the competencies and capacities for environmental mastery of cognitively impaired patients. For instance, as cognitive responses slow, the stress threshold decreases and capacities deteriorate. Staff often overwhelm sensory processing and coping abilities of elderly patients, leading to catastrophic reactions and other behavioral excesses. Finding a better fit between the patient's stress threshold and the demands of the environment can strengthen patient competencies and reduce behavioral excesses (Holmberg, 1997).

Relocation Stress Syndrome. This condition involves physical or psychosocial disturbances related to transfer from one environment to another. Since 1950 the care of many elderly mentally ill has shifted from state psychiatric hospitals to nursing homes. In fact, the number of mentally ill elderly residing in nursing homes greatly exceeds that in state psychiatric hospitals. This shift in treatment sites drew attention to the process and consequences of relocation.

Risk factors related to relocation stress syndrome include the following (North American Nursing Diagnosis Association [NANDA], 1999):

- Impaired psychosocial or physical health status
- Other recent losses
- Losses associated with the move
- Inadequate preparation for the move
- Feelings of powerlessness
- Moderate to great difference between the old and new environments
- Prior relocation experiences
- Inadequate support system

Behaviors associated with relocation stress syndrome are listed in Box 40-2.

The stress of relocation should be anticipated for all geriatric patients. Intervention should be planned to reduce the impact. In transfers between institutions, it may be helpful to arrange for the patient to visit the new location before the actual move. This allows the patient to meet other residents and staff, see the physical surroundings, and ask questions about the program. Posttransfer visits by staff from the transferring agency also ease the transition, as does offering staff from both agencies the opportunity to communicate about nursing approaches. Allowing the patient to have personal belongings, liberal visiting hours for family or friends, and careful explanations of the purpose and routines of the institution are a few of the ways in which the stress of change can be minimized. Establishing an effective support system within the new setting may prevent the negative behaviors often observed in isolated elders: apathy, depression, aggression, or hostility.

Box 40-2

Behaviors Associated with Relocation Stress Syndrome

- Anxiety, apprehension, restlessness, and verbalization of being concerned/upset about transfer
- Vigilance, dependency, increased verbalization of needs, insecurity, and lack of trust
- Increased confusion
- Depression, sad affect, withdrawal, and loneliness
- Sleep disturbance
- Change in eating habits, gastrointestinal disturbances, and weight changes
- Unfavorable comparison of posttransfer and pretransfer staff

Risk for Caregiver Role Strain. Disabled elderly people who live in the community rely on support and care from family members. As the percentage of elderly people in the population grows, family resources will be increasingly important to keep elders in the community and provide care that is less expensive than professional care. This role is stressful for people who care for frail elders. Providing elder care can result in emotional, physical, interpersonal, and occupational problems. Research has also demonstrated that stress to the caregiver increases over time. A caregiver under stress is at risk for problems in performing the caregiver role (NANDA, 1999). Risk factors for caregiver role strain are listed in Table 40-3.

Additionally, several other factors affecting the caregiver are predictors of institutionalization of the elder, including the following (Kelley et al, 1999):

- Safety concerns
- Incontinence
- Erratic sleep patterns of care recipient
- Critical health events (e.g., falls, wandering, hospitalization)

Nurses are in a unique position to identify and address the caregiver's needs for education, intervention, and support services. Such support can decrease caregiver role strain and premature institutionalization of the elder.

Table 40-3

Risk Factors for Caregiver Role Strain

Category	Risk Factors
Pathophysiological	Severe illness of elder
	Unpredictable illness course
	Addiction or co-dependency
	Elder discharged with serious home-care needs
	Caregiver health impairment
	Caregiver is female
Psychosocial	Psychosocial/cognitive problems in care receiver
	Family problems before caregiving
	Marginal caregiver coping patterns
	Poor relationship between caregiver and receiver
	Caregiver is spouse
	Care receiver has deviant or bizarre behavior
Situational	Abuse or violence
	Other sources of stress on family
	Need for long-term caregiving
	Inadequate physical environment
	Family/caregiver isolation
	Lack of caregiver respite or recreation
	Inexperience
	Competing role commitments
	Complex/demanding caregiving tasks

Behavioral Responses

Social Isolation. Multiple social losses or fear of loss may lead to social isolation. Prolonged grief after the loss of a spouse, sibling, child, or close friend may make the elder hesitant to become involved in other close relationships. The person who has been close only to a few family members or friends will have even more difficulty with loss.

Elderly patients experiencing organic cognitive impairment (such as Alzheimer's disease and related disorders) often withdraw from social contacts, daily routines, and ADLs. They may deny having a problem or fear the consequences of memory changes. Social isolation can become a defense mechanism, reinforcing denial of perceived disability, yet worsening the cognitive deficits. Sensory deficits such as hearing or vision impairment can also contribute to isolation for the elderly (Davis & Burgio, 1999).

Self-Care Deficit/Behavioral Deficit. Chronic illness is one aspect of aging that may result in the inability to care for oneself. With increasing years comes a greater chance of multiple chronic health problems. Affective illnesses such as major depression or bipolar disorder may cause psychomotor retardation, preventing elders from meeting their basic needs. Medications may cause forgetfulness, lethargy, and physical impairment. Because of increasing frailty or cognitive impairment, many elders are unable to converse or complete basic self-care activities such as bathing, toileting, grooming, and feeding. The underlying cause of the deficit must be determined and appropriate nursing interventions planned. Aphasia, agnosia, and apraxia contribute to self-care deficits. Admission to a nursing home often results in dependency in ADLs among those who previously were independent in such basic activities (Blair, 1999). Nurses are in a unique position to reduce the incidence of behavioral deficits and excess disability by enhancing self-efficacy and environmental competence.

Disruptive Behaviors/Behavioral Excess. The high incidence of disruptive behaviors is very troubling to caregivers. Even one resident displaying such behaviors can disrupt an inpatient unit or nursing home floor, setting off a chain reaction in other residents, and contributing significantly to caregiver stress. Nurses can assist staff to assess and intervene effectively using a variety of behavioral and environmental strategies, thus reducing use of physical and chemical restraints.

PLANNING AND INTERVENTION

Expected outcomes related to the nursing care of the geropsychiatric patient should be realistically based on the person's potential to change. If the person's behavioral problems result from a treatable disorder, expected outcomes and short-term goals may reflect a return to pre-illness functioning. For example, a goal for a patient with depression who is neglectful of personal hygiene might be:

The patient will bathe, dress, and brush his teeth independently.

Empirically validated treatments for depression and anxiety in the aged are summarized in Table 40-4.

If the condition is chronic and either no change or progressive deterioration is expected and current treatments do not effect change in target behaviors, then the outcomes of care focus on adaptation to the situation. For example, a goal for a patient with Alzheimer's disease who neglects personal hygiene might be:

The patient will help with bathing, dressing, and brushing one's teeth.

If the patient's condition is not expected to improve, the expected outcomes and goals may focus on the caregiver as well as the patient. For example, a goal for a caregiver of a person with Alzheimer's disease might be:

At least once a week the caregiver will participate in a recreational activity outside of the home while the home health aide is with the patient.

The plan of care must be developed with the active participation of the patient and the caregiver. It also must be reviewed frequently to ensure that it is relevant to the patient's current needs. Caregiver education is an important part of the plan.

Older adults respond well to both individual and group interventions. They need the opportunity to talk, be supported in their efforts to deal with day-to-day problems, and plan for a meaningful future. The type of nursing intervention selected depends on the nursing care problems identified, the interests and preferences of the elder, and the setting in which the care is to be provided. In the past, most geropsychiatric care was provided in state psychiatric hospitals. Nurses will now also find older patients with mental illness in acute psychiatric units, nursing homes, emergency rooms, and increasingly in community settings. Nursing care for cognitively impaired patients in inpatient settings is addressed in Chapter 24, including approaches to behaviors such as wandering, aggression, agitation, falls, and confusion.

Table **40-4**

Summarizing the Evidence on Depression and Anxiety in the Aged	
DISORDER:	Depression and anxiety in the aged
TREATMENTS:	■ The primary classes of antidepressant medications were effective in both the acute and maintenance phases of late-life depression, although they represented a heightened risk of adverse side effects.
	■ Electroconvulsive therapy (ECT) has shown its effectiveness and safety in the short-term management of late-life, severe psychotic depression and mania.
	■ Psychosocial interventions were efficacious in treating major depressive disorder in the aged.

From Nathan P, Gorman NP: *A guide to treatments that work,* New York, 1998, Oxford University Press.

Therapeutic Milieu

Whether in a hospital, nursing home, community program, or at home, the care environment should support effective interventions. There are several basic characteristics of a therapeutic milieu.

Cognitive Stimulation. Activities should be planned to maintain or improve the patients' cognitive functioning. Discussion groups help patients focus on topics of interest to them while they socialize. Projects can reinforce skills and offer an opportunity for success. Patients with dementia can participate in a wide variety of activities. The nurse can collaborate with the rehabilitation therapist in planning interesting and appropriate activities.

Promote a Sense of Calm and Quiet. Elders often do best in a setting that is designated for their care. In particular, inpatient units that admit all age groups may be too stimulating for confused elder patients. In general, the geropsychiatric setting should be decorated in soft colors. If music is played, it should be soothing and preferably familiar to the elderly. Bright lights that create glare should be avoided. Although the environmental background should be subdued, planned periods of increased activity help maintain interest and alertness. For elders who are not in their own home, personal articles such as family pictures, religious objects, favorite books, afghans, or decorative objects are reassuring and offer a sense of security.

Consistent Physical Layout. In residential or inpatient settings, room changes should be avoided as much as possible. Furniture arrangements should be stable; this helps disoriented people to locate themselves and adds to their security. Environmental barriers should be removed for wandering patients (Bellelli et al, 1998).

Structured Routine. The daily schedule should be as predictable as possible. Bedtime, waking time, nap times, and mealtimes should not vary. For elders who have recently moved to a new setting, it is helpful to give them and their families copies of the weekly schedule. Time should be allowed for reviewing the schedule with patients. Periodic reinforcement of the routines may be needed until patients adjust to the environment. A predictable routine can enhance an elder's capacity to function at his or her maximum level (Holmberg, 1997).

Focus on Strengths and Abilities. Most elders have strengths related to their past accomplishments. If the person is unable to communicate, family members can give information about the patient's life and suggest activities that are likely to be successful. Nursing creativity can be used to find ways to capitalize on elders' strengths by planning opportunities for them to help staff or other patients or participate in activities based on their abilities. Successful experiences can enhance perceptions of self-efficacy and control, decreasing premature dependency.

Minimize Disruptive Behavior. Understanding the patient's behavioral patterns can help to reduce agitation and behavioral crises. Observation reveals situations that lead to disruptions. Adhering to the person's usual lifestyle as closely as possible reduces conflicts. For instance, a person who has always taken a bath in the evening before bed should not be forced to shower before breakfast. Patients who agitate each other should be kept apart as much as possible. Distraction can often interrupt a conflict before it gets out of control. Understanding disruptive behavior or behavioral excesses from the perspective of the elder will strengthen the nurse's ability to design interventions that affect underlying causes.

Minimal Demands for Compliant Behavior. Elders who are cognitively impaired often resist demands from others. They may not understand what is being asked of them or they may be frightened of an unexpected change in activity. Some older adults resent being under the control of others and feel the need to assert themselves. It is best to avoid pressuring the patient to comply. Reapproaching the person after a few minutes is often successful. If the patient needs to be in control, it is helpful to negotiate a time of voluntary compliance.

> **?** *How would the therapeutic milieu differ if most patients were elderly and (a) depressed, (b) demented, (c) delusional, or (d) cognitively intact?*

Providing Safety. Safety is fundamental to a therapeutic milieu, thus safety needs should always be considered. The nurse should be alert for safety hazards and remove them. Because falls are a concern, floors should be free from slippery spots, obstacles, uneven surfaces, and loose rugs. Thresholds should be flush with the surrounding floor. Hand rails and grab bars are helpful for frail elders. Fire is also a concern. Open flames should be avoided. If smoking is allowed, it may be necessary to provide supervision in an area of the facility that permits smoking.

In many facilities restraints are still used in the mistaken notion that they enhance the patient's safety or control disruptive behavior. Physical restraints include a variety of devices such as mitts, posey vests, and geri chairs applied with a physician's order, although nurses are the most intimately involved professionals in decisions to restrain patients. Although such devices may help staff, they limit patient freedom of choice and movement, as well as threaten dignity. Six myths related to physical restraint of elderly patients are summarized in Table 40-5. In order to limit the use of restraints and to incorporate more appropriate methods to address safety concerning the elderly, nurses, in collaboration with other health care professionals, should develop a hospital or facility policy and protocol related to the use of restraints (Chien, 2000). National nursing efforts to expose these myths and realities led to federal regulations to implement less-restrictive alternatives, resulting in a decreased use of restraints (Ryden et al, 1999).

Somatic Therapies

Electroconvulsive Therapy. ECT has been found to be very effective in the treatment of depression in the older adult. Chapter 29 has a detailed discussion of ECT. Contraindications for this type of therapy are an intracranial

Table **40-5**

Myths and Realities about Physical Restraint	
Myths	**Realities**
Restraints reduce the risk of injury related to falls.	Restraints do not reduce the risk of injury from falls and may increase it. Falls do increase the likelihood of future restraint.
Restraining meets the nurse's moral duty to protect the patient from harm.	Restraints may increase the risk of injury and lead to problems related to immobility, confusion, aggression, depression, and incontinence.
Failure to restrain results in legal liability.	Federal and state laws and regulations prohibit the unnecessary use of restraint.
Older people do not mind being restrained.	Older people do not wish to be restrained. They feel angry, hurt, and embarrassed by the experience.
Inadequate staffing justifies restraining patients.	Federal and state laws and regulations forbid restraining patients for staff convenience. Providing adequate nursing care to a restrained patient takes at least as much time as caring for an unrestrained one.
There are no adequate alternatives to physical restraint.	Nursing care alternatives have been identified in several categories: Physical care: comfort, relief of pain, positioning Psychosocial care: remotivation, communication, attention Activities Environmental manipulation: improved lighting, removal of restraint devices, redesigned furniture Administrative support and staff training

Modified from Evans LK, Strumpf NE: *Image* 22:124, 1990.

space-occupying lesion with increased intracranial pressure, arrhythmias, and myocardial infarction within the last 3 months.

Psychotropic Medications. The addition of psychotropic medications to the care regimen of elders must be approached carefully and competently. Basic guidelines for medication administration for elders include the slow initiation of medications, preferably one at a time, using lower dosages: "start low and go slow" (Salzman, 1999). Special consideration must be given to psychotropic medications and elders because drugs that affect behavior also affect the central nervous system. Also, elderly patients are especially vulnerable to developing side effects. The nurse should remember that age-related pharmacokinetic and pharmacodynamic changes affect drug response and increase the risk for side effects in the elderly, making the atypicals the first-line treatments for psychosis in the elderly due to their more favorable side effect profile (Yeung et al, 2000; Massand, 2000). Table 40-6 describes recommended dosages of psychotropic medications for the elderly. (See Chapter 28 for a thorough discussion of psychopharmacology.)

Special attention must be given to the older adult when assessing medication use. Four factors place the elder at risk for drug toxicity and should be included in any assessment: advanced age, polypharmacy, decreased medication compliance, and comorbidity. Misuse of drugs by the elderly is also a factor in the rising cost of health care for this population.

Age. As a person ages, physiological responses to medications change. In the older-than 65 age group, drug dosages must be monitored carefully for continuing effectiveness. A medication dosage that is safe and effective at age 65 may be toxic at age 75. Gastrointestinal absorption, hepatic blood flow and metabolism, and renal clearance may all decline. Also, the ratio of fat to lean muscle mass increases with age.

Many psychoactive medications are lipophilic (attach to fat), which increases the risk of drugs building up in fatty tissue and causing toxicity. Experimental drugs are often tested on non-elderly adult populations. This does not allow evaluation of the differing effects of newly approved drugs on older people before their availability in the marketplace.

Polypharmacy. Several surveys report that older adults take an average of 8 to 10 medications daily. It is also suggested that the use of over-the-counter medicines is underreported because they are not thought to be significant. Drugs such as alcohol and acetaminophen (Tylenol) are not always reported but can be toxic in combination with other drugs.

Compliance. Many drugs take up to 6 weeks to effect a change in affective disorders. In the interim, elders may see no benefit to continued compliance and may abandon their medication regimen. Education regarding the time to effectiveness, the purpose, therapeutic value, and side effects (and their treatments) of medications should be provided to elders to enhance medication compliance and awareness.

Comorbidity. Acute and chronic illnesses and their treatments can alter the body's response to psychotropic medications. This includes chronic renal or liver failure, congestive heart failure, and structural and functional changes in the central nervous system. These conditions may result in heightened sensitivity to psychotropic drugs.

Interpersonal Interventions

Psychotherapy. Elderly patients should participate in both individual and group psychotherapy sessions. Nurses who have advanced degrees in psychiatric nursing are qualified to provide these services. The issue of the appropriateness of psychotherapy for this population is addressed in Critical Thinking about Contemporary Issues. The follow-

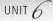

Table **40-6**

Psychoactive Medications	
Category	Recommended Dosage Range for Older Adults
SELECTIVE SEROTONIN REUPTAKE INHIBITORS (SSRIs) AND OTHER NEWER ANTIDEPRESSANTS	
fluoxetine (Prozac) (SSRI)	20–80 mg/day
citalopram (Celexa) (SSRI)	20 mg/day
fluvoxamine (Luvox) (SSRI)	50 mg/day
sertraline (Zoloft) (SSRI)	50 mg/day
paroxetine (Paxil) (SSRI)	20 mg/day
venlafaxine (Effexor) (SNRI)	37.5–225 mg/day
nefazodone (Serzone) (SARI)	100 mg/day
mirtazapine (Remeron) (NaSSA)	15–45 mg/day
bupropion (Wellbutrin) (SDRI)	200–300mg/day, divided doses
Tarazodone/Desyrel (SARI)	25–150 mg/day
TRICYCLIC ANTIDEPRESSANTS (TCAs)	
amitriptyline (Elavil)	10–75 mg/day
imipramine (Tofranil)	10–75 mg/day
desipramine (Norpramin)	10–150 mg/day
nortriptyline (Aventyl)	10–50 mg/day
MONOAMINE OXIDASE INHIBITORS (MAOIs)	
isocarboxazid (Marplan)	10–30 mg/day
phenelzine (Nardil)	15–45 mg/day
tranylcypromine (Parnate)	10–30 mg/day
MOOD STABILIZERS	
lithium	300 mg tid/qid
carbamazepine (Tegretol)	100–400 mg/day
valproate (Depakote)	125 mg/bid; titrate up slowly
ANXIOLYTIC AGENT	
buspirone (BuSpar)	5–30mg/day, divided doses
ANXIOLYTIC BENZODIAZEPINES	
clonazepam (Klonopin)	0.5–0.75 mg/day
oxazepam (Serax)	10–35 mg (divided in 3–4 doses)
lorazepam (Ativan)	0.5–1.0 mg bid to tid
SEDATIVE/HYPNOTIC BENZODIAZEPINES	
flurazepam (Dalmane)	15–30 mg qhs
temazepam (Restoril)	7.5–15 mg qhs
ANTIPSYCHOTICS: ATYPICAL (NOVEL)	
risperidone (Risperdal)	0.25–2 mg/day
olanzapine (Zyprexa)	5–10 mg/day
quetiapine (Seroquel)	25–50 mg/day
ANTIPSYCHOTICS: TYPICAL (CONVENTIONAL)	
haloperidol (Haldol)	0.25–15 mg/day
fluphenazine (Prolixin)	0.25–6 mg/day
trifluoperazine (Stelazine)	2–20 mg/day
thioridazine (Mellaril)	10–300 mg/day
chlorpromazine (Thorazine)	10–300 mg/day

? CRITICAL THINKING about CONTEMPORARY ISSUES

Is Psychotherapy an Appropriate Intervention for Geropsychiatric Patients?

Some believe that psychotherapy for elderly patients is inappropriate and not helpful. Psychotherapy requires confronting and working through basic personality traits. It is argued that the elderly do not have the capacity, stamina, or interest to take on such a challenging task. Is this based on an accurate estimate of the elder's cognitive ability and interpersonal potential? Psychotherapy may be a long-term process. Is it reasonable to ask a person who is nearing the end of life to make a commitment to an effort that might not be completed? People in therapy often change their relationships with others. Should the elderly be put in the position of possibly jeopardizing their support systems by changing their expectations of themselves and others?

Geropsychiatric nurse specialists have begun to document their experiences in providing psychotherapy to elders (Kim & Goldstein, 1997). These nurses believe that elderly patients benefit from this intervention. They describe the elder's ability to change and grow. Psychotherapists have noted that older patients are more focused on therapeutic work, perhaps because they know they do not have unlimited time to achieve their goals. Elders have a wealth of life experiences to bring to therapy and a need to find meaning in their lives that is often aided by therapeutic intervention. In groups, they also benefit from the mutuality and cohesion they find. Thus, is it worth the investment to improve the life experience of one who may or may not have enough time left to experience long-term rewards of psychotherapy?

ing three therapeutic approaches have demonstrated effectiveness in treating a variety of psychiatric problems:

- Interpersonal psychotherapy has been demonstrated to be effective in treating depression. The foci of treatment include: grief, role changes, multiple losses, bereavement, social isolation, and helplessness (Klausner & Alexopoulos, 1999).
- Cognitive therapy has a focus on identifying and changing thoughts and underlying belief systems and supports higher-level defense mechanisms such as rationalization and intellectualization. It encourages active participation of patients in the therapy and reinforces positive change within a time-limited framework.
- Cognitive-behavioral therapy has several goals, which include changing thoughts and behaviors, improving skills, and modifying emotional states (see Citing the Evidence).

Problem-solving therapy is also an effective treatment for elders with mild depression. Problem-solving therapy involves helping patients in identifying issues that are critical in their lives. These issues should be described in a measurable and observable format, appropriate solutions to these issues should be devised, and possible consequences should be predicted (Reynolds & Kupfer, 1999).

Citing the Evidence on

Memory Improvement with Cognitive Behavioral Therapy in the Elderly

BACKGROUND: This quasi-experimental study aimed to improve memory of 19 elderly (average are 85) using an eight session cognitive enhancement program called: "Memories, Memories, Can We Improve ours?", part of the Cognitive Behavioral Model of Everyday Memory (CNMEM).

RESULTS: Overall memory total score was not different at posttest, but there were significant improvements in some prospective items such as asking for an appointment, asking for a belonging, and delivering a message.

IMPLICATIONS: While additional studies are needed if a thorough model of memory enhancement in the elderly is to be devised, the prospective memory improvements found in this study have particular relevance for continued independent living, and the ability to maintain the status quo, without requiring greater supervision or service utilization.

McDougall G: Memory improvement in assisted living elders, *Issues Ment Health Nurs* 21:217, 2000.

Life Review Therapy. Life review therapy has a positive psychotherapeutic function, providing an opportunity for the person to reflect on life and resolve, reorganize, and reintegrate troubling or disturbing areas (Butler, 1961; Haight & Webster, 1995). Life review works well with groups or individuals. In a group, members may positively reinforce each other and stimulate mutual learning. Developing individual autobiographies to share with the group is one way to introduce common experiences and interests among the members and put them at ease. The group cohesion and sharing can build self-esteem and a feeling of belonging, in addition to the positive effect of the review itself.

Life review therapy is different from reminiscence (Haight & Bursnside, 1993). Both are planned interventions that are led by a mental health professional. Reminiscence is usually a pleasant experience in which the patient reviews life events without any particular structure and talks about meanings and feelings. The nurse listens and responds but does not try to interpret or probe for deeper meanings. The life review is structured, with the emphasis on analyzing life events. The nurse helps the patient to look for the meaning of experiences and to resolve conflicts and lingering feelings. Life review helps the elder to achieve the ego integrity and wisdom identified by Erikson (1963) as the goal of the last stage of life.

Reality Orientation. Both 24-hour and structured reality orientation can prevent confusion and keep patients oriented to time, place, person, and situation. The environment, when it is kept simple and focused, reinforces contact with reality, the here and now. Helpful physical props include clocks, directional signs, calendars, and orientation boards (season of the year, weather, and so on). Reality orientation groups can provide an opportunity to reinforce time, place, and person orientation with patients who have short attention spans and need extra verbal and visual stimulation. Reality orientation, along with a discussion of current events, stimulates patients to maintain contact with the real world and their place in it. Current events discussions, used alone, may be structured in various ways, such as sharing of newspaper articles or group viewing of television news programs. The scope of the group depends on the patients' abilities and the other therapeutic modalities at hand.

Validation Therapy. Although reality orientation is effective for many institutionalized and community-based elderly with confusion or disorientation, some evidence indicates that for some older adults, especially those with minimal organic impairment, disorientation may be a form of denial of unpleasant realities. These elders may become more anxious or agitated if constantly reminded of environmental realities. An alternate approach to confused and disoriented older adults was developed in relation to working with the patient who does not respond to reality orientation (Feil, 1993). This approach involves searching for the emotion and meaning in the patient's disoriented or confused words and behavior (such as wandering) and validating them verbally with the patient. A series of verbal cues or steps are involved that allow the patient to focus on key words or phrases in the confused interaction, and the nurse validates by asking for description, more detail, or clarification. What is sometimes identified as meaningless or incoherent conversation may often have significant meaning for the patient and can be related to current or past events. Validation is being used successfully with both mild and moderately impaired elders, providing an effective avenue for reaching older adults experiencing cognitive dysfunction.

Cognitive Training. Much research is under way using cognitive training and stimulation (see Chapter 32). Problem-solving situations, formal or didactic memory training, and selected memory exercises have been effective in increasing attention span, efficiency of recall, and the ability to learn new skills (such as mathematical calculations and vocabulary). Intelligence does not decline with age but may be dulled by depression, drugs, or lack of use. Cognitive training can keep older adults active mentally, which in turn enhances emotional well-being. The "use it or lose it" adage is as true for maintenance of intelligence as it is for physical functioning. Research suggests that cognitive retraining and memory cues can also be effective with demented elderly patients (Davis & Burgio, 1999). Such strategies can reduce behavioral deficits and excess disability.

Stimulating cognitive skills can challenge the nurse's creativity in relating to geropsychiatric patients. To be able to capitalize on the patient's interests and skills, the nurse must be familiar with the patient's past occupation, hobbies, and leisure activities. The nursing interview should focus on gathering as much of that information as possible on admission and adding it to the database as the nurse builds a trusting relationship with the patient and family.

Relaxation Therapy. Besides promoting a sense of physical well-being, relaxation can release tension and reduce stress, reducing barriers to communication. Additional information about relaxation therapy is presented in Chapters 17 and 32. Relaxation, combined with mild isometric exercises, increases cardiovascular output, energy, and mobility and reduces stress. Relaxation and exercise strategies, used in group or individual contexts, do not require advanced skills of the nurse or the patient. They may begin with simple tension-releasing muscle exercises, coupled with verbal instructions about breathing and concentration. Structured exercise programs are increasingly being used to meet patients' physical activity and social needs while reducing the incidence of behavioral excesses such as wandering (Holmberg, 1997).

Supportive and Counseling Groups. Geropsychiatric patients respond well to both supportive and counseling groups. These interventions may use either a nondirective or unstructured format or a more structured, didactic approach. Group members can ventilate feelings, try out problem-solving approaches, and resolve conflict in a rational, systematic manner. These groups may incorporate some aspects of cognitive training or reminiscence, described earlier in this chapter. Older adults respond well to a supportive group structure, which increases self-esteem, self-confidence, risk-taking, and empathy (Klausner & Alexopoulos, 1999).

Humor may be an effective way to reach the nonverbal or withdrawn elder. The ability to laugh at oneself and see the irony in everyday events provides an effective outlet for frustration, anger, stress, and anxiety. Promoting humor by telling jokes and stories and watching cartoons or situation comedies can be therapeutic in a group or with individual patients. Expressions of humor and active laughter allow older adults to step out of their situations, releasing some of the tension related to coping with changes accompanying aging.

Patient Education. Older adults often question the physiological and cognitive changes that occur naturally in aging. Slowed response time, benign memory loss, altered gait, and interrupted sleep patterns are a few of the normal changes of aging that elders may interpret as pathological. The nurse has an opportunity to teach patients about their own developmental changes during the assessment phase of the nurse-patient relationship. Dispelling myths and stereotypes related to aging is a primary goal for patient education. Exercises for promoting positive thoughts and images, visualization, and repetitive cognitive games can be used as a basis for teaching new patterns of behavior. Cognitive training, relaxation, and life review approaches are well-suited to patient education formats.

> *Your friend's grandfather is 85 years old and constantly complains of feeling tired and forgetful. He has been to many physicians without feeling better. Your friend asks what she should do next. How would you respond?*

Family Education and Support. Because 80% of the elders living at home are cared for by a spouse, sibling, their adult child or that child's spouse, education and support groups for family caregivers are essential. Many community agencies, clinics, and senior citizen centers are responding to the needs of family caregivers with special activities, classes, and support groups. Extensive nursing research demonstrates the effectiveness of nursing interventions in educating and empowering family caregivers (Kelley et al, 1999).

Family members often view nurses as the most approachable health-care professionals for understanding family relationships, conflicts, needs, and resources. Family education about aging processes, family dynamics, problem-solving, behavioral management, the caregiving trajectory, and stresses inherent in the caregiver role can be integrated into counseling sessions with family members, referral conferences, or part of the family history on admission of the patient (Schumacher et al, 1998).

A more formal approach to family education can be developed using the numerous books now available that address caring for older adults. These materials provide practical, step-by-step guidelines to handling common problems of the frail elderly, including agitation, wandering, withdrawal, resistance, anxiety, insomnia, incontinence, anorexia, and restlessness. These books, which have been written specifically for the consumer, supply the text for nurse-family teaching sessions and are excellent resource materials for use in the home (Mace & Rabins, 1999). Families genuinely wish that they can provide good caregiving for as long as possible. Thus they need to be the focus of nursing intervention and support if the caregiver role in the care of geropsychiatric patients is to be successful (Schumacher et al, 1998).

EVALUATING THE CARE OF THE GERIATRIC PATIENT

Implementing evidenced based care designed to promote optimum cognitive function and emotional well-being has been considered the role of the geropsychiatric nurse. Increasingly, research is being initiated to determine the most appropriate approach to meet the needs of patients and family caregivers and the most effective interventions to use.

Evaluation of patient care should be based on a model that explains the progression of behavior from adaptive to maladaptive. The type of care and the evaluation of outcome would be directly related to the level of behavior targeted for intervention.

The goal of nursing intervention is to promote maximum independence of the older adult, based on capacity and functional abilities. Evaluation of outcomes of nursing care would not be based on reversal of behaviors or elimination of patient needs but on the change the patient demonstrates based on individual abilities. This approach reinforces the emphasis on the individual as a unit for evaluation and allows for patient differences and for the process of change over time.

The effectiveness of family caregiver interventions must also be evaluated. Important dimensions include the caregiver's health and stress level, family coping strategies, caregiver knowledge and competence, status of the elder, and freedom from abuse.

Community geropsychiatric programs will become increasingly important to meet the impending demographic shift. Important evaluative criteria will include accessibility and coordination of services; patient, family, and systems outcomes and satisfaction; staff training; compliance with patient-centered regulatory systems; program goals; and cost-effectiveness.

In the final analysis, the most important evaluation criterion is the feedback from the patient and caregivers that nursing care was helpful and growth producing. The challenge to the nurse is to be creative in producing a positive experience for each elderly patient.

Summary

1. The demographics of aging continue to expand. The 21st century will see increasing longevity, geropsychiatric disability, and the need for evidence based, accessible, cost-effective programs.

2. The role of the geropsychiatric nurse includes providing primary mental health nursing care, including intervening with caregivers, providing case management, and consulting with other care providers. Advanced practice nurses provide individual and group psychotherapy, take leadership in program development, and prescribe medications in most states.

3. Biopsychosocial theories of aging were identified. No one theory can explain all aspects of aging. Biological, psychological, and sociocultural theories of aging guide the development of evidence based nursing practice.

4. A comprehensive geropsychiatric nursing assessment includes application of interviewing skills. The areas to be assessed include mental status, behavioral and functional abilities, physiological functioning, and social support.

5. NANDA nursing diagnoses related to geropsychiatric patients include altered thought processes, dysfunctional grieving, high risk for self-directed violence, situational low self-esteem, sleep pattern disturbance, altered nutrition, relocation stress syndrome, high risk for caregiver role strain, social isolation, self-care deficit (also called behavioral deficit), behavioral excess, and progressively lowered stress threshold.

6. Nursing interventions with geropsychiatric patients include creation of a therapeutic milieu, involvement in somatic therapies, and interpersonal interventions. Caregivers should be involved in planning, implementing, and evaluating nursing interventions.

7. Evaluation of geropsychiatric nursing care focuses on the patient's ability to reach maximum independence.

Competent Caring   A Clinical Exemplar of a Psychiatric Nurse

BETH GAGE GRECO, MSN, RN

A frail ghost of a man sat silently in his easy chair. He did not raise his head or speak as I entered the room with his wife. He made no eye contact as I introduced myself as his new home health nurse. He simply remained quiet, barely moving even as he breathed. I was struck by his appearance. He was not the person I had expected to meet that day.

Mr. R had been reported to be "very difficult," "demanding," "noncompliant," and "an impossible patient." Emergency visits by nurses were often necessary to fix a leaky catheter, assess a drastic decrease in urinary output, unclog a clogged feeding tube, and assess reported changes in cardiac and respiratory status. His wife and primary caretaker made numerous calls to the home health office and continually asked questions about Mr. R's medicines, diet, heart problems, breathing difficulties, and overall health. After meeting Mr. R, it occurred to me that caring for this patient would involve not only extensive medical management but also intensive psychiatric nursing care for him and his family. I was very glad that I had a few years of psychiatric nursing experience before I met this family.

My immediate response in assessing Mr. R's needs was to increase the frequency of home visits to three times per week. During these visits I carefully reviewed Mr. R's medications, diet, and treatments with him and his wife at the same time. I was very careful to include Mr. R in these discussions by asking him questions and providing him opportunities to make decisions about his care. At first he was very reluctant to participate in these teaching sessions, but gradually he began to show some interest. As he became more engaged in conversations with me, I began showing him how to take care of his feeding tube and catheter. I encouraged his wife to let Mr. R do his care when he felt up to it. I thought it would be very important for Mr. R to have some control over what was happening to him. I also thought it would be necessary for Mrs. R to let go of the total responsibility for her husband's care. Her anxiety level had reached almost unmanageable proportions several weeks before I had received the case.

I encouraged Mrs. R to arrange some time for herself away from the home on a regular basis. She agreed that she would have her daughter come in once a week so that she could spend time with her church friends. Mr. R stated that it would be good for his wife to get out more often and he would be all right in her absence. After a few weeks of concentrating on the tasks to be learned, Mr. R became more open to discussion of the impact of his illness on his life and his family. He talked about his past work and leisure activities and his disbelief over his current situation. He felt that his retirement years were supposed to be full of travel and leisure pursuits, and instead he was confined by his failing health to his home. He was very angry as he talked to me about these things, and as I glanced at a picture on his dresser of a broad-shouldered, confident military man, I better understood his anger and his pain. He had been that man in the picture, and his losses were great.

Grief work became an important focus of my nursing care in the remainder of the time that I worked with Mr. R and his

Continued

Competent Caring A Clinical Exemplar of a Psychiatric Nurse—cont'd

family. We talked about the changes in their lives, their disappointments over missed opportunities, their anger, and their fears. We explored ways to cope with Mr. R's limitations, and I was happy to hear one day that Mr. and Mrs. R had ventured out to dinner at a restaurant. A wheelchair and some courage were the necessary ingredients for an enjoyable evening.

As time went on, Mr. R's condition stabilized and weekly maintenance visits were all that was needed. His condition remained acute, but he and his wife were managing his care very well at home. Emergency visits were no longer needed, and this "difficult" patient was rarely heard from between home visits.

My last visit to Mr. R's home was prompted by an early morning telephone call from my office. There was an emergency at his home on that day. When I arrived at the house I found Mr. R in bed clutching his chest. His wife explained that he had awakened with chest pain. My quick physical assessment indicated that his pulse was rapid and thready and his blood pressure was lower than his normal baseline. He was alert but looked pale and was diaphoretic. I instructed Mrs. R to call EMS, and as she did so I sat with Mr. R. I held his hand and asked him whether he was afraid. He nodded and met my eyes with his. In them I saw only his courage. He remained conscious until EMS arrived, and they promptly started an IV line and provided oxygen and whisked him off to the nearest hospital. He died later that same day, but I will always remember him for the bravery of his struggle for life.

MERLIN **Visit MERLIN: www.mosby.com/MERLIN/Stuart** to find these additional materials and student activities.

- **Worksheets**
- **"Drug of the Month" Updates**
- **"Citing the Evidence" Updates**
- **Critical Thinking Activities and Exercises**
- **Annotated Suggested Readings**
- **Web Links**
- **More!**

Chapter Review Questions

1. Match each term in Column A with the correct description in Column B.

Column A

a. _____ Activity theory

b. _____ Cross-linkage theory

c. _____ Person-environment fit theory

d. _____ Biological programming theory

e. _____ Disengagement theory

f. _____ Life review theory

g. _____ Stability of personality

h. _____ Stress adaptation theory

Column B

A. The life span of a cell is stored within the cell itself.

B. Older adults and society mutually withdraw from active exchange.

C. Past experiences return to consciousness, and memories are examined and reintegrated.

D. Personality is viewed as unchanging from early adulthood through old age.

E. Collagen forms more rigid molecular bonds over time.

F. Older adults should find substitutes for work or participation in community organizations if they must stop these activities.

G. Positive and negative effects of stress on biopsychosocial development.

H. If capacities decrease, the environment may be threatening.

2. Fill in the blanks.

A. Increasing disorientation or confusion at night resulting from loss of visual accommodation is called _____.

B. Mitts, posey belts, and geri chairs are examples of _____ that should be used with caution with the elderly.

C. Contraindications for _____ therapy are increased intracranial pressure, arrhythmias, and a myocardial infarction within the last 3 months.

D. When older patients need antipsychotic medications, atypicals are usually used due to their _____.

E. _____ orientation can prevent confusion and keep patients oriented to time, place, person, and situation.

F. Intelligence is dulled by depression, drugs, or lack of use, but is stimulated by _____ therapy.

G. Evaluation of geropsychiatric nursing care focuses on the patient's ability to reach _____.

H. Doses of psychopharmacologic drugs for older patients are usually _____.

3. Provide short answers for the following questions.

A. Highlight important communication factors to consider when interviewing older patients.

B. List the risk factors for falls with older patients.

C. Some believe that the lack of regard shown by healthcare professionals for living wills and advanced directives of the elderly is related to their high suicide rate. Explore the many aspects of this complex issue.

REFERENCES

Bair B: Presentation and recognition of common psychiatric disorders in the elderly, *Clin Geriatr* 8(2):26, 2000.

Beck-Little R, Weinrich S: Assessment and management of sleep disorders in the elderly, *J Gerontol Nurs* 4:21, 1998.

Bellelli G et al: Special care units for demented patients: a multicenter study, *The Gerontologist* 38:456, 1998.

Blair C: Effect of self-care ADLs on self-esteem of intact nursing home residents, *Issues Ment Health Nurs* 20:559, 1999.

Butler R: Re-awakening interest, *Nurs Homes* 10:8, 1961.

Chien W: Use of physical restraints on hospitalized psychogeriatric patients, *J Psychosoc Nurs* 38(2):13, 2000.

Cohen G: Aging at a turning point in the 21st century, *Am J Geriatr Psychiatry* 8:1, 2000.

Davis L, Burgio L: Planning cognitive behavioral management programs for long-term care, *Issues Ment Health Nurs* 20:587, 1999.

Ebersole P, Hess P: *Toward healthy aging—human needs and nursing response*, ed 5, St Louis, 1998, Mosby.

Erikson E: *Childhood and society*, New York, 1963, WW Norton

Feil N: Communicating with the confused elderly patient, *Geriatrics* 39:131, 1993.

Friedland R, Summer L: *Demography is not destiny*, Washington, DC, 1999, National Academy Press.

Haight B, Burnside J: Reminiscing and life review: explaining the difference, *Arch Psychiatr Nurs* 7:91, 1993.

Haight B, Webster J: *Art and science of reminiscing: theory, research, methods, and application*, Washington, DC, 1995, Taylor & Francis.

Hegge M, Fischer C: Grief responses of senior and elderly widows: practice implications, *J Gerontol Nurs* 2:35, 2000.

Hirata E et al: Alcoholism in a geriatric outpatient clinic of Sao Paulo-Brazil, *Int Psychogeriatr* 9:95, 1997.

Holmberg S: Evaluation of a clinical intervention for wanders on a geriatric nursing unit, *Arch Psychiatr Nurs* 11:21, 1997.

Jeste D et al: Consensus statement on the upcoming crisis in geriatric mental health, *Arch Gen Psychiatry* 56:9, 1999.

Kelley L et al: Access to health care resources for family caregivers of elderly persons with dementia, *Nurs Outlook* 47:1, 1999.

Kim K, Goldstein M: Treating older adults with psychotic symptoms, *Psychiatr Serv* 48:9, 1997.

Klausner E, Alexopoulos G: The future of psychosocial treatments for elderly patients, *Psychiatr Serv* 50:9, 1999.

Krasucki C et al: Anxiety and its treatment in the elderly, *Int Psychogeriatr* 11:25, 1999.

Mace N, Rabins R: *The 36-hour day*, ed 3, New York, 1999, Warner Books.

Massand P: Side effects of antipsychotics in the elderly, *J Clin Psychiatry* 61(suppl 8):43, 2000.

Mulsant B, Ganguli M: Epidemiology and diagnosis of depression in late life, *J Clin Psychiatry* 60:20, 1999.

North American Nursing Diagnosis Association: *NANDA nursing diagnosis, definitions and classification*, 1999-2000, Philadelphia, NANDA, 1999.

Patterson T, Jeste D: The potential impact of the baby-boom generation on substance abuse among elderly persons, *Psychiatr Serv* 50(9): 1184, 1999.

Reynolds C, Kupfer D: Depression and aging: a look to the future, *Psychiatr Serv* 50:9, 1999.

Ryden M et al: Relationships between aggressive behavior in cognitively impaired nursing home residents and use of restraints, psychoactive drugs, and secured units, *Arch Psychiatric Nurs* 13:4, 1999.

Salzman C: Practical considerations for the treatment of depression in elderly and very elderly long-term care patients, *J Clin Psychiatry* 60, 1999.

Schumacher K et al: Conceptualization and measurement of doing family caregiving well, *Image: Journal of Nursing Scholarship* 30:1, 1998.

Targum S, Abbott J: Psychoses in the elderly: a spectrum of disorders, *J Clin Psychiatry* 60(suppl 8):4, 1999.

Yeung P et al: Quetiapine for elderly patients with psychotic disorders, *Psychiatric Ann* 30(3):197, 2000.

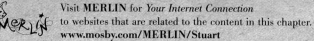
Visit **MERLIN** for *Your Internet Connection*
to websites that are related to the content in this chapter.
www.mosby.com/MERLIN/Stuart

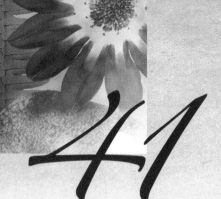

41 Care of Survivors of Abuse and Violence

Nancy Fishwick

Barbara Parker

Jacqueline C. Campbell

When I was a laddie I lived with my granny
And many a hiding my granny di'ed me.
Now I am a man and I live with my granny
And do to my granny what she did to me.

        Traditional rhyme, anonymous

Nurses encounter survivors of abuse and violence in many settings. However, because experiencing violence is generally devastating, survivors of abuse and violence are often seen in psychiatric settings. At times the violence is openly discussed and recognized as a precipitating factor for the current hospitalization, as when a survivor of sexual assault is treated in an emergency room. Often, however, violence is disclosed only after a trusting nurse-patient relationship is formed. Although there are various forms of violence, such as gang behavior and drug-related violence, the types most often described by psychiatric patients are family violence and nonfamily rape and sexual assault. Because the dynamics of these two forms of violence are different, they are covered in two separate sections of this chapter. Rape and sexual assault also can be forms of family violence. In addition, attention is given to populations that are particularly at risk for abuse. These include children, intimate partners, and the elderly.

The words used to describe people who have experienced violence are important. Traditionally the word **victim** has been used, along with discussions of syndromes. These labels distance nurses from the person who has been abused as they search for differences between themselves and the victims to decrease their feelings of vulnerability. In this chapter the word **survivor** is used to emphasize that the person who has experienced abuse has many strengths and coping strategies that can be incorporated into the plan of care.

Do you agree with the use of the word survivor *instead of* victim *in this chapter? What do you think of when you hear the words* victim *and* survivor*?*

DIMENSIONS OF FAMILY VIOLENCE

Family violence is a range of harmful behaviors that occur between family and other household members. It includes physical and emotional abuse of children, child neglect, abuse between adult intimate partners, marital rape, and elder abuse. Several different issues are related to abuse within families. Although each family is unique, some characteristics appear to be common to most violent families. Furthermore, regardless of the type of abuse occurring within a

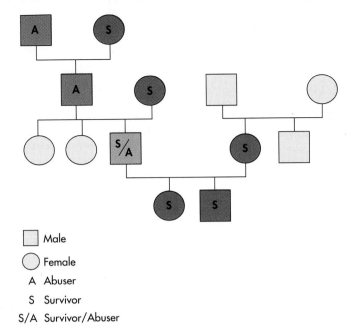

Male

Female

A Abuser

S Survivor

S/A Survivor/Abuser

Fig. 41-1   Genogram demonstrates the multigenerational transmission of family violence.

family, all members, including the extended family, are affected. Family violence, although often unnoted, is at the core of many family disturbances. Violence may be a family secret and often continues through generations.

Although many research studies and theories have been directed toward the causes, treatment, and prevention of family violence, there are more questions unanswered than answered. Some believe that the family is the training ground for violence and ask why the social group that is supposed to provide love and support is also the most violent group to which most people belong. Behaviors that would be unacceptable between strangers, co-workers, or friends are often tolerated within families.

Feminist authors note that most survivors of family violence are the most vulnerable and powerless family members: women, children, and the elderly. They say that the root cause of violence is the abuser's need for power and control, which is acted out by violent behavior. Social norms that support or at least allow male dominance and violence are considered crucial in feminist analysis.

Violence and abuse are caused by an interaction of personality, demographic, biological, situational, and sociocultural factors. Many of the unique characteristics of the family as a social group—time spent together, emotional involvement, privacy, and in-depth knowledge of each other—can lead to both intimacy and violence. Thus a given family can be loving and supportive as well as violent.

To understand violence in American families, the influence of society on the family must be examined. The United States has a high level of violence compared with other Western nations. Many believe that society's willingness to tolerate violence sets the stage for family violence. Social norms are sometimes used to justify violence to maintain the family system. For example, a husband's use of violence may be considered legitimate if the wife is having an extra-

marital affair. Historical attitudes toward women, children, and the elderly; economic discrimination; the nonresponsiveness of the criminal justice system; and the belief that women and children are property are social factors that promote violence. Changing norms about family privacy and when the government should intervene in family matters have also influenced the definition and recognition of family violence.

Why do you think more violence occurs in American society than in other Western nations? What societal factors influence the use of violence?

Characteristics of Violent Families

Factors common to violent families include the multigenerational family process, social isolation, the use and abuse of power, and the effect of alcohol and drug abuse.

Multigenerational Transmission. Multigenerational transmission means that family violence is often perpetuated through generations by a cycle of violence. Fig. 41-1 shows the multigenerational transmission of family violence. Social learning theory related to violence states that a child learns this behavior pattern in a family setting by taking a violent parent as a role model. In this case, violence and victimization are behaviors learned through childhood experience. The child learns both the means and the approval of violence. Children who witness violence not only learn specific aggressive behaviors but also come to believe that violence is a legitimate way to solve problems. When frustrated or angry as an adult, the person relies on this learned behavior and responds with violence.

Social learning theory was first applied to child abuse when it was noted that many child abusers were abused as children. Many studies have suggested the multigenerational

Table 41-1

Forms of Abuse within Families Reflecting Struggles for Power and Control

PHYSICAL

- **Inflicting or attempting to inflict physical injury or illness**—for example, grabbing, pinching, shoving, slapping, hitting, hair-pulling, biting, arm-twisting, kicking, punching, hitting with blunt objects, stabbing, shooting.
- **Withholding access to resources necessary to maintain health**—for example, medication, medical care, wheelchair, food or fluids, sleep, hygienic assistance.
- **Forcing alcohol or other drug use**.

SEXUAL

- **Coercing or attempting to coerce any sexual contact without consent**—for example, marital rape, acquaintance rape, forced sex after physical beating, attacks on the sexual parts of the body, bestiality, forced prostitution, unprotected sex, fondling, sodomy, sex with others, use of pornography.
- **Attempting to undermine the victim's sexuality**—for example, treating her or him in a sexually degrading manner, criticizing sexual performance and desirability. Also, accusations of infidelity, withholding sex.

PSYCHOLOGICAL

- **Instilling or attempting to instill fear**—for example, intimidation, threatening physical harm to self, victim, or others, threatening to harm or kidnap children, menacing, blackmail, harassment, destruction of pets and property, mind games.
- **Isolating or attempting to isolate victim from friends, family, school, or work**—for example, withholding access to phone or transportation, undermining victim's personal relationships, harassing others, constant "checking up," constant accompaniment, unfounded accusations, forced imprisonment.

EMOTIONAL

- **Undermining or attempting to undermine victim's sense of self-worth**—for example, constant criticism, belittling victim's abilities and competency, name calling, insults, put-downs, silent treatment, manipulating victim's feelings and emotions to induce guilt, subverting a partner's relationship with the children, repeatedly making and breaking promises.

ECONOMIC

- **Making or attempting to make the victim financially dependent**—for example, maintaining total control over financial resources, including victim's earned income or resources received through public assistance or social security, withholding money or access to money, forbidding attendance at school, forbidding employment, on-the-job harassment, requiring accountability and justification for all money spent, forced welfare fraud, withholding information about family finances, running up bills for which the victim is responsible for payment.

From New York State Office for the Prevention of Domestic Violence.

transmission of child abuse within families. However, other studies examining parental punishment history and current child abuse found no differences between abusive and non-abusive parents. Experiencing abuse as a child does not totally determine an adult's later behaviors. Many people who were abused as children are able to avoid violence with their own children. A key factor may be the age at which the child was abused or which parent was abusive. Experiencing abuse from a father at age 4 years may be totally different from experiencing abuse from a mother as an adolescent.

The incidence of violence in the families of both the survivors of wife abuse and their abusers also supports multigenerational transmission. A classic literature review identified witnessing parental violence during childhood or adolescence as one of the strongest risk factors for the abuse of wives in adulthood (Hotaling & Sugerman, 1986). It is less clear that women learn to tolerate wife abuse from childhood experiences with violence.

To date, there is limited evidence of multigenerational transmission of violence in elder abuse. However, elder abuse could be the result of formerly abused children displaying both retaliatory and imitative behavior or behavior modeled by their parents with their grandparents.

Many treatment modalities, especially cognitive-behavioral approaches, are based on the social learning model that violent reactions can be unlearned and replaced with constructive responses to conflict (Divitto, 1998).

Social Isolation. Violent families are also socially isolated. One reason may be that some types of violence are considered abnormal or illegitimate and become a family secret. Exposure of family violence can result in both formal and informal sanctions from other family members, neighbors, the police, or the judicial system; therefore, the abuser often purposely keeps the family isolated. Social isolation is a factor in elder abuse, intimate partner violence, and child abuse.

Use and Abuse of Power. Another common factor within the various forms of family violence is the use and abuse of power. In almost all forms of family violence the abuser has some form of power or control over the victim. For example, with the sexual abuse of children, the abuser is usually a male in an authority position victimizing a child in a subordinate position (U.S. Department of Health and Human Services, 2000).

Power issues appear to be a central factor in wife abuse. Although wife abusers justify the use of violence for trivial events such as not having a meal ready or not keeping the house tidy, violence often is related to the husband's need for total domination of his wife. Wife abuse often begins or escalates when the woman behaves more independently by working or attending school. Table 41-1 describes five forms of abuse within families that reflect domestic struggles for power and control.

Alcohol and Drug Abuse. Survivors of violence often report concurrent substance abuse by the abuser. However, one behavior is not necessary for the other to occur. That is, people who abuse alcohol are not consistently violent, and people who are violent are not always intoxicated. Instead, it has been suggested that the person uses alcohol as a socially

Box 41-1

Beyond the Myths: Recognizing Abuse Survivors

Myth: Family violence is most common among the lower class.

Reality: Family violence occurs at all levels of society without regard to age, race, culture, status, education, or religion. It may be less evident among the affluent because they can afford private physicians, attorneys, counselors, and shelters. In contrast, people with less money must turn to public agencies for help.

Myth: Violence rarely occurs between dating partners.

Reality: Estimates vary among studies, but violence occurs in a large percentage of dating relationships.

Myth: Abused spouses can end the violence by divorcing their abuser.

Reality: According to the U.S. Department of Justice, about 75% of all spousal attacks occur between people who are separated or divorced. In many cases, the separation process brings on an increased level of harassment and violence.

Myth: The victim can learn to stop doing things that provoke the violence.

Reality: In a battering relationship, the abuser needs no provocation to become violent. Violence is the abuser's pattern of behavior and the victim cannot learn how to control it. Even so, many victims blame themselves for the abuse, feeling guilty—even responsible—for doing or saying something that seems to trigger the abuser's behavior. Friends, family, and service providers reinforce this by laying the blame and the need to change on the shoulders of the victim.

Myth: Alcohol, stress, and mental illness are major causes of physical and verbal abuse.

Reality: Abusive people—and even their victims—often use those conditions to excuse or minimize the abuse. But abuse is a learned behavior, not an uncontrollable reaction. People are abusive because they have acquired the belief that violence and aggression are acceptable and effective responses to real or imagined threats. Fortunately, because violence is a learned behavior, abusers can benefit from counseling and professional help to alter their behavior. But dealing only with the perceived problem (for example, alcohol, stress, or mental illness) will not change the abusive tendencies.

Myth: Violence occurs only between heterosexual partners.

Reality: Increasing evidence suggests that gay and lesbian partners experience violence for varied but similar reasons as heterosexual partners do.

Myth: Being pregnant protects a woman from battering.

Reality: Battering often begins or escalates during pregnancy. According to one theory, the abuser who already has low self-esteem views his wife as his property. As a result, he resents the intrusion of the fetus as well as the extra attention his wife gets from friends, family, and health-care providers.

Myth: Abused women tacitly accept the abuse by trying to conceal it, not reporting it, or failing to seek help.

Reality: Many women, when they do try to disclose their situation, are met with denial or disbelief. This only discourages them from persevering.

---

acceptable explanation for the behavior. Family and friends may attribute the conduct to the effects of alcohol, which to some extent may decrease the degree of blame. The use of alcohol or drugs may also increase violent behavior by reducing fear or inhibitions and decreasing sensitivity to the impact of the behavior.

Cross-cultural studies suggest that behavior while drinking varies from culture to culture. In societies where it is believed that alcohol removes inhibitions, people become less inhibited. If they believe it is a depressant, they become depressed when drinking. If people in the United States believe that normal rules of behavior are suspended when one is drinking, people will behave antisocially.

Connections between drug abuse and family violence have been less well researched. Research on aggressiveness and illicit drugs has established that marijuana and heroin use are not related to violence. In contrast, drugs such as crack cocaine, amphetamines, mescaline, "angel dust" (PCP), and steroids have been associated with increased violence; but the specific relationships with various forms of family violence are not yet established.

Nursing Attitudes toward Survivors of Violence

It can be difficult and frustrating to provide nursing care for survivors of violence. The attitudes nurses bring to these situations shape their responses (Gallop et al, 1998). Studies of health-care professionals' attitudes indicate that myths about battered women are accepted even though there is sympathy toward the survivor. Nurses have been found not to blame rape survivors in general. However, the tendency to blame the survivor increases when a vignette describes the woman as having gone out late at night, not locked her car doors, or gone shopping for beer rather than milk for the baby. Box 41-1 describes common myths about survivors of abuse.

Although most nurses do not actually blame survivors for what has happened to them, they do dislike certain behaviors. They are not happy with sexual assault survivors who do not resist "enough." They have difficulty understanding abused children who want to return to abusive parents. They especially dislike battered women who do not leave their abusers. One study of psychiatric nurses found that attitudes toward sexuality were more positive and attitudes toward sexual assault included less victim-blaming than in previously reported studies of nurses in nonpsychiatric settings. Also, the younger the psychiatric nurses in the study, the more positive the attitudes, perhaps reflecting the societal norms in which they were raised, which have changed over time (Boutcher & Gallop, 1996).

Other studies describe how survivors find the health-care system to be unhelpful and even traumatizing when they go for help (see Citing the Evidence). Nurses often use a paternalistic and individualistic model of helping battered women. The paternalistic model may be contrasted with the empowerment model. Table 41-2 compares the characteristics of these models. When the paternalistic model is used, the nurse is more likely to be frustrated because the survivor does not follow the nurse's advice. Therefore, the empowerment model is not only more helpful to the survivor but also more professionally satisfying for the nurse.

Origins of Negative Attitudes. Several theories can help in understanding nurses' attitudes. The **just world hypothesis** proposes that people believe that others generally get what they deserve: Good things happen to good people and bad things happen to bad people. This belief helps one feel safe because one sees oneself as basically good and therefore protected. When a person is victimized by violence, there is a need to make sense of this horrible idea. The easiest way is not to see it at all, which explains some of the lack of recognition. However, when family violence is unmistakable, one needs to understand why that particular person is the victim. If bad things happen to bad people, the victimized person must have done something wrong or at least something stupid, something different from what oneself would have done.

The whole process of victim blaming is easier if the survivor is of "a type" who is already the focus of bias. It is easier to blame and distance oneself from women or minority groups if there is already bias against them. Conversely, the more the person resembles oneself, the harder it is to recognize the violence at all. Thus it is not reported as often; the abuse is just not seen when the people are middle class and especially professionals. Consequently, child abuse is more likely to be reported if the family is poor and of a racial minority.

Another example is the family member who has always been the most despised in cases of incest, the "collusive" mother. Despite the lack of evidence to support this notion, professionals are still eager to find out the mother's role in the sexual abuse of her child. Because it is difficult to blame the child, they have shifted the blame to the mother rather than trying to understand the mother's normal responses to a horrible dilemma. Even though some of the societal forces that lead to incest have been exposed, they are generally not addressed in recommendations for clinical interventions. The focus is on the "dysfunctional family unit" rather than the real issue: a criminal who has violated the safety and health of a child in a society uncomfortable with the attitudes that may encourage such behavior.

Yet another perspective is that of deviance theory, which proposes that making the survivors and perpetrators of violence into objects to be studied or diagnostic categories creates further distance between them and the nurse. This is the problem with a psychiatric diagnosis specific to survivors of violence. If adults receive diagnoses only because they were abused sometime in their past, the assumption of pathology becomes concrete. The survivor of family violence is officially sick and has the responsibility to become well. There is no chance that the person's responses will be seen as survival strategies or normal reactions; they become symptoms. Survivors become a "deviant group" to be studied and "fixed."

Citing the Evidence on

Women's Experiences with the Health-Care System

BACKGROUND: This survey was conducted to determine what experiences abused women have had in the health-care system including what discouraged or encouraged their disclosure of abuse and what interventions may improve detection and management of abuse in primary care.

RESULTS: Women's ability to access medical care was mainly affected by their partners who prevented them from receiving it. Women's attitudes about abuse that affected disclosure included feelings of shame, denial, and fear, and the lack of readiness to change the relationship with the abuser. Women did not disclose abuse if they perceived clinicians to be uncaring, too rushed, too busy, interested only in money, uncomfortable with the topic, or not listening. Leaflets and posters about domestic violence found in clinician offices helped women talk about their abuse. They found referral to women's groups and other agencies beneficial, but described having negative experiences with psychologists and psychiatrists.

IMPLICATIONS: Abused women often experience increased medical problems and barriers to health care. Clinician attitudes and behaviors can either facilitate or act as a barrier to disclosure of abuse.

McCauley J et al: Inside Pandora's box: abused women's experiences with clinicians and health services, *J Gen Intern Med* 13:549, 1998.

Table **41-2**

A Comparison of the Paternalistic and Empowerment Models of Intervention with Battered Women	
Paternalistic Model	**Empowerment Model**
Nurse is perceived to be more knowledgeable than the survivor.	There is mutual sharing of knowledge and information.
Responsibility for ending the violence is placed on the survivor.	The nurse strategizes with the survivor. Survivors are helped to recognize societal influences.
Advice and sympathy are given rather than respect.	The survivor's competence and experience are respected.

Because the nursing profession remains a predominantly female group, more nurses have been victimized by violence than other groups, which might explain nurses' negative attitudes toward other survivors. Research has not established whether there are more battered women among nurses than among other populations of women. One study found that nurses who were sexually abused as children had lower self-esteem and higher present distress scores than nurses who reported no sexual abuse in childhood. Additionally, the nurses who were abused reported that the abuse negatively influenced their private and professional relationships (Gallop et al, 1995). Regardless of the specific violence experience of nurses, power, control, and exploitation issues certainly have shaped the history of the nursing profession and continue to influence nurses' daily reality.

Overcoming Negative Attitudes. The first step in providing effective nursing care is exploring one's own attitudes toward survivors of family violence. Understanding the mechanisms that help create such attitudes is also helpful. Nurses who have had clinical experience with survivors and gotten to know them as people may be less blaming than nurses who have not. Therefore, it is important to gain this experience through educational programs or as a volunteer in programs such as rape crisis centers, battered women's shelters, or child protection programs. Formal continuing and in-service education on family violence should be directed toward recognizing and changing feelings as well as learning facts about violence. Nurses can also increase their own understanding and appreciation of the experience of survivors by reading books and watching media programs about these issues.

> *Many television shows and movies explore the issues of family abuse and violence. Do you think they have helped to change attitudes or reinforced fears and stereotypes?*

Responses of Survivors

There is a growing body of knowledge that describes how people respond to violence from other family members.

Physical Responses to Battering. One area of study has been the types and patterns of physical injuries received. A characteristic pattern of injuries, especially to the head, neck, face, throat, trunk, and sexual organs has been seen in all forms of family violence. For all groups experiencing family violence, sexual abuse often accompanies physical abuse. This has been best documented in battered women; several studies have found that approximately 40% were also sexually assaulted by their partners. All survivors of family violence tend to have injuries at multiple sites in various stages of healing.

Survivors of family violence often experience a range of physical symptoms not obviously related to their injuries, such as headaches, menstrual problems, chronic pain, and digestive and sleeping disturbances. Often, communicable diseases are a problem in shelters for battered women and their children.

Many characterize these symptoms as evidence of psychopathology, but similar symptoms occur after rape and other forms of violence, as well as in widows and divorcees. In addition, past injuries can cause such symptoms as headaches and other forms of chronic pain. Stress is also known to affect the immune system. Thus rather than labeling such symptoms "hysterical," "psychosomatic," or "evidence of somaticizing," they should be identified as part of a physical stress reaction that is common to those who have experienced many types of emotional trauma.

Behavioral Responses to Battering. There have been many attempts to understand the behavior of survivors of family violence, especially their continued involvement with an abuser. This has been especially damaging in literature addressing the question of why battered women remain in the relationship. It is assumed that she should leave rather than stay. In actuality, when a battered woman leaves, she is in the most danger of being killed by a partner obsessed with power and control. At the other end of the continuum, some battered women are able to end the violence but maintain their relationships using a variety of strategies.

However, family violence usually escalates in severity and frequency. In cases where the violence does not end, it is normal and healthy for a battered woman to consider her entire existence and that of her significant others for a long time before ending her most important attachment relationship (Byrne et al, 1999). Constraints that make it difficult to leave include cultural sanctions, an intense attachment to the man, and lack of resources. It has been observed that women usually make moral decisions by weighing the consequences to others more heavily than consequences to themselves (Gilligan, 1982). Thus concern for her children is a major issue in the woman's decision making.

Most battered women eventually leave a relationship that is continuously violent, but there is often a pattern of leaving and returning many times before making a final break. Rather than a sign of weakness, this can be seen as normal. It is influenced by the quality of social support and assistance to the woman and the batterer's behavior rather than the woman's psychological factors. Leaving and returning are purposeful and meant to pressure the abuser into meaningful change, test external and internal resources, or evaluate how the children react without their father.

Similar long processes of ending attachment relationships are seen with wives of alcoholics, divorced and separated women, and people experiencing anticipatory grief. In addition, grief can explain the denial that is often described in battered women. Clinical reports also describe the reluctance of abused children and elderly family members to view their families as pathological rather than normal. These responses seem more understandable and healthy if they are related to normal grief and fear of foster homes or nursing homes.

> *Discuss the issue of women remaining in abusive relationships. What factors keep them in these relationships? How do health professionals usually respond to a woman who has remained in an abusive relationship? What approach would be helpful to her?*

CRITICAL THINKING about CONTEMPORARY ISSUES

Can Adults Remember Repressed Episodes of Child Abuse or Are These Part of a "False Memory Syndrome"?

There has been considerable controversy about the validity of memories of childhood abuse. Some people have reported delayed recall of forgotten abuse that occurred during childhood, many years earlier. These reports of delayed recall of abuse have been challenged on a number of fronts, and in some cases people have retracted their allegations. Some experts claim that psychotherapists practicing "recovered memory therapy" created false memories of abuse through leading questions or excessive insisting. These therapists reportedly believe that psychopathology is related to childhood trauma and that the goal of therapy is to help patients remember incidents of previously forgotten abuse from childhood in order to get well.

That many people forget episodes of childhood abuse is well established. As many as 38% of trauma survivors who experienced abuse severe enough to result in a visit to a hospital emergency room had no memory of the event 20 or more years later. At issue is the meaning of these findings. Some investigators have explained the loss of memory of abuse as secondary to "repression" or dissociative amnesia: Memories of abuse, although present in the mind, may not be available to consciousness. The opposite viewpoint holds that the loss of memories of abuse is a process of "normal forgetting," arguing that there is a popular misconception that forgotten memories exist somewhere in the brain and are only awaiting the proper stimulus to bring them to consciousness.

A review of this literature found that neuropeptides and neurotransmitters released during stress can modulate memory function, acting in the limbic system at the level of the hippocampus (responsible for turning short-term memory into long-term memory), amygdala (responsible for emotion), and other brain regions involved in these functions. Such release may interfere with the accurate laying down of memory traces for incidents of childhood abuse. Also, childhood abuse may result in long-term alterations in the function of these neuromodulators (Bremner et al, 1996). Nurses can help these patients by keeping up to date with the neuroscientific research in this area and the impact of these findings on the controversy surrounding these issues.

Citing the Evidence on

PTSD in Abused Women

BACKGROUND: To describe the relationship between symptoms of posttraumatic stress disorder (PTSD) and severity of abuse, an ethnically stratified cohort of 131 abused women in a primary care setting was interviewed.

RESULTS: Symptoms of PTSD, both intrusion (i.e., trouble falling asleep, strong waves of feelings about the abuse) and avoidance (i.e., trying not to think or talk about the abuse, staying away from reminders of the abuse) were significantly related to severity of abuse, regardless of ethnicity. Childhood physical abuse was related to higher intrusion scores, while childhood sexual abuse was associated with higher avoidance scores.

IMPLICATIONS: Clinicians should ask all abused women about dreams, flashbacks, or terror attacks and assess for further symptoms of PTSD.

Silva C et al: Symptoms of post-traumatic stress disorder in abused women in a primary care setting, *J Womens Health* 6:543, 1997.

Attributions. Attributions are the reasoning processes people use to explain events. Attributions affect how people feel about their behavior and interpret life events. It is often said that survivors of violence tend to blame themselves, but research shows that only about 20% of battered women do so. Some believe that self-blaming attributions may be adaptive for survivors of violence as a way of maintaining control over their lives. Others think that self-blame may contribute to long-term depression. To date, research has not resolved this issue for battered women or for other survivors of family violence. There is insufficient evidence to assume that self-blame is either widespread among survivors or always pathological. Nurses who use the empowerment model when working with these patients believe it will help patients identify their attributions and explore the effect on their feelings and relationships .

Problem-solving techniques. Studies have found that battered women have trouble with problem solving. School problems have also been reported in abused children. In contrast, a variety of approaches are used by battered women that suggest appropriate decision making. Undoubtedly, some battered women, children, and elders are so frequently and severely beaten and controlled that their ability to solve problems is compromised.

Extreme difficulty in problem solving could be explained by posttraumatic stress disorder, with its symptoms of memory impairment and difficulty concentrating (see Citing the Evidence above). Problem-solving difficulties noted in widows and divorcees have been explained as normal responses to loss. Such problems could also be explained as one of the cognitive aspects of depression.

Psychological Responses to Battering. More work has been done to explore psychological responses to abuse in battered women than in either child abuse or elder abuse. Most of our knowledge about the emotional responses to incest describes delayed reactions rather than immediate ones. In addition, the question of "false memories" has complicated the diagnosis and treatment process (see Critical Thinking about Contemporary Issues). Psychological responses studied most often include the cognitive responses of attribution and problem solving and the emotional responses of depression and lowered self-esteem.

Depression. Depression is common among battered women, adult survivors of incest, abused children, and survivors of other forms of violence. Depression is discussed in detail in Chapter 20.

In summary, responses to family violence can be interpreted either as symptoms of pathology or as a way in which normal people respond to incredible physical and emotional trauma and yet survive. Research regarding this latter approach is beginning to document survivor mechanisms and a recovery process from abuse.

Preventive Nursing Interventions

Preventing family violence requires the use of primary prevention strategies of changing norms and values, preventive education with a variety of populations, and secondary prevention strategies of effective treatment.

Primary Prevention. Primary prevention is an activity that stops a problem before it occurs. Changing society's acceptance of violence and abuse is an important first step in prevention. Effective primary prevention includes eliminating cultural norms and values that accept and glamorize violence. This can begin by limiting the amount of violence permitted on television and in other media. The prevalence of violence on television plays a role in creating a social climate that says violence is exciting and appropriate. The average child watches television 20 hours a week. It has been estimated that American children observe 18,000 killings before they graduate from high school. Video and computer games are also popular with children, and there is a great deal of concern about the violence in these games.

A related area of primary prevention is the elimination of pornography, especially violent pornography, which has been associated with sexual violence. However, the rate of subscription to even a mild form of pornography such as *Playboy* magazine has been positively correlated with state rape rates.

Primary prevention of abuse also includes strengthening individuals and families so they can cope more effectively with stress. Nurses can conduct programs in the schools, workplace, or community. Strategies such as nurse-developed educational programs in high school parenting classes or childbirth education classes can be used to prepare families for the stress of child rearing. Topics could include normal child development and expectations, basic skills of infant care, and means of disciplining children that do not involve physical punishment. Additional educational strategies include teaching family members that conflict resolution does not always mean one party wins while the other loses and that they should respect individual differences among family members.

Nurses can be involved in teaching family life and sex education courses in elementary and middle schools. Child sexual abuse can be prevented or detected when children are taught about inappropriate sexual contact and what they should do if it occurs. Middle school students need information about how to have relationships in which jealousy is not viewed as a sign of love and domination of one partner over the other is not expected.

Family violence prevention also includes anticipatory guidance while working with families. For example, respite care is needed for families with chronically ill or incapacitated members, including the elderly and children. Planning in advance for relief from responsibility will prevent strained relationships and potential violence or abuse. Families also need to anticipate the difficult developmental stages of children. Parents need to know that infants are not intentionally frustrating to parents, that toddlers' obstinacy is necessary for independence in later childhood, and that bed-wetting is a signal for increased positive attention, not punishment.

A society must develop programs and policies that support families and reduce stresses and inequities. This includes adequate and appropriate day care for children and incapacitated elders, equity in salary and wages to make women less financially dependent, public education that ensures an adequate foundation for full employment of all, and sufficient financing of prevention and treatment programs.

> *Go to a computer store and search for the most popular games. Evaluate them for level of violence, sexual roles, and issues related to power and control.*

Secondary Prevention. Secondary prevention of family violence is aimed at its cyclic nature. Children raised in violent, noncaring homes are more likely to become spouse and child abusers. Therefore, one of the most effective methods of preventing violence and abuse in future generations is to stop current abuse.

Even when the violence has ended, those affected will need help. The children of battered women and siblings of abused children have witnessed violence and need help to counteract that learning. Often it is believed that abused children are "out of the woods" when they have been removed from the home or the family is no longer violent. Even if there are no identifiable long-term effects, there may have been trauma encapsulation, which may not be evident until many years afterward. In addition, these children may grow up believing that family members are normally violent to each other. Conscious resolve alone may not overcome this.

Secondary prevention also involves identification of families at risk or those who are beginning to use violence. Table 41-3 lists indicators of actual or potential abuse. These can be used for nursing assessment. Other early indicators of families at risk include violence in the family of origin of either partner, communication problems, and excessive family stress such as an unplanned pregnancy, unemployment, or inadequate family resources.

Pregnancy is an ideal time to identify women at risk to become battered or those in the early stages of an abusive relationship. This is also the best time to identify the infant's risk for abuse. Pregnancy is when healthy women are most often seen in the health-care system. A comprehensive assessment should include information about relationships and child-rearing beliefs and practices. When the nurse hears an indication of risk, immediate nursing intervention is required. Taking the time to explore the risk factors, discuss perceptions and attitudes, and brainstorm with the patient about possible alternatives is time well spent.

Table **41-3**

Indicators of Actual or Potential Abuse

NURSING HISTORY
Primary Reason for Contact

Vague information about cause of problem
Discrepancy between physical findings and description of cause
Minimizing injuries
Inappropriate delay between time of injury and treatment
Inappropriate family reactions (such as lack of concern, overconcern, threatening demeanor)

Information from Family Genogram

Family violence in history (child, spouse, elder)
History of violence outside of home
Incarcerations
Violent deaths in extended family
Alcoholism/drug abuse in family history

Health History

History of traumatic injuries
Spontaneous abortions
Psychiatric hospitalizations
History of depression
Substance abuse

Sexual History

Prior sexual abuse
Use of force in sexual activities
Venereal disease
Child with sexual knowledge beyond that appropriate for age
Promiscuity

Personal/Social History

Unwanted or unplanned pregnancy
Adolescent pregnancy
Social isolation (difficulty naming people available for help in a crisis)
Lack of contact with extended family
Unrealistic expectations of relationships or age-appropriate behavior
Extreme jealousy by spouse
Rigid traditional sex-role beliefs
Verbal aggression
Belief in use of physical punishment
Difficulties in school
Truancy, running away

Psychological History

Feelings of helplessness/hopelessness
Feeling trapped
Difficulty making plans for future
Tearfulness
Chronic fatigue, apathy
Suicide attempts

Financial History

Poverty
Finances rigidly controlled by one family member
Unwillingness to spend money on health care or adequate nutrition
Complaints about spending money on family members
Unemployment
Use of elders' finances for other family members

Family Beliefs/Values

Belief in importance of physical discipline
Autocratic decision making
Intolerance of differing views among members
Mistrust of outsiders

Family Relations

Lack of visible affection or nurturing between family members
Extreme dependency between family members
Autonomy discouraged
Numerous arguments
Temporary separations
Dissatisfaction with family members
Lack of enjoyable family activities
Extramarital affairs
Role rigidity (inability of members to assume nontraditional roles)

PHYSICAL EXAMINATION
General Appearance

Fearful, anxious, hyperactive, or hypoactive
Poor hygiene, careless grooming
Inappropriate dress
Increased anxiety in presence of abuser
Looking to abuser for answers to questions
Inappropriate or anxious nonverbal behavior (such as giggling at serious questions or questions related to abuse)
Flinching when touched

Vital Statistics

Overweight or underweight
Hypertension

Skin

Bruises, welts, edema
Presence of scars and indications of injuries in various stages of healing
Cigarette burns

Head

Bald patches on scalp from pulling hair
Subdural hematoma

Eyes

Subconjunctival hemorrhage
Swelling
Black eyes

Ears

Hearing loss from prior injury or untreated infections

Mouth

Bruising
Lacerations
Untreated dental caries
Venereal infection

Abdomen

Intraabdominal injuries
Abdominal injuries during pregnancy

Table **41-3**

Indicators of Actual or Potential Abuse—cont'd

Extremities
Bruising to forearms from attempts to protect self from blows
Broken arms
Radiological indications of previous fractures

Neurological
Developmental delays
Difficulty with speech or swallowing
Hyperactive reflex response

Genital/Urinary
Genital lacerations or bruising
Urinary tract infections
Sexually transmitted disease

Rectal
Rectal bruising
Bleeding
Edema
Tenderness
Poor sphincter tone

NURSING OBSERVATIONS
General Observations
Observations that differ significantly from history
Family members inadequately clothed or groomed

Home Environment
Inadequate heating
Inappropriate sleeping arrangements
Total household disorganization
Inadequate food
Spoiled food not discarded

Family Communication Pattern
One parent answers all questions
Looking for approval of other family members before answering questions
Members continually interrupt each other
Negative nonverbal behavior in other members when one member speaking
Members do not listen to each other
Taboo topics (family secrets)

Emotional Climate
Tense, secretive atmosphere
Unhappiness
Lack of affection
Apparent fear of other family members
Verbal arguing

High rates of family violence and low rates of detection, reporting, and therapeutic intervention by health-care professionals are well documented. The lack of educational content on child, spouse, and elder abuse in professional training programs for physicians, nurses, psychologists, social workers, and dentists underscores the need for educators to expand curricula on family violence and for legislators to examine the ineffectiveness of current mandatory reporting laws (Limandri & Tilden, 1996; Glass & Campbell, 1998).

SPECIAL POPULATIONS
Child Abuse

The earliest form of family violence recognized in the health professional literature was physical abuse to children. Although violence to children was identified as a social problem in the nineteenth century, it was not until the 1940s that it became a medical problem, even a unique "syndrome." By the end of the 1960s, every state had enacted legislation mandating the report of suspected child abuse and neglect. Under current laws, nurses and any other professionals are required to report suspected incidents of child and elder abuse and domestic violence (Freed & Drake, 1999).

There are many forms of child abuse including physical abuse or battering, emotional abuse, sexual abuse, and neglect. Children who witness family violence and abuse are themselves victimized (Mohr, 1999). Although they are often overlooked, they can be symptomatic as a result of this abuse (Table 41-4). Much is still unknown about the causes, treatment, or prevention of child abuse. In addition, research has failed to identify any factors that are present in all abusing and absent in all nonabusing parents.

Sexual Abuse of Children and Adolescents. Sexual abuse is the involvement of children and adolescents in sexual activities they do not fully comprehend and to which they do not freely consent. Physical problems related to sexual abuse include the following:

- Venereal disease or infection
- Vaginal or rectal bleeding, itching, or soreness
- Recurrent urinary tract infections
- Pregnancy

Emotional changes include the following:

- Sexual acting-out
- Physical aggression
- Excessive masturbation
- Withdrawal
- Low self-esteem
- Drop in school performance
- Disturbed sleep

The long-term effects of sexual abuse as a child include (Creedy et al, 1998; Painter & Howell, 1999) the following:

- Sexual problems
- Difficulty trusting others
- Anxiety and panic attacks
- Depression
- Substance abuse

Finally, sexually abused children experience more emotional distress and long-term effects when the perpetrator is

Table **41-4**

Effects of Witnessing Violence in Childhood			
Infant	Preschool	School-age	Adolescent
Disrupted attachment needs	Feeling that world is not safe or stable	Greater willingness to use violence	Feelings of rage, shame, betrayal
Disrupted routines (sleeping, eating)	Yelling, irritability, hiding, stuttering; signs of terror	Holding self responsible for violence at home	School truancy, early sexual activity, substance abuse, delinquency
Risk of physical injury	Many somatic complaints and regressive behaviors	Shame and embarrassment of the family secret	Unresponsiveness
Eating and sleeping problems in 50%	Anxious attachment behaviors: whining, crying, clinging	Distracted and inattentive, labile, and hypervigilant	Little memory of childhood
Decreased responsiveness to adults, increased crying	Increased separation and stranger anxiety	Limited range of emotional responses	Defensiveness
	Insomnia, sleepwalking, nightmares, bed-wetting	Psychosomatic complaints	Short attention span
		Uncooperative, suspicious, guarded behavior	

Modified from Rhea MH: The silent victims of domestic violence: who will speak?, *JCAPN* 9:7, 1996.

a person who was known and trusted by them, and thus their trust was violated (Johnson & Cheffer, 1996).

Nursing Assessment. Nursing assessment of actual or potential child abuse begins with a thorough history and physical examination. Gathering a history of child abuse can be a stressful experience for both the nurse and the family. It is essential for the nurse to examine personal values and past experiences to maintain a therapeutic and nonjudgmental clinical approach.

It is important to use an honest, open approach that does not punish or shame either the child or the parent. Most abusive parents are genuinely embarrassed about their behavior and would like help in developing alternative approaches to discipline. This knowledge can be used by the nurse to establish an environment that will facilitate honesty and sharing. The setting for the interview must be quiet, private, and uninterrupted.

In general, the child and the adults should be separated for the initial interview. However, this decision depends on the child's age and other factors. The nurse should honestly state the purpose of the interview and the type of questions being asked, and describe the subsequent physical examination. The approach must be calm and supportive because both the child and the family will be uneasy.

The interview with the parent can begin with a discussion of the problem that first brought the child to a healthcare facility. During this discussion the nurse should pay particular attention to the parent's understanding of the problem, discrepancies in the stories, and the parent's emotional responses. The interview can then be expanded to discussions of how the parent "disciplines" or spanks the child. The initial interview is not the time to confront a suspected abuser directly because measures must be taken to document and report the abuse in a way that will ensure the child's safety.

Nursing Interventions. When child abuse is suspected, the nurse must report it to protective services. An investigation by the state protective service agency is legally mandated and also reinforces to the family the seriousness of the problem. When protective services are involved, the nurse should explain to the family precisely what will happen in an investigation and the amount of time involved. The nurse should maintain frequent contact with the assigned worker to ensure a comprehensive, consistent approach. Nurses who work with violent families need to know exactly how protective services in their community operate. Ongoing professional relationships with colleagues at the agency will enable the nurse to remain informed about policies and reporting protocols and ensure successful coordination and continuity.

Intimate Partner Violence

The term "intimate partner violence" refers to a pattern of assaultive and coercive behaviors, including physical, sexual, and psychological abuse and violence, that adults or adolescents use against their intimate partners. "Intimate partnerships" include current or former dating, married, cohabiting relationships of heterosexuals, lesbian women, or gay men. It is purposeful behavior, directed at achieving compliance from, or control over, the targeted person (Ganley, 1995). The violence is part of a system of coercive control that may also include financial coercion, threats against children and other family members, and destruction of property.

Abuse of female partners is the most widespread form of family violence. One in three adult women experience at least one physical assault by a partner during adulthood, and at least one in six wives is hit by a husband sometime during their relationship. **Sexual abuse**, or marital rape, is part of the violence against female partners in almost half the cases. Although women do hit men, female violence is much more likely to be in self-defense. It seldom takes the intentional repeated, serious, and controlling form characteristic of abuse against female partners.

One of the most frightening realities of abuse of female partners is the potential for murder. The majority of female homicide victims in the United States are killed by a husband, lover, or ex-husband or ex-lover. The majority of these murders are preceded by abuse. There is evidence that a battered woman is in most danger of homicide when she leaves her abusive partner or makes it clear to him that she is ending the relationship. Some battered women kill their spouses. Many of the risk factors are similar. They include having a handgun in the house, a history of suicide threats or attempts in either partner, battering during pregnancy, sexual abuse, substance abuse, and extreme jealousy and controlling behavior (Oriel & Fleming, 1998). A frequent statement heard by potentially murderous abusers is, "If I can't have you, no one can."

Discuss social reaction to wife abuse in relation to the Lorena Bobbitt and O.J. Simpson trials.

Nursing Assessment. It has been documented that the most prevalent cause of trauma in women treated in emergency rooms is abuse by an intimate partner (Dearwater et al, 1998). It is also a common cause of female visits to psychiatric emergency departments and other mental health treatment centers. Thus a nursing assessment for all forms of violence is critical. Assessment for intimate partner violence should be mandatory in mental health settings, as well as in emergency rooms, prenatal settings, and primary care facilities (Feldhaus et al, 1997; Gondolf, 1998; Spielvogel & Floyd, 1997).

When there are no obvious injuries, assessment for abuse is best included with the history about the patient's primary intimate attachment relationship. Answers to general questions on the quality of that relationship should be assessed for feelings of being controlled or needing to control. A relationship characterized by excessive jealousy (of possessions, children, jobs, friends, and other family members, as well as potential sexual partners) is more likely to be violent.

The patient can be asked about how the couple solves conflicts; one partner needing to have the final say or frequent and forceful verbal aggression also can be considered risk factors. Finally, the patient should be asked whether arguments ever involve "pushing or shoving." Questions about minor violence within a couple relationship help to establish the unfortunate normalcy of wife abuse and to lessen the stigma of disclosure. If the patient hesitates, looks away, displays other uncomfortable nonverbal behavior, or reveals risk factors for abuse, she or he can be asked again later in the interview about physical violence.

If abuse is revealed, the nurse's first response is critical. It is important that an abused woman realize that she is not alone; important affirmation can be given with a statement about the frequency of abuse. The extent and types of the abuse must be identified and described in the record. Careful documentation using a body map identifying the locations of bruises, contusions, or cuts is necessary for potential legal actions, which are often child custody suits as well as criminal actions related to the violence.

The woman's responses to the violence are also a critical area for mental health assessment. It is important to interpret these responses to the woman as normal within the circumstances. Signs of posttraumatic stress disorder, depression, and low self-esteem must be assessed and recorded. Attribution regarding the abuse is also important. The nurse must carefully assess the woman's beliefs regarding the abuse and responsibility for the abuse. Because many abusive male partners find an excuse for the violence, the woman may be unnecessarily accepting the blame for his actions.

If the patient is an abuser, mental state is also important and the potential for further violence must be assessed carefully. The safety of the abused partner is a concern, as is treatment for the abuser. Consultation with legal advisors about the nurse's duty to warn may be needed (see Chapter 10).

Nursing Interventions. Most communities have treatment programs for abusive men. They have been found to be most effective when the court has ordered treatment, with punishment for noncompliance. Severely abusive men seldom admit they have a problem and often need to be mandated to enter and remain in treatment. The nurse needs to confront the violence and clarify that the responsibility lies with the abuser. A combination of strategies may be needed to get the abuser into treatment if he is not involved with the court.

The type of referral chosen is extremely important. Long-lasting change is more likely if the treatment combines behavioral therapy around anger control with a program designed to change attitudes toward women. Traditional marriage therapy or couple counseling as the only treatment is potentially dangerous to the woman because of the unequal power in the relationship and the possibility of retaliatory violence (Hattendorf & Tollerud, 1997).

Several themes expressed by women who have been in abusive relationships with men have been identified (Farrell, 1996; Weingourt, 1996; Draucker & Madsen, 1999). These themes, outlined in Table 41-5, can help the nurse in assessing and intervening with women who have been in abusive relationships.

To empower an abused woman, one must first make sure she has the information she needs. This includes knowledge of the related state and local laws and ordinances. She also needs to be aware of the local battered women's shelters available for advice, support, and group participation, even if she does not intend to enter the shelter at present.

Mutual goal setting is particularly important when working with abused women. Nurses can be frustrated if they impose their goals on the women, who may not be ready for drastic action. Ideally they will have an established relationship during which the nurse and patient can work through the normal denial and minimization that takes place when the primary attachment relationship is threatened. The nurse and patient can then consider all the options the woman has thought about and devise others. Dealing with an abusive situation is a recovery process that takes time and ongoing support. The nurse can help the patient mobilize natural, social, and professional support so that both her economic and emotional needs are addressed (see Citing the Evidence on Community-Based Advocacy for Abused Women).

Table **41-5**

Themes of Women Who Have Been in Abusive Relationships

THEMES OF DYSFUNCTION WHILE IN THE RELATIONSHIP

- **Lack of relational authenticity:** The women never felt emotionally real, never established relationships with themselves as individuals, and were uncertain about their own identities. This increased their perceived threat of rejection and their efforts to please the abuser in order to maintain the relationship. Leaving the abusive relationship was seen as a threat to one's personal identity.
- **Immobility:** Abuse permeated every aspect of the life of women in the study. Living in constant fear for their own well-being and that of their children created an appearance to outsiders that they were scattered, incapable, and indecisive. This fear created a barrier to others that increased their sense of isolation and decreased their ability to seek help.
- **Emptiness:** These women experienced multiple losses in their lives, including problems maintaining relationships with others, self-esteem, pride, a sense of control, and a sense of accomplishment. They eventually escaped the pain of abuse by having no feelings, not thinking, just constantly "doing" an intense schedule of the routines of daily living. This created a numbing effect that allowed them to continue to the next day.
- **Disconnection:** The women's sense of sexuality was adversely affected. They equated sex with love, so being sexually active was the only way they felt connected to another person. They lacked support from extended family members, who disapproved of the relationship. The abuse created physical illnesses because of the stress of the relationship. Many had indirect self-destructive behaviors (such as alcoholism and eating disorders), and some had suicidal or homicidal ideation as a means of escaping the abuse.

THEMES OF HEALING WHILE RECOVERING

- **Flexibility:** Women reported a readiness to alter the course of their lives in response to changing conditions and the acquiring of new behaviors. This included an acknowledgment of the past, resiliency with everyday events, increased self-awareness, and establishment of appropriate boundaries.
- **Awakening:** A turning point occurred within each woman when she realized there were choices and meaning in her life. This resulted in a sense of inner strength, hope, spirituality, and inner peace.
- **Relationship:** Women described an integration of all aspects of self, a sense of trust and connectedness between self and others, a feeling of harmony and contentment, and a linkage between internal and external events.
- **Empowerment:** Women related a new ability to make choices in their lives, which resulted in a valuing of the self, self-determination, and a sense of accomplishment.

Citing the Evidence on

Community-Based Advocacy for Abused Women

BACKGROUND: An intensive community-based advocacy intervention was designed and evaluated by randomly assigning 278 battered women to an experimental or control condition. The 10-week postshelter intervention involved providing trained advocates to work 1-on-1 with women, helping generate and access the community resources they needed to reduce their risk of future violence from their abusive partners.

RESULTS: Women who worked with advocates experienced less violence over time, reported higher quality of life and social support, and had less difficulty obtaining community resources. More than twice as many women receiving advocacy services experienced no violence across the 2 years postintervention compared with women who did not receive such services.

IMPLICATIONS: Innovative community advocacy programs have the potential for helping women with abusive partners. They can be cost-effective alternatives to more formal service options.

Sullivan C, Bybee D: Reducing violence using community-based advocacy for women with abusive partners, *J Consult Clin Psychol* 67:43, 1999.

Evaluation of nursing interventions is based on mutual goals, not on a preconceived notion of what a battered woman should do. Because most abused women eventually leave a seriously violent situation or end the violence in some other way and seek help when the violence becomes severe, the nurse can be optimistic about the eventual outcome. Interventions may not result in an immediately happy ending, but they can plant the seeds of empowerment that facilitate the woman's recovery process.

Elder Abuse

Estimates of the numbers of elderly people abused vary widely. Much of the abuse is committed by spouses; thus spouse abuse and **elder abuse** are often overlapping categories. Research has not found abused elders to be more functionally impaired than nonabused elders. Rather than the condition of the elder, characteristics of the abuser, such as mental and emotional problems including substance abuse, create a family situation at risk for elder abuse (Goldstein, 1995).

Nursing Assessment. It is important to assess for elder abuse in families where an emotionally ill person is financially dependent on aging parents. Family interviews should not focus exclusively on the patient but should also assess the interactions among family members for indications of verbal and physical aggression.

It is difficult for abused elders to admit being physically hurt by a child, spouse, or caregiver. Gentle inquiry about the family's usual approach to resolving interpersonal difficulties is useful. At least part of this assessment must take place with the elder alone. An elder may be reluctant to disclose abuse because of fear of being abandoned to a nursing home or a life of total isolation. Only by establishing a trusting relationship over time or using an already established relationship with someone else can the nurse completely explore the abusive situation.

Assessment is even more difficult when the elder is mentally or emotionally impaired. In those cases, physical assessment and careful attention to nonverbal behavior are critical. Bruises to the upper arms from shaking are especially common in elder abuse. Although bruises from abuse are difficult to differentiate from those normal in aging, bilateral upper outer arm bruises are definitive. Lacerations, especially to the face, are not usually caused by falls and should be regarded with suspicion. Vaginal lacerations or bruises and twisting bone fractures are particularly indicative of abuse. Signs of neglect are more common than those of physical abuse. Determining whether the neglect is intentional is the key to planning a nursing course of action.

Whenever a dependent elderly person is being cared for by another, their interaction will give important clues about the relationship. Flinching or shrinking away by the elder and rough physical treatment accompanied by verbal denigration by the caretaker are possible indicators of abuse. As with all types of family violence, the nurse needs to analyze the data from the history, physical examination, and direct observations to make an assessment of abuse. The decision to report is difficult, especially if it appears likely that the outcome will be a nursing home placement unwanted by the elder. However, most states have laws that require nurses to report suspected elder abuse.

> *You are providing home care services to an elderly person who shows evidence of physical abuse. The patient's caregiver handles her roughly and is impatient with her. The patient denies that she is unhappy or abused. Describe your response to this situation. What is your obligation to report your suspicions?*

Nursing Interventions. When the nurse must report elder abuse, it is usually less damaging to the therapeutic relationship to inform the family first. Deciding whether to discuss reporting beforehand is influenced by the likelihood of the abusing family member disappearing and the severity of the abuse. If the abuse is less severe or mainly a neglectful or caretaker stress situation, discussing the intent to report first makes the action seem less a condemnation, allows protective services to be perceived as a helping agency rather than a punitive one, and increases the chances that the nurse will be seen as a continuing source of help. Respite care or other stress relievers may be the key interventions for an overburdened caretaker.

In other cases the primary intervention may be therapeutic assistance for the abusers. This may include counseling, therapy for mental disorders, or substance abuse treatment. The success of various interventions for elder abuse is not yet known because research into this issue is scant. However, one should assume that the treatment will need to involve specific components aimed at the violence as well as at whatever other problems are involved.

RAPE AND SEXUAL ASSAULT

Rape and sexual assault are concerns for individuals, families, and the community. Sexual assaults against women and children (the most common survivors) result in physical trauma, psychic and spiritual disruptions, and deterioration of social relationships. In addition, fear of rape and sexual assault has major effects on women as they restrict their activities in attempts to ensure their safety. Survivors of sexual assaults include women and men of all ages, social classes, races, and occupations. Sexual assault disrupts every aspect of the survivor's life, including social activities, interpersonal relationships, employment, and career. Although males may be sexually assaulted and women may be sexual offenders, in this section the survivor is referred to as "she" and the offender as "he." It must be recognized, however, that men and young boys are also victimized and that assessment must not be limited to women and girls.

> *How would you respond to a roommate who returned from a date tearful and saying that her boyfriend forced her to have sex even though she refused? Would it make any difference if she had been sexually active with him in the past? Why or why not?*

Definition of Sexual Assault

Sexual assault is the forced perpetration of an act of sexual contact with another person without consent. Lack of consent could be related to the victim's cognitive or personality development, feelings of fear or coercion, or the offender's physical or verbal threats. Sexual assault is not a sexual act but is instead motivated by a desire to humiliate, defile, and dominate the victim. It has occurred for centuries but is now recognized as a social and public health problem.

A sexual assault occurs once every 6.4 minutes in the United States. One in every six women will be raped in her lifetime. Although a woman is four times more likely to be assaulted by someone she knows than by someone she does not know, the majority of these crimes go unreported even though rape is a felony.

Sexual consent can be thought of as a continuum, as seen in Box 41-2. This continuum demonstrates degrees of coercion, including bribery, taking advantage of one's position of power or trust in a relationship, or the victim's inability to consent freely.

Marital Rape

Marital rape is legally recognized in most states. It is often reported along with physical abuse. Many husbands of abused women believe it is their right to have sex whenever they want. Victims of marital rape describe forced vaginal intercourse; anal intercourse; being hit, burned, or kicked during sex; having objects inserted into their vagina and anus; or being forced to perform sexual acts with animals or while their children were present. Many of these women are threatened

Box **41-2**

Sexual Behavior: The Force Continuum

1. **Freely consenting.** Partners with equal power mutually choosing sexual activity. Equal power means each partner has equal status, knowledge, and ability to consent. This includes one partner agreeing to engage in sexual activity, even if not aroused, as an expression of love and caring for the other person.
2. **Economic partnership.** One person agrees to sexual activity as part of an economic agreement. The types of sexual behavior permitted are mutually determined as part of the economic agreement.
3. **Seduction.** One party attempts to persuade the other to engage in sexual activities.
4. **Psychic rape.** Assault to another person's dignity and self-respect, such as verbal abuse, street harassment, or the portrayal of violence or pornography in the media.
5. **Bribery or coercion.** The use of emotional or psychological force to persuade the other to take part in sexual activities. This includes situations of unequal power, especially when one person is in a position of authority.
6. **Acquaintance rape.** Sexual assault occurring when one party abuses the trust of a relationship and forces the other into sexual activities.
7. **Fear rape.** When one party engages in sexual activities out of fear of potential violence if she resists.
8. **Violent rape.** When violence is threatened or occurs. This includes forced sexual activity between spouses, acquaintances, or strangers.

Box **41-3**

Hotline Numbers for Survivors of Abuse Violence

National Center for Victims of Crime: 1-800-FYI CALL (394-2255)
Provides immediate referrals to the closet, most appropriate services in the victim's community (includes sexual assault).
National Domestic Violence Hotline: 1-800-799-7233 (TDD: 1-800-787-3224)
Provides crisis intervention, information, and referrals.
National Organization for Victim Assistance (NOVA): 1-800-TRY-NOVA (879-6682)
Provides advocacy, information, and referrals for crime victims (including sexual assault).

with weapons or beaten if they refuse to take part in these activities. Marital rape is especially devastating for the survivor who often must continue to interact with the rapist because of her dependence on him. In addition, many survivors do not seek health care or the support of family members or friends because of embarrassment or humiliation.

Nursing Care of the Sexual Assault Survivor

Nursing Assessment. The initial assessment is an important phase of the treatment of rape and sexual assault survivors. Although most nurses would quickly recognize the woman brought to the emergency department by the police after an attack by a stranger, many survivors of sexual assault are not so easily identified. Therefore, all nursing assessments must include questions to determine current or past sexual abuse. Because people have different definitions of rape, the assessment question must be broadly stated, such as "Has anyone ever forced you into sex that you did not wish to participate in?" This question may uncover other types of sexual trauma such as incest, date rape, or childhood sexual abuse. If the answer is yes, it can be gently followed with broad questions, such as "Can you tell me more about it?" or "How often has it happened?" Often the response may be hesitation, questioning, or an embarrassed

laugh. When this occurs, the nurse can increase the patient's comfort by explaining that the question is routine because sexual assault is common.

Nursing Interventions. When it is determined that abuse has occurred, it cannot be ignored. Disclosing sexual abuse is an indication of trust. If nurses immediately refer the patient elsewhere, they communicate that the problem is too distasteful or delicate to handle or that there are serious psychological implications. Therefore, an immediate response of nonjudgmental listening and psychological support is essential (Draucker, 1999). In addition, if a recent attack is disclosed, physical evidence will be needed. Evidence collection is an appropriate nursing responsibility and requires special training (Petter & Whitehill, 1998). Later interventions may include referrals to survivors' groups, shelters for battered women, or legal services. The organizations listed in Box 41-3 may be useful when helping survivors of abuse and violence organize their resources.

People respond to sexual assault differently depending on their past experiences, personal characteristics, and the amount and type of support received from significant others, health-care providers, and the criminal justice system. The acute stage, immediately after the attack, is characterized by extreme confusion, fear, disorganization, and restlessness. However, some survivors may mask these feelings and appear to be outwardly calm or subdued.

The second phase involves the long-term process of reorganization. It generally begins several weeks after the attack. This phase may include intrusive memories of the traumatic event during the day and while asleep, fears, or phobias such as extreme fears of being alone, being in a crowd, or traveling. The survivor often has a sense of living in a dangerous, unpredictable world and may become preoccupied with feelings of victimization and vulnerability. She may encounter difficulties in sexual relationships or her ability to relate comfortably to men. Some survivors develop secondary phobic reactions to people, places, or situations that remind them of the attack.

NURSING TREATMENT PLAN *Summary* *Survivors of Abuse and Violence*

NURSING DIAGNOSIS: Rape trauma syndrome
EXPECTED OUTCOME: The patient will resume his or her usual lifestyle and social relationships.

SHORT-TERM GOAL	INTERVENTION	RATIONALE
The patient will express feelings related to the assault, including guilt, fear, and vulnerability.	Allow patient to discuss feelings regarding assault. Communicate knowledge and understanding of emotional responses to sexual assault to help in identification of feelings. Provide anticipatory guidance regarding common physical, psychological, and social responses.	Women often experience various feelings, including guilt, shame, anger, and embarrassment. It is necessary to identify and express these feelings to develop coping skills. Knowing what to expect reassures the patient that her reactions are normal and can be managed.
The patient will identify supportive people to help in dealing with this crisis.	Explore relationships with significant others. Encourage the patient to discuss the situation with trusted and supportive people.	According to the principles of crisis intervention, it is important for the person in crisis to identify and use a social support system.
The patient will seek medical care for physical problems related to the assault.	Advise patient of the potential for sexually transmitted diseases or pregnancy. Help in identifying a medical care provider. Offer to accompany to the medical examination.	Early identification of physical problems provides the patient with the maximum number of treatment choices. Many women relive the assault during a gynecological examination. Support from a trusted person can be helpful.
The patient will be actively involved in mobilizing support systems.	Support decision making and active problem solving. Provide written information about community services and encourage use of them. Plan for a follow-up phone contact within a few days.	Active involvement in seeking resources gives the patient a sense of control over life, countering the helplessness related to the assault.

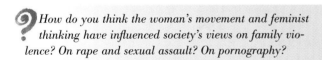
How do you think the woman's movement and feminist thinking have influenced society's views on family violence? On rape and sexual assault? On pornography?

Coping strategies may include changing one's phone number or residence, talking with friends or family, or taking classes in self-defense. Nursing actions to help the survivor of sexual assault include active listening, empathic responses, active concern and caring, assistance in problem solving, and referral to sexual assault crisis centers. A sample Nursing Treatment Plan for survivors of sexual assault is presented above.

Summary

1. Family violence refers to a range of behaviors occurring between family members and includes physical and emotional abuse of children, child neglect, intimate partner violence, marital rape, and elder abuse. Characteristics of violent families include multigenerational transmission, social isolation, abuse of power, and substance abuse.

2. Many nurses have a negative response to survivors of violence. It is important to identify and overcome these attitudes.

3. Physical responses to battering include a characteristic pattern of injuries and the occurrence of a variety of stress-related symptoms. Behavioral responses to battering include reluctance to leave the violent situation. Psychological responses to violence include attributions, problem-solving techniques, and depression.

4. Nursing actions related to the prevention of family violence include strategies to change norms and values, preventive education, and secondary prevention strategies of effective treatment.

5. Nursing interventions related to special populations including children, intimate partners, and the elderly are presented.

6. Nursing care of survivors of sexual assault include nonjudgmental listening, psychological support, evidence collection, and mobilization of community support such as shelters for battered women, survivor's groups, and legal services.

Competent Caring A Clinical Exemplar of a Psychiatric Nurse

PAT ENGDAHL, RN, C

When thinking about how I made a difference in a patient's life, I remembered an experience I had with a young woman just over 30 years of age who was admitted to the unit in a state of extreme panic, hardly able to process a simple request such as "I need you to please move away from the door." She told me this later, saying her first memories of being on our floor included a voice saying the above words "in the kindest, firmest, most caring tones" she had ever heard—and she felt safe. She said she didn't want to move away from the locked door, but she did it anyway and she said, "I think it was your voice."

We worked very hard together. She was a survivor of childhood sexual and physical abuse and, as often happens, married to a man who also abused her. She talked; I listened. She said she had shed enough tears and wasn't going to cry anymore. I replied she needed to "cry a river" for the therapeutic process to begin. We role-played. We practiced handling verbal abuse and daring to express anger—the latter frightened her more than the former. But she was not able to deal with issues related to her abusive husband and her angry feelings of victimization in the marriage.

The night before her discharge she began to discuss these feelings, as they had suddenly risen to the surface during a group meeting. In this meeting a male patient had boasted that he never struck his wife except when he was drunk, and then he "only slapped her around a few times, not enough to send her to the hospital or such—nothing like that." When my patient heard this, she got up in a rage and ran out of the group. Several hours later, during our one-on-one, she was finally able to discuss the episode. She berated herself for being "gutless" and not being able to say something right then. She paced and questioned whether she really was ready to go home and said that maybe she wasn't as strong as she thought.

We continued exploring her feelings of childhood helplessness. She talked until her rage was spent, but she did not seem to reach closure in her thoughts or feelings. She was discharged the next morning before I came to work for my evening shift. However, in my mailbox, I found a powerful note in which, among other things, she simply wrote, "I was able to confront that male patient in group today. . . . I guess I was ready for discharge after all. Thanks." It was now my turn to become a little emotional as my eyes filled with tears and I whispered, "You're welcome, you'll never know how welcome."

Merlin Visit **MERLIN: www.mosby.com/MERLIN/Stuart** to find these additional materials and student activities.

- **Worksheets**
- **"Drug of the Month" Updates**
- **"Citing the Evidence" Updates**
- **Critical Thinking Activities and Exercises**
- **Annotated Suggested Readings**
- **Web Links**
- **More!**

Chapter Review Questions

1. Match each term in Column A with the correct definition in Column B.

Column A

_____ Attributions

_____ Sexual assault

_____ Multigenerational transmission

_____ Myth about abuse

_____ Paternalistic model of health care

_____ Psychological abuse

_____ The force continuum

_____ Intimate partner violence

Column B

A. Family violence is often perpetuated from grandparents, to parents, to children.

B. Others generally get what they deserve in life.

C. Advice and sympathy are given rather than respect for a patient's competence and experience.

D. Reasoning processes people use to explain why certain events happen.

E. An intervention that stops an action before it occurs.

F. A view of sexual behavior that ranges from free consent to violent rape.

G. The victim can learn to stop doing things that provoke the violence.

H. A pattern of coercive and assaultive behaviors toward a partner in an ongoing intimate relationship.

_____ Just world view   **I.** Forced act of sexual contact with another person without consent.

_____ Primary prevention   **J.** Instilling fear or isolating victim from family, friends, school, or work.

_____ **D.** Witnessing parental violence during childhood or adolescence is one of the strongest risk factors for becoming an abuser in adulthood.

_____ **E.** Abusive people and their victims often excuse the abuse by blaming alcohol, stress, or drugs.

2. Identify whether the following statements are true (T) or false (F).

_____ **A.** Many nurses have a negative response to survivors of violence.

_____ **B.** Children who only witness family violence are usually safe from its effects.

_____ **C.** Family violence is most prevalent among the lower class.

3. Provide short answers for the following questions.

A. Briefly describe the four characteristics of violent families.

B. Compare the paternalistic model with the empowerment model used by nurses to help battered women.

C. Each culture and society has a different attitude toward and tolerance of violence. Compare the United States with another country in this regard.

REFERENCES

Boutcher F, Gallop R: Psychiatric nurses' attitudes toward sexuality, sexual assault/rape, and incest, *Arch Psychiatr Nurs* 10:184, 1996.

Bremner JD et al: Neural mechanisms in dissociative amnesia for childhood abuse: relevance to the current controversy surrounding the "false memory syndrome," *Am J Psychiatry* 153:71, 1996.

Byrne C et al: The socioeconomic impact of interpersonal violence on women, *J Consult Clin Psychol* 67:362, 1999.

Creedy D et al: A framework for practice with women survivors of childhood sexual abuse, *Aust N Z J Mental Health Nurs* 7:67, 1998.

Dearwater S et al: Prevalence of intimate partner abuse in women treated at community hospital emergency departments, *JAMA* 280:433, 1998.

Divitto S: Empowerment through self-regulation: group approach for survivors of incest, *J Am Psychiatr Nurs Assoc* 4:77, 1998.

Draucker C: The psychotherapeutic needs of women who have been sexually assaulted, *Perspect Psychiatric Care* 35:18, 1999.

Draucker C, Madsen C: Women dwelling with violence, *Image* 31:327, 1999.

Farrell M: The sense of relationship in women who have encountered abuse, *J Am Psychiatr Nurs Assoc* 2:46, 1996.

Feldhaus K et al: Accuracy of 3 brief screening questions for detecting partner violence in the emergency department, *JAMA* 277:1357, 1997.

Freed P, Drake V: Mandatory reporting of abuse: practical, moral, and legal issues for psychiatric home healthcare nurses, *Issues Mental Health Nurs* 20:423, 1999.

Gallop R et al: The impact of childhood sexual abuse on the psychological well-being and practice of nurses, *Arch Psychiatr Nurs* 9:137, 1995.

Gallop R et al: A survey of psychiatric nurses regarding working with clients who have a history of sexual abuse, *J Am Psychiatr Nurs Assoc* 4:9, 1998.

Ganley A: Understanding domestic violence. In Warshaw C, Ganley A, editors: *Improving the health care response to domestic violence: a resource manual for health care providers.* San Francisco, 1995, Family Violence Prevention Fund.

Gilligan C: *In a different voice,* Cambridge, Mass, 1982, Harvard University Press.

Glass N, Campbell J: Mandatory reporting of intimate partner violence by health care professionals: a policy review, *Nurs Outlook* 46:279, 1998.

Goldstein MZ: Maltreatment of elderly persons, *Psychiatr Serv* 46:1219, 1995.

Gondolf E: *Assessing woman battering in mental health services,* Thousand Oaks, Calif, 1998, Sage.

Hattendorf J, Tollerud T: Domestic violence: counseling strategies that minimize the impact of secondary victimization, *Perspect Psychiatric Care* 33:14, 1997.

Hotaling GT, Sugerman D: An analysis of risk markers in husband to wife violence: the current state of knowledge, *Violence Vict* 1:101, 1986.

Johnson L, Cheffer ND: Child sexual abuse: a case of intrafamilial abuse, *J Am Psychiatr Nurs Assoc* 2:108, 1996.

Limandri BJ, Tilden VP: Nurses' reasoning in the assessment of family violence during pregnancy: effects on maternal complications and birth weight in adult and teenage women, *Image J Nurs Sch* 28:247, 1996.

Mohr W: Family violence: toward more precise and comprehensive knowing, *Issues Ment Health Nurs* 20:305, 1999.

Oriel K, Fleming M: Screening men for partner violence in a primary care setting, *J Fam Pract* 46:493, 1998.

Painter S, Howell C: Rage and women' sexuality after childhood sexual abuse: a phenomenological study, *Perspect Psychiatric Care* 35:5, 1999.

Petter L, Whitehill D: Management of female sexual assault, *Am Fam Physician* 1998.

Spielvogel A, Floyd A: Assessment of trauma in women psychiatric patients. In Harris M, Landis C, editors: *Sexual abuse in the lives of women diagnosed with serious mental illness.* Amsterdam, 1997, Harwood Academic Press.

U.S. Department of Health and Human Services: *Child maltreatment: reports from the states to the National Child Abuse and Neglect Data System,* Washington, DC, 2000, U.S. Government Printing Office.

Weingourt R: Connection and disconnection in abuse relationships, *Perspect Psychiatric Care* 32:15, 1996.

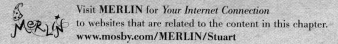

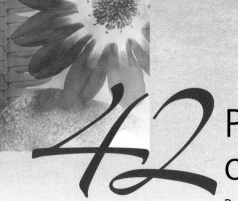

42 Psychological Care of the Patient with HIV/AIDS

Paula C. LaSalle

Arthur J. LaSalle

W̶hile we were fearing it, it came,
But came with less of fear
Because that fearing it so long
Had almost made it fair.
There is a fitting—dismay;
A fitting—a despair.
'Tis harder knowing it is due
Than knowing it is here.
The trying on the utmost,
The morning it is new,
Is terribler than wearing it
A whole existence through.

EMILY DICKINSON, "WHILE WE WERE FEARING IT, IT CAME"

HIV/AIDS is one of the most devastating global epidemics of the twentieth century. The human immunodeficiency virus (HIV) and the resulting acquired immunodeficiency syndrome (AIDS) include a variety of serious and debilitating disorders such as opportunistic infections resulting from a compromised immune system and significant co-occurring psychiatric illnesses. Care of patients with HIV/AIDS and their families, friends, and community involves the physical, psychological, emotional, and social aspects of people's lives from a variety of different population groups. What started as a disease predominantly affecting white homosexual men from industrialized nations in the late 1970s has spread rapidly to heterosexual men and women, children, intravenous drug users, and hemophiliacs of every ethnic and racial background in countries of every socioeconomic standing around the world.

HIV/AIDS is a blood-borne virus that requires body fluid-to-body fluid contact for transmission. This includes direct exposure to infected blood and blood derivatives (such as clotting factors), other body fluids, or blood-related equipment contaminated by these substances. The virus is transmitted through risky unprotected sexual behaviors with infected people, use of HIV-contaminated intravenous needles, transfusion of infected blood or blood derivatives, and from infected mother to fetus and breast-feeding infant.

Nearly 70 million people worldwide are carriers of the HIV virus, and more than 15 million have died from its effects. In the United States, it is estimated that about 2 million people have been infected with the virus and 688,200 cases have been reported to the Centers for Disease Control and Prevention (CDC, 1999). This includes almost 700,000 adults and adolescents (570,425 males and 109,311 females) and 8,461 children under 13 years of age. The total deaths from AIDS through June 1999 in the United States have exceeded 420,201 (Ruiz et al, 2000).

In the past several years, infection rates have stabilized in the United States and other developed countries. HIV continues to increase, however, in underdeveloped countries, with greatest prevalence in Africa. There, 25% to 40% of the population carries the virus, and AIDS is prematurely killing an entire generation of people (Ezzell, 2000). Additionally, HIV is one of the most rapidly adapting organisms ever described, and it mutates readily against antiretroviral therapies that have been used to contain it. Strains of drug-resistant HIV have spread in Brazil, Africa, and India (Shapshak et al, 2000). Thus additional research and public health vigilance will be critical well into the next century.

The number of women living with HIV continues to climb despite a decline in rates of infection for men in the United States. Among women ages 15 to 44 years, it is the third leading cause of death; among black women of the same age, it is the leading cause of death. Transmission route for most US women is from heterosexual contact. Heterosexual contact is the fastest growing category of AIDS in the United States (Schulte, 2000). The majority of HIV infected women are poor and socially disadvantaged. About one fourth of babies born to mothers with HIV will also have the virus. It is recommended that women with HIV not get pregnant because of the risk of transmitting HIV to the fetus, even though treatment with zidovudine (AZT) during pregnancy reduces the risk of transmission to the baby by two thirds. Women with HIV should not breastfeed since the breast milk is a mode of transmission of the virus (Bartlett & Finkbeiner, 1998).

Some public health changes in the past few years have reduced the risk of transmitting HIV. These include irradiating the blood supply and clotting factors; needle exchange programs for intravenous drug users; more comprehensive policies in health-care settings where needles, other sharps, and blood products are used; increased availability of free condoms in health-care, educational, and community settings; and increased educational programs regarding HIV transmission and safe sex practices.

Until 1978 studies indicated that most people with HIV developed a major life-threatening complication 8 to 10 years after infection and lived for 1 more year. By 1996, because of major research findings and changes in treatment, people with HIV/AIDS were living longer, making HIV/AIDS a chronic condition for many people. These changes include the following:

- New understanding that billions of new viruses are produced daily in HIV/AIDS infected individuals, requiring treatments focused on slowing down this process.
- Development of new drugs that could stop the progression of the disease for an indefinite time.
- Drug protocols that combine these drugs in ways that greatly enhance effectiveness.
- Development of the viral load test, which measures response to treatment.

Treatment for AIDS is complex and expensive. Most people require at least three different medications, which sometimes means taking 20 or more pills a day. These drugs have difficult side effects and can cost up to $12,000 a year for each patient (Bartlett & Finkbeiner, 1998). Thus although the incidence of AIDS increased by 10% in the United States between 1997 and 1998, the number of deaths resulting from AIDS decreased by 46% from 1996 to 1997 and another 20% from 1997 to 1998. As a result, the CDC reported in 1999 that AIDS is no longer among the top 10 causes of death in the general population of the United States.

CHARACTERISTICS OF HIV

HIV/AIDS is a lethal transmittable illness. It destroys cellular immunity by directly attacking the central nervous system (CNS) and helper T cells (lymphocytes that coordinate the responses of the immune system to biological invaders), specifically the subgroup of CD4 cells (a specific surface marker protein on T cells), leaving the body susceptible to opportunistic life-threatening infections. The virus itself is a protein capsule containing ribonucleic acid (RNA). In normal body cells, RNA is synthesized from DNA (deoxyribonucleic acid) to carry genetic information needed for the development of an organism. HIV is called a retrovirus because its genetic information passes in the reverse direction, from RNA to DNA. It assumes control of the infected cell's DNA and makes copies of itself that then enter the blood stream to attack other cells and make more copies of itself.

Have you known someone with HIV disease? What were your feelings about that person? Did you worry about becoming infected? Have your feelings changed since you began your nursing program?

ASSESSING THE PATIENT WITH HIV DISEASE

Psychiatric nurses are in a unique position to help diagnose, treat, and support patients affected by HIV/AIDS. These patients and their families experience significant losses as a result of this illness (Table 42-1). Because these patients' lives are affected in so many ways, assessment of each of these areas is an important aspect of nursing care planning. For example, a person's financial, transportation, and housing needs may directly relate to the ability to participate in treatment.

Psychiatric interventions with patients with HIV/AIDS can serve a number of important functions (Ruiz et al, 2000):

- Helping patients change risky behaviors, thus promoting prevention of HIV infection.
- Helping patients during the difficult process of HIV testing.
- Helping establish the diagnosis and treatment of other psychiatric illnesses commonly seen in patients with HIV.
- Implementing psychosocial interventions with patients at risk for HIV infection, or who are already suffering with HIV/AIDS.
- Helping patients, their families, and others in their lives with interpersonal problems related to HIV/AIDS.
- Assisting AIDS patients during the final phases of their illness.

The diagnostic criteria for AIDS require that the patient be HIV positive and have either a CD4 cell count below 200 per milliliter or the presence of a disease associated with

Table 42-1

Losses Associated with HIV Infection

Employment: Loss due to infection status, disability, stigma, or erratic work attendance related to illness or treatment requirements

Family: Fear, stigma, inability to cope, ignorance

Friends: Fear, stigma, inability to cope, ignorance, friends dying of AIDS

Health care: Inability to afford care or to obtain own or partner's insurance benefits

Financial: Cost of health care, loss of employment, cost of social resources and services, housing, food, and necessities

Social supports: Fear, stigma, inability to cope, ignorance, easily drained due to magnitude of need

Self-esteem/pride: Self-blame for personal infection and the epidemic in general, loss of autonomy, disfigurement, stigma, depression

Physical intimacy/sexual contact: Irrational fears of casual transmission, stigma, shame/blame

Future goals: Facing a life-threatening, chronic, painful, expensive illness

Physical functioning and autonomy: Disease progression, including disability, depression, dementia, dependency, and decreased sensory, cardiac, respiratory, musculoskeletal, reproductive, cognitive, and GI functioning

Lifestyle changes: Need to change sexual practices, improve nutrition, avoid smoking, alcohol, and other drugs, and give up pets (which may carry pathogens)

Modified from Kalichman S: *Understanding AIDS: a guide for mental health professionals*, Washington DC, 1995, American Psychological Association.

cellular immune dysfunction. Opportunistic infections such as toxoplasmosis (a parasitic infestation from cat feces or undercooked meat), *Pneumocystis carinii* pneumonia (a protozoa infection), and Kaposi's sarcoma (a neoplasm that was rare before the onset of AIDS) are common (Thomas & Java, 2000). Infections can develop in the CNS and cause dementia. Damage in the CNS is caused either directly through neuronal injury mediated by brain macrophages (which ingest and destroy microorganisms), or as a complication of opportunistic infection.

Many psychiatric syndromes are associated with HIV/AIDS. Depression, anxiety, paranoia, mania, irritability, psychosis, and substance abuse are common in HIV-positive persons. They complicate immune system function, adversely effect the patient's ability to fully participate in treatment, and negatively impact on quality of life (see Citing the Evidence). A thorough psychiatric history and complete neuropsychiatric evaluation are indicated when HIV-positive patients present with psychiatric symptoms. Patients with advanced HIV have a 30 times greater risk of suicide than age-matched control subjects; therefore a comprehensive assessment and treatment of suicidality is a necessity.

Psychosocial Behaviors

A number of social conflicts, such as fear of exposure of diagnosis and being a member of a stigmatized group, are

Citing the Evidence on

The Impact of Psychiatric Conditions on Quality of Life in HIV

BACKGROUND: This study estimates the burden on health-related quality of life associated with comorbid psychiatric conditions in a nationally representative sample of persons with HIV.

RESULTS: HIV subjects with probable mood disorder had significantly lower scores on health-related quality of life measures than did those without such symptoms.

IMPLICATIONS: Comorbid psychiatric conditions may serve as markers for impaired functioning and well-being in persons with HIV. A sufficient number of qualified mental health professionals to treat these symptoms may reduce unnecessary utilization of other health services as well as improve quality of life in these patients.

Shelbourne C et al: Impact of psychiatric conditions on health-related quality of life in persons with HIV infection, *Am J Psychiatry* 157:248, 2000.

commonly experienced by people who have HIV. Patients often need the nurse's support and assistance in deciding whom to tell about their disease status, as well as when and how to do so. Physical changes such as Kaposi's sarcoma, wasting, or rashes may force the patient to reveal the illness before feeling prepared to do so.

Conflict regarding sexual activity may leave the person socially isolated and alone. This is especially true for people who used sex to establish interpersonal contacts. Even people in stable relationships may find their sexual relationship dramatically changed, affecting feelings of closeness and the ability to give and receive love, comfort, and affection.

Employment and insurance issues are sources of stress because patients are often rejected and stigmatized. Although employers are not legally able to terminate someone from their job because of HIV status, because HIV is now a legally protected disability, subtle means may be used to force the person to leave the work setting. Reallocation of work, reassignment, poor evaluation, or redefinition of a job may result in a person with HIV/AIDS being terminated from a job. Others have lost positions because of being physically unable to work owing to their illness. Loss of a job often results in loss of health insurance. This can be problematic for many people, but especially for homosexuals because they are often unable to receive healthcare coverage under their partners' health benefits in most states.

Social support limitations are common, especially in a mobile society in which friends and family are scattered around the world. People who have chosen to keep their homosexual lifestyle secret often move away from their family of origin

CRITICAL THINKING about CONTEMPORARY ISSUES

Should a Person Be Obligated to Reveal HIV-Positive Status?

Some states require physicians to report all blood tests positive for HIV. All states require physicians to report every case of AIDS to the state public health department (Bartlett & Finkenbeiner, 1998). These data are used for statistical purposes and program development. Public health departments are legally barred from revealing the names of people reported to be HIV positive.

Nurses and other health-care workers are not under a legal obligation to report HIV cases. However, they do face the controversial issue of "duty to warn" the contacts of persons infected with HIV/AIDS. On the one hand the nurse has a duty to protect the confidentiality of patients. On the other hand, there is a duty to protect individuals who may come in contact with HIV-positive patients.

For example, a man who is HIV positive informs the nurse that he will not share the information with his wife, and he intends to continue having sexual relations with her. The patient claims that he will protect his wife from infection but will not be specific about the method he plans to use. The nurse is caught between maintaining a confidential relationship with the patient and protecting a third party, while being unsure of the degree of danger to the wife.

The law is not yet clear on the issue of disclosure of HIV status in order to warn potential victims, but the courts may apply the same principles used in cases involving dangerous psychiatric patients. Courts will likely decide that the right to privacy should be overridden to protect the rights of a larger group that might be in peril (Klink, 1999).

A similar conflict exists regarding the responsibility of health-care workers who know that they are HIV positive to inform their patients, supervisors, and co-workers. Since several patients were believed to have been infected by a Florida dentist a number of years ago, there has been political pressure to require reporting. Health-care workers fear that revealing HIV disease will result in job loss. They cite evidence that HIV is not transmitted in health-care situations as long as universal precautions are observed.

Because serious consequences exist for the patient in his or her personal relationships and continued employment, there are no easy answers to this question. The nurse should consider the facts related to each situation and help the patient to consider all of the alternatives, including the likely consequences. Additionally, the nurse should check with her state nurses association regarding state policy, think through the potential risks of each situation she encounters, and, if it seems most prudent to warn potential victims, she should first tell the patient and ask permission, carefully document the situation, and tell the caretakers about the patient's HIV status regardless of the patient's consent (Klink, 1999).

---

and may or may not have a group in whom they confide. For many people, work colleagues make up a major portion of their social support system. When the job is lost, the isolation increases. Resources that can be used to provide social support include community agencies that offer shopping, Meals on Wheels, and housekeeping services. Some clergy and churches have become involved in transportation or other services for people with AIDS. The homosexual community has also organized support services in many areas.

Nurses can help patients with psychosocial issues if a trusting, open-minded, confidential relationship is established. At times the boundaries of confidentiality are not clear (see Critical Thinking about Contemporary Issues). It is important for the nurse and all health-care providers of patients with HIV to address important ethical issues in their clinical supervision or peer review opportunities.

Stigma. Some of the psychosocial problems associated with HIV are a result of stigma. HIV stigma is closely connected to the risk behaviors that lead to infection. The illness was first identified in homosexual men, an already stigmatized group. Later, it became prevalent in intravenous drug users, another stigmatized population. Because of these risk behaviors, assumptions are often made about the lifestyles of people with HIV disease. Some believe these behaviors are immoral and that the illness is a punishment for them. Stigma may inhibit people from seeking HIV testing. It also fosters reluctance to inform others of their diagnosis and to adopt risk-reduction behaviors. It is reflected in the difficulty people with HIV face in keeping their jobs, getting insurance, finding housing, and obtaining health care.

Interventions with HIV-positive men and women who continue to engage in risky sexual behaviors include education about the importance of avoiding reinfection with HIV and exposure to sexually transmitted disease, and education about safe sex practices and the role of alcohol, cocaine, and other drugs in increasing the likelihood of risky sexual behaviors. Stigma is difficult to overcome, but the best way to confront it is through health education. Nurses can also model nonstigmatizing attitudes by providing sensitive and competent care to people with HIV disease.

Identify a situation in which you noticed stigmatizing behavior toward homosexuals, drug users, and people with HIV disease. What did you do (or could you have done) to change this behavior?

Crisis Points. Several potential crisis points occur during the course of HIV disease. The diagnosis of HIV may be the first crisis. However, the patient may already have had a crisis based on anticipation of the potential diagnosis. With the initial diagnosis the person often feels intense anxiety, fear, anger, and guilt and may act impulsively (Phillips & Morrow, 1998). High levels of anxiety and depression may continue for 2 to 3 months and may be exhibited in agitation, risky sexual behavior, crying, and suicidal ideation and attempts. In fact, symptoms of depression and anxiety may

Table 42-2

HIV and Overlapping Symptoms of Depression and Anxiety	
HIV Symptom	**Depression/Anxiety Symptom**
Fatigue	Fatigue, lethargy
Muscle aches	Muscle aches, pains
Night sweats	Insomnia, increased sweating
Weight loss	Appetite and weight changes
Diarrhea	GI distress
Neurological symptoms/dementia	Neurological symptoms: headaches, poor concentration and memory, dizziness
Hopelessness, helplessness, poor self-image	Hopelessness, helplessness, poor self-image
Social isolation, stigma	Isolation, stigma
Increased suicide risk	Increased suicide risk

overlap with HIV symptoms (Table 42-2), complicating diagnostic and treatment efforts.

The patient should not be left alone or expected to make decisions immediately after learning the diagnosis. Using safety precautions and taking the necessary time to allow the person to process the initial reaction are critical. The nurse should share information regarding HIV disease when the patient requests it. Helping the patient to recognize and talk about beliefs regarding HIV may be helpful.

During this phase the patient is learning to live with a disease whose prognosis is now likely to be one of a "chronic and manageable disease if treated aggressively" (Bartlett & Finkbeiner, 1998). It is essential to provide structure during this time by implementing crisis intervention techniques (see Chapter 14). Psychotropic medications may be indicated to enable the person to function, sleep, and cope during the crisis. The following clinical example highlights some of the issues around notification of the HIV diagnosis.

 CLINICAL EXAMPLE

Mr. and Ms. G are a prominent couple in the community. Mr. G was hospitalized for a severe case of herpes zoster (shingles). With his informed consent he was tested for HIV and was found to be positive. Mr. G is fearful of his wife's reaction to his diagnosis. They have been married for 24 years. He had one incident of homosexual marital infidelity 3 years ago while on a business trip. He is angry over the "unfairness" of how one experience will alter not only his health but also his relationship with his wife. He is also worried that his children will reject him and his employer will fire him. Another concern is that his high public profile will lead to negative publicity for him, his family, and the community organizations in which he has been active.

Selected Nursing Diagnoses

- Anxiety related to diagnosis of AIDS, as evidenced by verbalized concerns about impact of the diagnosis on relationships

- Altered family processes related to changed role of husband and father, as evidenced by concern over reactions of wife and children
- Altered role performance related to change in health status, as evidenced by concern that job and community activities will be affected

There may be a quiet phase between the initial diagnosis and the first opportunistic infection. There is a focus on learning about HIV disease and often the adoption of a healthier lifestyle, including attention to diet, exercise, and adequate rest. Attempts to cope may include denial of the illness. However, when the first opportunistic infection occurs, a crisis that is more intense than the first may be precipitated. Denial is no longer effective. The treatment phase may be characterized by alienation, depression, and discouragement. Patients may fear or experience disfigurement, pain, and loss of health. The process of treatment, which may include financial hardship, medical side effects, laboratory testing, and awaiting test results, may cause self-absorption, frustration, and irritability. Patients with HIV may experience a loss of control, especially in dealing with the medical system. They may become fearful, demanding, and dependent on health-care providers. As treatment continues, they may be frightened to be away from the close supervision of the hospital staff or health-care provider. They may become hypervigilant and seek reassurance that they will know what to do and when to ask for help.

The final phase for many patients may be marked by preparation for death. There is a gradual decline and deterioration of the person's functional ability. Recurrence and relapse are accompanied by feelings of depression, dependency, isolation, suicidal ideation, and fear of abandonment. There is usually ambivalence, dependence, and withdrawal from the world, combined with increased self-absorption. Patients often review their lives. They may finalize their wishes related to their death and postmortem arrangements. Support and physical assistance must be given because important decisions regarding the last phases of life are being made and important goodbyes being are shared. The person who is living with HIV disease often experiences conflict about the implications of the illness. These are summarized in Fig. 42-1. Concerns related to the person's lifestyle are illustrated in the next clinical example.

 CLINICAL EXAMPLE

Mr. J was diagnosed as HIV positive 4 years ago and has been asymptomatic. On his forty-fifth birthday he noticed a Kaposi's sarcoma spot on his cheek and is now in a state of panic. He has not told anyone about his discovery. His parents are scheduled to arrive on the next day to celebrate his birthday. They are not aware that he is HIV positive or that he is homosexual. He knows his mother will question him about the spot. His father is vehemently antihomosexual, consistent with his religious beliefs. Mr. J is anxious about how his father would accept this information. However, Mr.

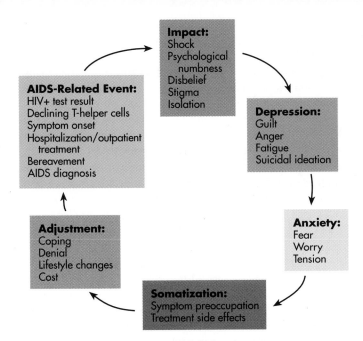

Fig. 42-1   Cycle of reactions to HIV disease. (Modified from Kalichman S: *Understanding AIDS: advances in research and treatments,* ed 2, Washington, DC, 1998, American Psychological Association.)

J's lover is pressuring him to tell his parents so that their relationship can be open.

Selected Nursing Diagnoses

- Anxiety related to parental response to sexual preference, as evidenced by secrecy about his homosexuality
- Body image disturbance related to discovery of facial lesion, as evidenced by not telling anyone
- Situational low self-esteem related to guilt about sexual preference, as evidenced by hiding relationship with lover

Behaviors Related to Depression

It has been well documented that the immune system is compromised in people with high levels of stress and with depression. In people with HIV, depression can confuse diagnostic and treatment issues of both illnesses because of the overlap between the vegetative symptoms of HIV and the neuropsychologic symptoms of depression. Depression is thought to be one of the most common psychiatric disorders in HIV-infected people, and is a potentially dangerous comorbid condition because it may hasten the course of HIV disease. It has been shown that there is a dramatic, sustained rise in depressive symptoms as AIDS develops, beginning as early as 18 months before clinical AIDS is diagnosed and that approximately 40% of hospitalized patients with HIV have clinical depression (Schulte, 2000).

Patients with HIV disease who are depressed experience the emotional pain and suffering common to depression, including depressed mood and decreased motivation, lowered self-esteem, guilt, increased isolation, lowered energy level, sleep disturbance, change in appetite, somatic complaints,

Citing the Evidence on

CBT Plus Medication for Depressed Gay Men with HIV/AIDS

BACKGROUND: This study evaluated the feasibility and effectiveness of 15 to 20 sessions of combination cognitive-behavioral therapy with antidepressants for 15 depressed gay men with HIV/AIDS.

RESULTS: Depression scores showed significant improvement from premeasurement to postmeasurement scores, and at 1-year follow-up evaluation. Subjects reported that the cognitive restructuring aspects of the treatment program were particularly valuable in alleviating their depression.

IMPLICATIONS: CBT (as modified in this study for the target population) plus antidepressants offer a reasonable option for treatment of this clinically challenging group of patients.

Lee M et al: Cognitive-behavioral therapy with medication for depressed gay men with AIDS of symptomatic HIV infection, *Psychiatric Serv* 50:948, 1999.

increased sense of hopelessness, increased risk for suicide, and increased social stigma in addition to the problems of having HIV. The nurse must be careful not to overlook or normalize depression in HIV-infected people, thus depriving them of treatment that could enhance their well-being and quality of life and increase their longevity. The critical components of a successful treatment program for HIV-infected people with depression are discussed next (Morris, 1996).

Psychotherapy. Treatment outcome studies identify cognitive behavioral therapy, stress reduction, psychoeducation, group therapy, psychosocial support, and combinations of therapy as the essential components of HIV-related psychotherapy (see Citing the Evidence above).

Psychopharmacology: In general, antidepressants with a low anticholinergic side effect profile (such as selective serotonin reuptake inhibitors) are effective and usually well tolerated. As with any antidepressant selection, attention to side effect profiles should be considered for individual patients. In depressed patients with HIV, low doses of the psychostimulant methylphenidate have been reported to improve the patient's well-being, reduce suicidal ideation, improve interaction with peers, and diminish vegetative symptoms. Most studies of the psychopharmacological treatment of psychiatric symptoms in HIV-positive people were done on men because HIV-positive women have been extremely difficult to enroll and retain in placebo-controlled clinical trials.

Nutrition. Nutritional deficiencies, commonplace in patients with HIV, may contribute to mood disturbance, cognitive difficulties, and neurological abnormalities. Research has shown that correction of nutritional deficits and supplementation beyond normal levels is associated with improvement in neuropsychiatric functioning in HIV patients, leading to improved quality of life (Baldewicz et al, 2000).

Testosterone. In HIV-positive male patients with signs of hypogonadism, testosterone was found to improve mood and energy level (Rabkin et al, 2000).

Electroconvulsive therapy (ECT): In severe HIV-related depression, ECT has been shown to be effective and should be considered as a therapeutic option.

Behaviors Related to Dementia

The difference between mild neurocognitive disorder, which usually occurs early in the disease and HIV-associated dementia, is the extent to which the cognitive deficits compromise the patient's daily functioning. Mild neurocognitive deficit (feeling mentally slowed, fatigue, difficulty concentrating) does not interfere in a major way with daily activities. People with HIV disease frequently worry about HIV-associated dementia (HAD). HAD occurs in 20% to 30% of people with AIDS, usually in late stages of the disease, and probably affects several brain structures (Table 42-3). Immune activation and an increase in the activity of cytokines (CKs) and chemokines (CCKs) (molecules of the immune system that are part of the host's protective response to tissue injury or a disease process but that can also cause damage in the brain under certain disease conditions) are implicated in the cognitive symptomatology of HIV (Shapshak et al, 2000). Additionally, the amount of viral load creates a stress for the infected cell and is increased in areas such as the basal ganglia, causing motor symptoms and contributing to the disease process.

HAD significantly disrupts the patient's daily functioning. Changes in mental ability (such as very slowed thinking and severe forgetfulness), difficulty performing complex tasks (multistage projects such as dressing) as a result of decreased muscle control, and poor cognition are evident in HAD. Initially, persons with HAD seem to need more time to organize their thoughts, but at other times they are clear and sharp. Eventually, they experience a decline in occupational performance, ultimately progressing to an inability to perform activities of daily living. Later, apathy, social withdrawal, and depression are seen. Most people with HAD will have muscle control problems resulting in unsteady walk and falling or weakness in their legs. They may have problems eating and writing. They eventually need full care and become bedridden. It is important to distinguish HAD diagnosis from depression or a CNS infection in order to plan appropriate interventions.

There is no specific therapy for HAD, and the triple therapy drug "cocktail" regimen for HIV is used. Some studies have shown that large doses of AZT have improved cognitive test scores, at least temporarily. Safety and supportive living measures should be incorporated as needed. Encouraging talk and decisions regarding resuscitation, power of attorney (for finances as well as health care), and living and end of life wills should be completed as soon as possible. The person with HAD may need support and help with decisions, such as when they can no longer work or drive or go places alone (Bartlett & Finkbeiner, 1998).

> *Do you believe that a person who is HIV positive should engage in sexual activity? Can any sexual activity with an HIV-positive person be safe? What types of sexual expression would you recommend? Do you feel comfortable discussing this with your patients?*

PLANNING AND IMPLEMENTING CARE

HIV disease and related opportunistic infections and illnesses affect multiple body systems. A complete nursing assessment will result in nursing diagnoses related to all of the identified behaviors discussed earlier. Nursing diagnoses related to physiological disruptions are discussed in medical-surgical nursing textbooks. Box 42-1 lists NANDA nursing diagnoses that are associated with the psychosocial aspects of HIV/AIDS.

The complexity of the biopsychosocial needs of the person with HIV/AIDS demands a team approach to health-care planning and implementation that includes the patient's entire health-care and social support system (Fig. 42-2). The physician or advanced practice registered nurse prescribes the course of medical treatment, often involving prophylactic medication or pharmacotherapy for identified physiological and psychological disorders. Occupational or physical therapy may be needed to help the patient to adjust to changing neuromuscular and cognitive functioning. Social workers help the patient and significant others to find and contact community resources. Nursing care centers provide support and counseling while helping the patient to conserve energy and set priorities for activities. Nurses are also responsible for ensuring that the patient is educated about the disease and the options related to intervention.

Nurses in HIV/AIDS care have opportunities to develop close relationships with patients and their significant others. The reaction to HIV and the AIDS disease process is unique to each patient. A common counseling issue is concern

Table **42-3**

HIV Symptoms Related to Brain Structures and Functions	
Brain Structure	**Clinical Symptoms**
Frontal lobes	Apathy, trouble concentrating and planning, loss of organizational skills, depression
Basal ganglia	Impaired movement, tremor
Limbic system	Emotional lability, memory loss, language impairment
Brainstem	Disturbances of gait, vision, and eye movement
Demyelination	Impaired fine motor skills, delayed information processing, impaired response time, incontinence

about the course of disease and the length of survival. This is reflected by a commonly asked question when people with HIV disease meet: "How long have you known your diagnosis?" This is a way of determining how far along the other person is in dealing with HIV. Also, there is the underlying hope that the question will identify a long-term survivor, serving as reassurance that a person with HIV disease can live a long and fruitful life.

Service Delivery

People with HIV disease are increasingly being treated in community-based health centers and at home. Efforts at cost containment for all health-care services have resulted in more outpatient care. Community mental health centers have a wide variety of patients. Nurses must include treatment of HIV/AIDS and the associated opportunistic infections in their patient case load and use their influence, education, and persuasion to obtain patient and family cooperation. With the increased availability of home health care, the nurse may be able to visit patients in their homes. The nurse must be skilled in dealing with family interactions and coordinating treatment with other home health-care providers (see Chapter 37).

Although many communities are attempting to organize the necessary services for people with HIV/AIDS, services and funds are usually not coordinated and are often difficult to find. The person who is struggling with the HIV diagnosis has the additional burden of locating needed help. Case management by the nurse, social worker, or other professional can help to locate available services. The case manager can help in identifying health-care providers, dentists, therapists, housing, and many other resources the person with HIV will need.

Medications and Treatment Issues

Although there is no cure for HIV/AIDS at this time, there has been an explosion of new drugs available to treat this illness. Antiretroviral drugs, usually in combinations, are used to slow viral replication. The Food and Drug Administration (FDA) has approved three classes of antiretroviral drugs (Box 42-2). It is important for the nurse to distinguish between psychiatric symptoms the patient may be experiencing and the side effects of the antiretroviral medications to competently treat patients taking these medications. Table 42-4 lists some of the antiretroviral drugs used in the treatment of HIV/AIDS and their common neuropsychiatric side effects.

Evidence of effectiveness of these combination antiretroviral drug regimens or "cocktails" include viral load reduction to a nondetectable level and CD4 lymphocyte count increase. To inhibit resistance to the antiretroviral drugs from developing, patients must adhere to strict schedules of drug administration as well as rigid food guidelines, often to the exclusion of other interests and pursuits because this regimen may be so time-consuming. People who have qualified for disability are concerned that their benefits will be lost as they have extended but unpredictable periods of wellness because new treatments change HIV infection from a disease progressing quickly to death to one with a more chronic, intermittent course. Even in the face of these difficulties, the advances in HIV/AIDS research have been remarkable in a short period; and new studies for more effective treatments,

Box 42-1

NANDA Diagnoses Related to Psychosocial Aspects of HIV Disease

- Adjustment, impaired
- Anxiety
- Body image disturbance
- Caregiver role strain, risk for
- Communication, impaired verbal
- Defensive coping
- Denial, ineffective
- Family processes, altered
- Fear
- Grieving, anticipatory
- Grieving, dysfunctional
- Health maintenance, altered
- Hopelessness
- Individual coping, ineffective
- Management of therapeutic regimen (individual), ineffective
- Parental role conflict
- Parenting, risk for altered
- Powerlessness
- Role performance, altered
- Self-esteem, situational low
- Sexual dysfunction
- Sexuality patterns, altered
- Social interaction, impaired
- Social isolation
- Spiritual distress
- Thought processes, altered

From North American Nursing Diagnosis Association: *NANDA nursing diagnoses: definitions and classifications 1999-2000,* Philadelphia, 1999, The Association.

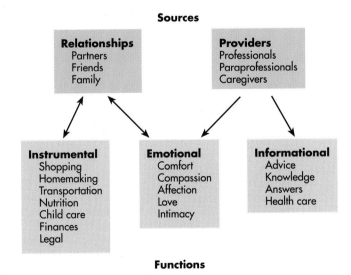

Fig. 42-2 Sources and functions of support needed by the person with HIV.

vaccines, and testing procedures are stimulating hope for the future of HIV-positive patients, their families, the health-care community, and society in general (St. Louis et al, 1997).

Interventions Related to Risk Reduction

Currently, the most effective way of combating HIV disease is by preventing it through risk reduction. Because of their credibility with the general public, nurses are in a good position to provide prevention education. Nurses should familiarize themselves with the routes of transmission of HIV (Table 42-5) and the currently recommended ways of preventing infection. For example, patients can be encouraged to inform sexual partners of their HIV status and to practice safe sex. Intravenous drug users can be referred to treatment programs, discouraged from sharing needles, and taught

how to disinfect used needles. Pregnant women who are HIV positive should be helped to find obstetrical care from a provider who understands the implications of the disease for the mother and infant. Clinical algorithms may help persons with HIV make decisions regarding timely treatment (Fig. 42-3).

People infected with HIV are often asymptomatic up to 10 years. Testing for the presence of HIV antibodies is the only way to determine whether a person is infected with the virus, and thus is at risk for infecting others. Stereotypes about HIV carriers based on sex, race, socioeconomic status, sexual preference, habits of cleanliness, nutrition, sexual practices, and drug behavior are not valid. Nurses should always use universal precautions when treating any patient, regardless of diagnosis, and when handling any equipment that may be contaminated by blood, blood products, or body fluids, regardless of their source.

Risk Reduction Strategies. People with mental illness are at increased risk for HIV owing to drug use and consensual and exploitive sexual behavior. Public health systems can take several actions to decrease risk of HIV infection among severely mentally ill. These include increasing the availability of free condoms, information about needle-exchange programs, and educating patients and family members about risk prevention measures (Kelly et al, 1997; Sullivan et al, 1999). A review of the literature and interviews with key informants regarding mental illness and HIV/AIDS risk reduction identified the following strategies for reducing HIV risk in this population (Brown & Jemmott, 2000):

- Health education/risk reduction strategies, provided by peer or nonpeer educators in one-to-one or group format, to enhance understanding and build self-esteem
- Institutionally based (e.g., partial day programs, residential programs, acute and long-term care centers) health-education/risk-reduction strategies, with an

---

Box 42-2

Drug Therapy for HIV/AIDS

Antiretroviral drugs are used to slow virus replication, slowing the progression of HIV/AIDS.

Three classes of retroviral drugs have been approved by the FDA:

1. NRTIs (Nucleoside Reverse Transcriptase Inhibitors): zidovudine (AZT), didanosine (ddI), zalcitabine (ddC), stavudine (d4T), lamivudine (3TC), Combivir (AZT+3TC), and abacavir (Ziagen)
2. PIs (Protease Inhibitors): saquinavir (Invirase & Fortovase), ritonavir (Norvir), indinavir (Crixivan), and nelfinavir (Viracept)
3. NNRTIs (non-nucleoside Reverse Transcriptase Inhibitors): nevirapine (Viramune), delavirdine (Rescriptor), and efavirenz (Sustiva)

The preferred treatment for HIV is a triple combination of drugs from more than one class (except pregnant women who should only take AZT).

Table 42-4

Neuropsychiatric Side Effects of Medications Used to Treat HIV/AID

Drug	Side Effects
Zidovudine (AZT)	Headache, restlessness, agitation, insomnia, mania, depression, irritability
Didanosine (ddI)	Insomnia, peripheral neuropathy, mania
Stavudine (d4T)	Mania
Cotrimoxazole	Depression, loss of appetite, insomnia, apathy, headache
Pentamidine	Hypoglycemia, hypotension
Steroids	Depression, euphoria, mania, psychosis
Acyclovir	Visual hallucinations, depersonalization, tearfulness, confusion, hyperesthesia, hyperacusia, thought insertion, insomnia, agitation
Gancyclovir	Mania, psychosis, agitation, delirium, irritability
Isoniazid	Depression, agitation, hallucinations, paranoia, impaired memory
Amphotericin B	Delirium, peripheral neuropathy, diplopia, anorexia
Thiabendazole	Hallucinations, olfactory disturbance
Vincristine	Depression, hallucinations, headache, ataxia, sensory loss, agitation
Vinblastine	Depression, anorexia, headache
Interferon	Depression, weakness (dose-dependent)
Methotrexate	Encephalopathy (with large doses)
Procarbazine	Mania, loss of appetite, insomnia, nightmares, confusion, malaise

From Schulte J: HIV infection: the quintessential biopsychosocial disease. In Kay J, Tasman A, editors: *Psychiatry: behavioral science and clinical essentials*, Philadelphia, 2000, WB Saunders.

emphasis on cognitive therapy techniques to increase knowledge, risk factors, and prevention strategies regarding HIV

- HIV counseling and testing, as many persons with mental illness engage in risky behaviors yet may not have an adequate support system in which they can address issues related to HIV
- Prevention case management, as many patients in this population tend not to be connected to comprehensive programs and services
- Strategies to educate and sensitize health-care professionals about HIV susceptibility of persons with mental illness, as patient HIV knowledge, status, prevention strategies, and participation in risky behaviors are not usually part of patient assessment by mental health professionals

Vaccines. The human immune system can control HIV under certain circumstances. For example, some people have no immune system deterioration after 15 or more years of infection, even without antiretroviral therapy. Other people remain uninfected after multiple exposures. The development of a safe and effective vaccine is the highest priority of AIDS research today (Fauci, 1999). Thus far, experimental vaccines have been protective in animal studies. HIV vaccine development is especially challenging because the virus continually mutates and recombines, necessitating the development of a vaccine that can protect from many strains of HIV.

> *Describe patient behaviors related to the psychiatric diagnoses of bipolar disorder and schizophrenia that might contribute to increased risk for HIV.*

Interventions Related to Changing Levels of Functioning

The unpredictability of the course of HIV disease is itself a stressor because people with the infection cannot prepare for disease events and often feel surprised by the onset of new symptoms. They cannot determine whether a common cold is the serious *Pneumocystis carinii* pneumonia that they have heard about or whether a new mole is actually Kaposi's sarcoma. With each opportunistic infection, they need to redefine what they can reasonably expect from themselves regarding energy output and physical and mental abilities.

People with HIV disease have been living longer because of medical breakthroughs and greater knowledge of the disease. This means that a person may have multiple opportunistic infections over the years. People may wonder, "Is all this worth it?" during periods of fatigue and discouragement. They may consider suicide. At this time it is helpful for nurses to listen receptively to patients' feelings and not discourage them from talking because of nurses' own discomfort or fear. Information about suicide assessment and inter-

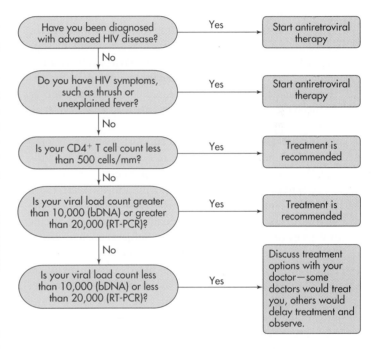

Figure 42-3 Clinical algorithm for HIV treatment. (From *HIV and its treatment: what you should know* (brochure), 1999, U.S. Department of Health and Human Services & Henry J. Kaiser Family Foundation, Washington, DC.)

Table **42-5**

Routes of HIV Transmission	
Risk Behavior	**Transmission Mechanism**
Anal intercourse	Infected semen or blood enters the anal/rectal mucosa or penis through absorption or micro-openings.
Vaginal intercourse	Infected vaginal fluids, semen, or blood enter the vaginal or penile mucosa or through micro-openings.
Oral-genital contact	Infected semen or vaginal fluids enter blood stream through micro-openings in oral cavity, or infected cells enter vagina or penis through micro-openings.
Perinatal transmission	Transplacental transfer of virus during gestation, transfer of virus or maternal blood during labor/delivery, breastfeeding.
Injection drug use	Use of needles and other injection equipment previously used by an infected person; virus or infected cells directly enter blood stream.
Blood transfusion—receiving blood products	Principal risk in United States occurred before 1984 blood-screening programs; blood or blood parts from an infected person enter blood stream.

Modified from Kalichman S: *Understanding AIDS: advances in research and treatment*, ed 2, Washington, DC, 1998, American Psychological Association.

vention is presented in Chapter 21. Nurses can remind patients that there is no need to go through this alone because others will be there to help. The respectful and careful use of physical touch may be a powerful intervention. People with HIV disease often express the feeling of being "lepers" and may isolate themselves at times. A touch on the hand or shoulder may convey the sense of being there for the patient.

> *The partner of a person who is terminally ill with AIDS asks for your opinion about assisted suicide. How would you respond?*

The link between psychosocial factors, the CNS and the immune system is the focus of psychoneuroimmunology. The fact that immune functioning can be enhanced by behavioral interventions is stimulating research in this area for patients with HIV. Interventions such as bereavement support groups, exercise, and cognitive-behavioral stress management have been proposed as having the potential for improved quality of life and increased longevity, as well as enhanced immune function for patients with HIV (Tyll et al, 2000).

Support Groups. Nurse-led support groups may provide the patient with a safe place to express feelings regarding HIV and the physical threats that are being experienced. The patient can give and receive information and learn more effective coping strategies. The group also serves as a social network for people who are gradually losing their sociocultural roles of worker and provider. Subjects such as living wills, new medications, suicide, responses of friends and family, and the future can be discussed. Group members grieve for themselves as well as their fellow members. Lifestyle and medical questions may be asked at this time. Education about exposing others to HIV and the dangers of re-exposure to themselves is important. Safer sex techniques and the responsibility to inform past sexual or needle-sharing partners must be addressed.

Encouraging Productive Activity. The course of HIV disease is characterized by periods of relative wellness, but inconsistent health may result in unstable employment. It is important for the nurse to help patients remain contributing members of society by offering outlets for their energy and skills. Such activities could include acting as a buddy for another person with HIV disease, regular physical exercise, joining political movements to promote legislation in which they believe, volunteering at a museum or library, and expanding talents in music, poetry, and other arts.

Interventions Related to Management of Pain Syndromes

Pain syndromes are common in patients with HIV/AIDS. The prevalence of pain in these patients is estimated at 30% to 80%, yet only 6% are treated for pain, and 97% of AIDS patients who are near death suffer significant pain (Shulte, 2000). Pain is associated with psychological and functional decline and is commonly undertreated. It is important for the nurse to know these statistics and to under-

stand principles of pain management for HIV/AIDS patients.

Pharmacological treatment of pain in patients with HIV/AIDS includes nonopioid analgesics such as nonsteroidal antiinflammatory drugs (NSAIDs), opioids such as codeine and morphine, and adjuvant agents such as tricyclic antidepressants, trazodone, and gabapentin.

Nonpharmacological treatments of pain include patient education, supportive psychotherapy, cognitive-behavioral therapy (including hypnotherapy and biofeedback), rehabilitation interventions, (massage, physiotherapy, acupuncture, transcutaneous electrical nerve stimulation called TENS units), regional nerve blocks, and neurosurgical interventions (cordotomy).

Interventions Related to Changes in Body Image

People with HIV disease often face the impairment of disfigurement such as the following:

- Kaposi's sarcoma, which may cause large, purple, bruiselike blotches on the face, hands, and legs
- "AIDS hair," which resembles the thinning, fine hair of people who have received chemotherapy
- Wasting, during which a person continuously loses weight and becomes skeletal in appearance

The nurse should offer opportunities for the patient and significant others to talk about feelings related to body changes. Encouraging the patient to consider himself or herself as a whole person with both strong, attractive components as well as less pleasing ones may be helpful in establishing perspective. Often, the visible changes caused by HIV disease are seen as evidence of approaching death. This idea must be discussed openly and accurate information about the cause and meaning of physical symptoms should be given.

Interventions Related to AIDS Dementia Complex

Nursing interventions for the person with HIV disease must address the limitations related to HAD if the patient has behaviors related to a cognitive disorder. The nursing care of patients with cognitive problems is addressed in Chapter 24. Memory problems may be especially troubling to young patients who want to remain actively involved in life, including work. The nurse may suggest ways to improve memory such as writing notes and establishing set routines for activities. Many patients are well informed about HIV/AIDS and may worry about cognitive changes. Some patients may interpret normal forgetfulness as a sign of pathological deterioration. The nurse must provide an opportunity for expression of fears and give accurate feedback about cognitive functioning. Significant others should also be provided with information about this aspect of the disease.

> *What is your reaction to the following statement? Patients should not be informed about potential cognitive changes related to HIV/AIDS; because these changes cannot be prevented, patients would worry unnecessarily.*

Interventions Related to Preparation for Death

Spiritual Concerns. Awareness of impending death often leads patients with HIV to think about the meaning of life and their spiritual belief system. For some, this means seeking comfort from a religion with which they are already connected. Others may wish to establish a connection with a member of the clergy or a lay representative of a religion. Some patients may choose not to become involved with a particular religion but may want to discuss spiritual and philosophical beliefs. The nurse should assess the patient's spiritual needs and preferences and help him or her access the desired manner of expression. Some patients appreciate the nurse sitting quietly while they think, providing reading materials, or discussing religious or philosophical writings. If the nurse is comfortable with praying with the patient, this may also be helpful. If the nurse is not comfortable, it is best to be candid and perhaps suggest a few moments of silent meditation, and a referral to someone who can help the patient with spiritual needs.

Advanced Directives. Taking charge of the practical aspects of their lives helps people with HIV disease feel in control. For example, making decisions about medical power of attorney, living will, and a last will helps patients take control during the later stages of their lives. For single parents, one of the most difficult decisions is selecting a custodian for their surviving children, as illustrated in the following clinical example.

 CLINICAL EXAMPLE

Ms. B is a 30-year-old divorced woman who is the mother of a 7-year-old boy. She was diagnosed as HIV positive 2 years ago but has had a rapid progression of opportunistic infections and is now in the acute phase of her illness. As part of trying to write her durable power of attorney, living will, and last will, she is trying to decide whom she will ask to care for her son. The child's father has had no contact with them, and Ms. B believes he is unfit and probably unwilling to assume responsibility for his child. Ms. B's parents are elderly and in frail health. Her older sister is married with four children. Her older brother is unmarried and travels a great deal for business. Ms. B's best friend, who is divorced and childless, has expressed a willingness to care for her son. Ms. B is depressed about leaving her son and highly anxious regarding the best situation for him.

Selected Nursing Diagnoses

- Anxiety related to conflict over arranging for son's care, as evidenced by indecision over completing will
- Anticipatory grieving related to expected loss of the relationship with her son, as evidenced by depressed mood

Many people wish to make decisions regarding their funeral. Some write their own obituaries; others design or even make their own quilt panel for the National AIDS Quilt. Some people prepare videotapes and letters for their family members, to be presented after their death. It is important that the nurse support these efforts to maintain control, allowing the person to live and die in his or her own style. Even though these decisions and activities may be difficult and emotional, the patient often feels a sense of relief and completion when these tasks are accomplished.

Interventions Related to Significant Others

Families, significant others, friends, co-workers, and others involved in the life of a person with HIV/AIDS need significant information and support to enable them to better help the patient. They can feel hopeful when the patient was asymptomatic and then hopeless when an opportunistic infection occurs. Interpersonal relationships often change in complex ways within families and support systems as a result of HIV/AIDS. Nurses should provide support and relevant information about the patient's changing condition, as well as a forum for the expression of feelings and concerns, and interventions or referrals for people who need or request it. Nurses can be helpful by inquiring about the status of relationships with family members and others and by exploring both positive and negative responses. Family meetings may facilitate the sharing of feelings and clarification of misconceptions.

Response of the Nurse to the Person with HIV Disease

As a progressive disease is discouraging to patients, it may also be discouraging to nurses (Sherman, 1996). The messages people receive when first diagnosed are extremely powerful and often set the stage for the course of the illness (Barroso, 1996). It is essential that nurses monitor their reactions and investment in patients. Professional nurses must allow themselves the necessary time and opportunities to grieve the multiple losses their patients experience and the death of patients they know well. Nurses may confront many challenges when working with patients with HIV.

Fear of Contagion. The nurse needs to know, understand, and use universal precautions. Careful planning during procedures and taking the time for necessary steps such as proper gloving and needle disposal will eliminate most opportunities for infection from contact with a patient.

As of Dec. 31, 1999, 56 health-care workers in the United States were documented to have seroconverted to HIV after occupational exposures. Of these, 23 were nurses. The vast majority of cases were due to puncture or cut injuries. There are 136 other cases for whom seroconversion after exposure was not documented. Since 1978, 16 cases of job-related transmission of HIV to nurses have been documented. They were exposed to the virus via percutaneous (such as needlesticks) or mucocutaneous routes. There are 68 additional instances of possible occupationally acquired HIV infection in the United States in health-care workers such as laboratory technicians, health aides, paramedics, surgeons, and dental workers.

Cultural and Behavioral Differences. Nurses work with patients whose backgrounds and behaviors may vary markedly from their own and challenge the nurse's beliefs and values. Although a nurse is entitled to have private views, there is an obligation to provide the best nursing care available to each patient. Disapproval of the patient's past behavior is the nurse's prerogative. The challenge is to keep that view from interfering with competent and needed care while accepting the patient as a person.

Identification. As HIV disease spreads throughout society, it will become increasingly common for the nurse to have many similarities with the patient including age, lifestyle, and socioeconomic status. In some cases it is difficult for the nurse to manage the feelings aroused by patients with HIV/AIDS and maintain an objective approach. For example, a pregnant nurse may care for a young woman who has recently delivered an HIV-infected baby. Anger, fear, confusion, disgust, and pity toward the patient are some of the reactions with which a nurse may have to cope to provide high-quality care.

Feeling emotionally involved with the patient and family, whom the nurse may know for years, may result in fatigue and diminished coping. Some signs of emotional fatigue include needing more energy than before to complete tasks, withdrawal from others, loss of humor, and feeling pressured, overwhelmed, and ineffective.

It is important that professionals be aware of their stress level and watch for signs of emotional fatigue to prevent exhaustion or burnout, allowing themselves to process the multiple losses one experiences in working with patients with AIDS. Methods of relieving or preventing stress overload include limit setting, relaxation, and exercise. The clinical example that follows illustrates this problem.

 CLINICAL EXAMPLE

TJ, a 2-year-old girl, entered the hospital with a broken wrist suffered during a fall from her porch. The treatment team was notified by her parents at the time of admission that TJ was HIV positive. She has had no opportunistic infections, has a T-cell count of 950, and is of normal weight and height for her age. She shows no symptoms of HIV disease. Ms. K, her primary nurse, has approached her senior clinical nurse with a dilemma. She believes that the only way TJ could have become infected was in utero. Ms. K is experiencing great anger toward TJ's parents, whom she believes should have taken precautions against the birth of children once they knew TJ's mother was HIV positive. Ms. K wants to be removed as TJ's primary nurse not only because of her anger against her parents, but also because Ms. K has a 2-year-old daughter and finds that she is too distressed to work with TJ.

When a nurse identifies that a patient is arousing strong feelings or if colleagues question one's objectivity, it is essential to seek out supervision or consultation from an experienced nurse or other health-care provider.

Fear of Death and Dying. For many nurses, dealing with death is an occasional stressor. But for the nurse caring for patients with HIV/AIDS, death and the preparation for it are still common issues. Nurses may get to know patients during the course of repeated hospitalizations or work with patients who are young and energetic but are showing signs of decreasing vitality. Unresolved grief on the nurse's part, lack of acceptance of death as an outcome, and the nurse's own religious and cultural values related to death are factors that may inhibit the nurse's ability to cope with the losses experienced while caring for patients with HIV.

> *Would you apply for a nursing position in a setting that specialized in the treatment of people with HIV disease? What considerations would influence your decision?*

Psychiatric Consultation Liaison Nursing. Of special note is the role of the psychiatric consultation liaison nurse in the general hospital setting. This nurse provides consultation to, collaborates with, and educates nurses and other members of the health team in addressing the biopsychosocial aspects of AIDS care. Among the services the nurse consultant can provide or coordinate are educational and informational programs on all aspects of HIV/AIDS, consistent policies and procedures for infection control practices, postexposure education and support, institutional resources and support for patients and staff, attention to work and personal stress-reduction techniques, encouragement of supervisor and peer recognition for work well done, regular and as-needed group meetings to provide emotional support for staff, and group forums for nurses to verbalize their feelings, attitudes, values, and concerns.

Nurses should recognize that complex and difficult challenges face patients and their families daily. Nurses may be burdened with their own feelings of helplessness and frustration. They do not have all the answers and may feel that they have failed the patient. It is often helpful to enlist the support of consultants who are experts at helping nurses cope with these difficult problems.

EVALUATING CARE OF THE PATIENT WITH HIV/AIDS

In working with the psychosocial aspects of HIV/AIDS, evaluation of nursing interventions focuses on the patient's reduction of maladaptive responses to the stressors associated with the disease. The primary issue for the patient is adjustment to loss. Self-esteem, social acceptance, employment and financial independence, family relationships, sexual relationships, and future goals may all be threatened for the patient who is HIV positive. The nurse's assessment and counseling skills, the teaching of coping skills, and referrals to support services are appropriate areas for evaluation. Nurses also should conduct periodic self-evaluation to prevent becoming overwhelmed by the stresses of working with patients with HIV disease.

Summary

1. HIV/AIDS includes all of the disorders resulting from infection with the human immunodeficiency virus. It has multiple effects on all aspects of biopsychosocial functioning.

2. Behaviors related to HIV/AIDS may be related to stigma, crisis, depression, or dementia.

3. Planning health care for the person with HIV/AIDS must involve the multidisciplinary team. Interventions include case management, medications, risk reduction, support groups, crisis intervention, encouragement of productive activity, enhancement of self-esteem, grief counseling, support during terminal stages, and support of significant others.

4. Evaluation focuses on the patient's adjustment to the multiple losses associated with HIV/AIDS.

Competent Caring   A Clinical Exemplar of a Psychiatric Nurse

DONNA GREEN, RN

A special moment for me happened many years ago at the beginning of the AIDS epidemic. It involved a relationship I formed with a patient who was diagnosed with AIDS. I spent time with him when others stayed away and allowed him to share his thoughts and feelings. I encouraged him to talk about his feelings concerning problems in his relationships in an atmosphere of unconditional acceptance of his sexuality. I promoted this by showing no fear of contracting the disease from him and no judgment of his life situation.

Slowly, he began to interact more on the unit by initiating conversations with the staff, although not with other patients.

When he consented to a case conference, he asked that I accompany him because he felt more at ease when I was with him.

At this point I realized the time that I spent with him and the efforts I made to reach out to him had made a difference in this man's hospital stay. My efforts were also recognized by my supervisor and were a large factor in my receiving a performance award. Such are the difficult challenges and special rewards of our profession and the specialty area in which we practice.

MERLIN Visit **MERLIN: www.mosby.com/MERLIN/Stuart** to find these additional materials and student activities.

- **Worksheets**
- **"Drug of the Month" Updates**
- **"Citing the Evidence" Updates**
- **Critical Thinking Activities and Exercises**
- **Annotated Suggested Readings**
- **Web Links**
- **More!**

Chapter Review Questions

1. Identify whether the following statements are true (T) or false (F).

_____ **A.** The AIDS virus cannot be spread through kissing, sneezing, or touching.

_____ **B.** A person can get AIDS by sharing kitchens and bathrooms with someone who has AIDS.

_____ **C.** The AIDS virus attacks the body's ability to fight off diseases.

_____ **D.** A person who got the AIDS virus from shooting up drugs cannot give the virus to someone by having sex.

_____ **E.** A pregnant woman can give the AIDS virus to her unborn baby.

_____ **F.** Most types of birth control also protect against getting the AIDS virus.

_____ **G.** A person must have many different sexual partners to be at risk for AIDS.

_____ **H.** Donating blood carries no AIDS risk for the donor.

_____ **I.** Most people who have AIDS look quite ill.

2. Fill in the blanks.

A. The most common way in which HIV is transmitted is through _____.

B. Symptoms of _____ and _____ may overlap with HIV symptoms, complicating diagnostic and treatment efforts.

C. A major complication of HIV disease is CNS involvement, which results in the clinical condition of _____.

D. _____ causes large, purple, bruise-like blotches on the face, hands, and legs.

3. Provide short answers for the following questions.

A. Describe changes in the incidence of HIV in the United States over the past 10 years. Consider gender, race, age, sexual preference, and socioeconomic status.

B. Briefly describe the three medication treatment classes for HIV discussed in the text. Are there newer ones at this time?

C. Your classmate tells you that she saw a computer printout from the laboratory during her clinical rotation that listed your clinical supervisor as HIV positive. Discuss the issues related to this situation, including potential losses, breaches of confidentiality, and potential stigmatizing reactions. How would you respond?

REFERENCES

Baldewicz T et al: Nutritional contributions to the CNS pathophysiology of HIV-1 infection and implications for treatment, *CNS Spectrums* 5:61, 2000.

Barroso J: Focusing on living: attitudinal approaches of long term survivors of AIDS, *Issues Ment Health Nurs* 17:395,1996.

Bartlett J, Finkbeiner A: *The guide to living with HIV infection,* Baltimore, 1998, Johns Hopkins University Press.

Brown E, Jemmott L: HIV among people with mental illness: contributing factors, prevention needs, barriers, and strategies, *J Psychosoc Nurs* 38:5, 2000.

Centers for Disease Control and Prevention: *HIV/AIDS surveillance report,* Washington, DC, 1999, CDC.

Ezzell C: Care for a dying continent, *Sci Am* 5:96, 2000.

Fauci A: The AIDS epidemic: considerations for the 21st century, *N Engl J Med* 341:1046, 1999.

Kelly J et al: Reduction in risk behavior among adults with severe mental illness who learned to advocate for HIV prevention, *Psychiatr Serv* 48:1283,1997.

Klink B: The patient is HIV positive. Do you protect his caretakers, or his privacy? *Med Econ* D5-K022:2, 1999.

Morris N: Depression and HIV disease: a critical review, *J Am Psychiatr Nurs Assoc* 2:154, 1996.

Phillips K, Morrow J: Nursing management of anxiety in HIV infection, *Issues Ment Health Nurs* 19:375,1998.

Rabkin J et al: A double-blind, placebo-controlled trial of testosterone therapy for HIV-positive men with hypogonadal symptoms, *Arch Gen Psychiatry* 57:141, 2000.

Ruiz P et al: Psychiatric considerations in the diagnosis, treatment, and prevention of HIV/AIDS, *J Psychiatr Pract* 5:129, 2000.

Schulte J: HIV infection: the quintessential biopsychosocial disease. In Kay J, Tasman A, editors: *Psychiatry: behavioral science and clinical essentials,* Philadelphia, 2000, WB Saunders.

Shapshak P et al: Dementia and the neurovirulence of HIV-1, *CNS Spectrums* 5:31, 2000.

Sherman D: Nurses' willingness to care for AIDS patients and spirituality, social support, and death anxiety, *Image J Nurs Sch* 28:205, 1996.

St. Louis M et al, editors: Janus considers the HIV pandemic: harnessing recent advances to enhance AIDS prevention, *Am J Public Health* 87:10, 1997.

Sullivan G et al: HIV and people with serious mental illness: the public sectors role in reducing HIV risk and improving care, *Psychiatric Serv* 50:5, 1999.

Thomas S, Java A: HIV-associated Kaposi's sarcoma, *Hosp Physician* 4:22, 2000.

Tyll M et al: Theory-driven interventions in psychoimmunology and HIV-2 infection, *CNS Spectrums* 5:25, 2000.

Glossary

A

abreaction The release of feelings that takes place as a patient talks about emotionally charged areas.

accountability To be answerable to someone for something, focusing responsibility on the individual for personal actions or lack of actions.

action cues A category of nonverbal communication that consists of body movements and is sometimes called kinetics.

addiction The biological and/or psychosocial behaviors related to substance dependence.

adolescence The period from the beginning of puberty to the attainment of maturity. The transitional stage during which the youth is becoming an adult man or woman. This period is described in terms of development in many different functions that may be reached at different times. Only conventional limits may be stated: 12 to 21 years for girls, 13 to 23 years for boys.

advanced directives Documents, written while a person is competent, that specify how decisions about treatment would be made if the person were to become incompetent.

advanced practice registered nurse (APRN) A licensed RN who has a master's degree and a depth of knowledge of psychiatric nursing theory, supervised clinical practice, and competence in advanced psychiatric nursing skills.

adventitious crisis An accidental, uncommon, and unexpected event that results in multiple losses and major environmental changes.

advocacy Helping people to receive available services and influencing providers to improve existing services and develop new ones.

affect Feeling, mood, or emotional tone.

affective Relating to a person's affect.

agnosia Difficulty recognizing well-known objects.

agonist In pharmacology, a substance that acts with, enhances, or potentiates a specific activity.

agoraphobia Fear of many situations, such as open spaces and the marketplace.

AIDS dementia complex Subcortical encephalopathy characterized by progressive dementia; believed to result primarily from direct infection with HIV.

akathisia A motor restlessness ranging from a feeling of inner disquiet, often localized in the muscles, to an inability to sit still or lie quietly; a side effect of some antipsychotic drugs.

alcohol hallucinosis A medical diagnosis referring to an alcohol withdrawal syndrome that is characterized by auditory hallucinations in the absence of any other psychotic symptoms.

alcohol withdrawal delirium A medical diagnosis for a serious alcohol withdrawal syndrome that is characterized by delirium and autonomic hyperactivity occurring within 1 week of reduction of alcohol intake.

alexithymia Difficulty naming and describing emotions.

altruism A concern for the welfare of others that can be expressed at the level of the individual or the larger social system.

amnesia Significant memory impairment in the absence of clouded consciousness or other cognitive symptoms.

amotivational syndrome A cluster of symptoms apparently related to prolonged marijuana use that includes apathy, lack of energy, loss of desire to work or be productive, diminished concentration, poor personal hygiene, and preoccupation with marijuana.

anaclitic depression A deprivational reaction in infants separated from their mothers in the second half of the first year of life. The reaction is characterized by apprehension, crying, withdrawal, psychomotor slowing, dejection, stupor, insomnia, anorexia, and gross retardation in growth and development.

anhedonia Inability or decreased ability to experience pleasure, joy, intimacy, and closeness.

anorexia nervosa An eating disorder in which the person experiences hunger but refuses to eat because of a distorted body image, leading to a self-perception of fatness. Starvation ensues.

antecedent The stimulus or cue that occurs before behavior that leads to its occurrence.

antisocial personality disorder A disorder occurring in adult patients with a history of conduct disorder; behavior is often characterized by poor work record, disregard for social norms, aggressiveness, financial irresponsibility, impulsiveness, lying, recklessness, inability to maintain close relationships or to meet responsibilities for significant others, and a lack of remorse for harmful behavior.

anxiety A diffuse apprehension vague in nature and associated with feelings of uncertainty and helplessness. It is an emotion without a specific object, is subjectively experienced by the individual, and is communicated interpersonally. It occurs as a result of a threat to the person's being, self-esteem, or identity.

apathy Lack of feelings, emotions, interests, or concern.

aphasia Difficulty finding the right word.

appraisal of stressor An evaluation of the significance of an event for one's well-being that takes place on the cognitive, affective, physiological, behavioral, and social levels.

apraxia Inability or difficulty in performing a purposeful organized task or similar skilled activities.

assertive community treatment An intensive community intervention program, undertaken by case managers with small caseloads and 24-hour responsibility for their patients, in which a multidisciplinary team works with patients in their homes, neighborhoods, and workplaces, providing varying intensities of services, depending on patient need.

assertiveness The midpoint of a continuum that runs from passive to aggressive behavior. Assertive behavior conveys a sense of self-assurance but also communicates respect for the other person.

attention The ability to focus on one activity in a sustained, concentrated manner.

attributions Reasoning processes used to explain events.

autogenic storytelling A therapeutic version of storytelling in which the child participates in creating the story.

autonomy Self-determination that fosters independence and self-regulation; the condition that allows for definition of and control over a domain.

aversion therapy Reduces unwanted but persistent maladaptive behaviors by applying an aversive or noxious stimulus when that maladaptive behavior occurs.

axon The presynaptic part of a neuron.

B

behavior Any observable, recordable, and measurable act, movement, or response.

behavioral Relating to a person's behavior.

bibliotherapy Use of literature to help patients identify and express feelings within the structure and safety of the nurse-patient relationship.

binge eating The rapid consumption of large quantities of food in a discrete period of time.

bioavailability How much of a drug reaches systemic circulation unchanged.

biofeedback The use of a machine to communicate physical changes; used to train a person to reduce anxiety and modify behavioral responses.

biological psychiatry A school of psychiatric thought that emphasizes physical, chemical, and neurological causes and treatment approaches.

bipolar disorder A subgroup of the affective disorders characterized by at least one episode of manic behavior, with or without a history of episodes of depression.

bisexuality A sexual attraction to people of both sexes and the engagement in both homosexual and heterosexual activity.

blood levels The concentration of a drug in the plasma, serum, or blood. In psychiatry the term is most often applied to levels of lithium or some tricyclic antidepressants. Maximum clinical responses to these agents have been correlated with specific ranges of blood levels.

body dysmorphic disorder A somatoform disorder characterized by a normal-appearing person's belief that he or she has a physical defect.

body image Sum of the conscious and unconscious attitudes the person has toward his or her body. It includes present and past perceptions as well as feelings about size, function, appearance, and potential.

borderline personality disorder A specific personality disorder with the essential features of unstable mood, interpersonal relationships, and self-image; characteristic behaviors may include unstable relationships, exploitation of others, impulsive behavior, labile affect, problems expressing anger appropriately, self-destructive behavior, and identity disturbances.

boundary violation When a nurse goes outside the limits of the therapeutic relationship and establishes a social, economic, or personal relationship with a patient.

brain electrical activity mapping (BEAM) Images brain activity and function by using CT techniques to display data derived from EEG recordings of brain electrical activity that has been sensory evoked by specific stimuli or cognitive evoked by specific mental tasks.

bulimia nervosa An eating disorder characterized by uncontrollable binge eating alternating with vomiting or dieting.

C

capitation A funding mechanism in which all defined services for a specific period of time are provided for an agreed-upon payment, payment is tied to the care of a particular person or group, and the provider agrees to be at risk for costs exceeding the agreed-upon amount.

case management Providing services aimed at linking the service system to the patient and coordinating the service components so that the patient can achieve successful community living.

catatonia A stuporous state.

catharsis Release that occurs when the patient is encouraged to talk about things that bother him or her most. Fears, feelings, and experiences are brought out into the open and discussed.

certification A formal review process of clinical practice.

certified specialist A nurse showing a high degree of proficiency in interpersonal skills, the use of the nursing process, and psychological, somatic, and milieu therapies who is prepared at least at the master's level and certified by ANCC.

child abuse Includes physical abuse or battering, emotional abuse, sexual abuse, and neglect. Children who witness family abuse or violence are also victimized.

circadian rhythms The correlation between human activities and behaviors and external environmental stimuli for a 24-hour period.

classical conditioning A theory describing the process by which involuntary behavior is learned, in which an event occurs when one stimulus, by being paired with another stimulus, comes to produce the same response as the other stimulus.

clinical pathway A shortened version of the plan of care for a particular patient that lists key nursing and medical processes and corresponding time lines to which the patient must adhere to achieve standard outcomes within a specified period.

cognition The mental process characterized by knowing, thinking, learning, and judging.

cognitive Relating to a person's cognition.

cognitive distortions Positive or negative distortions of reality that might include errors of logic, mistakes in reasoning, or individualized views of the world that do not reflect reality.

cohesion The strength of group members' desire to work together toward common goals.

collaboration The shared planning, decision making, problem solving, goal setting, and assumption of responsibilities by people who work together cooperatively and with open communication.

collegiality An essential aspect of professional practice that requires that nurses view their peers as collaborators in the caregiving, research, or educational process who are valued and respected for their unique contributions.

command hallucinations Hallucinations that tell the patient to take some specific action, such as to kill oneself, harm another, or join someone in afterlife.

commitment Involuntary admission in which the request for hospitalization did not originate with the patient. When committed, the patient loses the right to leave the hospital when he or she wishes. It is usually justified on the ground that the patient is dangerous to self or others and needs treatment.

communication Process of influencing the behavior of others by sending, receiving, and interpreting messages; feedback and consideration of the context complete the cycle.

community support systems Systems developed by community mental health centers to provide patients with necessary specialized mental health service. Includes such community-based components as crisis response services, health and dental care, rehabilitation services, and protection and advocacy.

compensation Process by which a person makes up for a deficiency in self-image by strongly emphasizing some other feature that the person regards as an asset.

competence building The health education strategy of primary prevention that involves the strengthening of individuals and groups and is based on the assumption that many maladaptive responses result from a lack of competence.

compulsion A recurring irresistible impulse to perform some act.

computed tomography (CT) Depicts brain structure with a series of radiographs that is computer-constructed into "slices" of the brain that can be stacked by the computer, giving a three-dimensional view.

concreteness Use of specific terminology rather than abstractions in the discussion of the patient's feelings, experiences, and behavior.

conduct disorder Disorder with the essential feature of behavior that violates the basic rights of others or societal norms and rules.

confidentiality Non-disclosure of specific information about another unless authorized by that person.

conflict Clashing of two opposing interests. The person experiences two competing drives and must choose between them.

confrontation An expression by the nurse of perceived discrepancies in the patient's behavior. It is an attempt by the nurse to bring to the patient's awareness the incongruence in feelings, attitudes, beliefs, and behaviors.

congruent communication A communication pattern in which the sender is communicating the same message on both the verbal and the nonverbal levels.

consequence The effect (positive, negative, or neutral) of a behavior on the individual.

consultation liaison nursing care Expert psychiatric consultation provided by a psychiatric mental health nurse in various other health-care settings.

context Setting in which an event takes place.

contingency contracting A formal contract between the patient and the therapist defining what behaviors are to be changed and what consequences follow the performance of these behaviors.

conversion disorder A somatoform disorder characterized by a loss or alteration of physical functioning without evidence of organic impairment.

coping mechanism Any effort directed at stress management. It can be problem, cognitive, or emotion focused.

coping resources Characteristics of the person, group, or environment that help people adapt to stress.

countertransference An emotional response of the nurse that is generated by the patient's qualities and is inappropriate to the content and context of the therapeutic relationship or inappropriate in the degree of emotional intensity.

crisis A disturbance caused by a stressful event or a perceived threat to self.

crisis intervention Short-term therapy focused on solving the immediate problem and allowing the patient to return to a precrisis level of function.

cultural sensitivity The ability to view each patient as a unique person, fully considering the patient's cultural experiences within the context of the common developmental challenges faced by all people.

culture-bound syndrome Recurrent, locality-specific patterns of aberrant behavior and troubling experience that may or may not be linked to a particular *DSM–IV–TR* diagnostic category.

cytochrome P-450 inhibition Some drugs, such as some SSRIs and TCAs, inhibit this liver enzyme, causing potentially dangerous changes in the metabolism of many drugs.

D

debriefing Therapeutic intervention that includes reviewing the facts related to an event and processing the response to them.

decatastrophizing Helping patients to evaluate whether they are overestimating the catastrophic nature of a situation.

decision making Arriving at a solution or making a choice.

defense mechanisms Coping mechanisms of the ego that attempt to protect the person from feelings of inadequacy and worthlessness and prevent awareness of anxiety. They are primarily unconscious and involve a degree of self-deception and reality distortion.

deinstitutionalization At the patient level, the transfer to a community setting of a patient hospitalized for an extended time, generally many years; at the mental health care system level, a shift in the focus of care from the large, long-term institution to the community, accomplished by discharging long-term patients and avoiding unnecessary admissions.

delinquency A minor violation of legal or moral codes, especially by children or adolescents. Juvenile delinquency is such behavior by a young person (usually younger than 16 or 18 years of age) that brings him or her to the attention of a court.

delirium The medical diagnostic term that describes an organic mental disorder characterized by a cluster of cognitive impairments with an acute onset and the identification of a specific precipitating stressor.

delirium tremens A medical diagnostic term that has been replaced with the diagnosis of alcohol withdrawal delirium.

delusion A false belief that is firmly maintained even though it is not shared by others and is contradicted by social reality.

dementia The medical diagnostic term that describes an organic mental disorder characterized by a cluster of cognitive impairments that are generally of gradual onset and irreversible. The predisposing and precipitating stressors may or may not be identifiable.

dendrite The postsynaptic part of a neuron.

denial Avoidance of disagreeable realities by ignoring or refusing to recognize them.

depersonalization A feeling of unreality and alienation from oneself. One has difficulty distinguishing self from others, and one's body has an unreal or strange quality about it. The subjective experience of the partial or total disruption of one's ego and the disintegration and disorganization of one's self-concept.

depression An abnormal extension or overelaboration of sadness and grief. The word depression can denote a variety of phenomena, a sign, symptom, syndrome, emotional state, reaction, disease, or clinical entity.

detoxification The removal of a toxic substance from the body, either naturally through physiological process, such as hepatic or renal functions, or medically by the introduction of alternative substances and gradual withdrawal.

differentiated practice Distinguishing among professionals with role descriptions and functional assignments based on education, experience, and competency; responsibilities reflect each person's unique knowledge base.

differentiation Sufficient separation between intellect and emotions so that one is not dominated by the reactive anxiety of the family's emotional system.

direct self-destructive behavior (DSDB) Suicidal behavior.

disadvantagement The lack of socioeconomic resources that are basic to biopsychosocial adaptation.

discrimination Differential treatment of individuals or groups not based on actual merit.

disengaged A transactional style in a family reflecting inappropriately rigid boundaries requiring a high level of individual stress to activate family response.

displacement Shift of an emotion from the person or object toward which it was originally directed to another, usually neutral or less dangerous person or object.

dissociation The separation of any group of mental or behavioral processes from the rest of the person's consciousness or identity.

diurnal mood variation Changes in mood that are related to the time of day.

double bind Simultaneous communication of conflicting messages in the context of a situation that does not allow escape. (See *incongruent communication*.)

drug interaction The effects of two or more drugs being taken simultaneously, producing an alteration in the usual effects of either drug taken alone. The interacting drugs may have a potentiating or additive effect, and serious side effects may result.

drug tolerance Repeated use of some substance or drug (such as narcotics) so that larger and larger doses are required to produce the same physiological or psychological effect.

drug trial The time it takes to administer a drug at adequate therapeutic doses for a long enough period to determine its efficacy for a particular patient. The trial culminates with acceptable clinical results, intolerable adverse effects, or poor response after an appropriate blood level is reached for an appropriate period of time.

DSM–IV–TR Commonly used abbreviation for the *Diagnostic and Statistical Manual of Mental Disorders*, which contains standard nomenclature of emotional illness used by all health-care practitioners. *DSM–IV–TR* is a text revision of the version published in 1994; it updates and classifies mental illnesses and presents guidelines and diagnostic criteria for various mental disorders.

dual diagnosis Simultaneous occurrence of a mental illness and a substance abuse disorder.

dyspareunia Recurrent or persistent genital pain occurring before, during, or after intercourse (male or female).

dystonia Acute tonic muscle spasms, often of the tongue, jaw, eyes, and neck but sometimes of the whole body. Sometimes occurs during the first few days of antipsychotic drug administration.

E

echopraxia Purposeless imitation of other's movements.

ego defense mechanisms See *defense mechanisms*.

ego fusion When the self borrows on the functioning of another person, and self-boundaries are blurred.

elder abuse A variety of behaviors that threaten the health, comfort, and possibly the lives of elderly people, including physical and emotional neglect, emotional abuse, violation of personal rights, financial abuse, and direct physical abuse.

electroconvulsive therapy (ECT) Artificial induction of a grand mal seizure by passing a controlled electrical current through electrodes applied to one or both temples. The patient is anesthetized and the seizure attenuated by administration of a muscle relaxant medication.

empathy Ability to view the patient's world from his or her internal frame of reference. It involves the nurse's sensitivity to the patient's current feelings and the verbal ability to communicate this understanding in a language attuned to the patient.

enabler The role that is often assumed by the significant others of substance abusers, characterized by covert support of the substance-abusing behavior.

encounter group therapy An application of the existential model of psychiatric care in a group setting. The focus is on here-and-now experience and the expression of real feelings, verbally and nonverbally, as members react to events in the group.

endogenous Developing or originating within the organism or arising from causes within the organism.

enmeshed A transactional style in a family reflecting diffuse subsystem boundaries, resulting in stress in one family member that emotionally reverberates quickly and intensely throughout the family system.

ethic A standard of behavior or a belief valued by an individual or group.

ethical dilemma Exists when moral claims conflict with one another, resulting in a difficult problem that seems to have no satisfactory solution because of the existence of a choice between equally unsatisfactory alternatives.

ethnicity A person's racial, national, tribal, linguistic, or cultural origin or background.

evidence based practice The ability to examine nursing practice patterns, evaluate the nature of the data supporting them, and demonstrate sound clinical decision making in a way that can be empirically supported.

exhibitionism Intense sexual arousal or desire and acts, fantasies, or other stimuli involving exposing one's genitals to an unsuspecting stranger.

existential (therapy) A school of philosophical thought that focuses on the importance of experience in the present and the belief that humans find meaning in life through their experiences.

exogenous Developing or originating outside the organism.

extinction The process of eliminating the occurrence of a behavior by ignoring or not rewarding that behavior.

extrapyramidal syndrome (EPS) A variety of signs and symptoms, including muscular rigidity, tremors, drooling, shuffling gait (Parkinsonism); restlessness (akathisia); peculiar involuntary postures (dystonia); motor inertia (akinesia); and many other neurological disturbances. Results from dysfunction of the extrapyramidal system. May occur as a reversible side effect of certain psychotropic drugs, particularly antipsychotics.

F

failure to thrive A syndrome consisting of weight loss, decreased appetite, poor nutrition, and inactivity.

family A group of people living in a household who are attached emotionally, interact regularly, and share concerns for the growth and development of individuals and the family.

family burden The impact of a family member's mental illness on the entire family.

family preservation Intensive home treatment modality for troubled youths and their families.

family projection process Transmission of anxiety of one or both parents onto a target child, establishing an overly protective or conflictual relationship with the child and resulting ultimately in impairment of the child.

family violence A range of behaviors occurring between family members, including physical and emotional abuse of children, child neglect, spouse battering, marital rape, and elder abuse.

fetishism Intense sexual arousal or desire and acts, fantasies, or other stimuli involving nonliving objects by themselves.

flight of ideas Overproductive speech characterized by rapid shifting from one topic to another and fragmented ideas.

flooding Exposure therapy in which the patient is immediately exposed to the most anxiety-provoking stimuli.

Food and Drug Administration (FDA) One of a number of health administrations under the assistant secretary of health of the U.S. Department of Health and Human Services to set standards for, to license the sale of, and in general to safeguard the public from the use of dangerous drugs and food substances.

free association The verbalization of thoughts as they occur, without any conscious screening or censorship.

frotteurism Intense sexual arousal or desire and acts, fantasies, or other stimuli involving rubbing against a nonconsenting person.

fusion A blurring of self-boundaries in a highly reactive emotional relationship with another.

G

gender identity A person's perception of one's maleness or femaleness.

gender role The cultural role characteristics attributed to one's gender, such as expectations regarding behavior, cognitions, occupations, values, and emotional responses.

genetic identity A person's chromosomal gender.

genogram A structured method of gathering family information and graphically symbolizing factual and emotional relationship data.

genuineness A quality of the nurse characterized by openness, honesty, and sincerity. The nurse is self-congruent and authentic and relates to the patient without a defensive facade.

Gestalt therapy A therapeutic approach based on the existential model of psychiatric care. It was developed by Perls and focuses on the development of enhanced self-awareness.

glial cells Support cells that form myelin sheaths; thought to remove excess transmitters and ions from the extracellular spaces in the brain, provide glucose to some nerve cells, and direct the flow of blood and oxygen to various parts of the brain.

grief A person's subjective response to the loss of a person, object, or concept that is highly valued. Uncomplicated grief is a healthy, adaptive, reparative response.

group A collection of people who have a relationship with one another, are interdependent, and may have common norms.

H

habeas corpus A right retained by all psychiatric patients that provides for the release of a person who claims that he or she is being deprived of liberty and detained illegally. The hearing for this determination takes place in a court of law, and the patient's sanity is at issue.

half-life The amount of time it takes the body to excrete approximately half of an ingested drug; after this time the effects of the drug usually begin to deteriorate.

hallucination Perceptual distortion arising from any of the five senses.

hallucinogens A class of abused drugs that cause a psychotic-like experience.

hardiness A measurement of a person's psychological capability to resist illness when faced with a stressful life event.

health education A teaching strategy related to health issues that involves the strengthening of individuals and groups through competence building.

heterosexuality Sexual attraction to members of the opposite sex.

HIV disease Describes all of the disorders resulting from infection with the human immunodeficiency virus.

home health care Delivery of health services in the home, including mental health services.

homophobia Persistent and irrational fear of homosexuals along with a negative attitude and hostility toward them.

homosexuality Sexual attraction to members of the same sex.

hypersomnia Disorders of excessive somnolence.

hypochondriasis A somatoform disorder characterized by the belief that one is ill without evidence of organic impairment, involving somatic overconcern with and morbid attention to details of body functioning.

hypomania A clinical syndrome that is similar to but less severe than that described by the term *mania* or *manic episode.*

hypoxia Inadequate oxygen at the cellular level, characterized by cyanosis, tachycardia, hypertension, peripheral vasoconstriction, dizziness, and mental confusion.

I

ideas of reference Incorrect interpretation of casual incidents and external events as having direct personal references.

identification Process by which a person tries to become like someone else whom he or she admires by taking on the thoughts, mannerisms, or tastes of that person.

identity Organizing principle of the personality system that accounts for the unity, continuity, uniqueness, and consistency of the personality. It is the awareness of the process of being oneself that is derived from self-observation and judgment. It is the synthesis of all self-representations into an organized whole.

identity confusion Lack of clarity and consistency in one's perception of the self, resulting in a high degree of anxiety.

identity diffusion A person's failure to integrate various childhood identifications into a harmonious adult psychosocial identity.

identity foreclosure Premature adoption of an identity that is desired by significant others without coming to terms with one's own desires, aspirations, or potential.

illusions False perceptions of or false responses to a sensory stimulus.

immediacy State that occurs when the current interaction of the nurse and the patient is the focus.

impulsivity A maladaptive social behavior characterized by unpredictability, unreliability, inability to plan or learn from experience, and overall poor judgment.

incompetency A legal status that must be proved in a special court hearing. As a result of the hearing, the person is determined incapable of making important decisions about himself or herself, and can thus be deprived of many civil rights. Incompetency can be reversed only in another court hearing that declares the person competent.

incongruent communication A communication pattern in which the sender is communicating a different message on the verbal and nonverbal levels and the listener does not know to which level he or she should respond. (See *double bind.*)

indirect self-destructive behavior (ISDB) Any activity that is detrimental to the person's well-being and could cause death, accompanied by lack of conscious awareness of the self-destructive nature of the behavior.

informed consent Disclosure of a certain amount of information to the patient about the proposed treatment and the attainment of the patient's consent, which must be competent, understanding, and voluntary.

insanity defense Legal defense proposing that a person who has committed an act that in a usual situation would be criminal should be held not guilty by reason of "insanity."

insight The patient's understanding of the nature of the problem or illness.

insomnia Disorder of initiating or maintaining sleep.

intellectualization Excessive reasoning or logic used to avoid experiencing disturbing feelings.

interdisciplinary team A team with members of different disciplines involved in a formal arrangement to provide patient services while maximizing educational interchange.

introjection An intense type of identification in which one incorporates qualities or values of another person or group into one's own ego structure.

K

Kaposi's sarcoma A malignant, multifocal neoplasm of reticuloendothelial cells that begins as soft, brownish or purple papules in the skin and slowly spreads; associated with AIDS.

L

learned helplessness A behavioral state and personality trait of people who believe they are ineffectual, their responses are futile, and they have lost control over the reinforcers in the environment.

lethality An estimation of the probability that a person who is threatening suicide will succeed on the basis of the method described, the specificity of the plan, and the availability of the means.

libido Freud's term for psychic energy.

life review Progressive return to consciousness of past experiences.

limbic system An area in the brain associated with the control of emotion and memory.

limit setting Nonpunitive, nonmanipulative act in which the patient is told what behavior is acceptable, what is not acceptable, and the consequences of behaving unacceptably.

living will Determining in advance one's participation in heroic measures during the dying process.

logotherapy An approach to psychotherapy based on the existential model and developed by Frankl. The focus is on the search for meaning in present experiences.

loose associations Lack of a logical relationship between thoughts and ideas that renders speech and thought inexact, vague, diffuse, and unfocused.

M

magical thinking Belief that thinking equates with doing, characterized by lack of realistic understanding of cause and effect.

magnetic resonance imaging (MRI) Depicts brain structure using a magnetic field that surrounds the head and induces brain tissues to emit radio waves that are then computerized for clear and detailed construction of sections of the brain.

malingering Deliberate feigning of an illness.

malpractice Failure of a professional person to give the type of proper and competent care provided by members of his or her profession. This failure causes harm to the patient.

mania A condition characterized by a mood that is elevated, expansive, or irritable. It is a component of bipolar illness.

manipulation A maladaptive social response in which people treat others as objects, enter relationships that are centered around control issues, and are self-oriented or goal oriented rather than other oriented.

masochism Intense sexual arousal or desire and acts, fantasies, or other stimuli involving being humiliated, beaten, bound, or otherwise made to suffer (real or simulated).

maturational crisis A developmental event requiring a role change.

medical diagnosis A physician's or advanced practice nurse's independent judgment of the patient's health problems or disease states.

memory The retention or storage of knowledge learned about the world.

mental health Indicators of mental health include positive attitudes toward self, growth, development, self-actualization, integration, autonomy, reality perception, and environmental mastery.

mental status examination Represents a cross-section of the patient's psychological life and the sum total of the nurse's observations and impressions at the moment, serving as a basis for future comparison to track the progress of the patient.

message A unit of communication.

methadone maintenance A treatment program in which methadone is given to a patient recovering from heroin abuse to prevent the characteristic withdrawal symptoms, as methadone substitutes for the heroin without causing withdrawal symptoms or impaired functioning.

modeling Strategy used to form new behavior patterns, increase existing skills, or reduce avoidance behavior in which the patient observes a person modeling adaptive behavior and is then encouraged to imitate it.

mood The patient's self-report of prevailing emotional state and a reflection of the patient's life situation.

mourning Includes all the psychological processes set in motion by a loss. The process of mourning is resolved only when the lost object is internalized, bonds of attachment are loosened, and new object relationships are established.

multidisciplinary team A team with members of different disciplines, each providing specific services to the patient.

multigenerational transmission process The repetition of relationship patterns and anxiety associated with toxic issues passed through generations in a family.

multiple personality disorder The existence within an individual of two or more distinct personalities or personality states, with each having its own pattern of perceiving, feeling, and thinking.

myelin sheath Provides insulation to the cells of the nervous system. (See *glial cells*.)

N

narcissism A maladaptive social response characterized by egocentric attitude, fragile self-esteem, constant seeking of praise and admiration, and envy.

narcissistic personality disorder A specific personality disorder having the essential features of a pattern of grandiosity, lack of empathy, and hypersensitivity to the evaluation of others, beginning in early adulthood; characteristic behaviors may include rageful reactions to criticism, exploitation of others, inability to recognize how others feel, sense of entitlement, envy, belief that one's problems are unique, preoccupation with grandiose fantasies, and search for constant attention and admiration.

narcolepsy A condition characterized by brief attacks of deep sleep.

National Institute of Mental Health (NIMH) Responsible for programs dealing with mental health, NIMH is an institute under the U.S. Department of Health and Human Services that provides leadership, policies, and goals for the federal effort to ensure the treatment and rehabilitation of people with alcohol, drug abuse, and mental health problems; this agency is also responsible for administering grants to support research, training, and service programs.

negative identity Assumption of an identity that is at odds with the accepted values and expectations of society.

negative reinforcement Increases the frequency of a behavior by reinforcing the behavior's power to control an aversive stimulus.

neologisms New word or words created by the patient; often a blend of other words.

neurosis Category of health problems distinguished by the following characteristics: recognized by the person as unacceptable, reality testing is intact, behavior is overall consistent with social norms, problem is enduring or recurrent, and there is no apparent organic cause.

neurotransmission The process whereby neurons communicate with each other through chemical messengers called neurotransmitters.

neurotransmitters Chemical messengers of the nervous system, manufactured in one neuron and released from the axon into the synapse and received by the dendrite of the next neuron.

nihilistic ideas Thoughts of nonexistence and hopelessness.

noncompliance The failure of a patient to carry out the self-care activities prescribed in a health-care plan.

nonverbal communication Transmission of a message without the use of words. It involves all five senses.

norms Standards of behavior.

nuclear family emotional system Patterns of interaction between family members and the degree to which these patterns promote fusion.

nursing diagnosis A nurse's judgment of the patient's behavioral response to stress. It is a statement of the patient's problems, which may be overt, covert, existing, or potential, and includes the behavioral disruption or threatened disruption, the contributing stressors, and the adaptive or maladaptive health responses.

nursing process An interactive, problem-solving process; a systematic and individualized way to achieve the outcomes of nursing care. The phases of the nursing process as described by the *Standards of Psychiatric–Mental Health Clinical Nursing Practice* are assessment, diagnosis, outcome identification, planning, implementation, and evaluation.

O

object cues A category of nonverbal communication that includes the speaker's intentional and unintentional use of all objects, such as dress, furnishings, and possessions.

obsession An idea, emotion, or impulse that repetitively and insistently forces itself into consciousness; unwanted, but cannot be voluntarily excluded from consciousness.

operant conditioning A theory concerned with the relationship between voluntary behavior and the environment that states that behaviors are influenced by their consequences and that operant behaviors are cued by environmental stimuli.

orgasm Peaking of sexual pleasure and the release of sexual tension accompanied by rhythmic contractions of the perineal muscles and pelvic reproductive organs.

outreach clinical services Delivery of health services in which health workers reach out to patients wherever they are in the community.

P

pain disorder A preoccupation with pain in the absence of physical disease to account for its intensity.

panic An attack of extreme anxiety that involves the disorganization of the personality. Distorted perceptions, loss of rational thought, and inability to communicate and function are evident.

paraphilia Characterized by sexual arousal in response to objects or situations that are not normally arousing for affectionate sexual activities with human partners (such as pedophilia, exhibitionism, or zoophilia).

parasomnia Disorder associated with sleep stages, such as sleepwalking, night terrors, nightmares, and enuresis.

patient classification system Designed to determine the amount or intensity of nursing services needed by each patient based on patient acuity or severity of illness.

pedophilia Intense sexual arousal or desire and acts, fantasies, or other stimuli involving children 13 years of age or younger.

perception Identification and initial interpretation of a stimulus based on information received through the five senses of sight, hearing, taste, touch, and smell.

perseveration Involuntary, excessive continuation or repetition of a single response, idea, or activity; may apply to speech or movement, but most often verbal.

personality fusion A person's attempt to establish a sense of self by fusing or belonging to someone else.

pharmacodynamics The study of the effects of the drug on the body, particularly the interaction of the drug on the targeted receptor site.

pharmacokinetics The study of the process and rates of drug absorption, metabolism, distribution, and excretion in the organism.

phobia A morbid fear associated with extreme anxiety.

phototherapy Light therapy that consists of exposing patients to artificial therapeutic lights about 5 to 20 times brighter than indoor lighting and more consistent with the light spectrum of natural sunlight.

physical abuse Harm or threatened harm to a person's health or welfare that occurs through nonaccidental physical or mental injury, sexual abuse, or maltreatment.

physical dependence A characteristic of drug addiction that is present when withdrawal of the drug results in physiological disruptions.

polypharmacy Use of combinations of psychoactive drugs in a patient at the same time without determining whether one drug by itself is effective; can cause drug interactions, and may increase the incidence of adverse reactions.

positive reinforcement Increases the frequency of a behavior by reinforcing the behavior's power to achieve a rewarding stimulus.

positron emission tomography (PET) Depicts brain activity and function using an injected radioactive substance that travels to the brain and shows up as a bright spot on the scan; different substances are taken up by the brain in different amounts depending on the type of tissue and activity level.

postpartum blues Brief episodes lasting 1 to 4 days of labile mood and tearfulness that occur in about 50% to 80% of women within 1 to 5 days of delivery.

postvention Therapeutic intervention with the significant others of a person who has committed suicide.

power The member's ability to influence the group and its other members.

precipitating stressors Stimuli that the person perceives as challenging, threatening, or harmful. They require the use of excess energy and produce a state of tension and stress.

predisposing factors Conditioning factors that influence both the type and the amount of resources that the person can elicit to cope with stress. They may be biological, psychological, or sociocultural.

prejudice A preconceived, unfavorable belief about individuals or groups that disregards knowledge, thought, or reason.

premature ejaculation Ejaculation that occurs with minimal sexual stimulation or before, on, or shortly after penetration and before the person wishes it.

primary prevention Biological, social, or psychological intervention that promotes health and well-being or reduces the incidence of illness in a community by altering the causative factors before they have an opportunity to do harm.

projection Attributing one's own thoughts or impulses to another person. Through this process the person can attribute intolerable wishes, emotional feelings, or motivations to another person.

pseudodementia A depressive condition of the elderly characterized by impaired cognitive function.

psychiatric nursing An interpersonal process that strives to promote and maintain patient behavior that contributes to integrated functioning. It uses the theories of human behavior as its science and the purposeful use of self as its art. Psychiatric nursing is directed toward both preventive and corrective effects on mental disorders and their sequelae and is concerned with the promotion of optimum mental health for society, the community, and individuals.

psychoanalysis A therapeutic approach based on the belief that behavioral disorders are related to unresolved, anxiety-provoking childhood experiences that are repressed into the unconscious. The goal of psychoanalysis is to bring repressed experiences into conscious awareness and to learn healthier means of coping with the related anxiety.

psychobiological resilience A concept that proposes that there is a recurrent human need to weather periods of stress and change throughout life. The ability to weather successfully each period of disruption and reintegration leaves the person better able to deal with the next change.

psychoeducation The teaching of a patient and family about the mental illness and the coping skills that will help with successful community living.

psychological autopsy A retrospective review of the person's behavior for the time preceding death by suicide.

psychological dependence A characteristic of drug addiction that is manifested in a craving for the abused substance and a fear that it will not be available in the future.

psychological factors affecting physical condition A category of psychophysiological disruptions in which organic impairment is evident. Examples include migraine headache, asthma, hypertension, colitis, and duodenal ulcer.

psychoneuroimmunology The scientific field exploring the relationship between psychological states and the immune response.

psychopharmacology Drugs that treat the symptoms of mental illness and whose actions in the brain provide us with models to better understand the mechanisms of mental disorders.

psychosis A category of health problems that are distinguished by regressive behavior, personality disintegration, reduced level of awareness, great difficulty in functioning adequately, and gross impairment in reality testing.

punishment Decreases the frequency of a behavior by causing an aversive stimulus to occur after that behavior.

purging A variety of maladaptive behaviors intended to prevent weight gain, including vomiting, excessive exercise, and use of diuretics, diet pills, laxatives, and steroids.

Q

quality improvement The process of evaluating treatment outcomes in clinical settings, usually monitored by an interdisciplinary body.

R

racism The belief that inherent differences between races determine individual achievement and that one race is superior over others.

rational-emotive therapy (RET) A therapeutic approach based on the existential model of psychiatric care and developed by Ellis. The emphasis is on risk taking and the assumption of responsibility for one's behavior.

rationalization Offering a socially acceptable or apparently logical explanation to justify or make acceptable otherwise unacceptable impulses, feelings, behaviors, and motives.

reaction formation Development of conscious attitudes and behavior patterns that are opposite to what one really would like to have.

reality orientation Formal process of keeping a person alert to events in the here and now.

reality therapy A therapeutic approach based on the existential model of psychiatric care developed by Glasser. The focus is on recognition and accomplishment of life goals, with emphasis on development of the capacity for caring.

receptor A specialized area on a nerve membrane, blood vessel, or muscle that receives the chemical stimulation that activates or inhibits normal action of the nerve, blood vessel, or muscle.

recurrence Return of a new episode of illness.

reframing To change the conceptual or emotional viewpoint in how a situation is experienced and to place it in a different frame that fits the "facts" of the concrete situation equally well; this changes the situation's entire meaning. Attributing positive motivations behind undesirable behavior often constitutes reframing.

regression A retreat in the face of stress to behavior that is characteristic of an earlier level of development.

rehabilitation The process of enabling a mentally ill person to return to the highest possible level of functioning.

relapse Return of symptoms.

relaxation response A protective mechanism against stress that brings about decreased heart rate, lower metabolism, and decreased respiratory rate. It is the physiological opposite of the fight-or-flight, or anxiety, response.

relaxation training Training a person to relax and thus reduce anxiety. Procedures include rhythmic breathing, reduced muscle tension, and an altered state of consciousness.

reminiscence Thinking about or relating past experiences, especially those that are personally significant.

remission Occurs when a patient is symptom-free at the end of a phase of pre-illness functioning, which generally lasts 6 to 12 weeks.

repression Involuntary exclusion of a painful or conflictual thought, impulse, or memory from awareness. It is the primary ego defense, and other mechanisms tend to reinforce it.

residual Remaining, or left behind; the symptoms that remain after treatment has reached its maximum effect.

resistance Attempt of the patient to remain unaware of anxiety-producing aspects within the self. Ambivalent attitudes toward self-exploration in which the patient both appreciates and avoids anxiety-producing experiences that are a normal part of the therapeutic process.

respect An attitude of the nurse that conveys caring for, liking, and valuing the patient. The nurse regards the patient as a person of worth and accepts the patient without qualification.

response Improvement with treatment.

response cost Decreases the frequency of a behavior through the experience of a loss or penalty following the behavior.

response prevention Patient is encouraged to face a particular fear or situation without engaging in the accompanying behavior.

restraint The use of mechanical or manual devices to limit the physical mobility of the patient.

reuptake The process of neurotransmitters returning to the presynaptic cell after communication with receptor cells.

risk management Assessment of activities related to situations that could result in legal action involving patients, families, the hospital, or the health-care provider.

role playing Acting out of a particular situation. It functions to increase the person's insight into human relations and can deepen one's ability to see a situation from another point of view.

role strain Stress associated with expected roles or positions and experienced as frustration.

roles Set of socially expected behavior patterns associated with one person's function in various social groups. Roles provide a means for social participation and a way to test identities for consensual validation by significant others.

room program A titration of the amount of time patients are allowed in the unit milieu, with patients asked to stay in their rooms for certain lengths of time, and conversely allowed out of their rooms for a specific amount of time.

S

sadism Intense sexual arousal or desire and acts, fantasies, or other stimuli involving the infliction of real or simulated psychological or physical suffering (including humiliation).

schizoaffective disorder Diagnosis given to a patient who meets the diagnostic criteria for schizophrenia as well as one or both of the major mood disorders of bipolar disorder and major depression.

seasonal affective disorder (SAD) Depression that comes with shortened daylight in winter and fall and that disappears during spring and summer.

seclusion Separating the patient from others in a safe, contained environment with minimal stimulation.

secondary prevention A type of prevention that seeks to reduce the prevalence of illness by interventions that provide for early detection and treatment of problems.

self-actualization Process of fulfilling one's potential.

self-concept All the notions, beliefs, and convictions that constitute a person's knowledge of self and influence relationships with others.

self-disclosure Revelation that occurs when a person reveals information about self, ideas, values, feelings, and attitudes.

self-esteem The person's judgment of personal worth obtained by analyzing how well his or her behavior conforms to self-ideal.

self-help groups Groups composed of members who organize to solve their own problems; the members share a common experience, work together toward a common goal, and use their strengths to gain control over their lives.

self-ideal The person's perception of how he or she should behave on the basis of certain personal standards. The standard may be either a carefully constructed image of the type of person one would like to be or merely various aspirations, goals, or values that one would like to achieve.

self-inflicted injury The act of deliberate harm to one's own body.

sensory integration A category of perceptual behaviors including pain recognition, stereognosis, graphesthesia, right/left recognition, and recognition and perception of faces.

serotonin syndrome Hyperserotonergic state (confusion, autonomic dysfunction, muscle rigidity, ataxia) that occurs when SSRIs are given concurrently with other serotonin-enhancing drugs, causing an excess of serotonin in the system.

sexual abuse The involvement of children, adolescents, and adults in sexual activities that they do not fully comprehend and/or to which they cannot or do not fully consent.

sexual assault Forced perpetration of an act of sexual contact with another person without consent.

sexual orientation The gender to which one is romantically attracted.

shaping Introduces new behaviors by reinforcing behaviors that approximate the desired behavior.

situational crisis Occurs when a life event upsets an individual's or group's psychological equilibrium.

sleep deprivation therapy A possible therapy for depressed and bipolar patients based on reports that as many as 60% of depressed patients improve immediately after a night of sleep deprivation.

social skills training Teaching smooth social functioning to those who do not manifest social skills, using the principles of guidance, demonstration, practice, and feedback, resulting in the acquisition of behaviors that will support community living.

somatization disorder A somatoform disorder characterized by multiple physical complaints with no evidence of organic impairment.

somatoform disorder A category of psychophysiological disruptions with no evidence of organic impairment.

splitting Viewing people and situations as either all good or all bad. Failure to integrate the positive and negative qualities of oneself and of objects.

steady state Exists when the body has reached a state of drug level equilibrium: a drug has been taken long enough that the amount of drug excreted equals the amount ingested. This occurs in approximately four to six half-lives.

stereotype A depersonalized conception of individuals within a group.

stigma An attribute or trait deemed by the person's social environment as negative, different, and diminishing.

sublimation Acceptance of a socially approved substitute goal for a drive whose normal channel of expression is blocked.

substance abuse The use of any mind-altering agent to such an extent that it interferes with the person's biological, psychological, or sociocultural integrity.

substance dependence A severe condition of addictive behaviors often resulting in physical problems as well as serious disruptions of work, family life, and social life; usually considered a disease.

subsystems Smaller components of the larger system composed of individuals or dyads, formed by generation, gender, interest, or function.

suicide Self-inflicted death.

suicide attempt A deliberate action that, if carried to completion, will result in death.

suicide gesture A suicide attempt that is planned to be discovered in an attempt to influence the behavior of others and to indirectly seek help.

suicide threat A warning—direct or indirect, verbal or nonverbal—that the person plans to attempt suicide.

sundowning syndrome Cognitive ability diminishing in the late afternoon or early evening.

sunrise syndrome Unstable cognitive ability upon rising in the morning.

supervision Guidance provided through a mentoring relationship between one nurse and a more experienced, skilled, and educated nurse.

suppression A process that is the conscious analogy of repression. It is the intentional exclusion of material from consciousness.

synapse The gap between the membrane of one neuron and the membrane of another. The synapse is the point at which the transmission of nerve impulses occurs.

systematic desensitization Designed to decrease avoidance behavior linked to a specific stimulus by helping the patient change the response to a threatening stimulus.

T

tardive dyskinesia Literally, "late-appearing abnormal movements," a variable complex of choreiform or athetoid movements developing in patients exposed to antipsychotic drugs. Typical movements include tongue writhing or protrusion; chewing; lip puckering; choreiform finger movements; toe and ankle movements; leg jiggling; and movements of neck, trunk, and pelvis.

target symptoms Symptoms of an illness that are most likely to respond to a specific treatment, such as a particular psychopharmacological drug.

tertiary prevention Rehabilitative measures designed to reduce the severity, disability, or residual impairment resulting from illness.

testamentary capacity Competency to make a will, which requires that people know they are making a will, the nature and extent of their property, and who their friends and relatives are.

testimonial privilege A term used in court-related proceedings to refer to the communication between two parties. The right to reveal information belongs to the person who spoke, and the listener cannot disclose the information unless the speaker gives permission. This includes communication between husband and wife, attorney and patient, and clergy and church member.

themes Underlying issues or problems experienced by the patient that emerge repeatedly during the course of the nurse-patient relationship.

therapeutic community The inpatient environment described as a community with cultural norms for behaviors, values, and activity.

therapeutic impasses Roadblocks in the progress of the nurse-patient relationship. They arise for a variety of reasons and may take different forms, but they all create stalls in the therapeutic relationship.

therapeutic milieu The controlled environment of treatment facilities that shelters patients from what they perceive to be painful and frightening stressors, thus providing patients with a stable and coherent social environment that facilitates the development and implementation of treatment.

therapeutic nurse-patient relationship A mutual learning experience and corrective emotional experience for the patient in which the nurse uses self and specified clinical techniques in working with the patient to bring about behavioral change.

therapeutic touch The nurse's laying of hands on or close to the body of an ill person for the purpose of helping or healing.

thought blocking Sudden stopping in the train of thought or in the midst of a sentence.

thought stopping Teaching a patient to interrupt dysfunctional thoughts.

time-out Short-term removal of the patient from overstimulating and sometimes reinforcing situations.

token economy A form of positive reinforcement in which patients are rewarded with tokens, which they can use for desired purchases or activities, for performing desired target behaviors.

tolerance A characteristic of some potentially addictive drugs that refers to the progressive need for more of the drug to achieve the desired effect.

transactional analysis A model of communication developed by Eric Berne that consists of the study of the communication or transactions between people and the sometimes unconscious and destructive ways ("games") in which people relate to each other.

transference An unconscious response of patients in which they experience feelings and attitudes toward the nurse that were originally associated with significant figures in their early life.

transsexual A person who is anatomically a male or female but who expresses, with strong conviction, that he or she has the mind and emotions of the opposite sex, lives as a member of the opposite sex part time or full time, and seeks to change his or her sex legally and through hormonal and surgical sex reassignment.

transvestism Condition in which a male (less often a female) has a sexual obsession for or addiction to women's (men's) clothes.

triangle A predictable emotional process that takes place when there is difficulty in a relationship. Triangles represent dysfunctional efforts to reduce fusion or conflict in a relationship. The three corners of a triangle can be composed of three people, or two people and an object, group, or issue.

U

undoing An act or communication that partially negates a previous one.

unidisciplinary team A team with members of the same discipline.

unipolar depression Patients with an affective disorder who only have had recurrent episodes of depression and no history of manic episodes.

utilization review A three-part process intended to ensure that resources are appropriately used. It includes a review of the initial request to hospitalize the patient, the length of the patient's stay, and a retrospective review after discharge.

V

vaginismus Recurrent or persistent involuntary spasm of the musculature of the outer third of the vagina that interferes with coitus.

validation Reflection of the content of the patient's communication back to the patient.

value clarification A method whereby a person can assess, explore, and determine personal values and what priority they hold in personal decision making.

values The concepts that a person holds worthy in personal life. They are formed as a result of one's life experiences with family, friends, culture, education, work, and relaxation.

visualization The conscious programming of desired change with positive images.

vocal communication Spoken transmission of a message.

vocal cues A category of nonverbal communication that includes all the noises and sounds other than speech. They are sometimes called paralinguistic cues.

voyeurism Intense sexual arousal or desire and acts, fantasies, or other stimuli involving the observation of unsuspecting people who are naked, in the act of disrobing, or engaging in sexual activity.

W

wife abuse Includes all forms of emotional and/or physical violence toward a female partner in an ongoing intimate relationship, as well as emotional degradation and intimidation.

withdrawal symptoms Result from a biological need that develops when the body becomes adapted to having an addictive drug or substance in the system. Characteristic symptoms occur when the level of the substance in the system decreases.

word salad Series of words that seem totally unrelated.

DSM–IV–TR Classification*

NOS = not otherwise specified.

An *x* appearing in a diagnostic code indicates that a specific code number is required.

An ellipsis (. . .) is used in the names of certain disorders to indicate that the name of a specified mental disorder or general medical condition should be inserted when recording the name (e.g., 293.0 Delirium Due to Hypothyroidism).

If criteria are currently met, one of the following severity specifiers may be noted after the diagnosis:

Mild

Moderate

Severe

If criteria are no longer met, one of the following specifiers may be noted:

In Partial Remission

In Full Remission

Prior History

Disorders Usually First Diagnosed in Infancy, Childhood, or Adolescence

Mental Retardation

Note: These are coded on Axis II.

317	Mild Mental Retardation
318.0	Moderate Retardation
318.1	Severe Mental Retardation
318.2	Profound Mental Retardation
319	Mental Retardation, Severity Unspecified

Learning Disorders

315.00	Reading Disorder
315.1	Mathematics Disorder
315.2	Disorder of Written Expression
315.9	Learning Disorder NOS

Motor Skills Disorder

315.4	Developmental Coordination Disorder

Communication Disorders

315.31	Expressive Language Disorder
315.31	Mixed Receptive-Expressive Language Disorder
315.39	Phonological Disorder

307.0	Stuttering
307.9	Communication Disorder NOS

Pervasive Developmental Disorders

299.00	Autistic Disorder
299.80	Rett's Disorder
299.10	Childhood Disintegrative Disorder
299.80	Asperger's Disorder
299.80	Pervasive Developmental Disorder NOS

Attention-Deficit and Disruptive Behavior Disorders

314.xx	Attention-Deficit/Hyperactivity Disorder
.01	Combined Type
.00	Predominantly Inattentive Type
.01	Predominantly Hyperactive-Impulsive Type
314.9	Attention-Deficit/Hyperactivity Disorder NOS
312.8	Conduct Disorder
	Specify type: Childhood-Onset Type/Adolescent-Onset Type
313.81	Oppositional Defiant Disorder
312.9	Disruptive Behavior Disorder NOS

Feeding and Eating Disorders of Infancy or Early Childhood

307.52	Pica
307.53	Rumination Disorder
307.59	Feeding Disorder of Infancy or Early Childhood

TIC Disorders

307.23	Tourette's Disorder
307.22	Chronic Motor or Vocal Tic Disorder
307.21	Transient Tic Disorder
	Specify if: Single Episode/Recurrent
307.20	Tic Disorder NOS

Elimination Disorders

___.__	Encopresis
787.6	With Constipation and Overflow Incontinence
307.7	Without Constipation and Overflow Incontinence

*Reprinted with permission from the *Diagnostic and statistical manual of mental disorders,* Fourth Edition, Text Revision. Copyright 2000. American Psychiatric Association.

307.6   Enuresis (Not Due to a General Medical Condition)
Specify type: Nocturnal Only/Diurnal Only/Nocturnal and Diurnal

Other Disorders of Infancy, Childhood, or Adolescence

309.21   Separation Anxiety Disorder
Specify if: Early Onset

313.23   Selective Mutism

313.89   Reactive Attachment Disorder of Infancy or Early Childhood
Specify type: Inhibited Type/Disinhibited Type

307.3   Stereotypic Movement Disorder
Specify if: With Self-Injurious Behavior

313.9   Disorder of Infancy, Childhood, or Adolescence NOS

Delirium, Dementia, and Amnestic and Other Cognitive Disorders

Delirium

293.0   Delirium Due to . . . *[Indicate the General Medical Condition]*

___.__   Substance Intoxication Delirium *(refer to Substance-Related Disorders for substance-specific codes)*

___.__   Substance Withdrawal Delirium *(refer to Substance-Related Disorders for substance-specified codes)*

___.__   Delirium Due to Multiple Etiologies *(code each of the specific etiologies)*

780.09   Delirium NOS

Dementia

290.xx   Dementia of the Alzheimer's Type, with Early Onset *(also code 331.0 Alzheimer's disease on Axis III)*
  .10   Uncomplicated
  .11   With Delirium
  .12   With Delusions
  .13   With Depressed Mood
Specify if: With Behavioral Disturbance

290.xx   Dementia of the Alzheimer's Type, with Late Onset *(also code 331.0 Alzheimer's disease on Axis III)*
  .0   Uncomplicated
  .3   With Delirium
  .20   With Delusions
  .21   With Depressed Mood
Specify if: With Behavioral Disturbance

290.xx   Vascular Dementia
  .40   Uncomplicated
  .41   With Delirium
  .42   With Delusions
  .43   With Depressed Mood
Specify if: With Behavioral Disturbance

294.9   Dementia Due to HIV Disease *(also code 043.1 HIV infection affecting central nervous system on Axis III)*

294.1   Dementia Due to Head Trauma *(also code 854.00 head injury on Axis III)*

294.1   Dementia Due to Parkinson's Disease *(also code 332.0 Parkinson's disease on Axis III)*

294.1   Dementia Due to Huntington's Disease *(also code 334.4 Huntington's disease on Axis III)*

290.10   Dementia Due to Pick's Disease *(also code 331.1 Pick's disease on Axis III)*

290.10   Dementia Due to Creutzfeldt-Jakob Disease *(also code 046.1 Creutzfeldt-Jakob disease on Axis III)*

294.1   Dementia Due to . . . *[Indicate the General Medical Condition not listed above] (also code the general medical condition on Axis III)*

___.__   Substance-Induced Persisting Dementia *(refer to Substance-Related Disorders for substance specific codes)*

___.__   Dementia Due to Multiple Etiologies *(code each of the specific etiologies)*

294.8   Dementia NOS

Amnestic Disorders

294.0   Amnestic Disorder Due to . . . *[Indicate the General Medical Condition]*
Specify if: Transient/Chronic

___.__   Substance-Induced Persisting Amnestic Disorder *(refer to Substance-Related Disorders for substance-specific codes)*

294.8   Amnestic Disorder NOS

Other Cognitive Disorders

294.9   Cognitive Disorder NOS

Mental Disorders Due to General Medical Condition Not Elsewhere Classified

293.89   Catatonic Disorder Due to . . . *[Indicate the General Medical Condition]*

310.1   Personality Change Due to . . . *[Indicate the General Medical Condition]*
Specify type: Labile Type/Disinhibited Type/Aggressive Type/Apathetic Type/Paranoid Type/Other Type/Combined Type/Unspecified Type

293.9   Mental Disorder NOS Due to . . . *[Indicate the General Medical Condition]*

Substance-Related Disorders

[a]*The following specifiers may be applied to Substance Dependence:*

With Physiological Dependence/Without Physiological Dependence
Early Full Remission/Early Partial Remission
Sustained Full Remission/Sustained Partial Remission
On Agonist Therapy/In a Controlled Environment

The following specifiers apply to Substance-Induced Disorders as noted:

[I]With Onset During Intoxication/[W]With Onset During Withdrawal

Alcohol-Related Disorders
Alcohol Use Disorders

303.90	Alcohol Dependence[a]
305.00	Alcohol Abuse

Alcohol-Induced Disorders

303.00	Alcohol Intoxication
291.8	Alcohol Withdrawal
	Specify if: With Perceptual Disturbances
291.0	Alcohol Intoxication Delirium
291.0	Alcohol Withdrawal Delirium
291.2	Alcohol-Induced Persisting Dementia
291.1	Alcohol-Induced Persisting Amnestic Disorder
291.x	Alcohol-Induced Psychotic Disorder
.5	With Delusions[I,W]
.3	With Hallucinations[I,W]
291.8	Alcohol-Induced Mood Disorder[I,W]
291.8	Alcohol-Induced Anxiety Disorder[I,W]
291.8	Alcohol-Induced Sexual Dysfunction[I]
291.8	Alcohol-Induced Sleep Disorder[I,W]
291.9	Alcohol-Related Disorder NOS

Amphetamine (or Amphetamine-Like)-Related Disorders
Amphetamine Use Disorders

304.40	Amphetamine Dependence[a]
305.70	Amphetamine Abuse

Amphetamine-Induced Disorders

292.89	Amphetamine Intoxication
	Specify if: With Perceptual Disturbances
292.0	Amphetamine Withdrawal
292.81	Amphetamine Intoxication Delirium
292.xx	Amphetamine-Induced Psychotic Disorder
.11	With Delusions[I]
.12	With Hallucinations[I]
292.84	Amphetamine-Induced Mood Disorder[I,W]
292.89	Amphetamine-Induced Anxiety Disorder[I]
292.89	Amphetamine-Induced Sexual Dysfunction[I]
292.89	Amphetamine-Induced Sleep Disorder[I,W]
292.9	Amphetamine-Related Disorder NOS

Caffeine-Related Disorders
Caffeine-Induced Disorders

305.90	Caffeine Intoxication
292.89	Caffeine-Induced Anxiety Disorder[I]
292.89	Caffeine-Induced Sleep Disorder[I]
292.9	Caffeine-Related Disorder NOS

Cannabis-Related Disorders
Cannabis Use Disorders

304.30	Cannabis Dependence[a]
305.20	Cannabis Abuse

Cannabis-Induced Disorders

292.89	Cannabis Intoxication
	Specify if: With Perceptual Disturbances
292.81	Cannabis Intoxication Delirium
292.xx	Cannabis-Induced Psychotic Disorder
.11	With Delusions[I]
.12	With Hallucinations[I]
292.89	Cannabis-Induced Anxiety Disorder[I]
292.9	Cannabis-Related Disorder NOS

Cocaine-Related Disorders
Cocaine Use Disorders

304.20	Cocaine Dependence[a]
305.60	Cocaine Abuse

Cocaine-Induced Disorders

292.89	Cocaine Intoxication
	Specify if: With Perceptual Disturbances
292.0	Cocaine Withdrawal
292.81	Cocaine Intoxication Delirium
292.xx	Cocaine-Induced Psychotic Disorder
.11	With Delusions[I]
.12	With Hallucinations[I]
292.84	Cocaine-Induced Mood Disorder[I,W]
292.89	Cocaine-Induced Anxiety Disorder[I,W]
292.89	Cocaine-Induced Sexual Dysfunction[I]
292.89	Cocaine-Induced Sleep Disorder[I,W]
292.9	Cocaine-Related Disorder NOS

Hallucinogen-Related Disorders
Hallucinogen Use Disorders

304.50	Hallucinogen Dependence[a]
305.30	Hallucinogen Abuse

Hallucinogen-Induced Disorders

292.89	Hallucinogen Intoxication
292.89	Hallucinogen Persisting Perception Disorder (Flashbacks)
292.81	Hallucinogen Intoxication Delirium
292.xx	Hallucinogen-Induced Psychotic Disorder
.11	With Delusions[I]
.12	With Hallucinations[I]
292.84	Hallucinogen-Induced Mood Disorder[I]
292.89	Hallucinogen-Induced Anxiety Disorder[I]
292.9	Hallucinogen-Related Disorder NOS

Inhalant-Related Disorders
Inhalant Use Disorders

304.60	Inhalant Dependence[a]
305.90	Inhalant Abuse

Inhalant-Induced Disorders

292.89	Inhalant Intoxication
292.81	Inhalant Intoxication Delirium
292.82	Inhalant-Induced Persisting Dementia
292.xx	Inhalant-Induced Psychotic Disorder
.11	With Delusions[I]
.12	With Hallucinations[I]
292.84	Inhalant-Induced Mood Disorder[I]
292.89	Inhalant-Induced Anxiety Disorder[I]
292.9	Inhalant-Related Disorder NOS

Nicotine-Related Disorders

Nicotine Use Disorder

305.10	Nicotine Dependence[a]

Nicotine-Induced Disorders

292.0	Nicotine Withdrawal
292.9	Nicotine-Related Disorder NOS

Opioid-Related Disorders

Opioid Use Disorders

304.00	Opioid Dependence[a]
305.50	Opioid Abuse

Opioid-Induced Disorders

292.89	Opioid Intoxication
	Specify if: With Perceptual Disturbances
292.0	Opioid Withdrawal
292.81	Opioid Intoxication Delirium
292.xx	Opioid-Induced Psychotic Disorder
.11	With Delusions[I]
.12	With Hallucinations[I]
292.84	Opioid-Induced Mood Disorder[I]
292.89	Opioid-Induced Sexual Dysfunction[I]
292.89	Opioid-Induced Sleep Disorder[I,W]
292.9	Opioid-Related Disorder NOS

Phencyclidine (or Phencyclidine-Like)-Related Disorders

Phencyclidine Use Disorders

304.90	Phencyclidine Dependence[a]
305.90	Phencyclidine Abuse

Phencyclidine-Induced Disorders

292.89	Phencyclidine Intoxication
	Specify if: With Perceptual Disturbances
292.81	Phencyclidine Intoxication Delirium
292.xx	Phencyclidine-Induced Psychotic Disorder
.11	With Delusions[I]
.12	With Hallucinations[I]
292.84	Phencyclidine-Induced Mood Disorder[I]
292.89	Phencyclidine-Induced Anxiety Disorder[I]
292.9	Phencyclidine-Related Disorder NOS

Sedative-, Hypnotic-, or Anxiolytic-Related Disorders

Sedative, Hypnotic, or Anxiolytic Use Disorders

304.10	Sedative, Hypnotic, or Anxiolytic Dependence[a]
305.40	Sedative, Hypnotic, or Anxiolytic Abuse

Sedative-, Hypnotic-, or Anxiolytic-Induced Disorders

292.89	Sedative, Hypnotic, or Anxiolytic Intoxication
292.0	Sedative, Hypnotic, or Anxiolytic Withdrawal
	Specify if: With Perceptual Disturbances
292.81	Sedative, Hypnotic, or Anxiolytic Intoxication Delirium
292.81	Sedative, Hypnotic, or Anxiolytic Withdrawal Delirium
292.82	Sedative-, Hypnotic-, or Anxiolytic-Induced Persisting Dementia
292.83	Sedative-, Hypnotic-, or Anxiolytic-Induced Persisting Amnestic Disorder
292.xx	Sedative-, Hypnotic-, or Anxiolytic-Induced Psychotic Disorder
.11	With Delusions[I,W]
.12	With Hallucinations[I,W]
292.84	Sedative-, Hypnotic-, or Anxiolytic-Induced Mood Disorder[I,W]
292.89	Sedative-, Hypnotic-, or Anxiolytic-Induced Anxiety Disorder[W]
292.89	Sedative-, Hypnotic-, or Anxiolytic-Induced Sexual Dysfunction[I]
292.89	Sedative-, Hypnotic-, or Anxiolytic-Induced Sleep Disorder[I,W]
292.9	Sedative,-, Hypnotic-, or Anxiolytic-Related Disorder NOS

Polysubstance-Related Disorder

304.80	Polysubstance Dependence[a]

Other (or Unknown) Substance-Related Disorders

Other (or Unknown) Substance Use Disorders

304.90	Other (or Unknown) Substance Dependence[a]
305.90	Other (or Unknown) Substance Abuse

Other (or Unknown) Substance-Induced Disorders

292.89	Other (or Unknown) Substance Intoxication
	Specify if: With Perceptual Disturbances
292.0	Other (or Unknown) Substance Withdrawal
	Specify if: With Perceptual Disturbances
292.81	Other (or Unknown) Substance-Induced Delirium
292.82	Other (or Unknown) Substance-Induced Persisting Dementia
292.83	Other (or Unknown) Substance-Induced Persisting Anonestic Disorder
292.xx	Other (or Unknown) Substance-Induced Psychotic Disorder
.11	With Delusions[I,W]
.12	With Hallucinations[I,W]

292.84 Other (or Unknown) Substance-Induced Mood Disorder[I,W]

292.89 Other (or Unknown) Substance-Induced Anxiety Disorder[I,W]

292.89 Other (or unknown) Substance-Induced Sexual Dysfunction[I]

292.89 Other (or Unknown) Substance-Induced Sleep Disorder[I,W]

292.9 Other (or Unknown) Substance-Related Disorder NOS

Schizophrenia and Other Psychotic Disorders

295.xx Schizophrenia

The following Classification of Longitudinal Course applies to all subtypes of Schizophrenia:

Episodic with Interepisode Residual Symptoms (*specify if:* With Prominent Negative Symptoms)/Episodic with No Interepisode Residual Symptoms/Continuous (*specify if:* With Prominent Negative Symptoms)

Single Episode in Partial Remission (*specify if:* With Prominent Negative Symptoms)/Single Episode in Full Remission

Other or Unspecified Pattern

.30 Paranoid Type
.10 Disorganized Type
.20 Catatonic Type
.90 Undifferentiated Type
.60 Residual Type

295.40 Schizophreniform Disorder
Specify if: Without Good Prognostic Features/With Good Prognostic Features

295.70 Schizoaffective Disorder
Specify type: Bipolar Type/Depressive Type

297.1 Delusional Disorder
Specify type: Erotomanic Type/Grandiose Type/Jealous Type/Persecutory Type/Somatic Type/Mixed Type/Unspecified Type

298.8 Brief Psychotic Disorder
Specify if: With Marked Stressor(s)/Without Marked Stressor(s)/With Postpartum Onset

297.3 Shared Psychotic Disorder

293.xx Psychotic Disorder Due to . . . *[Indicate the General Medical Condition]*
.81 With Delusions
.82 With Hallucinations

___.__ Substance-Induced Psychotic Disorder (*refer to Substance-Related Disorders for substance-specific codes*)
Specify if: With Onset during Intoxication/With Onset during Withdrawal

298.9 Psychotic Disorder NOS

Mood Disorders

Code current state of Major Depressive Disorder or Bipolar I Disorder in fifth digit:
1 = Mild
2 = Moderate
3 = Severe without Psychotic Features
4 = Severe with Psychotic Features
Specify: Mood-Congruent Psychotic Features/Mood-Incongruent Psychotic Features
5 = In Partial Remission
6 = In Full Remission
0 = Unspecified

The following specifiers apply (for current or most recent episode) to Mood Disorders as noted:
[a]Severity/Psychotic/Remission Specifiers
[b]Chronic
[c]With Catatonic Features
[d]With Melancholic Features
[e]With Atypical Features
[f]With Postpartum Onset

The following specifiers apply to Mood Disorders as noted:
[g]With or without Full Interepisode Recovery
[h]With Seasonal Pattern
[i]With Rapid Cycling

Depressive Disorders

296.xx Major Depressive Disorder,
.2x   Single Episode[a,b,c,d,e,f]
.3x   Recurrent[a,b,c,d,e,f,g,h]
300.4 Dysthymic Disorder
Specify if: Early Onset/Late Onset
Specify: With Atypical Features
311 Depressive Disorder NOS

Bipolar Disorders

296.xx Bipolar I Disorder,
.0x   Single Manic Episode[a,c,f]
Specify if: Mixed
.40 Most Recent Episode Hypomanic[g,h,i]
.4x Most Recent Episode Manic[a,c,f,g,h,i]
.6x Most Recent Episode Mixed[a,c,f,g,h,i]
.5x Most Recent Episode Depressed[a,b,c,d,e,f,g,h,i]
.7 Most Recent Episode Unspecified[g,h,i]
296.89 Bipolar II Disorder[a,b,c,d,e,f,g,h,i]
Specify (current or most recent episode): Hypomanic/Depressed
301.13 Cyclothymic Disorder
296.80 Bipolar Disorder NOS
293.83 Mood Disorder Due to . . . *[Indicate the General Medical Condition]*
Specify type: With Depressive Features/With Major Depressive-Like Episode/With Manic Features/With Mixed Features
___.__ Substance-Induced Mood Disorder (*refer to Substance-Related Disorders for substance-specific codes*)
Specify type: With Depressive Features/With Manic Features/With Mixed Features
Specify if: With Onset During Intoxication/With Onset During Withdrawal
296.90 Mood Disorder NOS

Anxiety Disorders

300.01	Panic Disorder without Agoraphobia
300.21	Panic Disorder with Agoraphobia
300.22	Agoraphobia without History of Panic Disorder
300.29	Specific Phobia

Specify type: Animal Type/Natural Environment Type/Blood-Injection-Injury Type/Situational Type/Other Type

300.23	Social Phobia

Specify if: Generalized

300.3	Obsessive-Compulsive Disorder

Specify if: With Poor Insight

309.81	Post-traumatic Stress Disorder

Specify if: Acute/Chronic
Specify if: With Delayed Onset

308.3	Acute Stress Disorder
300.02	Generalized Anxiety Disorder
293.89	Anxiety Disorder Due to . . . *[Indicate the General Medical Condition]*

Specify if: With Generalized Anxiety/With Panic Attacks/With Obsessive-Compulsive Symptoms

___.__	Substance-Induced Anxiety Disorder *(refer to Substance-Related Disorders for substance-specific codes)*

Specify if: With Generalized Anxiety/With Panic Attacks/With Obsessive-Compulsive Symptoms/With Phobic Symptoms
Specify if: With Onset During Intoxication/With Onset During Withdrawal

300.00	Anxiety Disorder NOS

Somatoform Disorders

300.81	Somatization Disorder
300.81	Undifferentiated Somatoform Disorder
300.11	Conversion Disorder

Specify type: With Motor Symptom or Deficit/With Sensory Symptom or Deficit/With Seizures or Convulsions/With Mixed Presentation

307.xx	Pain Disorder
.80	Associated with Psychologic Factors
.89	Associated with Both Psychologic Factors and a General Medical Condition

Specify if: Acute/Chronic

300.7	Hypochondriasis

Specify if: With Poor Insight

300.7	Body Dysmorphic Disorder
300.81	Somatoform Disorder NOS

Factitious Disorders

300.xx	Factitious Disorder
.16	With Predominantly Psychological Signs and Symptoms
.19	With Predominantly Physical Signs and Symptoms
.19	With Combined Psychological and Physical Signs and Symptoms
300.19	Factitious Disorder NOS

Dissociative Disorders

300.12	Dissociative Amnesia
300.13	Dissociative Fugue
300.14	Dissociative Identity Disorder
300.6	Depersonalization Disorder
300.15	Dissociative Disorder NOS

Sexual and Gender Identity Disorders

Sexual Dysfunctions

The following specifiers apply to all primary Sexual Dysfunctions:

Lifelong Type
Acquired Type
Generalized Type
Situational Type Due to Psychologic Factors
Due to Combined Factors

Sexual Desire Disorders

302.71	Hypoactive Sexual Desire Disorder
302.79	Sexual Aversion Disorder

Sexual Arousal Disorders

302.72	Female Sexual Arousal Disorder
302.72	Male Erectile Disorder

Orgasmic Disorders

302.73	Female Orgasmic Disorder
302.74	Male Orgasmic Disorder
302.75	Premature Ejaculation

Sexual Pain Disorders

302.76	Dyspareunia (Not Due to a General Medical Condition)
306.51	Vaginismus (Not Due to a General Medical Condition)

Sexual Dysfunction Due to a General Medical Condition

625.8	Female Hypoactive Sexual Desire Disorder Due to . . . *[Indicate the General Medical Condition]*
608.89	Male Hypoactive Sexual Desire Disorder Due to . . . *[Indicate the General Medical Condition]*
607.84	Male Erectile Disorder Due to . . . *[Indicate the General Medical Condition]*
625.0	Female Dyspareunia Due to . . . *[Indicate the General Medical Condition]*
628.89	Male Dyspareunia Due to . . . *[Indicate the General Medical Condition]*
625.8	Other Female Sexual Dysfunction Due to . . . *[Indicate the General Medical Condition]*
608.89	Other Male Sexual Dysfunction Due to . . . *[Indicate the General Medical Condition]*

___.__   Substance-Induced Sexual Dysfunction *(refer to Substance-Related Disorders for substance-specific codes)*
Specify if: With Impaired Desired/With Impaired Arousal/With Impaired Orgasm/With Sexual Pain
Specify if: With Onset During Intoxication
302.70   Sexual Dysfunction NOS

Paraphilias

302.4   Exhibitionism
302.81   Fetishism
302.89   Frotteurism
302.2   Pedophilia
Specify if: Sexually Attracted to Males/Sexually Attracted to Females/Sexually Attracted to Both
Specify if: Limited to Incest
Specify type: Exclusive Type/Nonexclusive Type
302.83   Sexual Masochism
302.84   Sexual Sadism
302.3   Transvestic Fetishism
Specify if: With Gender Dysphoria
302.82   Voyeurism
302.9   Paraphilia NOS

Gender Identity Disorders

302.xx   Gender Identity Disorder
.6   in Children
.85   in Adolescents or Adults
Specify if: Sexually Attracted to Males/Sexually Attracted to Females/Sexually Attracted to Both/Sexually Attracted to Neither
302.6   Gender Identity Disorder NOS
302.9   Sexual Disorder NOS

Eating Disorders

307.1   Anorexia Nervosa
Specify type: Restricting Type; Binge-Eating/Purging Type
307.51   Bulimia Nervosa
Specify type: Purging Type/Nonpurging Type
307.50   Eating Disorder NOS

Sleep Disorders

Primary Sleep Disorders

Dyssomnias

307.42   Primary Insomnia
307.44   Primary Hypersomnia
Specify if: Recurrent
347   Narcolepsy
780.59   Breathing-Related Sleep Disorder
307.45   Circadian Rhythm Sleep Disorder
Specify if: Delayed Sleep Phase Type/Jet Lag Type/Shift Work Type/Unspecified Type
307.47   Dyssomnia NOS

Parasomnias

307.47   Nightmare Disorder
307.46   Sleep Terror Disorder
307.46   Sleepwalking Disorder
307.47   Parasomnia NOS

Sleep Disorders Related to Another Mental Disorder

307.42   Insomnia Related to . . . *[Indicate the Axis I or Axis II Disorder]*
307.44   Hypersomnia Related to . . . *[Indicate the Axis I or Axis II Disorder]*

Other Sleep Disorders

780.xx   Sleep Disorder Due to . . . *[Indicate the General Medical Condition]*
.52   Insomnia Type
.54   Hypersomnia Type
.59   Parasomnia Type
.59   Mixed type
___.__   Substance-Induced Sleep Disorder *(refer to Substance-Related Disorders for substance-specific codes)*
Specify type: Insomnia Type/Hypersomnia Type/Parasomnia Type/Mixed Type
Specify if: With Onset During Intoxication/With Onset During Withdrawal

Impulse-Control Disorders Not Elsewhere Classified

312.34   Intermittent Explosive Disorder
312.32   Kleptomania
312.33   Pyromania
312.31   Pathological Gambling
312.39   Trichotillomania
312.30   Impulse-Control Disorder NOS

Adjustment Disorders

309.xx   Adjustment Disorder
.0   With Depressed Mood
.24   With Anxiety
.28   With Mixed Anxiety and Depressed Mood
.3   With Disturbance of Conduct
.4   With Mixed Disturbance of Emotions and Conduct
.9   Unspecified
Specify if: Acute/Chronic

Personality Disorders

Note: These are coded on Axis II.

301.0   Paranoid Personality Disorder
301.20   Schizoid Personality Disorder
301.22   Schizotypal Personality Disorder
301.7   Antisocial Personality Disorder
301.83   Borderline Personality Disorder
301.50   Histrionic Personality Disorder
301.81   Narcissistic Personality Disorder
301.82   Avoidant Personality Disorder

301.6	Dependent Personality Disorder
301.4	Obsessive-Compulsive Personality Disorder
301.9	Personality Disorder NOS

Other Conditions That May Be a Focus of Clinical Attention

Psychological Factors Affecting Medical Condition

| 316 | . . . [Specified Psychologic Factor] Affecting . . . [Indicate the General Medical Condition] Choose name based on nature of factors: Mental Disorder Affecting Medical Condition Psychologic Symptoms Affecting Medical Condition Personality Traits or Coping Style Affecting Medical Condition Maladaptive Health Behaviors Affecting Medical Condition Stress-Related Physiologic Response Affecting Medical Condition Other or Unspecified Psychologic Factors Affecting Medical Condition |

Medication-Induced Movement Disorders

332.1	Neuroleptic-Induced Parkinsonism
333.92	Neuroleptic Malignant Syndrome
333.7	Neuroleptic-Induced Acute Dystonia
333.99	Neuroleptic-Induced Acute Akathisia
333.82	Neuroleptic-Induced Tardive Dyskinesia
333.1	Medication-Induced Postural Tremor
333.90	Medication-Induced Movement Disorder NOS

Other Medication-Induced Disorder

| 995.2 | Adverse Effects of Medication NOS |

Relational Problems

V61.9	Relational Problem Related to a Mental Disorder or General Medical Condition
V61.20	Parent-Child Relational Problem
V61.1	Partner Relational Problem
V61.8	Sibling Relational Problem
V62.81	Relational Problem NOS

Problems Related to Abuse or Neglect

V61.21	Physical Abuse of Child (code 995.5 if focus of attention is on victim)
V61.21	Sexual Abuse of Child (code 995.5 if focus of attention is on victim)
V61.21	Neglect of Child (code 995.5 if focus of attention is on victim)
V61.1	Physical Abuse of Adult (code 995.81 if focus of attention is on victim)
V61.1	Sexual Abuse of Adult (code 995.81 if focus of attention is on victim)

Additional Conditions That May Be a Focus of Clinical Attention

V15.81	Noncompliance with Treatment
V65.2	Malingering
V71.01	Adult Antisocial Behavior
V71.02	Child or Adolescent Antisocial Behavior
V62.89	Borderline Intellectual Functioning *Note: This is coded on Axis II.*
780.9	Age-Related Cognitive Decline
V62.82	Bereavement
V62.3	Academic Problem
V62.2	Occupational Problem
313.82	Identity Problem
V62.89	Religious or Spiritual Problem
V62.4	Acculturation Problem
V62.89	Phase of Life Problem

Additional Codes

300.9	Unspecified Mental Disorder (nonpsychotic)
V71.09	No Diagnosis or Condition on Axis I
799.9	Diagnosis or Condition Deferred on Axis I
V71.09	No Diagnosis on Axis II
799.9	Diagnosis Deferred on Axis II

Axis II: Personality Disorders

301.0	Paranoid Personality Disorder
301.20	Schizoid Personality Disorder
301.22	Schizotypal Personality Disorder
301.7	Antisocial Personality Disorder
301.83	Borderline Personality Disorder
301.50	Histrionic Personality Disorder
301.81	Narcissistic Personality Disorder
301.82	Avoidant Personality Disorder
301.6	Dependent Personality Disorder
301.4	Obsessive-Compulsive Personality Disorder
301.9	Personality Disorder NOS

Axis III: ICD-9-CM General Medical Conditions

Infectious and Parasitic Diseases (001-139)

Neoplasms (140-239)

Endocrine, Nutritional, and Metabolic Diseases and Immunity Disorders (240-279)

Diseases of the Blood and Blood-Forming Organs (280-289)

Diseases of the Nervous and Sense Organs (320-389)

Diseases of the Circulatory System (390-459)

Diseases of the Respiratory System (460-519)

Diseases of the Digestive System (520-579)

Diseases of the Genitourinary System (580-629)

Complications of Pregnancy, Childbirth, and the Puerperium (630-676)

Diseases of the Skin and Subcutaneous Tissue (680-709)

Diseases of the Musculoskeletal System and Connective Tissue (710-739)

Congenital Anomalies (740-759)

Certain Conditions Originating in the Perinatal Period (760-779)
Symptoms, Signs, and Ill-Defined Conditions (780-799)
Injury and Poisoning (800-999)

Axis IV: Psychosocial and Environmental Problems

Problems with Primary Support Group (Childhood [V61.9], Adult [V61.9], Parent-Child [V61.2]). These include death of a family member; health problems in family; disruption of family by separation, divorce, or estrangement; removal from the home; remarriage of parent; sexual or physical abuse; parental overprotection; neglect of child; inadequate discipline; discord with siblings; birth of sibling.

Problems Related to the Social Environment (V62.4). These include death or loss of friend, social isolation, living alone, difficulty with acculturation, discrimination, adjustment to life cycle transition (e.g., retirement).

Educational Problems (V62.3). These include illiteracy, academic problems, discord with teachers or classmates, inadequate school environment.

Occupational Problems (V62.2). These include unemployment, threat of job loss, stressful work schedule, difficult work conditions, job dissatisfaction, job change, discord with boss or coworkers.

Housing Problems (V60.9). These include homelessness, inadequate housing, unsafe neighborhood, discord with neighbors or landlord.

Economic Problems (V60.9) These include extreme poverty, inadequate finances, insufficient welfare support.

Problems with Access to Health Care Services (V63.9). These include inadequate health care services, transportation to health care facilities unavailable, inadequate health insurance.

Problems Related to Interaction with the Legal System/Crime (V62.5). These include arrest, incarceration, litigation, victim of crime.

Other Psychosocial and Environmental Problems (V62.9). These include exposure to disasters, war, other hostilities; discord with non-family caregivers (e.g., counselor, social worker, physician); unavailability of social service agencies.

Axis V: Global Assessment of Functioning (GAF) Scale*

Consider psychological, social, and occupational functioning on a hypothetical continuum of mental health–illness. Do not include impairment in functioning due to physical (or environmental) limitations.

Code (Note: Use intermediate codes when appropriate, e.g., 45, 68, 72.)

100 Superior functioning in a wide range of activities, life's problems never seem to get out of hand, is sought out by others because of his many positive qualities. No symptoms.
91

90 Absent or minimal symptoms (e.g., mild anxiety before an exam), good functioning in all areas, interested and involved in a wide range of activities, socially effective, generally satisfied with life, no more than everyday problems or concerns (e.g., an occasional argument with family members).
81

80 If symptoms are present, they are transient and expectable reactions to psychosocial stressors (e.g., difficulty concentrating after family argument); no more than slight impairment in social, occupational or school functioning (e.g., temporarily falling behind in school work).
71

70 Some mild symptoms (e.g., depressed mood and mild insomnia) OR some difficulty in social, occupational, or school functioning (e.g., occasional truancy, or theft within the household), but generally functioning pretty well, has some meaningful interpersonal relationships.
61

60 Moderate symptoms (e.g., flat affect and circumstantial speech, occasional panic attacks) OR moderate difficulty in social, occupational, or school functioning (e.g, no friends, unable to keep a job).
51

50 Serious symptoms (e.g., suicidal ideation, severe obsessional rituals, frequent shoplifting) OR any serious impairment in social, occupational, or school functioning (e.g., no friends, unable to keep a job).
41

*The rating of overall psychological functioning on a scale of 0-100 was operationalized by Luborsky in the Health-Sickness Rating Scale (Luborsky L: Clinicians' judgments of mental health, *Arch Gen Psychiatry* 7:407-417, 1962). Spitzer and colleagues developed a revision of the Health-Sickness Rating Scale called the Global Assessment Scale (GAS) (Endicott J, Spitzer RL, Fleiss JL, Cohen J: The global assessment scale: a procedure for measuring overall severity of psychiatric disturbance, *Arch Gen Psychiatry* 33:766-771, 1976). A modified version of the GAS was included in *DSM-III-R* as the Global Assessment of Functioning (GAF) Scale.

40 Some impairment in reality testing or communication (e.g., speech is at times illogical, obscure, or irrelevant) OR major impairment in several areas, such as work or school, family relations, judgment, thinking, or mood (e.g., depressed man avoids friends, neglects family, and is unable to work; child frequently beats up younger children, is defiant at home, and is failing at school).

31

30 Behavior is considerably influenced by delusions or hallucinations OR serious impairment in communication or judgment (e.g., sometimes incoherent, acts grossly inappropriately, suicidal preoccupation) OR inability to function in almost all areas (e.g., stays in bed all day; no job, home, or friends).

21

20 Some danger of hurting self or others (e.g., suicide attempts without clear expectation of death, frequently violent, manic excitement) OR occasionally fails to maintain minimal personal hygiene (e.g., smears feces) OR gross impairment in communication (e.g., largely incoherent or mute).

11

10 Persistent danger of severely hurting self or others (e.g., recurrent violence) OR persistent inability to maintain personal hygiene OR serious suicidal act with clear expectation of death.

1

0 Inadequate information.

Chapter Review Questions Answer Key

Chapter 1

1. A. Linda Richards
   B. Hildegard Peplau
   C. Direct care, communication, management
   D. Basic (RN), advanced (APRN)
   E. American Psychiatric Nurses' Association
2. A. True C. True
   B. True D. True
   E. False: There are more than 82,000 psychiatric nurses working in mental health organizations.
   F. False: There are few studies in this important area of psychiatric nursing.
3. A. The development of psychotropic drugs allowed patients to become more treatable, and fewer environmental constraints were needed to contain patient behavior. Also, the introduction of medications gave new hope to psychiatric patients and allowed psychiatric nurses to spend more time with patients in therapeutic activities.
   B. The five core mental health disciplines are psychiatric nursing, marriage and family therapy, psychiatry, psychology, and social work.
   C. The six dimensions of the nurse-patient partnership are clinical competence, patient-family advocacy, fiscal responsibility, interdisciplinary collaboration, social accountability, and legal-ethical parameters.

Chapter 2

1. A. Preinteraction   F. Orientation
   B. Orientation   G. Preinteraction
   C. Orientation   H. Working
   D. Termination   I. Working
   E. Working   J. Termination
2. A. Incongruent
   B. Validation
   C. Empathy
   D. Boundary violation
3. A. Will the self-disclosure enhance the patient's (1) cooperation, (2) learning, (3) catharsis, or (4) support?
   B. Names of individuals, roles of nurse and patient, responsibilities of nurse and patient, expectations of nurse and patient, purpose of the relationship, meeting location and time, conditions for termination, confidentiality

C. Purpose
   Social: Pleasure
   Therapeutic: Patient insight and behavior change
Use of feelings
   Social: Variable
   Therapeutic: Patient encouraged to share feelings
Content of interaction
   Social: Social and spontaneous
   Therapeutic: Goal-directed and purposeful
Confidentiality
   Social: Not an issue
   Therapeutic: Protected for the patient
Termination
   Social: Open-ended
   Therapeutic: Mutually predetermined and honored

4. G. Altruism
   B. Catharsis
   F. Confrontation
   D. Countertransference
   E. Resistance
   C. Role-playing
   A. Transference

Chapter 3

1. D. Freud   C. Spitzer
   F. Rockland   B. Sullivan
   A. Rogers   E. Szasz
2. A. Difficulty in earlier stages of development
   B. Free association
   C. Faulty interpersonal relationships
   D. Satisfaction, security
   E. Social conditions that culturally define what is acceptable
   F. Social
   G. One is out of touch with one's self or the environment
   H. Existential
   I. Problems in living from biopsychosocial causes
   J. Active, partner
   K. Disorders of the central nervous system
   L. Continuous learning about the brain and nervous system using the scientific process
   M. *DSM–IV–TR*

3. A. Psychoanalysis proposes that dreams provide insight into areas of unresolved conflict in thoughts or feelings. Dream analysis or dream work is a common notion in contemporary society, and dreams play an important role in the belief system of various cultures.

   B. Stranger, resource person, teacher, leader, surrogate, counselor

Chapter 4

1. A. True
   B. False: One out of every two people will do so.
   C. True
   D. False: The sympathetic division is stimulated.
   E. True
   F. True
2. A. Reality perception/reality testing
   B. Psychobiological resilience
   C. Psychological
   D. Social attribution
   E. Harm/loss, threat, challenge
   F. II
   G. Culture-bound syndromes
3. A. The three parts of a hardy personality are commitment, challenge, and control. They help people cope with stress by transforming events to their advantage and reframing problems as opportunities for growth and learning.
   B. The three types of coping mechanisms are problem-focused, cognitive-focused, and emotion-focused.
   C. Nurses assess risk factors and look for vulnerabilities; physicians assess disease states and look for causes. Nursing diagnoses focus on the adaptive-maladaptive coping continuum of human responses; medical diagnoses focus on the health-illness continuum of health problems. Nursing intervention consists of caregiving activities; medical intervention consists of curative treatments.
   D. The four stages of psychiatric treatment and related level of prevention are crisis, secondary prevention; acute, secondary prevention; maintenance, tertiary prevention; and health promotion, primary prevention.

Chapter 5

1. A. True
   B. False: Randomized controlled clinical trials are the gold standard.
   C. True
   D. False: Practice guidelines vary greatly in clinical orientation, clinical purpose, complexity, format, and intended users.
   E. True
   F. False: Studies show that very few psychiatric nurses routinely use behavioral rating scales in their practice.

2. A. The efficacy of mental health treatments is well-documented; a range of treatments exists for most mental disorders.
   B. Defining the clinical question, finding the evidence, analyzing the evidence, using the evidence, and evaluating the outcome.
   C. Meta-analysis
   D. Practice guidelines
   E. Algorithms
   F. Clinical, functional, satisfaction, and financial
3. A. Central to this accountability is the ability to examine nursing practice patterns, evaluate the nature of the data supporting them, and demonstrate sound clinical decision making in a way that can be empirically supported. This is the essence of evidence based practice.
   B. There are four bases for nursing practice. The lowest level is the **traditional basis** for practice, which includes rituals, unverified rules, anecdotes, customs, opinions, and unit culture. The second level is the **regulatory basis** for practice, which includes state practice acts and reimbursement and other regulatory requirements. The third level is the **philosophical** or **conceptual basis** for practice, which includes the mission, values and vision of the organization, professional practice models, untested conceptual frameworks, and ethical frameworks and professional codes. The fourth and highest level is **evidence based practice,** which includes research findings, performance data, and consensus recommendations of recognized experts. Apart from situations requiring a philosophical or regulatory basis, the best basis to substantiate clinical practice is the evidence of well-established research findings. Such evidence reflects verifiable, replicable facts and relationships that have been exposed to stringent scientific criteria.

Chapter 6

1. G. Tryptophan   L. DST
   H. PET   E. Locus ceruleus
   J. Eugenics   I. Basal ganglia
   C. Synapse   F. Challenge tests
   D. REM   B. Kindling
   K. Hippocampus   A. Hypothalamus
2. A. Blood-brain, blood-CSF barriers
   B. Neurotransmission
   C. Neurosciences
   D. Circadian rhythms
   E. Cholinergic
3. A. False: Only perhaps 10% of cases.
   B. True
   C. False: This has been replaced by more complex biochemical theories.
   D. False: CT scans have found enlargement of ventricles.
   E. True

4. A. Axon: Presynaptic cell; stores and releases neurotransmitter. Dendrite: Post-synaptic cell; contains receptor cells. Receptor cell: Recognizes the neurotransmitter, receives it, and reacts to it. Second messengers: Chemicals within the cell that continue the process of neurotransmission. Reuptake: Neurotransmitter is taken back up into the presynaptic cell. Enzymatic degradation: Neurotransmitter is metabolized and inactivated.

B. It is the emotional brain, concerned with both subjective emotional experiences and body functions associated with emotional states, such as aggressive and submissive behavior, sexual behavior, pleasure, memory, learning, mood, motivation, and sensations, all central to preservation.

C. Stage one, falling asleep; stage two, sleep (50% of sleep time); stages three and four: deep sleep (15% of sleep time); stage five, rapid eye movement (REM) sleep, or dream sleep (20% to 25% of sleep time). REM latency is the period of time (60 to 90 minutes) it usually takes the normal person to enter the first REM period. Decreased REM latency (5 to 30 minutes) is a biological marker for depression that occurs in approximately 90% of people with depression, thus indicating that there is sleep dysregulation in depression.

D. Challenge testing is a procedure that causes panic attacks under controlled conditions to study the biology of the attack. Vulnerable people are more likely to have a panic attack when given challenges such as lactate, carbon dioxide, and caffeine than are people who do not have panic disorder. They are also less likely to have another attack when challenged again after adequate treatment with antipanic medications. PET studies show that these people also tend to have an abnormality in the parahippocampal region of the brain, an area of the cerebral cortex that is associated with the limbic system, and may be implicated in panic attacks.

Chapter 7

1. C. Affect
   A. Delusion
   E. Flight of ideas
   F. Hallucinations
   B. Illusions
   H. Insight
   D. Loose associations
   G. Mood
2. A. Flat affect
   B. Command hallucinations
   C. Sound or hearing
   D. Confabulation
3. A. The major categories of information in a mental status examination are general description, emotional state, experiences, thinking, and sensorium and cognition.

B. Person (What is your name?), place (Where are you today?), and time (What is today's date?)

C. To measure the extent of the patient's problem. Make an accurate diagnosis, track patient progress over time, and document the efficacy of treatment.

Chapter 8

1. A. Risk factors
   B. Ethnicity
   C. Substance abuse, antisocial personality
   D. Affective, anxiety
   E. Schizophrenia, manic depression
   F. Increase, decrease
2. F. Disadvantagement
   D. Discrimination
   G. Intolerance
   B. Prejudice
   E. Racism
   A. Stereotype
   C. Stigma
3. A. Cultural sensitivity is the ability to view each patient as a unique individual, fully considering the patient's cultural experiences within the context of the common developmental challenges faced by all people.

Chapter 9

1. A. Access
   F. Capitation
   E. Case rate
   B. Clinical appropriateness
   D. Outcomes
   C. Utilization review
2. A. Behavioral
   B. Person, population
   C. Quality, costs
   D. Employee assistance program
   E. Patient characteristics, nature of the therapeutic relationship, treatment intervention, placebo effect
   F. Telepsychiatry
3. A. HMOs are organized delivery systems that provide care to a defined population, usually for a predetermined fixed amount (capitation rate). Consumers enrolled in HMOs are restricted to using HMO providers.
   POSs are plans that contract with a limited number of clinicians, most often physicians, and hospitals that provide care at discounted rates.
   PPOs allow consumers to choose between delivery systems at the time they seek care.

B. Medicare and Medicaid were designed to help those who were medically in need. The law passed in 1996 implies that chemical dependency problems are not medical conditions but rather the result of personal choice or weakness. In this way it further stigmatizes people with these debilitating conditions.

Chapter 10

1. A. True
   B. False: The police power is currently emphasized.
   C. False: The profile is that of a young, unmarried black male.
   D. False: People with mental illness are not more violent or more dangerous than people in the general population.
   E. True
   F. True
   G. False: The patient's right of confidentiality does not allow police or lawyers access to information about patients without the patient's expressed consent.
   H. True
   I. False: Patient records belong to the treatment facility or clinician, and the original should remain on file and never be given to patients.
   J. False: Back problems are the most often cited disability.
   K. False: Three states—Montana, Idaho, and Utah—have abolished the insanity defense.
2. A. 48 to 72
   B. History of violent behavior, noncompliance with medications, current substance abuse, and an antisocial personality
   C. Outpatient commitment
   D. Competent, understanding, voluntary
   E. Protection and advocacy
   F. Advanced directives
   G. American Law Institute's test
3. A. Dangerous to self or others, mentally ill and in need of treatment, and unable to provide for own basic needs
   B. Confidentiality involves the disclosure of certain information to another person, but it is limited to authorized people. It applies to all patients at all times. Privilege or testimonial privilege applies only in court-related proceedings, and it exists only if established by law.
   C. The duty to warn obliges the clinician to assess the threat of violence to another, identify the person being threatened, and implement some affirmative and preventive action.

Chapter 11

1. C. Data collection   E. Nursing diagnosis
   A. Evaluation   D. Outcome identification
   B. Implementation   F. Planning
2. A. Specific   D. Current
   B. Measurable   E. Adequate
   C. Attainable   F. Mutual
   G. Psychotherapy, prescription of medications, consultation
   H. Health promotion, maintenance, acute, crisis
   I. Develop insight, change behavior
   J. Patient
   K. Costs/disadvantages, benefits/advantages

3. A. Phenomena relate to the range of actual or potential mental health problems that can be experienced by patients; theory maintains that psychiatric nurses need a conceptual model and research basis for their practice; action includes the nursing interventions used in the nursing process; and effects identifies the need to evaluate the outcomes of care.
   B. *DSM–IV–TR* diagnoses are used in most mental health settings to describe and classify the symptoms of mental disorders. Nurses should use both NANDA and *DSM–IV–TR* diagnoses to conceptualize patient problems, needs, and treatment strategies.
   C. Goal setting with psychiatric patients can be difficult for a number of reasons, including issues such as resistance, confusion, lack of insight, denial, vagueness about problem areas, and inability to articulate ideas. The nurse needs to clarify the reason and develop specific strategies to address it, which is part of the therapeutic process.

Chapter 12

1. A. True
   B. False: As of 1998 a baccalaureate degree is required to become certified as a generalist in psychiatric nursing.
   C. True
   D. False: The statement describes utilitarianism. Fairness is based on the concept of justice and benefit to the least advantaged in society.
   E. True
2. A. Accountability
   B. Autonomy
   C. Nurse-patient relationship
   D. Internet
   E. Ethic
   F. Interdisciplinary
3. A. The nursing process and the quality improvement process have similar steps. Each involves identifying or assessing a situation, analyzing the data to define the situation, developing a plan, implementing it, and then evaluating the results. Both of these processes are similar to the scientific process used in research.
   B. The aim of supervision is to teach psychotherapeutic skills. The goal of therapy is to alter a person's patterns of coping to enable the person to function more effectively in all areas of life.

Chapter 13

1. A. Primary prevention
   B. Secondary prevention
   C. Tertiary prevention
2. A. Work with people to avoid or better cope with stressors; change the resources, policies, or agents of the environment to enhance individual functioning
   B. Competence building or self-efficacy
   C. *Healthy People 2010*
   D. Stigma
   E. Environmental change

F. All three (primary, secondary, and tertiary)

3. A. The medical prevention model focuses on mental illness prevention and the importance of genetic and biochemical and brain research to discover the specific causes of mental illness. The nursing prevention model assumes that problems are multicausal, that everyone is vulnerable to stressful life events, and that any disability can arise in response to them. It focuses on intervention based on stressful events and vulnerable groups with known risk factors.

B. Universal interventions are targeted to the general population without consideration of risk factors. Selective interventions are targeted to individuals or groups with a significantly higher risk of developing a particular disorder. Indicated interventions are targeted to high-risk individuals who indicate a predisposition for developing the disorder.

C. Increasing a person's awareness of issues related to health and illness; increasing understanding of potential stressors and adaptive and maladaptive coping responses; increasing knowledge of where and how to acquire needed resources; and increasing the actual abilities such as the problem-solving skills, social skills, or self-esteem of the individual or group.

Chapter 14

1. G. Catharasis
   A. Clarification
   C. Exploration of solutions
   E. Raising self-esteem
   D. Reinforcement of behavior
   F. Suggestion
   B. Support of defenses
2. A. Crisis
   B. Precipitating events
   C. Precrisis
   D. Assessment
   E. Health educator
3. A. True
   B. False: A crisis is a short-term event requiring short-term treatment.
   C. True
   D. False: The patient's perception of the precipitating event is critically important.
   E. False: The generic approach is the correct answer.
4. A. Maturational crises are social and biological developmental events requiring role changes. These types of crises can be influenced by role models, interpersonal resources, and the acceptance of others. Situational crises occur when a life event upsets an individual's or a group's psychological equilibrium. This can cause feelings of inadequacy, bereavement, role change, financial stress, fear of loss, and feelings of helplessness and guilt. They can also be accidental, uncommon, and unexpected events.

   B. Cultural factors to be considered in crisis intervention are migration and citizen status, gender and family roles, religious belief systems, child-rearing practices, and use of extended family and support systems.

   C. Identify your own behaviors, precipitating events, perception of the event, support systems and coping resources, and previous strengths and coping mechanisms.

Chapter 15

1. A. True
   B. False: The career potential of people with mental illness, as with anyone else, depends on the person's talents, abilities, experience, motivation, and health status.
   C. True
   D. False: Consumers of mental health services can be productive as providers of mental health services. They can provide positive staff-recipient relationships, good knowledge of mental health resources and ways to overcome barriers, and positive role modeling.
   E. True
2. A. Rehabilitation
   B. Family burden
   C. Deinstitutionalization
   D. Social skills training
   E. Psychoeducation
3. A. Grief, anger, powerlessness, and fear
   B. Helping people develop their strengths and potential, learn living skills, and access environmental support
   C. Ways in which nurses can share power with families include clarifying mutual goals, not expecting families to fit a specific model, acknowledging one's own limitations, pointing out family strengths, working with families as a team, learning to respond to intense feelings, encouraging family enrichment, providing psychoeducation, offering practical advice, making a personal commitment, acknowledging diverse beliefs, and developing one's own supports.

Chapter 16

1. The preventive strategies of health education, environmental change, and social support can be used with a sibling of a patient who is mentally ill.
2. Families can influence each of the following balancing factors available to a person with mental illness who is in crisis: the nature of the precipitating event or stressor, the person's perception of the event, the nature and strength of the patient's support systems and coping resources, and the patient's previous strengths and coping mechanisms.
3. Family members can work with health professionals to assist patients with mental illness by using the three basic interventions used in psychiatric rehabilitation: helping the patient to develop strengths and potential, learn living skills, and access environmental supports.

Chapter 17

1. G. Affective responses
   A. Anxiety
   C. Cognitive responses
   I. Ego-oriented reactions
   F. Fear
   J. Moderate anxiety
   E. Neurosis
   D. Panic
   H. Psychosis
   B. Task-oriented reactions
2. A. Anxiety, depression
   B. Obsessions
   C. Emotional seduction
   D. Physical integrity and self-esteem
   E. Benzodiazepines and antidepressants
3. A. Conflict is the clashing of two opposing interests. The person experiences two competing drives and must choose between them. A reciprocal relationship exists between conflict and anxiety. Conflict produces anxiety, and anxiety increases the perception of conflict by producing feelings of helplessness.
   B. Allow the patient to determine the amount of stress he can handle at any given time. Do not force the patient into situations that he is not able to handle. Do not attack the patient's coping mechanisms or try to strip him of these. Do not ridicule the nature of his defense. Do not argue with the patient or try to talk him out of the defense. Do not reinforce the defense by focusing too much attention on it. Know when to eventually place some limits on the defense as more adaptive coping mechanisms fall into place. Assess for suicidal ideation as appropriate.

Chapter 18

1. E. Body dysmorphic disorder
   C. Conversion disorder
   H. Hypersomnia
   D. Hypochondriasis
   I. Insomnia
   F. Pain disorder
   G. Parasomnia
   J. Sleep pattern disturbance
   A. Somatization disorder
   B. Somatoform disorders
2. A. Alarm, resistance, exhaustion
   B. Repression, denial, compensation, regression
   C. Verbally, physical
   D. Conversion disorder
   E. Psychoneuroimmunology
3. A. Supportive therapy, insight therapy, group therapy, cognitive-behavioral strategies, stress reduction, relaxation training, and psychopharmacology
   B. Secondary gain is an indirect benefit, usually obtained through an illness or disability. Such benefits may include personal attentions, release from unpleasant situations and responsibilities, or monetary and disability benefits.

Chapter 19

1. A. True
   B. False: Research indicates that self-esteem has a genetic component.
   C. True
   D. False: The development of insight is not the desired outcome; the ultimate goal is to take action to effect lasting behavioral changes.
   E. False: Sympathetic responses by the nurse do not help patients assume responsibility for their own behavior. In fact, they can reinforce the patient's self-pity.
2. A. Self-ideal
   B. Self-esteem
   C. Roles
   D. Identity
   E. Depersonalization
   F. Child abuse
   G. Reminiscence
3. A. Provide the child with success, instill ideas, encourage the child's aspirations, and help the child build defenses against attacks to one's self-perceptions.
   B. In adolescence, the crisis of identity versus identity diffusion occurs. The task is one of self-definitions as the adolescent strives to integrate previous roles into a unique and reasonably consistent sense of self.
   C. Positive and accurate body image, realistic self-ideal, positive self-concept, high self-esteem, satisfying role performance, clear sense of identity

Chapter 20

1. C. Behaviors related to emotional responses
   A. Coping mechanisms
   D. *DSM–IV–TR* diagnoses
   B. Precipitating stressors
   E. Predisposing factors
   F. Seasonal affective disorder
2. A. ECT
   B. Serotonin
   C. Bipolar, unipolar
   D. Risk
   E. Prefrontal cortex
   F. Anxiety disorders, substance abuse disorders
   G. 75, 85
   H. Response, 6, 12, remission
   I. Relapse, recovery, 4, 9
   J. Recurrence, indefinitely
3. A. Emotional responsiveness: The person is affected by and is an active participant in both internal and external worlds. Uncomplicated grief reaction: The person is facing the reality of the loss and is immersed in the work of grieving. Suppression of emotions: This is the denial of feelings, detachment from them, or the internalization of all aspects of one's affective world. Delayed grief reaction: This is a prolonged suppression of emotion that ultimately interferes with effective functioning. Depression/mania: The most maladaptive emotional responses, recognized by their intensity, pervasiveness, persistence, and interference with usual functioning.

B. To increase the patient's sense of control over goals and behavior, increase the patient's self-esteem, and help the patient modify negative thinking patterns

Chapter 21

1. A. False: The highest rate of suicide is among white men older than 65 years.
   B. True
   C. False: All suicidal behavior is serious and, whatever the intent, must be given full consideration.
   D. True
   E. True
   F. False: The tricyclics have the higher rate of death by overdose.
   G. True
   H. False: A person already has the suicidal idea, and asking about it gives the person an opportunity to talk about how he or she feels.
2. A. Psychological autopsy
   B. Mood disorders, substance abuse, schizophrenia
   C. Serotonin (5HT)
   D. Communicating hope
   E. Hostility, impulsivity, depression
   F. Contracting for safety
   G. Surgeon General
3. A. Patients often appear less depressed immediately before attempting suicide because they feel relief at having made a decision and developed a plan to do so.
   B. Circumstances of the attempt, presenting symptoms, psychiatric diagnosis, personality factors, psychosocial history, family history, biochemical factors
   C. Suicidal patients can be treated in a variety of settings. Factors that should be considered in deciding on the best setting relate to your assessment of overall risk and should include whether the patient is resolute or ambivalent about suicide, has impaired judgment, and has dependable social supports available in the home.

Chapter 22

1. C. Attention   H. Anhedonia
   D. Perception   I. Affect
   E. Hallucinations   J. Decision-making
   G. Mood   B. Memory
   A. Cognition   F. Soft signs
2. A. Cognition, perception, emotion, behavior and movement, socialization
   B. Apraxia
   C. Dysregulation hypothesis
   D. Symptom triggers
   E. Overextension, restricted consciousness, disinhibition, psychotic disorganization, psychotic resolution
3. A. True
   B. False: The majority are auditory.
   C. False: Atypical antipsychotics often provide a better response and fewer side effects and should be considered first-line treatments.
   D. True

E. False: It is called Family to Family.
4. A. Nursing interventions should address the positive symptoms of schizophrenia, which include delusions, hallucinations, thought disorders, and bizarre behaviors, as well as the negative symptoms of flat affect, alogia, avolition, anhedonia, and attentional impairment. Positive symptoms respond well to typical and atypical antipsychotic medications. Negative symptoms respond best to atypical antipsychotic medications.
   B. The specific genetic defects that cause schizophrenia have not been identified yet, but family studies show increased risk for the disease and other psychiatric illnesses in people with a first-degree relative with schizophrenia. Children with a biological parent with schizophrenia have a 15% risk of developing the disorder. If both of the child's parents have schizophrenia, the risk increases up to 35%.
   C. Things you may notice are facial expressions, style of dress, mannerisms, tone of voice, behaviors, use of language, and body contact with others.

Chapter 23

1. A. Cluster B   F. Cluster B
   B. Cluster C   G. Cluster C
   C. Cluster B   H. Cluster A
   D. Cluster C   I. Cluster A
   E. Cluster B   J. Cluster A
2. A. Adolescence, adulthood
   B. Borderline personality disorder
   C. Serotonin
   D. Splitting
   E. Projective identification
   F. Countertransference
   G. Behavioral contract
3. A. Distinguishing characteristics of personality disorders include chronic and long-standing, not based on a sound personality structure, and difficult to change.
   B. Two levels of evaluation necessary when working with patients with personality disorders are evaluation of the nurse and the nurse's participation in the relationship and evaluation of the patient's behavior and the behavioral changes that the nurse works to facilitate.

Chapter 24

1. C. Delirium   H. Sundown syndrome
   D. Denial   A. Amygdala
   F. Dementia   G. Aphasia
   B. Agnosia   J. Apraxia
   E. Pseudodementia   I. Excess disability
2. A. Neurotic plaques, neurofibrillary tangles
   B. Alzheimer's disease
   C. Catastrophic reaction
   D. Delirium

3. A. Working memory, the ability to keep in mind recent events or the moment-to-moment results of mental processing, is mediated by the prefrontal cortex, which is responsible for executive functions. Long-term memory: Declarative memory (facts and events) is mediated by the hippocampus (in the limbic system), which consolidates new memories into long-term memories. Procedural memory (skills and procedures) is mediated by several brain structures: the striatum, motor cortex, and cerebellum (skills and habits); the amygdala (emotional associations); and the cerebellum (conditional reflexes).

B. Understand the possible causes of the cognitive impairment, adjust communication approaches to the person who is cognitively impaired, assist with self-care of the individual as needed, obtain available community services, engage in stress reduction activities, use respite care, participate in a peer support group, access social supports.

Chapter 25

1. A. False: Substance abuse affects all races.
   B. False: Only 1 in 10 people progress from use to abuse to dependence.
   C. True
   D. True
   E. False: In the addicted population there is no greater prevalence of psychiatric illness than in the general population.
   F. True
   G. False: Shorter half-lives result in more withdrawal.
   H. True
   I. False: Most people have one or more slips in their attempt at recovery.
   J. True
2. A. Substitution of a medication from the same drug class for gradual tapering
   B. Dual diagnosis
   C. Gateway drugs
   D. CAGE
   E. Breathalyzer
   F. Co-dependence
   G. Endorphins or enkephalins
   H. CNS depressants
   I. Detoxification
   J. Antabuse, naltrexone
3. A. Patients in maintenance methadone programs may object to the following: (1) they must remain on stable doses of the drug for years—some even for the rest of their lives, and (2) they must report to the clinic daily or they may be given take-home doses for certain days if they qualify.
   B. The advantages of having treatment programs staffed by counselors who have also recovered from substance abuse include that they may have a heightened sense of empathy for the patient population, a greater understanding of the realities of the abuse, and provide positive recovery-based role modeling. There is

controversy in the field, however, about what proportion of the staff should be recovered individuals. Some believe that a critical number of staff who have not been substance abusers is necessary to provide a professional balance to the treatment program. More research is needed in this area.

Chapter 26

1. C. Maladaptive eating regulation responses
   D. SSRIs
   A. Adaptive eating regulation responses
   E. Predisposing factors
   B. Serotonin
2. A. Females, 1, 4
   B. Binge eating
   C. Avoidance, intellectualization, isolation of affect, denial
   D. Anxiety, body image disturbance, fluid volume deficit, risk for self-mutilation, altered nutrition, powerlessness, self-esteem disturbance
   E. Cognitive behavioral therapy
3. A. Amount of bingeing
      Obese nonbingers: Once per month
      Obese bingers: High amount
      Nonobese bulimics: Very high amount
      Purging obese nonbingers: Rare
      Obese bingers: Infrequent
      Nonobese bulimics: High level
      Mood disturbance
      Obese nonbingers: Same as general population
      Obese bingers: One third chronic
      Nonobese bulimics: One third to one half chronic and up to 80% lifetime
   B. The patient will restore healthy eating patterns and normalize physiological parameters related to body weight and nutrition.

Chapter 27

1. I. Bisexuality   H. Homosexuality
   B. Gender identity   E. Orgasm
   J. Gender role   K. Sexual orientation
   A. Genetic identity   C. Transsexualism
   G. Heterosexuality   D. Transvestism
   F. Homophobia
2. A. Cognitive dissonance
   B. XX, XY
   C. Oedipus/Electra
   D. Childhood sexual abuse
   E. Education
   F. Acceptance
3. A. Between two consenting adults, mutually satisfying to both, not psychologically or physically harmful to either party, lacking in force or coercion, and conducted in private
   B. Safe sex practices include using condoms, reducing the number of sexual partners, and promoting sexual behaviors that decrease the exchange of body fluids.

Chapter 28

1. J. Barbiturates
   H. Selective serotonin reuptake inhibitors
   I. Antianxiety drugs
   K. Cytochrome P-450 inhibition
   L. Anti-Parkinsonian drugs
   E. Tricyclics
   A. Serotonin syndrome
   D. Sedative-hypnotics
   B. Atypical antidepressants
   C. Hypertensive crisis
   G. Typical neuroleptic antipsychotics
   F. Mood stabilizers
2. C. 5HT reuptake inhibition
   E. $5HT_2$ receptor blockade
   B. ACh receptor blockade
   D. $Alpha_1$ receptor blockade
   F. $Alpha_2$ receptor blockade
   A. DA reuptake inhibition
   H. H_1 receptor blockade
   G. NE reuptake inhibition
3. A. Role of the nurse
   B. Drug co-administration
   C. Pharmacokinetics
   D. Dysregulation hypotheses
   E. Neurosciences, psychopharmacology, clinical management
4. A. False: Serotonin syndrome is a life-threatening emergency caused by combining 5HT-enhancing drugs.
   B. False: With NMS, all drugs should be discontinued.
   C. True
   D. True
   E. True
5. A. Positive symptoms include delusion, hallucinations, formal thought disorder, and bizarre behavior. Negative symptoms include affective flattening, alogia, avolition/apathy/anhedonia, asociality, and attentional impairment. These symptoms respond better to the atypical antipsychotics than they do to the typical or conventional neuroleptic antipsychotics.
   B. Reuptake inhibition occurs when drugs such as TCAs and SSRIs prevent the presynaptic cell from reabsorbing the neurotransmitter after it has been released into the synapse. It is thought that this strategy produces an antidepressant effect by making more neurotransmitter available to the receptors in illnesses such as depression, in which increasing the effects of some neurotransmitters appears to exert a therapeutic effect.

   Receptor blockade occurs when drugs such as antipsychotics prevent a postsynaptic receptor from receiving a neurotransmitter after it has been released into the synapse. It is thought that this strategy produces an antipsychotic effect by making less neurotransmitter available to receptors in illnesses such as schizophrenia, in which decreasing the effects of some neurotransmitters appears to exert a therapeutic effect.

   C. When receiving antidepressants for the treatment of depression, patients begin to look better and sleep and eat better, and they feel more energy and motivation before the remission of subjective depressive feelings and suicidal thoughts. Objectively, they appear to be less depressed at a time when their safety must still be assessed because they now have the energy to act on suicidal impulses that have not responded to treatment.

Chapter 29

1. A. True
   B. False: ECT may be followed by antidepressant medication to prevent relapse.
   C. False: There is no evidence that ECT causes structural brain damage.
   D. True
   E. True
   F. False: The long-term efficacy of light therapy has not been fully evaluated.
   G. False: Light therapy appears to be insufficient for severely ill patients.
   H. True
   I. False: TMS is a noninvasive procedure using magnetic fields.
2. A. 6, 12
   B. 20, 30
   C. Major depression
   D. 80%
   E. Surgical
   F. Headache, muscle soreness, nausea
   G. 50, 60
   H. Mania
   I. Mood
   J. Vagus nerve stimulation
3. A. ECT is a treatment in which a grand mal seizure is artificially induced in an anesthetized patient by passing an electrical current through electrodes applied to the patient's temples.
   B. Avoiding medications is often recommended for women who are in their first trimester of pregnancy. ECT allows the depression of the woman to be treated while avoiding the need to expose the fetus to antidepressant medications.

Chapter 30

1. A. Complementary and alternative medicine (CAM)
   B. 1998
   C. St. John's wort
   D. Melatonin
   E. Progressive muscle relaxation
   F. Therapeutic touch
   G. Kava-kava
   H. Ginko biloba
2. A. False: Use of CAM therapies has increased 65% from 1993 to 1997.
   B. True
   C. True

D. False: Drug interactions have been reported, and it should not be taken with other antidepressants.

E. True

F. False: Most studies on the use of acupuncture for cocaine and other substance use disorders have failed to detect differences between experimental (real) and control (sham) acupuncture groups.

3. A. Enhanced public health education had heightened health-care awareness and interest in making lifestyle changes. CAM therapies often seem to be more available, accessible, and therefore more appealing to the health-care consumer. In addition, the benefits of CAM therapies may include less cost, more convenience, fewer side effects, more individualized care, and more contact with practitioners.

B. Ethical concerns about CAM therapies include issues of safety and effectiveness, as well as the expertise and qualifications of the practitioner. Of equal importance is the communication between the CAM and traditional health-care provider. Other concerns are related to effective symptom management, potential for drug interactions, possible side effects, and the lack of regulation of herbal products for purity and potency.

C. It is believed that acupuncture may stimulate the synthesis and release of endorphins, serotonin, and norepinephrine.

Chapter 31

1. A. False: Research suggests that this intervention may actually increase the patient's potential for aggressive behavior.

B. True

C. False: A patient's diagnosis is complicated by many factors and is at best merely suggestive of potentially violent behavior.

D. True

E. True

2. A. Assertive behavior
   F. Debriefing
   B. Limit-setting
   E. Passive behavior
   G. Restraint
   D. Seclusion
   C. Token economy

3. A. Areas of the brain include the limbic system, frontal lobe, and temporal lobe.

B. Preventive strategies include self-awareness, patient education, and assertiveness training. Anticipatory strategies include communication, environmental change, behavioral action, and psychopharmacology. Containment strategies include crisis management, seclusion, and restraint.

C. You should assume a supportive stance at least one leg length or 3 feet away from the patient. You should be at an angle to the patient, with hands kept open and out of pockets.

Chapter 32

1. B. Behavior
   G. Biofeedback
   F. Contingency contracting
   H. Extinction
   D. Flooding
   A. Punishment
   E. Shaping
   J. Social skills training
   C. Systematic desensitization
   I. Reframing

2. A. Classical conditioning
   B. Operant conditioning or negative reinforcement
   C. Punishment, response cost, extinction
   D. Perception or interpretation
   E. Hierarchy
   F. Direct patient care, planning treatment programs, teaching others cognitive behavior therapy techniques
   G. Homework

3. A. A cognitive behavioral assessment would include collecting data about a patient's actions, thoughts, and feelings; identifying problems from the data, defining the problem behavior, deciding how to measure the problem behavior, and identifying environmental variables that influence the problem behavior. It includes a review of the patient's strengths and deficits and minimizes the use of assumptions and unvalidated inferences.

B. The ABCs of behavior are **antecedent, behavior,** and **consequence.** The ABCs of treatment are **affective, behavioral,** and **cognitive.**

C. Use of the form allows patients to distinguish between thoughts and feelings and to identify adaptive responses that would be alternatives to the situation.

Chapter 33

1. E. Follower   G. Questioner
   C. Moralist   B. Facilitator
   H. Truant   I. Leader
   A. Gatekeeper   F. Complainer
   J. Encourager   D. Summarizer

2. A. Power
   B. Orientation
   C. 60-120 minutes, 20-40 minutes
   D. Forming, storming, norming, performing
   E. Universality, altruism

3. A. A group is a collection of individuals who have a relationship with one another, are independent, and may have common norms. Eight components of small groups are structure, size, length of sessions, communication, roles, power, norms, and cohesion.

B. Psychoeducational groups are designed to teach symptom identification, symptom management, and recovery planning skills.
   Intensive problem-solving groups are designed for 6 to 10 patients, each working on the identification and resolution of specific target problems, goals, and

problem-solving strategies identified in an individual treatment plan.

Activity groups are designed to enhance the psychological and emotional well-being of psychiatric patients. These groups are a combination of group psychotherapy and remotivation therapy that stimulates interaction among members by focusing on simple tasks that encourage members to focus on group rather than individual goals.

C. Group norms facilitate the accomplishment of the group's goals or tasks, control interpersonal conflict, interpret social reality, and foster group interdependence.

Chapter 34

1. A. False: It is not a problem to be in a triangle, and it is impossible to stay out of all triangles.
   B. True
   C. False: The third leg of a triangle may be a person, an issue, or an object, and they or it may not be a willing part of the emotional system of a family.
   D. False: Therapists must avoid becoming part of a triangle in a family system.
   E. True
2. A. Strengths, resources or competencies; deficits, pathological states, and dysfunction
   B. Educate, support
   C. National Alliance for the Mentally Ill (NAMI)
   D. Bowen
   E. Thinking, feeling
   F. Ego fusion
   G. Interactional patterns
   H. Reframe
   I. Obtain a clear description of the presenting problem in specific and concrete terms
3. A. A person with high differentiation of self has personal autonomy, distinguishes between thoughts and feelings, and retains objectivity when stressed. A person with low differentiation is fused with others, blends thoughts and feelings, and is emotionally reactive when stressed.
   B. A family genogram is a structured method of gathering information and graphically symbolizing factual and emotional relationship data related to the family.

Chapter 35

1. a. C   f. D
   b. E   g. C
   c. D   h. E
   d. B   i. B
   e. A   j. A
2. A. Crisis, stabilization
   B. Institutionalization
   C. Multidisciplinary
   D. Therapeutic community
   E. Florence Nightingale
   F. JCAHO

3. A. Crisis stabilization and intermediate-term treatment
   B. The exact nature of the crisis bed concept is dependent on the structure of the health system in which it operates. Common goals include a focus of issues of suicidality, homicidality, and violence; assessment; rapid resolution of the crisis; decreased dependency on the hospital; prevention of regressive behaviors; and improved functioning of the inpatient environment.

Chapter 36

1. a. C   e. A
   b. D   f. D
   c. A   g. B
   d. C   h. B
2. A. Epidemiological
   B. Tertiary
   C. Case management
   D. Primary
   E. Assertive community treatment
   F. Secondary
   G. Multisystemic therapy
   H. Forensic
3. A. Common elements of ACT and MST include using a social-ecological framework, pragmatic treatment approaches, home-based interventions, individualized treatment goals, and emphasis on outcomes and innovation.

Chapter 37

1. A. True
   B. False: The patient must be unable to access psychiatric follow-up independently and consistently.
   C. True
   D. False: Medicare is a retrospective payer.
   E. True
2. A. Be homebound, have a diagnosed psychiatric disorder, require the skills of a psychiatric nurse
   B. Homebound
   C. Case management
   D. Medicare
   E. People older than 65 years who may have a history of mental illness or a newly diagnosed mental illness and people younger than 65 years who qualify for Medicare because of their disabilities
   F. Standardized rating scales
   G. Clinical pathways
3. A. The advantages of home care in relationship to inpatient treatment involve its ability to serve as an alternative to hospitalization by maintaining a patient in the community, a facilitator of an impending hospital admission through preadmission assessment, an enhancement of inpatient treatment through integration of home issues in the inpatient treatment plan, a way to shorten inpatient stay while keeping the patient engaged in active treatment, and a part of the discharge planning process by assessing potential problems and issues upon discharge into the community.

B. Psychiatric nursing home care is reminiscent of the early days of public health nursing, which included home visits.

Chapter 38

1. A. False: 9% to 13% of children have some type of psychiatric disorder
   B. True
   C. True
   D. False: Young children exhibiting sexual behavior may have been abused. They should be dealt with in an open and honest way and reported to child protective services for investigation into possible abuse.
   E. False: To avoid aggression, nurses should make a consistent schedule that is developmentally based, keep staff highly visible and engaged with the children, and carefully prepare children for activities.
2. A. 25% to 36%
   B. Handling separation and independent decision making
   C. Working for delayed gratification
   D. Bibliotherapy
   E. Autogenic storytelling
   F. Inability of the family to control the child at home
   G. Legal, ethical
   H. Anxiety, depression, conduct disorder, ADHD
3. A. Dealing with frustration and unfavorable events, celebrating good things, and feeling pleasure
   B. Parents can enhance a child's self-esteem by having realistic caregiver expectations; demonstrating positive personal values; communicating clearly, tolerantly, and respectfully; using appropriate ways to discipline; offering guidance and support; and promoting the child's autonomy.

Chapter 39

1. A. False: Brain growth continues into adolescence, and there is also additional fine tuning of the neural system.
   B. False: Chronological age is not a good indicator of physical maturation during adolescence because growth often occurs in spurts and individual differences exist.
   C. True
   D. True
   E. False: It is best for the nurse to have the initial contact directly with the adolescent because he or she is often concerned that the nurse will be aligned with the parents rather than with the adolescent.
   F. Truew
2. A. Identity versus identity diffusion
   B. Formal operational thought
   C. Males, females
   D. 50%
   E. Hypochondriasis
   F. Coping with stress and anxiety, involvement in personally meaningful activities

3. A. Female teenagers delay seeking and using contraceptives either because they are unwilling or unable to make conscious decisions about their sexual and contraceptive behavior or because they either do not mind becoming pregnant or do not think it will happen to them.
   B. They are called gateway drugs because their use often precedes the use of marijuana and other illegal substances.
   C. Curiosity, experimentation, regular use, psychological or physical dependence, and using drugs to feel "normal"
   D. Medication with adolescents necessitates comprehensive family involvement; developmental differences in adolescence affect psychopharmacological assessment, treatment alliance, management, and compliance; difficulty in diagnosing emerging first episodes versus adjustment disorders in adolescents; and lack of controlled clinical drug trials in adolescents

Chapter 40

1. F   5. B
2. E   6. C
3. H   7. D
4. A   8. G
2. A. Sundown syndrome
   B. Physical restraints
   C. Electroconvulsive
   D. More favorable side effects profile
   E. Reality
   F. Cognitive
   G. Maximal independence
   H. Lower than for younger patients
3. A. Show respect by addressing the patient by his or her last name, reinforce the amount of time left in the interview, give sufficient time for response, tie the interview to historical events, choose words that are based on the sociocultural background of the patient, use touch to convey support and interest, and give careful and repeated explanations to increase understanding and cooperation.
   B. Environmental hazards, patient variables, assistive devices, medications, and physical or mental disorders

Chapter 41

1. D. Attributions
   I. Sexual assault
   A. Multigenerational transmission
   G. Myth about abuse
   C. Paternalistic model of health care
   J. Psychological abuse
   F. Force continuum
   H. Intimate partner abuse
   B. Just world view
   E. Primary prevention

2. A. True
   B. False: Children who witness abuse are also victimized.
   C. False: Family violence occurs at all levels of society regardless of income, age, race, education, or religion.
   D. True
   E. True
3. A. Violent families have the following characteristics: multigenerational transmission (family violence is often perpetuated through generations within a family by a cycle of violence), social isolation (violent families are often isolated by the abuser to keep the "family secret," thus avoiding formal and informal sanctions from others in the community), use and abuse of power (the abuser almost always has some form of power or control over the victim), and alcohol and drug abuse (survivors often report concurrent substance abuse by the abuser, although one behavior is not necessary for the other to occur).

B. Paternalistic model	Empowerment model
Nurse is perceived to be more knowledgeable than the survivor.	There is mutual sharing of knowledge and information.
Responsibility for ending the violence is placed on the survivor.	The nurse strategizes with the survivor. Survivors are helped to recognize societal influences.
Advice and sympathy are given rather than respect.	The survivor's competence and experience are respected.

   C. American social norms that maintain violence include historical attitudes toward women, children, and the elderly; the belief that violence is justified to maintain the family system; economic discrimination; the nonresponsiveness of the criminal justice system; and the belief that women and children are property.

Chapter 42

1. A. True
   B. False: AIDS requires body fluid-to-body fluid contact for transmission.
   C. True
   D. False: The virus is transmitted through risky unprotected sexual behaviors.
   E. True
   F. False: Only condoms protect against getting the AIDS virus.
   G. False: Contact with only one partner can pass the AIDS virus.
   H. True
   I. False: There may be no signs of illness for many years after being diagnosed with AIDS.
2. A. Heterosexual contact
   B. Depression, anxiety
   C. AIDS dementia complex (ADC)
   D. Kaposi's sarcoma
3. A. The incidence of HIV infection in the United States has decreased for men in general, greatly decreased for homosexual men, and decreased for babies born to HIV-positive mothers. It has increased for women, particularly poor women, and for racial minorities.
   B. There are three classes of retroviral drugs approved by the FDA: (1) NRTIs (nucleoside reverse transcriptase inhibitors), (2) PIs (Protease inhibitors), (3) NNRTIs (non-nucleoside reverse transcriptase inhibitors) combination of drugs from more than one class (except pregnant women who should only take AZT). Although there are newer drugs in clinical trials, they are not approved by the FDA at this time.

Special features

Citing the Evidence*

CRITICAL THINKING ABOUT CONTEMPORARY ISSUES

* Partial List